THE MERCK MANUAL OF GERIATRICS

Second Edition

First Edition – 1990
Second Edition – 1995

OTHER
MERCK PROFESSIONAL HANDBOOKS

THE MERCK INDEX
First Edition, 1889

THE MERCK MANUAL OF DIAGNOSIS AND THERAPY
First Edition, 1899

THE MERCK VETERINARY MANUAL
First Edition, 1955

Merck Professional Handbooks
are published on a nonprofit basis
as a service to the scientific community.

THE MERCK MANUAL OF GERIATRICS

Second Edition

Editors
William B. Abrams, M.D.; Mark H. Beers, M.D.; and Robert Berkow, M.D.
Senior Assistant Editor: Andrew J. Fletcher, M.B., B.Chir.

Published by

MERCK RESEARCH LABORATORIES

Division of
MERCK & CO., INC.
Whitehouse Station, N.J.

1995

MERCK & CO., INC.
Whitehouse Station, N.J.
U.S.A.

First Printing—January 1995
Second Printing—December 1995
Third Printing—July 1996

Library of Congress Catalog Card Number 89-63495
ISBN 0-911910-66-2

Printed in the U.S.A.

CONTENTS

§1. A PROBLEM–ORIENTED APPROACH

§2. SPECIFIC APPROACHES

§3. ORGAN SYSTEMS

INTRODUCTION

CARDIOVASCULAR DISORDERS

CARDIOVASCULAR DISORDERS *(Continued)*

PULMONARY DISORDERS

GASTROINTESTINAL DISORDERS

GASTROINTESTINAL DISORDERS *(Continued)*

GENITOURINARY AND GYNECOLOGIC DISORDERS

HEMATOLOGIC DISORDERS

MUSCULOSKELETAL DISORDERS

MUSCULOSKELETAL DISORDERS *(Continued)*

METABOLIC AND ENDOCRINE DISORDERS

INFECTIOUS DISEASE

NEUROLOGIC DISORDERS

PSYCHIATRIC DISORDERS

PSYCHIATRIC DISORDERS *(Continued)*

SKIN DISORDERS

EYE DISORDERS

EAR, NOSE, AND THROAT DISORDERS

§4. SPECIAL ISSUES

§5. REFERENCE GUIDES

GUIDE FOR READERS

- The **Contents** (p. v) shows the pages where readers will find listings of Editorial Board members, consultants, and contributors; explanations of abbreviations and symbols; titles of sections, subsections, and chapters; and the index.

- **Thumb tabs** with appropriate abbreviations mark each section, selected subsections, and the index. Each section, designated by the symbol §, and each subsection in Section 3 has its own table of contents, listing chapters and subchapters in that section.

- **Chapters** are numbered serially from the beginning to the end of the book.

- The **Index** contains many cross-entries; page numbers in boldface type signify major discussions of the topics. In addition, the text gives numerous cross-references to other sections and chapters.

- **Page numbers** run serially from the beginning to the end of the book. **Running heads** on left-hand pages give the section or subsection title and on right-hand pages, the chapter number and title.

- **Abbreviations and symbols**, used throughout the book as essential space savers, are listed on pp. xvii and xviii. Other abbreviations in the text are explained at their first use in the chapter or subchapter.

- The **Tables** and **Figures** found throughout the text are referenced appropriately in the index but are not listed in a table of contents.

- **Drugs** are designated in the text mainly by generic (nonproprietary) names.

- The authors, reviewers, editors, and publisher of this book have made extensive efforts to ensure that treatments, drugs, and dosage regimens are accurate and conform to the standards accepted at the time of publication. However, constant changes in information resulting from continuing research and clinical experience, reasonable differences in opinions among authorities, unique aspects of individual clinical situations, and the possibility of human error in preparing such an extensive text require that the reader exercise individual judgment when making a clinical decision and, if necessary, consult and compare information from other sources. In particular, the reader is advised to check the product information provided by the manufacturer of a drug product before prescribing or administering it, especially if the drug is unfamiliar or is used infrequently.

PREFACE TO THE SECOND EDITION

In the five years since the first edition of THE MERCK MANUAL OF GERIATRICS was published, geriatric medicine has evolved and THE MANUAL has evolved with it. Coverages of Medicare, nursing home and home care, and the roles of nursing, social services, and rehabilitation have been expanded. New information about normal and abnormal aging, diagnosis, management, and treatment of disease and important updates on the legal and ethical issues relevant to clinicians have been added. New chapters provide information on breast, gynecologic, pulmonary, and gastroenterologic disorders and cancer. In addition, this edition has been completely redesigned and includes more than 50 new illustrations and more than 100 new tables.

THE MERCK MANUAL OF GERIATRICS builds on the tradition of THE MERCK MANUAL OF DIAGNOSIS AND THERAPY, which has been continuously published since 1899 and is the world's most widely used general medical text. Yet readers will find THE MERCK MANUAL OF GERIATRICS a very different book. Although both books are concise and include only clinically relevant material, geriatrics requires longer discussions to explain the differences between normal and abnormal changes and to describe the multidisciplinary approach and the many complications, nuances, and differences in caring for older persons.

The proportion of elderly persons—especially very elderly persons—is growing rapidly. Yet education for health care professionals in geriatrics remains inadequate: Many doctors, nurses, and pharmacists receive only several hours or less of formal geriatric training. THE MERCK MANUAL OF GERIATRICS is intended to help meet the need for additional information on geriatric care. It is published by Merck & Co., Inc., on a nonprofit basis to make information available at a modest cost.

An editorial board of outstanding experts in geriatrics has reviewed all manuscripts, and more than 125 experts have supplied manuscripts and served as consultants. There is no way to adequately thank all these people for their contributions and cooperation. Their reward comes from helping the elderly persons who we hope will be the ultimate beneficiaries of this book.

We welcome your comments and will carefully consider all suggestions for improvement.

William B. Abrams, M.D.
Mark H. Beers, M.D.
Robert Berkow, M.D.

Merck Research Laboratories
West Point, PA 19486-0004

PREFACE TO THE FIRST EDITION

THE MERCK MANUAL OF GERIATRICS is intended to provide information of clinical relevance to all physicians involved in the care of elderly patients. It follows the tradition set by THE MERCK MANUAL, which has been continuously published since 1899 and is the world's most widely used medical text.

The concept of a geriatric medical book was under consideration for several years. There was concern about whether there were sufficient important data to warrant a separate book on geriatric medicine. However, we became convinced that there is so much new information on both the structural and physiologic changes of normal aging and the clinical aspects of caring for elderly patients that it was not possible to include all that a practicing physician should know in a general textbook of medicine. Furthermore, even experienced clinicians are often not fully aware of much of this valuable information. Hence, this separate text seemed warranted.

The demographic imperative is clear: America, and indeed the entire world, is experiencing a dramatic increase in the number and proportion of persons over the age of 65. People over 65 now represent about 13% of the US population and utilize about 30% of all health care resources; these figures are projected to reach over 20% and 50%, respectively, by 2030. It is also clear that gerontology, which includes the sciences describing the changes of normal aging as distinguished from disease effects, is becoming more sophisticated and prolific, while the practice of geriatrics is becoming increasingly specialized. Interest within the medical community is evidenced by the popularity of the examination, first offered in 1988, leading to a certificate of special competence in geriatrics.

In many individuals certain physiologic processes decline with age (eg, renal blood flow and glomerular filtration rate, maximal heart rate and cardiac output with exercise, glucose tolerance, cellular immunity), but other processes (eg, most liver functions and total lung capacity) remain unchanged. Secretion of ADH and response to osmolar stimuli actually increase with advancing age. The striking differences in how disease processes manifest themselves in the elderly, as compared to younger patients, are particularly important. For example, it has long been recognized that disorders such as hyperthyroidism may present in a masked or "apathetic" form, and that inflammatory intra-abdominal disorders such as appendicitis may not evoke typical symptoms and signs, requiring adjustments in the diagnostician's thinking. However, it is far less recognized that presenting symptoms in the elderly, while indicating that the patient is sick, may be totally misleading with regard to the nature and the primary location of the disease process. For example, when a patient presents with confusion, one thinks immediately of psychoactive drugs or a disease process primarily affecting the brain as a possible cause. In an elderly person, one must also consider such diverse factors as simple dehydration due to a wide variety of etiologies, infection, cardiac disorders producing subtle failure, intra-abdominal organ disease, etc. In short, diagnostic logic is different.

Similarly, the approach to therapeutics is far more complex in the elderly. Drug pharmacokinetics may be significantly different from those in younger adults, depending on the drug and the individual patient. Drug disposition may be altered by declines in kidney function and some liver metabolic activities, as well as by changes in body composition such as increased fat, decreased lean body mass, and reduced serum albumin levels. In addition, fluid stores such as plasma volume and total body water decline with age.

Nondrug therapy is more complex in this population and must take into account many factors; eg, rehabilitation strategies and the mobilization of a variety of community services. Furthermore, consideration of specific sites for optimal care and of the social, cultural, legal, financial, and ethical issues is important, complex, and evolving. Clearly, care of the elderly requires a substantially different approach to case management.

We have tried to provide a practical handbook covering all aspects of disease and the clinical management of elderly patients in a readily usable format. The book begins with a problem-oriented diagnostic approach to common presentations of illness in older patients. The second section deals with broad management approaches specific to the elderly. The third section addresses individual organ systems, with emphasis on age-related concerns. This is followed by a section dealing with epidemiologic, social, ethical, financial, and legal issues. Reference guides, with laboratory values and other data unique to the older population, are provided in the final section.

This book is designed to be comprehensive and authoritative, yet tightly edited to provide a large amount of information in a compact, handbook format. It is published by MERCK SHARP & DOHME RESEARCH LABORATORIES, a division of MERCK & CO., INC., on a not-for-profit basis in order to make the information available at a very modest cost, and thus accessible to students and nonmedical professionals involved in the care of older patients.

In developing this book, we have continued the tradition of THE MERCK MANUAL in seeking outstanding experts to serve as members of the Editorial Board, consultants, authors, and reviewers. We cannot adequately thank these contributors for the enormous effort and cooperation they provided to produce this book, but we know that they will feel sufficiently rewarded if their efforts serve your needs and those of the elderly for whom you care.

We hope THE MERCK MANUAL OF GERIATRICS will be compatible with your needs and worthy of frequent use. Suggestions for improvements will be warmly welcomed and carefully considered.

William B. Abrams, M.D., and Robert Berkow, M.D., *Editors*
MERCK SHARP & DOHME RESEARCH LABORATORIES
West Point, Pa. 19486

ABBREVIATIONS AND SYMBOLS

ACE	angiotensin converting enzyme
ADL	activities of daily living
AIDS	acquired immunodeficiency syndrome
ALT	alanine aminotransferase (formerly SGPT)
AST	aspartate aminotransferase (formerly SGOT)
bid	two times a day
BUN	blood urea nitrogen
C	Celsius; centigrade; complement
CBC	complete blood cell (count)
Ch.	chapter
Cl	chloride; chlorine
cm	centimeter
CNS	central nervous system
CO_2	carbon dioxide
CPR	cardiopulmonary resuscitation
CSF	cerebrospinal fluid
CT	computed tomography
dL	deciliter (= 100 mL)
DNA	deoxyribonucleic acid
D/W	dextrose in water
ECF	extracellular fluid
ECG	electrocardiogram
EEG	electroencephalogram
ESR	erythrocyte sedimentation rate
F	Fahrenheit
FDA	Food and Drug Administration
ft	foot; feet (measure)
GFR	glomerular filtration rate
GI	gastrointestinal
gm	gram
GU	genitourinary
h	hour
H_2	histamine
Hb	hemoglobin
Hct	hematocrit
HDL	high-density lipoprotein
Hg	mercury
HIV	human immunodeficiency virus
HLA	human leukocyte antigen
Hz	hertz (cycles per second)
IADL	instrumental activities of daily living
ICF	intracellular fluid
Ig	immunoglobulin
IM	intramuscular(ly)
in.	inch; inches
IPPB	intermittent positive pressure breathing
IV	intravenous(ly)
kcal	kilocalorie (food calorie)
kg	kilogram
L	liter
LDH	lactate dehydrogenase
LDL	low-density lipoprotein
m	meter
mEq	milliequivalent
mg	milligram
min	minute
mL	milliliter

mm	millimeter
mo	month
mOsm	milliosmole
MRI	magnetic resonance imaging
Na	sodium
ng	nanogram (= millimicrogram)
NSAID	nonsteroidal anti-inflammatory drug
OTC	over-the-counter
oz	ounce
pH	hydrogen ion concentration
po	orally
prn	as needed
q	every
qid	four times a day
RBC	red blood cell
s.c.	subcutaneous(ly)
SD	standard deviation
sec	second
SLE	systemic lupus erythematosus
sq	square
TB	tuberculosis
tid	three times a day
u.	unit
UTI	urinary tract infection
WBC	white blood cell
wk	week
yr	year
μL	microliter
μm	micrometer; micron
μg	microgram
μU	microunit
/	per
$<$	less than
$>$	more than
$\leq$	equal to or less than
$\geq$	equal to or more than
$\pm$	plus or minus
§	section

EDITORS

William B. Abrams, M.D.
Consultant,
Merck Research Laboratories
and
Adjunct Professor of Medicine,
Jefferson Medical College of
Thomas Jefferson University

Mark H. Beers, M.D.
Senior Director of Geriatrics,
Merck Research Laboratories
and
Associate Clinical Professor of Medicine,
Medical College of Pennsylvania;
Adjunct Associate Professor of Medicine,
University of Pennsylvania

Robert Berkow, M.D.
Senior Director of Medical Literature,
Merck Research Laboratories
and
Clinical Professor of Medicine and of Psychiatry,
Hahnemann University

Senior Assistant Editor

Andrew J. Fletcher, M.B., B.Chir.
Merck Research Laboratories
and
Adjunct Professor of Pharmaceutical Health Care,
Temple University

EDITORIAL BOARD

CONSULTANTS

T. H. D. Arie, B.M., F.R.C.P., F.R.C.Psych., F.F.P.H.M.
Professor and Head, Department of Health Care of the Elderly, University of Nottingham, England

Psychiatric Disorders

Marquette Leona Cannon-Babb, Pharm.D.
Professor of Pharmacy Practice, Temple University

Pharmaceutical Preparations and Dosages

Harvey J. Cohen, M.D.
Professor of Medicine, Chief of Geriatrics Division, and Director of Center for the Study of Aging, Duke University; Director, Geriatric Research, Education, and Clinical Center, VA Medical Center, Durham

Oncologic and Hematologic Disorders

Edward G. Lakatta, M.D.
Professor of Medicine (Cardiology), Johns Hopkins University; Professor of Physiology, University of Maryland; Chief, Laboratory of Cardiovascular Science, Gerontology Research Center, National Institute on Aging

Cardiovascular Disorders

Marvin M. Schuster, M.D.
Professor of Medicine and Psychiatry, Johns Hopkins University; Chief, Division of Digestive Diseases, Johns Hopkins Bayview Medical Center

Gastrointestinal Disorders

ACKNOWLEDGMENTS

We wish to express our appreciation to the following persons for their expert assistance in reviewing specific chapters: Yung-Ping Chen, Ph.D. (*Health Insurance*); L. Jack Faling, M.D. (*The Effects of Age on the Lung*); Stephen C. Goss (*Health Insurance*); Alan M. Laties, M.D. (*Ophthalmologic Disorders*); Richard A. Marottoli, M.D. (*The Older Driver*); Timothy Moon, M.D. (*Disorders of the Lower Genitourinary Tract*); Donald Morgan, Ph.D. (*Ear Disorders*); Mary C. Newton (*Home Health Care*); John W. Rowe, M.D. (*Water and Electrolyte Disorders*).

W.B.A., M.H.B., and R.B.

Editorial and Business Staff

Executive Editor	**Shirley Claypool**
Senior Staff Editors	**William J. Kelly, Keryn A.G. Lane**
Staff Editor	**Susan T. Schindler**
Textbook Production Coordinator/Copy Editor	**Catherine J. Humber**
Medical Textbook Coordinator	**Dorothy A. Bailey**
Senior Secretary	**Diane C. Zenker**
Designer	**Lynn Foulk**
Illustrator	**Bob Neumann**
Computer Graphics	**Kevin Curry**
Publisher	**Gary Zelko**
Advertising and Promotion Administrator	**Pamela J. Barnes**

CONTRIBUTORS

Ronald D. Adelman, M.D.
Chief, Division of Geriatrics, Winthrop-University Hospital, New York

Elder Abuse and Neglect

T. H. D. Arie, B.M., F.R.C.P., F.R.C.Psych., F.F.P.H.M.
Professor and Head, Department of Health Care of the Elderly, University of Nottingham, England

Acute Confusional State

Shirley P. Bagley, M.S.
Assistant Director for Special Programs, National Institute on Aging, National Institutes of Health

Preventive Strategies

Lodovico Balducci, M.D.
Professor of Medicine, University of South Florida; Program Leader, Senior Adult Oncology Program, H. Lee Moffitt Cancer Center and Research Institute

Breast Cancer

John G. Bartlett, M.D.
Professor of Medicine and Chief, Division of Infectious Diseases, Johns Hopkins University

Pneumonia and Tuberculosis

Bruce J. Baum, D.M.D., Ph.D.
Clinical Director and Chief, Clinical Investigations and Patient Care Branch, National Institute of Dental Research

Dental and Oral Disorders

Michael K. Bay, M.D.
Assistant Professor, Department of Medicine, University of Texas Health Science Center at San Antonio

The Aging Liver

Mark H. Beers, M.D.
Editor, THE MERCK MANUAL OF GERIATRICS; Senior Director of Geriatrics, Merck Research Laboratories; Associate Clinical Professor of Medicine, Medical College of Pennsylvania; Adjunct Associate Professor of Medicine, University of Pennsylvania

Behavior Disorders; Male Hypogonadism and Impotence

Robert Berkow, M.D.
Editor, THE MERCK MANUAL OF GERIATRICS; Senior Director of Medical Literature, Merck Research Laboratories; Clinical Professor of Medicine and of Psychiatry, Hahnemann University

Cognitive Failure: Delirium and Dementia

Richard W. Besdine, M.D.
Director, Travelers Center on Aging; Travelers Professor of Geriatrics and Gerontology; Professor of Internal Medicine and of Community Medicine, University of Connecticut

Introduction; Hyperthermia and Accidental Hypothermia; Establishing Therapeutic Objectives: Quality of Life Issues

Dan G. Blazer, M.D., Ph.D.
Professor of Psychiatry, J. P. Gibbons Professor of Community and Family Medicine, and Dean of Medical Education, Duke University

Depression; Anxiety Disorders; Hypochondriasis; Schizophrenia and Schizophreniform Disorders; Alcohol Abuse and Dependence

Risa Breckman, C.S.W.
Staff Psychotherapist, Institute for Rational-Emotive Therapy, New York

Elder Abuse and Neglect

Reginald C. Bruskewitz, M.D.
Professor of Surgery/Urology, University of Wisconsin Hospitals

Disorders of the Lower Genitourinary Tract: Bladder, Prostate, and Testicles

Robert N. Butler, M.D.
Brookdale Professor of Geriatrics and Adult Development and Chairman, Henry L. Schwartz Department of Geriatrics and Adult Development, The Mount Sinai School of Medicine

Sexuality; Cognitive Failure: Delirium and Dementia; Living Alone

Enrico M. Camporesi, M.D.
Professor and Chairman of Anesthesiology and Professor of Physiology, State University of New York, Health Science Center at Syracuse

Anesthesia Considerations

Louis R. Caplan, M.D.
Professor and Chairman, Department of Neurology, Tufts University; Neurologist-in-Chief, New England Medical Center

Cerebrovascular Disease

Donald O. Castell, M.D.
Kimbel Professor and Chairman, Department of Medicine, The Graduate Hospital, Philadelphia

Upper Gastrointestinal Tract Disorders

Jane E. Castle, R.N., M.S.N.
Clinical Associate, Duke University Medical Center and School of Nursing

Ethical Issues

Maxwell M. Chait, M.D.
Assistant Clinical Professor of Medicine, Division of Gastroenterology, College of Physicians and Surgeons of Columbia University

Gastrointestinal Neoplasms

A. Mark Clarfield, M.D.
Professor, McGill University, and Attending Physician, Division of Geriatrics, Sir Mortimer B. Davis–Jewish General Hospital, Montreal, Canada; Director, Academic Affairs, Sarah Herzog Memorial Hospital, and Head, Division of Geriatrics, Ministry of Health, Jerusalem, Israel

A Cross-National Perspective

Gene D. Cohen, M.D., Ph.D.
Director, Center for Aging and Health, School of Medicine and Health Sciences, George Washington University; Director, Washington DC Center on Aging

Normal Changes of Aging and Patterns of Psychiatric Disease

Barry S. Collet, D.P.M., M.P.H.
Consultant, Hebrew Rehabilitation Center for Aged, Boston

Foot Problems

Eugene Coodley, M.D.
Professor of Medicine, University of California, Irvine; Chief of Internal Medicine Section, VA Medical Center, Long Beach

Laboratory Values

Morton C. Creditor, M.D.
Professor Emeritus of Internal Medicine, University of Kansas

Hospitalization

Barry J. Cusack, M.D.
Associate Professor of Medicine, Division of Gerontology/Geriatric Medicine, University of Washington; Chief, Section of Gerontology and Geriatric Medicine, VA Medical Center, Boise

Clinical Pharmacology

Mayer B. Davidson, M.D.
Professor of Medicine, University of California, Los Angeles; Director, Diabetes Program, Cedars-Sinai Medical Center

Diabetes Mellitus and Other Disorders of Carbohydrate Metabolism

Catherine E. DuBeau, M.D.
Instructor in Medicine, Harvard University; Staff Physician, Gerontology Division, Brigham and Women's Hospital

Urinary Incontinence

Nancy N. Dubler, LL.B.
Professor of Bioethics, The Albert Einstein College of Medicine; Director, Division of Bioethics, Department of Epidemiology and Social Medicine, Montefiore Medical Center

Legal Issues

Jennie D. Dulac
Research Associate, Center for the Evaluative Clinical Sciences, Dartmouth Medical School

Care of the Dying Patient

Theodore C. Eickhoff, M.D.
Professor of Medicine, Division of Infectious Disease, University of Colorado

Vaccines and Immunization

Walter H. Ettinger, M.D.
Professor, Departments of Internal Medicine and Public Health Sciences, and Associate Chairman, Department of Internal Medicine, Bowman Gray School of Medicine of Wake Forest University

Bone, Joint, and Rheumatic Disorders

David Fellows, M.D.
Assistant Professor, Department of Anesthesiology, State University of New York, Health Science Center at Syracuse

Anesthesia Considerations

Michael Feltes, M.D.
Assistant Professor of Medicine and Family Medicine, University of Connecticut

Human Immunodeficiency Virus Infection

Jerome L. Fleg, M.D.
Associate Professor of Medicine, Johns Hopkins University; Staff Cardiologist, Laboratory of Cardiovascular Science, Gerontology Research Center, National Institute on Aging

Diagnostic Evaluation; Arrhythmias and Conduction Disorders

Marshal F. Folstein, M.D.
Professor and Chairman, Department of Psychiatry, Tufts University; Psychiatrist-in-Chief, New England Medical Center

Mental Status Examination

Susan E. Folstein, M.D.
Professor of Psychiatry, Tufts University

Mental Status Examination

Michael L. Freedman, M.D.
The Diane and Arthur Belfer Professor of Geriatric Medicine and Director, Division of Geriatrics, New York University

Age-Related Hematologic Changes; Anemias; Malignancies and Myeloproliferative Disorders

Sandor A. Friedman, M.D.
Professor of Medicine, State University of New York, Health Science Center at Brooklyn; Chairman, Department of Medicine, Coney Island Hospital

Peripheral Vascular Diseases; Aneurysms

Edward D. Frohlich, M.D.
Alton Ochsner Distinguished Scientist and Vice President for Academic Affairs, Alton Ochsner Medical Foundation

Hypertension

Terry T. Fulmer, Ph.D., R.N.
Anna C. Maxwell Professor and Associate Dean for Research, Columbia University School of Nursing

Geriatric Nursing

Philip P. Gerbino, Pharm.D.
Vice President of Academic Affairs and Dean, School of Pharmacy, Philadelphia College of Pharmacy and Science

The Role of the Pharmacist

Tobin N. Gerhart, M.D.
Clinical Assistant Professor, Harvard University; Orthopaedic Surgeon, Department of Orthopaedic Surgery, Beth Israel Hospital

Fractures

Bernard J. Gersh, M.B., Ch.B., D. Phil.
W. Proctor Harvey Teaching Professor of Cardiology and Chief, Division of Cardiology, Georgetown University

Cardiovascular Surgery and Percutaneous Interventional Techniques

Gary Gerstenblith, M.D.
Professor of Medicine and Director of Clinical Trials, Cardiology Division, Johns Hopkins University

Coronary Artery Disease

Barbara A. Gilchrest, M.D.
Professor and Chairman, Department of Dermatology, Boston University

Skin Changes and Disorders

Charles J. Glueck, M.D.
Director, Cholesterol Center, The Jewish Hospital of Cincinnati, Inc.

Lipoprotein Disorders

A. Julianna Gulya, M.D.
Associate Professor of Otolaryngology–Head and Neck Surgery, Georgetown University

Ear Disorders

Jack M. Guralnik, M.D., Ph.D.
Chief of Epidemiology and Demography Office, Epidemiology, Demography, and Biometry Program, National Institute on Aging

Epidemiology and Demographics

Richard J. Havlik, M.D.
Associate Director, Epidemiology, Demography, and Biometry Program, National Institute on Aging

Epidemiology and Demographics

Charles O. Herrera, M.D.
Adjunct Associate Professor and Medical Director, Sleep Disorders Center, City College of New York; Clinical Associate Professor of Medicine, University of Miami

Sleep Disorders

Bruce Hirsch, M.D.
Assistant Professor of Medicine, Cornell University; Attending Physician, Infectious Disease, North Shore University Hospital

Normal Changes in Host Defense

Kathryn Hyer, M.D.
Department of Geriatrics and Adult Development, The Mount Sinai Medical Center

Living Alone

Masayoshi Itoh, M.D.
Associate Professor of Clinical Rehabilitation Medicine, New York University; Associate Deputy Director, Department of Rehabilitation Medicine, and Deputy Director, Nursing Facility, Goldwater Memorial Hospital

Rehabilitation

Robert J. Joynt, M.D., Ph.D.
Professor of Neurology, University of Rochester

Normal Aging and Patterns of Neurologic Disease

Robert J. Just, M.D.
Fellow in Gastroenterology, The Graduate Hospital, Philadelphia

Upper Gastrointestinal Tract Disorders

Donald Kaye, M.D.
Professor and Chairman, Department of Medicine, Medical College of Pennsylvania

Infective Endocarditis; Influenza; Meningitis

B. J. Kennedy, M.D.
Regents' Professor of Medicine (Emeritus) and Masonic Professor of Oncology (Emeritus), Division of Medical Oncology, University of Minnesota

Cancer in the Elderly

Edmond S. Klausner, M.D.
Attending Psychiatrist, Department of Psychiatry, Jewish Home and Hospital for Aged, New York

History and Physical Examination

Mary Jane Koren, M.D.
Adjunct Associate Professor of Public Administration, Wagner Graduate School of Public Service, New York University; Adjunct Assistant Professor, Department of Geriatrics, The Mount Sinai School of Medicine

Care in Nursing Homes and Other Long-term Care Facilities; Home Health Care

O. Dhodanand Kowlessar, M.D.
Professor of Medicine and Director of Nutrition Education, Department of Medicine, Thomas Jefferson University

Diarrhea; Malabsorption Syndromes

Carl Kupfer, M.D.
Director, National Eye Institute, National Institutes of Health

Ophthalmologic Disorders

Edward G. Lakatta, M.D.
Professor of Medicine (Cardiology), Johns Hopkins University; Professor of Physiology, University of Maryland; Chief, Laboratory of Cardiovascular Science, Gerontology Research Center, National Institute on Aging

Normal Changes of Aging

James E. Lang, M.D.
Associate Director, Cholesterol Center, The Jewish Hospital of Cincinnati, Inc.

Lipoprotein Disorders

Mathew H. M. Lee, M.D.
Professor and Chairman (Acting), Department of Rehabilitation Medicine, Rusk Institute, New York

Rehabilitation

Myrna I. Lewis, M.S.W.
Assistant Professor, Department of Community Medicine, The Mount Sinai School of Medicine

Sexuality

Leslie S. Libow, M.D.
Anna A. Greenwall Professor, The Mount Sinai School of Medicine; Chief of Medical Services, The Jewish Home and Hospital for Aged

History and Physical Examination

Lewis A. Lipsitz, M.D.
Associate Professor of Medicine, Harvard University; Co-Director, Research and Training Institute, Hebrew Rehabilitation Center for Aged

Syncope; Hypotension

David T. Lowenthal, M.D., Ph.D.
Professor of Medicine, Pharmacology, and Exercise Science, University of Florida; Director, Geriatric Research, Education, and Clinical Center, VA Medical Center, Gainesville

Exercise

Marjorie M. Luckey, M.D.
Assistant Professor and Director of Osteoporosis and Metabolic Bone Disease Program, Department of Obstetrics, Gynecology, and Reproductive Science, The Mount Sinai Medical Center

Metabolic Bone Disease

Joanne Lynn, M.D.
Senior Associate and Professor, Center for the Evaluative Clinical Sciences, Dartmouth-Hitchcock Medical Center

Care of the Dying Patient; Ethical Issues

William J. MacLennan, M.D., F.R.C.P.
Professor, Geriatric Medicine Unit, Department of Medicine of the Royal Infirmary, University of Edinburgh, Scotland

Giant Cell (Temporal) Arteritis and Polymyalgia Rheumatica

Diana Eve Meier, M.D.
Associate Professor, Departments of Geriatrics and Medicine, and Co-Director of Osteoporosis and Metabolic Bone Disease Program, The Mount Sinai Medical Center

Metabolic Bone Disease

Geno J. Merli, M.D.
Clinical Professor of Medicine and Vice Chairman and Director, Division of Internal Medicine, Thomas Jefferson University

Geriatric Emergencies

John R. Michael, M.D.
Professor of Medicine, University of Utah

Pulmonary Embolism

Myron Miller, M.D.
Professor and Vice-Chairman, Department of Geriatrics and Adult Development, and Professor of Medicine, Department of Medicine, The Mount Sinai School of Medicine

Water and Electrolyte Disorders

John E. Morley, M.B.
Dammert Professor of Gerontology, Department of Internal Medicine, St. Louis University Health Sciences Center; Director, Geriatric Research Education and Clinical Center, VA Medical Center, St. Louis

Nutrition

Richard T. Moxley, M.D.
Professor of Neurology and of Pediatrics and Director,Neuromuscular Disease Center, University of Rochester

Muscular Disorders

S. Ragnar Norrby, M.D., Ph.D.
Professor and Chairman, Department of Infectious Diseases, University of Lund, Sweden

Urinary Tract Infection; Antimicrobial Agents

Colleen E. O'Leary, M.D.
Assistant Professor, Department of Anesthesiology, State University of New York, Health Science Center at Syracuse

Anesthesia Considerations

René Oliverio, B.S.N., R.N.
Clinical Trials Coordinator, Cardiology, Duke University

Care of the Dying Patient

Marilyn Pajk, R.N., M.S.
Gerontological Clinical Nurse Specialist, Home Medical Service, Boston University Medical Center

Pressure Sores

Russell K. Portenoy, M.D.
Associate Professor of Neurology, Cornell University; Director of Analgesic Studies, Pain Service, and Associate Attending Neurologist, Memorial Sloan-Kettering Cancer Center

Pain

Lawrence G. Raisz, M.D.
Professor of Medicine and Head, Division of Endocrinology and Metabolism, University of Connecticut

Disorders of Mineral Metabolism

Neil M. Resnick, M.D.
Assistant Professor, Harvard University; Chief of Gerontology Division, Brigham and Women's Hospital

Urinary Incontinence

Sheldon M. Retchin, M.D.
Professor of Internal Medicine, Virginia Commonwealth University; President and Chief Executive Officer, MCV Associated Physicians, Richmond

The Older Driver

Joel E. Richter, M.D.
Chairman, Department of Gastroenterology, The Cleveland Clinic Foundation

Functional Disorders of the Gastrointestinal Tract

Deborah W. Robin, M.D.
Assistant Professor of Medicine, Vanderbilt University

Falls and Gait Disorders

Joan C. Rogers, Ph.D.
Professor of Occupational Therapy, School of Health and Rehabilitation Sciences, and Assistant Professor of Psychiatry, School of Medicine, University of Pittsburgh

Occupational Therapy

John W. Rowe, M.D.
President, The Mount Sinai School of Medicine and The Mount Sinai Medical Center

Aging Processes; Renal Changes and Disorders

Laurence Z. Rubenstein, M.D.
Professor of Geriatric Medicine, University of California, Los Angeles; Director, Geriatric Research Education and Clinical Center, VA Medical Center, Sepulveda

Comprehensive Geriatric Assessment

Malvin Schechter, M.S.
Assistant Professor, Henry L. Schwartz Department of Geriatrics and Adult Development, The Mount Sinai School of Medicine

Health Insurance

Steven Schenker, M.D.
Professor of Medicine and of Pharmacology, University of Texas; Staff Physician, VA Hospital, San Antonio

The Aging Liver

Isaac Schiff, M.D.
Joe Vincent Meigs Professor of Gynecology, Harvard University; Chief of Vincent Memorial Obstetrics and Gynecology Service, Massachusetts General Hospital

Menopause and Ovarian Hormone Therapy

Edward L. Schneider, M.D.
Dean, Andrus Gerontology Center, University of Southern California

Aging Processes

Marvin M. Schuster, M.D.
Professor of Medicine and Psychiatry, Johns Hopkins University; Chief, Division of Digestive Diseases, Johns Hopkins Bayview Medical Center

Effects of Aging on the Gastrointestinal System

Hugh M. Shingleton, M.D.
National Vice President for Detection and Treatment, American Cancer Society

Female Genitourinary Disorders

Gary W. Small, M.D.
Associate Professor of Psychiatry, University of California, Los Angeles; Chief, Geriatric Psychiatry, West Los Angeles VA Medical Center

Geriatric Psychiatric Consultation Services

David H. Solomon, M.D.
Professor-Emeritus of Medicine/Geriatrics and Director, Center on Aging, University of California, Los Angeles

Age-Related Endocrine and Metabolic Changes; The Normal and Diseased Thyroid Gland

Perry J. Starer, M.D.
Assistant Professor, Department of Geriatrics and Adult Development, The Mount Sinai School of Medicine; Attending Physician, The Jewish Home and Hospital for Aged

History and Physical Examination

Trey Sunderland, M.D.
Chief, Section on Geriatric Psychiatry, Laboratory of Clinical Science, National Institute of Mental Health

Cognitive Failure: Delirium and Dementia

Peter B. Terry, M.D.
Professor of Medicine, Environmental Health Sciences, Anesthesiology, and Critical Care Medicine, The Johns Hopkins Medical Institutions

Chronic Obstructive Pulmonary Disease

Randall C. Thompson, M.D.
Assistant Professor of Medicine, Mayo Medical School; Consultant in Cardiovascular Disease, Mayo Clinic, Jacksonville

Cardiovascular Surgery and Percutaneous Interventional Techniques

Melvyn S. Tockman, M.D., Ph.D.
Associate Professor of Environmental Health Sciences, Johns Hopkins University

The Effects of Age on the Lung; Lung Cancer

Ronald G. Tompkins, M.D., Sc.D.
Associate Professor of Surgery, Harvard University; Visiting Surgeon, Massachusetts General Hospital

Surgery: Preoperative Evaluation and Intraoperative and Postoperative Care; Surgery of the Gastrointestinal Tract

Allan R. Tunkel, M.D., Ph.D.
Associate Professor of Medicine, Medical College of Pennsylvania

Infective Endocarditis; Influenza; Meningitis

Jürgen Unützer, M.D.
Research Fellow and Acting Instructor, Department of Psychiatry, University of Washington

Geriatric Psychiatric Consultation Services

Robert E. Varner, M.D.
Associate Professor and Director, Division of Medical and Surgical Gynecology, University of Alabama at Birmingham

Female Genitourinary Disorders

Robert E. Vestal, M.D.
Associate Chief of Staff for Research and Development and Chief, Clinical Pharmacology and Gerontology Research Unit, VA Medical Center, Boise; Professor of Medicine and Adjunct Professor of Pharmacology, University of Washington

Clinical Pharmacology

Arnold Wald, M.D.
Professor of Medicine, Division of Gastroenterology and Hepatology, University of Pittsburgh; Chief, Gastroenterology Division, Montefiore University Hospital

Lower Gastrointestinal Tract Disorders; Constipation

Brian Walsh, M.D.
Assistant Professor, Obstetrics, Gynecology, and Reproductive Biology, Harvard University

Menopause and Ovarian Hormone Therapy

John Wasson, M.D.
H.O. West Professor of Geriatrics, Dartmouth Medical School

Disorders of the Lower Genitourinary Tract: Bladder, Prostate, and Testicles

Kara Watne, R.N., M.P.H.
Clinical Nurse Coordinator, University of California, Los Angeles Medical Center

Ethical Issues

Jerome D. Waye, M.D.
Chief, Gastrointestinal Endoscopy Unit, Mount Sinai Hospital

Gastrointestinal Endoscopy

Jeanne Y. Wei, M.D., Ph.D.
Director, Division on Aging, Harvard University; Chief, Gerontology Division, Beth Israel Hospital

Heart Failure and Cardiomyopathy

Howard H. Weitz, M.D.
Director of Clinical Cardiology and Clinical Associate Professor of Medicine, Thomas Jefferson University

Geriatric Emergencies

Marc E. Weksler, M.D.
Wright Professor of Medicine, Cornell University

Normal Changes in Host Defense

Claude E. Welch, M.D.
Clinical Professor of Surgery (Emeritus), Harvard University; Senior Surgeon, Massachusetts General Hospital

Surgery: Preoperative Evaluation and Intraoperative and Postoperative Care; Surgery of the Gastrointestinal Tract

Nanette K. Wenger, M.D.
Professor of Medicine (Cardiology), Emory University; Director, Cardiac Clinics, Grady Memorial Hospital, Atlanta

Valvular Heart Disease

Terrie Wetle, Ph.D.
Associate Professor of Community Medicine, University of Connecticut; Director, Braceland Center for Mental Health and Aging, Institute of Living

Social Issues

T. Franklin Williams, M.D.
Professor of Medicine (Emeritus), University of Rochester; Attending Physician, Monroe Community Hospital, Rochester

Preventive Strategies

William R. Wilson, M.D.
Chief, Division of Otolaryngology-Head and Neck Surgery, The George Washington University

Nose and Throat Disorders

Sidney J. Winawer, M.D.
Professor of Medicine, Cornell University; Chief, Gastroenterology and Nutrition Service, and Member and Head, Laboratory for Gastrointestinal Cancer Research, Memorial Sloan-Kettering Cancer Center

Gastrointestinal Neoplasms

Melvin D. Yahr, M.D.
Aidekman Family Professor of Neurological Research and Chairman Emeritus, Department of Neurology, The Mount Sinai School of Medicine

Movement Disorders

Arie Ben Yehuda, M.D.
Attending Physician, Department of Medicine, Geriatric Unit, Hadassah University Hospital, Jerusalem, Israel

Normal Changes in Host Defense

Robert A. Zorowitz, M.D.
Assistant Professor of Medicine, Emory University; Associate Chief of Medicine, Wesley Woods Geriatric Center at Emory University

Metabolic Bone Disease

§1. A PROBLEM–ORIENTED APPROACH

§1. A PROBLEM–ORIENTED APPROACH

1. INTRODUCTION

One distinguishing characteristic of geriatric medicine is the prominence of certain recurring clinical problems that can originate in various organ system disorders. These problems—anorexia, weight loss, fluid and electrolyte abnormalities, heat regulation disorders, syncope, gait disturbance, falls, immobility, confusion, incontinence, pain, sleep abnormalities, and pressure sores—bedevil the elderly. Because the presenting symptoms or syndromes often do not help identify the locus of disease, a thorough, comprehensive evaluation is needed. Elucidation and treatment are critical to the well-being of elderly people, and a thorough understanding of age-dependent changes in their associated organ systems is the blueprint to successful patient care for a geriatrician.

In the elderly, the common outcome of many disorders is **functional impairment,** *a decreased ability to meet one's needs*. In elderly people, unlike in younger ones, the first sign of a new illness or a recurring chronic one is rarely a single, specific complaint that helps to localize the diseased organ system or tissue. Rather, presentation is more likely to include one or more nonspecific problems, which themselves are only manifestations of impaired function. These problems quickly impair independence in an elder, but do not necessarily produce the typical signs of illness.

The reasons that disease in the elderly manifests itself first as functional loss, often in organ systems unrelated to the locus of illness, are not well understood. Apparently, when disease disrupts homeostasis in a functionally independent elder, the most vulnerable, delicately balanced systems are likely to be affected first. For example, heart failure that produces peripheral edema may lead to worsening gait and an inability to walk before it produces obvious shortness of breath. The result is a loss of independent function in activities of daily living (ADL) or instrumental activities of daily living (IADL).

Deterioration of functional independence in active, previously unimpaired elders is an early, subtle sign of untreated illness, usually without the typical symptoms and signs of the disease. Thus, difficulty with mobility, cognition, continence, and nutrition require a problem-oriented approach, linking **functional assessment** with traditional clinical evaluation (see also Ch. 17). Maintaining the quality of life requires a rapid, thorough clinical evaluation as soon as functional impairments develop. Disease-generated impairments are usually reversible—if they are detected and treated promptly.

Although early functional assessment and prompt treatment are often called preventive medicine, they are tertiary prevention at best. They do not replace primary and secondary prevention, often overlooked in the elderly; nevertheless, they are crucial to restoring independence. Periodic formal reassessment and rapid response to detected declines in independence are essential for providing adequate geriatric care.

A **problem-oriented approach** to the impaired elderly person illuminates another phenomenon common in geriatric medicine—a discrepancy between the disease problem list and the type and severity of functional disability. Because the burdens of illness and functional loss increase with age, practitioners often assume that the number of diseases or conditions on the problem list correlates with the type and degree of functional disability. However, an accumulation of diseases does not necessarily result in serious loss of function. More common is the elderly person who despite a very long list of serious diseases remains independent and vigorous.

Another erroneous assumption is that the diseased organ or tissue determines the specific functional impairment in the elderly. For example, the assumption that mobility problems are caused by musculoskeletal or neurologic disorders, that confusion arises from brain disease, or that incontinence results from bladder dysfunction is usually valid in young and middle-aged patients, but not in elderly patients. Certain vulnerable tissues and systems responsible for functional integrity in the elderly are likely to decompensate as a result of a systemic influence elsewhere in the body. For example, evaluation of an elderly man with urinary incontinence may show that his urinary tract is normal but that his diuretic medication is causing the problem.

The discovery of disease in an organ system does not necessarily indicate that the cause of functional loss can be attributed to that organ system. If prostatitis is found in an incontinent man, treating the infection may not alleviate the incontinence. Only after treatment of the disease in that body system restores normal organ function can a causal relationship be confirmed.

The severity of illness, as measured by objective data, does not necessarily determine the presence or severity of functional impairment. For example, routine ECG or Holter monitoring may detect cardiac arrhythmias, or multiphasic screening may show chronic elevation of alkaline phosphatase levels in an independent, fully functional elderly person. When a patient's laboratory study results are notably abnormal but functional disability is minimal, the functional evaluation can support a decision to avoid further evaluation or withhold treatment, particularly if it involves considerable cost, discomfort, or health risk.

The lessons of these noncorrelations between function and diagnoses are crucial. The following chapters in this section explore the functionally related problems to which the elderly are most vulnerable. Each chapter maintains a clinical focus on etiology of the presenting problem and considers the most useful approaches to diagnosis and management. Many of the disease states provoking these problems are considered in detail in Section 3, in which diseases are discussed in relation to organ systems. The physician, however, should consider the problems discussed in this section, along with those described in Section 3, to ensure that elderly patients are receiving adequate care.

2. NUTRITION

The primary nutritional problems affecting the elderly are protein-energy undernutrition, vitamin deficiencies, trace mineral deficiencies, and obesity. The physiologic changes of aging place older persons at risk for undernutrition. Mild vitamin deficiencies are very common in older persons, particularly those in institutions, and have been associated with cognitive impairment, poor wound healing, anemia, bruising, and an increased propensity for developing infections and some cancers (eg, vitamin A deficiency is associated with lung cancer). Trace mineral deficiencies are associated with immune dysfunction and many other disorders. Though a less serious problem in older persons than protein-energy undernutrition, obesity can impair functional status, increase the risk of pulmonary embolus and pressure sores, and aggravate chronic diseases such as diabetes mellitus and hypertension.

AGE–RELATED CHANGES

Body mass increases between ages 20 and 50, then remains stable until about age 65, when weight loss occurs as a result of both lean and adipose tissue loss. The percentage of body fat increases around age 40 and then decreases after age 70. Intra-abdominal and intramuscular fat increases with aging. Older women have a lower waist-to-hip ratio than older men, and these lower ratios indicate a fat distribution that is less likely to be associated with hyperinsulinemia, hypertension, and diabetes.

Compared with younger men, older men experience a 20% decrease in total energy expenditure. Older women, however, experience only a minimal change in total energy expenditure. The explanation for this is that men tend to markedly reduce their physical activity with retirement, while women continue doing the bulk of the housework throughout their life. Resting metabolic rate decreases by 20% in men and 13% in women. These age-related reductions in resting metabolic rate result from a small decrease in triiodothyronine levels, reduced responsiveness to norepinephrine, reduced muscle tone and strength of muscle contraction, and reduced Na^+K^+ATPase activity. However, the major factor affecting resting metabolic rate is decreased food intake with aging. Nonsmoking women ages 55 to 74 consume 300 kcal/day less than women ages 19 to 29; for men, the decrease is 950 kcal/day. Older persons also have a decreased thermic response to food.

PROTEIN–ENERGY UNDERNUTRITION

Protein-energy undernutrition (malnutrition) results from a deficient supply or absorption of nutrients or an excessive utilization of nutrients by the body. Marasmus and kwashiorkor are two forms of protein-energy undernutrition.

Marasmus is a condition of borderline nutritional compensation in which a patient has a marked depletion of muscle mass and fat stores but normal visceral protein and organ function. Because the patient has depleted nutritional reserves, any additional metabolic stress (eg, surgery, infection, burn) may rapidly lead to **kwashiorkor** (hypoalbuminemic protein-energy malnutrition). Characteristically, elderly patients deteriorate to this state more rapidly than young patients; even relatively minor stress may be the cause. Usually, susceptible elderly patients are underweight, but even those who appear to have ample fat and muscle mass are susceptible if they have a recent history of rapid weight loss.

About 16% of elders living in the community consume < 1000 kcal/day, an amount that cannot maintain adequate nutrition. Undernutrition also occurs in 3% to 12% of older outpatients, 17% to 65% of older persons in acute care hospitals, and 26% to 59% of older persons living in long-term care institutions. Studies show that being underweight in middle age and later places a person at greater risk of death than being overweight. As TABLE 2–1 shows, protein-energy undernutrition can lead to many conditions.

Etiology

An elderly person may eat less food for several reasons (see TABLE 2–2). Diminished senses of smell and taste may decrease the pleasure of eating. Changes in taste are variable and are often associated with lifelong cigarette smoking, poor dental hygiene, and disease. Aging is associated with a decrease in the opioid (dynorphin) feeding drive and an increase in the satiety effect of cholecystokinin. Recent studies suggest that the early satiety in older persons may be caused by a nitric oxide deficiency, which decreases the adaptive relaxation of the fundus of the stomach in response to food.

Certain **medications** can produce weight loss by causing anorexia (eg, digoxin, quinidine, hydralazine, vitamin A, fluoxetine and other psychoactives); causing nausea (eg, antibiotics, theophylline, aspirin); increasing energy metabolism (eg, thyroxine, theophylline); or causing malabsorption (eg, sorbitol vehicle in theophylline elixir, cholestyramine). Also, withdrawal from certain drugs (eg, alcohol, anxiolytics, other psychoactives) may be associated with weight loss.

TABLE 2–1. CONDITIONS RESULTING FROM PROTEIN–ENERGY UNDERNUTRITION

Cognitive dysfunction	Decreased serum antibody response to antigen challenge
Anergy	Anemia
Fatigue	Infections
Decreased muscle strength (frailty)	Altered thyroid function (euthyroid sick syndrome)
Hip fracture	Increased drug-drug interactions (decreased albumin binding and fat depots)
Orthostatic hypotension	
Pressure sores	
Pedal edema	
Decreased natural killer cell activity	
Decreased CD4+:CD8 ratio	

Depression is one of the most common reversible causes of weight loss in older persons. When depressed, they are more likely to lose weight than depressed younger persons. Some very old persons may stop eating because of the "unbearable weight of continued life." Management of this condition depends on the patient's ethical beliefs. **Alcoholism** in late life is often associated with weight loss, squalor syndrome, and depression.

The recurrence of **anorexia nervosa** in older persons who had an episode in their teens is being increasingly recognized. Abnormal attitudes about food intake and body image are not rare in underweight older persons. When these abnormal attitudes are associated with severe weight loss, the condition is called **anorexia tardive.** Late-life **paranoia** and late-life onset of **mania** may also be associated with weight loss.

Dementia usually produces weight loss because the person forgets to eat. Those who are wanderers can use large amounts of calories in a single day; consuming sufficient calories may be difficult. Demented persons may have a number of picas, including coprophagia. Recent studies show that patients with Alzheimer's disease do not have increased metabolism. On the other hand, persons with Parkinson's disease have a markedly increased metabolic rate, presumably because of their continuous tremors.

Dysphagia from a stroke or another neurologic disorder or from esophageal pain caused by candidiasis may result in decreased food intake. **Dental problems** may decrease food intake by up to 100 kcal/day. **Xerostomia** can also decrease food intake.

Medical causes of weight loss include hyperthyroidism, hypercalcemia, pheochromocytoma, and chronic infections (eg, tuberculosis, cancers). Malabsorption syndromes, particularly a late onset of celiac disease, should also be considered. Tremors and other physical problems with eating (eg, an inability to cut food after a stroke) can be

TABLE 2–2. CAUSES OF PROTEIN–ENERGY UNDERNUTRITION IN THE ELDERLY

Diminished sense of smell	Dental problems
Diminished sense of taste	Xerostomia
Early satiety	Hyperthyroidism
Use of medications (eg, digoxin, theophylline)	Hypercalcemia
	Pheochromocytoma
Withdrawal from medications (eg, anxiolytics, psychoactives)	Chronic infection
	Cancer
Alcoholism	Chronic obstructive pulmonary disease
Depression	Malabsorption syndrome
Anorexia nervosa, anorexia tardive	Physical disability (eg, tremors)
Late-life paranoia	Difficulty shopping for or preparing food
Mania	Low-salt, low-fat diet
Dementia	Poverty
Dysphagia	Loneliness

corrected with adaptive utensils, such as a heavy-handled spoon or a rocker-bottom knife. Older persons tend to tolerate medically prescribed diets poorly and thus lose weight.

Poverty is a major cause of low food intake. Elders on fixed incomes may have to choose between filling their drug prescriptions or buying food.

Problems with shopping and food preparation may result in insufficient food being available in the home. **Loneliness** can diminish the desire to prepare meals.

Diagnosis

No screening battery has been shown to have good sensitivity and specificity for identifying persons at risk for undernutrition. One screening device based on the acronym SCALES has been used to identify persons at risk, but it still needs to be validated (see TABLE 2–3).

Weight loss is the single best factor for predicting persons at risk for malnutrition. Adequate height and weight tables for optimum body mass are not available, but a body mass index below 20 kg/m^2 (weight/height^2) suggests a problem. Midarm circumference or arm muscle circumference (which corrects for triceps skinfold thickness) can be useful in following muscle mass changes in persons with a fluid retention problem. Skinfold thickness measurements have little diagnostic value.

In persons with **marasmus,** edema is absent; serum albumin and hemoglobin levels, total iron-binding capacity, and tests of cell-mediated immune function are usually normal. When **hypoalbuminemic protein-**

TABLE 2–3. "SCALES" PROTOCOL FOR EVALUATING RISK OF MALNUTRITION IN THE ELDERLY

Item Evaluated	*Assign One Point*	*Assign Two Points*
Sadness (as measured on Yesavage Geriatric Depression Scale; see TABLE 95–2)	10–14	≥ 15
Cholesterol level	< 160 mg/dL	——
Albumin level	3.5–4 gm/dL	< 3.5 gm/dL
Loss of weight	1 kg (or 1/4 in. midarm circumference) in 1 mo	3 kg (or 1/2 in. midarm circumference) in 6 mo
Eating problems	Patient needs assistance	——
Shopping and food preparation problems	Patient needs assistance	——

A total score ≥ 3 indicates that the patient is at risk.
Modified from Morley JE, Miller DK: "Malnutrition in the elderly." *Hospital Practice* 27(7):95–116, 1992; used with permission.

energy malnutrition occurs, the serum albumin level is < 3.5 gm/dL, and anemia, lymphocytopenia, and hypotransferrinemia (evidenced by a total iron-binding capacity < 250 µg/dL) are likely. Often, anergy and edema are present.

Albumin, which has a 21-day half-life, is an excellent measure of protein status. Normal ambulatory elders should have serum albumin levels > 4 gm/dL; only when a person is recumbent do fluid shifts result in a normal albumin level of 3.5 gm/dL. Albumin levels < 3.2 gm/dL in hospitalized older persons are highly predictive of subsequent mortality. Cholesterol levels < 160 mg/dL in nursing home residents predict mortality, presumably because such levels reflect malnutrition. Acute illness associated with cytokine release can also lower cholesterol levels. Anergy (failure to respond to common antigens, such as mumps, injected into the skin) can occur in healthy as well as malnourished older persons. The combination of anergy and signs of malnutrition correlates more strongly with a poor outcome than either one alone.

Treatment

Some evidence indicates that the mortality rate for *all* hospitalized older persons would decrease if calorie supplements were given. Also, recent studies clearly show that older persons with hip fractures benefit from either oral calorie supplements or, when their albumin level is < 3 gm/dL, from short-term tube feeding. Total parenteral nutrition should be reserved for severely undernourished persons (those with an albumin level < 2 gm/dL) and for those who cannot tolerate enteral feedings. Peripheral vein parenteral nutrition appears to be underused in acutely ill older persons, in part because its role has not been adequately studied.

The use of specific types of nutrient supplements has little scientific basis. High-protein supplements are generally used for persons with infections. High-fat, high-fiber diets may smooth the glycemic response in persons with diabetes. High-fiber diets may reduce tube-feeding diarrhea but may also result in fecal impaction in immobile persons. In most cases, the choice of a supplement should be based on the patient's preference. For a tube feeding, the choice should be the most cost-effective supplement.

For long-term tube feedings, most patients prefer percutaneous enteral gastrostomy tubes to nasogastric tubes. Demented patients appear to pull out gastrostomy tubes less often than nasogastric tubes. All types of tube feedings carry the risk of aspiration.

When a malnourished older person is fed, food may produce side effects, including electrolyte abnormalities, hyperglycemia, and aspiration pneumonia. Food can cause a significant drop in blood pressure, which is associated with falls. The decrease in blood pressure results from carbohydrate, which releases the vasodilatory gene-related peptide, calcitonin gene-related peptide.

Recently, recombinant growth hormone has been used to retain nitrogen and increase weight in severely malnourished older persons. Medroxyprogesterone acetate has produced weight gain in older persons with lung cancer.

Overall, undernutrition is poorly recognized and treated in older persons. Thorough examination for treatable causes of weight loss is essential. Appropriate use of short-term aggressive food supplementation can save lives. The ethical questions regarding the appropriate withdrawal of nutritional support is beyond the scope of this chapter (see Chs. 108 and 109).

VITAMIN DEFICIENCIES

Noninstitutionalized older persons in Newfoundland who took a daily vitamin and trace mineral supplement had improved immune function compared to a control group who did not take a supplement. Older men who took vitamin C were shown to live longer than those who did not; older women had no such advantage. Increasing evidence indicates that free radical damage may play a role in the pathogenesis of many diseases in older persons, including atherosclerosis, cancer, arthritis, and Parkinson's disease. This has reopened the question of the pharmacologic use of free radical scavengers (vitamins and minerals) to prevent a diverse group of degenerative diseases.

About 25% of older Americans take a vitamin and mineral supplement, with women more likely to do so than men. Vitamin deficiencies are common in institutionalized older persons, but vitamin replacement studies have failed to show any major effects except for a decreased hip fracture rate with vitamin D replacement.

Vitamin A deficiency is rarely a problem in older persons. This vitamin should be avoided because it can produce hypercalcemia, liver dysfunction, and pseudotumor cerebri.

Thiamine (vitamin B_1) deficiency occurs mainly in alcoholics. Thiamine replacement can result in hypoglycemia in persons with liver dysfunction because they have inadequate glycogen reserves. Glucose administration can precipitate acute thiamine deficiency with delirium, ataxia, and bilateral sixth nerve palsies (Wernicke's syndrome). Thus, in alcoholics, thiamine and glucose should always be administered together.

Riboflavin (vitamin B_2) and pyridoxine (vitamin B_6) deficiencies are common among nursing home residents. Signs of vitamin B_2 deficiency include cheilosis, glossitis, angular stomatitis, seborrheic dermatitis, and a magenta tongue; signs of vitamin B_6 deficiency include sideroblastic anemias. A vitamin B complex is indicated for those with signs of vitamin B_2 deficiency; pyridoxine is indicated for those with signs of vitamin B_6 deficiency.

Niacin deficiency occurs in older persons who are alcoholics, are receiving isoniazid, or have carcinoid syndrome. Characteristically, the patient develops pellagra, ie, dermatitis on areas exposed to the sun, dementia, and diarrhea or constipation. High doses of nicotinic acid, but not nicotinamide, lower the cholesterol level. Nicotinic acid is complexed with chromium to produce glucose tolerance factor and may play a minor role in the hyperglycemia of aging. However, the practice of taking these agents as supplements is not recommended for older persons.

Vitamin B_{12} deficiency can lead to dementia, megaloblastic anemia, incontinence, orthostatic hypotension, or posterior column disease (loss of position and vibration sense). Up to 5% of persons over age 80 have vitamin B_{12} deficiency. The most common cause is pernicious anemia, which results from a lack of instrinsic factor. The diagnosis of vitamin B_{12} deficiency is made by documenting a vitamin B_{12} level < 200 μg/dL. However, 25% of persons with levels between 200 and 300 μg/dL are deficient, as demonstrated by elevated methylmalonic acid and homocysteine levels in the urine. Thus, patients who are suspected clinically of vitamin B_{12} deficiency and who have vitamin B_{12} levels between 200 and 300 μg/dL should have their urine methylmalonic acid and homocysteine levels checked. Traditionally, the Schilling test has been used to diagnose pernicious anemia. However, it is now recognized that when older persons develop gastric achlorhydria, they may be able to absorb vitamin B_{12} that is not bound to food but cannot liberate vitamin B_{12} that is bound to food and therefore absorb it. Thus, in most cases, the Schilling test is not clinically useful. Although oral vitamin B_{12} has been used to treat this deficiency, most authorities recommend vitamin B_{12} 1000 μg IM every month.

Vitamin C deficiency is associated with increased bruising, poor wound healing, and the development of pressure sores. Ingesting vitamin C at any dose results in false-negative fecal and urinary occult blood tests; ingesting megadoses can interfere with serum and urine glucose tests and may result in oxalate kidney stones, increased serum salicylate levels, and rebound scurvy (bleeding after withdrawal).

TRACE MINERAL DEFICIENCIES

Zinc deficiency, as indicated by plasma zinc levels < 70 μg/dL, occurs in institutionalized, shut-in, and ambulatory elderly persons. Zinc loss in the urine occurs in persons with diabetes, cirrhosis, and alcoholism and in those using a diuretic. Zinc deficiency is associated with poor wound healing, impaired immune function, night blindness, and hypogonadism. High doses of zinc have been reported to slow the progression of age-related macular degeneration.

Selenium deficiency reportedly occurs in patients receiving long-term tube feedings. The major features are muscle weakness and pain.

Copper deficiency is associated with anemia and possibly mild glucose intolerance.

OBESITY

Fat acts as a storage organ for excess calories, providing protection for older persons with acute illnesses. Fat also protects vital organs from injury during falls and plays an important role in maintaining core body temperature.

Persons who weigh 120% to 130% of their desirable weight are considered moderately obese; those who weigh more than 130% of their desirable weight are considered morbidly obese.

In men, the prevalence of obesity peaks during middle age, and then declines to 26% by age 65 to 74. In white American women, the prevalence of obesity peaks at 36% between ages 65 and 74; 60% of African American women are overweight at these ages. In older persons, obesity may cause certain medical complications (see TABLE 2–4). However, low waist-to-hip ratios protect against obesity-associated diseases.

TABLE 2–4. COMPLICATIONS OF OBESITY IN THE ELDERLY

Moderate Obesity (120% to 130% of desirable weight)	*Morbid Obesity (> 130% of desirable weight)*
Impaired functional status	Decreased longevity
Hypertension	Diagnostic problems
Diabetes mellitus	Increased surgical risk
Coronary artery disease	Immobility
Gallbladder disease	Pickwickian syndrome (alveolar hypoventilation)
Gout	Intertrigo
Sleep apnea	
Deep vein thrombosis	
Pulmonary embolism	
Osteoarthritis	
Decubitus ulcers	
Uterine, breast, cervical, and ovarian cancer (in women)	
Colon and prostate cancer (in men)	

Etiology

In older men, obesity appears to result from a decrease in physical activity; in older women, from the loss of estrogens; and in both sexes, from decreased growth hormone. Genotype appears to account for 25% of visceral body fat. Acquired causes of obesity include hypothyroidism, Cushing's syndrome, tumors of the ventromedial hypothalamus, glucocorticoid therapy, monoamine oxidase inhibitors, and moderate doses of phenothiazines. Overeating remains the most common cause.

Treatment

Generally, obesity is a less important problem in older persons than in younger persons, and management should involve evaluation of the risk-benefit ratio of any therapeutic intervention.

Since the major identifiable cause of weight gain in older persons is lack of physical activity, an exercise program represents the most reasonable approach to weight reduction. Walking 1 mile burns about 100 calories. Thus, a mall-walking program in which a person walks 2 to 3 miles four times a week may produce gradual weight loss. For persons with osteoarthritis, an upper body exercise program is recommended.

Diets in older persons should provide at least 800 kcal/day and should always be supplemented with vitamins and trace elements. Older persons on a diet should drink at least 1 L of fluid daily. Any dietary program should be associated with a behavior modification program because in many cases starting a diet is an attempt to change lifetime habits.

Drugs such as fenfluramine or fluoxetine are not recommended for weight loss in older persons because they are associated with irreversible malnutrition, and the possible benefits do not outweigh the side effects. Similarly, any operation that decreases stomach size is contraindicated in older persons unless obesity is associated with sleep apnea.

3. WATER AND ELECTROLYTE DISORDERS

Many diseases common to the elderly present with water and electrolyte disorders. Both water overload and plasma volume depletion, which are common in the hospitalized elderly, are often accompanied by changes in serum sodium levels, especially by hyponatremia. Various diseases and drugs can affect serum potassium levels and acid-base balance.

PHYSIOLOGIC REGULATION OF WATER AND SODIUM

The ability to regulate the volume and tonicity of extracellular fluid (ECF) within narrow limits is essential to the health of elderly persons, but aging is associated with impaired water conservation and sodium balance maintenance—the two primary factors that determine the volume and tonicity of ECF. Among the homeostatic mechanisms are **thirst perception;** secretion of **antidiuretic hormone (ADH,** or **vasopressin),** the major hormonal regulator of water balance; secretion of **aldosterone** and **atrial natriuretic peptide,** hormonal regulators of sodium excretion; **renal hemodynamics** (blood pressure, renal blood flow, and glomerular filtration rate; **renal sympathetic nerve activity;** and the **renal response system** (proximal and distal tubules). When these intake, hormonal, and effector systems function normally, wide variations in water or sodium intake are modulated to maintain a consistent ECF volume and tonicity. When any mechanism is impaired, however, water or sodium balance may be seriously disturbed, producing clinical consequences.

In young healthy adults, total body water (TBW) is about 60% of body weight, with ECF and plasma volumes being about 20% and 5%, respectively. With aging, however, total body water decreases to about 45% of body weight because of a proportionate increase in fat and decrease in lean body mass.

The principal hormonal regulator of body water is ADH secretion by the neurohypophyseal system. Such secretion varies in response to several stimuli, including changes in blood tonicity, blood volume, and **blood** pressure, as well as nausea, pain, emotional stress, and many drugs. Osmoreceptors in the hypothalamus respond to small changes in blood tonicity, resulting primarily from changes in serum sodium. Increased tonicity stimulates ADH release, producing antidiuresis; decreased tonicity inhibits ADH release, producing diuresis. These changes in ADH release help maintain plasma osmolality in the narrow range between 292 mOsm/kg (at which maximum urine concentration occurs) and 282 mOsm/kg (at which full diuresis occurs).

Via volume receptors in the left atrium, a decrease in blood volume stimulates ADH release; an increase in blood volume inhibits it. Similarly, ADH secretion responds to blood pressure changes via baroreceptors in the aorta and carotid arteries. A fall in blood pressure triggers ADH secretion; a rise in blood pressure inhibits it.

Sodium and its accompanying anions are the major solutes of ECF, accounting for more than 90% of osmolality. Serum osmolality can be estimated by using the following formula:

$$\text{Osmolality} = 2[\text{Na}] + \frac{\text{BUN}}{2.8} + \frac{\text{glucose}}{18}$$

Body sodium content is determined by the balance between dietary intake and renal excretion because extrarenal losses in sweat and stool are normally minimal. Within 2 to 4 days of stopping sodium intake, urinary excretion normally decreases to < 5 mEq/L; increasing sodium intake is followed promptly by an increase in excretion.

In extreme circumstances, a change in sodium intake may result in hyponatremia or hypernatremia. *However, because serum sodium concentration is determined primarily by body water balance, hyponatremia usually results from excessive water retention, and hypernatremia usually results from water loss.* The amount of sodium intake can influence the ECF volume: Excessive sodium expands ECF volume, and decreased sodium reduces ECF volume. Therefore, serum sodium concentration alone rarely provides information on the clinical state of sodium balance.

AGE-RELATED CHANGES IN WATER AND SODIUM REGULATION

Normal aging is accompanied by certain changes that can affect water and sodium regulation: impaired renal ability to concentrate urine, increased ADH sécretion, impaired renal ability to conserve sodium, increased secretion of atrial natriuretic peptide, and impaired thirst perception.

Impaired renal ability to concentrate urine: Studies in healthy men between ages 40 and 101 show an impaired renal ability to concentrate urine as age increases. After 24 h of water deprivation, the maximum attainable urine specific gravity declines. The decrease is slight in those ages 60 to 65, greater in those > 65 yr, and even greater in those > 75 yr. Other studies in healthy men ages 26 to 86 show a progressive age-related decline in renal ability to concentrate urine in response to IV vasopressin. Thus, age predisposes a person to water loss when fluid intake is limited, increasing the risk of dehydration, even without clinically identifiable renal disease. The cause appears to be resistance to the renal action of ADH, ie, a form of **acquired partial nephrogenic diabetes insipidus.** In a patient with coexisting renal disease, this condition may lead to a clinically significant impaired ability to conserve fluid.

Increased ADH secretion: With age, the ability of the neurohypophyseal system to secrete ADH increases. In response to the osmotic stimulus of an IV hypertonic sodium chloride infusion, plasma ADH increases more at any level of serum osmolality in persons ages 54 to 92 than in persons ages 21 to 49. Similarly, IV ethanol is less effective in inhibiting ADH release in older persons. These observations suggest that osmoreceptor sensitivity increases with age. Some evidence indicates that this increased sensitivity may result from an impaired baroreceptor function, which decreases normal inhibitory activity on ADH release. Several studies also show that the basal concentration of ADH in blood may increase with age, becoming most evident in those > 60 yr. This increased ADH concentration and the increased secretion in response to osmotic and perhaps other stimuli elevate the risk of hyponatremia when fluid intake increases, leading to the **syndrome of inappropriate secretion of ADH (SIADH).**

Impaired renal ability to conserve sodium: A study of 89 healthy men ages 18 to 76 shows that the ability to decrease renal sodium excretion is impaired with age. When dietary sodium intake was restricted, those < 30 yr decreased urinary sodium excretion by 50% in a mean of 17.6 h, but those > 60 yr required a mean of 30.9 h. The cause of this decline is not fully understood, but it may result partly from an age-related decrease in circulating renin and aldosterone and partly from decreased responsiveness to acute stimuli. Another factor is nephron loss with a resulting increase in osmotic load per nephron and consequent osmotic diuresis.

In the elderly, basal blood levels of atrial natriuretic peptide are increased, and blood levels of this hormone increase more than in young persons after atrial stretch receptors are stimulated by acute volume expansion or increased heart rate. Atrial natriuretic peptide inhibits aldosterone secretion and is a likely factor in the age-associated decrease in aldosterone blood levels. These age-related changes may play a role in the impaired ability to conserve sodium and account for the continued renal loss of sodium when intake is reduced because of illness or dietary modification. The consequences are sodium depletion, decreased plasma volume, and the risk of hyponatremia.

Impaired thirst perception: Decreased thirst perception is not as well recognized as the other age-related factors discussed above. After being deprived of fluid intake for 24 h, healthy elderly persons are less thirsty than younger persons. When fluid is offered, the older persons ingest a strikingly lower amount, despite evidence that fluid deprivation increases plasma osmolality to a significantly higher level in this group. This loss of thirst perception again places older people at increased risk for volume depletion and dehydration.

VOLUME DEPLETION AND DEHYDRATION

Volume depletion is *a loss of body water and sodium, resulting in decreased ECF volume*. **Dehydration** is *a relatively pure depletion of water alone*.

Symptoms and Signs

Volume depletion and dehydration may present in several ways, but altered mental status, lethargy, light-headedness, and syncope are particularly common in elderly patients. Physical examination may disclose decreased skin turgor, dry mucous membranes, tachycardia, and orthostatic hypotension, but these findings may also appear in elderly persons with normal volume status. Increased hematocrit, blood urea nitrogen (BUN), and serum creatinine levels also point to significant volume depletion. The serum sodium level may be high, normal, or low, depending on the cause of the volume depletion. Urinary sodium excretion is usually < 20 mEq/L when sodium intake has been chronically reduced or losses have occurred from vomiting or diarrhea.

Diagnosis

A history of decreased food or fluid intake, febrile illness, diabetes mellitus, vomiting, diarrhea, chronic renal disease, use of diuretics, or nasogastric suction should alert the physician to the possibility of volume depletion or dehydration. Adrenal insufficiency must always be considered, especially if the physician notes evidence of a malignancy with a propensity toward metastasis to the adrenal gland. A urinary sodium concentration > 20 mEq/L is consistent with this disorder, as well as with chronic renal disease, which results in an impaired ability to conserve sodium. Hypercalcemia, hypokalemia, and hyperglycemia, with consequent glycosuria leading to osmotic diuresis, must be excluded as causes of the impaired renal ability to conserve water.

Treatment

When decreased ECF volume results almost entirely from water loss alone, the water deficit can be estimated using this calculation:

$$\text{Total body fluid volume (L)} = \frac{140 \text{ mEq/L} \times \text{basal body wt(kg)} \times 0.45}{\text{current serum Na (mEq/L)}}$$

In this formula, 0.45 represents the approximate proportion of body weight that is water. Total body fluid volume is subtracted from the patient's estimated normal total body water (0.45 × body weight) to give the value for approximate water deficit. This calculation is *not* valid if the person has also lost a large amount of sodium, resulting in hyponatremia.

When the volume deficit is modest (1 to 2 L), oral fluid intake can correct it, provided the patient does not have an accompanying GI disorder or impaired mental status. If the patient does have such a problem or if the volume deficit is more significant, IV fluid therapy is required, preferably with isotonic fluid (0.9% sodium chloride), provided the patient is not hypernatremic from dehydration. If the patient is hypernatremic, hypotonic fluid (0.45% sodium chloride) should be used. The administration rate should be such that once orthostatic hypotension and tachycardia resolve, the remaining deficit will be corrected over 2 to 3 days to avoid precipitating heart failure. Useful clinical indications of therapeutic effectiveness are increases in skin turgor and urine output and decreases in heart rate, orthostatic blood pressure, and BUN and creatinine levels. The patient should be evaluated for other deficits (including hypokalemia, hypomagnesemia, hypophosphatemia, and metabolic acidosis) and treated as necessary.

HYPONATREMIA

A serum sodium level of < 136 mEq/L that occurs with an excess of water relative to total sodium. Total ECF volume may be increased, normal, or decreased.

Older persons are at increased risk for developing hyponatremia. An analysis of 139 sets of plasma electrolyte values for healthy persons revealed an age-related decrease of 1 mEq/L/decade from a mean value of 141 ± 4 mEq/L in younger persons. In another study, 7% of ambulatory persons ≥ 65 yr who were living at home and showed no evidence of acute illness had serum sodium levels ≤ 137 mEq/L. An increased prevalence of hyponatremia has also been found in hospitalized patients. An analysis of 5000 consecutive sets of plasma electrolyte values from hospitalized patients with a mean age of 54 yr revealed a mean serum sodium level of 134 mEq/L, with values skewed toward the hyponatremic end of the frequency distribution curve. Among elderly patients in long-term care facilities, an 18% to 22% prevalence of serum sodium levels ≤ 135 mEq/L was noted. In a longitudinal study over 12 mo, the incidence of hyponatremia in this population was about 50%. While hyponatremia is common in the elderly, it often does not produce clinically apparent symptoms, especially when it is mild.

Etiology and Pathophysiology

Hyponatremia may occur in association with combined sodium and ECF volume depletion, as with vomiting, diarrhea, GI suction, renal disorders, and diuretic therapy. In such cases, volume depletion stimulates ADH release so that excess water is retained in excess of sodium. Hyponatremia resulting from these events is usually mild—rarely being < 125 mEq/L.

Disorders producing edematous states, eg, heart failure, cirrhosis, nephrotic syndrome, or acute glomerulonephritis, are associated with an *elevated* total body sodium content and normal or increased ECF volume. However, effective plasma volume is reduced, restricting the delivery of sodium and water to the diluting segments of the nephron. Consequently, sodium-retaining mechanisms are activated as ADH release increases. Over time, a net gain of water relative to sodium leads to dilutional hyponatremia.

In a form of hyponatremia common among the elderly, total body sodium content is *normal* but water is retained because of increased ADH secretion, ie, the **syndrome of inappropriate secretion of ADH (SIADH).** This syndrome, which has many causes, is defined by inappropriate hypertonicity of the urine, often with hypotonicity of the plasma; increased excretion of sodium in the urine; plasma volume dilution, as suggested by normal or low BUN and creatinine levels; and no edema. Elderly patients with underlying disorders that may lead to SIADH often have normal serum sodium levels because fluid intake may not be sufficient to produce a dilutional hyponatremia. However, when fluid intake increases (eg, when IV fluids are administered or when oral intake is encouraged to treat febrile illness), the increase in body water may lead to rapid development of hyponatremia. This condition is especially likely to occur in institutionalized patients, whose fluid intake is not primarily determined by thirst or custom (see TABLE 3–1).

Another common cause of hyponatremia in elderly patients is the use of nutritional supplements such as Isocal, Ensure, or Osmolite. Such formulas are almost universally low in sodium content, containing about 20 to 30 mEq/1000 calories. These dietary sources should be supplemented with sodium to provide a total intake of about 100 mEq daily.

Symptoms, Signs, and Diagnosis

The severity of the symptoms and signs depends on the severity of the hyponatremia and the rapidity with which the serum sodium level declined. Mild chronic hyponatremia may be asymptomatic. When serum levels fall to < 125 mEq/L, lethargy, fatigue, and muscle cramps may occur. Such GI symptoms as anorexia and nausea may also occur early.

TABLE 3–1. CAUSES OF SIADH

CNS disorders	Acute intermittent porphyria Infectious diseases Systemic lupus erythematosus Trauma Tumor Vascular diseases
Malignancy with ectopic hormone production	Hodgkin's disease Lymphosarcoma Pancreatic carcinoma Reticulum cell sarcoma Small cell carcinoma of lung Thymoma
Pulmonary disease	Lung abscess Pneumonia Tuberculosis
Drugs	Carbamazepine Chlorpropamide Cyclophosphamide General anesthetics Narcotics Oxytocin Phenoxybenzamine Serotonin reuptake inhibitors (eg, fluoxetine) Thiazide diuretics Tricyclic antidepressants Vinblastine Vincristine
Other	Hypothyroidism Positive-pressure breathing

SIADH = syndrome of inappropriate secretion of antidiuretic hormone.

The CNS manifestations of hyponatremia—ranging from disorientation to confusion, coma, and seizures—are often related to the severity of the hyponatremia. Severe hyponatremia may be accompanied by depressed sensorium, depressed deep tendon reflexes, hypothermia, Cheyne-Stokes respiration, and pathologic reflexes. *Serum sodium values < 115 mEq/L may result in sudden death.* The overall mortality rate in patients with symptomatic hyponatremia and a serum sodium level < 120 mEq/L is about 40%; with coexisting alcoholism or cachexia, the rate reaches about 70%.

When hyponatremia results from volume depletion, the physical examination may reveal signs of hypovolemia; when hyponatremia results from sodium retention and decreased effective plasma volume, the examination may reveal edema. Edema rarely occurs in patients with SIADH.

Measurements of serum BUN and creatinine levels also help determine the type of hyponatremia. These values are usually elevated in patients with combined sodium and ECF volume depletion and in those with decreased effective plasma volume. Serum BUN and creatinine values are usually normal or low in patients with dilutional hyponatremia or SIADH. The urinary sodium level is usually < 20 mEq/L in patients with volume depletion or edema; it is usually > 20 mEq/L in patients with expanded ECF volume, such as occurs in SIADH.

An **oral water-loading test** may help diagnose SIADH. *However, this test should not be performed on patients who have serum sodium levels < 125 mEq/L or those who have symptomatic hyponatremia regardless of the serum sodium level.* A patient undergoing the test receives an oral water load of 20 mL/kg of body weight over 15 to 30 min. The patient is then kept recumbent for 5 h, except when voiding. Urine is collected hourly for 5 h, and the volume and osmolality of each specimen are measured. A normal response is excretion of > 80% of the water load in 5 h and a decrease in urine osmolality to < 100 mOsm/kg in at least one specimen, usually that collected for the second hour. Patients with SIADH have an impaired ability to excrete the water load and dilute the urine. A normal response in a hyponatremic person whose clinical and laboratory findings indicate a normal or expanded ECF volume suggests that the hyponatremia may result from primary polydipsia or a low-set osmoreceptor mechanism.

Other possible causes of hyponatremia, such as hyperglycemia from diabetes mellitus, must be excluded. With hyperglycemia, the glucose-induced hyperosmolar state produces a shift of body water into the intravascular space, diluting serum sodium by about 1.6 mEq/L for each 100 mg/dL increase in blood glucose above normal. Correcting the hyperglycemia returns the serum sodium level to normal.

Pseudohyponatremia may occur in patients with marked hyperlipidemia or hyperproteinemia. In these conditions, the increased lipid or protein replaces a portion of sodium-containing plasma so that the measured sodium concentration per liter of plasma is reduced. However, a plasma osmolality determination will reveal a normal value for solute concentration because this measurement reflects solute concentration of plasma water.

A summary of the differentiating features of various types of hyponatremia appears in TABLE 3–2.

Treatment

In patients with hyponatremia from sodium and ECF volume depletion, treatment is based on correcting the volume deficit with 0.9% sodium chloride. If the serum sodium level is < 125 mEq/L, some of the IV fluid should be hypertonic sodium chloride solution. In hypona-

TABLE 3–2. DIFFERENTIATING FEATURES OF HYPONATREMIA

Type of Hyponatremia	*Edema*	*BUN and Serum Creatinine Levels*	*Urine Sodium Level (mEq/L)*	*Response to Water Load*
Sodium and ECF volume depletion	–	↑	< 20	Impaired
Decreased effective plasma volume	+	↑	< 20	Impaired
Dilutional SIADH	–	NL or ↓	> 20	Impaired
Primary polydipsia	–	NL or ↓	> 20	Normal
Low-set osmoreceptor	–	NL	> 20	Normal

ECF = extracellular fluid; SIADH = syndrome of inappropriate secretion of antidiuretic hormone; NL = normal limits

tremic patients who have decreased effective plasma volume and edema, treatment should be directed at the underlying cause—ie, heart failure, cirrhosis, or nephrotic syndrome. Although diuretics (eg, furosemide) can often reduce edema, they may cause a natriuresis that further decreases the serum sodium level. In such cases, moderate fluid restriction (eg, 1000 to 1500 mL/24 h) may be sufficient to correct the hyponatremia.

Symptomatic hyponatremia, particularly that resulting from a dilutional state, warrants prompt intervention. In the mildly symptomatic patient with a serum sodium level > 125 mEq/L, restricting fluid to 800 to 1000 mL/day is usually sufficient. In a patient with more severe symptoms, serum sodium should be increased more rapidly by infusing hypertonic sodium chloride solution until symptoms begin to clear and the serum sodium level reaches about 120 to 125 mEq/L. A goal is to elevate the serum sodium level at a rate of 1 to 2 mEq/L/h. This can usually be accomplished by administering 200 to 300 mL of 3% sodium chloride solution over 4 to 6 h. Patients with serum sodium levels < 105 mEq/L and symptoms of seizure or coma may benefit from simultaneous administration of IV furosemide to promote diuresis. These patients may require larger amounts of hypertonic sodium chloride solution to compensate for the enhanced natriuresis, and serum electrolyte levels must be monitored to avoid diuretic-induced hypokalemia and hypomagnesemia.

Overcorrection of hyponatremia must be avoided. Usually, restoring the serum sodium level to about 120 to 125 mEq/L corrects the major symptoms. In severely malnourished patients and especially in alcoholics, **central pontine myelinolysis** may result from rapidly increasing the level to > 140 mEq/L.

Chronic management of hyponatremia is based on identifying and correcting the underlying cause. Fluid intake may also be restricted (usually 1000 to 1500 mL/day) to maintain a serum sodium level > 130 mEq/L. In patients who do not respond to or are unable to comply with fluid restriction, the tetracycline antibiotic demeclocycline 600 to 1200 mg/day can induce mild nephrogenic diabetes insipidus with polyuria of 2 to 4 L/24 h. Patients treated with this drug require careful monitoring of fluid balance to avoid excessive fluid loss. Also, some patients have markedly elevated serum BUN levels as a result of demeclocycline treatment.

HYPERNATREMIA

A serum sodium level of > 146 mEq/L that results from decreased body water relative to total body sodium content.

Common in the elderly, hypernatremia has a prevalence of about 1% in hospitalized patients ≥ 60 yr of age. A similar prevalence was noted among elderly residents of a long-term care facility, with the incidence increasing to 18% when the population was evaluated over 12 mo.

Hypernatremia in the elderly poses a high risk of morbidity and mortality; often, the more severe the predisposing factor, the higher the risk. The CNS manifestations are common, often leading to a depressed sensorium and chronic functional decline in those who survive the acute episode. In one study of elderly hospitalized patients who developed hypernatremia with serum sodium levels > 148 mEq/L, the mortality rate was about 40%. The mortality rate was highest in those with a rapid onset and those with a serum sodium level > 160 mEq/L.

Etiology

The most common mechanism underlying hypernatremia is an excessive loss of body water relative to the loss of sodium in association with inadequate fluid intake (see TABLE 3–3). The water deficit can reach 11 L or 30% of the total body water volume. Disorders leading to such severe water depletion include febrile illness with increased insensible losses, tachypnea with increased water loss from the lungs, fever-related obtundation or debilitating illness with decreased oral fluid intake, diarrhea from hyperosmolar tube feedings, and polyuria from uncontrolled diabetes mellitus with glycosuria. Rarely, dehydration and hypernatremia occur in elderly patients with central diabetes in-

TABLE 3–3. CAUSES OF HYPERNATREMIA

Decreased water intake	Physical impairment Mental impairment Obtundation Hypodipsia, adipsia
Increased water loss	Increased insensible loss Fever Tachypnea Sweating Diarrhea Dialysis Renal water loss Loop diuretics Osmotic diuresis—glucose, mannitol, sodium, urea Diabetes insipidus Nephrogenic diabetes insipidus Chronic renal disease Hypercalcemia Hypokalemia
Increased sodium intake	Sodium bicarbonate therapy IV administration of isotonic or hypertonic sodium chloride solution

sipidus or with acquired vasopressin resistance resulting from chronic renal disease, hypercalcemia, or hypokalemia. Excessive water depletion commonly results from potent loop diuretics.

Occasionally, hypernatremia occurs without accompanying dehydration because of a high sodium intake. This may occur after sodium bicarbonate administration for cardiac arrest or metabolic acidosis or after an infusion of 0.9% sodium chloride solution for fluid loss or shock.

Symptoms and Signs

The symptoms of moderate hypernatremia may be nonspecific; weakness and lethargy are common. More severe hypernatremia (serum sodium levels > 152 mEq/L) may be accompanied by obtundation, stupor, coma, and seizures. The clinical signs are those of volume depletion and dehydration—weight loss, decreased skin turgor, dry mucous membranes, and orthostatic hypotension. Besides an increased serum sodium level, the laboratory findings are those of hemoconcentration—increased hematocrit, serum osmolality, BUN, and creatinine values. Urine osmolality may not be greatly increased because of age-associated impairment in renal concentrating capacity.

Treatment

Early recognition and treatment of mild hypernatremia and maintenance of fluid balance are especially important in hospitalized elderly patients. Many cases of severe hypernatremia develop after admission and evolve rapidly as a result of therapeutic interventions or progression of the underlying disease.

Correcting hypernatremia requires replacing body water deficits with hypotonic fluid. The severity of the water deficit can be estimated as described under VOLUME DEPLETION AND DEHYDRATION, above. Either 0.45% sodium chloride solution or 5% dextrose in water should be administered at a rate that will correct the hypernatremia in about 48 h. The serum sodium level should be lowered no more rapidly than 2 mEq/L/h. *Excessively rapid correction may lead to cerebral edema with either permanent brain damage or death.* In the elderly patient with coexisting cardiac disease, caution must be used to avoid heart failure.

When the cause of hypernatremia is identified (eg, diabetes insipidus, diuretic therapy, increased sodium intake), specific treatment measures should be implemented.

PHYSIOLOGIC REGULATION OF POTASSIUM

Normal total body stores of potassium are about 3500 to 4000 mEq, most of which is within the cells, where levels range from 120 to 160 mEq/L. Only about 2% of total body potassium is in the ECF, where levels are 4 to 5 mEq/L. Thus, a serum potassium measurement is often inadequate for estimating total body potassium. However, small shifts of potassium between the extracellular and intracellular compartments can have profound effects on the serum potassium level with marked functional consequences.

Several homeostatic mechanisms help maintain serum potassium levels within a relatively narrow range. The usual dietary intake of potassium is 70 to 100 mEq/day, of which about 90% is taken up into the ECF and subsequently excreted by the kidney. The kidney can respond to variations in dietary potassium intake because most is filtered at the glomerulus, and about 90% of this potassium is passively reabsorbed at the level of the proximal tubule and loop of Henle. At the level of the distal tubule and collecting duct, potassium is secreted into the tubular lumen, partly through the action of aldosterone; the amount excreted daily is similar to the amount of oral intake. In response to severe potassium depletion, urinary potassium levels will fall but rarely to < 5 to 10 mEq/L. Besides the kidney, the distal colon also can increase potassium excretion in response to increased intake.

Transcellular flux is also important in regulating the serum potassium level. Cellular uptake is stimulated by insulin, aldosterone, epinephrine, and alkalosis and can modulate the impact of high oral potassium intake on serum levels. Thus, the intracellular mass of potassium serves as a buffer system to help maintain consistency in the ECF.

With normal aging, total body potassium decreases. This decrease reflects the decline in lean body muscle mass, which contains about 75% of intracellular potassium. Although cross-sectional data generally do not show that age influences serum potassium levels, several studies of healthy elderly people and longitudinal data suggest a slight increase, especially in men, but not to values above normal. The kidney's ability to regulate potassium excretion is unaffected by aging, even though an age-associated decline in aldosterone secretion has been documented.

HYPOKALEMIA

A serum potassium level of < 3.5 mEq/L. Total body potassium may be normal or decreased.

Etiology

Common in the elderly, hypokalemia can result from decreased dietary intake of potassium, increased renal or GI losses caused by diseases of these organs, use of drugs that interfere with normal regulatory mechanisms, and excessive mineralocorticoid or glucocorticoid levels (see TABLE 3–4). Hypokalemia may also result when potassium shifts from the ECF into the cells, as may occur in response to alkalosis, insulin administration, or use of β-adrenergic agonists. In diabetic acidosis, potassium shifts from the intracellular compartment to the extracellular compartment and is subsequently excreted in the urine. The resulting potassium depletion is usually masked by the intercompartmental shift, so that when the acidosis is corrected by insulin administration and fluid deficits are corrected, marked hypokalemia may occur.

One of the most common causes of hypokalemia is treatment with thiazide or loop diuretics. About 20% of patients receiving thiazide diuretics develop hypokalemia, but serum potassium levels rarely fall below 3 mEq/L.

Symptoms and Signs

Common symptoms of hypokalemia in the elderly are fatigue, confusion, and muscle weakness and cramps from impaired skeletal muscle function. Severe hypokalemia (< 2.5 mEq/L) can result in frank paralysis, as occurs in periodic paralysis. Smooth muscle function of the GI tract can also be affected, leading to adynamic ileus.

Potassium deficiency can affect cardiac function, resulting in atrial and ventricular ectopic beats, atrial and ventricular tachycardia, ventricular fibrillation, and sudden death—particularly in patients who have preexisting heart disease or those taking digitalis preparations.

TABLE 3–4. CAUSES OF HYPOKALEMIA IN THE ELDERLY

Inadequate dietary potassium intake

Increased gastrointestinal loss
- Vomiting
- Diarrhea
- Laxative use
- Fistulas
- Tube drainage

Increased renal loss
- Renal tubular acidosis (proximal and distal)
- Thiazide diuretic use
- Loop diuretic use (furosemide, bumetanide, ethacrynic acid)
- Antibiotic use (gentamicin, penicillins, amphotericin B)
- Primary hyperaldosteronism
- Secondary hyperaldosteronism (heart failure, cirrhosis)
- Cushing's syndrome
- Exogenous glucocorticoids
- Exogenous mineralocorticoids
- Hyperreninemic renovascular hypertension
- Postobstructive diuresis

Transcellular shift
- Alkalosis
- Insulin administration
- β-Adrenergic agonists

Hematologic disorders
- Vitamin B_{12} treatment of megaloblastic anemia
- Acute myeloid leukemia

Hypomagnesemia

The ECG often shows ST segment depression, T wave flattening, and a prominent U wave. With severe potassium depletion, atrioventricular conduction disturbances can develop.

Polyuria and secondary polydipsia can result from hypokalemic nephropathy, which is characterized by a vasopressin-resistant impairment in urinary concentrating capacity that makes the isotonicity of urine about that of plasma. Potassium depletion increases renal ammonia synthesis and acid excretion, resulting in metabolic alkalosis and elevated serum bicarbonate levels. Hypokalemia can impair insulin secretion without altering peripheral glucose use. Thus, about 33% of patients receiving long-term thiazide therapy develop glucose intolerance, most likely from hypokalemia. However, overt diabetes mellitus is uncommon.

Treatment

Treatment consists of correcting the underlying cause if possible, correcting total body deficits, and restoring normal serum potassium levels. When no cause (ie, use of a diuretic or chronic diarrhea) is apparent, measuring urinary potassium excretion helps establish whether urinary loss is abnormal. In a patient with hypokalemia, urinary excretion of > 20 mEq/L suggests an excessive urinary loss.

When urgent treatment is not required, potassium chloride 10 to 15 mEq orally q 4 to 8 h should be given until the serum potassium level is normal. Using timed-release preparations decreases local exposure of the GI mucosa to high concentrations of potassium and thus reduces the risk of irritation and ulceration. If hypokalemia is caused by a thiazide diuretic, adding a potassium-sparing agent such as triamterene, amiloride, or spironolactone may maintain normal blood potassium levels once the deficit has been corrected. Magnesium depletion may need to be corrected before hypokalemia responds to treatment. In patients with severe diarrhea or ureteral diversions such as an ileal bladder, hypokalemia may be accompanied by a hyperchloremic metabolic acidosis. In such cases, potassium replacement should be accomplished with potassium bicarbonate.

When urgent treatment is needed (ie, when the patient has serious symptoms or an arrhythmia), potassium chloride should be given IV. The potassium concentration in the IV fluid usually should not exceed 40 mEq/L, and the administration rate should not exceed 10 to 20 mEq/h with a total dose of 100 to 300 mEq/24 h. In rare emergencies when a patient has a serious cardiac arrhythmia and the serum potassium level is < 2 mEq/L, the infusion can be given in a concentration of 60 mEq/L at a rate up to 40 mEq/h. Such therapy should be given for only a few hours and requires continuous ECG monitoring and frequent measurement of serum potassium levels.

HYPERKALEMIA

A serum potassium level of > 5 mEq/L. Total body potassium is normal, but distribution between intracellular and extracellular compartments is abnormal.

Etiology

An elevated serum potassium level may result from **pseudohyperkalemia** caused by hemolysis or the release of potassium from platelets during sample storage. Platelets are rich in potassium, and with thrombocytosis, enough potassium may be released during the clotting process to raise serum levels above normal. However, plasma potassium levels remain normal.

Normally, potassium from excessive intake is excreted in the urine. Only in patients with renal disease or impaired tubular function does excessive intake lead to hyperkalemia. Patients with acute oliguric renal failure are at especially high risk. Chronic renal disease with hyperkalemia may result from hyporeninemic hyperaldosteronism, particularly in patients with diabetes mellitus. The possibility of primary or secondary adrenal insufficiency must also be considered. Active GI bleeding, especially in a patient with a reduced glomerular filtration rate, can also lead to hyperkalemia.

In the elderly, hyperkalemia can be caused by several common medications, including potassium-sparing diuretics (triamterene, amiloride, and spironolactone) and nonsteroidal anti-inflammatory drugs. Angiotensin converting enzyme inhibitors and β-adrenergic blockers, which interfere with potassium excretion, can also cause hyperkalemia. A relatively small shift of potassium from the intracellular compartment to the extracellular compartment can result in marked hyperkalemia. This may occur in metabolic acidosis, especially diabetic ketoacidosis. Rhabdomyolysis from trauma can also shift potassium into the ECF.

Symptoms and Signs

Hyperkalemia may be asymptomatic until evidence of cardiac toxicity develops. Initial ECG changes—shortened QT_C interval and tall, narrow T waves—usually signify a serum potassium level of > 5.5 mEq/L. A further rise in the serum potassium level causes nodal and ventricular arrhythmias along with widened QRS complexes and prolonged PR intervals. Ultimately, ventricular fibrillation or asystole can develop.

Nonspecific neuromuscular symptoms, including vague weakness and paresthesias, may occur. With severe hyperkalemia, flaccid paralysis may occur.

Treatment

In patients with mild hyperkalemia (5.0 to 5.5 mEq/L), decreasing potassium intake to 40 to 60 mEq/day may correct the serum values. Potentially causative drugs and foods should be discontinued. If the patient has chronic renal disease or another clinical disorder in which hypoaldosteronism is a suspected cause, trial therapy with fludrocortisone acetate 0.05 to 0.2 mg/day may produce a normal serum potassium level in several days.

A patient with moderate hyperkalemia (5.5 to 6.0 mEq/L) and no significant ECG changes can be given the ion exchange resin sodium polystyrene sulfonate 15 to 20 gm orally. Administering 30 mL of a 50% solution of sorbitol orally enhances the effectiveness of the sodium polystyrene sulfonate and prevents constipation. If oral intake is not possible, sodium polystyrene sulfonate can be given as a retention enema of 50 to 60 gm in 200 mL of tap water at 4-h to 6-h intervals. Furosemide in doses of 40 to 100 mg IV may also help by rapidly increasing potassium excretion in the urine. Intravascular volume repletion with 0.9% sodium chloride is essential in ensuring the maximum renal capacity for excreting potassium.

Severe hyperkalemia (> 6.0 mEq/L) or a rising serum potassium level in a patient with renal insufficiency warrants prompt, aggressive therapy and may constitute a medical emergency. The first priority is to reverse cardiac toxicity. Thus, if an atrioventricular block or changes in the QRS complex or P wave appear on the ECG, 10 to 20 mL of 10% calcium gluconate should be given IV along with 50 to 100 mL of 7.5% sodium bicarbonate solution. Calcium gluconate must be given cautiously to patients receiving digitalis preparations. An infusion of 100 to 300 mL of 50% glucose containing 1 u. of regular insulin per 3 gm of glucose given over 30 min will shift potassium to the intracellular space. Sodium polystyrene sulfonate and sorbitol in the doses described above will facilitate potassium excretion. If these emergency measures do not adequately control severe hyperkalemia, hemodialysis should be initiated promptly.

ACID–BASE REGULATION

The pH of the ECF (normal range 7.35 to 7.45) is unaffected by normal aging, although age-associated changes do occur in certain respiratory and renal regulatory processes involved in maintaining a normal pH. Thus, the ability to respond to a challenge may be limited. For example, the ability to hyperventilate in response to acute metabolic acidosis may be blunted, leading to a further decline in pH. The aging kidney is slower to respond to an acid load, so that the blood pH may recover more slowly. Many disorders common in the elderly can overwhelm the regulatory systems and contribute to acid-base disturbances. Such disorders include heart failure, anemia, sepsis, renal disease, pulmonary disease, and diabetes mellitus. Also, many common drugs—including salicylates, diuretics, and laxatives—may precipitate acid-base disturbances.

The combination of impaired homeostatic mechanisms and the high prevalence of drug use and disease in the elderly make disturbances of acid-base balance common. Metabolic and respiratory acidosis and alkalosis can occur as simple disorders or, frequently in the elderly, as mixed disorders. For example, metabolic acidosis with concomitant respiratory acidosis can occur with heart failure, pneumonia, and acute respiratory failure. Similarly, a patient with heart failure may have a metabolic acidosis from poor tissue perfusion and a metabolic alkalosis from diuretic therapy. In general, changes in serum bicarbonate (HCO_3^-) concentration reflect metabolic acidosis or alkalosis, and $PaCO_2$ changes reflect respiratory acidosis and alkalosis. Characterizing the disturbance requires measurements of arterial pH, Pa_{O_2}, and Pa_{CO_2} along with serum electrolyte, BUN, and creatinine levels. Urinary electrolyte levels and pH may also be helpful.

METABOLIC ACIDOSIS

Metabolic acidosis is *a primary decrease in ECF HCO_3^-; pH and carbon dioxide content are decreased.* Metabolic acidosis with no increase in the anion gap (normal 8 to 15 mEq) can result from renal tubular acidosis or from a loss of bicarbonate or organic acid anions in patients with diarrhea; the condition is characterized by hyperchloremia. Acidosis with an increased anion gap (such as occurs with lactic acidosis, diabetic ketoacidosis, salicylate toxicity, and renal failure) is more common.

The history; physical examination findings such as hyperpnea; and laboratory measurements such as blood gas determinations, urine pH, and BUN, creatinine, blood glucose, and ketone levels usually establish the diagnosis and point to the underlying disease process. A urine pH > 5.5 with metabolic acidosis occurs in renal tubular acidosis.

Initial treatment is directed toward correcting the underlying disease process. When severe acidosis (pH < 7.2) is accompanied by symptoms such as anorexia, nausea, lethargy, and hyperventilation, treatment should be started with IV sodium bicarbonate. The sodium bicarbonate requirement can be estimated with this formula: mEq of sodium HCO_3^- required = (HCO_3^- desired − HCO_3^- observed) × 40% body weight in kilograms. Acute complete correction of arterial pH is not a goal of therapy, and caution must be used to avoid volume and sodium overload.

METABOLIC ALKALOSIS

Metabolic alkalosis is a *primary increase in blood HCO_3^-; pH and carbon dioxide content are increased.* Acid loss can result from vomiting, prolonged gastric suctioning, and diuretic-induced renal potassium loss. Alkalosis can also result from increased renal bicarbonate reabsorption in the proximal tubule as a consequence of plasma volume contraction and primary or secondary aldosteronism. Potassium depletion further enhances the renal tubular reabsorption of bicarbonate stimulated by volume contraction. Metabolic alkalosis may also develop in patients who have respiratory failure and hypercapnia after mechanical ventilation therapy.

The goal of therapy is to eliminate the factors maintaining the alkalosis. Plasma volume expansion with 0.9% sodium chloride solution should be initiated, and potassium deficits should be corrected. Acetazolamide 500 to 1000 mg/day given orally in divided doses may help in chronic alkalosis.

RESPIRATORY ACIDOSIS

Respiratory acidosis is *a primary increase in* Pa_{CO_2}*; pH is decreased and carbon dioxide content increased if renal function is intact.* Caused by carbon dioxide retention from alveolar hypoventilation, respiratory acidosis may result from disorders that depress the central respiratory center, restrict chest wall mobility, reduce pulmonary alveolar surface area, or narrow the upper airway. In the elderly, reduced vital capacity and ventilatory responses to hypoxia and hypercapnia predispose patients to acid-base disorders. Common causes are drugs that can produce respiratory depression, neuromuscular disorders that affect chest wall muscle function, and pulmonary disorders including emphysema, chronic bronchitis, pneumonia, asthma, and pneumothorax. Respiratory acidosis is often accompanied by hypoxia.

Progressive respiratory failure often results in a metabolic encephalopathy with headache, drowsiness, and ultimately stupor and coma. Asterixis and myoclonus may develop. Treatment aims at improving the underlying pulmonary disorder and may include intubation and assisted mechanical ventilation. Hypoxia must be corrected with the lowest possible oxygen concentration to avoid further depression of respiratory drive. Many patients also have concomitant metabolic alkalosis.

RESPIRATORY ALKALOSIS

Respiratory alkalosis is *a primary decrease in* Pa_{CO_2}*; pH is increased and carbon dioxide decreased.* The hyperventilation usually present leads to an excessive loss of carbon dioxide. Common causes include mechanical overventilation, hypoxemia, sepsis, pulmonary embolism, heart failure, hepatic failure, primary CNS disorders, and salicylate toxicity. Anxiety can cause a mild, acute respiratory alkalosis with a characteristic hyperventilation syndrome including facial flushing, finger and circumoral paresthesias, light-headedness, tachycardia, and a sense of suffocation. Physiologic consequences of respiratory alkalosis include cerebral vasoconstriction with resulting cerebral hypoxia and decreased ionized serum calcium levels leading to tetany and hypophosphatemia.

When the patient is hypoxemic, inspired oxygen should be used to correct abnormal gas exchange. Hyperventilation symptoms from anxiety usually resolve when the patient rebreathes expired carbon dioxide from a paper bag.

4. GERIATRIC EMERGENCIES

Rapid diagnosis and treatment of medical emergencies is often impaired in older persons because they respond differently to the stress of illness and have coexisting medical and social problems. Some elderly persons are unable to give complete histories and to cope with the bustle of the emergency department. Hearing and visual impairment, dementia, delirium, and a patient's inadequate knowledge of his medical history may present special problems for both the patient and the health care providers. Because presbycusis and other hearing disorders decrease auditory discrimination in noisy places, the history should be obtained in a quiet area whenever possible. Because the bright lights used in examinations may be frightening to persons with dementia and cause visual disturbances in persons with cataracts, lighting should be adjusted to allow adequate examination without distracting the patient. Taking a little extra time to calm and comfort an older patient can save time in the long run and increase the yield from the history and examination.

Supplementing the patient interview with an interview of family members and caregivers is often necessary to obtain relevant information. The family is usually the best source of information on baseline function, the onset of illness, and chronic medical conditions and treatment. These interviews are best performed before transferring the patient from the emergency department to the hospital floor because family members often leave before the patient is admitted to a hospital room. When available, a patient's previous records should be reviewed, and the existence of advance medical directives should be sought. When a patient arrives in the emergency department from a nursing home, a nurse or doctor should call the nursing home to obtain relevant data rather than rely on the sparse information provided on a transfer record.

This chapter addresses the following common emergencies: chest pain, syncope, gastrointestinal bleeding, infections, heatstroke, and hypothermia. Other important emergencies—such as cardiac arrhythmias, changes in mental status, hyperosmotic-hyperosmolar nonketotic coma, perforation of peptic ulcer, and socially determined crises (eg, "elder dumping")—are discussed elsewhere in THE MANUAL.

CHEST PAIN

Many diseases cause acute chest pain, and therefore the specific cause is often difficult to identify. Chronic illnesses, dementia, delirium, and atypical presentations of illness may contribute to the difficulty. Because treatment of chest pain in the elderly is similar to that in younger patients, this discussion focuses on diagnosis.

Coronary artery disease: Although coronary artery disease is the most common cause of death in the elderly, older patients often do not have (or do not report) the associated pain of angina pectoris. Chest pain accompanies an acute **myocardial infarction** in less than 50% of older patients compared with 80% of younger patients. Dyspnea, confusion, paresthesias, or syncope may be the initial manifestations of myocardial infarction, and physical findings are nonspecific. Electrocardiographic findings are similar to those in younger persons (see also Ch. 37).

Thoracic aortic dissection: Usually characterized by sudden, severe, tearing chest pain, thoracic aortic dissection is suspected in patients with a history of hypertension. Supportive diagnostic criteria include the murmur of aortic regurgitation (proximal aortic dissection), pulse deficits of the upper extremities (brachiocephalic vessel involvement), chest x-ray evidence of mediastinal widening, and an ECG without evidence of acute myocardial infarction (see also AORTIC DISSECTION in Ch. 43).

The diagnosis of thoracic aortic dissection can be confirmed using a variety of studies. For the unstable patient who requires rapid diagnosis, transesophageal echocardiography should be used when available. For the stable patient, MRI scanning is acceptable. Though CT scanning may also be used, it is less accurate than other imaging modalities and requires the use of IV contrast agents. While aortography was once the gold standard, the other diagnostic modalities are now preferred. However, aortography is often required before surgical repair to define involvement of vessels that arise from the aorta.

Pulmonary embolism: Signaled by chest pain that is typically pleuritic and usually associated with acute dyspnea, pulmonary embolism is suspected in patients who have been immobilized, have recently undergone surgery, are taking estrogen therapy, have a history of deep venous thrombosis or pulmonary embolism, or have a malignancy. Tachycardia is common but may be absent if the patient is taking a β-blocking drug or has cardiac conduction system disease (eg, sick sinus syndrome). A pleural friction rub is characteristic but often difficult to detect. Suggestive laboratory findings are hypoxia with hypocapnia and an ECG indicating right ventricular strain. The chest x-ray is nonspecific and may demonstrate diaphragmatic elevation; basal, platelike atelectasis; pleural effusion; pulmonary infiltrate; or, in massive embolism, decreased vascularity of the affected lung. The diagnosis is supported by a high-probability radionuclide lung scan, but definitive diagnosis requires a pulmonary angiogram (see also Ch. 49).

Pneumothorax: Defined as the spontaneous rupture of the pleura with air from the lung entering the pleural space, pneumothorax may cause acute chest pain with dyspnea. Emphysema is the most common cause, but pulmonary fibrosis, chronic bronchitis, and asthma can also lead to pneumothorax. The diagnosis is supported by decreased breath sounds over the affected lung and is confirmed by evidence of lung collapse on an expiration chest x-ray.

Pneumonia: Patients with pneumonia may have sharp, pleuritic chest pain and an atypical presentation (see Ch. 46 and INFECTION, below).

Pericarditis: The pain of pericarditis is a stabbing sensation that increases with inspiration and decreases while the patient is sitting up and leaning forward. Idiopathic or viral pericarditis (which may follow an upper respiratory infection) is the most common cause of this type of chest pain, but tuberculosis, collagen-vascular disease, metastatic tumor, and acute myocardial infarction must be considered. An electrocardiogram typically reveals diffuse, concave upward ST-segment elevations in all leads (except aVR and V_1); these changes persist for several days.

Acute cholecystitis, peptic ulcer disease, and esophagitis: These disorders are common, and the initial presentation may be nonspecific, including referred chest pain. The medical history often suggests the diagnosis, and a relationship between meals and pain provocation can be identified. The physical examination may be nonspecific or may reveal right upper quadrant tenderness (cholecystitis) or epigastric tenderness (peptic ulcer disease, esophagitis). Laboratory and x-ray studies include testing stool for occult blood (peptic ulcer disease), upper GI series (peptic ulcer disease, esophagitis), oral cholecystogram (cholecystitis), abdominal ultrasonography (cholecystitis), and occasionally endoscopy.

Herpes zoster: This disorder is readily diagnosed by the characteristic vesicular eruption on an erythematous base along a dermatome. Occasionally, pain along the dermatomal distribution *precedes* the skin rash by 3 to 4 days. This may cause chest pain, sometimes with chills, fever, and malaise.

Musculoskeletal disease: While usually chronic, the chest pain caused by musculoskeletal disease may be acute and difficult to differentiate from that of more serious visceral causes. Diagnostic clues include generalized tenderness of the chest wall, reproducibility of the pain by palpating local areas of the chest wall, and relief of pain after injecting local anesthetics.

SYNCOPE

(See also Ch. 6)

Syncope, a transient loss of consciousness, is a common reason for a visit to the emergency department and, depending on its cause, may be a medical emergency. Syncope usually results from acutely diminished cerebral blood flow, which may be precipitated by cardiac arrhythmias, orthostatic hypotension, hypovolemia, vasodilation, cerebrovascular disease, cardiac outflow obstruction, or decreased cardiac output from left ventricular dysfunction (often because of a myocardial infarction).

Diagnosis

The history of the episode, including precipitating events, symptoms, coexisting medical problems, and drug use (see TABLE 4–1), is crucial to presumptive diagnosis. Information from family members or witnesses can also be helpful.

Clues to the cause of syncope are outlined in TABLE 4–2. Syncope preceded by sudden weakness, nausea, sweating, and warmth (especially in circumstances involving pain, fear, or prolonged standing, or when urinating, defecating, coughing, or swallowing) is usually due to enhanced vasovagal tone, resulting in bradycardia and/or peripheral vasodilation. This form of syncope does not occur in the supine position, and recovery is rapid. However, weakness, nausea, and sweating could indicate myocardial ischemia, which can cause syncope in any position and is often associated with chest pain. Loss of consciousness without warning suggests a cardiac arrhythmia or a seizure disorder that often has a prolonged recovery time or is followed by a postictal state.

Questioning about the position of the neck before the episode (ie, whether it was hyperextended) may provide a clue to carotid sinus hypersensitivity. Exertional syncope suggests a specific group of causes: aortic stenosis, hypertrophic cardiomyopathy, pulmonary hypertension, and exercise-induced arrhythmias. Syncope that develops within

TABLE 4–1. CATEGORIES OF DRUGS THAT CAN CAUSE SYNCOPE

Diuretics	Antidepressants
Most antihypertensives	Antipsychotics
Nitrates	β-blockers (including ophthalmics)
Calcium channel blockers	Digitalis
Antiarrhythmics	

TABLE 4–2. CLUES TO THE CAUSE OF SYNCOPE

	Most Common Cause
Symptoms and signs	
Nausea, sweating, anxiety, fever, warmth	Vasovagal syncope or myocardial infarction
Loss of consciousness without warning	Cardiac arrhythmia or other causes of poor cardiac output
Prolonged confusion, fatigue, postsyncope syndrome	Seizure
Precipitating event	
Neck turning	Hypersensitive carotid sinus
Exertion	Aortic stenosis, hypertrophic cardiomyopathy, pulmonary hypertension
Change to standing position	Orthostatic hypotension

a few seconds after standing indicates orthostatic hypotension (see Ch. 36), which may be associated with autonomic dysfunction or certain drugs (eg, vasodilators, diuretics).

The additive effect of coexisting diseases (eg, heart failure, chronic renal failure, angina pectoris, anemia, chronic obstructive pulmonary disease, venous and arterial insufficiency in the legs, and diabetes) and multiple drug regimens may result in a critical threshold for CNS dysfunction. Antihypertensive and antianginal drugs, as well as those with arrhythmogenic effects, often cause hypotension with syncope because of volume depletion, inadequate cardiac output, or peripheral vasodilation.

Some 60% to 85% of assignable diagnoses are based on the history, physical examination, and 12-lead ECG. **The physical examination** begins with measurement of blood pressure and pulse in the supine and standing positions. Orthostatic hypotension is more common in the elderly, although hypertension may be the primary cause of syncope. To implicate orthostatic hypotension, symptoms of syncope must appear with the postural drop in blood pressure. The carotid arteries should be examined for evidence of obstruction (bruits or delayed upstroke) and aortic stenosis (transmitted murmur and delayed upstroke). Aortic stenosis is particularly difficult to detect because the loss of vascular elasticity may mask typical physical findings (ie, delayed carotid upstroke and pulsus parvus et tardus). An ECG should be obtained to rule out acute myocardial infarction. If heart disease with arrhythmia is found or suspected, continuous cardiac monitoring should be initiated. An IV access should be maintained, and supplemental oxygen should be given by nasal cannula at 2 to 4 L/min. All patients should have a CBC and measurement of blood glucose, electrolytes, BUN, and creatinine levels.

Prognosis

The need for hospital admission can best be determined by reviewing the mortality rates of specific risk groups. At lowest risk are patients < 60 yr of age with a noncardiac or undetermined cause of syncope; these patients have a 2-yr mortality rate of 2% to 5%. Intermediate-risk patients are > 60 yr of age with a noncardiac or an unknown cause of syncope; they have a 2-yr mortality rate of 20%. Patients at highest risk are those of all ages whose syncope has a cardiac origin; their 2-yr mortality rate is 32% to 38%. However, *the underlying diseases that cause syncope determine mortality risk, not the syncope per se*. Patients whose syncope is suspected of being of cardiac origin *must* be admitted for evaluation. Lower-risk patients may require hospitalization, depending on the presumed cause of syncope.

GASTROINTESTINAL BLEEDING

(See also GASTROINTESTINAL BLEEDING in Ch. 62)

In the USA, GI bleeding in the elderly has a mortality rate that approaches 10%. Clinical manifestations are diverse, ranging from change in mental status to syncope with hemodynamic collapse. Rapid assessment of blood loss, cardiac status, and cause of hemorrhage is essential. Bleeding in the upper GI tract can lead to hyperkalemia, especially in those with renal failure or those receiving drugs that inhibit potassium excretion.

TABLE 4–3. ESTIMATION OF BLOOD VOLUME LOSS

Blood Volume Loss (%)	*Blood Pressure (mm Hg)*	*Pulse*	*Shock Status*
10–20	> 90	110/min	Mild
20–30	> 70–90	110–130/min	Moderate
> 30	< 70	> 130/min	Severe

TABLE 4–4. TREATMENT OF GASTROINTESTINAL BLEEDING

Categorize bleeding as severe, moderate, or occult
Insert large-bore (16- to 18-gauge) IV catheter, administer isotonic (0.9%) sodium chloride or lactated Ringer's solution
Type and crossmatch 4 units packed red blood cells (monitor fluid status closely)
Determine CBC (including platelets), PT, and PTT, and measure electrolyte, glucose, and creatinine levels
Insert nasogastric tube (No. 16 French or Ewald)
Consult with surgeon

CBC = complete blood count; PT = prothrombin time; PTT = partial thromboplastin time

Blood loss can be estimated by serial determinations of pulse and degree of shock. However, pulse rate may not be a sensitive indicator of hypovolemia because of baroreflex blunting. Hemoglobin and hematocrit levels may not reflect the degree of blood loss because of insufficient intravascular equilibration. Therefore, blood volume loss is perhaps best estimated as shown in TABLE 4–3.

Gastrointestinal bleeding may be described as follows: **severe** (active hematemesis or hematochezia with shock); **moderate** (active hematemesis or hematochezia with orthostatic change in blood pressure); or **occult** (positive result for occult blood in stool, decreased hemoglobin and hematocrit levels, fatigue, weakness, and stable blood pressure). Patients with severe or moderate bleeding require emergency evaluation and stabilization. Those with occult blood loss may receive outpatient evaluation if they are hemodynamically stable.

Treatment

Treatment is directed at replacing intravascular volume, achieving hemodynamic stabilization, and localizing the bleeding site (see TABLE 4–4). A large-bore (16- to 18-gauge) IV catheter is inserted, and blood or fluids are administered. If bleeding is severe or there is evidence of cardiac dysfunction, a pulmonary artery catheter may be needed to monitor fluid therapy. The following laboratory studies should also be performed: CBC (including platelet count); partial thromboplastin time; blood type and crossmatch; and measurement of electrolyte, glucose, and creatinine levels.

TABLE 4–5. CAUSES OF UPPER AND LOWER GASTROINTESTINAL TRACT BLEEDING

Cause	%
Upper GI tract	
Gastric ulcer	29
Duodenal ulcer	21
Gastritis	17
Esophagitis	14
Esophageal varices	12
Other	7
Lower GI tract	
Diverticulosis	43
Vascular ectasia of right colon	20
Undetermined	11
Radiation proctitis	6
Colorectal carcinoma	5
Colonic polyps	4
Other (inflammatory bowel disease, infections, hemorrhoids)	11

A nasogastric tube (No. 16 French or Ewald) is placed to assess upper GI tract bleeding, the major causes of which are listed in TABLE 4–5. If the nasogastric aspirate is bloody or has a coffee-ground appearance, the stomach is lavaged with 1 to 2 L room-temperature water or saline until the aspirate clears. The nasogastric tube can be removed after the diagnostic aspirate is obtained, but it should remain in place if the patient has an obstruction or protracted nausea and vomiting (see also Ch. 54).

If bright red blood from the rectum is noted, bleeding from the lower GI tract is likely. Causes of lower GI tract bleeding are listed in TABLE 4–5; diverticulosis and vascular ectasias (angiodysplasia) are most often implicated (see also Ch. 55). Surgical consultation is obtained for possible immediate intervention.

After achieving hemodynamic stabilization, the cause of bleeding should be determined. Additional history of drug use, abdominal vascular surgery, bleeding problems, or concomitant illness is obtained.

INFECTION

Infection is a common problem needing emergency evaluation. Most infections occur in the urinary tract or lungs, but diagnosis is often difficult because of atypical presentations.

URINARY TRACT INFECTIONS

(See also Ch. 65)

Urinary tract infections are very common, with an incidence of substantial bacteriuria as high as 15% in the elderly. Bacteremia may occur in up to ⅓ of these cases. Several factors—some age-related, some disease-related, and others iatrogenic—contribute to this high infection rate: bladder outlet obstruction from benign prostatic hyperplasia in men, atrophic vaginitis in women, diabetes, upper urinary tract stones, neuropathy resulting in poor bladder emptying, dementia with poor perianal hygiene, stroke, immobilization, and instrumentation of the urinary tract and use of indwelling bladder catheters.

Symptoms, Signs, and Diagnosis

In younger patients, the usual manifestations of urinary tract infection are frequency, dysuria, suprapubic discomfort, fever, and flank pain; in the elderly, incontinence, confusion, vague abdominal pain, anorexia, nausea, vomiting, azotemia, and loss of glycemic control in diabetics may also occur. On occasion, the initial manifestation of urosepsis may be septic shock, which has a mortality rate of 50% to 70% in the elderly.

When the patient arrives in the emergency department, a history is obtained and a physical examination is performed. In most cases, a CBC, measurement of serum creatinine level, and blood cultures are obtained. Urinalysis, urine culture and sensitivity, and Gram stain of sediment should be performed. Five organisms per high-power field corresponds with 95% confidence to bacteriuria at 10^5 organisms. Pyuria *without* bacteriuria should prompt consideration of renal calculi, papillary necrosis due to obstruction, diabetes, analgesic nephropathy, chronic prostatitis, or tuberculosis.

Fever, chills, abdominal discomfort, or signs of cardiopulmonary compromise strongly suggest sepsis. When these signs are present, a large-bore IV catheter is placed for administration of 5% dextrose in water and isotonic (0.9%) sodium chloride solution. If the urinary bladder is distended, an indwelling catheter is inserted and drained slowly to prevent bladder wall hemorrhage.

Treatment

Therapy may be initiated in the emergency department on the basis of the Gram stain findings. If gram-negative organisms are noted, one of the third-generation cephalosporins (cefotaxime, cefoperazone, moxalactam) or an aminoglycoside (gentamicin or tobramycin) may be administered. Gram-positive cocci in chains may represent enterococci, and a penicillin (ampicillin) or vancomycin (for the penicillin-allergic patient) is necessary. Gram-positive cocci in clumps suggest *Staphylococcus,* and the patient should be treated with a first-generation cephalosporin (cefazolin). Hospital admission for a 10-day course of therapy and further evaluation of underlying problems is warranted in those with suspected pyelonephritis or sepsis. If the patient is afebrile and the white blood cell count is normal with no bands present, oral therapy with ampicillin or ciprofloxacin is indicated and the patient may be discharged.

PNEUMONIA

(See also Ch. 46)

Bacterial pneumonias are the principal cause of death from infectious disease in the elderly and overall the fourth or fifth leading cause in the USA of death in patients > 65 yr of age.

Symptoms, Signs, and Diagnosis

The older patient with pneumonia may present with lethargy, confusion, anorexia, and deterioration of a preexisting medical condition. Typical features—fever, chills, and productive cough—may also occur. After the history and physical examination are completed, the following laboratory tests should be performed: CBC; measurement of serum electrolyte, serum creatinine, and arterial blood gas levels; blood cultures; chest x-ray; and ECG. If an adequate sputum specimen (< 10 epithelial cells and > 25 polymorphonuclear leukocytes per low-power field) can be obtained, a Gram stain is useful to guide initial antibiotic therapy.

Treatment

If the patient appears to have cardiopulmonary compromise, IV fluids and oxygen by nasal cannula should be given. Antibiotic therapy may be initiated in the emergency department, depending on the clinical situation. If the Gram stain of a sputum sample shows gram-positive cocci in pairs or chains, *Streptococcus pneumoniae* is the most likely cause, and penicillin or erythromycin may be given. Gram-negative infections can be treated with a second-generation cephalosporin or an aminoglycoside. If the results of a sputum sample are unavailable, broad antibiotic coverage (eg, ampicillin, a second- or third-generation cephalosporin, or erythromycin) should be provided. If the patient resides in a long-term care facility, an aminoglycoside plus a cephalosporin is required. These drugs are needed because the organisms that usually cause pneumonia in nursing homes are more like those in hospitals than like those in the community.

Because of the associated mortality, an elderly patient with pneumonia and a coexisting illness must be hospitalized for monitoring of vital signs, hydration status, and IV antibiotic therapy. (More information on pneumonia and the drugs used in its treatment is given in Chs. 46 and 86.)

HEATSTROKE

(See also HYPERTHERMIA in Ch. 5)

Nonexertional heatstroke is a disorder of thermoregulation usually occurring during summer heat waves and typically affecting elderly persons who are debilitated or taking drugs that alter fluid balance or temperature regulation. The mortality rate reaches 80% in persons > 65 yr of age.

Diagnosis

The diagnosis is established when the clinical features of **hyperpyrexia** (temperature of 37.8° to 41.1° C [100° to 106° F]), **severe CNS dysfunction** (altered mental status, seizures, focal neurologic defects), and **anhidrosis** are present. Also common are hyperventilation, vomiting, diarrhea, fatigue, weakness, and headaches.

Diagnostic tests to assess the degree of thermal injury include all or most of the following: CBC, partial thromboplastin time and prothrombin time, platelet count, potassium and serum creatinine levels, urinalysis for myoglobulinuria, arterial blood gas levels, ECG, and chest x-ray.

Treatment

Treatment is directed initially at immediate reduction of core temperature and support of vital organ systems. Vital signs are checked periodically to assess the degree of cardiovascular impairment secondary to thermal stress. A large-bore (16- to 18-gauge) IV catheter is placed to deliver isotonic (0.9%) sodium chloride or lactated Ringer's solution. A pulmonary artery catheter may be of value in the patient who requires close monitoring of cardiac parameters during fluid therapy. Oxygen at 4 to 6 L/min is provided by nasal cannula or mask.

Ice packs placed in the groin and axillae and on the chest will reduce core body temperature. Ice-water immersion may not be readily available and could interfere with other resuscitation measures. Constant misting of the patient with tepid (20° to 25° C) water with concurrent cooling by a fan is also useful for reducing core temperature. If these measures fail, nasogastric ice-water lavage may be used. The temperature should be reduced to only 38.8° C (102° F) to avoid overcooling and hypothermia. Seizures and aspiration may occur during cooling, so the airway must be closely monitored. Seizures are treated with diazepam or phenytoin, and the patient should be admitted to the intensive care unit for cardiovascular monitoring.

HYPOTHERMIA

(See also ACCIDENTAL HYPOTHERMIA in Ch. 5)

Hypothermia (core temperature < 34.4° C [94° F]) generally occurs with prolonged exposure to ambient temperatures < 60° F. However, elderly persons may develop hypothermia after only modest exposure to low temperatures because of decreased thermal regulation, impaired mobility, and coexisting disease.

Diagnosis

Symptoms are often nonspecific and include confusion, sleepiness, slurred speech, and dilated pupils. In more severe cases, seizures, paralysis, and arrhythmias may occur. Laboratory findings are likewise nonspecific. Diagnosis is made by measuring core temperature with a thermometer capable of recording low body temperatures. Unfortunately, emergency department physicians and nurses often miss the diagnosis because they do not thoroughly shake down glass thermometers before measuring temperature, or they interpret low readings on tape or electronic thermometers as an inadequate measurement.

Treatment

Rewarming is essential but should not be accomplished too rapidly. Rapid rewarming may precipitate profound hypotension, arrhythmias, and metabolic derangement. Rewarming is generally best accomplished slowly, at a rate of about 0.6° C (1° F)/h, using blankets or other insulating materials to retain body heat. If slow spontaneous rewarming does not raise body temperature, core rewarming using heated, moist inspired air, and warmed IV therapy is necessary. In more severe cases, warmed heated peritoneal dialysis may be needed. Core rewarming must be done with scrupulous comprehensive intensive care.

5. HYPERTHERMIA AND ACCIDENTAL HYPOTHERMIA

HYPERTHERMIA

Abnormally high body temperature due to inadequate or inappropriate responses of heat-regulating mechanisms.

Hyperthermia represents an important health risk for older people, because heat exacerbates chronic diseases and because heatstroke causes many pathophysiologic changes. The number of deaths resulting from most diseases increases during hot, humid weather, particularly among elderly persons. About 80% of heatstroke deaths occur in those > 50 yr of age.

NORMAL AGING AND TEMPERATURE REGULATION

Under usual environmental conditions, convection and radiation account for 65% of heat loss; evaporation from skin and lungs contributes another 30%. The hypothalamus regulates heat loss through neuroendocrine and autonomic mechanisms. Heat causes blood vessels in the skin to dilate, and sweating increases as a result of cholinergic discharge. Vasodilation, in turn, reflexly increases heart rate and cardiac output.

When environmental temperature exceeds body surface temperature, heat is no longer lost through convection and radiation but begins to be absorbed. Evaporation of sweat becomes the last major mechanism by which to lose heat, but increased humidity can prevent cooling by this mechanism.

Aging appears to reduce the effectiveness of sweating in cooling the body. Many eccrine glands become fibrotic, and surrounding connective tissue becomes less vascular. In addition, the remaining anatomically normal eccrine glands may not function properly. Older persons initiate sweating at higher core temperatures and have less maximal sweat output per gland.

Heart disease increases the risk for heat stress. Under experimental conditions, increased ambient heat and humidity exacerbate heart failure. The greater the degree of cardiac impairment, the less a person is able to withstand the environmental stress. Thus, physiologic changes resulting from normal aging and from diseases more common in the elderly combine to impair optimal heat regulation.

DISORDERS CAUSED BY HEAT

HEAT CRAMPS

Heat cramps (muscle cramps), preceded by profuse sweating and polydipsia without an elevation in body temperature, often occur during intense physical activity in hot, humid weather. Heat cramps probably result from sweat-induced fluid and electrolyte loss, followed by oral fluid replacement mainly with water. Electrolyte-rich beverages such as Gatorade for oral replacement, or normal saline with potassium supplement, are likely to prevent heat cramps.

HEAT EXHAUSTION

Heat exhaustion is characterized by anorexia, nausea, vomiting, disorientation, and postural hypotension. Cramping may occur, and body temperature may be normal or elevated. Patients may be thirsty and weak; they generally have some CNS signs—usually light-headedness, dizziness, or loss of consciousness. Two major forms of heat exhaustion are recognized: **water depletion,** which produces hypertonic dehydration, and **salt depletion,** which results when fluid and sodium chloride lost by sweating are replaced with electrolyte-free water (similar to what happens when patients suffer from heat cramps). Death and major complications are rare.

HEATSTROKE

Heatstroke is a syndrome characterized by fever (generally > 41° C [> 106° F], although a lesser degree of fever is accepted if other criteria are met), absence of sweating, and severe CNS disturbance. Prodromal light-headedness, dizziness, headache, weakness, dyspnea, and nausea may appear transiently, but loss of consciousness may be the first manifestation. Heatstroke has a bimodal population distribution, occurring in younger people who overexert at high ambient temperatures and in older people, in whom it develops insidiously as the ability to dissipate heat declines.

Two patterns of **cardiovascular response** may occur with heatstroke. In the **hyperdynamic response,** generally seen in younger persons, pulse is typically very rapid (160 to 180 beats per minute), cardiac output is normal or increased, blood pressure is usually normal, and central venous pressure is commonly elevated. In the **hypodynamic response,** more typical in the elderly, pulse is usually slow and thready, blood pressure may be low or imperceptible, hypovolemia is often present, and capillary wedge pressure is normal. The hypodynamic response may be due to an inability to respond to heat stress by sufficient rise in heart rate or appropriate change in peripheral vascular resistance. In addition, the slower development of heatstroke in older patients may result in greater fluid loss. Other cardiovascular manifestations include

ECG changes in ST segments and T waves, premature ventricular contractions, supraventricular tachycardias, and conduction abnormalities.

Signs of CNS involvement may include lethargy, stupor, or coma. The electroencephalogram is usually normal initially, in the absence of seizures, and CSF is unremarkable. Cerebellar symptoms may be permanent in a small number of those who recover. At autopsy, edema, patchy congestion, and diffuse petechial hemorrhages are found in the brain.

Renal manifestations range from mild proteinuria to acute tubular necrosis in 10% to 30% of cases. Rhabdomyolysis, which causes acute renal failure, has been described in both exercise-induced heatstroke and heatstroke from other causes. Generally, heatstroke is accompanied by metabolic acidosis and an elevated lactate level, with compensatory respiratory alkalosis. **Severe hypokalemia** is common and is thought to be secondary to increased aldosterone secretion.

Although **transient elevations of transaminases** are common and **jaundice** may be seen, there is usually no residual hepatic damage. **Coagulation defects** include elevated prothrombin and partial thromboplastin times and a decreased fibrinogen level; the full-blown syndrome of disseminated intravascular coagulation is rare.

Specific prognostic signs remain undefined, but elderly patients with the highest fever, the most severe hypotension, or the deepest neurologic impairment have the highest mortality rate.

Risk Factors

During the summer of 1980, the hottest in two decades in the USA, the incidence of heatstroke in persons ≥ 65 yr of age was 12 to 13 times that in younger persons. Risk factors for heatstroke in older persons include low socioeconomic status, impaired self-care ability, alcoholism, mental illness, unavailability of air-conditioning, and concomitant medical disorders (eg, cardiovascular or cerebrovascular disease, diabetes, or chronic obstructive pulmonary disease). Deaths attributed to diabetes, lung disease, and hypertension increase by > 50% during heat waves; thus, the risk of hyperthermia-related death may depend more on severity of associated disease than on severity of heat stress.

Many illnesses common in old age, particularly psychiatric problems, are treated with drugs that predispose the patient to heatstroke (see TABLE 5–1). Anticholinergic agents, phenothiazines, tricyclic antidepressants, antihistamines, and synthetic and belladonna alkaloids impair hypothalamic function centrally and sweat output peripherally. These drugs, as well as narcotics, sedative-hypnotics, and alcohol, alter a person's awareness of heat and diminish the ability to respond to heat stress. Amphetamines can increase body temperature by acting directly on the hypothalamus. Diuretics (by causing additional fluid loss) and β-adrenergic blockers (by impairing cardiovascular responsiveness) can also increase the risk of heatstroke. Therefore, a thorough drug history can be helpful in elucidating the cause of heatstroke and preventing it.

TABLE 5–1. TYPES OF DRUGS THAT IMPAIR RESPONSE TO HEAT

Drugs That Cause Hypohidrosis	*Drugs That Cause Hypovolemia*
Anticholinergics	Diuretics
Antihistamines	
Antiparkinsonian drugs	
Butyrophenones	
Monoamine oxidase (MAO) inhibitors	
Phenothiazines	
Thioxanthenes	
Tricyclics	

Prevention

Heatstroke in the elderly, like many conditions, results from an interaction of adverse environmental factors with the normal physiologic changes of aging, often complicated by concomitant diseases and the effects of certain drugs. Prevention is preferable to treatment, since morbidity and mortality rates are high.

Those who care for high-risk older persons should be alert to the symptoms of heatstroke and, in very hot weather, should move them to an air-conditioned environment, even if only for brief periods. At times of greatest risk, these older persons may need to be moved to temporary shelters. Elderly persons should wear light clothing; windows should be opened at night and shaded during the day. Ensuring adequate fluid intake and avoiding exercise are important. Decreasing the doses of drugs that predispose one to heatstroke is advised.

Primary care physicians should be aware of the nonspecific presentation of heatstroke. In times of heat stress, routine temperature monitoring is advisable. Heatstroke is both a public and an individual health problem; morbidity and mortality rates can be reduced by increased awareness and action.

Treatment

Heatstroke is a medical emergency requiring hospitalization and continuous monitoring (see also HEATSTROKE in Ch. 4). Normal body temperature must be restored as quickly as possible, since many metabolic and cardiovascular problems are temperature-dependent. Core temperature should be continuously monitored with a thermocouple while the patient is immersed in cool water. To avoid overcooling and hypothermia, the patient should be removed from the bath when body temperature reaches 38.8° C (102° F). The cooling process can then continue with wet sponging.

Since heatstroke may be either hyperdynamic, often associated with pulmonary edema, or hypodynamic, with major fluid loss, central venous pressure or pulmonary capillary wedge pressure monitoring to guide fluid replacement is advisable. Close monitoring of hematologic and renal parameters during the acute event is mandatory, as is a search for predisposing factors, including infection.

ACCIDENTAL HYPOTHERMIA

The unintentional decrease in body temperature to ≤ 34.4° C (94° F).

Most episodes of hypothermia are initiated by ambient temperatures near 15.5° C (60° F), but older persons may become hypothermic while at home in mildly cool environments.

Current prevalence, incidence, and mortality data for accidental hypothermia are scanty, particularly in the USA. In one study, temperatures of elderly patients admitted to two London hospitals during three winter months revealed a 3.6% incidence of hypothermia in those ≥ 65 yr of age. In a large community survey conducted in Great Britain during the winter of 1972, 10% of the elderly population had early morning core temperatures of ≤ 35.5° C (96° F). There was no correlation between low body temperature and living alone, being housebound, or being without central heating or indoor plumbing. The only available US data are from a study done in Maine, in which 97 elderly persons (average age, 74 yr) from an internal medicine clinic were surveyed. Many persons were poor or lived in subsidized housing; none had a basal body temperature < 35.5° C (96° F).

Estimates of deaths due to hypothermia are difficult to calculate, since no definitive clinical or pathologic findings are available. Also, since most corpses are cold when discovered, attributing the death to hypothermia is difficult. Accordingly, figures indicating that only a few hundred deaths each year in the USA are caused by hypothermia probably underestimate the problem.

In the USA, about 75,000 "excess winter deaths" occur among the elderly, including deaths from hypothermia and deaths associated with many other winter risks, such as influenza and pneumonia. Among identified cases of hypothermia, the mortality rate is disturbingly high at 50%. Persons > 75 yr of age are five times more likely to die from hypothermia than are those < 75 yr. Mortality correlates more closely with the presence and severity of associated illness than with the degree of hypothermia.

Hypothermia may also result in substantial morbidity. One British study showed a midwinter peak in the incidence of hip fracture in malnourished patients and a higher mortality rate after hip fracture. Malnourished patients were frequently hypothermic on admission to the hospital, whereas well-nourished patients had normal body temperatures. Malnutrition presumably led to impaired heat generation and retention, which caused hypothermia; the hypothermia resulted in lack of coordination and subsequent injury.

Additionally, elderly patients with diabetes have a sixfold greater risk of hypothermia, probably due to vascular disease that alters thermoregulatory mechanisms.

Etiology and Pathophysiology

The factors usually implicated in the genesis of accidental hypothermia are a cold environment, age-related physiologic changes in thermoregulation, drugs, and the diseases that decrease heat production, increase heat loss, or impair thermoregulation (see TABLE 5–2).

Ambient temperature only a few degrees cooler than body temperature can cause hypothermia in severely debilitated elderly persons. Also, a number of physiologic changes predispose elderly persons to hypothermia, including a diminished perception of cold. Changes in response to endogenous catecholamines reduce the vasoconstrictor and shivering responses to cold. A decrease in lean body mass reduces the efficiency of shivering for heat production. Less physical activity and reduced caloric intake affect the ability to generate heat.

Pathologic conditions in older patients add to the physiologic risks. Decreased heat production occurs with hypopituitarism, hypoglycemia, starvation, and malnutrition. Forced or involuntary inactivity (eg, as in Parkinson's disease, arthritis, paralysis, and dementia) decreases heat production and increases the risk of hypothermia. Increased heat loss can occur secondary to inflammatory skin disease, Paget's disease, alcohol-induced vasodilation, cold exposure, and reduction in insulating subcutaneous fat. Central hypothalamic temperature regulation can be disturbed by stroke, subarachnoid hemorrhage, subdural hematoma, and brain tumor. Uremia and carbon monoxide poisoning may also affect thermoregulation.

TABLE 5–2. CAUSES OF ACCIDENTAL HYPOTHERMIA

Exposure to environmental cold

Physiologic changes with age
- Autonomic nervous system deterioration
  - Decreased shivering
  - Low resting peripheral blood flow
  - Nonconstrictor response to cold
  - Orthostatic hypotension
- Diminished perception of cold

(continued)

TABLE 5–2. CAUSES OF ACCIDENTAL HYPOTHERMIA *(Continued)*

Drugs
- Alcohol
- Antidepressants
- Sedative-hypnotics
- Tranquilizers

Diseases
- Decreased heat production
  - Diabetic ketoacidosis
  - Hypoglycemia
  - Hypopituitarism
  - Malnutrition or starvation
  - Myxedema
- Diminished activity
  - Arthritis
  - Dementia
  - A fall
  - Paralysis or stroke
  - Parkinsonism
- Impaired thermoregulation
  - Neuropathy
    - Alcoholism
    - Diabetes
  - Primary CNS disease
    - Head trauma
    - Polio
    - Stroke
    - Subarachnoid hemorrhage
    - Subdural hematoma
    - Tumor
    - Wernicke's encephalopathy
  - Systemic disease influencing hypothalamus
    - Carbon monoxide poisoning
    - Uremia
- Increased heat loss
  - A-V shunt
  - Inflammatory dermatitis
    - Exfoliation
    - Ichthyosis
    - Psoriasis
  - Paget's disease

From Besdine RW: "Accidental hypothermia in the elderly." *Medical Grand Rounds* 1:36, 1982; used with permission of Plenum Publishing Corporation.

Many drugs, including phenothiazines, tricyclic antidepressants, benzodiazepines, barbiturates, reserpine, and narcotics, depress central thermoregulation and predispose patients to accidental hypothermia. Chlorpromazine, which inhibits shivering, is the best-known offender.

Symptoms and Signs

The symptoms of hypothermia are insidious and may be transient. Although elderly people with body temperatures between 35° C (95° F) and 36.1° C (97° F) often complain of being cold, patients with established hypothermia usually do not. Clinical findings are nonspecific; they can suggest stroke or metabolic disorder. The patient feels cool to the touch and has a history of confusion and sleepiness, which may progress to coma.

Neurologic findings include thick, slow speech; ataxic gait; and depressed deep tendon reflexes. Pathologic reflexes and plantar responses may be present, and pupils may be dilated and sluggishly reactive. Focal signs, seizures, paralysis, and sensory loss may also occur.

Although shivering may occur at temperatures > 35° C (> 95° F), it is absent in most hypothermic elderly patients. Instead, marked rigidity accompanied by a generalized increase in muscle tone and, occasionally, a fine tremor may be found.

Although many people have cold hands or feet in winter, hypothermic patients also have cold abdomens and backs. The **skin** has a cadaveric pallor and chill, and pressure points show erythematous, bullous, or purpuric patches. Subcutaneous tissues are firm, probably from edema, which also produces a puffy appearance, especially of the face.

The **cardiovascular system** is initially stimulated by cold, resulting in peripheral vasoconstriction, tachycardia, and elevation of blood pressure. As hypothermia progresses, the myocardium is depressed, producing hypotension and progressive sinus bradycardia. Severe hypothermia can reduce blood pressure and heart beat to barely detectable levels, sometimes leading to an erroneous pronouncement of death. Various other cardiac arrhythmias are associated with cold temperatures, including atrial fibrillation and flutter, premature ventricular beats, and idioventricular rhythm. Cardiac arrest, from either ventricular fibrillation or asystole, is increasingly likely as body temperature falls below 30° C (86° F).

The **gastrointestinal response** to hypothermia consists of decreased peristalsis or even ileus, producing abdominal distention and diminished or absent bowel sounds. Less often, acute gastric dilation occurs with vomiting. Pancreatitis may also occur but is usually not apparent until rewarming has been achieved. Because hepatic metabolism is depressed, drug metabolism may be sharply reduced.

Pulmonary findings include depression of respiration and cough reflex. Atelectasis is almost universal, and pneumonia is common. Pulmonary edema during recovery may be related to increased vascular permeability as well as to heart failure.

Early in hypothermia, there is an increase in heart rate, cardiac output, and renal blood flow with diuresis. In addition, cold suppresses antidiuretic hormone secretion and diminishes tubular responsiveness to its action, further increasing diuresis. As volume depletion reduces glomerular filtration and renal blood flow, oliguria and tubular necrosis follow.

Diagnosis

Hypothermia is often missed; the usual clinical practice is to search for and exclude fever, not to search for and exclude hypothermia. Hypothermia should be suspected if the history or physical examination is suggestive, and core temperature should be recorded using a low-reading thermometer. The diagnosis of accidental hypothermia depends on the ability to measure body temperature $< 34.4°$ C ($94°$ F). Standard clinical thermometers are calibrated from $34.4°$ to $42.2°$ C ($94°$ to $108°$ F), and hypothermic patients have temperatures $\leq 34.4°$ C. Since these thermometers are usually shaken down to only between $35°$ and $35.5°$ C ($95°$ and $96°$ F) before measuring temperature, they probably will not detect hypothermia. Rectal thermometers calibrated from $28.9°$ to $42.2°$ C ($84°$ to $108°$ F) are available from most hospital suppliers, although they are not commonly used. A special low-reading thermometer can be obtained from Becton Dickinson, 1 Becton Drive, Franklin Lakes, NJ 07417 (201-847-4000). If a low-reading thermometer is unavailable, more expensive thermistors or thermocouples can be used.

Most **clinical laboratory data** are not specific for hypothermia. Hemoconcentration, leukocytosis, lactic acidosis, and thrombocytopenia are all common. The ECG can provide a major diagnostic clue. A junctional (J), or Osborn, wave is a small deflection early in the ST segment, positive in the left ventricular leads and negative in the right ones. Although present in only about ⅓ of hypothermic patients, this finding always indicates hypothermia. Another, more common ECG finding frequently seen in the nonshivering patient is a fine regular oscillation of the baseline produced by increased muscle tone with an imperceptible tremor.

Blood glucose findings in hypothermia can be confusing. Usually, hyperglycemia is found. Hypothermia triggers hyperglycemia by corticosteroid- and catecholamine-induced gluconeogenesis. Although insulin secretion is also stimulated, cold interferes with its action, further raising blood glucose levels. Less commonly, hypothermic patients are hypoglycemic, in which case it is the hypoglycemia, usually drug-induced, that produces the hypothermia.

Prevention

Preventing accidental hypothermia is preferable to treating it. Older persons with identifiable predisposing problems should have their household thermostats set at $\geq 18.3°$ C ($\geq 65°$ F) and should keep a reliable thermometer available (separate from the thermostat) for determining room temperature. This should be checked daily, especially during very cold weather. Extra clothing, particularly for hands, feet, and head, should be worn indoors. Frequent periods of exercise can increase heat production, and adequate caloric intake is of primary importance. Drugs that may alter thermoregulatory mechanisms should be discontinued whenever possible.

Treatment

An elderly patient with accidental hypothermia usually is treated initially for some other disorder—either a cause or complication of hypothermia is the exclusive focus, or the symptoms and signs of hypothermia are erroneously attributed to some disease common in the elderly. In either case therapy is delayed.

Once the temperature falls into the hypothermic range, thermoregulation becomes progressively impaired; indeed, early during the temperature fall, regulatory mechanisms fail altogether and the patient reacts like a poikilotherm. Accordingly, *even mild accidental hypothermia should be considered a medical emergency, and patients should be monitored under hospital conditions* (usually in an intensive care setting) until recovery is complete.

Therapy can be divided into two foci: (1) primary treatment by rewarming and (2) secondary treatment of the direct effects and complications of hypothermia. General medical care demands comprehensive evaluation, close monitoring, and anticipation of likely complications. Laboratory evaluation should include CBC count; platelet count; clotting studies; measurements of BUN, creatinine, electrolytes, blood glucose, and serum and urine amylase levels; thyroid and liver function tests; arterial blood gas studies; ECG with constant monitoring; chest and abdominal x-rays; and constant monitoring and recording of core temperature.

Primary measures aim to restore normal body temperature and to abort the pathophysiologic consequences of hypothermia. In young, physiologically vigorous persons who suffer hypothermia, especially as a result of exposure, **rapid active rewarming** is carried out by active heating. Elderly persons with accidental hypothermia, *when rewarmed actively and rapidly, often develop a syndrome of profound hypotension, new cardiac arrhythmias, and deteriorating metabolic abnormalities, culminating in death.* For this reason, **slow spontaneous rewarming** is recommended for older victims of hypothermia. By preventing further heat loss and conserving the heat still being produced by the patient, slow spontaneous rewarming allows the body temperature to rise slowly, at a rate of about 0.6° C (1° F)/h. A more rapid rise in core temperature, even when slow spontaneous rewarming is used, has been associated with rewarming hypotension. The environmental temperature is kept > 21.1° C (> 70° F), and blankets or more sophisticated insulating materials are used to retain body heat.

If slow spontaneous rewarming does not produce a rise in body temperature, **rapid active rewarming of the core** is necessary. Techniques for core rewarming include the use of heated, moist inspired air, warmed IV fluids at 37° C (98.6° F), and heated peritoneal dialysis. *If rapid active rewarming of the core or periphery is used in elderly patients, scrupulous, comprehensive intensive care must be taken.* When ventricular fibrillation or cardiac standstill occurs at temperatures < 29.4° C (85° F), warming must be accomplished as quickly as possible because the heart is unresponsive to electrical defibrillation at temperatures below this level. Bradycardia resulting from myocardial depression is not influenced by atropine. The need for ventilatory assistance, intracardiac monitoring and pacing, and full circulatory support should be anticipated, since collapse and profound hypotension associated with warming are common under such conditions.

Ventricular arrhythmias, if not rapidly responsive to rewarming, should be suppressed with lidocaine. Both countershock and pacing are less effective at low temperatures; if critical arrhythmias appear, appropriate therapy should be administered while the patient is rewarmed. If cardiac arrest or ventricular fibrillation is unresponsive to usual measures, cardiopulmonary resuscitation should be continued until rewarming has been accomplished; treatment then should be repeated. All IV fluids should be warmed to normal or slightly above normal body temperature.

Although some studies have recommended the routine use of such drugs as corticosteroids, thyroid hormone, anticoagulants, antibiotics, and digitalis, none of these agents has proved effective unless specifically indicated. Myxedema is, of course, a well-known cause of hypothermia; when hypothermia and hypothyroidism occur together, they result in a very high mortality rate.

Although hyperglycemia is common in hypothermic patients, insulin is rarely given unless glucose levels are very high (> 400 mg/dL) because insulin is ineffective at low temperatures. Any previously administered insulin, combined with endogenous insulin, can produce severe hypoglycemia during rewarming. In general, most drugs are less active during hypothermia but have exaggerated pharmacologic effects as body temperature rises.

Death usually results from cardiac arrest or ventricular fibrillation. The temperature at which each cardiac event appears varies, but at temperatures < 29.4° C (85° F), risk of death is high, particularly in patients with underlying heart disease. Movement or excessive stimulation of hypothermic patients may provoke arrhythmias and should be performed cautiously. *Resuscitation during rewarming should be aggressive and prolonged in patients who are profoundly hypothermic;* remarkable recoveries have been reported in such cases. Most authorities agree that patients should not be pronounced dead until cardiopulmonary resuscitation is shown to be ineffective after body temperature has been raised to at least 35.8° C (96.5° F).

6. SYNCOPE

A sudden, transient loss of consciousness characterized by unresponsiveness and loss of postural control. Usually, recovery is spontaneous. Syncope is not a disease but a symptom.

The prevalence and incidence of syncope in the elderly have not been thoroughly investigated, but studies indicate that about 25% of institutionalized elderly patients have experienced syncope within 10 yr and that 6% to 7% experience it each year. In about 33% of cases, syncope is recurrent.

Syncope alone does not increase the risk of death, but it is associated with physical disability and subsequent functional decline. Syncope and falls may be signs of a serious underlying disorder associated with high morbidity and mortality rates.

Etiology and Pathophysiology

Syncope results from inadequate delivery of oxygen or metabolic substrate to the brain or from disorganized electrical activity in the brain. The elderly are subject to many age-related and disease-related conditions that threaten cerebral blood flow or blood oxygen content. An accumulation of these conditions may diminish cerebral oxygen delivery, pushing it dangerously close to the threshold needed to maintain consciousness. Early literature suggests that this threshold is about 3.5 mL of oxygen per 100 gm of brain tissue per minute. Although this threshold is difficult to quantify and has never been confirmed, the accumulation of conditions that reduces cerebral blood flow or blood oxygen content certainly brings cerebral oxygen delivery close to this value. Any additional stress further reducing cerebral blood flow or blood oxygen content may precipitate syncope.

For example, the many cardiovascular and neuroendocrine homeostatic mechanisms that normally maintain blood pressure decline with age, thus reducing the ability to maintain adequate cerebral perfusion during hypotensive stress. Heart failure with dyspnea and hyperventilation can further decrease cerebral blood flow by as much as 40%. Other common conditions, such as chronic obstructive pulmonary disease or anemia, can reduce cerebral oxygen delivery still further. At this point, pneumonia, a cardiac arrhythmia, a hypotensive drug, or even situational stress that reduces blood pressure may produce syncope. Seemingly minor stresses, such as taking medications, eating a meal, defecating, urinating, or changing posture, can precipitate syncope (see Ch. 36).

Baroreflex sensitivity to both hypertensive and hypotensive stimuli also decreases with age. Additionally, the heart rate response to postural change becomes blunted in many elderly patients. Thus, after changing position, an elderly person is likely to experience hypotension, leading to syncope.

Progressive age-related decreases in basal and stimulated renin levels and aldosterone production along with increases in atrial natriuretic peptide predispose the elderly to syncope by impairing renal sodium conservation and intravascular volume maintenance. Therefore, the elderly are more likely to become dehydrated and experience hypotension in response to diuretics, acute febrile illness, or limited salt and water intake. Also, healthy elderly persons are less likely to experience thirst in response to hypertonic dehydration. This impairment in their ability to defend intravascular volume can lead to rapid volume depletion, orthostatic hypotension, and syncope.

Conditions causing syncope: **Cardiovascular causes** of syncope are more prevalent in elderly patients than in younger patients. Any cardiac illness that abruptly diminishes cardiac output can produce syncope. Cardiac output may be transiently compromised by anatomic, myocardial, or electrical abnormalities (see TABLE 6–1).

Orthostatic hypotension, *a drop in systolic blood pressure of 20 mm Hg or greater upon standing,* occurs in 15% to 20% of noninstitutionalized elderly persons. Although usually asymptomatic, orthostatic hypotension is an important risk factor for syncope and falls, accounting for about 4% of falls among the noninstitutionalized elderly. Causes include the age-related physiologic changes mentioned above, drugs, and autonomic insufficiency syndromes, such as pure autonomic failure **(idiopathic orthostatic hypotension), Shy-Drager syndrome** (distinguished by brain and spinal cord degeneration leading to parkinsonian symptoms and failure of the central nervous system to activate the autonomic nervous system), and **multiple cerebral infarctions.** Elderly persons can usually maintain adequate postural blood pressure for central nervous system function, but when mild volume depletion occurs—during diuretic therapy, for instance—postural blood pressure may drop profoundly, resulting in syncope.

Postprandial hypotension is also common among the elderly. In some elderly persons, blood pressure declines an average of 11 mm Hg within an hour after a meal. Such a decline usually does not cause symptoms, but a more profound decline may produce syncope. Postprandial hypotension may be related to impaired peripheral vasoconstriction and abnormal sympathetic nervous system control of heart rate in response to splanchnic blood pooling.

When syncope occurs a few seconds after urination or defecation, it is called **micturition or defecation syncope.** Similarly, syncope after strenuous coughing or swallowing is called **coughing or swallowing syncope. Carotid sinus syncope** occurs when neck movement, a tight collar, or a tumor or other lesion at the carotid bifurcation stimulates baroreceptors in the carotid sinus, resulting in excessive cardiac slowing (a sinus pause longer than 3 sec) or hypotension (a drop in systolic blood pressure of $>$ 50 mm Hg or to a value of $<$ 90 mm Hg). **Vasovagal syncope** (more common in younger people than in the elderly) occurs when the vagus nerve is stimulated, eg, by nauseous stimuli, fright, or pain.

TABLE 6–1. CAUSES OF SYNCOPE

Cardiac conditions
- Anatomic
  - Aortic stenosis
  - Mitral prolapse and regurgitation
  - Hypertrophic cardiomyopathy
  - Myxoma
- Myocardial
  - Ischemia and infarct
  - Cardiomyopathy
- Electrical
  - Tachyarrhythmia
  - Bradyarrhythmia
  - Heart block
  - Sick sinus syndrome

Vasomotor stimuli
- Vasomotor instability
  - Orthostatic hypotension
  - Postprandial hypotension
  - Carotid sinus syndrome
  - Micturition, defecation, coughing, swallowing
  - Vasovagal reflex
  - Autonomic insufficiency syndromes
- Drugs (vasodilators, α-antagonists)

Volume depletion

Blood metabolic abnormalities
- Hypoxemia
- Hypoglycemia

Cerebral disorders
- Vascular insufficiency
- Seizures

Pulmonary embolism

Anemia may threaten cerebral oxygen delivery. When transient hypotension occurs, the anemic patient may not have sufficient oxygen in the blood to maintain cerebral function.

Syncope can be attributed to **cerebrovascular disease,** but only if transient focal neurologic deficits are associated with the episode. Syncope may result from a **seizure disorder;** however, syncope can also cause seizure activity. Clinical features such as the occurrence of syncope while a person is supine, an olfactory or gustatory aura, tongue biting, fecal incontinence, and postictal confusion support a diagnosis of epilepsy.

Studies of institutionalized elderly patients show that syncope is more likely in those who have two or more contributing factors, such as coronary artery disease, postural hypotension, aortic stenosis, or a need for insulin therapy.

Diagnosis

Because syncope in elderly persons usually results from several interacting abnormalities rather than a single disease, the clinician must search for age-related and disease-related abnormalities that impede cerebral oxygen delivery. The evaluation should begin with a thorough history and a physical examination, which in most cases are sufficient to identify the underlying causes.

History: All witnesses should be asked to describe what the patient was doing just before fainting. Major precipitating causes include eating, taking medications, and straining while defecating or urinating. Vasovagal syncope is usually preceded by hunger, fatigue, emotional stress, or a typical autonomic prodrome. Family members or others close to the patient should also be asked about recent changes in clinical condition that may point to the underlying pathophysiology.

The history should determine if any prescription or over-the-counter drugs, including eye medications, were used. Many over-the-counter drugs have anticholinergic properties that cause tachyarrhythmias, precipitating syncope. Prescription drugs with anticholinergic activity (such as phenothiazines and tricyclic antidepressants) and those with sympatholytic activity (such as prazosin, guanethidine, and reserpine), volume-contracting agents (such as diuretics), and vasodilators (such as nitrates and alcohol) may cause syncopal episodes. Certain eye medications have autonomic effects, and topical ophthalmic β-blockers have systemic effects (such as bronchospasm, bradycardia, and heart failure) that may cause syncope.

The nature of the recovery can also provide important clues. Recovery from syncope is usually rapid; however, when syncope results from a seizure, recovery is usually slow.

Physical examination: Evaluating **postural vital signs** to rule out orthostatic hypotension consists of checking blood pressure and heart rate with the patient supine after resting for 5 min, then after standing for 1 min and 3 min, if the patient is able to do so. Although the standing position is best for detecting immediate and delayed orthostatic hypotension, the patient may sit if necessary. A small increase or no increase in heart rate upon standing may suggest baroreflex impairment. An exaggerated increase in heart rate upon standing, uncommon in the elderly, may indicate volume depletion.

The carotid arteries should be auscultated for bruits to rule out conditions contraindicating carotid sinus massage (see below) as well as to determine the quality of the carotid upstroke. With normal aging, the upstroke usually becomes brisker because of increased vascular rigidity. When an older person develops **aortic stenosis,** the amplitude of the upstroke may slow to a level that would be considered normal in a younger person, but it is slow for the older patient.

The heart should be auscultated for murmurs of **aortic stenosis, mitral regurgitation,** or **hypertrophic cardiomyopathy,** all of which are common in elderly patients. An apical heave; a loud, late-peaking aortic systolic murmur; and a diminished second aortic sound suggest significant aortic stenosis. Mitral regurgitation is marked by a holosystolic murmur at the apex, but such a murmur may also occur in elderly patients who have aortic stenosis or hypertrophic cardiomyopathy. An accentuation of the systolic murmur while the patient performs Valsalva's maneuver helps distinguish hypertrophic cardiomyopathy from aortic stenosis or mitral regurgitation.

Neurologic examination is essential to search for focal abnormalities that may indicate cerebrovascular disease or space-occupying lesions.

Diagnostic tests: Specialized studies generally are undertaken only if indicated by findings in the history and physical examination. **Screening tests** are often useful because disease presentations can be atypical in elderly patients. These tests include a white blood cell count to detect occult sepsis (which rarely causes syncope) and a hematocrit measurement to diagnose anemia. Electrolyte, blood urea nitrogen (BUN), and creatinine studies help in assessing hydration status and ruling out electrolyte disorders. Serum glucose measurements help exclude hyperglycemia. The first sign of hyperosmolar dehydration with hyperglycemia may be syncope.

If the patient is taking an antiarrhythmic, anticonvulsant, bronchodilator, or lithium, the drug concentration should be measured to determine if it is subtherapeutic, therapeutic, or toxic. If it is subtherapeutic, syncope may have resulted from inadequate treatment of a known, predisposing condition, such as seizure disorder.

An **ECG** should also be obtained. If it reveals ischemia or if the patient has a history of chest pain associated with syncope, the patient should be admitted to a hospital, and cardiac enzyme and isoenzyme measurements should be obtained to rule out myocardial infarction.

Arrhythmias commonly cause syncope in elderly patients. Although **24-h ambulatory cardiac monitoring** (Holter monitoring) is often used to evaluate syncope, the results are difficult to interpret because they usually show many arrhythmias whose relationship to syncope is uncertain. Also, empiric treatment of these arrhythmias with an antiarrhythmic drug is often complicated by severe toxic effects. Thus, an ambulatory ECG should be obtained only in patients whose arrhythmias will be treated despite the risk of toxic reactions; eg, patients with underlying cardiovascular disease and patients who have had a recent myocardial infarction and are at highest risk for sudden death.

Because symptomatic arrhythmias occur sporadically and are often missed during ambulatory monitoring, self-activated loop recorders may be useful when serious arrhythmias are suspected. These recorders can be worn continuously for 1 mo and activated when symptoms develop. A memory function captures several minutes of cardiac rhythm *before* the recorder is activated; thus, an arrhythmia can be documented by activating the recorder after recovering from syncope.

Carotid sinus massage can be performed to detect carotid sinus syndrome. However, this technique should be used only when no other cause of syncope is apparent and when the patient has *no* evidence of cerebrovascular disease (a carotid bruit, previous stroke, or transient ischemic attacks) or cardiac conduction abnormalities. Serious complications resulting from carotid sinus massage have been reported, although hundreds of elderly patients have undergone it without complication. The proper technique consists of a gentle, circular, 5-sec massage of one carotid sinus at a time, while monitoring the patient by ECG. Before and immediately after each massage, blood pressure is measured.

Carotid sinus syndrome, *a sinus pause longer than 3 sec (cardioinhibitory response) or a drop in systolic blood pressure of > 50 mm Hg (vasodepressor response) during carotid sinus massage,* occurs more often with advanced age and cardiovascular disease. Patients with carotid sinus syndrome usually can be helped by discontinuing cardioinhibitory or hypotensive drugs, such as β-blockers, calcium channel blockers, digoxin, and methyldopa. If this intervention is not effective (or if these drugs are not implicated), patients with a cardioinhibitory response can be treated with cardiac pacing, and those with associated hypotension may benefit from vasopressors such as phenylephrine.

Although an **EEG** and a **brain CT scan** are often ordered to evaluate syncope, studies suggest that they have little value unless underlying focal abnormalities are found on neurologic examination.

Cardiac ultrasonography and **Doppler echocardiography** are often used to detect hemodynamically significant valvular heart disease as well as hypertrophic cardiomyopathy in patients with a cardiac murmur.

Recently, **tilt tests** (with and without isoproterenol infusions) have gained popularity for evaluating unexplained syncope. A 60° to 80° head-up tilt for up to 45 min can precipitate vasovagal syncope with associated bradycardia and hypotension—the **Bezold-Jarisch reflex,** provoked by vigorous cardiac contraction around a relatively empty ventricular chamber. Using isoproterenol to strengthen cardiac contraction can increase the test's sensitivity. However, isoproterenol is often contraindicated in elderly patients with known or suspected coronary artery disease. The development of vasovagal syncope during the tilt test suggests, but does not prove, it was the cause of the unexplained episode. Most episodes of vasovagal syncope can be readily diagnosed without the tilt test, based on the history of a typical vagal prodrome (nausea, light-headedness, and pale, cold, clammy skin). When delayed orthostatic hypotension is the suspected cause of syncope, the tilt test may help detect it.

Invasive tests: Tests such as cerebral angiography, cardiac catheterization, and cardiac electrophysiologic studies should not be used in the initial evaluation. Electrophysiologic studies have detected occult sinus node disorders, conduction disorders, or inducible ventricular arrhythmias in more than 50% of patients with unexplained syncope. Treatment of these abnormalities significantly reduces but does not eliminate recurrences of syncope, thus suggesting but not proving they are the cause.

The value of electrophysiologic studies is difficult to determine because even elderly patients who do not have syncope are likely to have electrophysiologic abnormalities and because those who do have syncope often spontaneously stop having episodes. Thus, electrophysiologic studies should be reserved for elderly patients with ECG or other clinical evidence of heart disease and recurrent episodes of unexplained syncope.

Treatment

The first step is to identify and treat all likely causes and all predisposing pathologic conditions. Age alone is rarely a contraindication to therapy. Major interventions, such as aortic valve repair, are relatively well tolerated in otherwise healthy elderly persons and can significantly improve their quality of life. Similarly, pacemaker insertion, coronary artery bypass grafting, and carotid endarterectomy should be considered when appropriate. The patient's coexisting conditions rather than age should be the decisive factor in determining therapy.

When no primary cause of syncope is apparent, potential predisposing conditions should be treated. For example, anemic patients may benefit from vitamin or iron supplements or transfusions, depending on the cause of anemia. A patient with orthostatic hypotension may benefit from increasing salt intake, wearing support hose, and elevating the head of the bed (see also Ch. 36). If orthostatic hypotension persists despite these measures, fludrocortisone may be added. Usually, the dose is increased gradually from 0.1 mg/day to as much as 1.0 mg/day until orthostatic hypotension resolves or a trace of pedal edema develops. During therapy, patients must be monitored for supine hypertension and hypokalemia. If hypertension develops, the dose may need to be reduced; if hypokalemia develops, the patient may need potassium supplements.

Adjusting the time of hypotensive drug administration to avoid a peak effect after a meal may ameliorate postprandial hypotension. A patient with ischemic heart disease and angina should be given antianginal therapy, as long as it does not severely reduce blood pressure. The drug regimens of patients with carotid sinus hypersensitivity or cardiac conduction disorder should be evaluated to ensure that cardioinhibitory or hypotensive drugs, such as β-blockers, calcium channel blockers, digoxin, or methyldopa are not contributing to their condition.

Also, patients should be taught to avoid common precipitants of syncope. For example, they should not rise from bed quickly, particularly in the middle of the night. Patients with orthostatic hypotension should sit on the edge of the bed and flex their feet before standing. Those with postprandial hypotension may benefit from eating small, frequent meals and lying down after each meal. Walking after a meal may prevent postprandial hypotension, but this approach should be undertaken only with supervision. Elderly patients should learn to avoid Valsalva's maneuver (straining) during defecation by using stool softeners and altering their diet.

7. FALLS AND GAIT DISORDERS

Falls among the elderly represent a major public health problem with substantial medical and economic consequences. The elderly have the highest mortality and experience the greatest degree of disability and dysfunction from falls. The cost of fall-related injuries among the elderly has been estimated at more than $7 billion per year.

The average primary care physician sees daily one or two older patients who have fallen recently, many of whom have not sustained an obvious injury. Often, these falls go unrecognized, probably because the routine history and physical examination does not usually include an evaluation for falls. Also, older persons may be reluctant to report falls for fear of having their activities restricted or being placed in a nursing home. Even when the fall is brought to light, both the physician and patient are likely to attribute it to the normal aging process and not proceed with a thorough evaluation for treatable causes.

Medical personnel usually define a fall as an event in which a person comes to rest on the ground or some other lower level after losing balance during walking or some other activity. Generally, falls that result from medical causes such as syncope, a cerebrovascular accident, or a seizure or from events such as a motor vehicle accident or violence are discussed separately.

Etiology

The factors responsible for falls can be classified as intrinsic (eg, related to the host) or extrinsic (eg, related to the environment). Intrinsic factors include age-related physiologic changes in balance and gait, cognitive impairment, medical conditions, and the use of certain medications. Intrinsic factors may be chronic, predisposing the older person to repeated falls, or acute, increasing the risk of falls only transiently. Extrinsic factors include environmental hazards such as slippery floors, inadequate lighting, and a lack of handrails. Falls usually have more than one cause, and distinguishing between intrinsic and extrinsic ones is difficult (eg, a frail older woman with osteoarthritis and Parkinson's disease trips over the edge of a rug). In older patients, a fall may be a nonspecific presenting sign of many acute illnesses—such as pneumonia, urinary tract infection, or myocardial infarction—or an acute exacerbation of a chronic disease.

Intrinsic factors: Both age-related and disease-related **abnormalities in balance and gait** have been implicated in falls among older persons. The normal physiology of balance and gait requires intact sensory inputs, central integration, and a motor response. Sensory inputs come from vision, hearing, vestibular function, and proprioception. These inputs are processed in the cerebellum, brain stem, and cerebrum. The motor response involves the large muscle groups of the trunk and legs.

The normal corrective movements associated with maintaining upright posture, known as postural sway, increase with age. Also, righting reflexes diminish, and reaction time increases. Age-related changes in vision, hearing, vestibular function, and proprioception also contribute to falls (See TABLE 7–1). As age and disease impair sensory inputs and the body's ability to correct postural perturbations, falls become more likely. Diabetes mellitus, vitamin B_{12} deficiency, alcoholism, cervical and lumbar spondylosis, and other less common conditions such as vasculitis and multiple myeloma may further impair vision, hearing, vestibular function, or proprioception.

The visual system provides the most accurate and sensitive information about the position of the body in space and helps a person detect and avoid environmental hazards. Visual acuity, adaptation to darkness, peripheral vision, contrast sensitivity, depth perception, glare tolerance, and accommodation can be impaired with age and by diseases such as cataracts, macular degeneration, and glaucoma.

The vestibular system contributes to spatial orientation at rest and during movement. With age, peripheral vestibular excitability decreases. Acute labyrinthitis, Meniere's disease, and benign positional vertigo are more common in older persons; these conditions not only decrease sensory input but also send inappropriate afferent stimuli, causing vertigo. Medications such as aminoglycosides, aspirin, furosemide, and quinine can also cause vestibular dysfunction.

With age, a person's gait changes. Older men tend to have a wide-based gait; older women adopt a narrow-based, waddling gait. Older persons may walk slower with reduced stride, toe-floor clearance, arm swing, and hip and knee rotation. Both feet are on the ground for a greater part of the gait cycle. This kinematic profile of walking is often referred to as **senile gait.**

Significant gait disturbances occur in more than 15% of older persons, and up to 25% need a walking aid such as a cane, walker, or leg brace. Some 40% to 50% of patients in nursing homes have difficulty walking. Many older persons assume that gait disorder and diminished mobility are part of old age, but an abnormal gait may result from treatable underlying musculoskeletal or neurologic disorders.

TABLE 7–1. AGE–RELATED PHYSIOLOGIC CHANGES THAT PREDISPOSE THE ELDERLY TO FALLS

Visual System	*Auditory–Vestibular System*	*Nervous System*
Decreased accommodation	Impaired speech discrimination	Slower reaction time
Decreased visual acuity	Increased pure tone threshold (high-frequency sounds predominantly affected)	Possible diminished position sense
Decreased adaptation to darkness	Decreased peripheral vestibular excitability	Increased postural sway
Decreased peripheral vision		Impaired righting reflexes
Decreased glare tolerance		Senile gait
Decreased contrast sensitivity		

Cognitive impairment is associated with an increased risk of falling. Confusion, impaired judgment, distraction, agitation, and lack of awareness increase a person's exposure to hazardous situations. Also, neurologic deficits, which frequently occur in dementia, can cause balance and gait abnormalities and psychomotor retardation.

The risk of falling appears to increase as the number of chronic **medical conditions** increases (see TABLE 7–2). Orthostatic hypotension, a common chronic condition in older persons, is probably not a common cause of falls; frequently, it causes elders to sit down because of lightheadedness. Falls related to standing up from a sitting or lying position are more likely to result from physical instability rather than changes in blood pressure. About 80% of older persons experience nocturia, and frequent nocturia has been associated with falls, probably because of the physical difficulties of getting up and walking to the bathroom quickly at night. Neurologic conditions, such as Parkinson's disease, normal pressure hydrocephalus, and hemiparesis, cause gait disorders and commonly are associated with falls. Parkinson's disease, for example, increases the risk of falling tenfold.

Muscle and joint abnormalities also contribute to the risk of falling. Many older persons have reduced muscular strength and tone. Also, proximal muscle weakness can result from thyroid disease, polymyositis, or corticosteroid use, making it difficult to arise from a chair and climb stairs. Both osteoarthritis and inflammatory joint diseases, especially involving the knees and hips, can lead to pain and joint instability. Foot deformities such as corns, calluses, and bunions can lead to pain on ambulation, destabilizing gait.

A **drop attack** is a sudden unexpected loss of balance without a loss of consciousness that often results in a fall. In the past, this term was used

TABLE 7–2. DISORDERS AND MEDICATIONS THAT PREDISPOSE THE ELDERLY TO FALLS

Neurologic disorders	Stroke Transient ischemic attack Parkinsonism Delirium Myelopathy Seizures Vertebrobasilar insufficiency Carotid sinus supersensitivity Cerebellar disorders Peripheral neuropathy Dementia
Cardiovascular disorders	Myocardial infarction Orthostatic hypotension Arrhythmia
Gastrointestinal disorders	Bleeding Diarrhea Defecation syncope Postprandial syncope
Metabolic disorders	Hypothyroidism Hypoglycemia Anemia Hypokalemia Dehydration Hyponatremia
Genitourinary disorders	Micturition syncope Incontinence Nocturia
Musculoskeletal disorders	Arthritis Proximal myopathy Deconditioning
Psychologic disorders	Depression Anxiety
Medications	Benzodiazepines Phenothiazines Tricyclic antidepressants Some antihypertensives Diuretics Narcotics

to describe an unexpected fall with no identifiable cause, and it was considered one of the most common causes of falls. By the newer, more limited definition, drop attacks are considered a much less common cause of falls.

Medications are associated with an increased risk of falls and fall-related injuries. The risk of falling increases with the number of prescribed medications. In epidemiologic studies, psychoactive drugs such as long-acting benzodiazepines, phenothiazines, and tricyclic antidepressants have been reported to increase the risk of falls and hip fractures among elders in the community and nursing homes. About 14% of hip fractures are attributed to psychoactive medications. Codeine and propoxyphene have also been shown to increase the risk of hip fractures. Drug effects such as decreased alertness, impaired judgment, compromised neuromuscular function, and dizziness may be the mechanisms. Diuretics may contribute to falls by causing somnolence, volume depletion, electrolyte disturbance, or an urgency to rush to the bathroom. Antihypertensives may cause decreased alertness, postural hypotension, or somnolence.

At least 40% of older persons are alcohol users, and 5% to 10% are heavy drinkers. Alcohol is a risk factor for falls in people < 60 yr, and the assumption that alcohol's effects on cognition, gait, and balance would be more pronounced in the elderly and contribute significantly to falls seems sensible. However, the association has not been convincingly shown in studies. This failure to show a clear association may result from underreporting of alcohol consumption or premature mortality from alcohol consumption.

Extrinsic factors: Environmental hazards are implicated in 33% to 50% of falls. Common extrinsic hazards in the home are clutter, electrical cords in pathways, inadequate lighting, throw rugs, low chairs, soft chairs, uneven surfaces, raised thresholds, and slippery surfaces. Stairs are a common site of falls, and the first and last steps are the most dangerous. Indoor falls occur most often in the bathroom, bedroom, and kitchen. Frequent sites of outdoor falls are curbs and steps. The most frequent sites of falls in institutions are the bedside (during transfers into or out of bed) and the bathroom. Although institutions are generally considered safer environments, the patients are frailer, and therefore, subtle environmental hazards may pose greater risks.

Epidemiology

Falls are the leading cause of accidental death (and the seventh leading cause of death) in persons > 65 yr. In the USA, 75% of deaths caused by falls occur in the 12% of the population > 65 yr. The rate of death from falls rises exponentially with increasing age for both sexes and all racial groups > 75 yr. Falls occur more often in women until age 75; after age 75, the frequency is similar in both sexes. However, white men > 85 yr have the highest death rate associated with falls.

The incidence and prevalence of falls vary according to the population. About 33% of generally healthy community-dwelling elders fall each year, as do about 67% of nursing home residents, despite their limited activity and protection from many environmental risk factors. The rate of falls for elderly hospital patients is between those for elders in the community and elders in nursing homes. The higher rates of falls in nursing homes and hospitals are partially explained by the greater frailty of these populations but may also reflect increased reporting. Also, the use of restraints may actually increase the risk of falls because patients struggle to free themselves and accidentally fall. Similarly, bedrails may increase the risk of falls because patients try to climb over them.

Most falls occur indoors. No specific time of day, time of the year, or location is associated with falling. In older persons, most falls occur during usual activities such as walking. About 5% of falls occur during hazardous activities such as standing on chairs, climbing ladders, or participating in sports. About 10% of falls occur on stairs, with descent being more hazardous than ascent.

Complications

Children and young adults, who have a higher incidence of falls than all but the very frail elderly, rarely sustain substantial injury or die from a fall. In the elderly, the propensity for injury is associated with age-related osteoporosis and slowed protective reflexes, which can make even a relatively mild fall dangerous.

About 5% of falls in older persons, whether community-dwelling or institutionalized, result in a fracture. Another 10% to 20% result in severe soft tissue trauma, such as lacerations, hematomas, sprains, and joint dislocations; about half of these injuries require medical care. About 7% of persons > 75 yr visit hospital emergency departments for fall injuries each year, accounting for 70% of emergency department visits for injuries in this age group. Older persons have the highest rate of acute care hospitalization for injuries. Of elders hospitalized for a fall, only 50% live for 1 yr thereafter.

The humerus, wrist, pelvis, and hip are the most common sites of fractures caused by the combination of osteoporosis and falls. Hip fractures are the most serious, and more than 250,000 of them occur each year in persons > 65 yr. The rate of hip fracture increases exponentially with age and is highest among white women. Whites have about twice the rate of hip fractures as persons of all other races. About 20% of women who reach age 80 have suffered a hip fracture. The risk of falling and fracturing a hip doubles with the use of certain psychoactive drugs, such as antipsychotics and long-acting benzodiazepines.

About 5% of hip fractures result in death during hospitalization; the overall mortality in the 12 mo following a hip fracture ranges from 12% to 67%, depending on the population studied. At least half of those who could walk before sustaining a hip fracture cannot walk afterward, and half are unable to live independently; thus, their quality of life drastically deteriorates. An older person who remains on the floor for a time after a fall may suffer serious physical and psychologic effects. Dehydration, pressure sores, rhabdomyolysis, hypothermia, and pneumonia can develop from lying for prolonged periods after a fall.

Even the 90% of falls that do not result in injury may have serious consequences. The fear of another fall can make elders lose confidence, self-esteem, and a sense of well-being and thus impose restrictions on their mobility. About 40% of older persons have a fear of falling, and about 20% avoid activities such as shopping and cleaning because of this fear. This reduced mobility after a fall is referred to as **postfall syndrome.** Decreased activity can lead to increased joint stiffness and weakness, further compromising mobility. Functional decline increases the burden on caregivers, which partially explains why falls are a contributing factor in 40% of admissions to nursing homes.

Evaluation

Because elderly persons frequently fail to report falls, they should be asked about them as a routine part of screenings. When a patient does report a fall, the first step is to assess and, if necessary, treat any acute injury. Then the fall should be evaluated like any symptom, with a history and physical examination (see TABLE 7–3). The routine use of laboratory tests, electrocardiograms, and Holter monitoring is not recommended unless a specific clinical indication exists. The evaluation of a fall may also include an assessment of environmental hazards. The evaluation of falls associated with syncope differs from that of falls without syncope (see also Ch. 6).

History: The initial inquiry concerning the circumstances of a fall should be made using open-ended questions. Then more specific questions should be asked about when and where the fall occurred and what the patient was doing. Did the patient experience any symptoms such as palpitations, shortness of breath, chest pain, vertigo, or lightheadedness at the time of the fall? Did the patient lose consciousness? Were any obvious environmental hazards involved? Does the patient have a history of falls? The history should also explore present and past medical problems and medication use. Any witnesses to the fall should be questioned as well.

Physical examination: The physical examination should be comprehensive enough to exclude obvious intrinsic causes of falling and to help distinguish syncope from other causes, such as tripping. The pattern of injury is useful, but not conclusive, evidence in determining the cause.

Emphasis should be placed on examining the cardiovascular, musculoskeletal, and neurologic systems. Blood pressure should be measured with the patient both supine and standing to rule out orthostatic hypotension. Examining the cardiovascular system helps exclude arrhythmia, valvular heart disease, and heart failure. The extremities should be evaluated for arthritis and podiatric problems that could impair gait. Neurologic findings may suggest cerebrovascular disease, tumor, Par-

TABLE 7–3. EVALUATION OF THE FALL

Assessment and treatment of acute injury

History

- Activity at time of fall
- Premonitory symptoms—ie, light-headedness, palpitations, dyspnea, chest pain, vertigo, confusion, incontinence, loss of consciousness, tongue biting
- Location of fall
- Witnesses to fall
- History of previous falls (of same or different character)
- Past medical history
- Medications

Physical examination

- Visual acuity, visual fields, low-vision evaluation
- Cardiovascular system
  - Blood pressure and pulse, supine and standing
  - Arrhythmia, murmur, bruits
- Extremities
  - Arthritis, edema, podiatric problems, poorly fitting shoes
- Neurologic system
  - Mental status testing
  - Gait and balance assessment—ie, getting in and out of chair, walking, bending, turning, reaching, ascending and descending stairs, standing with eyes closed (Romberg test), sternal push

kinson's disease, myelopathy, peripheral neuropathy, or proximal myopathy. Mental status testing may suggest dementia, delirium, or depression. Vision and hearing should be checked as well. Because falling may be an atypical presentation of an acute illness, occult problems such as infection, myocardial infarction, dehydration, and anemia also should be reasonably evaluated.

A set of simple clinical tests, in which patients perform position changes and gait maneuvers during daily activities, can identify those at greatest risk of falling. This type of evaluation is more likely than a formal neurologic examination to detect fall-related risk factors. The patient is observed getting into and out of a chair, turning around, bending down and picking up objects from the floor, and reaching up to get something from a shelf. Aside from revealing abnormalities that might not have been apparent on a routine inspection of gait (eg, proximal muscle weakness that may be apparent only when the patient rises from a chair), this testing also helps establish functional abilities.

Gait should be observed with the patient rising from a chair, walking at least 20 ft, turning, returning, and sitting down. The clinician can walk alongside the patient for safety. In the **circumduction gait,** the lower extremity assumes triple extension at the hip, knee, and ankle, and the person swings the leg in an outward arc to ensure ground clearance. This type of gait occurs in patients with hemiplegia. Bilateral upper motor neuron lesions may cause a **scissoring gait,** which is essentially a bilateral circumduction gait.

The **festinating gait** is a symmetric shuffling of the feet with poor ground clearance, typically seen in Parkinson's disease. Frequently, festination is seen only when the person starts to walk and when the person reaches an obstacle or attempts to turn. The parkinsonian patient also tends to assume a forward-flexed posture and have little or no arm movement while walking. Severe postural instability in the parkinsonian patient leads to an inability to maintain balance when pushed from the back or front, known as propulsion and retropulsion, respectively.

The **cerebellar gait** is a broad-based gait with irregular steps. The patient veers to either side, forward, or backward. In severe cases, the patient is not able to stand unsupported, even with open eyes. This form of ataxia is common in chronic alcoholics and in persons with paleocerebellar atrophies, progressive supranuclear palsy, multiple sclerosis, and cerebellar tumors. When such ataxia has an acute onset in an older person, the cause is almost always vascular.

Frontal lobe apraxia causes a **broad-based gait** that in many respects resembles the parkinsonian gait. The person assumes a forward-flexed posture, and the steps are short, slow, and shuffling; at times, the feet appear to be glued to the floor. However, a bedside examination reveals normal power in the legs, and the patient may be able to perform complex movements with the legs, such as drawing a figure 8 on the floor. This gait disorder frequently precedes the dementia and incontinence that complete the triad of normal-pressure hydrocephalus. Because this neurologic condition is potentially treatable with a shunt procedure, it should be considered when a patient presents with an apraxic gait.

Sensory ataxia is a broad-based, foot-stamping gait. The person constantly looks at his feet as he walks to compensate for the lack of proprioception from visual input. When asked to stand with his feet together and eyes open, the patient can maintain the stance, but when asked to close the eyes, the patient loses balance—a positive Romberg test. In the elderly, this condition is caused by disorders affecting the posterior columns, such as vitamin B_{12} deficiency (posterolateral sclerosis), cervical spondylosis, and paleocerebellar degeneration.

Assessment of environmental hazards: A physician, visiting nurse, physical or occupational therapist, family member, or the patient may assess the home for hazards. A patient home assessment checklist is presented in TABLE 7–4.

Treatment

The management plan should include an approach to both intrinsic and extrinsic causes. Also, patients should be taught what to do if they fall and cannot get up. Turning from the supine position to the prone position, crawling to a strong support surface, and pulling themselves

TABLE 7–4. HOME ASSESSMENT CHECKLIST FOR FALL HAZARDS

Hazard	*Correction*	*Rationale*
General household		
Lighting		
Too dim	Provide ample lighting in all areas	Increased illumination improves visual acuity
Too direct, creating glare	Reduce glare with evenly distributed light, indirect lighting, translucent shades	
Light switches inaccessible	Install so switches are immediately accessible on entering room	Reduces risk of falling when walking across dark room
Carpets, rugs		
Torn	Repair or replace torn carpet	Prevents tripping and slipping by persons with decreased stepping ability
Slippery	Provide rugs with nonskid backs; tack down to prevent curling	
Chairs, tables		
Unstable	Must be stable enough to support weight of person leaning on table edges or chair arms and backs	Balance-impaired persons use furniture for support
Lack of armrests	Provide chairs with armrests that extend forward enough for leverage in getting up or sitting down	Assists persons with proximal muscle weakness
Low-back chairs	Provide high-back chairs	High back provides support for neck and while transferring weight; parkinsonian patients often begin rocking movement to assist in getting up; high chair back prevents falling backward

(continued)

TABLE 7–4. HOME ASSESSMENT CHECKLIST FOR FALL HAZARDS *(Continued)*

Hazard	*Correction*	*Rationale*
General household *(continued)*		
Furniture		
Obstructs path	Arrange furnishings so that pathways are not obstructed; avoid cluttered hallways	Aids mobility in persons with impaired peripheral vision
Heating		
Too cool	Maintain temperature at 22.2° C (72° F) in winter	Prevents falls secondary to hypothermia
Kitchen		
Cabinets, shelves		
Too high	Keep frequently used items at waist level; install shelves, cupboards at accessible height	Reduces risk of falling because of frequent reaching or standing on unstable ladders or chairs
Floor		
Wet or waxed	Place rubber mat on floor in sink area; wear rubber-soled shoes in kitchen; use nonslip wax or buff paste wax thoroughly	Prevents slipping, especially if person is gait-impaired
Gas range		
Dial difficult to see	Clearly mark "on" and "off" positions on dials	Prevents a fall from gas asphyxiation, especially if sense of smell is impaired
Chair		
Armrests lacking	Provide chairs with armrests and sturdy legs	Armrests assist in transfer
Legs unsound	Avoid chairs with wheels; repair legs that are loose	Sturdy, stable chairs do not slide away when transferring
Table		
Wobbly, unstable	Install table with sturdy legs of even length; avoid tripod or pedestal tables	Gait-impaired persons often use table for support

(continued)

TABLE 7–4. HOME ASSESSMENT CHECKLIST FOR FALL HAZARDS *(Continued)*

Hazard	*Correction*	*Rationale*
Bathroom		
Bathtub		
Slippery tub floor	Install skid-resistant strips or rubber mat; use shower shoes or bath seat	Prevents sliding on wet tub floor; if balance is impaired, sitting while showering prevents falls
Side of bathtub used for support or transfer	Use portable grab bar on side of tub	Aids transfers; portable grab bar can be taken along on trips
Towel racks, sink tops		
Unstable for use as support while transferring from toilet	Fasten grab rails to wall studs next to toilet	Aids transfer to and from toilet
Toilet seat		
Too low	Use elevated toilet seat	Aids transfer to and from toilet
Medicine cabinet		
Inadequate lighting	Install brighter lighting	Helps avoid incorrect administration of medication, especially for visually impaired
Drugs improperly labeled	Label all drugs according to need for internal or external use; keep magnifying glass in or near cabinet	
Door		
Locks	Remove locks from bathroom doors, or use locks that can be opened from both sides of door	Permits access by others if fall occurs
Stairways		
Height		
Rise between steps is too high	Correct step height to less than 6 in.	Reduces risk of tripping for persons with decreased stepping ability

(continued)

TABLE 7–4. HOME ASSESSMENT CHECKLIST FOR FALL HAZARDS *(Continued)*

Hazard	*Correction*	*Rationale*
Stairways *(continued)*		
Handrails		
Missing	Install and anchor well on both sides of stairway; use cylindric rails placed 1 to 2 in. away from wall	Person can grasp rail with either hand
Improper length	Extend beyond top and bottom step, and turn ends inward	Signals that top or bottom step has been reached
Configuration		
Too steep, or too long	Provide stairways with intermediate landings	Rest stop especially convenient for cardiac or pulmonary patients
Condition		
Slippery	Place nonskid treads securely on all steps	Prevents slipping
Lighting		
Inadequate	Install adequate lighting at both top and bottom of stairway; night lights or bright-colored adhesive strips can be used to clearly mark steps	Outlines location of steps, especially for persons with vision or perception impairment

Modified from Tideiksaar R: "Preventing falls: Home hazard checklist to help older patients protect themselves." *Geriatrics* 41:26–28, 1986; used with permission.

up may help. Frequent contact with family or friends, a phone that is reachable from the floor, or a remote alarm system can decrease the likelihood of an older person lying on the floor for a prolonged period. Such strategies may be particularly appropriate for frequent fallers.

Intrinsic factors: Although some intrinsic risk factors are reversible, many are not. Still, modifying even a few risk factors may be all that is needed. Falls from Parkinson's disease may improve with dopaminergic drugs. Falls from osteoarthritis may improve with pain management, physical therapy, and surgery. Correcting visual impairment may help. Also, any medication that may increase the risk of falls should be discontinued or the dosage should be adjusted, if possible. However, risk factors such as cognitive impairment or severe peripheral neuropathy from diabetes are generally irreversible.

Physical therapy can improve mobility, strength, and balance. However, increased mobility may expose an older person to more environmental hazards. Assistive devices such as canes and walkers provide additional stability and safety. Proper training in the use of assistive devices is important (see also Ch. 29).

Extrinsic factors: The major environmental hazards are floors, lighting, stairs, bathrooms, beds, chairs, and shelves. Floors should not be wet or highly waxed; thick pile carpet or area rugs without nonskid backings should be avoided. All lighting should be controlled by easily accessible wall switches, and the color of the switch plates should contrast with the color of the wall so they are more visible. Glare from sunlight through a window or from highly polished floors should be eliminated.

Stairways should be adequately illuminated, and light switches should be positioned at the top and bottom. Placing night lights at the first and last steps provides additional safety. Worn step runners and carpet should be repaired or replaced. Placing nonslip adhesive strips along the step edges helps define the steps, and installing handrails on both sides of the stairs helps older persons negotiate the stairs safely. The handrails should be round, about 30 in. higher than the stairs, attached to the wall, and set out far enough from the wall to permit a good grasp. The ends of the handrails should be specially shaped to signal that the top or bottom of the stairs has been reached.

In the bathroom, towel bars should be replaced with nonslip grab bars. The grab bars must be securely fixed to the studs of the walls, so they will not easily give way. Using an adjustable, raised toilet seat and toilet grab bars or grab bars located on the wall next to the toilet helps to minimize falls. Slip-resistant grab bars should be installed on the rim of the bathtub or in the shower. Nonslip adhesive rubber strips or a rubber mat with suction cups should be attached to the shower or bathtub floor. Tub or shower chairs or benches should be used if the patient lacks the ability to rise after bathing or is unable to stand for long periods of time.

A bed height of about 18 in. from the top of the mattress to the floor allows for the safest transfer. Chair heights should be adjusted so that the patient can sit with feet firmly on the floor and knees flexed at 90°. Armrests should be horizontally placed about 7 in. above the seat and should extend beyond the edge of the seat by 1 to 2 in. to allow for maximum leverage.

Using shelves that are too high or too low may contribute to a loss of balance. Frequently used items should be placed so they can be retrieved without excessive bending, reaching, or climbing. Shelf storage in kitchens and closets should be between hip and eye level. The use of hand-held reachers or grabbing devices helps patients retrieve objects from high and low shelves without compromising safety.

8. FRACTURES

In the elderly, fractures are a major cause of morbidity and mortality. Most result from low-energy injuries and involve bone weakened by osteoporosis or other pathologic processes. Compared with fractures in younger people, fractures in the elderly occur more often, in different locations within the bone, and in different patterns. The prognosis for uncomplicated healing also differs in the elderly, who have a greater tendency to develop joint stiffness from immobilization and medical complications from enforced bed rest. Consequently, treatment goals in the elderly emphasize a rapid return to the activities necessary for independent living rather than a restoration of perfect limb alignment or length using prolonged casting or traction.

Most elderly people do not need to perform strenuous work, and high-strength functional capabilities are not a priority. Because they place less stress on the musculoskeletal system, many older people do well with a fracture alignment or a prosthetic replacement that would be unsuitable in younger patients.

Descriptive and Anatomic Terms

A typical long bone is divided into three anatomic regions: the **diaphysis,** or shaft, consists of a tube of cortical bone surrounding a medullary cavity of hematopoietic or fatty marrow; the **epiphysis** lies at the end of the bone between the growth plate, or physis, and the articular surface; the **metaphysis** is the intermediate, flared region joining the other two. The skeleton consists of two forms of bone: **trabecular** and **cortical.** Most of the metaphysis and epiphysis is composed of trabecular, or porous, bone, which varies widely in density and strength, depending on age, skeletal location, and associated pathologic conditions (eg, osteoporosis). The diaphysis is composed of cortical, or lamellar, bone. Its dense histologic architecture of parallel haversian systems gives it great strength.

Standard terminology facilitates the description of fracture patterns. Proximal, midshaft, and distal describe the location. The orientation of a fracture line may be transverse, oblique, or spiral. Comminution refers to fragmentation. Open or closed indicates whether or not the fracture communicates to the outside through a soft tissue wound. (The archaic terms "simple" and "compound" should be avoided.) Alignment refers to the relative position of the main fracture fragments. Their apex may point anteriorly, posteriorly, laterally (varus angulation), or medially (valgus angulation). The bone ends may be overriding, distracted, or impacted.

Incidence and Epidemiology

In 1990, about 281,000 hip fractures occurred in the USA. As the population ages, the problem continues to grow. Census projections indicate that by 2000, about 340,000 hip fractures will occur annually, about half of them in those age 85 and older. One in three women and one in six men who live to age 90 will sustain a hip fracture. In the year following the fracture, the mortality rate increases by 15%. Of functionally independent patients who live at home before the fracture, 20% require institutional care for more than a year, and another 30% become dependent on mechanical aids or assistive personnel.

With advancing age, the incidence of certain kinds of fractures increases. Long bone shaft fractures, which involve predominantly cortical bone, do not correlate with age. In contrast, the incidence of vertebral body and hip fractures is low until the fifth and sixth decades of life, when it increases dramatically. Fractures of the proximal humerus and tibia, wrist, and pubic rami follow a similar pattern. These fractures that occur increasingly with age involve predominantly trabecular bone.

Etiology and Pathophysiology

The most common cause of fractures, **falls** account for about 90% of geriatric hip, forearm, and pelvic fractures (see also Ch. 7). The frequency of falls among the elderly results in part from a high incidence of underlying medical conditions: failing vision, neurologic diseases and their sequelae, arthritis that impairs leg function, orthostatic hypotension, and the use of sedatives and other medications. Also, slowed reflexes, decreased muscle strength, and impaired coordination may reduce older people's ability to protect themselves from the impact of falls, increasing the likelihood of fractures. Most fractures in the elderly result from the relatively low-energy trauma incurred by a fall on level ground.

Pathologic fracture refers to *any fracture involving abnormal (weakened) bone,* eg, from underlying malignancy, benign bone tumor, metabolic disorder, infection, or osteoporosis. Thus, a pathologic fracture should be suspected in any patient who sustains a fracture after minimal trauma. Usually, the patient will have a history of progressively increasing pain in the affected region, especially noticeable at night and on weight bearing. Diagnosing pathologic fracture is important because the choice of treatment and prognosis may depend on the underlying pathologic condition.

Occasionally, patients present with an impending pathologic fracture, in which the bone has not yet broken entirely. Such patients feel pain in the affected area when using the limb. For instance, a patient with a lesion of the femur may feel thigh pain when rising out of a chair. Prophylactic internal fixation of such fractures with metal plates, rods, or prostheses is often indicated to prevent displacement, provide pain relief, and preserve function. If the impending fracture breaks through completely and becomes displaced, treatment can be considerably more difficult, with decreased function and increased morbidity.

Most skeletal malignancies are **metastatic lesions,** with the breast, lung, prostate, gastrointestinal tract, kidney, and thyroid being the most common primary sites. The typical x-ray shows multiple lytic lesions. All these tumors can produce lucencies on x-ray; prostatic and breast metastases may also produce sclerosis. **Primary bone malignancies** occur much less frequently. Multiple myeloma and lymphoma are the most common; osteosarcoma, fibrosarcoma, and chondrosarcoma are rare. Osteosarcoma occurs more commonly in people with Paget's disease, however.

Osteopenia, or abnormally decreased bone density, results from four conditions that are indistinguishable on x-ray but involve different pathologic processes: **osteoporosis,** due to too little bone; **osteomalacia,** due to decreased mineralization; **hyperparathyroidism,** which causes increased resorption; and **myeloma,** which destroys bone. Thus, patients with osteopenia require laboratory evaluation to identify the underlying condition.

Biomechanics

The force required to break a bone depends on both its material properties and its geometry. Material properties determine the force per unit area required to cause material failure. These properties are referred to as ultimate tensile or ultimate compressive strength (expressed in megapascals [MPa], with 1 MPa equal to 145 lb/sq in).

The ultimate tensile strength of cortical bone decreases only slightly with aging from about 140 MPa in the second decade to about 120 MPa in the eighth decade. With age, the diameter of the diaphysis increases as bone is resorbed from the inner, or endosteal, surface and is added to the outer, or periosteal, surface. This change increases the resistance of the diaphysis to bending forces and compensates for the decreased strength of the cortical bone. Thus, fractures of the diaphysis do not occur more frequently with advancing age.

The ultimate compressive strength of trabecular bone is proportional to its density and ranges between 1 and 10 MPa. Since normal cancellous bone has a density > 1.4 gm/cm^3, a density of 1 gm/cm^3 represents a halving of strength. An increased rate of fracture of the vertebrae and ends of the femur does not occur until bone density falls below 1 gm/cm^3. This loss of bone density is usually caused by osteoporosis (see Ch. 73). Most fractures in the elderly occur in the metaphyseal region, which does not remodel with age and thus does not compensate for the decreased density of the trabecular bone.

Normal Healing

Clinical management of fractures is based on an understanding of the physiology of bone repair. Fracture healing can be divided into three overlapping phases: inflammation, repair, and remodeling.

The **inflammatory phase** includes the initial response to injury and lasts several days. The trauma that fractures the bone also injures the surrounding blood vessels, muscles, and other soft tissues. Hemorrhage at the fracture site results in a hematoma. Traumatic devascularization of the fractured ends and bony fragments may result in nonviable or necrotic bone. This necrotic material elicits an immediate and intense acute inflammatory reaction. The fracture site is swollen and tender.

The **reparative phase** begins within 24 h after the injury and reaches peak activity after 1 to 2 wk. Diaphyseal fractures that are not rigidly stabilized heal by formation of rapidly created new bone around the fracture site called the **external callus.** External callus is not visible radiographically until about 3 to 6 wk after the injury. Until sufficient external callus forms and provides stability—a process that can take several months in long-bone fractures—collapse and displacement of the fracture can occur. Metaphyseal fractures heal by direct union of the trabecular bone, a faster process that begins within 2 to 3 wk.

During the **remodeling phase,** the rapidly formed callus is slowly resorbed and replaced by mechanically stronger bone distributed to best resist load-bearing stresses. These events proceed slowly in the elderly and may result in many months of discomfort after a fracture.

DIAGNOSIS

Physical Examination

Most fractures cause swelling, deformity, and pain on attempted movement. Minimally displaced, stress, or impending fractures cause tenderness on palpation and pain on weight bearing or loading of the involved bone. In noncommunicative patients, refusal to move an extremity may be the only sign of a fracture or dislocation. Thorough assessment of the sensory, motor, and circulatory status of the injured extremity is important before starting therapy. After application of a cast, splint, or traction or after manipulation of a fractured extremity, the neurovascular status of the limb should always be reevaluated.

When injury or lack of cooperation makes physical examination unreliable, x-rays are required to detect a fracture. For instance, a hip fracture may make examining the contralateral side difficult. Because coexisting injuries and preexisting abnormal conditions may be present, the physician should obtain x-rays of both hips and the pelvis in any patient with a femoral or pelvic fracture.

In patients with suspected hemarthrosis, joint aspiration is useful. Aspiration of fluid suggests acute effusion secondary to gout, pseudogout, or infection, which can be confirmed by laboratory test. Aspiration of blood confirms an intra-articular injury (eg, fracture or torn ligament or meniscus). Fat globules in the blood, which can be seen easily when the aspirate is viewed in an open container, imply a fracture that allows fat from the marrow cavity to enter the joint.

Diagnostic Tests

X-rays: Radiographs remain the most important tool for diagnosing and treating fractures. Routine x-ray evaluation of suspected fractures should always include both anteroposterior and lateral views. On a single view, the characteristic displacement, discontinuity in contour, or altered alignment of a fracture may be hidden because of overlap or projection. When standard views are equivocal, as sometimes occurs with minimally displaced spiral fractures, oblique views can be helpful. Fractures may be missed if the x-ray shows too small an area. A patient complaining of thigh and knee pain, for instance, may actually have a hip fracture causing referred pain; unless x-rays of the entire femur are taken, the fracture may be missed.

Computed tomography: Although not routinely needed, computed tomography is a useful adjunct to plain x-rays in several circumstances. It allows visualization of occult fractures, particularly in areas difficult to image with x-rays because of overlying bony structures (eg, the cervical spine). Computed tomography helps in determining the extent of articular surface disruption in joint fractures and in assessing suspected pathologic fractures for bone destruction and soft tissue masses.

Magnetic resonance imaging: In special circumstances, magnetic resonance imaging offers advantages, providing excellent tomography, soft tissue contrast, and spatial resolution using noninvasive and nonionizing radiation technology. Magnetic resonance imaging helps in evaluating pathologic fractures and in diagnosing osteonecrosis and osteomyelitis, both of which can mimic fractures. Often, magnetic resonance imaging can show occult fractures before an x-ray can detect them. Magnetic resonance imaging cannot directly show calcification or bone mineral and thus does not visualize bone structure as well as x-ray or computed tomography.

Bone scan: Total-body scanning, using ^{99m}Tc-labeled pyrophosphate or similar radioactive analogs, is performed to detect focal injury to bone from any cause. Uptake occurs wherever new bone forms, which can occur in response to infection, arthritis, tumor, or fracture. Occult fractures not yet visible on x-ray can often be detected on bone scan 3 to 5 days after injury. Patients with suspected pathologic fractures require bone scans for evaluation of metastatic and metabolic bone disease, which involve areas other than the fracture site.

Blood tests: Fractures, especially those of the hip, can result in substantial bleeding into soft tissues. The most widely used clinical test for evaluating blood loss from fractures is hematocrit measurement. A 3 mL/dL drop in hematocrit corresponds to the loss of roughly 500 mL (1 u.) of blood in a normally hydrated patient. Patients with *acute* bleeding or dehydration may initially have a falsely normal or elevated hematocrit; when intravascular volume is replenished with IV fluids, hematocrit will fall. Since elderly patients are often at high risk for developing myocardial ischemia, their RBC volume should not be allowed to drop below a level that maintains sufficient oxygen-carrying capacity. As a clinical guideline, a hematocrit < 30 mL/dL usually indicates the need for blood transfusion, especially preoperatively. In hip fracture patients, the hematocrit should be monitored for at least 4 days after injury or surgery, since a 4- to 8-mL/dL drop can occur because of continued bleeding or equilibration.

A low or falling hematocrit can also warn of a serious underlying medical condition with important implications in the fracture patient. For instance, gastrointestinal bleeding can be exacerbated by anticoagulants routinely given to immobilized patients for prophylaxis of deep venous thrombosis. Anemia may be the first sign of multiple myeloma or another malignancy that has led to a pathologic fracture.

Serum alkaline phosphatase rises when bone turnover increases. This occurs with normal fracture healing as well as with malignancy and metabolic abnormality (eg, Paget's disease). Serum calcium rises with some endocrine disturbances (eg, hyperparathyroidism) and with metastatic disease, especially breast carcinoma. When patients with Paget's disease are on bed rest, excessively rapid bone resorption can also elevate the serum calcium level.

TREATMENT

Immobilization of Fractures

Initial immobilization of injured extremities prevents further damage before definitive stabilization can be achieved. Movement of sharp fracture ends can cause serious soft tissue trauma and even skin puncture, converting a closed injury to an open one. Immobilization also facilitates transport of patients and relieves pain, thus decreasing the need for narcotic analgesics.

Injuries located about or distal to the knee or elbow can usually be immobilized initially with splints. A wide variety of splints are available, including those made of preformed aluminum or plastic, those made of inflatable clear plastic, and those that are easily adjustable with Velcro closures. Plaster of Paris (calcium sulfate hemihydrate) splints molded individually for patients provide the best support. All splints are best applied by an assistant while the injured extremity is held with gentle longitudinal traction.

Most injuries of the shoulder, upper arm, and elbow can be immobilized effectively with a sling. If needed, the arm can be kept close to the body with an elastic wrap or swath. Hip fractures can be immobilized by careful positioning with pillows or by light skin traction.

Casts are used to control the alignment of a fracture while it heals. Traditionally, casts are made of rolls of stiff muslin impregnated with plaster of Paris. Inexpensive and easy to mold, plaster is often used for initial casts and for those that need frequent changing. Plaster casts are relatively heavy, deteriorate with excessive or prolonged use, and weaken when wet. Cast materials made of polymeric resins and fiberglass are stronger, stiffer, and half as heavy as plaster casts. Water will not weaken the cast itself, but if the underlying padding becomes wet, the cast must be changed to prevent skin maceration.

To provide complete immobilization, the cast must extend across one joint above and one joint below the fracture site. Thus for a distal radial fracture, the cast should extend from above the elbow to just proximal to the metatarsal joint; however, because joint stiffness is a major problem in the elderly, the cast is often made to end below the elbow, allowing joint motion.

Patients with casts must be given detailed instructions. For the first 24 to 48 h after the injury, the extremity should be elevated to prevent swelling. Rhythmic flexion and extension of the fingers or wiggling of the toes should be encouraged to facilitate venous return. The patient should immediately report progressive or unrelenting pain, pressure, or numbness in the affected extremity because swelling within an unyielding circular cast can cause enough pressure to stop tissue perfusion, creating compartmental syndrome (see below).

Traction is used in the elderly only when no satisfactory alternative exists, eg, if the fracture is too fragmented for a cast or surgical stabilization or if the patient's medical condition will not permit surgery. Complications of traction include pressure sores, deep venous thrombosis, pulmonary embolism, depression, disorientation, loss of appetite, deconditioning, atelectasis, and pulmonary infection. Meticulous, aggressive nursing care is required during traction.

Skin traction is particularly hazardous in the elderly. Its only indication is to provide temporary, gentle restraint of the extremity for comfort. Such traction is applied using foam boots or carefully wrapped moleskin strips, a sash cord, and a pulley with a 5-lb weight. A weight > 5 lb should never be used. Vigilant monitoring is required. The strong, prolonged traction needed to maintain bone alignment must not be applied with skin traction but rather with the use of skeletal pins. The proximal tibia is the most common traction pin site for femoral and acetabular fractures.

Operative stabilization of fractures can offer dramatic benefits in elderly patients. Those with hip fractures, for instance, can usually begin walking within days after surgery. The risks of surgery are small compared with those of prolonged traction, especially for leg fractures.

Despite these advantages, surgical treatment of most fractures should be postponed until acute medical problems can be corrected. Only fractures associated with such limb-threatening conditions as impending compartmental syndrome, neurovascular compromise, or open wounds require urgent treatment. Furthermore, some conditions are relative contraindications to surgery. Sepsis could lead to infection of the operative site and prohibits the use of metallic implants. Severely osteoporotic bone has poor mechanical properties, and the hardware used in operative stabilization will become displaced if it does not have a secure hold in the bone.

A deep postoperative wound infection, a serious complication, frequently requires removal of all implanted hardware, prolonged daily dressing changes, and weeks of IV antibiotics. Prophylactic antibiotics can reduce the incidence of postoperative infections in hip fracture patients to about 1%. A cephalosporin is the agent of choice; an appropriate regimen is cefazolin 1 gm given IV during the hour before surgery, followed by 1 gm q 8 h for the next 24 h.

Ambulatory Aids

Orthotic and self-help devices are described in Ch. 29.

COMPLICATIONS OF FRACTURES

Compartmental Syndrome

Compartmental, or closed-space, syndrome is the most frequent limb-threatening complication associated with extremity trauma. Swelling of injured muscle within a compartment surrounded by an unyielding envelope, such as fascia or a cast, leads to elevated tissue pressures that block normal perfusion. The resulting ischemia leads to further muscle injury and swelling and higher tissue pressures. The only solution to this ever-intensifying cycle is to remove all confining envelopes around the swollen muscular compartment. Thus, whenever patients complain of increasing pain or distal numbness in an immobilized, injured extremity, their casts, splints, and dressings must be thoroughly loosened immediately. If the muscle swelling has increased to the point that the surrounding fascia has become a constricting envelope, an emergency fasciotomy must be performed. Even a few hours of muscle ischemia can lead to irreversible injury and necrosis.

The most reliable clinical signs of impending compartmental syndrome are progressively increasing pain in an immobilized extremity, pain with passive flexion or extension of the toes or fingers, and numbness in a specific peripheral nerve distribution. The presence of distal pulses in a limb does not exclude compartmental syndrome; muscle necrosis and irreversible nerve damage occur at tissue pressures much lower than those required to obliterate arterial inflow. A definitive diagnosis of compartmental syndrome can be made using a device that percutaneously measures intramuscular pressures.

Thromboembolism

(See also Chs. 42 and 49)

Pulmonary embolism is the most frequent fatal complication following leg trauma. Autopsies have shown that 38% of patients who die after hip fracture die of pulmonary embolism. Among patients with hip fractures who are not given anticoagulant therapy, about 50% develop deep venous thrombosis; about 10%, pulmonary emboli; and about 2%, fatal pulmonary emboli. The major predisposing factors for deep venous thrombosis are advanced age, leg trauma or surgery, history of deep venous thrombosis, immobilization, malignancy, and obesity. The associated clinical findings—pain, swelling, tenderness, Homans' sign (pain on forced dorsiflexion of the foot), fever, and leukocytosis—are unreliable criteria for making a diagnosis. Venography remains the standard test, while ultrasonography has become the most effective noninvasive study for detecting deep venous thrombosis.

Ideally, patients with a femoral or pelvic fracture should begin prophylactic anticoagulant therapy for thromboembolic disease on admission and continue therapy until they are ambulatory. For orthopedic patients at high risk for deep venous thrombosis (eg, those with hip fractures), warfarin and dextran have traditionally been considered the most effective prophylactic agents. Neither aspirin, low-dose heparin, nor external pneumatic boot compression provides as much protection. If warfarin is used, the initial dose should be between 2.5 and 10 mg, depending on the patient's age and weight. Subsequent daily doses are given to maintain prothrombin time at about 1.2 to 1.4 times control. A history of recent gastrointestinal bleeding, malignancy, bleeding tendencies, or stroke is a relative contraindication to anticoagulation. Newer agents such as low-molecular-weight heparin and heparinoids may be as effective as warfarin with a lower incidence of bleeding.

Fat Embolism Syndrome

Although microscopic fat emboli accompany most femoral fractures, overt symptoms and signs develop in only about 2%. Usually occurring 2 to 3 days after fracture, **fat embolism syndrome** includes at least one of these major signs: respiratory insufficiency, drowsiness and confusion, petechial rash. Minor signs include pyrexia, tachycardia, retinal changes, jaundice, renal changes, thrombocytopenia, and an elevated erythrocyte sedimentation rate. Chest x-ray shows variable streaks and infiltrates associated with overt pulmonary edema in 33% of patients. Prothrombin time and activated partial thromboplastin time are also mildly elevated. In some patients, **adult respiratory distress syndrome** with noncardiac pulmonary edema and clinically significant **disseminated intravascular coagulation** occur. A **hyperacute syndrome** may result in death secondary to emboli of the coronary arteries and brain.

Treatment of fat embolism syndrome is aimed at respiratory support. Corticosteroids are often used, although their efficacy is unproved. Fortunately, the mortality rate is only about 8%, compared with that of 50% for most other causes of adult respiratory distress syndrome.

SPECIFIC FRACTURES

Fractures of the proximal humerus, distal radius, pelvic ramus, proximal femur, proximal tibia, and thoracic and lumbar vertebral bodies occur more commonly in the elderly. These sites consist of predominantly trabecular bone, often seriously weakened by osteoporosis.

Most of these fractures, except those involving the hip, are treated nonoperatively. Nonetheless, rehabilitation is often prolonged, and recovery is incomplete (see also Ch. 29). Usually, several months to a year passes before patients regain their preinjury capabilities.

PROXIMAL HUMERUS FRACTURES

Symptoms, Signs, and Diagnosis

The most common mechanism of injury is a fall on an outstretched hand. Patients present with shoulder pain and an inability to move the arm. On x-ray, the proximal humerus may show as many as four separate fragments: eg, an articular fragment containing the humeral head, a greater tuberosity fragment, a lesser tuberosity fragment, and a distal fragment including the humeral shaft. These fragments are prone to displacement because of the pull of the supraspinous, subscapular, and pectoral muscles. Displaced fractures are classified according to increasing order of severity into two-, three-, and four-part patterns. Fortunately, about 80% of proximal humerus fractures are minimally displaced, with < 45° angulation and < 1 cm displacement of any fragment. When displaced, the articular fragment may not lie in a satisfactory posture above the humeral shaft, as shown on anteroposterior and lateral x-rays. Fractures associated with a glenohumeral dislocation usually result from major trauma and constitute the most severe injuries.

Treatment and Prognosis

Treatment and prognosis depend on the number of fragments and the extent of displacement. Patients should be told to expect considerable swelling and discoloration that will spread to the lower arm and hand. If the alignment and position of the fragments are satisfactory, the arm may simply be immobilized in a sling. Otherwise, an orthopedist may attempt closed reduction. If satisfactory alignment cannot be achieved by manipulation, open reduction with internal fixation or insertion of a prosthetic replacement may be indicated.

Beginning range-of-motion exercises as soon as possible is essential (see Ch. 29). The most common complication after a shoulder fracture is adhesive capsulitis, which results from approximation of the inflamed surfaces of the joint capsule. Capsulitis can cause chronic pain and functional disability because of restricted motion.

For a stable two-part fracture, active motion and use of the hand and wrist should be encouraged immediately. A physical therapist should give instructions and monitor exercises. At 1 wk, pendulum exercises in the sling should begin. The patient leans forward and, using the noninjured arm to assist, swings the injured arm like a pendulum, making circles with the elbow. The sling may be removed daily to allow bathing and elbow motion. By 2 wk, the patient should begin active and passive arm elevation. Regaining the ability to perform overhead activities, such as combing hair, may take several months.

DISTAL RADIUS FRACTURES

In 1814, Abraham Colles first described the classic silver fork deformity of the wrist. A Colles fracture occurs when the dorsal trabecular bone of the distal radius impacts into itself, resulting in angulation and shortening. Patients present with pain, tenderness, and swelling of the wrist. The mechanism of injury is usually a fall on an outstretched hand.

Treatment and Prognosis

The severity of the fracture and need for reduction are assessed radiographically. Ideally, on the anteroposterior view, shortening of the radial styloid should be < 0.5 cm compared with the ulna. On the lateral view, dorsal tilting of the distal radius articular surface should not go beyond neutral. Patients with minimally displaced fractures or low functional demands are treated with a short arm cast or splint. When a fracture requires closed reduction, anesthesia is necessary. A local lidocaine injection with hematoma aspiration may be sufficient, but regional or IV general anesthesia is superior for relaxation and analgesia. Fractures with severe shortening or intra-articular comminution may require external fixation. In the operating room, pins are inserted through the skin into the metacarpals and proximal radius or ulna. Next, a metal external frame or plaster cast is applied to the pins to maintain the fracture reduction.

The most frequent complication of distal radius fractures is finger and shoulder stiffness. Thus, active motion of the fingers, elbow, and shoulder should be strongly encouraged. Elevating the hand above the level of the heart minimizes swelling. Cast immobilization is usually maintained for 3 to 8 wk, depending on the fracture's stability. Patients can expect pain to gradually diminish and wrist weakness to remain for 6 to 12 mo after the injury. Physical therapy may help speed recovery. Most patients eventually regain satisfactory pain-free function.

PELVIC RAMUS FRACTURES

Symptoms, Signs, and Diagnosis

The usual mechanism of injury is a fall on level ground. Patients present with pain and are unable to walk. Physical examination reveals localized tenderness in the groin and pain on leg movement. The clinical appearance mimics a proximal femoral fracture; diagnosis is made by x-ray. Usually, only a single ramus is fractured, with the pubic ramus breaking twice as often as the ischiatic ramus. Less commonly, two or more rami fracture, either on the same or on opposite sides of the symphysis pubis.

Normally, the pelvis bears weight mainly on the strong bony arches in the ilium, with the pubic and ischiatic rami acting as secondary tie arches. When the pelvis suffers trauma, the rami tend to fracture first, weakening the secondary tie arches but leaving the main iliac weight-bearing arches intact.

Treatment and Prognosis

Hospitalization is usually required because most patients are initially unable to stand or sit without considerable pain. Analgesics and nonsteroidal anti-inflammatory drugs help. To avoid the complications associated with bed confinement, patients should be encouraged to begin full weight-bearing ambulation as soon as possible. Most are able to walk with a walker by 1 wk. Pubic ramus fractures typically heal without causing permanent functional disabilities.

HIP FRACTURES

(See also Hip Fracture Rehabilitation in Ch. 29)

Hip fractures involve the femoral neck or the trochanteric processes.

Femoral Neck Fractures

Symptoms, Signs, and Classification

These fractures can be classified as occult, impacted, displaced, or nondisplaced. Occult fractures may occur in the elderly after little or no apparent trauma. The patient complains of persistent groin pain on weight bearing. A crack, initially undetectable on x-ray, can continue to propagate across the femoral neck with the cyclic stresses of walking. Weight bearing must be avoided, or eventually, complete displacement can occur. Bone scans or magnetic resonance imaging reveals the fracture before x-rays.

Patients with impacted and nondisplaced femoral neck fractures also present with groin pain and no deformity on physical examination. The Garden classification system describes the extent of impaction and displacement of hip fractures. X-rays of impacted fractures (Garden I) show the femoral head slightly tilted inward (valgus deformity) with an incomplete fracture line, leaving the medial cortex intact. Nondisplaced fractures extending across both cortices of the femoral neck (Garden II) are more unstable. Patients with displaced femoral neck fractures (Garden III and IV) present with groin pain and a shortened, externally rotated leg that is too painful to move (see Fig. 8–1).

The Garden classification reflects the degree of disruption of the blood supply to the femoral head and has crucial implications for treatment and prognosis. Because the femoral head is intra-articular, its sole

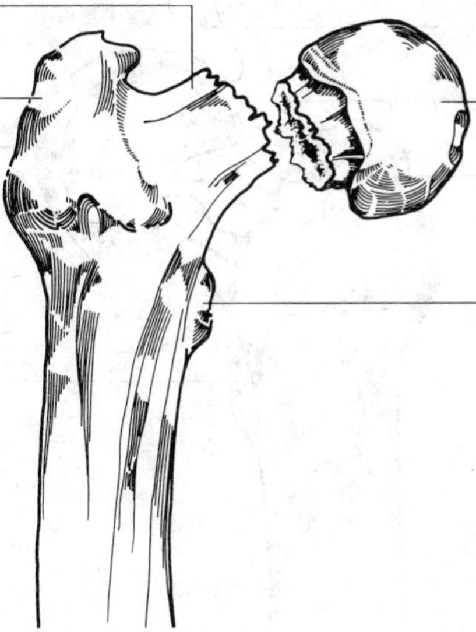

FIG. 8–1. Subcapital femoral neck fracture.

blood supply comes from vessels traversing three structures: the bone of the femoral neck, the surrounding hip capsule, and the ligamentum teres (see FIG. 8–2). A displaced fracture completely disrupts the blood vessels of the femoral neck and can tear those of the hip capsule. The vessels in the ligamentum teres do not function in ⅔ of adults. Thus, a displaced fracture often completely devascularizes the femoral head. Although a devascularized femoral head can heal if securely stabilized, poor healing is common. Nonunion occurs in 15% to 20% of patients, and osteonecrosis of the femoral head occurs in another 15% to 30%.

Treatment and Prognosis

Occult, impacted, and nondisplaced femoral neck fractures are usually treated by internal fixation with multiple pins (see FIG. 8–3). This stabilization permits immediate full weight-bearing ambulation and prevents later displacement. Since the blood supply to the femoral head is not significantly disrupted, these fractures usually heal well. Nonambulatory, demented patients who have limited pain perception can be treated with bed rest followed by transfer from bed to chair.

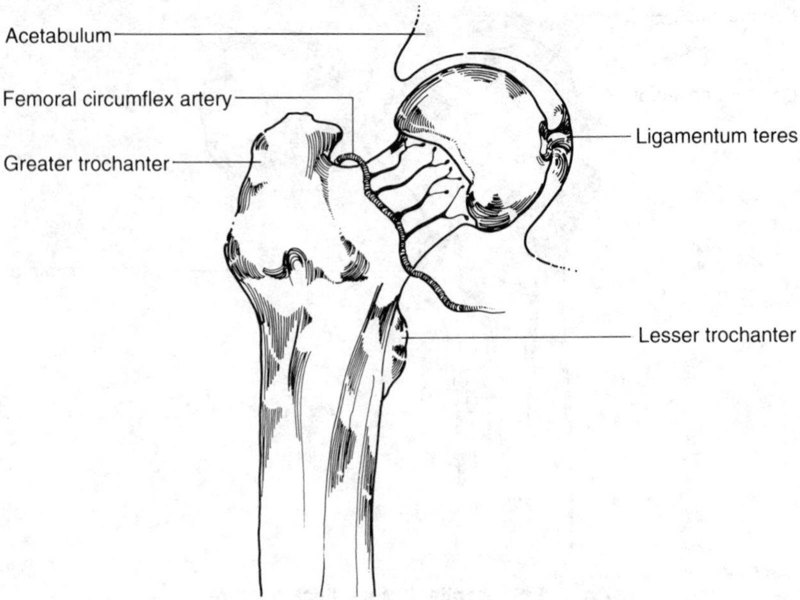

FIG. 8–2. Blood supply to femoral head.

Displaced fractures have two main treatment options—operative stabilization and prosthetic replacement. Each has advantages and disadvantages. Open reduction and internal fixation is usually reserved for vigorous patients $<$ 70 yr of age who are able to comply with a postoperative regimen of limited weight bearing using crutches. The procedure preserves the femoral head, and with successful healing, the hip is nearly normal. However, if osteonecrosis or nonunion occurs, the result is a painful, nonfunctional joint that requires total hip replacement. For this reason, less active elderly patients with displaced fractures often undergo primary prosthetic replacement of the femoral head (hemiarthroplasty). This permits immediate, full weight bearing and a faster return to independent functioning with a minimum chance of needing a second procedure.

The simplest prosthesis (the Moore prosthesis) consists of a smooth metal sphere attached to a stem that is wedged into the medullary canal

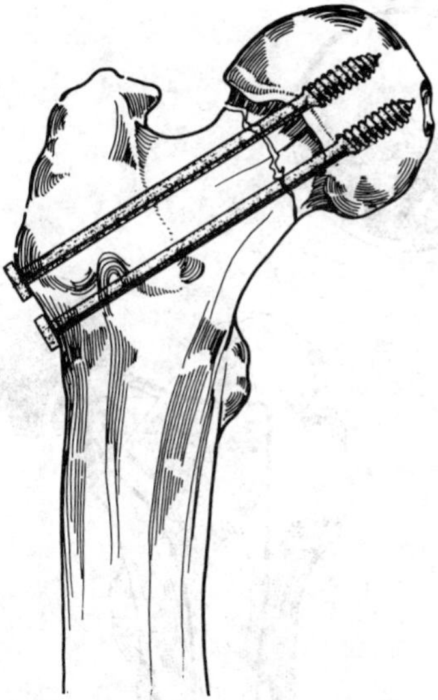

FIG. 8–3. Internal fixation of subcapital fracture with pins.

of the femur (see FIG. 8–4). Drawbacks include a tendency to wear away the acetabular articular surface and pain from a loose fit of the stem in the femoral medullary canal. A loose fit can be remedied by a prosthesis designed to be stabilized inside the femur with either acrylic cement or a special coating of hydroxyapatite or porous metal that facilitates direct bone fixation. A bipolar prosthesis with an internal metal-polyethylene bearing can reduce acetabular wear. Patients who develop acetabular arthritis may require total hip replacement. Primary total hip replacement in acute femoral neck fractures is reserved for patients with severe preexisting arthritis because this more extensive operation has a higher morbidity than either hemiarthroplasty or internal fixation with pins.

INTERTROCHANTERIC HIP FRACTURES

Symptoms, Signs, and Classification

These fractures usually result from a fall, often on level ground. Physical examination of a displaced fracture shows the leg to be shortened and externally rotated from the pull of the leg muscles and gravity.

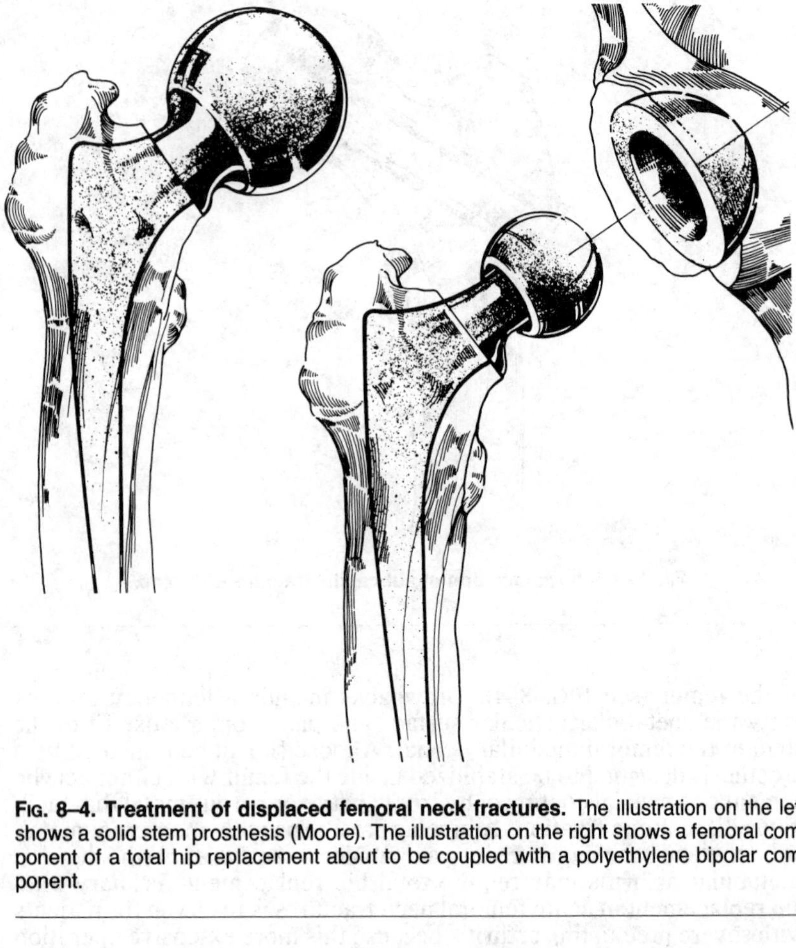

FIG. 8–4. Treatment of displaced femoral neck fractures. The illustration on the left shows a solid stem prosthesis (Moore). The illustration on the right shows a femoral component of a total hip replacement about to be coupled with a polyethylene bipolar component.

Hemorrhage from multiple bone fragments and associated soft tissue injuries can be extensive and may cause hypovolemic shock.

Intertrochanteric hip fractures are classified by the number of bony fragments and by the inherent stability (the ability to maintain continuity of the weight-bearing medial femoral cortex). Typically with two-part fractures, a single break slopes obliquely between the greater and lesser trochanters on the anteroposterior x-ray view (see FIG. 8–5). Three-part fractures also have a lesser trochanteric fragment, and four-

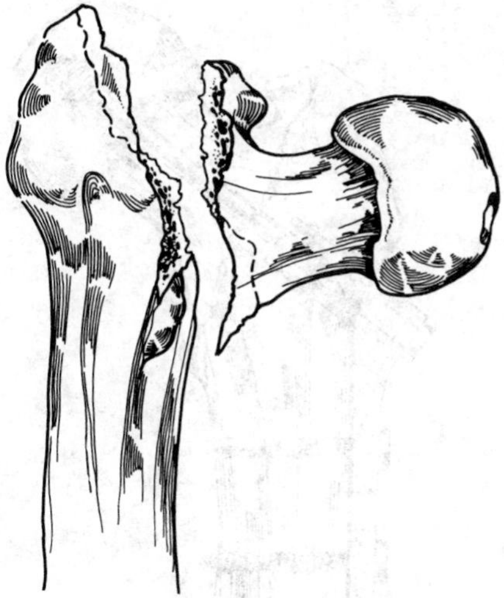

FIG. 8–5. Intertrochanteric fracture.

part fractures have a greater trochanteric fragment. As a rule, three- and four-part fractures are inherently unstable because of comminution of the medial femoral cortex. Fractures in the intertrochanteric region of the proximal femur usually allow adequate blood supply to all fragments; thus, osteonecrosis and nonunion rarely occur.

Treatment and Prognosis

Intertrochanteric hip fractures are treated by surgical stabilization unless an absolute medical contraindication exists or the patient is nonambulatory and demented, with limited pain perception. Traction does produce healing, but it usually takes 4 to 8 wk and introduces the risks of prolonged bed rest. Also, traction may not adequately control the deforming muscle forces around the hip, so that the bone may heal in a shortened and externally rotated position, producing a poor functional result.

The most common fixation device is the sliding compression hip screw, which provides rigid stabilization while impacting the fracture fragments, thus ensuring healing (see FIG. 8–6). Postoperatively, most patients can immediately begin full weight-bearing ambulation with a walker. Usually, they are able to use a cane in 6 to 12 wk.

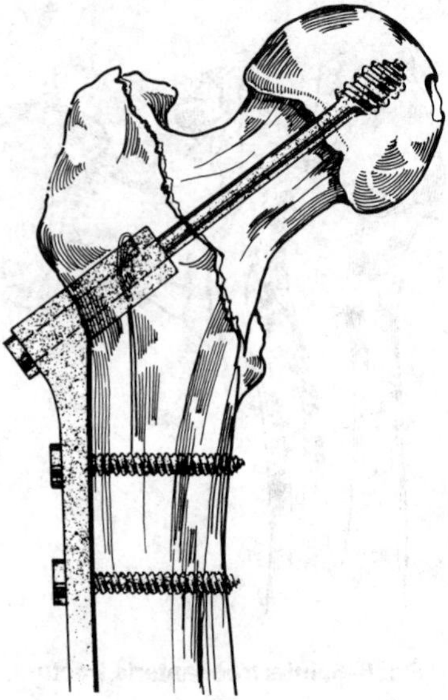

FIG. 8–6. Fixation of intertrochanteric fracture with compression screw and sideplate.

TIBIAL PLATEAU FRACTURES

Symptoms, Signs, and Classification

Fractures of the proximal tibia usually result from a lateral bending force (eg, as when a car strikes a pedestrian from the side). As the leg bends, the femoral condyle drives the tibial articular surface down into the underlying metaphyseal bone, which gives way easily in the elderly because of osteoporotic weakness. Patients present with knee pain and effusion, proximal tibial tenderness, and an inability to bear weight. Although standard anteroposterior and lateral x-rays typically show displaced fractures, oblique views may be needed to see occult fractures. Fat globules in blood aspirated from the knee joint are also diagnostic of an occult fracture.

Treatment and Prognosis

Because soft tissue swelling can cause neurovascular complications, patients are usually hospitalized so the leg can be elevated and observed. Following initial traction or continuous passive motion to help mold the fragments, patients are placed on a regimen of restricted weight bearing in a long leg brace or cast for 8 to 12 wk. Patients need physical therapy to learn to walk using ambulatory aids (eg, crutches or walkers). In the elderly, articular surface displacement of $\leq$ 1 cm is usually acceptable, but severe displacement requires operative reduction of the articular surface with a bone graft to fill the void left by the impacted trabecular bone. Unfortunately, weight bearing must be prohibited for 2 to 3 mo postoperatively, until healing occurs.

Elderly patients have a lower risk than young, active patients of developing osteoarthritis from joint surface disruption. When it does develop, total joint replacement is a good option.

THORACIC AND LUMBAR VERTEBRAL–BODY COMPRESSION FRACTURES

Symptoms and Signs

Injury usually results from an activity that increases the compressive load on the spine (eg, lifting, bending forward, or misstepping while walking). In the elderly, osteoporosis weakens the trabecular bone of the vertebral bodies and leaves the posterior elements relatively unaffected. Excessive loads then compress the vertebral bodies into a wedge-shaped configuration as the trabecular bone impacts into itself.

Patients often present with acute pain that is exacerbated by sitting or standing. Percussion over a specific spinal region reveals well-localized tenderness. Associated neurologic deficits are rare.

Many vertebral-body fractures occur silently, however. Elderly patients often have x-ray evidence of fractures without a history of symptoms or injury.

Treatment and Prognosis

Vertebral-body compression fractures always heal, because the trabecular bone is only impacted into itself, and the blood supply is not impaired. These fractures are relatively stable because the intact posterior elements prevent translational displacement. Neurologic deficits from bony impingement rarely occur. The primary clinical sign is progressive kyphosis due to wedging and loss of height of the vertebral bodies.

Initially, hospitalization for bed rest may be needed to relieve pain. Analgesics, nonsteroidal anti-inflammatory drugs, and laboratory screening tests for other causes of osteopenia may be indicated. Patients should be encouraged to sit up and walk for short periods as soon as possible to prevent deconditioning and accelerated bone loss. They may not be able to walk independently for a week or so and may have considerable back pain for 6 to 12 wk. Sometimes, a month or more later, the pain shifts from the fracture site to a higher or lower site, probably because of altered mechanical stresses caused by the deformity.

Bracing probably does little to prevent deformity, but it can help relieve pain and allows a quicker return to activities. Bracing is useful only for fractures of the lumbar and lower thoracic spine because adequate support cannot be achieved above these regions. While hyperextension braces (eg, the Jewett) are the most effective biomechanically, they are not the most comfortable. They apply three-point stabilization of the spine through an anterior abdominal pad, a chest pad, and a posterior pad at the level of the fracture. Corsets or abdominal binders are effective and better tolerated alternatives in patients with lumbar fractures.

---

9. ACUTE CONFUSIONAL STATE

(Delirium; Acute Brain Syndrome)

An alteration of mental status characterized by an inability to appreciate and respond normally to the environment, often with altered awareness, disorientation, inability to process visual and auditory stimuli, and other signs of cognitive dysfunction.

Terms such as confusion, delirium, and acute brain syndrome are often used without being clearly defined. Sometimes they are used synonymously, but often the user has very specific (and often subtle) distinctions in mind. In fact, all of these terms refer to aberrations in cognitive mental processes, the ways by which we perceive, think, and remember. The emphasis in this chapter is on *acute* dysfunction of these mental processes.

Confusion is not a disease or even a single syndrome; rather it is a sign of a whole spectrum of diseases and syndromes. Confusion is often the presenting or most prominent sign in cognitive failure syndromes, all of which are characterized by impaired cerebral function (see also Ch. 90). When acute, confusion is usually caused by medical illness or drugs and can be reversed in most cases.

Etiology

An acute confusional state presumably reflects a disturbance in cerebral metabolism, probably mediated through disturbed arousal systems or structural damage to brain cells. The brain of an aging (particularly very elderly) person, like the immature brain, tends to respond to such disturbances by demonstrating confusion at a lower threshold.

Almost any **physical derangement,** and even a **sudden environmental change,** may precipitate acute confusion (see TABLE 9–1). Some psychologic disturbances, most notably **depression,** can provoke a confusional state in the brain of a very elderly person. Bereavements, actual or symbolic, are among the life events that most commonly precipitate depression. Patients with depression may present with subacute confu-

TABLE 9–1. COMMON CAUSES OF ACUTE CONFUSION

Intracranial	*Extracranial*
Infections (eg, meningitis, encephalitis)	Anesthesia
Seizures, postictal states	Giant cell arteritis
Stroke	Hip fracture
Subdural hematomas	Hypercapnia
Tumors	Hypothermia
	Hypoxia
	Infections (eg, respiratory, urinary tract)
	Intoxication or withdrawal of alcohol or drugs*
	Metabolic disturbances (eg, liver or kidney failure, electrolyte disturbances, hyper- or hypoglycemia)
	Myocardial infarction
	Psychologic or environmental changes

*Drugs, particularly psychoactive agents, are a common cause.

sion (possibly through arousal disorders). Some cases of depressive **pseudodementia,** in which depression *mimics* dementia, would be better labeled **depressive confusion,** because the depression actually worsens the underlying (often unrecognized) dementia, precipitating an acute confusional state.

Drugs, *prescription or over the counter, are among the most common causes of confusional states.* Anticholinergic agents are involved particularly often; because many psychoactive (psychotropic) drugs are anticholinergic, these drugs should always be suspected as potential causes of the acute confusion. In addition, many patients have problems complying with standard drug regimens and cannot be assumed to be taking their drugs as prescribed. Self-medication with over-the-counter or shared drugs must not be overlooked.

Sometimes drugs used in treating the early stages of a confusional state actually exacerbate or perpetuate it. Antipsychotic and sedative-hypnotic drugs may be potent precipitants of confusion. Drug metabolism in the elderly is often altered, even without disease, leading to high blood levels in patients taking normal or low doses of drugs. Because polypharmacy is common, the elderly are at increased risk for drug interactions that potentiate confusion. Confusional states often are dramatically reversed or alleviated by changing or eliminating drug therapy. Eliminating nonessential drugs should be one of the first steps in determining the cause of and treating a confusional state.

Symptoms and Signs

The acute confusional state is characterized by **clouding of consciousness,** *a diminished level of awareness that fluctuates between the extremes of alertness and coma*. Alertness, awareness, and ability to pay attention are generally diminished; drowsiness is common. One or more of the following other key features are likely to occur (but rarely do they all occur): a relatively acute onset, clouded sensorium, disorientation, agitation, impaired memory, anxiety, and suspicion (see TABLE 9–2). Frank hallucinations and disrupted or delusional thinking may occur, and speech abnormalities are common. However, many acutely confused elderly persons are not hyperactive and may even become withdrawn and quietly paranoid. Symptoms such as dyspnea and chest pain may provide clues to the cause of the acute confusion. Impaired cardiopulmonary performance or neurologic findings may also provide clues.

Early in its course, acute confusion is characterized by **changes in attentiveness.** An acutely confused patient will not be able to pay attention to an interviewer, register names, or remember objects even long enough to repeat them. The patient may appear to be following conversations or visual cues that are not part of the interview, as if he were somewhere else. Changes in attentiveness may be subtle and measurable only on thorough testing, or they may be obvious, accompanied by clouded consciousness and obvious hallucinations.

Typically, the acute confusional state has a waxing and waning course. At one moment a patient may appear nearly normal, and just a few minutes later he may appear completely and obviously confused. Thus, conducting more than one evaluation is important before determining that mental status is normal. Confusion often becomes worse at dusk, a phenomenon known as **sundowning** (see Ch. 11).

Diagnosis

Diagnosing an acute confusional state may be difficult. Although acute confusion is usually identifiable in its florid form, physicians and nurses may be unaware that it exists if the patient is withdrawn and quiet.

Since virtually any medical or psychologic condition could cause acute confusion, a meticulous history taking and physical examination are essential. The causes of acute confusion are myriad, and confusional states are often accompanied by other major, nonspecific presentations of disease in the elderly (eg, incontinence or instability and falls). The patient may be smelly and unprepossessing, inspiring little therapeutic optimism. Such patients must be viewed with an open mind, *since the results of thorough appraisal may mean the difference between life and death*. The initial evaluation usually focuses on drug toxicity, cardiovascular changes, infection, and metabolic abnormalities.

TABLE 9–2. COMMON SYMPTOMS AND SIGNS OF THE ACUTE CONFUSIONAL STATE*

Acute onset
Clouding of consciousness
Reduced wakefulness
Disorientation of time and space
Increased motor activity: restlessness, plucking, and picking
Impaired attention and concentration
Impaired memory (especially new learning and recall)
Anxiety, suspicion, agitation
Variability of symptoms over time
Worsening of symptoms at night
Misinterpretation, illusions, hallucinations
Disrupted thinking
Delusions (usually transient and primitive)
Speech abnormalities
Diffuse EEG slowing

*Symptoms and signs may occur in any combination and may be intermittent.

Acute confusion may be difficult to separate from baseline cognitive impairment, especially in persons with chronic conditions such as **dementia.** *Differentiating between an acute confusional state and dementia is essential* (see also Ch. 90). Dementia is chronic, progressive, and generally irreversible. It is not a medical emergency, and evaluation can be performed slowly and when convenient. Confusion in an elderly patient should not be presumed to be dementia, unless the history documents a chronic, progressive disorder. Acute confusional reactions occur suddenly, are more common in demented patients, and are more often due to nonspecific or mild disorders, but serious disorders are also common.

The mental status examination follows standard lines (see Ch. 89); there is no specific test for clouding of consciousness. Observing the total clinical picture—in which some, but rarely all, of the features listed in TABLE 9–2 occur—is necessary.

If the patient is hospitalized, detailed observations should be sought from nurses, who are present around the clock. **Depressive confusion** may be manifested by occasional facial expressions or utterances in an otherwise expressionless or virtually mute patient; these behaviors are likely to occur when the physician is not there. For example, a withdrawn disoriented patient may make revealing, self-deprecating utterances such as "I don't deserve this food" or "I'm a trouble to everyone."

History: Because a confused patient rarely gives a useful history, another information source is essential. Potential sources may be difficult to find, especially after the patient has been admitted to the hospital. Whenever possible the initial examination and history should be taken when such sources are most likely to be available (ideally in the patient's home). Persons who may have accompanied the patient to the hospital (relatives, friends, police, or neighbors) should be interviewed before they leave; their names, addresses, and telephone numbers should be noted in case further information is needed.

The principles of history taking are routine, but certain factors must be considered. **Onset:** Was the onset sudden or insidious? Was it associated with any possibly related events (eg, trauma, illness, development of specific symptoms such as cough, urinary tract infection, changes in medication)? **Duration:** When did the changes first become apparent? Has the duration of confusion been very short? Brief duration strongly suggests a specific precipitating cause. **Course:** Has the patient's condition been constant or variable? Is there a diurnal pattern? Are relatively lucid periods associated with any specific factors? What makes the patient worse? **Recurrence:** Has the patient been confused before? If so, what caused the confusion? What treatment did it respond to? Has the patient been depressed before? **Lifestyle:** Does the patient use alcohol or prescribed or illicit drugs? A thorough drug review is essential. What is the patient's nutritional status? Has the patient been exposed to infection? Are the patient's living conditions, including heating, adequate?

Laboratory findings: The EEG is the only regularly abnormal test in acute confusion, but it is rarely necessary because it usually provides no more information than can be determined clinically. The value of other laboratory tests depends on the clinical findings. The tests most often ordered are CBC, blood chemistry profile, urinalysis, and chest x-ray. Specific tests may be required for certain conditions (see TABLE 9–1) or for diagnosing other suspected disorders (eg, thyroid function tests, vitamin B_{12} measurements, toxicology screening, or lumbar puncture). Brain imaging by CT, MRI, or single photon emission computed tomography may be indicated after discussion with the radiologist.

Treatment

Two tasks must be accomplished quickly: protecting the patient from harm and, if possible, treating the cause of the confusion. Nurses should be alerted so that they can assess the need for close observation or continuous sitters. Increased supervision is almost always needed, and both mental status and medical status should be frequently reevaluated. Restraints are almost always unacceptable; human, not mechanical, care is needed. The environment should be stable, with the same caregivers if possible, because frequent changes can exacerbate confusion. The room should be either well lighted or, at night, dark; ambiguous lighting can induce illusions and even hallucinations.

Confused patients need information repeated frequently; patience is important. Many elderly persons have impaired hearing, which makes communication more difficult, but shouting is inappropriate because a hearing impaired person responds to clear enunciation rather than to loud voices. Caregivers should speak slowly, be prepared to repeat their remarks several times, and use the patient's name, which can be an important point of reference in the midst of confusion.

Dehydration and electrolyte imbalance, which are ever-present threats to ill older persons, may occur rapidly. Fluid intake must be charted meticulously (especially if the patient is febrile), and urinary output must be estimated, even if the patient is incontinent. Blood chemistry reports must be obtained *promptly* from the laboratory. *In the short term, hydration is much more important than nutrition.*

Specific treatment depends on the cause of the confusional state (eg, infections require specific drug therapy). Often, the symptoms must be treated. Sedatives may break the vicious circle of confusion, anxiety, and more confusion, but these drugs can also worsen confusion. Occasionally, a patient is so restless that sedation is needed to allow hydration and feeding; however, this is always a difficult course, for heavy sedation may worsen mental status. Treatment should be limited to a small, familiar range of drugs. A regular regimen and close observation is the best approach; drugs should almost never be prescribed on an as-needed basis. Proper dose titration is the responsibility of physicians, not nurses.

All drugs have risks, but phenothiazines (eg, thioridazine 10 to 25 mg tid) or butyrophenones (eg, haloperidol 1 mg tid initially) are useful in most cases of acute confusion. These drugs are all antipsychotics and are indicated for treating acute confusion, hallucinations, delusions, and paranoia; generally they should not be used solely for their sedating effects. (For the caveats in using these drugs in patients with chronic confusion and behavior disorders, see Ch. 10.) Butyrophenones are less sedating but more likely than phenothiazines to cause dystonic reactions. Promazine 25 mg tid is an antipsychotic with mild sedating effects that rarely causes dystonia. All these drugs usually should be given orally; liquid forms are sometimes easier to administer. Occasionally, an IM injection (eg, haloperidol 2.5 mg) may be required. Benzodiazepines are purely sedative and do not alter confusion.

For sleep, chloral hydrate (eg, as syrup, 500 mg in 10 mL) may be given alone or combined with a phenothiazine in low doses. Occasionally, a short-acting oral benzodiazepine hypnotic (eg, oxazepam 10 to 15 mg, temazepam 7.5 to 15 mg, lorazepam 0.5 to 1 mg, or lormetazepam [not available in the USA] 0.5 to 1 mg) may be needed.

Effective treatment of a confusional state may leave other disabilities or care needs unresolved. Proper management includes attending to *all* of the patient's needs and making appropriate arrangements for continuing care.

When medical or drug-related causes are treated successfully, most patients will recover to their baseline mental status. However, not all patients recover fully, particularly when the confusion was caused by hypotension or hypoxia. Yet, even when the cause is something less obviously toxic to the central nervous system, recovery may not be complete. The extent of recovery cannot be predicted. However, a slow recovery is not necessarily cause for despair because many elderly patients require several weeks to return to their baseline status.

Failure of a confusional state to resolve after successful treatment of an underlying cause calls for a thorough review. Several causes may be involved, only one of which was treated, or a new cause may have developed.

---

10. BEHAVIOR DISORDERS

Intolerable actions, such as wandering, yelling, throwing, and hitting, which disrupt the environment and generally occur in persons with dementia.

Although behavior disorders can occur at any age, they are remarkably common in elderly persons with dementia. A large majority of elderly persons admitted to acute care hospitals have behavior disorders. In addition, behavior disorders account for up to 50% of nursing home admissions; as a result, behavior disorders are one of the most costly disorders affecting older adults. Despite the prevalence of behavior disorders and the cost of caring for persons with such disorders, little research has been done in this area. Neither the epidemiology nor the natural history of behavior disorders in dementia has been well characterized, and optimal treatment has not been determined.

Because tolerability defines whether or not an action is a behavior disorder, deciding what constitutes a behavior disorder is highly subjective. If an adult living alone wanders around his apartment or sleeps during the day and is awake all night, his behavior might be considered eccentric but not intolerable. However, in a family setting, such behavior could be considered intolerable because it disrupts normal activities. In a nursing home or hospital, the staff might consider such behavior intolerable because it could disturb other patients and interfere with the orderly operation of the institution. Within an institution, staff members may have different degrees of tolerance. For example, one attendant or nurse may readily tolerate frequent, repetitive questioning, but another may become frustrated and annoyed by the constant interruption. The time of day also affects tolerance. During the day, the number of staff members and the high level of activity make many behaviors (such as wandering, repeated questioning, and being uncooperative) relatively tolerable. However, during the evening and night, when the number of staff members is reduced and many activities

TABLE 10–1. TYPES OF BEHAVIOR DISORDERS

Psychologic	Perceived anxiety Mania Perceived depression
Physically dangerous	Hitting others Harming self Wandering (when patient is at risk of harm) Throwing objects
Disruptive	Yelling or screaming Asking repeated questions Wandering (without danger) Undressing Hypersexuality Being uncooperative regarding treatments and care Insomnia
Psychotic	Paranoia Delusions Hallucinations (auditory or visual)

cease, the staff may not tolerate these behaviors. Frustration may cause a caregiver (either at home or in an institution) to punish or abuse the elder. Therefore, with behavior disorders, the caregiver must often be the focus of intervention.

Classification

Behavior disorders are often collectively referred to as agitation; yet, the term agitation has so many different meanings that it is useless in the management of behavior disorders. Identifying a person's specific action or affect and classifying the behavior disorder as shown in TABLE 10–1 is more useful. In addition, factors associated with the identified behaviors, such as events that appear to stimulate behavior, duration of behavior, the time that behavior occurs, and response to treatment, should be described. With this information, planning a management strategy is considerably easier. FIG. 10–1 shows one system for charting the characteristics of behavior disorders.

Identifying psychotic behavior is particularly important because treatment varies, depending on whether or not a person has signs of psychosis. There is clear evidence that the management of psychotic persons differs substantially from that of persons without psychosis. An estimated 10% of demented persons with behavior disorders show signs of psychosis; the percentage may be somewhat higher in nursing homes.

FIG. 10–1. BEHAVIOR CHART

*Behavior**	*Date*	*Time Started*	*Time Resolved*	*Precipitating Event†*	*Type of Treatment‡*	*Time of Treatment*	*Response to Treatment*	*Additional Comments*
Screaming	5/7	9:00 PM	10:00 PM	Bedtime	Glass of milk; turned light on	9:30 PM	Quieted with visit	

* Examples are hitting, throwing, refusing treatment, yelling, interrupting staff, wandering, restlessness, insomnia, crying, or other specific behaviors.

† Examples are feeding, toileting, medication administration, or visits.

‡ Include both nonpharmacologic and pharmacologic treatment, including dose.

The three major psychotic features to look for are paranoia, delusions, and hallucinations. These must be differentiated from fearfulness, disorientation, and misunderstanding, all of which occur commonly in demented adults and none of which indicates psychosis. Paranoid patients may appear frankly terrified or quietly withdrawn; however, when questioned, they usually claim that others are trying to harm them, often in specific terms, such as by poisoning. Delusions may or may not involve paranoia and are particularly difficult to distinguish from disorientation in demented persons. Usually, delusional behavior is fixed; that is, it remains the same. Thus, a delusional patient repeatedly calls the nursing home a prison. In contrast, the disoriented person may first call the nursing home a prison, then a restaurant, and later a home. Hallucinations, which involve hearing or seeing something that has no external source, must be differentiated from misunderstanding (illusions), which involves misinterpreting external sensory stimuli, such as sounds from the public address system or beepers. Hallucinations may occur with either dementia or separately as part of paraphrenia.

Exacerbating Factors

At least four functional changes related to dementia result in behavior disorders. (1) Demented persons lose the capacity to conform their behavior to the sociologic norms of their environment. For example, yelling is acceptable at a baseball game but unacceptable in a restaurant; sexual encounter and nudity are acceptable in the privacy of a home but generally unacceptable in public places. (2) Demented persons misunderstand visual and auditory cues. They may lash out at a nurse who has come to help them because they think that the nurse meant to harm them. (3) Demented persons have impaired short-term memory, so they are unable to remember directions or avoid repetition. They may ask the same questions repeatedly, demand attention constantly, and ask for things (such as meals) that they have already received. (4) Demented persons are unable to express their needs clearly, and severely demented persons cannot make their needs known at all. Thus, demented persons may yell when in pain or when short of breath, wander when lonely or frightened, or urinate in public when their bladder feels full.

Institutional living is highly regimented and restrictive. Many elders without dementia find it difficult and frustrating to live in a place where mealtimes, bedtimes, and toileting times are scheduled and where social and sexual relations are restricted or forbidden. Therefore, demented people, who frequently lack the ability to control their frustrations and to conform to rules and routines, are often poorly served by institutional regimentation. In fact, in many cases, behavior deteriorates when demented elders are moved from a less restrictive to a more restrictive environment.

Behavior disorders generally follow a pattern in many demented persons, and changes in the pattern should be thoroughly evaluated. A physical examination can help determine if pain, shortness of breath, urinary retention, constipation, or some other medical condition has caused the change in behavior. Additionally, patients should be examined for signs of abuse, which sometimes results if the caregiver feels frustrated. Behavior disorders can be exacerbated by acute confusion (delirium) superimposed on chronic dementia; acute confusion may be the first indication of a new pathophysiologic process (see Ch. 90).

Sometimes a report of a variation in the frequency or intensity of the behavior disorder reflects a change in the caregiver (whether a nurse, attendant, or family member) rather than in the patient. The caregiver's tolerance threshold may change because of stress or frustration from providing care as well as from other factors.

Treatment

The management of behavior disorders in the elderly is one of the most controversial areas of geriatric medicine. A few controlled, small-scale studies have examined the effectiveness of treatments. No acceptable studies comparing different types of pharmacologic treatments exist. The drugs, mostly antipsychotics, used ubiquitously for nearly three decades are notoriously toxic, and their use has been based on anecdote and tradition without scientific evidence to support their effectiveness.

Nonpharmacologic: Manipulating the environment of the demented person is often the most successful, least expensive, and safest form of treatment. Yet, because of traditional medical training and reimbursement policies, physicians rarely exhaust nonpharmacologic treatments before they prescribe drugs.

Instructional materials are available to teach nursing home staff how to work with demented elders who have behavior disorders and how to structure institutional care to best meet their needs. Doors equipped with locks or alarms and stripes painted on floors can help ensure the safety of patients who wander; signs can help patients find their way; flexible sleeping hours can make insomnia tolerable; and reorganization of beds can make even noisy nursing home residents tolerable. In many instances, providing orientation and explanation before delivering care can forestall violent outbursts, and frequent brief visits by staff can prevent yelling. Involving patients in physical activity often helps induce sleep without medication and may reduce wandering and episodes of noisiness, hitting, and throwing.

For the most part, environmental changes are best implemented by nursing staff in collaboration with social workers and physical and occupational therapists. When an institution cannot provide an appropriate environment for a patient, a move to another institution may be necessary. For example, if a nursing home cannot provide doors with locks or alarms for a patient who wanders, transferring the patient to another home may be better than attempting to use medication to prevent ambulation.

Pharmacologic: Drugs should be used only when nonpharmacologic approaches have failed and when absolutely necessary to maintain the safety of the patient and those around him. When used, drugs should be selected to target the specific behaviors that are most intolerable. The need for continued therapy should be reassessed periodically, at least every month.

The two classes of drugs most commonly prescribed for treating behavior disorders are **sedative-hypnotics** and **antipsychotics**; drugs from both classes are among those most commonly used in nursing homes. Nearly 1/3 of nursing home residents receive sedative-hypnotics, and > 1/4 receive antipsychotics. Usually, sedative-hypnotics are used to treat insomnia and antipsychotics to treat most other behavior-related disorders. Antidepressants should not be used for their sedating properties; rather, they should be reserved for persons with signs of depression.

Despite the widespread use of antipsychotic drugs in treating behavior disorders, little evidence supports their effectiveness, except perhaps as potent sedatives. Worldwide literature on the subject includes only several hundred patients. Although a recent meta-analysis supports the use of antipsychotics for treating behavior disorders, no single well-designed study has ever shown statistically significant differences between antipsychotics and placebo in controlling nonpsychotic behaviors associated with dementia. On the other hand, studies examining the withdrawal of antipsychotics have shown that when these drugs are withdrawn, behavior does not deteriorate in most patients and, in fact, improves considerably in many. No good data exist comparing the effectiveness of benzodiazepines with that of antipsychotics in patients with behavior disorders.

The **toxicity of antipsychotic drugs** is well documented. At least 40% of elderly patients who use antipsychotics chronically develop extrapyramidal symptoms. Anticholinergic drugs, such as diphenhydramine or benztropine, may relieve these symptoms but tend to cause sedation and anticholinergic side effects, especially worsening confusion. Patients may also develop tardive dyskinesia or tardive dystonia from antipsychotics; these conditions often do not respond to dose reduction or drug withdrawal. Because of the toxic nature of antipsychotics, informed consent should be obtained from families before they are prescribed chronically.

Because of the paucity of data on effectiveness, recommending the use of these highly toxic agents in the routine treatment of nonpsychotic demented persons is difficult. Yet, the frustration of caring for persons with behavior disorders often prompts physicians to prescribe them. Less toxic sedating agents, such as short-acting benzodiazepines, seem preferable when drugs are needed, ie, if environmental manipulation fails to make behavior tolerable. In persons with psychotic behaviors, antipsychotics are usually the drug of choice.

No study has ever shown an advantage of one antipsychotic drug over another. The choice is usually based on relative toxicity. Haloperidol is relatively nonsedating and has less potent anticholinergic side effects, but it is most likely to cause extrapyramidal side effects. Thioridazine and thiothixene are less likely to cause extrapyramidal side effects but are more sedating and have more anticholinergic effects than haloperidol. All of these drugs should be used in very small doses (eg, haloperidol 0.5 to 1 mg one or two times a day or thioridazine 2.5 to 10 mg one to three times a day).

Some evidence suggests that **β-blockers** can be useful in treating persons with violent physical outbursts. In these cases, a lipophilic agent, such as propranolol, seems to be most effective. The dose should be started low, at 10 mg bid, and increased slowly, and the patient should be monitored for hypotension, bradycardia, and depression. Other drugs, such as carbamazepine, may be useful in controlling violent outbursts in persons who have not responded to less toxic treatments.

11. SLEEP DISORDERS

Complaints about sleep are common among the elderly. Older people have difficulty falling and staying asleep, and sleep is less refreshing for the elderly than for younger people. Hypnotics are widely sought and used. Yet, relatively little about aging and sleep is well understood.

SLEEP AND AGING

Patterns of Sleep

Sleep patterns change with aging, but authorities disagree as to which changes are a natural part of aging and which are pathologic. Normal differences among people complicate this distinction. Some data on elderly urban populations suggest an association between poor quality of sleep, physical disease, and decreased social activities; other data show that increased socialization and community involvement are associated with better sleep quality. Additional contributors to sleep disturbances include bereavement, posttraumatic stress, anxiety, depression, and forced retirement.

Self-reports of sleep disturbances can be confounding. Two people sleeping the same amount of time may assess their sleep differently. For example, one person who sleeps 6 h may feel refreshed and able to function; another person may have 6 h of fragmented sleep that impedes daytime performance and optimal functioning. Chronic medical or psychiatric conditions can also make sleep disorders difficult to evaluate. An even more difficult dilemma to evaluate is the overlap between pathologic aging (ie, dementia in its early stages) and the various manifestations of sleep disturbances as expressions of early depression, effects of psychoactive drugs, concurrent medical illnesses, or psychologic stressors.

Environmental factors greatly influence sleep. In nursing homes, patients are usually required to go to bed according to personnel shift changes. Because such scheduling is often not conducive to good sleep, sleep disorders are common in nursing homes. In hospitals, patients often are awakened for checks or medication throughout the night, and many find it difficult to resume sleep without sedation. Noise, lack of privacy, uncomfortable beds, and rooms that are either too warm or too cold further contribute to sleeping difficulties. Thus, separating sleep changes that result from disease or environment from those that are a normal concomitant of aging becomes difficult. **Institutionally induced insomnia** is often perpetuated after discharge through ongoing use of hypnotics. The drugs lose effectiveness after a short time, and patients become psychologically dependent on them.

Sleep efficiency (the ratio of time spent sleeping to total time spent in bed) decreases from 95% in adolescence to < 80% in old age. **Nocturnal sleep latency** (the time it takes to fall asleep once the lights are turned off) may not be prolonged in the elderly, as once believed. Another widely held belief—that the elderly require less sleep—is also a misconception. Although many studies show that elderly persons spend less time sleeping, other studies suggest that **sleep time** does not change or actually increases with age. Daytime napping and redistribution of sleep through the 24-h day may compensate for poor nocturnal sleep. However, elderly persons do have a tendency to fall asleep and awaken earlier and to be less tolerant of shifts of the sleep-wake cycle (eg, jet lag).

Stages of Sleep

Sleep progresses from stage 1 (the lightest level during which a person can easily be awakened) to stage 4 (the deepest level). The amount of time spent in stage 1 sleep increases with age, from 5% in younger adults to between 12% and 15% in the elderly, perhaps because older persons awaken more often during the night. The number of transient arousals (consisting of alpha intrusions into sleep that last between 2 and 15 sec) increases. Muscle tone, heart and breathing rates, and blood pressure are lowest in stage 4 sleep. Slow wave activity (stages 3 and 4 sleep) in the first non–REM cycle decreases, although recent data suggest a decline may be seen by age 20. In extreme old age, stages 3 and 4 may disappear completely. Older women may have better preserved slow wave sleep than men.

Rapid-eye-movement **(REM)** sleep is separate from these four stages and is characterized by unusual electrical activity in the brain. During a normal night's sleep, REM sleep follows five or six cycles of non-REM sleep. Both the rate and depth of breathing increase during REM sleep, but muscle tone is depressed even further than it is in stage 4 sleep. Most dreaming occurs during REM and stage 3 sleep, while most night terrors, sleepwalking, and sleeptalking occur during stages 3 and 4. Some studies report no appreciable change in REM sleep with aging; others show low REM percentages in the elderly. Overall, the proportion of REM sleep may be well preserved through senescence, although the absolute amount decreases as a result of reduced nocturnal sleep time.

INSOMNIA

Insomnia, *the inability to sleep,* is a symptom complex, not a diagnostic entity. An evaluation is necessary to exclude illnesses or problems that can impair sleep, such as orthopnea, pain, reflux, nocturia, sleep apnea, anxiety, and depression. Patients may complain of difficulty falling asleep and maintaining sleep, frequent nocturnal awakenings, early morning awakening with inability to resume sleep, daytime fatigue, irritability, or problems concentrating or performing under stress. Insomnia is often accompanied by unwanted daytime naps. Many persons spend 10 to 12 h in bed at night trying to sleep.

Insomnia may be transient, short-term, or chronic (see the decision tree in FIG. 11–1).

TRANSIENT INSOMNIA

Transient insomnia usually results from an acutely stressful situation (eg, hospitalization, surgery, bereavement, or retirement). Additionally, the elderly are less tolerant of phase shifts in the sleep-wake cycle, and a change in time zones can produce temporary insomnia, as in jet lag. This condition is benign and generally resolves in less than 1 wk.

Transient situational distress affecting sleep usually requires no **treatment,** but hypnotics used judiciously can help prevent the condition from becoming chronic, a common phenomenon in geriatrics. Hypnotics should be used for no more than 2 or 3 nights, followed by intermittent use and early discontinuation (see HYPNOTICS, below). The lowest effective dose of the safest drug—usually a short- or intermediate-acting benzodiazepine—(eg, temazepam 7.5 mg) should be used. Adverse effects of hypnotics (even in small doses) are discussed below. Stimulants such as caffeine should also be avoided within 12 h of bedtime.

CHRONIC INSOMNIA

Chronic insomnia lasts > 1 mo and results both from age-related changes in sleep and from chronic stressors such as forced retirement, nursing home placement, bereavement, concurrent illness, use of drugs with sleep-disrupting side effects, poor sleep hygiene, or primary sleep disorders. About 1/3 to 1/2 of patients who suffer from chronic insomnia are found to have psychiatric disorders. **Adjustment sleep disorder** usually occurs in fair to good sleepers who are under stress. Symptoms include anxiety, irritability, fatigue, impaired cognition, and hypersensitivity about perceived sleeplessness. The more severe the stress, the longer the adaptation period. Chronic insomnia is difficult to evaluate and treat in patients who have been using a hypnotic chronically, because the drug's side effects may be indistinguishable from the sleep disorder.

A focused **medical history** is essential to determine the effect on insomnia of chronic disease, such as pain from osteoarthritis, nocturnal dyspepsia, nocturnal exacerbations of chronic obstructive pulmonary disease, nocturia (from medications, urinary incontinence, or infection), thyroid disease, or nocturnal headache. Complaints of insomnia in the elderly often center around sleep maintenance or early morning awakening (common in depression). More difficult to uncover is an older person's poor sleep habits. Sleep can be adversely affected by an erratic sleep-wake schedule, unpleasant bedroom environment (extreme temperature, uncomfortable bed, excessive noise, inappropriate lighting, or a restless, snoring bed partner), poor timing of meals, lack of regular exercise, and inappropriate or excessive use of caffeine, alcohol, or medications.

Treatment

Informing a patient about the normal changes that occur with aging can change the patient's expectations about a good night's sleep (eg, sleep can be less refreshing at 80 than it was at 40, without indicating a serious problem). An occasional sleepless night does not signal poor health. A short, refreshing daytime nap may not necessarily disrupt nocturnal sleep, especially when included as part of a comprehensive treatment plan. Social isolation and daytime inactivity should be discouraged; interaction with friends and family and social activities should be encouraged.

Patients should be weaned from hypnotics, alcohol, and over-the-counter sleep preparations, with special attention given to withdrawal symptoms and rebound insomnia (see HYPNOTICS, below). Patients and their families or caregivers should be warned that sleep patterns initially may worsen. Successful treatment requires withdrawal before a solution can be found.

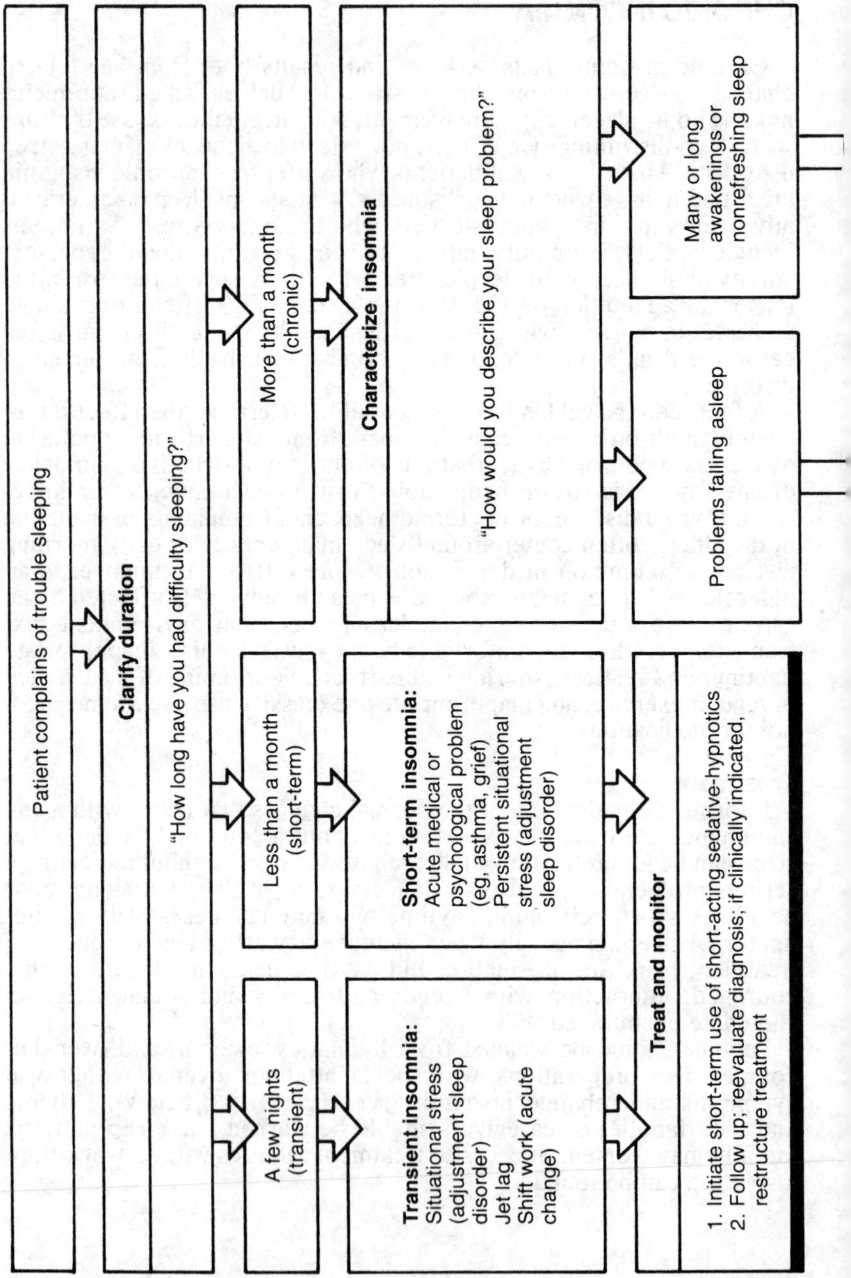
Patient complains of trouble sleeping
Clarify duration
"How long have you had difficulty sleeping?"
A few nights (transient)
Less than a month (short-term)
More than a month (chronic)
Transient insomnia:
Situational stress (adjustment sleep disorder)
Jet lag
Shift work (acute change)
Short-term insomnia:
Acute medical or psychological problem (eg, asthma, grief)
Persistent situational stress (adjustment sleep disorder)
Characterize insomnia
"How would you describe your sleep problem?"
Treat and monitor
1. Initiate short-term use of sedative-hypnotics
2. Follow up; reevaluate diagnosis; if clinically indicated, restructure treatment
Problems falling asleep
Many or long awakenings or nonrefreshing sleep

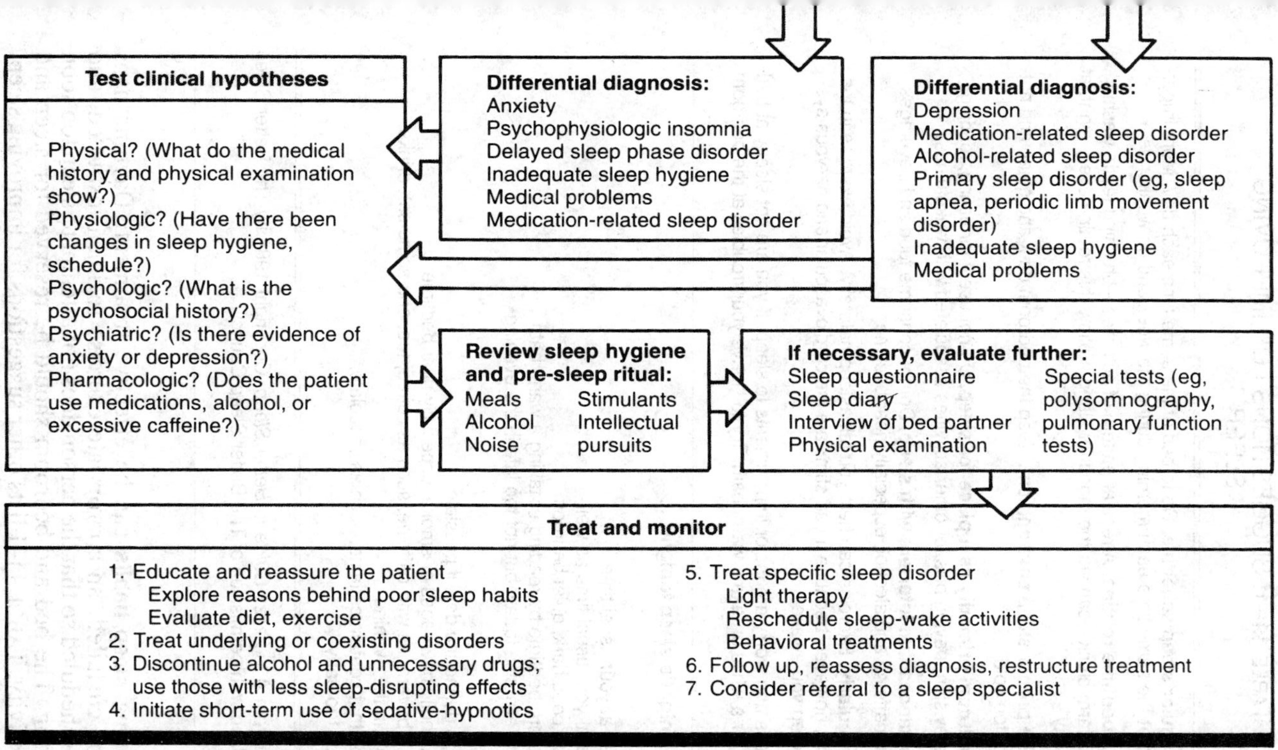
Test clinical hypotheses
Physical? (What do the medical history and physical examination show?)
Physiologic? (Have there been changes in sleep hygiene, schedule?)
Psychologic? (What is the psychosocial history?)
Psychiatric? (Is there evidence of anxiety or depression?)
Pharmacologic? (Does the patient use medications, alcohol, or excessive caffeine?)
Differential diagnosis:
Anxiety
Psychophysiologic insomnia
Delayed sleep phase disorder
Inadequate sleep hygiene
Medical problems
Medication-related sleep disorder
Differential diagnosis:
Depression
Medication-related sleep disorder
Alcohol-related sleep disorder
Primary sleep disorder (eg, sleep apnea, periodic limb movement disorder)
Inadequate sleep hygiene
Medical problems
Review sleep hygiene and pre-sleep ritual:
Meals
Alcohol
Noise
Stimulants
Intellectual pursuits
If necessary, evaluate further:
Sleep questionnaire
Sleep diary
Interview of bed partner
Physical examination
Special tests (eg, polysomnography, pulmonary function tests)
Treat and monitor
1. Educate and reassure the patient
Explore reasons behind poor sleep habits
Evaluate diet, exercise
2. Treat underlying or coexisting disorders
3. Discontinue alcohol and unnecessary drugs; use those with less sleep-disrupting effects
4. Initiate short-term use of sedative-hypnotics
5. Treat specific sleep disorder
Light therapy
Reschedule sleep-wake activities
Behavioral treatments
6. Follow up, reassess diagnosis, restructure treatment
7. Consider referral to a sleep specialist

Fig. 11–1. Decision tree for evaluating and treating sleep disorders. (Adapted from *The Management of Insomnia: Guidelines for Clinical Practice.* Chicago, Pragmaton, 1992. © 1992 The Upjohn Company.)

TABLE 11–1. SUGGESTIONS FOR IMPROVING SLEEP

Follow a regular sleep schedule. Go to bed at the same time each day. More important, get up at the same time each morning during the week and on weekends

Establish a bedtime routine. A regular pattern of activities—brushing teeth, washing, setting the alarm clock—can set the mood for sleep. Follow this routine every night, at home or away

Maintain the proper sleep environment. Keep the bedroom dark and quiet, and not too warm or too cold

Use the bedroom primarily as a place for sleep. Do not use it for eating, reading, watching television, paying bills, or other activities associated with wakefulness

Avoid substances that interfere with sleep. Do not consume food and beverages that contain caffeine and alcohol, especially near bedtime

Exercise regularly. Exercise can help you fall asleep naturally. Avoid exercise in the late evening, however, because it can stimulate the cardiovascular and nervous systems and keep you awake

Relax. Stress and worry are major impediments to sleep. If you are not sleepy at bedtime, read for a while or take a warm bath. Try to "leave your troubles at the bedroom door"

For a good night's sleep tonight . . .

Do

Go to bed at your usual time
Wake up at your usual time as well
Sleep in a cool, dark, quiet bedroom
Relax before bedtime by reading or taking a warm bath
Get some exercise today, but not too late in the evening

Don't

Take naps during the day, if possible
Drink alcoholic beverages or smoke, especially near bedtime
Consume beverages with caffeine, such as coffee, tea, and some soft drinks, especially in the evening
Eat foods that contain caffeine, such as chocolate
Go to bed too early

Adapted from *A to Zzzzz Guide to Better Sleep.* Copyright 1988 by The Better Sleep Council. Used with permission of The Better Sleep Council.

Improving **sleep habits** can be effective treatment. Daytime naps should be curtailed, an appropriate exercise regimen instituted, and meals rescheduled so that the person does not attempt to sleep too soon after eating. The bed and bedroom should be reserved for sleep and sexual activity. TABLE 11–1 lists other suggestions for improving sleep.

Referral to a sleep specialist is recommended if the sleep disturbance cannot be explained; if sleep apnea, restless leg syndrome, periodic leg movements, or a circadian rhythm disturbance is suspected; or if the insomnia resists treatment.

SPECIFIC SLEEP DISORDERS
(Dyssomnias)

Disorders producing difficulty in initiating or maintaining sleep.

INSOMNIA ASSOCIATED WITH DEPRESSION

Insomnia is often associated with psychiatric disturbances; the most common is depression. Early morning awakening with inability to return to sleep is typical of depression; patients with atypical depression may complain of hypersomnolence or problems initiating sleep. Successful therapy depends on treatment of the primary depression (see Ch. 95). When medication is indicated, a sedating antidepressant (eg, doxepin or trazodone) taken at bedtime is preferable to a more stimulating antidepressant.

Winter or seasonal depression is related to increased secretion of melatonin by the pineal gland. Melatonin production is stimulated by darkness and inhibited by light. Melatonin may be a timekeeper in setting the circadian cycle for sleep. In younger patients, seasonal depression is treated with bright light therapy to suppress the production of melatonin. Controversy has recently arisen over an oral preparation of melatonin being sold as an OTC soporific. The American Sleep Disorders Association discourages the use of melatonin to promote sleep. The drug has not been approved or classified by the Food and Drug Administration.

INSOMNIA ASSOCIATED WITH DRUGS

Many drugs can cause sleep problems. Discontinuing sedatives often leads to **rebound insomnia,** a condition that is generally transient but may lead to reinstituting sedatives, thus creating a vicious circle. Antipsychotics can produce akathisia, sometimes resulting in behavioral disturbances and wakening. In most cases, the behavior abates when the antipsychotics are discontinued.

Decongestants that contain stimulants such as ephedrine, β-agonists, and methylxanthines can prolong initiation of sleep, especially when they are taken at bedtime. β-Blockers such as propanolol can cause nocturnal wheezing and breathlessness in persons with asthma and chronic obstructive pulmonary disease. Antihypertensives such as reserpine can cause depression and insomnia, and other centrally acting agents such as the α_1-blockers can disrupt sleep. H_2-blockers may cause nocturnal delirium in the elderly. Caffeine can prolong latency and interfere with maintenance of sleep. Levodopa-carbidopa can cause nightmares. Diuretics given at night produce nocturia.

RESTLESS LEG SYNDROME AND PERIODIC LIMB MOVEMENT DISORDER

Restless leg syndrome and periodic limb movement disorder, common in the elderly, make initiating or maintaining sleep difficult, leading to excessive daytime sleepiness. Nocturnal leg myoclonus is discussed under MYOCLONUS in Ch. 93.

Restless leg syndrome, which occurs at bedtime, is described as a sensation like running in bed or a vague sensation that requires that the limb be moved for relief. Relief occurs with movement, and symptoms recur when the legs are stationary. Restless leg syndrome is different from nocturnal leg and hand cramps, in which the patient awakens from sleep with calf pain and muscle spasms. Bromocriptine and L-dopa are effective in relieving the long-term symptoms of restless leg syndrome; opioids should be restricted to patients with severe symptoms who do not respond to other drugs.

Periodic limb movement disorder occurs only during sleep and involves unilateral or bilateral flexion of the big toe, rapid ankle flexion, and partial flexion of the knee and hip. Movement lasts 2 to 4 sec and occurs continually, sometimes as often as every 20 to 40 sec, throughout the night. The age-related decrease in dopamine receptors may be the cause of periodic limb movement disorder; L-dopa administration decreases the number of leg movements. Incidence increases with age; about 45% of community-dwelling persons > 65 yr have some degree of periodic limb movement disorder, but most persons are unaware that these movements occur. Persons who have frequent periodic limb movements complain of insomnia or excessive daytime sleepiness, fatigue, or asthenia.

Periodic limb movement disorder is difficult to treat, and referral to a sleep specialist may be indicated. Several drugs are effective, but all pose risk of toxicity and should be used cautiously. Among them are clonazepam, L-dopa (carbidopa-levodopa), bromocriptine, and opioids. L-Dopa may be the safest if used in low doses, but the drug must be given both in the evening and during the day to prevent rebound periodic limb movement disorder. Propoxyphene is less effective than L-dopa in relieving periodic limb movement disorder.

SLEEP APNEA SYNDROME

Sleep apnea syndrome in the elderly is mostly of the obstructive type, consisting of complete cessation of breathing for > 10 sec during sleep resulting from obstruction of the upper airway. Diaphragmatic efforts persist in attempting to overcome the airway obstruction; nevertheless, periods of profound oxygen desaturation may occur with systemic and pulmonary hypertension or cardiac arrhythmias (eg, tachycardia, bradycardia, atrial arrhythmias, ventricular arrhythmias). Sleep apnea syndrome has been associated with sudden death at night and can lead to or exacerbate angina, renal dysfunction, stroke, myocardial infarction, cognitive impairment, impotence, or depression.

Sleep apnea syndrome is characterized by partial (hypopnea) or complete (apnea) cessation of respiration during sleep. In order to resume breathing, a person awakens (unknowingly) and spends excessive time in the lighter stages of sleep, restless and unrefreshed. Cacophonous snoring and grunting accompany the respiratory collapse. The site of obstruction is in the oropharyngeal wall. Pharyngeal collapse begins at the junction of the lower part of the soft palate, the posterosuperior part of the tongue's base, and the posterior pharyngeal wall and spreads retrocaudally.

The number of apneic or hypopneic episodes per hour **(apnea/hypopnea index)** can help predict mortality. A causal relationship has not been found between mortality and morbidity with an apnea/hypopnea index of < 10/h. Mild sleep apnea (an apnea/hypopnea index of ≤ 5/h) is quite common in the elderly, occurring in 24% of persons who live independently, 33% of those in acute care settings, and 42% of those in nursing homes. However, hypertension occurs in about 50% of these patients. An apnea/hypopnea index of ≥ 15/h suggests a more serious sleep-related respiratory disturbance that requires intervention.

Patients suspected of having obstructive sleep apnea should be referred to a sleep disorders center for evaluation. Criteria for referral include unexplainable excessive daytime sleepiness, witnessed episodes of apnea, and lack of response to treatment such as avoiding alcohol and sedatives. **Diagnosis** is made by overnight polysomnography with measurement of sleep, respiratory, muscular, and cardiac parameters. **Treatment** options are listed in TABLE 11–2. They begin with common sense measures (eg, weight loss or termination of hypnotic, drug, or alcohol use). Continuous positive airway pressure resolves the apnea but must be continued indefinitely. The only measure that achieves total success is tracheostomy, a procedure reserved for the most severe cases. Procedures such as uvulopalatopharyngoplasty, in which excess pharyngeal tissue is removed, help less than 50% of those who undergo the procedure and are not effective long term. Laser surgery to reduce or obliterate pharyngeal tissue has been shown to alleviate snoring but may not reduce the number of apnea episodes. Little information is available to help decide who would benefit from this new procedure.

CIRCADIAN RHYTHM SLEEP DISORDERS

Circadian rhythm disorders result from alterations in the day-night sleep cycle. In younger adults, they are generally caused by jet lag and shift work; in the elderly, they are more likely to be caused by hospital-

TABLE 11–2. TREATMENTS FOR SLEEP–RELATED RESPIRATORY DISTURBANCES

Avoidance of supine position	Tongue-retaining device
Weight loss	Tracheostomy
Continuous positive airway pressure	Uvulopalatopharyngoplasty
Mandibular advancement	Intrapalatine resection
Nasal surgery or adenotonsillectomy	Hyoid bone suspension
Patient-managed nasopharyngeal intubation	Tongue surgery
	Laryngeal surgery

From Crampette L, Carlander B, Mondain M, et al: "Surgical alternatives to uvulopalatopharyngoplasty in sleep apnea syndrome." *Sleep* 15(6 Suppl):S63–S68, 1992; used with permission.

ization in an intensive care unit. People in their 60s and 70s who travel by air are more affected by jet lag than younger persons and take longer to recover. Even without an obvious cause, circadian rhythm disorders are common in the elderly.

The increased incidence of sleep-wake schedule disturbances in persons > 50 yr old suggests loss of circadian control of the sleeping process. People tend to fall asleep and wake up progressively earlier as they age. Older persons who have no complaints of disturbed sleep are better able to adapt to internal changes in the sleep-wake cycle.

Therapy with the short-term use of hypnotics attempts to restore the integrity of circadian rhythm by resetting the biologic clock to consolidate sleep into one nocturnal episode. Sedatives should be used as an adjunct to other treatments and only for limited time periods (7 to 10 days at most) before being tapered.

ADVANCED SLEEP PHASE SYNDROME

In advanced sleep phase syndrome, the onset and awakening times of habitual sleep occur earlier than desired, leading to an inability to adhere to a standard sleep schedule. Although this syndrome does not meet the strict criteria of a disabling sleep disorder, sufferers complain of fatigue during the day and tend to use excessive amounts of hypnotics or alcohol. In the elderly, this syndrome may be more sociologic than physiologic.

Treatment includes all aspects of sleep hygiene (see TABLE 11–1), especially gradually reducing the total time spent in bed and avoiding chronic use of hypnotics. Contributory factors (eg, depression, concomitant medical illness, drugs that alter sleep physiology) should be ruled out or dealt with.

SLEEP DISORDERS ASSOCIATED WITH DEMENTIA

The suprachiasmatic nucleus and other neuroanatomic areas involved in the control of sleep (eg, the locus ceruleus and the nucleus basalis of Meynert) are affected by Alzheimer's disease. Patients with Alzheimer's disease have low sleep efficiency, spend a high percentage of sleep time in stage 1 and less time in stages 3 and 4 sleep, and experience more arousals and awakenings, all of which parallel the severity of dementia. The percentage of REM sleep (as compared with total sleep time) decreases, the reduction becoming more pronounced as dementia progresses. Many persons with Alzheimer's disease or multi-infarct dementia also have sleep-related respiratory disturbances.

Sundowning, a poorly understood phenomenon associated with dementia, has been defined as the nocturnal exacerbation of disruptive behaviors in which agitation is a prominent feature. Between 12% and 14% of demented nursing home patients demonstrate agitated behavior (eg, pacing and verbal aggression) more often at night than during the day. Demented patients are unlikely to sleep between 3 and 7 PM, the time such agitation usually occurs during winter months in northern regions when the sun sets earlier.

Treatment

Reversible causes of sleep disorders associated with dementia, such as drug-related toxicity, infections, dehydration, drug-drug interactions, pressure necrosis, malnutrition, and anemia, should be sought. Commonly used **pharmacologic treatment** includes benzodiazepines and antipsychotics. No drug has been shown to be particularly effective, and antipsychotics have many adverse effects. **Nonpharmacologic treatment** includes scheduling activities at a time when the patient seems to be affected by sundowning. Napping during the day may help consolidate the sleep schedule, but a long nap may interfere with nighttime sleep. Other approaches include manipulating the environment (eg, providing adequate light and temperature), evaluating and treating pain, correcting hearing and visual deficits, and treating metabolic illnesses (see also DEMENTIA in Ch. 90).

SLEEP DISORDERS ASSOCIATED WITH MEDICAL CONDITIONS

Medical illnesses and their drug treatments can adversely affect sleep. Drugs can blunt nocturnal breathing, exacerbate or cause apnea, produce unwanted arousals, and otherwise alter sleep physiology. In addition, some disease symptoms are worse during sleep.

Musculoskeletal disorders: Patients with osteoarthritis may awaken with stiffness and pain, then have difficulty falling asleep again. Fibromyositis, polymyalgia rheumatica, recent fractures, and flexion contractures all can cause pain and impair sleep. Treatment consists of effecting behavioral change with the judicious use of analgesics, exercise, and other forms of physical activity.

Cardiovascular disorders: Many drugs for **hypertension** can adversely affect sleep. Diuretics can awaken a person to urinate, who then may have difficulty resuming sleep. β-Blockers, clonidine, reserpine, and α-methyldopa act on the CNS, altering sleep physiology. Patients who have insomnia related to antihypertensive use may need to have their drug regimens altered. **Heart failure** can lead to orthopnea; demented patients with orthopnea may be unable to explain their complaint, becoming agitated instead. **Angina pectoris** can prolong sleep latency, reducing the deep sleep of stages 3 and 4. This disruption of sleep integrity can lead to chronic insomnia and dependency on hypnotics.

Pulmonary disorders: Chronic obstructive pulmonary disease can cause frequent awakenings, increase the amount of time spent in lighter (stage 1) sleep, markedly reduce stages 3 and 4 and REM sleep, and decrease total sleep time. Sympathomimetic bronchodilators (the mainstay of treatment for reversible bronchospasm) are CNS stimulants that can exacerbate insomnia.

Gastrointestinal disorders: Acid secretion increases during the night, which can awaken patients with ulcer disease or cause difficulty initiating sleep. Recent studies support nocturnal use of H_2-receptor blockers, although some (eg, cimetidine) can penetrate the CNS and cause side effects. Esophageal reflux, which can cause discomfort, may be prevented by elevating the head of the bed.

Renal disease: Patients undergoing renal dialysis experience chronic sleep disturbances. In uremic patients, long awakenings from all stages of sleep are common, deep sleep time is proportionally shorter, and total sleep time is decreased. Elevated BUN levels correlate with the severity of the disturbance; dialysis alleviates the disturbance, increasing stages 3 and 4 sleep.

Metabolic disorders: Sleepiness during the day and decreased functional capacity are prominent symptoms of **hypothyroidism.** Stages 3 and 4 sleep are reduced significantly but return to normal with thyroid replacement. **Hyperthyroidism** increases stages 3 and 4 sleep to almost 70% of total sleep time (25% is normal), but hyperthyroid patients often complain of insomnia. When a euthyroid state returns, sleep stages become normal.

Neurologic disorders: Parkinson's disease compromises both initiation and maintenance of sleep. The effects of levodopa on REM and deep sleep vary, depending on dosage, and the drug can cause nightmares. Amantadine improves quantitative sleep.

HYPNOTICS
(Soporifics)

Hypnotics provide only symptomatic relief and rarely treat specific disturbances. Many classes of drugs can promote sleep, such as benzodiazepines, antidepressants, antihistamines, barbiturates, analgesics (including narcotics), phenothiazines, antihypertensives, alcohol, and over-the-counter medications.

The use of sedative-hypnotics increases with age; 10% of elderly men and 50% of women use such drugs. Despite concerns about side effects, most elderly patients are very satisfied with the effects of hypnotics and plan to continue taking them.

Complications and Contraindications

Objections to a drug-oriented approach to sleep disturbances include the following: (1) The changes in sleep physiology associated with aging are not improved by hypnotics, nor are the discrete entities that disturb sleep eliminated. (2) Use of CNS depressants may adversely affect the already compromised physiologic function causing the sleep disturbance (eg, sleep apnea). (3) The elderly are at increased risk for potentially harmful drug interactions (eg, with tranquilizers, alcohol, β-blockers, β-agonists, antihistamines, analgesics). (4) Because the elderly may metabolize and excrete drugs less effectively, they often experience prolonged pharmacologic effects (eg, daytime sedation and cognitive deficits). (5) The data on long-term effects suggest that other therapies (see TABLE 11–3) may be more effective than long-term use of sedative-hypnotics. (6) Use of hypnotics is associated with increased risk of death.

Other complications associated with hypnotics include addiction, dependence, and tolerance. **Contraindications** to hypnotics include sleep apnea syndrome, severe depression, and untreated drug or alcohol abuse.

Rebound insomnia is a transient increase in insomnia that occurs when hypnotics are abruptly withdrawn. Withdrawal should be done through gradual weaning rather than abrupt discontinuation. Reassurance that the effects of withdrawal are temporary is essential for success. Continuation or escalation of dosage is not recommended.

Choice of Drug

Benzodiazepines are preferred for the treatment of insomnia because side effects are predictable and dose related, half-life effects can be controlled by drug selection, and fatal overdoses are rare. The risk of abuse is low except in those with a history of drug or alcohol abuse.

In the USA, five benzodiazepines (estazolam, flurazepam, quazepam, temazepam, and triazolam) are approved for treating insomnia. The main differences among them are related to half-life. Short- or intermediate-acting drugs are less likely to cause daytime sedation and

TABLE 11–3. BEHAVIORAL TREATMENTS FOR INSOMNIA

Progressive muscle relaxation	Tense and relax specific muscle groups (eg, forearms, biceps, neck) systematically; focus on feelings of relaxation; do this before bedtime
Muscle tension release only	Administer progressive resistance; follow instructions on how not to focus on tension and relaxation in muscles
Desensitization	Learn to avoid sleep-disturbing and anxiety-arousing images
Autogenic training	Systematically focus on specific muscle groups (eg, arms, legs) to induce feelings of warmth or heaviness in those muscles
Metronome-conditioned relaxation	Listen to metronome each night upon retiring; follow verbal relaxation instructions paired with sounds of metronome
Metronome-induced relaxation	Follow verbal relaxation instructions paired with sounds of metronome
Meditation	Focus on single mental stimulus (eg, word, phrase, image, or sound) sub-vocalized repeatedly, usually before bedtime
Hypnotic relaxation	Listen to person giving a suggestion to relax
Stimulus control	Associate bed and bedroom only with sleep; in bedroom, eliminate or reduce activities incompatible with sleep while in bed and at bedtime; leave bed and bedroom if not sleeping or engaged in sexual activity
Biofeedback	Undergo electromyelography to relax specific muscles (usually frontalis) or electroencephalography to increase central or occipital alpha or theta activity
Sensorimotor rhythm biofeedback	Increase sensorimotor rhythm to improve sleep spindles and delta waves at night

Adapted from Killen J, Coates T: "The complaint of insomnia: What is it and how do we treat it?" in *New Developments in Behavior Therapy: From Research to Clinical Application*, edited by CM Franks. Binghamton, NY, Haworth Press, 1984, pp 337–408; used with permission.

accumulate in serum than are longer-acting drugs. Also, short-acting benzodiazepines without active metabolites have less risk of drug-drug interactions. Reasonable choices are temazepam 7.5 to 15 mg or estazolam 0.5 to 1 mg.

Patients > 65 yr old who use longer-acting benzodiazepines are twice as likely to fracture a hip as those using short- or intermediate-acting benzodiazepines. Long-term use of flurazepam or quazepam in persons > 75 yr old can produce a syndrome mimicking Alzheimer's disease.

Barbiturates, chloral hydrate, antihistamines, and over-the-counter preparations are generally not recommended because of their side effects such as prolonged daytime sedation, risk of drug-drug interactions, and risk of physical dependence and addiction. In particular, antihistamines produce anticholinergic side effects such as confusion, memory loss, dry mouth, blurred vision, constipation, and urinary retention. Barbiturates, methyprylon, ethchlorvynol, and chloral hydrate can cause delirium. Barbiturates have prolonged duration of action, induce hepatic enzymes, and are highly addictive. Chloral hydrate may be used for occasional insomnia, but it can cause gastrointestinal upset.

12. PAIN

Traditionally, little attention has been given to the influence of aging on the incidence, clinical manifestations, and treatment of pain. However, information is now available to provide a framework for rational nosology and therapeutic strategy.

EPIDEMIOLOGY

Although one study reports a threefold *increase* in persistent pain between 18 and 80 yr of age, another larger study reveals an age-related *reduction* in pain at all anatomic sites other than joints. Other studies have shown that analgesic use declines with age, the elderly constitute a relatively small proportion of pain-clinic admissions, and fewer pain complaints are recorded in older than in younger patients with myocardial infarction.

A shift occurs in the relative frequency of disorders commonly associated with pain. Osteoarthritis is by far the most common painful disorder in the elderly. Some types of neuropathic pain, notably trigeminal and postherpetic neuralgia, occur often; and some common, chronic nonmalignant pain syndromes (eg, atypical facial, failed low back, and myofascial pain) appear to occur infrequently.

The age-related reduction in pain prevalence is unexplained but may be associated with alterations in neural pathways involved in **nociception** (ie, *the sensory processing initiated by a noxious stimulus*) or with differences in the psychologic disposition to report pain. The latter may reflect either reticence in responding to any stimuli or stoicism toward pain. If neural changes are the cause, the lower prevalence of pain may accurately represent the experience of these patients. If less frequent pain reporting occurs, however, pain may be underrecognized and inadequately assessed and treated. The latter conclusion is supported by studies suggesting that the neural apparatus involved in nociception does *not* decline with age. Comprehensive pain assessment is necessary to ensure that pain is not undertreated and underlying conditions are not missed.

Chronic pain has a major impact on quality of life, and associated affective and behavioral disturbances may become particularly problematic. Depression often complicates pain in these patients, who may deny overt mood disturbance but manifest profound vegetative signs (eg, sleep abnormalities and lassitude). The terms **abnormal illness behavior** and **chronic pain syndrome** are used to characterize the behavioral changes commonly accompanying chronic pain (including social isolation, loss of interest in avocations, and inability to perform activities of daily living). Such consequences of chronic pain are especially important in older persons, who can rapidly become hopeless and disabled.

ASSESSMENT

The **history** is central. However, stoicism or slowness to respond, at times compounded by mild cognitive deficits, compromises its reliability. The clinician must be alert to this, spend adequate time with the patient, and obtain additional information from others.

The assessment of pain includes its location, severity, quality, duration and course, palliative and provocative factors, and associated somatic and psychosocial symptoms. A medical and drug history should attempt to evaluate compliance. A family history of chronic pain may provide insight into the patient's complaints. The patient's level of cognitive, psychologic, and social functioning must also be assessed.

Nociception should be distinguished from **pain,** a perception only loosely related to nociception. The nociceptive focus (eg, an arthritic joint) must be identified so primary therapy can be instituted. However, pain can exist without a nociceptive focus, and conversely, profound tissue damage can be present without the *perception* of pain. An attempt should be made to identify all the salient factors, both nociceptive and nonnociceptive, that contribute to the pain. Nonnociceptive factors can be pathophysiologic (eg, neuropathic mechanisms that persist without ongoing tissue damage) or psychopathologic.

The concept of **suffering** must also be distinguished from both pain and nociception. Suffering is *the aversive emotional state derived from the aggregate of negative perceptions, only one of which is pain.* Treatment directed only at pain or its nociceptive components will be ineffective in a patient whose complaints express more pervasive suffering (eg, loss of friends, withdrawal of family, financial concerns, or physical impairments).

Physical examination should attempt to identify underlying nociceptive and neuropathic factors; it includes observation and palpation of the painful region and functional testing, if indicated. The need for laboratory and special studies is clarified by findings in the history and physical examination.

CLASSIFICATION

Acute pain usually has a readily identifiable cause (eg, hip fracture) and signals tissue damage, enforcing immobility that may be essential for healing. The associated affect is often anxiety, and the concomitant physiologic findings are those of sympathetic stimulation (eg, tachycardia, tachypnea, diaphoresis). An important subgroup of acute pain syndromes is characterized by **recurrence;** eg, recurrent acute pain from arthritis, intermittent claudication, or decubitus ulcers.

Chronic pain can be defined as (1) pain that persists ≥ 1 mo beyond the usual course of an acute illness or injury, (2) pain that recurs at intervals over months or years, or (3) pain that is associated with a chronic pathologic process. In contrast to acute pain, chronic pain loses its adaptive biologic function. Depression is common, and abnormal illness behavior often compounds the patient's impairment.

Chronic pain can be divided broadly into that which is inferred to be **predominantly somatogenic** and that which is inferred to be **predominantly psychogenic.** A similar classification based on inferred pathophysiology designates chronic pain as **nociceptive** (commensurate with ongoing activation of pain-sensitive nerve fibers), **neuropathic** (due to aberrant somatosensory processing in afferent neural pathways), or **psychogenic** (see TABLE 12–1). Although these distinctions may blur in an individual patient, this classification provides a practical framework that aids diagnosis and management.

Nociceptive pain can be somatic or visceral. Most chronic pain in the elderly is nociceptive and somatic; arthritis, cancer pain, and myofascial pain are most common. Relief is likely with removal of the peripheral cause (eg, reducing periarticular inflammation), and analgesic drugs are often effective. Therapeutic interruption of afferent nerve pathways may ameliorate the pain but is usually impractical and risky.

A common subtype of neuropathic pain, known collectively as **peripheral neuropathic pain,** is presumably sustained by mechanisms that involve disturbances in the peripheral nerve or nerve root; neuroma formation after axonal injury and nerve compression are the two major

TABLE 12–1. PROPOSED PATHOPHYSIOLOGIC CLASSIFICATION OF PAIN

Type	*Subtype*	*Example*	*Comment*
Nociceptive	Somatic	Bone metastases	Due to chronic activation of nociceptive afferent neurons
	Visceral	Bowel obstruction	
Neuropathic			
Deafferentation	Peripheral	Phantom limb	Due to central reorganization of sensory processing after injury to an afferent pathway
	Central	Thalamic pain	
Sympathetically maintained		Causalgia Reflex sympathetic dystrophy	
Peripheral neuropathic	Compressive	Carpal tunnel pain	
	Neuromatous	Stump pain	
	Neuralgic	Trigeminal neuralgia	
Psychogenic	Somatoform Chronic nonmalignant pain syndrome	Psychogenic pain Failed low back pain Atypical facial pain	Does not include factitious disorders (eg, malingering)

processes. Another subtype of neuropathic pain is related to the reorganization of nociceptive information processing by the CNS; it persists without ongoing activation of pain-sensitive fibers. This type of pain, known collectively as the **deafferentation syndromes,** includes postherpetic neuralgia, central pain (which can result from a lesion at any level of the CNS), phantom limb pain, and others. A third subtype of neuropathic pain, often called **sympathetically maintained pain,** can be ameliorated by interruption of sympathetic nerves to the painful area; the prototypic disorder is reflex sympathetic dystrophy. The precise mechanisms involved in these disorders are conjectural, but all can produce an unfamiliar pain, often described as burning and stabbing. They may respond poorly to analgesics.

Some patients have persistent pain without either nociceptive foci or evidence of a neuropathic mechanism for the pain. Many others have nociceptive lesions that do not sufficiently explain the degree of pain and disability. Psychopathologic processes account for these complaints in some patients. If no evidence for a psychologic cause is found, the pain should be called **idiopathic.**

Many patients have an idiopathic pain syndrome that is best described by the generic diagnosis **chronic nonmalignant pain syndrome,** a term denoting pain and disability disproportionate to an identifiable somatic cause and usually related to a more pervasive set of abnormal illness behaviors. Some of these patients may be labeled by the more formal psychiatric diagnosis of **somatoform pain disorder.** Others have complaints that constitute a specific pain diagnosis, most commonly the failed low back syndrome or atypical facial pain. Still others have significant organic lesions (eg, lumbar arachnoiditis) but also have a clear psychologic contribution associated with excessive disability. Diagnosis may be difficult, but the relative contributions of both organic and psychologic components of the pain must be defined.

The chronic nonmalignant pain syndrome appears to be relatively rare in the elderly, whose persistent pain is usually associated with an organic lesion, either nociceptive (eg, osteoarthritis) or neuropathic (eg, postherpetic neuralgia). Nonetheless, profound psychosocial impairment is common and can have a devastating impact on function, regardless of whether it causes or is a reaction to the pain.

Another clinically useful classification of chronic pain is broadly syndromic. For example, chronic pain may be part of a medical illness (eg, cancer or arthritis). A mixture of pathophysiologic mechanisms may be involved; eg, tumor invasion of nerve and bone may cause neuropathic and somatic nociceptive pains, respectively, and psychologic factors may be prominent. The relationship between the pain and the underlying disease must be clarified to permit optimal management. Alternatively, specific organic syndromes exist that are characterized only by pain (eg, postherpetic neuralgia). Each diagnosis suggests specific therapeutic options.

PRINCIPLES OF TREATMENT

The general principles of pain treatment—pharmacologic and nonpharmacologic—are outlined briefly below.

1. Treat the underlying problem, if possible. Particularly in cancer pain, recognition of the pain syndrome can lead to diagnosis of the cause and, possibly, to effective primary therapy. Although elimination of the underlying cause in nonmalignant pain syndromes is seldom feasible, primary treatment is often available for nociceptive pain (eg, prosthetic joint replacement for intractable hip or knee pain from osteoarthritis).

2. Address psychologic factors and functional impairment concurrently. This requires an accurate diagnosis.

3. Consider a multimodal approach. While some patients respond to only one form of therapy (eg, > 80% of patients with trigeminal neuralgia respond to carbamazepine), many require several concomitant analgesic approaches. Therapeutic modalities can be categorized as pharmacologic, neurostimulatory, anesthetic, surgical, physiatric, and psychologic.

PHARMACOLOGIC THERAPY

Pharmacotherapy, the mainstay of analgesia, involves three categories of drugs: nonsteroidal anti-inflammatory drugs **(NSAIDs)**, opioid analgesics, and the so-called adjuvant analgesics (see TABLE 12–2).

The aging process may dramatically alter the clinical pharmacologic dynamics of all classes of analgesic drugs (see Ch. 21). Studies of several opioids have demonstrated some combination of diminished volume of distribution, prolonged half-life, and reduced clearance for each, *in every case leading to higher plasma levels than the same dose given to a younger patient*. Although the data on NSAIDs are less conclusive and those on adjuvant analgesics almost nonexistent, similar observations have been made about several compounds in each class.

Increased sensitivity to the adverse effects of all classes of analgesic drugs has been noted among the elderly. The relative contributions of pharmacokinetic factors (leading to higher plasma drug levels) and pharmacodynamic factors (increased sensitivity to drug effects independent of plasma level, presumably involving changes at a receptor level) remain undetermined.

General principles of pharmacologic management are as follows.

Choose an appropriate drug. Such choice depends on the severity and type of pain. In cancer pain, for example, mild pain is treated with an NSAID, moderate pain usually requires the addition of an opioid conventionally used to treat mild to moderate pain (eg, codeine), and severe pain mandates the selection of an opioid conventionally used in this setting (eg, morphine)—see Pain in Ch. 19. Patients with neuropathic pain may be less likely to respond to NSAIDs or opioids and should be treated early with adjuvant drugs, often beginning with a tricyclic antidepressant. Patients with pain associated with marked inflammation should be treated with an NSAID.

Choose a short-acting drug. Four to five half-lives are required to achieve steady-state plasma drug levels. This applies to initiation, discontinuance, or change in dosage. A drug with a long half-life thus has a longer period before its effects stabilize. For example, steady-state plasma levels are approached after 12 to 24 h with morphine, but more than a week may be required with methadone, which therefore has a far greater risk of delayed toxicity.

Prescribe one drug at a time. When combinations of drugs are needed, they should be started one at a time to avoid cumulative toxicity and to allow identification of the offending agent if an adverse effect occurs.

TABLE 12–2. ANALGESIC DRUGS

Nonsteroidal anti-inflammatory drugs

Opioid analgesics

Adjuvant analgesics
- Antidepressants
- Anticonvulsants
- Oral local anesthetics
- Antipsychotics (neuroleptics)
- Sympatholytic drugs
- Calcium channel blockers
- Corticosteroids
- Antihistamines
- Miscellaneous drugs
  - Baclofen
  - Clonidine

Begin with low doses. *For all analgesic drugs, starting doses administered to older patients should be lower than those administered to younger patients.* For example, for an opioid equivalent to morphine, an initial dose of 5 mg IM or 10 to 15 mg orally q 4 h is reasonable. Ibuprofen should be started at 400 mg tid or qid. The initial dose of analgesic antidepressants (amitriptyline, doxepin, or imipramine) should be 10 mg orally at bedtime.

Increase the dose incrementally until therapeutic effects or side effects occur, or until some upper limit based on the drug's known pharmacology is reached. Dose escalation to efficacy or toxicity is fundamental for opioid drugs. Given the **ceiling effect** (ie, a dose beyond which incremental increases fail to provide additive analgesia) and dose-related toxicity of the NSAIDs, upward titration of doses is finite. A useful empiric guideline for the NSAIDs is that the maximum reasonable dose is 1.5 to 2 times the starting dose; if analgesia is not achieved after an adequate trial at this level, an alternative drug should be considered.

Be aware of additive effects from combinations of drugs. Sedation and confusion are the greatest problems, usually related to shared central depressant, antihistaminic, and anticholinergic effects of many drugs. Similarly, the hypotensive effects of antihypertensives and the vasodilating effects of many agents used in ischemic heart disease may be exaggerated by the α-blockade produced by tricyclic antidepressants or the venodilation produced by opioids.

Continue drug trials for an adequate duration. Virtually all nonopioid analgesic drugs require a minimum trial of 2 wk at an adequate dose to judge efficacy.

Nonsteroidal Anti-inflammatory Drugs

Although there is evidence for a central mechanism as well, NSAIDs are generally believed to act peripherally, with varying and possibly disproportionate anti-inflammatory and analgesic effects. They can be classified into a weak acidic group and a nonacidic group (see TABLE 12–3). Acetaminophen is usually considered together with these drugs, despite minimal anti-inflammatory effects and a mechanism of action that is presumably central. All of these drugs share a ceiling effect, as noted above. Except for acetaminophen, all are anti-inflammatory, with variable potency. Although all are used empirically for pain, only some (eg, acetaminophen, aspirin, diflunisal, ibuprofen, naproxen, and several others) are currently approved as analgesics in the USA. Little data are available on NSAID use in the elderly. Therefore, proper use depends on understanding their pharmacologic implications and clinical experience, as follows.

Ensure that the indication is appropriate. The NSAIDs are generally used to treat mild to moderate pain, particularly that caused by an inflammatory lesion. An NSAID also provides additive analgesia to chronic opioid therapy. The NSAIDs should be prescribed cautiously in patients with preexisting renal disease, heart failure, hypertension, gastroduodenopathy, and bleeding diatheses because of the risks of interstitial nephritis, sodium retention, peptic ulcer disease, and platelet dysfunction shared to some degree by most of these drugs.

Choose an appropriate drug. Patient response to an individual agent varies widely, and the initial choice of NSAID is largely empiric. However, several factors influence this choice. For the elderly, a drug with a short half-life is generally preferred, although this guideline is less applicable to these analgesics than to others. A better guide is favorable prior experience with a specific drug. A history of ulcer disease or risk of ulcer or bleeding from any cause is an indication for selecting a drug that least affects the gastric mucosa and platelet function (ie, acetaminophen, or if anti-inflammatory effects are desirable, choline magnesium trisalicylate or salsalate).

Begin with a low initial dose and titrate to ceiling. This approach is described under the general principles of pharmacologic management, above. Intervals between dose escalations should be long enough to ensure that steady-state effects can be observed at one dose before a higher dose is administered. Dose escalation before steady state is ap-

TABLE 12–3. NONSTEROIDAL ANTI-INFLAMMATORY DRUGS

Class	*Drug*	*Comment*
Anti-inflammatory, antipyretic, acidic analgesics		
Salicylates	Aspirin Choline magnesium trisalicylate Diflunisal Salsalate	Choline magnesium trisalicylate and salsalate have less effect on GI tract and platelet aggregation than do other NSAIDs
Propionic acids	Fenoprofen Flurbiprofen Ibuprofen Ketoprofen Naproxen Naproxen Na Oxaprozin	Ibuprofen and naproxen are available over the counter
Pyroles	Diclofenac Etodolac Indomethacin Ketorolac Sulindac Suprofen Tolmetin	Potent anti-inflammatory effects; higher incidence of side effects
Fenamates	Meclofenamate Mefenamic acid	Use not recommended beyond 1 wk
Oxicams	Piroxicam	Very long half-life
Pyrazoles	Phenylbutazone	Considered to be most toxic; use supplanted by newer agents
Nonacidic, antipyretic analgesics		
p-Aminophenyl derivatives	Acetaminophen	Minimally anti-inflammatory; no effect on GI tract or platelet aggregation
Nonacidic pyrazoles	Dipyrone Phenacetin	No longer used in USA
Naphthyl-alkanones	Nabumetone	Long half-life; can be administered once daily

proached may lead to delayed toxicity as plasma drug concentration continues to rise beyond the targeted therapeutic range. The risks of rapidly titrating long-acting drugs are particularly great in populations predisposed to adverse effects, such as the elderly.

Switch to another NSAID if the response is unsatisfactory. Patients who fail to respond to a 2- to 3-wk trial of one drug at adequate doses should be switched to another. The selection of subsequent drugs during these sequential trials is empiric.

Opioid Analgesics

Opioid analgesics are indicated primarily to relieve moderate to severe acute pain and chronic pain due to cancer. Response to these drugs is enhanced in the elderly, partly because of elevated plasma levels and prolonged clearance and partly because of increased tissue sensitivity. Therapeutic guidelines for this population are summarized as follows.

Ensure that the indication is appropriate. Severe acute pain, such as that accompanying fractures, is the clearest indication. For chronic cancer pain, a so-called **analgesic ladder** has been advocated; mild pain is managed with acetaminophen or an NSAID, moderate pain with the addition of an opioid conventionally used for this indication (eg, codeine), and severe pain with an opioid usually used to treat intense pain (eg, morphine). For nonmalignant pain, chronic opioid therapy is controversial and should be considered only after all other reasonable attempts at analgesia have failed.

Choose an appropriate drug. Opioid selection is based on empiric factors such as favorable prior experience, cost, availability of a certain formulation, and specific pharmacologic properties. Pharmacologic issues include the class of opioid, side effects of specific drugs, and pharmacokinetic differences among drugs.

The opioid analgesics can be divided into pure **agonists** and **agonist-antagonists** (see TABLE 12–4). The latter are characterized by a balance of agonism and competitive antagonism at one or more types of opioid receptor site. Clinical characteristics of the agonist-antagonist opioids include a ceiling effect for respiratory depression, a lesser tendency to cause physical dependence, a relatively high incidence of psychotomimetic effects in the mixed agonist-antagonist subclass, and the ability to reverse opioid agonist effects and precipitate withdrawal in physically dependent patients. Because they reverse agonist effects, agonist-antagonists should be given only to patients not already receiving opioid drugs (ie, as first-line agents only). The only drug in this class available in the USA in an oral formulation is pentazocine, which is relatively likely to cause psychotomimetic effects.

Agonist-antagonist drugs are *not* currently recommended for the treatment of chronic cancer pain and should be used for severe acute pain only when parenteral administration is necessary. None has compelling advantages over the agonists. The clinical usefulness of a new intranasal formulation of butorphanol has not yet been determined. Older patients with pain requiring opioid analgesics usually can be adequately managed with pure agonists.

Of the agonist drugs, **meperidine** causes a relatively high incidence of CNS hyperexcitability, including agitation, tremulousness, myoclonus, seizures, and dysphoria. This effect is caused by the accumulation in plasma of normeperidine, a toxic metabolite with a long half-life. Renal insufficiency is the major predisposing factor for this effect, suggesting that the elderly may be at particular risk. Thus, meperidine should generally be *avoided.*

The most important pharmacokinetic consideration is half-life. The preferred opioids are those that rapidly approach steady state and, therefore, are more easily monitored (eg, morphine, hydromorphone, and oxycodone).

Begin with the lowest dose that produces analgesia. In the nontolerant older patient, initial doses should be lower than those prescribed in younger patients. For example, opioid-naive patients with postoperative pain can be given morphine 5 mg or hydromorphone 0.75 mg IM q 3 to 4 h. Patients already receiving opioids require an initial dose based on prior opioid exposure and converted to an equianalgesic dose as described below.

Titrate the dose to desired analgesic effect or to intolerance of side effects. If analgesia is *entirely* inadequate after the initial dose in the naive patient, the next dose should be doubled. If *partial* analgesia follows the initial dose of an opioid with a short half-life, succeeding doses should be increased by a smaller amount q 12 to 24 h, as steady-state plasma levels are approached. A useful technique for dose titration involves the concurrent prescription of a fixed dose and a "**rescue dose**" as needed (q 2 or 3 h). The latter should be a drug with a short half-life, the same as the drug used for fixed dosing, if possible. This technique gives the patient some control over pain, allows transitory exacerbations of pain to be managed expeditiously, and can be the basis for upward titration of the fixed dose. The increment can equal the total of the rescue dose administered during the previous period or can be empirically chosen to be 25% to 50% of the current fixed dose. Analgesia provided by agonist opioids has no ceiling effect; upward titration of doses should continue until analgesia occurs or limiting side effects develop.

Be aware of analgesic duration. Although methadone is sometimes effective with dosing q 6 to 8 h, other opioids usually require dosing q 4 h. The controlled-release oral morphine formulation can be administered q 8 to 12 h, and the new fentanyl transdermal system can be administered q 48 to 72 h.

Administer analgesics regularly. Generally, opioid drugs should be administered around the clock to provide consistent analgesia and to reduce anticipatory anxiety and clock watching. Exceptions to this are as follows: (1) In patients requiring long-term opioid use, several days of dosing on an as-needed basis can determine the analgesic requirement. (2) With drugs possessing a long half-life, particularly methadone, dos-

TABLE 12–4. THE OPIOID ANALGESICS: EQUIANALGESIC DOSES, HALF–LIVES, AND DURATIONS

Drug	*Route*	*Equianalgesic**	*Half-life (h)*	*Duration (h)*
Opioid agonists				
Morphine	IM, IV, sc	10	2–4	3–5
	Oral, rectal	30–60†	——	8–12‡
Methadone	IM, IV, sc	10	15–>100	4–6
	Oral	20		
Levorphanol	IM, IV, sc	2	12–16	4–6
	Oral	4		
Hydromorphone	IM, IV, sc	1.5	2–3	3–5
	Oral	7.5		
Meperidine	IM, IV, sc	75	3–4	3–5
	Oral	300		
Oxymorphone	IM, IV, sc	1	2–3	3–5
	Rectal	10		
Oxycodone	IM, IV, sc	15	——	3–5
	Oral	30		
Codeine	IM, IV, sc	130	3–4	3–5
	Oral	200		
Fentanyl	Transdermal	——	——	48–72
Opioid agonist-antagonists				
Mixed agonist-antagonists				
Pentazocine	IM, IV, sc	60	2–3	3–5
	Oral	180		
Nalbuphine	IM, IV, sc	10	5	3–5
Butorphanol	IM, IV, sc	2	2–4	3–5

(continued)

TABLE 12–4. THE OPIOID ANALGESICS: EQUIANALGESIC DOSES, HALF-LIVES, AND DURATIONS *(Continued)*

Drug	*Route*	*Equianalgesic**	*Half-life (h)*	*Duration (h)*
Opioid agonist-antagonists *(continued)*				
Partial agonists				
Buprenorphine	IM	0.4	4–5	4–8
	Sublingual	0.3		
Dezocine	IM, IV, sc	——	2–3	3–4

IM = intramuscular; IV = intravenous; sc = subcutaneous.
* Equianalgesic doses based on single-dose relative-potency assays.
† An IM-oral relative potency of 1:6 is reported in single-dose studies of morphine, but uncontrolled data and clinical experience suggest that this changes to 1:2-3 with chronic dosing.
‡ Controlled-release formulation.

ing could be initiated on an as-needed basis to reduce the risk of accumulation and toxicity as steady state is approached. (3) When the degree of nociception is likely to change rapidly (eg, following certain operations or radiotherapy), dosing as needed allows the patient to adjust the amount of analgesic needed. (4) A rescue dose as needed is combined with a fixed dose during chronic opioid administration.

Choose an appropriate route of administration. Opioids have a wide range of potential routes of administration (see TABLE 12–5). The oral route is preferred for safety, ease of administration, and longer duration of action. If this route is unavailable or if pain is very severe and rapid titration of doses is desired, a parenteral route should be used. Parenteral administration is *not* more effective than oral administration; if *equianalgesic* doses are used and all orally administered drug is absorbed, efficacy is the same although onset of action is faster via the parenteral route.

Be aware of equianalgesic doses. TABLE 12–4 lists the equianalgesic doses for most opioid analgesics, relative to morphine 10 mg IM. This information must be used when switching drugs or routes of administration. For example, in switching a postoperative patient from 50 mg of meperidine IM to 50 mg orally, analgesic potency is abruptly reduced by 75%, resulting in undermedication. Conversely, if a patient with can-

TABLE 12–5. ROUTES OF ADMINISTRATION FOR OPIOID DRUGS

Route	*Comment*
Oral	Preferred for chronic use
Rectal	Morphine, oxymorphone, and hydromorphone suppositories are available; although very few studies have been done, the rectal route is believed to be approximately equianalgesic with the oral route
Transdermal	Patch for chronic pain releases fentanyl over 72 h
Subcutaneous Repetitive bolus Continuous infusion Patient-controlled analgesia	Ambulatory pumps allow outpatient continuous subcutaneous infusion, with or without patient-controlled analgesia
Intramuscular	——
Intravenous Repetitive bolus Continuous infusion Patient-controlled analgesia	Patient-controlled administration provides analgesia with less drug in the postoperative setting; however, cost and need for manual dexterity and intact cognition may limit its usefulness in the elderly and severely ill
Epidural Repetitive bolus Continuous infusion	Spinal administration is now well accepted and used for both cancer pain and postoperative pain; many controversies remain, especially in cancer pain, including indications, best drug, timing of therapy, and best site of administration
Intrathecal	Administered as a continuous infusion
Intraventricular	Rarely used technique for cancer pain

cer pain receiving oral hydromorphone 8 mg q 3 h develops a bowel obstruction and 8 mg IM is prescribed, potency is increased five times, with a serious risk of toxicity. Similar considerations apply when switching from one drug to another. Because cross-tolerance between drugs is incomplete, the equianalgesic dose should be reduced by 30% to 50%, and clinical experience indicates that a switch to methadone should be accompanied by a 75% reduction of the equianalgesic dose.

Anticipate and treat side effects. Constipation and sedation or confusion are the most common opioid side effects in older persons. **Constipation** should be addressed at the start of therapy and can be managed by (1) an osmotic (saline) laxative q 3 days (eg, magnesium citrate, magnesium sulfate, sodium citrate); (2) a daily contact laxative (senna, bisacodyl, or phenolphthalein); (3) a daily dose of stool softener (docusate); and (4) daily administration of lactulose or sorbitol 15 to 30 mL bid initially. Doses of these drugs and the use of combinations may be necessary in patients receiving chronic therapy. **Sedation and confusion** are often transient and may improve if other contributing factors (eg, the use of nonopioid drugs with sedative effects) are reduced; if they persist, a switch to an alternative opioid may be salutary. Using a psychostimulant (eg, methylphenidate or dextroamphetamine) to manage opioid-induced sedation may be relatively more risky in the elderly, but clinical experience is generally sanguine. Both drugs should be started at 2.5 to 5 mg orally once or twice daily, and the dose should be escalated every other day as needed.

Although **respiratory depression** is a serious potential adverse effect, tolerance to it develops rapidly, and it is rarely a problem if doses are increased cautiously. If respiratory depression does develop, an alternative cause such as pulmonary embolism or pneumonia should be sought. **Nausea** may be treated with antiemetic drugs (metoclopramide 10 mg orally qid or prochlorperazine 10 mg orally qid or 25 mg rectally bid, followed by dose escalation, if needed). **Side effects** such as dry mouth, urinary retention, and accommodation difficulties occur occasionally, particularly in patients receiving other drugs with similar effects. Nonessential drugs should be discontinued and a switch to an alternative opioid considered. **Pruritus,** an uncommon side effect, usually responds to antihistamines (eg, hydroxyzine 25 mg orally qid).

Use analgesic combinations cautiously. Drug combinations can enhance pain relief. If there are no contraindications, an NSAID may be added to the opioid. One or more of the adjuvant analgesics may also be appropriate, depending on the nature of the pain. However, because *the older patient is at increased risk for side effects, particularly sedation or confusion,* these drugs should be added cautiously, at low initial doses and one drug at a time. Guidelines for their use are listed below.

Watch for the development of **tolerance,** *the need for increasing doses to maintain the same analgesic effect.* This phenomenon is poorly understood. Although it can be reproducibly demonstrated in animals, tolerance has a far more variable course in humans. The need to escalate doses usually signals progressive disease or increased distress rather than the development of pharmacologic tolerance per se. The earliest indication of tolerance is the complaint of decreasing duration of analgesia after a dose. Clinically, tolerance is seldom a problem, since pain relief recurs with an increase in dose or a reduction in the dosing interval. If rapid escalation of doses becomes problematic, a switch to an alternative drug or route of administration may be useful.

Observe for signs of physical and psychologic dependence. **Physical dependence** is a *pharmacologic phenomenon in which a specific abstinence (withdrawal) syndrome occurs after abrupt discontinuance of an opioid drug or administration of an opioid antagonist.* Clinically, phys-

TABLE 12–6. GUIDELINES FOR OPIOID THERAPY IN PATIENTS WITH NONMALIGNANT PAIN

Should be used only after all reasonable nonopioid therapies are exhausted
Formal consent should be obtained, specifically noting possibilities of side effects, minimal risk of addictive behaviors, and implications of physical dependence
Agreed-upon titration period should be determined, aiming for at least partial pain relief
After titration, agreed-upon monthly quantity of drug should be determined, with some leeway in daily dose but return to maintenance dose by month's end
Monthly visits should be established, at least initially
Return of function should continue to be the major emphasis
Drug hoarding and acquisition elsewhere should not be tolerated; if they occur, opioid drugs should be tapered and therapy should be discontinued
Rapid dose escalation or escalation without subsequent decrement suggests need for hospitalization

ical dependence poses no problem unless withdrawal is produced by noncompliance or inadvertent administration of a drug with antagonistic effects. In contrast, **psychologic dependence or addiction** is a *psychologic and behavioral syndrome in which there is drug craving and aberrant drug-related behaviors characterized by loss of control, compulsive use, and continued use despite harm.* Although psychologic dependence is a risk with opioid drugs, the overwhelming majority of patients with acute pain and pain due to cancer do not develop such aberrant behaviors.

Chronic opioid therapy in patients with chronic nonmalignant pain syndrome is controversial, but some patients benefit substantially from long-term use of opioids without developing clinically significant tolerance, toxicity, or psychologic dependence. Guidelines for the management of opioid therapy are shown in TABLE 12–6.

ADJUVANT ANALGESICS

Adjuvant analgesics have other primary indications but are analgesic in certain settings. They are used as initial therapy in many nonmalignant pain syndromes and in combination with opioid drugs in patients receiving chronic opioid therapy.

Tricyclic Antidepressants

Tricyclics are used in patients with neuropathic pain (eg, diabetic neuropathy and postherpetic neuralgia), chronic back pain, chronic headache, psychogenic pain, and others; one study has shown that imipramine is effective in relieving the pain of arthritis. Of those available in the USA, **amitriptyline, clomipramine, desipramine, doxepin, imipramine,** and **nortriptyline** have shown efficacy in clinical trials. Data are most compelling for amitriptyline, but like the other tertiary amines (clomipramine, imipramine, and doxepin), this drug has strong anticholinergic and sedative effects and may cause orthostatic hypotension. The secondary amine tricyclic antidepressants desipramine and nortriptyline are usually better tolerated than any of the tertiary amines. One of these drugs is often selected as first-line therapy in the elderly.

The regimens for all the tricyclic antidepressants are similar: initially, 10 mg at bedtime, increasing over several weeks to 50 to 150 mg at bedtime. Although analgesia often occurs at doses substantially lower than those required for depression, higher doses may be needed by some patients. Plasma levels can be monitored to determine whether poor results may be related to compliance or pharmacokinetic factors and to provide guidance during dose escalation.

These drugs should *not* be prescribed in patients with symptomatic urinary retention, narrow-angle glaucoma, or greater than first-degree heart block. They should be *used cautiously* in patients with mild dementia and in those receiving other drugs with similar side effects. A baseline ECG should be obtained, and another ECG should be obtained when the daily dose reaches about 150 mg; conduction or rhythm disturbances mandate dose reduction or discontinuance of the drug.

Structurally unrelated compounds (eg, fluoxetine, maprotiline, paroxetine, or trazodone) are sometimes administered as analgesics in patients unable to tolerate the first-line drugs or in those with relative contraindications to them. All have less anticholinergic effects, and fluoxetine and paroxetine do not cause weight gain, are much less sedating, and, in fact, can induce a CNS stimulatory effect. The literature provides less support for the use of these drugs. Since the analgesic effects of paroxetine have been demonstrated in controlled trials, it is most reasonable to select this drug as an alternative antidepressant for pain.

Anticonvulsants

Anticonvulsants are advocated in neuropathic disorders characterized by paroxysmal or lancinating pain, a use supported largely by controlled studies of carbamazepine in trigeminal neuralgia. There are also some studies and many anecdotal reports of phenytoin, valproate, and clonazepam use in a wide variety of similar pain disorders, prescribed in the same dosage as that used to treat seizures.

Carbamazepine dosing in the elderly should be started at 100 mg orally bid, then increased gradually (by 100 mg/day) to the usually effective range of between 600 and 1800 mg/day in divided doses. A CBC count should be performed before initial dosing and again at 2 to 4 wk, 6 to 8 wk, and periodically thereafter. **Phenytoin,** with an oral loading dose of 500 mg once, 300 mg that night, and 300 mg on subsequent nights, may also be used. The initial dose of **clonazepam** is 0.5 mg/day, which is gradually increased; the usual effective dose is 0.5 to 3.0 mg bid. **Valproate** may be given at 250 mg once or twice daily and increased slowly (about every week by 250 mg/day in divided doses) to the usual range of 750 to 2500 mg/day in divided doses.

For all these drugs, doses should be increased until clinical efficacy or intolerance of side effects is achieved, or until plasma concentration exceeds the upper anticonvulsant range by a modest amount. Plasma drug levels should also be monitored, if possible, to judge compliance, to identify patients who rapidly metabolize the drug, to evaluate changes when other drugs are taken, and to document an effective plasma level. Although not an anticonvulsant, **baclofen** is classified with these agents because of its documented efficacy in trigeminal neuralgia. When it is used for lancinating pain in the elderly, treatment should begin at 5 mg orally bid, and dosage should be increased by 10 mg/day every other day until the patient is pain-free or side effects occur. While the neuroleptic **pimozide** can also be used for this indication, it is not preferred because of its high incidence of side effects.

Other Neuroleptic Drugs

Other drugs have been used in a variety of neuropathic pain states, despite little evidence of efficacy in controlled clinical trials. *The risk of adverse effects, including parkinsonism and tardive dyskinesia, is relatively high in the elderly. Neuroleptics should be viewed only as second-line agents,* to be considered in refractory neuropathic pain such as postherpetic neuralgia or painful neuropathy. Clinical experience is greatest with fluphenazine 1 to 2 mg orally bid to tid; haloperidol 0.5 to 2.0 mg orally bid to tid is sometimes used.

Oral Local Anesthetic Drugs

Local anesthetics have become accepted for the treatment of diverse types of neuropathic pain. The preferred agent is **mexiletine** because of its relatively low risk of serious toxicity. Mexiletine is often tried as a second- or third-line drug after trials of antidepressants or anticonvulsants have failed. Treatment is initiated at 150 mg orally once daily. The dose is gradually increased (usually every 3 to 7 days) by 150 mg/day to a usual maximum of 300 mg tid. Conduction block is a contraindication, and the ECG should be monitored during dose escalation. Plasma concentration monitoring can also guide dosing.

Sympatholytic Drugs

These drugs have been used effectively in patients with sympathetically maintained pain—specifically causalgia or reflex sympathetic dystrophy—according to anecdotal evidence. The oral drugs phenoxybenzamine, prazosin, propranolol, and guanethidine *should be considered only in unequivocal cases of reflex sympathetic dystrophy that have failed to respond to other measures.*

Calcium Channel Blockers

These drugs may be used for analgesia. Nifedipine has been used in refractory reflex sympathetic dystrophy, and both nifedipine (usually 10 mg orally tid) and verapamil (80 mg orally tid or qid) may have efficacy in migraine prophylaxis. Recurrent migraine is rare in the elderly, and experience with these agents in this population is limited.

Corticosteroids

Corticosteroids have been used in reflex sympathetic dystrophy (prednisone 60 mg daily in divided doses, tapered over 2 wk), in acute herpetic neuralgia in the immunocompetent host (see POSTHERPETIC NEURALGIA, below), and in malignant pain due to tumor invasion of bone or nerve trunks (empirically chosen as methylprednisolone, prednisone, or dexamethasone at a dose equivalent to 80 mg prednisone daily). The risks of short-term therapy with these agents are generally low. Concurrent diseases such as diabetes or heart failure may change these considerations.

Antihistamines

Antihistamines (eg, hydroxyzine, diphenhydramine, and orphenadrine) may have analgesic activity, although supporting data are limited. One of these agents may be selected for patients with pain and an associated indication for antihistamine therapy; eg, those with pain from a malignancy and anxiety or nausea may be given a trial of hydroxyzine 25 to 50 mg orally qid. The anticholinergic and sedative effects of these drugs in the elderly patient should always be considered.

OTHER ANALGESIC APPROACHES

(See also TREATMENT OF PAIN AND INFLAMMATION in Ch. 29)

Integration of pharmacologic approaches with other analgesic techniques is the foundation of the multidisciplinary team approach successfully used by pain clinics in the treatment of refractory pain. Some elements of each of these approaches fall within the purview of nonspecialists (see TABLE 12–7).

NEUROSTIMULATORY TECHNIQUES

Neurostimulatory techniques enhance afferent stimulation to provide segmental analgesia. They are useful for localized pain, particularly that of neuropathic origin. **Counterirritation,** or *brisk rubbing of the painful part,* often preceded by application of a vapocoolant spray (Fluori-Methane or Fluro-Ethyl) and **transcutaneous electrical nerve stimulation (TENS),** now widely available, can be applied by the nonspecialist. Although the analgesia provided is usually short-lived, and cognitive deficits and lack of manual dexterity may preclude their use

TABLE 12–7. SOME NONPHARMACOLOGIC TECHNIQUES OF PAIN CONTROL

Approach	*Treatment*	*Indication*
Neurostimulatory	Counterirritation Transcutaneous electrical nerve stimulation (TENS)	Localized pain; neuropathic pain
Anesthetic	Trigger point injections	Myofascial pain with trigger points
Physiatric	Some physical therapy techniques, such as range-of-motion exercise programs	Myofascial or joint pain; inactivity
Psychologic	Some cognitive techniques, such as relaxation, distraction; behavioral programs	Predictable pain; muscle spasm; inactivity and abnormal illness behavior

in many older patients, the inherent safety of these techniques recommends their use. Other neurostimulatory techniques, including **acupuncture, percutaneous electric nerve stimulation, dorsal column stimulation,** and **deep brain stimulation,** require special expertise.

ANESTHETIC TECHNIQUES

Anesthetic approaches include trigger point injection, nitrous oxide inhalation in patients with advanced cancer, and a variety of somatic and sympathetic nerve blocks. **Trigger point injection** with saline or a local anesthetic is useful for myofascial pain. If palpation of a painful region reveals focal tenderness, injection may provide transitory relief, leading to improved physical activity, and occasionally, long-term analgesia. **Nerve blocks** (temporary or permanent, depending upon the solution injected) are most useful in managing sympathetically maintained pain and cancer pain and should be performed only by experienced personnel.

SURGICAL TECHNIQUES

Joint replacement may cure intractable arthritic pain. Surgical lesions to manage cancer pain have been placed at every level of the nervous system, from peripheral nerve to cortex. The most common approach is cordotomy. Both chemical and surgical transsphenoidal pituitary ablation have been used to relieve cancer pain. These procedures should be considered only after analgesic drugs have failed and should be performed only by clinicians with expertise in cancer pain management.

Neuroablative surgery for providing analgesia is rarely appropriate in patients with nonmalignant pain syndromes. Occasionally, patients with reflex sympathetic dystrophy who obtain short-term relief from repeated temporary nerve blocks may be candidates for surgical sympathectomy. A new procedure, the dorsal root entry zone lesion, has been developed for the treatment of selected deafferentation pain syndromes. Data suggest this procedure should be considered particularly in patients with pain from nerve root avulsion.

Physiatric Techniques

Many rehabilitative modalities may directly ameliorate pain as well as increase the level of activity and reduce secondary myofascial complications that often contribute to chronic pain. Orthoses may be useful in splinting the painful region, reducing so-called **incident pain** that occurs with movement or the assumption of certain positions. Participation in physical therapy and exercise programs often improves psychologic outlook and social interaction, if not always the pain.

Psychologic Techniques

Psychologic modalities include formal psychotherapy, cognitive techniques (eg, relaxation training, distraction, biofeedback, and hypnosis), and behavioral therapy to reverse dysfunctional behaviors such as physical inactivity and social withdrawal. Many of these techniques can be applied by nonphysicians. However, the elderly do not easily engage in these activities and are often not given the opportunity to do so. There may be clinician bias against such techniques, and elderly patients may have subtle cognitive deficits or be disinclined to trust psychologic procedures. For older patients who are willing to participate and appear capable of benefiting, a psychologic approach should be offered.

COMMON PAIN SYNDROMES

Certain pain syndromes are particularly common in the elderly. Their recognition and management should be viewed as a central focus of geriatric care.

NOCICEPTIVE SYNDROMES

Many pain syndromes are best understood as a consequence of ongoing nociceptive stimulation, eg, chronic lumbar pain due to degenera-

TABLE 12–8. COMMON CANCER PAIN SYNDROMES

Associated with disease	Bone
	  Local pain at site of metastasis
	  Generalized pain from multiple metastases
	  Base-of-skull syndromes
	  Vertebral body syndromes
	Nerve
	  Epidural spinal cord compression
	  Leptomeningeal metastasis
	  Radiculopathy
	  Lumbosacral or brachial plexopathy
	  Painful polyneuropathy (eg, in paraproteinemias)
	  Painful mononeuropathies
	Soft tissue infiltration
	Blood vessel infiltration
	Hollow viscus obstruction

Associated with therapy	Postsurgical syndromes
	  Post-thoracotomy
	  Postmastectomy
	  Phantom limb pain
	  Postradical neck dissection
	Postchemotherapy syndromes
	  Painful polyneuropathy
	  Aseptic necrosis of femoral head
	  Steroid pseudorheumatism
	Postradiation syndromes
	  Radiation fibrosis of nerve plexus
	  Radiation myelopathy
	  Radiation necrosis of bone

tive arthritis. They must be distinguished from others that result from similar organic lesions but are associated with such a degree of psychologic impairment that they are classified with the psychologic syndromes described below. Psychosocial features are important but less compelling in the nociceptive syndromes than in other syndromes.

CANCER PAIN

This pain is usually nociceptive. A peripheral lesion activates pain-sensitive fibers, even in patients with mixed syndromes also characterized by a neuropathic component (usually caused by tumor infiltration of nerve trunks) or a prominent psychologic component.

Many cancer pain syndromes have been described (see TABLE 12–8). Primary therapy should be directed at the underlying cause, if possible.

TABLE 12–9. INVASIVE PROCEDURES USED IN CANCER PAIN MANAGEMENT

Site	*Anesthetic Procedures*	*Neurosurgical Procedures**	*Purpose (neurostimulatory)*
For localized pain			
Pelvis or perineum†	Chemical rhizotomy	Bilateral cordotomy; midline myelotomy	Dorsal column stimulation
Epigastrium	Celiac plexus block‡	——	——
Abdomen or chest†	Chemical neurectomy; chemical rhizotomy	Neurectomy; rhizotomy; cordotomy	Dorsal column stimulation; percutaneous electrical stimulation
Arms or legs†	Chemical rhizotomy	Neurectomy; rhizotomy; cordotomy	Dorsal column stimulation; percutaneous electrical stimulation
Head or neck	Chemical rhizotomy; chemical gangliolysis	Rhizotomy	——
For generalized pain	Chemical hypophysectomy	Bilateral cordotomy	Deep brain stimulation

* Other surgical procedures directed at the brain stem, specifically tractotomy and thalamotomy, are rarely done but may be useful for unilateral pain, especially that involving the face; other procedures (eg, lobotomy and cingulumotomy) are now seldom done and were designed to reduce suffering.

† Spinal opioids commonly used in this setting.

‡ The risk:benefit ratio of celiac plexus block is such that it is often used early in the management of epigastric visceral pain without prior extensive trials of opioid drugs.

Most cancer pain can be managed pharmacologically (see OPIOID ANALGESICS, above). Patients who fail to respond to pharmacologic management may be candidates for invasive anesthetic, neurosurgical, or neurostimulatory approaches (see TABLE 12–9). In addition, newer techniques of opioid administration (see TABLE 12–5) may be effective (eg, intraspinal administration is commonly used to relieve pain below mid-thorax). All these techniques require the guidance of persons with special expertise.

OSTEOARTHRITIS

Degenerative arthritis is the most common cause of nociceptive pain in the elderly (see also Ch. 75). Several specific syndromes may occur. (1) Diffuse and focal joint pain is frequent, but some patients develop pain at only a single joint or bilaterally at only one level (usually, hips), while others develop only diffuse large and small joint pain. (2) Refractory low-back pain may be related to degenerative processes affecting facet joints and the intervertebral space. (3) An often unrecognized syndrome of occipital headache may occur, related to cervical osteoarthritis.

Since both anti-inflammatory and analgesic effects are desirable, NSAIDs are the primary treatment (see NONSTEROIDAL ANTI-INFLAMMATORY DRUGS, above). Occasionally, patients whose pain is virtually continuous or is compounded by sleeplessness or depression will benefit from the addition of a tricyclic antidepressant. Patients with refractory pain can be considered for opioid therapy (see TABLE 12–6).

Physical therapy may forestall the development of secondary progressive ankylosis and contractures and also helps prevent inactivity (see TREATMENT OF PAIN AND INFLAMMATION in Ch. 29). Orthoses (eg, a corset for lumbar pain, a soft collar for occipital or cervical pain, or a knee brace) may be useful.

Injections of local anesthetics and corticosteroids into joints, or into the epidural space for lumbar pain, are widely used despite a lack of well-controlled clinical trials establishing their efficacy. Dramatic benefits are often reported anecdotally, and the procedures should be considered if experienced personnel are available to perform them.

Joint replacement surgery is an option for intractable pain in some joints.

OTHER NOCICEPTIVE SYNDROMES

Myofascial pains, common in the elderly, may be acute or recurrent and may conform to clear-cut causes; eg, bursitis, tendinitis, or sprains. Management usually relies on NSAIDs and local injection. Less well characterized is the **myofascial pain syndrome,** which typically involves painful trigger points in muscle. Pathogenesis is obscure, but the syndrome may be related to overuse of a muscle. Pain may be referred and is usually reproduced by palpating the causative trigger points. These trigger points can be inactivated by injection (dry needling, saline, or local anesthetic) or by a spray-and-stretch technique, in which a vapocoolant (Fluori-Methane or Fluro-Ethyl) is applied until the skin is numb and the muscle then stretched through a full range of motion. Physical therapy and transcutaneous electrical nerve stimulation may also reduce acute discomfort in these syndromes; continued activity without muscle overuse prevents recurrence.

NEUROPATHIC PAIN SYNDROMES

These syndromes are less common than nociceptive pain syndromes in the elderly. Postherpetic neuralgia, painful polyneuropathies, compressive mononeuropathies, and trigeminal neuralgia are usually encountered by clinicians; rare causes are central pain, phantom limb pain, pain from root avulsion, and sympathetically maintained pains (eg, reflex sympathetic dystrophy). Adjuvant analgesics are the primary pharmacologic modalities for all of these disorders.

POSTHERPETIC NEURALGIA

Persistent pain following resolution of acute herpes zoster. The pathogenesis of this pain is unclear but is presumed to involve central reorganization of afferent neural pathways. Persistent pain is present 1 yr after onset in 50% of patients 70 yr of age. Precisely when the pain of acute zoster neuralgia becomes postherpetic neuralgia is controversial and has been variably defined as from the time of lesion clearing to 6 mo. About 2 mo after the onset of the acute disease, treatment should be directed specifically to postherpetic neuralgia.

Primary prevention of postherpetic neuralgia may become possible with widespread use of a varicella vaccine. In patients with acute herpes zoster, corticosteroids and sympathetic blockade have been tried for prevention, but their efficacy has not been confirmed. However, the data suggest the following management scheme.

Immunocompromised patients who develop acute herpes zoster should be treated with antiviral agents (usually acyclovir); these agents prevent viral dissemination and reduce acute pain but have not been shown to reduce the incidence of postherpetic neuralgia. Immunocompetent patients with very severe eruptions, corneal involvement, or intense pain that has not responded to an opioid should also be considered for acyclovir therapy. If the pain is severe and does not respond to NSAIDs or opioids, corticosteroids (eg, prednisone 60 mg daily tapered over 2 wk, or longer if pain flares on dose reduction) can be administered in immunocompetent patients. Sympathetic block with a local anesthetic may also help reduce the pain of acute herpetic neuralgia. Other drugs that have been reported to clear the rash or reduce acute pain include amantadine 100 mg orally bid, levodopa, and adenine monophosphate. The risk:benefit ratio of levodopa and adenine monophosphate in the older patient is unknown, and they are not recommended. The data for amantadine are limited to a single study, and its role remains undetermined. The pain of acute herpetic neuralgia should be managed with NSAIDs and opioids, and local skin care is important.

For postherpetic neuralgia, the mainstay of pharmacologic therapy is an antidepressant. Controlled trials with amitriptyline and maprotiline have been conducted, but as noted anecdotally, some of the tricyclic antidepressants (eg, desipramine) appear to be better tolerated than others in the elderly. Oral local anesthetics, specifically mexiletine, are often used as second-line agents. Patients whose pain has a prominent lancinating component may benefit from the addition of an anticonvulsant. Dosing guidelines for these drugs are described above. NSAIDs appear to have little effect on this and other neuropathic pains, but they help occasionally and are reasonable to try. Opioid therapy is controversial but may ameliorate the pain in some patients. Trials of topical capsaicin and topical local anesthetic (specifically EMLA—eutectic mixture of lidocaine and prilocaine) should be considered despite modest supporting data.

A neurostimulatory technique, usually transcutaneous electrical nerve stimulation, and physical therapy for prevention of secondary myofascial complications should be considered, particularly if the pain affects an extremity. Psychologic interventions are often useful for secondary affective disturbances and abnormal illness behavior. Therapeutic goals should be individualized to restore normal day-to-day function, even when pain relief is incomplete.

Patients with refractory pain should be considered for a trial of temporary sympathetic blocks or subcutaneous injection of a local anesthetic and corticosteroid, although these techniques are supported only by uncontrolled survey data. All anesthetic and surgical neurolytic procedures carry too much risk to be considered except in the most unusual circumstances of profound functional impairment caused by intractable pain alone. The dorsal root entry zone lesion is currently the procedure most accepted.

Painful Polyneuropathies

Diabetes is the most common cause of neuropathic pains. **Diabetic polyradiculopathy,** a subtype of which is **diabetic amyotrophy,** can cause excruciating pain along multiple nerve roots, usually lumbar, at times accompanied by weight loss and lassitude suggestive of underlying malignancy. The pain is usually self-limited. In contrast, painful **diabetic polyneuropathy** is characterized by dysesthesias of the feet and calves that may be persistent and intractable.

The *acute* pain of diabetic polyradiculopathy can usually be managed with opioid drugs. Adjuvant analgesics are considered if the pain persists for more than several weeks. The diagnosis usually is reassuring to the patient, and the severe pain is self-limited.

Chronic painful polyneuropathy is a far greater management problem. Psychologic interventions should be considered early to maintain activity and prevent abnormal illness behavior. Pharmacologic management is similar to that of other continuous neuropathic pains (see above). Occasionally, patients may benefit from the application of transcutaneous electrical nerve stimulation to both calves.

Compressive Mononeuropathies

In addition to the pharmacologic approaches described above, splinting (eg, a nocturnal wrist splint for carpal tunnel syndrome) and, occasionally, injection of a local anesthetic and a corticosteroid into the site of compression may benefit these neuropathies. Oral corticosteroids (prednisone 60 mg daily tapered over 1 to 2 wk) are used for acute carpal tunnel syndrome, although no controlled studies support this course. Surgical release of the median nerve is considered the treatment of choice in the elderly patient with chronic carpal tunnel syndrome.

Trigeminal Neuralgia

This disorder is believed to be caused by cross-compression of the proximal part of the trigeminal nerve (usually by an aberrant blood vessel), because an offending lesion is usually identified during surgery and its removal or mechanical protection of the nerve is followed by pain relief. Other causes, including multiple sclerosis, are relatively rare, especially in the elderly.

Medical treatment of trigeminal neuralgia is usually successful. Carbamazepine and baclofen have been effective in controlled studies; the other anticonvulsants described above and mexiletine are used in patients who fail to respond to these agents or cannot tolerate them. Patients for whom drug treatment fails are candidates for an invasive procedure. Trigeminal gangliolysis by a radiofrequency lesion or by injection of glycerol or other neurolytic solution provides relief to about 80% of these patients for at least a year. Glycerol injection is now considered the safest of these procedures. Suboccipital craniectomy with microvascular decompression of the trigeminal nerve has a similar success rate but is a major operation requiring general anesthesia.

Central Pain

Persistent painful dysesthesias can complicate a lesion at any level of the CNS. In the elderly, such central pain usually follows a stroke; the thalamic syndrome is the best example (unilateral dysesthesias, often accompanied by sensory loss and sometimes by weakness and abnormal involuntary movements, occurring after a vascular insult to the contralateral thalamus). Lesions can be too small to be detected with current imaging techniques, and the diagnosis often depends solely on clinical criteria.

Pharmacologic treatment of central pain is similar to that of postherpetic neuralgia. Maintenance of activity, physical therapy for retaining the function of affected extremities, and treatment for concomitant psychologic disturbances are essential. Peripheral neurostimulatory techniques are seldom useful since the pain is diffuse (often throughout half the body), although deep brain stimulation has been used in specialized centers. Neurolytic techniques are not useful.

PSYCHOGENIC PAIN

Chronic pain existing without any organic explanation or with an explanation insufficient to account for the degree of pain and disability.

The presenting complaint may be headache, low back, atypical facial, pelvic, or other pain. Some organic component (eg, degenerative arthritis of the spine in chronic lumbar pain) also is usually present. *These pains are unequivocally experienced,* but psychologic factors predominate in their genesis. The term **chronic nonmalignant pain syndrome** is a general appellation for these conditions, which implies considerable associated disability (see CLASSIFICATION, above).

From the start, the therapist must recognize the interrelatedness of physical impairment and psychologic state. While psychologic consultation is often needed, the nonspecialist can use principles of behavioral psychology to reduce the abnormal illness behavior and enhance function. The patient should keep a diary, recording the activities performed and the pain experienced (on a scale of 0 to 10) every hour during selected periods. Specific recommendations for increasing activity should be made that are contingent on time rather than on pain. If pain is limiting, the amount of activity can be reduced and again be made contingent on time. *The goal is to reduce the intense focus on symptoms and provide the patient with functional goals that can be achieved.*

Simultaneously, maladaptive behaviors can be addressed with specific suggestions for gradual change; eg, for social withdrawal, a telephone call to a friend may be prescribed first, followed by a once-a-week outing, then by a visit to a senior center, and so on. The cooperation of the elderly patient may be difficult to obtain, but repeated interventions may yield small changes, with self-reinforcing cumulative improvement. Interventions aimed at similar maladaptive behaviors on the part of others in the patient's environment may be useful; eg, advising family members or caregivers to encourage the patient to perform self-care activities and not to constantly ask the patient about pain, which only adds to the patient's ruminations.

Attempts to provide pain relief should not be neglected; nonpharmacologic methods should be stressed. Cognitive approaches (eg, relaxation training and distraction), transcutaneous electrical nerve stimulation and counterirritation, trigger point injection, spray-and-stretch techniques, and physical therapy may all be useful. Therapy with an NSAID and perhaps a tricyclic antidepressant may help. Opioid therapy is occasionally considered in responsible patients willing to conform to strict management guidelines (see TABLE 12–6). Patients with profound abnormal illness behavior often benefit from referral to a pain clinic, which applies the same principles with greater resources.

13. CANCER IN THE ELDERLY

(See also Chs. 50, 60, 67, 71, 72, and 101)

The probability of developing cancer increases rapidly with advancing age. More than 50% of new cases of cancer and 67% of all cancer deaths occur in people > 65 yr. The enormous, cumulative lifetime risk of cancer and the impact of cancer in the rapidly growing, older population suggest a forthcoming major health care problem.

In the past 20 yr, the incidences of lung, breast, and prostate cancer; malignant melanoma; and non-Hodgkin's lymphoma have increased. Until age 50, the incidence of cancer is higher in women, but after age 60, the incidence increases remarkably among men (see FIG. 13–1). However, lung cancer, common in elderly men, is becoming increasingly common in women. In the USA, it is the leading cause of death from cancer among women, killing more women than breast cancer.

Because of the increased incidence and prevalence of cancer in older persons and the high mortality rate from cancer, some have implied that little progress has been made in the fight against cancer in the USA. This is not true. But the major advances have benefited children and younger adults. The cure rates are high for acute leukemia in children, testicular cancer, and Hodgkin's disease; among persons < 55 yr, all cancer mortality has decreased by 23%. In contrast, among persons > 55 yr, cancer mortality has increased by 17%. Survival rates are lower in older adults than in younger adults for most types of cancer, even within the same stage at diagnosis.

Etiology

Whether the increased incidence of cancer in the elderly results primarily from the biological changes of aging or from prolonged exposure to carcinogens is not known. Observations support both theories. Age-dependent decreases in mitochondrial activity lead to an impaired ability to fight cancer. Changes in the immune system, often called immune senescence, include decreased interleukin-2 levels, decreased T-cell function, and impaired mitogen responsiveness, which are thought to lead to a decreased ability to recognize and destroy cancerous mutations at the microscopic stage. Decreased immune function may also place older persons at risk of viral infections that lead to cancer, such as Kaposi's sarcoma and lymphoma.

However, prolonged exposure is also likely to play a role. Some cancers (eg, gastric, lung, skin, colon) are clearly related to exposure to carcinogens. These cancers rarely occur in younger adults, and when they do, exposure has usually been extraordinary or a genetic defect has impaired the ability to detoxify the carcinogen. Moreover, the incidence of these cancers, even within the elderly population, has been closely associated with the duration and degree of exposure to toxic substances.

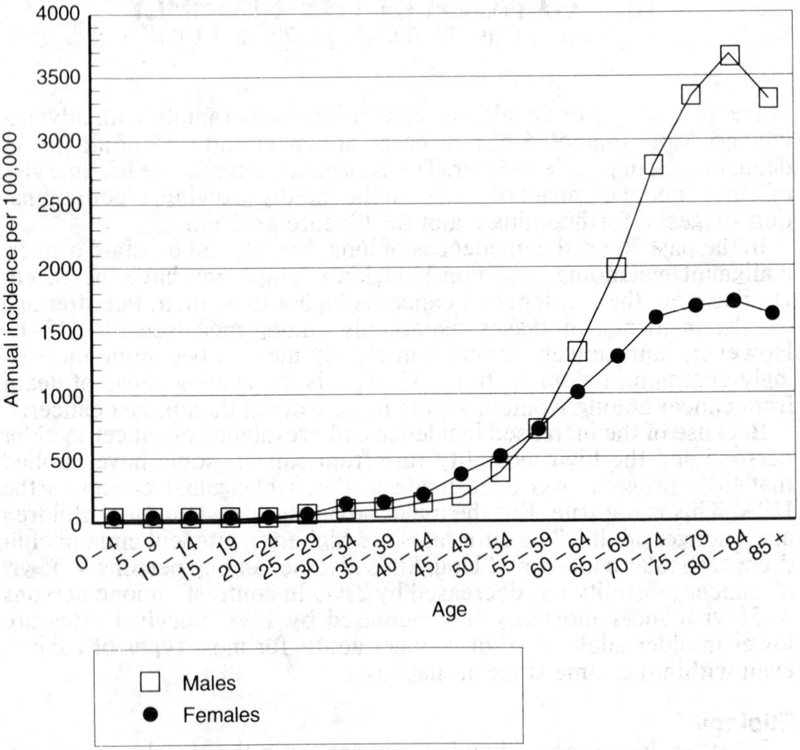

FIG. 13–1. Annual incidence of cancer by age. (Modified from Kennedy BJ, Bushhouse SA, Bender AP: "Minnesota population cancer risk." *Cancer* 73(3):724–729, 1994; used with permission.)

Management

Attitudes toward the older patient have affected the management of cancer. Many health care professionals associate chronologic age with poor prognosis, cognitive impairment, decreased quality of life, limited life expectancy, and decreased social worth. Thus, the elderly receive less screening for cancer, less staging of diagnosed cancer, less aggressive therapy, and often no treatment at all.

In the elderly, mammography, breast self-examination, and thorough clinical breast examination are performed less often than recommended. Likewise, prostate examination and stool guaiac testing are not performed yearly on most elders. Also, older patients may attribute the symptoms of cancer to the aging process, delaying medical attention even further. When older patients do seek medical attention, physicians tend to pursue a diagnosis less aggressively than they would with younger patients. Thus, for these reasons alone, the higher mortality rates among the elderly are not surprising. Screening for cancer in the elderly should follow the guidelines in TABLE 20–1.

Diagnostic and treatment decisions should not be based on a person's age alone. However, age-related reductions in organ function—including losses in renal, pulmonary, and immune function—and the patient's ability to tolerate procedures and treatment must be considered. Treatment regimens and dose adjustments should be based on physiology, health status, and the patient's wishes, not age alone.

Currently, older persons receive treatment less often than younger people; when older persons do receive treatment, often it is less aggressive. One reason is that the risks associated with aggressive therapy and the best modifications to standard protocols when applied to the elderly are not fully understood. As a result, a great need exists for basic and clinical research of cancer in older persons to guide clinical practice. Another reason is that older patients may decline diagnostic and therapeutic procedures because they do not understand the advances in medical care and believe that cancer is hopeless. Sometimes, the decision to forgo treatment or to accept less aggressive treatment is appropriate. Patients and families should receive honest, detailed explanations of the risks and benefits along with advice on support programs such as family counseling, group counseling, and home health care services.

14. PRESSURE SORES

(Decubitus Ulcers; Bedsores)

Ischemic damage and subsequent necrosis affecting the skin, the subcutaneous tissue, and often the muscle covering bony prominences, resulting from exertion of intense pressure for a short time or low pressure for a long time.

The terms **decubitus ulcer** and **bedsore** have been used to describe this problem. Translated literally from Latin, decubitus means "a lying down," which implies a specific positional predisposition to pressure sores. Although pressure sores usually occur from the waist down on bedridden patients, they can develop anywhere on the body (eg, in the nares or in the corners of the mouth from nasogastric or endotracheal tubes) and with the patient in any position. They may also occur interdigitally in patients whose hands are gnarled from rheumatoid arthritis and are common over the ischial tuberosities of patients who sit for prolonged periods. Therefore, **pressure sore** is the preferred term to describe this condition.

TABLE 14–1. COMMON PRESSURE POINTS

Most common sites	Sacrum Greater trochanters Ischium Medial and lateral condyles Malleolus Heels
Less common sites	Elbows Scapulae Vertebrae Ribs Ears Back of head

INCIDENCE AND ETIOLOGY

In the USA, as many as 10% to 20% of patients are admitted to the hospital with a pressure sore or develop one during hospitalization. Most pressure sores occur in patients > 70 yr. Among nursing home residents, the prevalence of pressure sores has been reported to be as high as 23%.

When a patient develops pressure sores, the cost of medical and nursing care may increase by $2,000 to $10,000, although this increase is difficult to estimate. Complications such as sepsis and osteomyelitis add to the length of the hospital stay and the time needed for rehabilitation. Moreover, pressure sores increase mortality in older patients.

Four physical factors contribute to skin breakdown: pressure, friction, shearing, and maceration.

Pressure is the primary external factor causing ischemic damage and tissue necrosis. Normal capillary blood pressure at the arteriolar end of the vascular bed averages 32 mm Hg. When tissues are externally compressed, that pressure may be exceeded; blood supply to and lymphatic drainage of the affected area are reduced. When a patient sits or lies supine, the surface of the seat or bed puts excessive pressure on bony prominences, or **pressure points** (see TABLE 14–1). For a patient in the sitting position, pressures > 300 mm Hg can be exerted against the ischial tuberosities, a common area of breakdown in those who sit for long periods or are confined to a wheelchair.

Friction occurs when the skin rubs against another surface, resulting in the loss of epidermal cells. This may happen when a patient slides down in bed or is pulled up in bed without a pull sheet.

Shearing occurs when two layers of skin slide on each other, moving in opposite directions and causing damage to the underlying tissue. This may happen when a patient is transferred from bed to stretcher or when a patient slides down in a chair.

Maceration, caused by excessive moisture, softens the skin and reduces its resistance. This can occur with excessive perspiration, urinary or fecal incontinence, or grossly exudative wounds.

Additional risk factors for pressure sores include immobility, inactivity, fecal and urinary incontinence, poor or borderline nutritional status, and decreased level of consciousness. Medical conditions associated with these risk factors and with pressure sore formation include anemia, infections, peripheral vascular disease, edema, diabetes mellitus, stroke, dementia, alcoholism, fractures, and malignancies. Other relevant factors include low body weight, smoking, and corticosteroid use.

CLASSIFICATION

Staging or classification systems are commonly used to describe the severity of skin breakdown. Similar to the system for burn assessment, the following classification provides a clear, objective way to describe the degree of tissue breakdown, a common language for all members of the health care team, and a basis for developing treatment protocols for each stage.

Stage 1: Nonblanchable erythema of intact skin; the heralding lesion of skin ulceration. Reactive hyperemia should not be confused with a stage 1 pressure ulcer. This stage is reversible.

Stage 2: Partial-thickness skin loss involving epidermis and/or dermis. The ulcer is superficial and presents clinically as an abrasion, blister, or shallow crater. This stage is also reversible.

Stage 3: Full-thickness skin loss involving damage or necrosis of subcutaneous tissue that may extend down to, but not through, underlying fascia. The ulcer presents clinically as a deep crater with or without undermining of adjacent tissue. This stage may be life threatening.

Stage 4: Full-thickness skin loss with extensive destruction, tissue necrosis, or damage to muscle, bone, or supporting structures (eg, tendon or joint capsule). Undermining and sinus tracts may also be associated with stage 4 pressure ulcers. Osteomyelitis or septic arthritis in contiguous joints may prove fatal.

LABORATORY FINDINGS

Routine culturing of pressure sores in the absence of clinical symptoms and signs of infection (elevated temperature, inflamed wound margins, malodorous exudate) is of questionable value. Growth of common pathogens (eg, *Staphylococcus aureus, Escherichia coli, Proteus mirabilis*) in such cultures does not necessarily indicate an infection requiring antibiotic therapy. If, however, there are symptoms and signs of bacteremia or systemic infection or if healing of the pressure sore is delayed, a wound culture and sensitivity test are indicated. Bacterial counts of 100,000/gm of tissue (determined by biopsy in special situations) represent a critical value for wound infection, correlating with the inability of the wound to heal normally.

An untreated pressure sore may lead to cellulitis or a chronic infection. A diagnosis of **osteomyelitis** in the bone under the pressure sore must be considered. Although frequently overlooked, osteomyelitis is associated with high morbidity and mortality rates. It usually occurs in long-standing pressure sores but may also occur in those that have developed within 2 wk. A **technetium Tc 99m medronate scan,** alone or in combination with an **x-ray,** is recommended to detect osteomyelitis. If either test is abnormal, a biopsy of the bone under the pressure sore should be obtained, and antibiotic therapy should be initiated based on the culture results.

Other laboratory values that may be abnormal in patients at risk for or with pressure sores include a low hemoglobin level (< 12 gm/dL), a low total lymphocyte count (< 1200 μL), a low serum albumin level (≤ 3.3 gm/dL), and a low serum transferrin level (< 170 mg/dL).

PREVENTION AND MODIFICATION OF RISK FACTORS

Identifying **risk factors** and examining the patient's skin, especially over bony prominences, at least daily are essential for preventing pressure sores. A systematic risk assessment should be documented, using a validated assessment tool such as the Norton Scale or the Braden Scale (see FIG. 14–1). These tools help identify and rate such potential risk factors as poor sensory perception, incontinence, immobility, poor nutrition, friction, and shearing. After risk factors have been identified and rated, a preventive regimen should be initiated and documented in the patient's record.

1. Institute a written turning schedule adapted to the patient's activity level and daily routine. The patient's position should be changed q 2 h. High-risk patients should be turned from the supine position to the right or left 30° oblique position because such changes relieve pressure on all major pressure points. Patients should not be placed in a 90° lateral position because it puts intense pressure on the greater trochanter and lateral malleolus.

2. Limit the time the patient sits up in a chair to no more than 2 h. This position creates intense pressure on the ischial tuberosities. A chair that will not allow the patient to slide down should be used to avoid friction and shearing forces. A seat cushion made with high-density foam or plastic or silicone gel pads should be used to reduce pressure against bony prominences. However, no cushion uniformly distributes and relieves pressure entirely. *Pillows and rubber rings (donuts) should not be used* because they may cause compression and decrease blood supply to the area.

3. Avoid elevating the head of the bed more than 30° (except when the patient is eating) to reduce shearing forces. For the same reason, a pull sheet should be used to help move the patient up in bed.

4. Teach the patient to change position and make frequent small body shifts, if possible, to help redistribute body weight and promote blood flow to the tissues. Range-of-motion exercises and ambulation at least q 8 h, if possible, help prevent contractures, improve circulation, and maintain joint integrity, mobility, and muscle mass.

5. Select the appropriate bed surface. The following bed surfaces are listed in order of effectiveness, from minimal to maximal pressure relief.

Convoluted foam pad. This high-density, solid, 3- to 4-in. foam pad is less likely to be compressed by the patient's weight and may redistribute body weight effectively. **Advantages:** The foam pad is (1) inexpensive, (2) lightweight, and (3) comfortable. **Disadvantages:** It (1) provides minimal pressure relief and thus limited protection, (2) may cause retention of body heat, thereby increasing perspiration and the potential for maceration, and (3) is a fire hazard and may emit lethal fumes if ignited. **Indications** include patients whose activity is limited for a short time, such as postoperative patients and those in the operating room undergoing lengthy surgical procedures.

Alternating pressure mattress. This vinyl, air-filled mattress inflates and deflates small air cells at regular intervals via an electric pump. Some models have vents that allow air to circulate between the mattress and the patient. **Advantages:** The mattress (1) mechanically alters the points of pressure against the body, (2) provides a moderate degree of protection against pressure, (3) decreases maceration (models with air vents), (4) is lightweight, and (5) is easy to clean if wet or soiled. **Disadvantages:** It (1) minimizes but does not completely prevent pressure, (2) may be uncomfortable because it feels lumpy, and (3) is more costly because an electric pump is needed. **Indications** include patients at high risk for skin breakdown and those with stage 1 or 2 pressure sores.

Water mattress. This heavy, vinyl, water-filled mattress is placed on top of the bed mattress. **Advantages:** The water mattress (1) distributes the patient's weight evenly over the greatest possible surface, (2) provides moderate protection against pressure, (3) is comfortable, (4) is easy to maintain (no pumps required), and (5) is easy to clean if wet or soiled. **Disadvantages:** It (1) minimizes but does not prevent pressure, (2) is heavy (130 to 150 lb when filled), and (3) costs about the same as an air mattress. **Indications** include patients at high risk for and patients who already have stage 1, 2, or 3 pressure sores.

Patient's Name		*Evaluator's Name*		*Date of Assessment*				
Sensory perception Ability to respond meaningfully to pressure-related discomfort	**1.** *Completely limited:* Unresponsive (does not moan, flinch, or grasp) to painful stimuli, owing to diminished level of consciousness or sedation or limited ability to feel pain over most of body surface	**2.** *Very limited:* Responds only to painful stimuli; cannot communicate discomfort except by moaning or restlessness or has a sensory impairment that limits the ability to feel pain or discomfort over half of body	**3.** *Slightly limited:* Responds to verbal commands but cannot always communicate discomfort or need to be turned or has some sensory impairment that limits ability to feel pain or discomfort in 1 or 2 extremities	**4.** *No impairment:* Responds to verbal commands; has no sensory deficit that would limit ability to feel or voice pain or discomfort				
Moisture Degree to which skin is exposed to moisture	**1.** *Constantly moist:* Skin is kept moist almost constantly by perspiration, urine, etc; dampness is detected every time patient is moved or turned	**2.** *Moist:* Skin is often but not always moist; linen must be changed at least once a shift	**3.** *Occasionally moist:* Skin is occasionally moist, requiring extra linen change about once a day	**4.** *Rarely moist:* Skin is usually dry; linen changes required only at routine intervals				
Activity Degree of physical activity	**1.** *Bedfast:* Confined to bed	**2.** *Chairfast:* Ability to walk severely limited or nonexistent; cannot bear own weight or must be assisted into chair or wheelchair	**3.** *Walks occasionally:* Walks occasionally during day but for very short distances, with or without assistance; spends most of each shift in bed or chair	**4.** *Walks frequently:* Walks outside the room at least twice a day and inside room at least once every 2 h during waking hours				

Mobility Ability to change and control body position	**1.** *Completely immobile:* Does not make even slight changes in body or extremity position without assistance	**2.** *Very limited:* Makes occasional slight changes in body or extremity position but unable to make frequent or significant changes independently	**3.** *Slightly limited:* Makes frequent though slight changes in body or extremity position independently	**4.** *No limitations:* Makes major and frequent changes in position without assistance				
Nutrition Usual food intake pattern	**1.** *Very poor:* Never eats a complete meal; rarely eats > ⅓ of any food offered; eats ≤ 2 servings of protein (meat or dairy products) per day; takes fluids poorly; does not take a liquid dietary supplement or is NPO or maintained on clear liquids or IV for > 5 days	**2.** *Probably inadequate:* Rarely eats a complete meal and generally eats only about half of any food offered; protein intake includes only 3 servings of meat or dairy products per day; occasionally takes a dietary supplement or receives less than optimum amount of liquid diet or tube feeding	**3.** *Adequate:* Eats > ½ of most meals; eats a total of 4 servings of protein (meat, dairy products) each day; occasionally refuses a meal, but usually takes a supplement if offered or is on a tube feeding or TPN regimen, which probably meets most of nutritional needs	**4.** *Excellent:* Eats most of every meal; never refuses a meal; usually eats a total of ≥ 4 servings of meat and dairy products; occasionally eats between meals; does not require supplementation				

FIG. 14–1. Braden Scale for predicting pressure sore risk. To use the Braden Scale, assess and score a patient in the six categories described: sensory perception, moisture, activity, mobility, nutrition, and friction and shear. (Modified from Braden B, Bergstrom N: "Pressure ulcers in adults: Prediction and prevention." *Clinical Practice Guideline*, Number 3, May 1992. US Department of Health and Human Services.) *(continued)*

Friction and shear	**1.** *Problem:* Requires moderate to maximum assistance in moving; complete lifting without sliding against sheets is impossible; frequently slides down in bed or chair, requiring frequent repositioning with maximum assistance; spasticity, contractures, or agitation leads to almost constant friction	**2.** *Potential problem:* Moves feebly or requires minimum assistance; during a move skin probably slides to some extent against sheets, chair, restraints, or other devices; maintains relatively good position in chair or bed most of the time but occasionally slides down	**3.** *No apparent problem:* Moves in bed and in chair independently and has sufficient muscle strength to lift up completely during move; maintains good position in bed or chair at all times					
NPO = nothing by mouth; TPN = total parenteral nutrition.				*Total Score*				

Fig. 14–1 *(continued)*. **Braden Scale for predicting pressure sore risk.**

Air-fluidized bed (eg, Clinitron, Fluid Air, Mediscus Heavy Duty System). This mattress filled with ultrafine silicone-coated beads has warm air flowing through a compressor. A loose polyester sheet separates the patient from the beads, allowing air to circulate around the skin and body fluids to drain into the bed. When the compressor is turned off, the beads firmly mold around the patient, facilitating positioning for dressing changes, transfers, or cardiopulmonary resuscitation. **Advantages:** The bed (1) supports the patient at subcapillary closing pressures (< 15 to 33 mm Hg), (2) provides maximum protection against pressure, friction, shearing, and maceration, and (3) is usually considered comfortable. **Disadvantages:** It (1) has a fixed height and immovable head, making patient transfers in and out of bed difficult, (2) cannot maintain a patient in the semi-Fowler's or Fowler's position, causing difficulty when the patient eats or has pulmonary problems, (3) weighs about 1800 lb, (4) circulates warm air that may dehydrate the patient and the wound, (5) moves and molds, so that turning the patient is difficult (although the manufacturer claims the patient needs to be turned less often, turning and range-of-motion exercises are needed to prevent pulmonary and renal complications and flexion contractures), (6) has an expensive rental fee ($50 to $100/day), and (7) has complexities that make it difficult to adapt for home use. **Indications** include patients with any stage pressure sore, particularly stages 3 and 4 and patients undergoing graft or flap surgery.

Low-air-loss bed (eg, Flexicair, Mediscus Air Support Therapy). This bed consists of air-filled cushions arranged in a segmented configuration and fitted onto a hospital bed frame. The cushions are filled to exert the lowest possible pressure for the patient's height, weight, and body type. The distribution of air pressure supports the patient uniformly over a maximum area with minimum pressure on bony prominences. **Advantages:** The bed (1) may be raised or lowered, easing patient transfers in and out of bed, (2) provides low pressure, (3) decreases friction and shear, (4) prevents moisture buildup, (5) reduces patient dehydration, and (6) allows patients to be placed in the semi-Fowler's position. **Disadvantage:** It is expensive (rental fee up to $150/day). **Indications** are the same as for the air-fluidized bed.

6. Select the appropriate adjunctive devices, such as sheepskin, protective pads for heels, elbow protectors, and trapezes.

Sheepskin is not thick or dense enough to reduce pressure but may be useful if the patient is predisposed to skin breakdown from friction. For example, a sheepskin at the foot of the bed may decrease friction against the heels of patients with vascular disease.

Heel and elbow protectors (pads made of sheepskin or a synthetic equivalent) are effective primarily in decreasing friction. Some models offer protection from pressure as well.

A **trapeze** enables the patient to move or shift weight while in bed.

7. Evaluate and manage incontinence. An assessment of the patient's patterns of incontinence should be followed by a medical evaluation to identify causes, such as a urinary tract infection or side effects of a medication (see Ch. 15). A bowel and bladder management program that involves the patient and family should be developed.

8. Keep the skin clean and dry. The following regimen is suggested.

Gently wash the area with plain water or a small amount of mild soap and water, applying minimal force and friction to the skin. Soap removes the skin's natural protective oils, and cleaning the soap residue may mean massaging already damaged tissues. Next, apply a thin layer of moisturizing lotion, massaging gently around, rather than over, the reddened area or bony prominence. Vigorous massage may increase tissue damage by creating shearing forces.

After moisturizing the area, apply a thin layer of a petroleum-based product. These water-resistant products provide a protective barrier against urine and feces. Heavier agents, such as zinc oxide and aluminum paste, are not recommended; although protective, they are difficult to remove.

Do not place plastic-lined paper bed pads directly against the patient's skin because they can cause drying and irritation. Use as few pads as possible to protect the bedding, and cover them with a draw sheet or pillowcase. Apply a light dusting of a noncaking body powder (eg, commercially prepared cornstarch baby powder) to the skin folds to reduce friction and shearing and to absorb moisture.

Use absorbent incontinence briefs, indwelling bladder catheters, or condom catheters judiciously. They may be indicated for some patients but should not be substituted for efforts to help a patient regain continence through bowel and bladder management programs.

9. Monitor nutritional status at least twice a month. A nutritional consultation is recommended for patients who have a borderline or poor nutritional status (see Ch. 2). Anthropometric measurements and laboratory data (serum albumin level, serum transferrin level, and total lymphocyte count) should be obtained. If serum albumin is < 3.3 gm/dL, serum transferrin is < 170 mg/dL, and total lymphocyte count is $< 1200/\mu L$, oral supplements should be given. Canned oral supplements are relatively inexpensive and provide additional protein, calories, essential fatty acids, and trace elements needed for wound healing. In general, patients at high risk of developing pressure sores should be given supplements with vitamin C and zinc because they promote skin growth.

Functional disabilities affecting intake (eg, poor dentition, poorly fitting dentures) should be identified and modified when possible. If oral supplementation cannot meet a patient's nutritional requirements, alternative methods (eg, nasogastric feedings, gastrostomy feedings, or total parenteral nutrition) must be considered.

TREATMENT

Specific treatment of a pressure sore is based on its stage. With all stages, identifying and reducing risk factors and performing appropriate interventions are essential. Specific types of dressings and topical agents are described under DRESSINGS AND TOPICAL AGENTS, below.

GENERAL PRINCIPLES

NOTE: *Heat lamps are not recommended for treating a pressure sore at any stage.* Besides posing a risk of injury, these lamps dehydrate wounds, inhibiting the healing process.

Stage 1

Cleaning the wound with normal saline solution only is safe and effective. Selection of the dressing may be dictated by location of the wound; either a liquid barrier, a film dressing, or a hydrocolloid dressing may be used. All decrease friction, shearing, and maceration.

Stage 2

The wound should be cleaned with normal saline solution. The dressing choices include film, hydrocolloid, and hydrogel dressings. Moist normal saline dressings may be used, although they require more frequent changes and tend to be less comfortable. Dry sterile dressings are not recommended because they dry out the wound and delay healing.

Stage 3

The intense focus on local care may mean that risk factors are overlooked. However, risk factors must be assessed and modified. For healing to occur, the wound must be free of infection and necrotic tissue. If signs of infection are present (elevated temperature, malodorous exudate, inflamed tissue surrounding the wound), culture and sensitivity studies should be performed. Until the results are known, wound and skin precautions should be taken.

If necrotic tissue is present, mechanical, surgical, or chemical debridement may be performed to attain a clean wound base. For **mechanical debridement,** irrigation with normal saline is used to clean the wound of purulent drainage or necrotic debris. Antiseptic agents (eg, 1% povidone-iodine, 3% hydrogen peroxide, 0.5% sodium hypochlorite, and 0.25% acetic acid) are not recommended as irrigating agents because they have been found to adversely affect wound healing unless carefully diluted to specific noncytotoxic concentrations. The wound may be irrigated with a catheter-tipped syringe, using aseptic technique. Alternatively, a high-pressure dental irrigation device provides a pulsating stream that both aids debridement and stimulates circulation. A wet-to-dry dressing, consisting of plain loosely woven gauze without cotton filling, moistened with normal saline is then gently packed to conform to the wound without extending onto the intact skin, since this may cause tissue irritation or maceration. The packing material should be appropriate to the wound size and depth, and care must be taken not to pack the wound too tightly, since this inhibits the absorptive capability of the dressing and applies pressure on the area. Loose necrotic tissue and wound drainage are absorbed into the dressing and removed with each dressing change (usually q 8 h). Other packing materials include the absorption and calcium alginate dressings described below.

An appropriately sized outer dressing should be applied over the packed wound to prevent contamination from the environment. This dry, sterile dressing should be secured with hypoallergenic tape or other devices, such as Montgomery straps or stockinette. The intact surrounding skin should be protected.

For local control of infected wounds (as evidenced by a bacterial count > 10^5/gm of tissue), 1% silver sulfadiazine can be used to reduce bacterial counts and establish a clean wound. A sterile glove should be worn during application, and the agent should be worked into the crevices of the wound. Then the wound should be covered with a fine mesh gauze.

Mechanical debridement is minimally effective on eschar. **Surgical debridement** is the quickest way to remove necrotic tissue and the only effective way to remove eschar. However, surgical debridement may increase the risk of hemorrhage, infection, wound enlargement, and pain. **Chemical debridement** (using enzymatic agents) is most effective when used in combination with mechanical or surgical debridement.

After debridement, a moist environment should be maintained to facilitate granulation and wound healing. Either a moist normal saline dressing (changed every 6 to 8 h) or an absorption or calcium alginate dressing may be used.

Care of a stage 3 pressure sore is costly and labor-intensive. Although many such wounds heal slowly by secondary intention, surgical closure is often needed to shorten hospitalization and rehabilitation.

Stage 4

Care of a stage 4 pressure sore is similar to that of a stage 3 pressure sore. Variations may be indicated in the presence of sinus tracts or exposed bone. Irrigation should be performed as described for stage 3. If sinus tracts are present, an appropriately sized red rubber catheter attached to an irrigating syringe may be used to direct the flow of irrigant. All exudate and necrotic debris must be removed from narrow pathways.

The wound, including crevices and sinuses, should be packed loosely. If used, gauze should be kept in one piece for easy removal and to ensure that no dressing material will be left in the wound. Rolled gauze is available in various widths; if more than one roll is needed, the rolls should be tied together. Exposed bone should be covered with a wet, normal saline dressing, which should be changed q 4 h to avoid drying and maintain viability of the bone tissue. An outer dressing should be applied as with a stage 3 wound.

Surgical debridement to thoroughly excise infected or necrotic tissue usually is followed by a musculocutaneous flap procedure. Postoperative care includes monitoring the patient for infection and keeping pressure off the flap site.

DRESSINGS AND TOPICAL AGENTS

The dressings and topical agents most commonly used to treat pressure sores include liquid barriers, film dressings, hydrocolloid dressings, debriding enzymes, absorption dressings, hydrogels, and calcium alginate dressings.

Liquid Barriers

These barriers (eg, United Skin Prep, Bard Protective Barrier Film) contain plasticizing agents and alcohol; they provide a protective waterproof coating over affected areas, reducing maceration and shearing. Liquid barriers may be applied using a spray, wipe, or roll-on method. Generally, they do not irritate the skin and are not affected by urine, perspiration, or digestive acids. Although insoluble in water, they can be dissolved by a soap solution. NOTE: *Tincture of benzoin should not be used on reddened areas.* Because of its high alcohol content, it becomes sticky when dry, and fragile skin may be inadvertently pulled.

Guidelines for use: (1) The skin must be gently cleaned and then rinsed and dried. (2) The liquid barrier should be applied and allowed to dry for one minute. (3) The patient may feel a momentary sting when the barrier is applied to excoriated skin.

Film Dressings

Polyurethane dressings (eg, Biocclusive, Tegaderm, Op-Site) are permeable to gases and vapors but not to fluids; thus, oxygen can reach the healing tissues, but contaminating fluids can not. These dressings work on the principle that healing occurs more quickly in a moist environment. Usually left in place for 5 to 7 days, the dressing maintains the wound exudate against the wound surface, promoting epithelial cell migration across the wound.

The exudate that collects under the dressing varies in color and consistency from thin, clear, and serous to thick, cloudy, and brown. This variation is normal, and the exudate should not be drained. If exudate leaks to the surrounding skin, the dressing may need to be changed or a different product used. If wound infection is suspected, the dressing should be changed daily. As the amount of exudate decreases, the exudate becomes darker and begins to dry. When healing is completed, the dressing may be removed or may be used to protect the new skin from shearing, friction, and maceration.

Guidelines for use: (1) The wound and surrounding skin must be cleaned, and the surrounding skin must be dry so the dressing will adhere. (2) The dressing should cover at least a 1-in. margin around the wound. (3) The dressing should not be stretched tightly over the wound; such stretching exerts shearing forces against the tissues. (4) Dressings may be cut or overlapped without reducing effectiveness. (5) If excessive exudate threatens to loosen the dressing, the exudate may be aspirated through the dressing, using a small-bore needle. The dressing may reseal itself or may need to be patched with another piece of dressing.

Hydrocolloid Dressings

These opaque, gas-impermeable occlusive dressings (eg, DuoDERM, Comfeel Ulcer Care Dressing, Restore) consist of inert hydrophobic polymers containing fluid-absorbent hydrocolloid particles. When these particles come in contact with wound exudate, they swell, forming a moist gel that promotes cell migration, cleaning, debridement, and granulation. These dressings work on the principle that optimal wound healing occurs in a closed, moist environment. The lack of atmospheric oxygen is not thought to prevent healing in superficial wounds.

Guidelines for use: (1) The wound and surrounding skin should be cleaned before applying the dressing. The surrounding skin must be dry so the dressing will adhere. (2) The dressing should cover the wound and extend at least 1½ in. beyond its edges. (3) The dressing is not recommended if signs of infection (elevated temperature, purulent malodorous exudate, inflamed borders) are present. (4) The dressing may initially enlarge the wound because of its debriding action. (5) The dressing may be left on for up to 7 days unless exudate leakage occurs.

Debriding Enzymes

These proteolytic and fibrinolytic agents (eg, Travase, Elase, Santyl) act against devitalized tissue. They are most useful on superficial wound layers. Because these agents must be in contact with the substrate of the wound, they are ineffective on dense, dry eschar. They should be used as an adjunct to mechanical or surgical debridement.

Guidelines for use: (1) All hardened or dry eschar should be removed or crosshatched so the enzyme can come in contact with the wound substrate. (2) Because some preparations, such as Elase powder, become inactive in 24 h, they must be reconstituted for each use. (3) Antibacterials and antiseptics (eg, povidone-iodine, hexachlorophene, silver nitrate, hydrogen peroxide, and benzalkonium chloride) may inhibit the action of Travase.

Absorption Dressings

These dressings (eg, Debrisan, Bard Absorption Dressing, Hydra-Gran) consist of hydrophilic beads, grains, or flakes that absorb excess wound exudate and necrotic debris, which may inhibit tissue regeneration. The dressings also keep the wound moist enough to encourage healing and deodorize the wound.

Guidelines for use: (1) The products, reconstituted according to the manufacturer's instructions, are gently packed into the wound and covered with a dry outer dressing. (2) The absorption dressings usually must be changed once or twice a day.

Hydrogels

These polymers (eg, Vigilon, Gel-Syte) absorb wound exudate to form water-soluble gelatinous substances. Semitransparent and nonadhesive, these dressings provide a moist environment for wound healing.

Guidelines for use: (1) The dressing may be refrigerated to promote patient comfort. (2) After the wound has been gently cleaned with normal saline, the dressing (which should extend 1½ in. beyond the wound edges) is applied directly over the wound. (3) The dressing occasionally causes maceration of the surrounding skin. (4) If intact, the dressing may be left on for 1 to 3 days.

Calcium Alginate Dressings

Made of natural polysaccharides found in brown seaweed, the dressing (eg, Sorbsan, Kaltostat) is a high-quality textile fiber pad capable of absorbing 20 times its weight in exudate. On contact with exudate, the dressing forms a soft gas-permeable gel, thereby maintaining a moist environment for wound healing.

Guidelines for use: (1) After the wound is irrigated with normal saline, the dry dressing is applied. (2) As the alginate turns into a gel in the wound, it may produce an unpleasant odor of seaweed, which can be controlled by placing a charcoal pad over the outer gauze dressing. (3) If wounds have heavy exudate, the dressing may need to be changed once or twice daily. As the wound heals, the dressing may be left on longer, up to several days.

---

15. URINARY INCONTINENCE

Urinary incontinence affects 15% to 30% of community-dwelling elderly persons, 30% of those in hospitals, and 50% of those in long-term care institutions. Its burdens are substantial. Incontinent older persons are frequently embarrassed, isolated, stigmatized, depressed, and regressed; they also are predisposed to institutionalization because incontinence is such a significant burden for caregivers. Incontinent persons are also predisposed to perineal rashes, decubitus ulcers, urinary tract infections, urosepsis, falls, and fractures. The economic costs of incontinence are startling. Over $15 billion was spent on the management of incontinence in the USA in 1993, more than the annual amount spent on dialysis and coronary artery bypass surgery combined.

Despite its considerable prevalence, morbidity, and expense, incontinence remains largely a neglected problem. Many incontinent elderly persons dismiss incontinence as a normal part of aging; only a minority consult a health care professional. Even when incontinence is brought to a doctor's attention, it is often inadequately evaluated. Incontinence is abnormal at any age, and regardless of an incontinent person's age, mobility, mental status, or frailty, the condition is highly treatable and often curable.

IMPACT OF AGE ON CONTINENCE

Continence requires not only the integrity of lower urinary tract function but also adequate mentation, mobility, motivation, and manual dexterity.

The lower urinary tract changes with age, even without disease. Bladder capacity, the ability to postpone voiding, and urinary flow rate appear to decline in both sexes. Uninhibited contractions become more prevalent. The postvoiding residual volume increases but probably to no more than 50 to 100 mL. Maximum urethral closure pressure and urethral length probably decline in women, and prostate size increases in most men. The pattern of fluid excretion also changes: younger persons excrete most of their daily ingested fluid before bedtime, whereas many elderly people—even those who do not have peripheral venous insufficiency, renal disease, heart failure, or prostatism—excrete most of theirs during the night. Because of this and an increased prevalence of sleep disorders, most healthy elderly persons have one or two episodes of nocturia every night.

Although none of these age-related changes causes incontinence, each predisposes to it. And an older person is more likely to encounter additional pathologic, physiologic, or pharmacologic insults, which further increase the risk of incontinence. The corollary is equally important. The new onset or exacerbation of incontinence in an older person is likely due to a precipitant outside the lower urinary tract that is often amenable to medical intervention. Treatment of the precipitant alone may be sufficient to restore continence, even if a urinary tract abnormality coexists. For example, in a woman with age-related detrusor overactivity, a flare-up of hip arthritis that impairs mobility may convert urinary urgency to incontinence. Treating the arthritis rather than the uninhibited contractions may not only restore continence but will lessen pain and improve mobility.

CLASSIFICATION OF URINARY INCONTINENCE

Incontinence can be categorized by duration of symptoms, by clinical presentation, or by physiologic abnormality. Determining whether incontinence is of recent onset (transient) or chronic (established) is important because, although some overlap exists, the differential diagnosis of each differs. Categorizing the problem as urge incontinence, stress incontinence, or overflow incontinence offers a framework around which to organize the differential diagnosis, diagnostic evaluation, and treatment options. The clinical presentation may point to an underlying physiologic abnormality as the actual cause of the incontinence, knowledge of which offers the clearest guide to treatment.

TRANSIENT INCONTINENCE

Transient incontinence is common in the elderly, accounting for up to one third of the incontinence in community-dwelling persons and up to half of the incontinence in hospitalized patients. Transient incontinence becomes persistent if its cause is left untreated; the incontinence cannot be considered chronic merely because it is of long-standing duration. The risk of transient incontinence is increased if an older person suffers from a pathologic condition or is taking a medication that could cause incontinence. For example, a person with a weak bladder who takes an anticholinergic agent is more likely to develop overflow incontinence; a person with detrusor overactivity or impaired mobility who is taking a loop diuretic is more likely to develop urge incontinence.

Etiology

The eight reversible causes of transient incontinence can be recalled using the mnemonic DIAPPERS (misspelled with an extra P; see TABLE 15–1). These causes should be assiduously sought in *every* incontinent elderly patient. Identification of these factors is important in all settings because they are easily treatable and contribute to other morbidity. Continence often can be regained by those who become incontinent in the context of acute illness.

Delirium: In a delirious patient, incontinence is merely an associated symptom that abates once the underlying cause of delirium is identified and treated.

Infection: Symptomatic urinary tract infection causes transient incontinence when dysuria and urgency are so severe that the person is unable to reach the toilet before voiding. Asymptomatic infection, which is much more common in the elderly and occurs even in noncatheterized persons, is usually not a cause of incontinence. However, because

TABLE 15–1. CAUSES OF TRANSIENT INCONTINENCE

D	elirium
I	nfection—urinary (symptomatic)
A	trophic urethritis and vaginitis
P	harmaceuticals
P	sychologic disorders, especially depression
E	xcessive urine output (eg, from heart failure or hyperglycemia)
R	estricted mobility
S	tool impaction

Adapted from Resnick NM: "Urinary incontinence in the elderly." *Medical Grand Rounds* 3:281–290, 1984, used with permission.

older patients can present atypically, incontinence is occasionally the only symptom of a urinary tract infection. Thus, if an otherwise asymptomatic urinary tract infection is found on the initial evaluation of incontinence, bacteriuria should be treated and the result documented in the patient's record to prevent futile and unnecessary therapy in the future. However, because treatment may lead to the emergence of resistant organisms, bacteriuria should be treated only when it occurs with otherwise unexplained new onset incontinence, fever, leukocytosis, dysuria, or (particularly in demented or debilitated patients) inanition or agitation. Sexually active women with persistent dysuria, despite negative urinalysis and adequate estrogen treatment, may have *Chlamydia trachomatis* infection and should be tested or treated with doxycycline. Pyuria without bacteriuria should be further evaluated with a urine culture for mycobacteria and with a purified protein derivative (PPD) skin test for tuberculosis.

Atrophic urethritis and vaginitis: These disorders are often a source of lower urinary tract symptoms, including incontinence, in women. As many as 80% of elderly women attending an incontinence clinic have physical evidence of atrophic vaginitis characterized by mucosal atrophy, friability, erosions, and telangiectasia. Atrophic urethritis leads to epithelial and submucosal thinning of the urethra, which may cause local irritation and loss of the mucosal seal. Incontinence associated with atrophic urethritis is characterized usually by urgency and occasionally by a sense of "scalding" dysuria. In demented persons, atrophic urethritis may produce agitation.

Atrophic urethritis and vaginitis can be treated with systemic or topical low-dose estrogen (eg, conjugated estrogen 0.3 to 0.625 mg orally once a day or vaginally in a cream containing 0.625 mg estrogen per gram). While the duration of therapy is not well established, one approach is to administer a low dose of estrogen daily for 1 to 2 mo and then to taper it. Eventually, most patients can be treated as infrequently as two to four times per month. After 6 mo, estrogen can be discontinued entirely in some patients, although recurrence of atrophy is common. Treatment has another benefit: it may ameliorate recurrent cystitis and dyspareunia. Since the estrogen dose is low and given briefly, it has little or no carcinogenic effect. However, if long-term estrogen therapy is required and the patient has an intact uterus, a progestin probably should be added to the regimen (see Ch. 83). Mammography should be performed before initiating hormone therapy, which is contraindicated in women with a history of breast cancer.

Pharmaceuticals: Drugs are a major cause of transient incontinence in the elderly (see TABLE 15–2). Many of these agents also are used to treat incontinence, underscoring the fact that most medications used by the elderly are "double-edged swords." The **long-acting sedative-hypnotics,** such as diazepam and flurazepam whose half-lives can exceed 100 h, can cloud an older patient's sensorium. **Alcohol** has the double effect of clouding the sensorium and inducing a diuresis. **Loop diuretics** such as furosemide or bumetanide can provoke leakage by inducing a brisk diuresis; **methylxanthine agents** such as theophylline and caffeine may have a similar effect in frail persons.

Drugs with anticholinergic side effects present particular problems and include major tranquilizers, most antidepressants, some antiparkinsonian agents (not L-dopa or selegiline but trihexyphenidyl and benztropine mesylate), antihistamines, disopyramide, and gastrointestinal antispasmodics. Opioids are not anticholinergic but nonetheless decrease detrusor contractility. A reduction in detrusor contractility can lead to urinary retention and overflow incontinence. Anticholinergic properties occur in many nonprescription preparations (eg, antihistamines for colds or insomnia) that people take without consulting a physician, and elderly persons often may take more than one.

As direct smooth muscle relaxants, **calcium channel blockers** may increase residual volume and lead to overflow incontinence, particularly in older women with detrusor weakness and a weak urethral sphincter or in men with urethral obstruction. The dihydropyridine class of these drugs also may cause peripheral edema, which exacerbates nocturia and nocturnal incontinence.

By blocking receptors for smooth muscle contraction at the bladder neck, **α-adrenoceptor antagonist antihypertensives** may induce stress incontinence in older women in whom urethral length and closure pressure have decreased. Thus, before interventions for stress incontinence are considered in such women, an alternative antihypertensive drug should be tried and the incontinence should be reevaluated.

In men with otherwise asymptomatic prostatic enlargement, **α-adrenoceptor agonists** in nonprescription preparations such as decongestants may provoke acute retention, especially if the preparation also contains an antihistamine (anticholinergic). For example, uri-

TABLE 15–2. DRUGS THAT CAN CAUSE INCONTINENCE

Type of Drug	*Examples*	*Potential Effects on Continence*
Potent diuretics	Bumetanide, furosemide	Polyuria, frequency, urgency
Anticholinergics	Antihistamines, benztropine, dicyclomine, disopyramide, trihexyphenidyl	Urinary retention and overflow, delirium, fecal impaction
Psychoactives		
Antidepressants	Amitriptyline, desipramine	Anticholinergic actions, sedation
Antipsychotics	Haloperidol, thioridazine	Anticholinergic actions, sedation, rigidity, immobility
Sedatives and hypnotics	Diazepam, flurazepam	Sedation, delirium, immobility
Narcotic analgesics	Opioids	Urinary retention, fecal impaction, sedation, delirium
α-Adrenergic blockers	Prazosin, terazosin	Urethral relaxation
α-Adrenergic agonists	Nasal decongestants	Urinary retention in men
Calcium channel blockers	All	Urinary retention
Alcohol	——	Polyuria, frequency, urgency, sedation, delirium, immobility
Vincristine	——	Urinary retention

Adapted from Kane RL, Ouslander JG, Abrass IB: *Essentials of Clinical Geriatrics*. New York, McGraw-Hill, 1989; p 149; used with permission.

nary retention may be precipitated in an older man who takes a cold capsule, long-acting nose drops, and a hypnotic (usually an antihistamine). How often this results in an unnecessary or premature prostatectomy is unknown.

Vincristine can cause a partially reversible neuropathy that leads to urinary retention. The prostaglandin E_1 analog **misoprostol** has been associated with stress incontinence, possibly through its action on urethral smooth muscle tone. The cough associated with **angiotensin converting enzyme inhibitors** may exacerbate what otherwise would be mild or not bothersome stress incontinence.

Psychologic disorders: Although psychologic causes of incontinence have not been well studied in any age group, they are probably less common in older persons than in younger ones. Initial intervention is directed at the psychologic disturbance, usually depression or lifelong neurosis. Persistent incontinence warrants further evaluation.

Excessive urine output: Causes of excessive urine output include high fluid intake; diuretics (including caffeine and alcohol), metabolic abnormalities (eg, hyperglycemia and hypercalcemia); and disorders associated with fluid overload, including heart failure, peripheral venous insufficiency, hypoalbuminemia (especially in malnourished debilitated elderly), and drug-induced peripheral edema (eg, that associated with nonsteroidal anti-inflammatory drugs and some calcium channel blockers). Factors associated with peripheral edema are likely to be present when incontinence occurs at night.

Restricted mobility: Incontinence can result from not being able to get to the toilet. Many treatable conditions can restrict mobility, including arthritis, hip deformity, physical deconditioning, postural or postprandial hypotension, claudication, spinal stenosis, heart failure, poor eyesight, fear of falling, a stroke, foot problems, and drug-induced disequilibrium or confusion. Restricted mobility may simply be a matter of the patient being restrained in a bed or a chair. A diligent search often identifies these or other correctable causes. If it does not, a urinal or bedside commode may improve or resolve the incontinence.

Stool impaction: Impacted stool is implicated as a cause of urinary incontinence in up to 10% of older patients seen in hospitals or referred to incontinence clinics. The mechanism may involve stimulation of opioid receptors or a mechanical disturbance of the bladder or urethra. Patients usually present with symptoms of either urge or overflow incontinence and typically have associated fecal incontinence as well. Removing the impacted stool restores continence.

ESTABLISHED INCONTINENCE

If leakage persists after transient causes of incontinence have been addressed, lower urinary tract causes must be considered (see TABLE 15–3). Lower urinary tract malfunction generally is similar in older and younger patients, although older persons rarely develop fistulas or impaired detrusor compliance.

TABLE 15–3. LOWER URINARY TRACT CAUSES OF ESTABLISHED INCONTINENCE

Urodynamic Diagnosis	*Some Neurogenic Causes*	*Some Nonneurogenic Causes*
Detrusor overactivity	Multiple sclerosis Stroke Parkinson's disease Alzheimer's disease	Urethral obstruction or incompetence Cystitis Bladder carcinoma Bladder stone
Detrusor underactivity	Disk compression Plexopathy Surgical damage (eg, anteroposterior resection) Autonomic neuropathy (eg, from diabetes mellitus, alcoholism, vitamin B_{12} deficiency)	Idiopathic (common in women) Chronic outlet obstruction
Outlet incompetence	Radical prostatectomy* Lower motor neuron lesion (rare)	Urethral hypermobility (type 1 and 2 SUI) Sphincter incompetence (type 3 SUI) Prostate surgery
Outlet obstruction	Spinal cord lesion with detrusor-sphincter dyssynergia (rare)	Prostate enlargement Prostate carcinoma Large cystocele Anterior urethral stricture Following bladder neck suspension

SUI = stress urinary incontinence.
* Other prostate surgery rarely causes *neurogenic* incontinence.
Adapted from Resnick NM: "Urinary incontinence—A treatable disorder," in *Geriatric Medicine,* ed. 2, edited by JW Rowe. Boston, Little, Brown and Company, 1988, p 250; used with permission.

Etiology

Detrusor overactivity: The leading urinary tract cause of incontinence in older persons is detrusor overactivity, a generic term for uninhibited bladder contractions. The distinction between detrusor overactivity associated with a CNS lesion (detrusor hyperreflexia) and that which is not (detrusor instability) is often less clear in older patients. Uninhibited contractions may occur incidental to normal aging, a past stroke, prostatic outlet obstruction, or stress incontinence—even in persons with Alzheimer's disease. No reliable way is known to determine the source of such contractions. While detrusor overactivity is the primary urinary tract cause of incontinence in demented patients, it is also the most common cause in nondemented patients. Two studies have failed to find a definite association between cognitive status and detrusor overactivity. Moreover, demented patients may also be incontinent because of transient causes (see TRANSIENT INCONTINENCE, above) or other urinary tract abnormalities.

Detrusor overactivity is characterized by **frequent and precipitant voiding.** The urge to void comes on abruptly. The volume of leakage is usually moderate to large, nocturnal frequency and incontinence are common, sacral sensation and reflexes are preserved, voluntary control of the anal sphincter is intact, and the postvoiding residual volume is generally low. A residual volume > 50 to 100 mL in a patient with detrusor overactivity suggests outlet obstruction (although the residual may be nil in early obstruction), detrusor hyperactivity with impaired contractility, or pooling of urine in a cystocele (in a woman) or large bladder diverticulum. A large residual volume is also found in patients with Parkinson's disease, spinal cord injury, or diabetic neuropathy.

Detrusor overactivity in the elderly exists as two physiologic subsets: one in which contractile function is preserved and one in which it is impaired. The latter condition is termed **detrusor hyperactivity with impaired contractility (DHIC)** and is the most common cause of established incontinence in frail elderly persons. Because the bladder is weak in DHIC, urinary retention is common. Even without urinary retention, DHIC mimics virtually every other lower urinary tract cause of incontinence. For example, if the uninhibited contraction is triggered by or occurs coincidentally with a stress maneuver, DHIC may be misdiagnosed as stress incontinence. Alternatively, because DHIC is associated with urgency, frequency, a weak flow rate, significant residual urine, and bladder trabeculation, it may mimic prostatism in men. Finally, bladder weakness may interfere with anticholinergic therapy of DHIC if urinary retention is induced. Thus, alternative therapeutic approaches are often required (see TREATMENT CONSIDERATIONS, below).

Outlet incompetence: The second most common cause of incontinence in older women is outlet incompetence, which is manifested as **stress incontinence.** Leakage without a bladder contraction occurs coincidentally with stress maneuvers such as coughing, laughing, bending, and lifting.

In women, stress incontinence is usually caused by **pelvic muscle laxity.** A less common cause is **intrinsic sphincter deficiency,** also known as type 3 stress incontinence, which is usually due to operative trauma but also can result from nothing more than urethral atrophy. Women with intrinsic sphincter deficiency may leak even when sitting or standing quietly. This is a helpful diagnostic and therapeutic point, since many women become dry when bladder volume is kept below the leakage threshold (eg, 200 to 400 mL). A third but rare cause of stress incontinence is **urethral instability,** in which the sphincter abruptly and paradoxically relaxes without an apparent detrusor contraction. Most older women who are thought to have urethral instability probably have DHIC instead.

In men, stress incontinence is usually due to **sphincter damage** after transurethral or radical prostatectomy. In both sexes, stress-associated leakage also can occur in association with urinary retention, but in this situation, leakage is not the result of outlet incompetence.

Outlet obstruction: Although outlet obstruction is the second most common cause of incontinence in older men, most men with obstruction are not incontinent. Common causes of outlet obstruction include benign prostatic hyperplasia, prostate cancer, and urethral stricture. Outlet obstruction can also occur in women, but anatomic obstruction is uncommon in women who have not had previous surgery for incontinence or who do not have a large cystocele that prolapses and kinks the urethra when straining to void. Patients who are incontinent because of obstruction most often present with postvoid dribbling. However, if secondary detrusor overactivity develops, urge incontinence may result, and if detrusor decompensation supervenes, overflow incontinence may ensue.

Obstruction that results from neurologic disease is invariably associated with a spinal cord lesion. In this situation, interruptions occur in pathways to the **pontine micturition center** (see FIG. 15–1), where outlet relaxation is coordinated with bladder contraction. Then, rather than relaxing when the bladder contracts, the outlet contracts simultaneously, leading to severe outlet obstruction (causing severe trabeculation, diverticula, and a "Christmas tree" deformation of the bladder; hydronephrosis; and renal failure—a constellation termed **detrusor-sphincter dyssynergia).**

Detrusor underactivity: An underactive detrusor sufficient to cause urinary retention and overflow incontinence is found in only about 5% to 10% of incontinent older persons. Injury may have occurred to the nerves supplying the bladder (eg, by disk compression or tumor involvement). Detrusor underactivity is also caused by the autonomic neuropathy of diabetes, pernicious anemia, Parkinson's disease, alcoholism, or tabes dorsalis. Alternatively, the detrusor may be replaced by fibrosis and connective tissue in men with chronic outlet obstruction, so that the bladder fails to empty normally even when the obstruction is removed. Detrusor weakness may also occur in women, but the cause is unknown.

Symptoms of severe detrusor underactivity (eg, urgency, frequency, and nocturia) may mimic those of detrusor overactivity, and urinary retention must be excluded before initiating treatment for detrusor overactivity. Less severe degrees of bladder weakness are common in older women. Although mild weakness does not cause incontinence, it can complicate treatment when it occurs with other causes of incontinence.

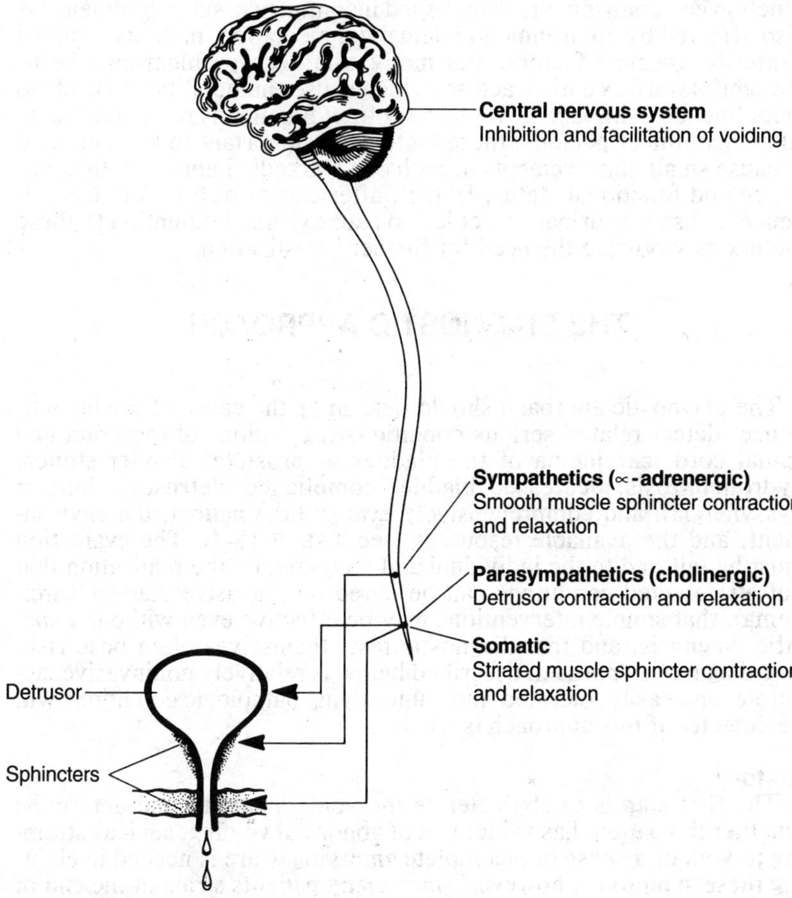

FIG. 15–1. Normal micturition occurs when bladder contraction is coordinated with urethral sphincter relaxation. Four nervous system components are involved: (1) The *central nervous system* inhibits voiding until the appropriate time; it also coordinates and facilitates input from the bladder to start and complete voiding. (2) The *sympathetic system* contracts the smooth muscle sphincter through α-adrenergic fibers from the hypogastric nerve. (3) The *parasympathetic system* contracts the bladder detrusor muscle through cholinergic fibers from the pelvic nerve. (4) The *somatic nervous system* contracts the striated muscle sphincter through cholinergic fibers from the pudendal nerve. (Adapted from DuBeau CE, Resnick NM, with the Massachusetts Department of Health EDUCATE project collaborators. Urinary Incontinence in the Older Adult: An Annotated Speaker/Teacher Kit, 1993; used with permission of the authors.)

Functional incontinence: Factors other than lower urinary tract dysfunction can contribute to established incontinence, since continence is also affected by environmental demands, mentation, mobility, manual dexterity, medical factors, and motivation. The problem may be as straightforward as a hip fracture, which causes immobility and leads to incontinence. Although lower urinary tract function is rarely normal in such incontinent persons, these factors are important to keep in mind because small improvements in each can markedly improve both continence and functional status. In fact, after causes of transient incontinence and severe urinary tract lesions are excluded, attention to these factors may obviate the need for further investigation.

THE DIAGNOSTIC APPROACH

The diagnostic approach should determine the cause of the incontinence; detect related serious conditions (eg, lesions of the brain and spinal cord, carcinoma of the bladder or prostate, bladder stones, hydronephrosis, decreased bladder compliance, detrusor-sphincter dyssynergia); and comprehensively evaluate the patient, the environment, and the available resources (see TABLE 15–4). The evaluation must be tailored to the individual and tempered by the realization that not all detected conditions can be cured (eg, invasive bladder carcinoma), that simple interventions may be effective even without a specific diagnosis, and that diagnostic tests themselves often pose risk. The diagnostic approach described below is relatively noninvasive, accurate, and easily tolerated; most underlying pathologic conditions will be detected if this approach is used.

History

The first step is to characterize the voiding pattern and determine whether the patient has symptoms of abnormal voiding, such as straining to void or a sense of incomplete emptying. Care is needed in eliciting these symptoms, however, since many patients strain at the end of voiding to empty the last few drops. On the other hand, many patients have been straining for so long that they fail to acknowledge it. Thus, observations by the physician and family members are extremely useful. The doctor or nurse then elicits a detailed description of the incontinence, focusing on its onset, frequency, severity, pattern, precipitants, palliating features, and associated symptoms and conditions.

Voiding record: One of the most helpful components of the history is the voiding record kept by the patient or caregiver during a 48- to 72-h period. The chart notes the volume and time of each void or incontinent episode. A measuring cup, coffee can, jar, or other large container can be used at home to measure and record the volume voided. Many voiding records have been devised; a sample is shown in TABLE 15–5.

TABLE 15–4. CLINICAL EVALUATION OF THE INCONTINENT PATIENT

History	Type (urge, reflex, stress, overflow, or mixed) Frequency, severity, duration Pattern (diurnal, nocturnal, or both; also, for example, after taking medications) Associated symptoms (straining to void, incomplete emptying, dysuria, hematuria, suprapubic or perineal discomfort) Alteration in bowel habit or sexual function Other relevant factors (eg, cancer, diabetes, acute illness, neurologic disease, urinary tract infections, pelvic or lower urinary tract surgery or radiation therapy) Medications, including nonprescription drugs Functional assessment
Physical examination	Identify other medical conditions (eg, heart failure, peripheral edema) Test for stress-induced leakage when bladder is full Observe or listen to voiding Palpate for bladder distention after voiding Conduct pelvic examination (looking for atrophic vaginitis, pelvic muscle laxity, pelvic mass) Examine the rectum (looking for skin irritation, resting tone and voluntary control of anal sphincter, prostate nodules, fecal impaction) Perform a neurologic examination (mental status and elemental examination, including sacral reflexes and perineal sensation)
Initial investigation	Voiding record or chart of episodes of incontinence Metabolic survey (measurement of electrolytes, calcium, glucose, and BUN) Measurement of postvoiding residual volume Urinalysis and culture Renal ultrasound* Urine cytology* Uroflowmetry* Cytoscopy?*

* See text.

Adapted from information appearing in Resnick NM, Yalla SV: "Management of urinary incontinence in the elderly." *New England Journal of Medicine* 313:800–805, 1985; used with permission.

The **volume voided** provides an index of functional bladder capacity and, together with the **pattern of voiding and leakage,** can be quite helpful in pointing to the cause of the leakage. For example, incontinence that occurs only between 8 AM and noon may be caused by a morning

TABLE 15–5. SAMPLE VOIDING RECORD OF INCONTINENT 75–YR–OLD

Date	*Time*	*Volume Voided (mL)*	*Patient Wet or Dry*	*Approximate Volume of Leakage*	*Comments*
4/5	3:50 PM	240	Wet	Slight	
	6:05 PM	210	Dry		
	8:15 PM	150	Dry		
	10:20 PM	150	Wet	15 mL	Sound of running water precipitated episode
	10:30 PM	30	Dry		Bowel movement
4/6	3:15 AM	270	Dry		
	6:05 AM	300	Dry		
	7:40 AM	200	Dry		
	9:50 AM	?	Dry		
	11:20 AM	200	Dry		
	12:50 PM	180	Dry		
	1:40 PM	240	Dry		
	3:35 PM	160	Wet	Slight	
	6:00 PM	170	Wet	Slight	Sound of running water precipitated episode
	8:20 PM	215	Wet	Slight	
	10:25 PM	130	Dry		

Notes: Urodynamic evaluation confirmed a diagnosis of detrusor hyperactivity with impaired contractility. However, note the 24-h urine output of nearly 3 L. The patient drank 10 glasses of fluid daily, believing it was good for her health. (Patient did not mention this until queried about the voiding record.) Given the typical voided volume of 150 to 250 mL and a measured postvoiding residual volume of 150 mL, the excessive fluid intake was overwhelming the (normal) bladder capacity of 400 mL (150 + 250 mL). Although uninhibited bladder contractions were present, the easily reversible volume component of the problem—coupled with the risk of precipitating urinary retention with an anticholinergic agent—prompted treatment with volume restriction alone. After daily urinary output dropped to 1500 mL, frequency abated and incontinence resolved.

Adapted from DuBeau CE, Resnick NM: "Evaluation of the causes and severity of geriatric incontinence: A critical appraisal." *Urologic Clinics of North America* 18:243–256, 1991; used with permission.

diuretic. Incontinence that occurs at night in a demented person with heart failure, but does not occur during a 4-h daytime nap in the wheelchair, is probably attributable to the postural diuresis associated with heart failure. A woman with volume-dependent stress incontinence may leak only on the way to void after a full night's sleep when her bladder contains > 400 mL—more than it ever does during her continent waking hours. A patient may also void frequently because of polyuria.

Specific symptoms: **Urge** is neither a sensitive nor a specific symptom; 20% of patients with detrusor overactivity (and an even higher percentage of patients who also have dementia) do not have urge. Although urge incontinence is most often associated with detrusor overactivity, it is also common in patients with outlet incompetence (stress incontinence), outlet obstruction, and detrusor underactivity (overflow incontinence).

Precipitancy is the *abrupt sensation that urination is imminent, whatever the interval and amount of leakage that follows.* Defined in this way, precipitancy is both sensitive and specific for detrusor overactivity. For patients with no warning of imminent urination (often called reflex or unconscious incontinence), an abrupt gush of urine in the absence of a stress maneuver also can be considered precipitant leakage and is almost invariably due to detrusor overactivity. For those who do sense a warning, it is of less value to focus on the leakage; whether and how much the patient leaks depends on bladder volume, the amount of warning, the accessibility of a toilet, the patient's mobility, and whether the relative sphincter relaxation that accompanies detrusor contraction can be overcome.

Urinary frequency (more than seven diurnal voids) is common in the elderly. It may be due to preemptive voiding habits, overflow incontinence, sensory urgency, a stable but poorly compliant bladder, depression, anxiety, or excessive urine production (eg, because of diabetes, hypercalcemia, or high fluid intake). Conversely, incontinent persons may severely restrict their fluid intake, so that even if they have detrusor overactivity they do not void frequently. Thus, the significance of urinary frequency (or its absence) can be determined only in the context of more information.

Nocturia, another common symptom in the elderly, can be misleading (eg, two episodes may be normal for the person who sleeps 10 h but not for one who sleeps 4 h). It must be evaluated systematically. The three general reasons for true nocturia—excessive urine output, sleep-related difficulties, and bladder dysfunction—can be differentiated by thorough questioning and a voiding record that includes voided volumes (see above discussion and TABLE 15–5). Voided volumes help determine the functional bladder capacity (the largest single voided volume) and should be compared with the volume of each nighttime void. For example, if the functional bladder capacity is 400 mL and each of three nightly voids is about 400 mL, the nocturia is due to excessive production of urine at night. If the volume of most nightly voids is much

TABLE 15–6. CAUSES OF NOCTURIA

Volume-related	Age-related changes in nocturnal urine output
	Excess or late intake of fluids or alcohol
	Ingestion of diuretic, caffeine, theophylline
	Peripheral edema
	  Heart failure
	  Hypoalbuminemia
	  Peripheral vascular disease
	  Drugs (eg, indomethacin, nifedipine)

Sleep-related	Insomnia Pain (eg, arthritis) Dyspnea Depression Drugs (eg, caffeine, a short-acting hypnotic such as triazolam)
Lower urinary tract–related	Small bladder capacity Detrusor overactivity Prostate disease Overflow incontinence Decreased bladder compliance Sensory urgency

Adapted from Resnick NM: "Noninvasive diagnosis of the patient with complex incontinence." *Gerontology* 36 (Suppl 2):8–18, 1990; used with permission of S. Karger AG, Basel.

smaller than bladder capacity, the patient has either a sleep-related problem (the patient voids because he is awake anyway) or a bladder problem. Sleep-related and bladder-related causes of nocturia are listed in TABLE 15–6. Whatever the cause, however, the nocturnal component of incontinence is often treatable.

Neither **obstructive nor irritative symptoms** are specific for either benign prostatic hyperplasia (BPH) or bladder outlet obstruction, especially in the elderly. About one third of patients referred for prostatectomy because of obstructive symptoms actually are not obstructed. Usually, the problem is an overactive detrusor, which, if unaccompanied by outlet obstruction, may be exacerbated or at least unimproved by operative intervention. Thus, symptoms of prostatism are a clue to the diagnosis but warrant careful evaluation for other contributing medical and urologic factors. Prostatism symptom scores may be used to assess symptom severity (see TABLE 64–3) but should not be used to screen for or diagnose BPH.

All patients (or their caregivers) should be asked which voiding symptoms are the most bothersome. For example, although a woman may have mixed stress and urge incontinence, the urge component may be the truly bothersome one and should be the focus of evaluation and treatment. A man with prostatism may be most bothered by nocturia, which may be remedied without treating the enlarged prostate.

Physical Examination

Like the history, the physical examination is important not only to detect causes of established incontinence but also to rule out transient causes and to evaluate comorbid disease and functional ability. Functional impairment and general medical illnesses (such as heart failure and peripheral edema) can cause incontinence. A **neurologic examination,** as well as the standard urologic examination, is important because neurologic diseases, such as delirium, dementia, stroke, Parkinson's disease, cord compression, and neuropathy (autonomic or peripheral), are more common in older persons. Additionally, spinal column deformities or dimples suggestive of dysraphism, bladder distention (indicative of bladder weakness or outlet obstruction), and stress leakage (see below) should be explored.

Rectal examination: The rectal examination includes a check for fecal impaction, masses, prostate nodules, sacral reflexes, and symmetry of the gluteal creases. Prostate size, as determined by palpation, correlates poorly with outlet obstruction. The rest of the rectal examination is actually a detailed neuro-urologic examination, since the same sacral roots (S2-4) innervate both the external urethral sphincter and the anal sphincter. Placing a finger in the patient's rectum, the physician or nurse assesses motor innervation by asking the patient to volitionally contract and relax the anal sphincter. The other hand is placed on the patient's abdomen to check for abdominal straining, which can mimic sphincter contraction. Many neurologically intact elderly patients are unable to volitionally contract the sphincter. However, successful sphincter contraction is evidence against a cord lesion. Motor innervation is assessed further by testing the anal wink (S4-5) and bulbocavernosus (S2-4) reflexes (see FIG. 15–2). However, the absence of these reflexes (especially the anal wink) is not necessarily pathologic, nor does their presence exclude an underactive detrusor (due to diabetic neuropathy, for example). Finally, afferent nerve supply is assessed by testing perineal sensation.

Pelvic examination: A pelvic examination should be performed on all incontinent women. **Pelvic muscle laxity** may cause a cystocele, enterocele, rectocele, or uterine prolapse. After removing one blade of the vaginal speculum (or using a tongue blade), the physician should apply the remaining blade sequentially to the anterior and posterior vaginal walls and ask the patient to cough or strain. Bulging of the anterior wall when the posterior wall is stabilized indicates a cystocele. Conversely, bulging of the posterior wall indicates a rectocele or enterocele. Laxity

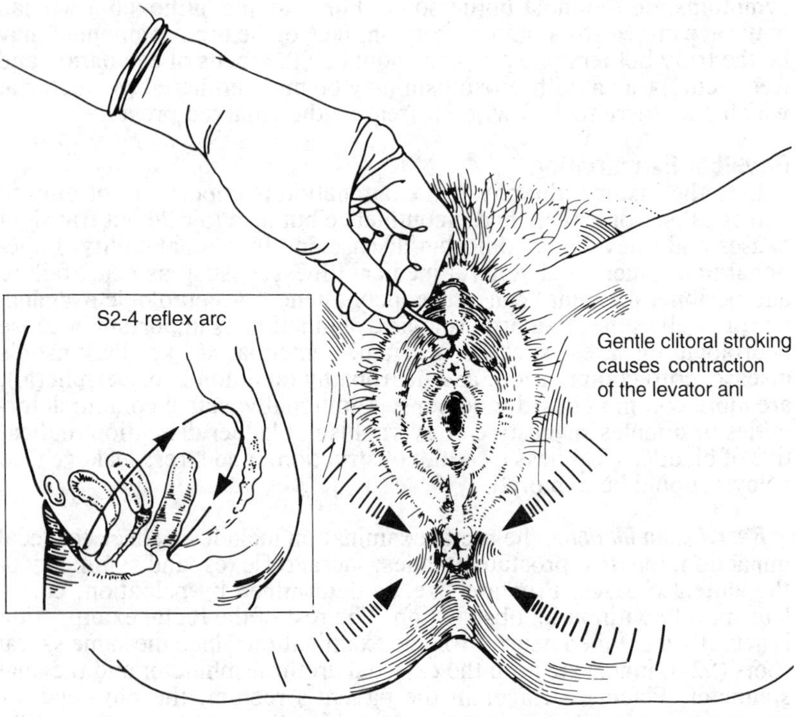
S2-4 reflex arc
Gentle clitoral stroking causes contraction of the levator ani

FIG. 15–2. Bulbocavernosus reflex—determination of the integrity of the sacral cord reflex arc.

can be determined in any position, although its extent may be underestimated if the patient is examined only in the supine position. Pelvic floor muscle laxity indicates little about the cause of leakage. Detrusor overactivity may exist in addition to a cystocele, and stress incontinence may exist without a cystocele. Thus, knowledge of pelvic muscle laxity is useful primarily to the surgeon in choosing the best type of operation. The one exception occurs in the woman with a large cystocele; its descent may kink the urethra and cause obstruction.

The **Q-tip test** for pelvic floor laxity is not helpful in the assessment of incontinence. The **Bonney (or Marshall) test** is also of limited usefulness. The test is used to determine whether leakage can be prevented by stabilizing (but not occluding) the bladder base and thereby preventing its herniation through the urogenital diaphragm. Two fingers are placed in the lateral vaginal fornices, and the patient is asked to cough. Urethral hypermobility is likely if leakage is prevented. However, vaginal stenosis is common, and inaccurate finger placement may occlude the urethra and thereby lead to a false-positive result. Even if the test is performed correctly, a false-positive result may occur if leakage was due to a cough-induced detrusor contraction and (when the bladder is empty) does not recur when the bladder base is elevated.

Stress incontinence is best assessed with a **provocative stress test.** When performed properly, this test has a sensitivity and specificity exceeding 90%, even in the elderly. With a full bladder, the patient assumes a position as close to upright as possible, spreads the legs, relaxes the perineal area, and provides a single, vigorous cough. A false-negative result may occur if the patient does not relax, if the bladder is not full, if the cough is not strong, or if the test is conducted in the upright position in a woman with a large cystocele. In the last case, the test should be repeated in the supine position with the cystocele reduced, if possible.

Whether leakage occurs coincidentally with the stress maneuver or is delayed for a few seconds or more should be noted. Delayed leakage suggests detrusor overactivity (triggered by coughing) rather than outlet incompetence. A stress test should not be performed when the patient has an abrupt urge to void, because the urge may be due to an uninhibited contraction. If the contraction is accompanied by physiologic sphincter relaxation and the patient then coughs, she will leak instantaneously, prompting the physician to misdiagnose a detrusor abnormality as outlet incompetence.

The vagina should be inspected for signs of **atrophic vaginitis,** which is characterized by indications of inflammation such as mucosal friability, petechiae, telangiectasia, and vaginal erosions. Loss of rugal folds and a thin, shiny mucosa are signs of vaginal atrophy rather than the inflammation of atrophic vaginitis (see also GENITAL ATROPHY in Ch. 83). A cytologic maturation index showing 100% parabasal cells also indicates atrophy but not necessarily atrophic vaginitis. Treatment of atrophic vaginitis is discussed under TRANSIENT INCONTINENCE, above.

Finally, the pelvic examination provides an opportunity to obtain a Papanicolaou smear; many elderly women have never been screened for cervical carcinoma.

Observation of micturition: An observation of how a patient voids is part of the physical examination and provides much information about bladder and urethral function. When feeling full, the patient should first forestall voiding for several minutes to see if the sensation passes or if precipitant leakage occurs. The examiner should explain the reason for observing micturition and accompany the patient to a toilet that is equipped with a receptacle to measure the volume voided. If the patient will not allow the examiner to observe voiding, then the flow rate can be assessed either by using a uroflow machine (uroflowmeter) or by audibly monitoring the flow with a portable audio monitor (such as that used to monitor a baby's room at home) and then asking the patient to place a hand on the abdomen to check for straining during urination.

Straining should be searched for especially if stress incontinence is suspected and surgery is contemplated, since straining suggests detrusor weakness that might predispose the patient to postoperative retention. If detrusor overactivity is suspected, it may be triggered by offering fluids; by having the patient change posture, cough, or hop; or by jouncing the heels (if the patient is unable to stand). If detrusor overactivity is precipitated, whether and how quickly the patient can interrupt the urine stream should be determined; rapid and complete interruption augurs well for bladder retraining.

The examination concludes with determination of the **postvoiding residual volume,** either by catheterization or ultrasound estimate. Adding the postvoiding residual volume to the voided volume provides an estimate of total bladder capacity (if the patient felt full before voiding) and a crude assessment of bladder proprioception. A postvoiding residual volume > 50 to 100 mL suggests either bladder weakness or outlet obstruction, but smaller amounts do not exclude either diagnosis, especially if the patient strained to void or double voided. Thus, observation of micturition or listening to the voided stream is important. If straining is observed, the patient is asked whether it is typical.

Incidentally, relying on the ease of catheterization to establish the presence of obstruction can be misleading. Difficult catheter passage may be caused by urethral tortuosity, a false passage, or catheter-induced spasm of the distal sphincter, whereas catheter passage may be easy even in severely obstructed patients.

Laboratory Tests

Electrolyte, BUN, and creatinine levels should be measured, and a urinalysis and urine culture should be obtained in all patients. If the voiding record suggests polyuria, serum concentrations of glucose and calcium (and albumin, to allow calculation of free calcium levels in sick, malnourished patients) are measured as well. The age-associated decline in glomerular filtration rate—30% by the eighth decade—is not associated with an increase in serum creatinine because of a concomitant decrease in muscle mass; thus normal creatinine levels do not imply a normal glomerular filtration rate (see Ch. 63).

In any patient with sterile hematuria or suprapubic or perineal discomfort or in a patient at high risk for bladder carcinoma (eg, unexplained recent onset of urgency or urge incontinence, exposure to industrial dyes), urine cytology or cystoscopy should be performed.

Urodynamic Testing

If the cause of the incontinence still cannot be determined, urodynamic evaluation should be considered. Urodynamic evaluation is reproducible and safe, even in frail and debilitated people. Although its precise role remains to be determined, multichannel urodynamic testing is probably warranted in older patients when diagnostic uncertainty may affect therapy, when empiric therapy has failed and other approaches could be tried, or when surgical correction is being contemplated. Unfortunately, although simple to perform and up to 75% sensitive for detrusor overactivity with normal contractility, bedside cystometry cannot differentiate primary detrusor overactivity from that secondary to stress incontinence or obstruction (and therefore not of primary importance). Moreover, sensitivity and reproducibility are lower in nursing home patients, and the test is neither sensitive nor specific for detrusor hyperactivity with impaired contractility, the most common cause of incontinence in the nursing home population for whom this test might be the most useful.

TREATMENT CONSIDERATIONS

Treatment must be individualized because factors outside the lower urinary tract often affect the feasibility and efficacy of the intervention. For example, a severely demented and bedridden person is treated differently from one who is ambulatory and cognitively intact, although both may have detrusor overactivity that can be managed successfully. Treatment guidelines are given in TABLE 15–7; serious underlying conditions and transient causes of incontinence should already have been excluded or treated. It cannot be overemphasized that successful treatment of established incontinence is multifactorial.

Detrusor Overactivity

The initial approach to detrusor overactivity is to identify and treat its causes when possible. Unfortunately, since many of its specific causes are not reversible, treatment is usually symptomatic. Simple measures such as treating peripheral edema, adjusting the timing or amount of fluid ingested (see TABLE 15–5), or providing a bedside commode or urinal are often successful. However, the cornerstone of treatment is behavioral therapy.

If the patient can cooperate, **bladder retraining** regimens, including techniques to suppress precipitancy, will extend the voiding interval. For example, if the voiding record shows that the patient is wet every 3 h, he should void every 2 h and suppress urgency in between. Once dry for three consecutive days, the patient can extend the interval by a half hour, repeating the process until a satisfactory result or continence is achieved. Patients need not follow this regimen at night; once they are dry during the day, they generally become dry at night. Biofeedback may be added, but its additional benefit is unclear.

If the patient cannot cooperate (eg, the patient has dementia), a technique of **prompted voiding** is used. The patient is asked at 2-h intervals whether he needs to void and, if the answer is yes, is escorted to the toilet. Positive behavioral reinforcement is used, and negative reinforcement is avoided. Prompted voiding can reduce incontinence frequency in nursing home patients by up to 50%. Moreover, the 75% of

TABLE 15–7. TREATMENT OF ESTABLISHED INCONTINENCE

Condition	*Clinical Type of Incontinence*	*Treatment**
Detrusor overactivity with normal contractility	Urge	1. Try bladder retraining or prompted voiding regimens 2. Consider a bladder relaxant medication (anticholinergic, smooth muscle relaxant, calcium channel blocker) if needed and not contraindicated 3. Indwelling catheterization alone is often unhelpful because detrusor spasms often increase, leading to leakage around the catheter 4. In selected cases, induce urinary retention pharmacologically and add intermittent or indwelling catheterization
Detrusor hyperactivity with impaired contractility	Urge†	1. If bladder empties adequately with straining, use behavioral methods (as above) ± bladder relaxant medication (low doses; especially if sphincter incompetence coexists) 2. If residual urine is high (eg, > 150 mL), bladder relaxant medication is contraindicated. Instead, use augmented voiding techniques‡ or intermittent catheterization (± bladder relaxant medication). If neither is feasible, undergarment or indwelling catheter may be used. Antimicrobial prophylaxis can be given for recurrent symptomatic urinary tract infections if catheter is not indwelling
Outlet incompetence	Stress	1. Try conservative methods (weight loss if obese; treating cough or atrophic vaginitis; rarely, use of pessary or tampon) 2. Prescribe pelvic muscle exercises ± biofeedback or weighted intravaginal cones 3. Prescribe imipramine (or doxepin) or α-adrenergic agonists—± estrogen—if not contraindicated 4. Consider surgery
Outlet obstruction	Urge or overflow§	1. Try conservative methods (eg, adjustment of fluid intake, bladder retraining or prompted voiding ± bladder relaxants) if hydronephrosis, elevated residual urine, recurrent symptomatic urinary tract infection, and gross hematuria have been excluded

(continued)

TABLE 15–7. TREATMENT OF ESTABLISHED INCONTINENCE *(Continued)*

Condition	*Clinical Type of Incontinence*	*Treatment**
Outlet obstruction *(continued)*		2. Prescribe α-adrenergic antagonists if not contraindicated 3. Prescribe bladder relaxants if detrusor overactivity coexists, postvoiding residual volume is small (< 50–100 mL), and surgery is not desired or feasible 4. If above fail, prescribe finasteride, antiandrogens, or luteinizing hormone–releasing hormone analogs if not contraindicated and the patient either prefers them or is not a surgical candidate 5. Consider surgery
Detrusor underactivity	Overflow	1. If duration is unknown, decompress for several weeks and perform a voiding trial 2. If this fails or retention is chronic, try augmented voiding techniques§ ± α-adrenergic antagonist, *if* any voiding is possible; bethanechol rarely is useful unless bladder weakness is due to an anticholinergic agent that cannot be discontinued 3. If this fails or voiding is not possible, use intermittent or indwelling catheterization

* These treatments should be initiated only after access to a toilet has been ensured, contributing conditions (eg, atrophic vaginitis, heart failure) have been treated, fluid management has been optimized, and unnecessary medications have been stopped. See text for additional details, recommendations, and drug doses.

† Detrusor hyperactivity with impaired contractility may also mimic stress or overflow incontinence.

‡ Augmented voiding techniques include Credé (application of suprapubic pressure—see Fig. 15–3) and Valsalva (straining) maneuvers and double voiding.

§ Outlet obstruction in men can cause postvoid dribbling alone, which is treated conservatively (eg, by sitting to void and allowing more time, double voiding, or gently milking the urethra after voiding).

Adapted from Resnick NM: "Voiding dysfunction and urinary incontinence," in *Geriatrics Review Syllabus: A Core Curriculum in Geriatric Medicine*, edited by JC Beck. New York, American Geriatrics Society, 1991, pp 141–154; used with permission.

such patients who will respond to prompted voiding can be identified within a few days. These are patients who, when asked every 2 h, can recognize the intermittent need to void and can urinate into a toilet or commode at least half the time. With prompted voiding, patients who once leaked four times or fewer in a 12-h daytime period will leak less than once; 60% of these patients (25% of all incontinent nursing home residents) will actually become dry for two or more consecutive days. Improvement persists in most patients. For those who leaked more than four times in the 12-h baseline period, prompted voiding generally decreases the frequency of incontinence by about two episodes, but these patients will still be wet more than once a day. For the 25% of patients who do not respond to prompting at baseline, little benefit is obtained by further prompting.

If incontinence is worse at night and the voiding record shows an inappropriately large **nocturnal diuresis,** the cause of the diuresis should be determined (see TABLE 15–6). Diuresis attributable to heart failure should improve with diuretic therapy. Diuresis due to peripheral edema without heart failure and hypoalbuminemia (eg, venous insufficiency) may respond to treatment with pressure gradient stockings and daytime leg elevation. Diuresis not associated with peripheral edema may respond to a change in the pattern of fluid intake or to the administration of a rapidly acting diuretic in the late afternoon or early evening. For the patient with detrusor hyperactivity with impaired contractility whose voiding record and postvoiding residual volume reveal that uninhibited contractions are provoked only at high volumes, catheterization just before bedtime will remove the residual urine, increasing functional bladder capacity and probably restoring both continence and sleep.

Pharmacotherapy can augment behavioral therapy but not replace it, since drugs generally do not abolish uninhibited contractions (see TABLE 15–8). Data regarding these drugs' efficacy and toxicity in the elderly are scarce, and comparative or controlled trials are rare. Since available studies generally show equivalent results (except for flavoxate, which fares poorly in controlled trials), the decision of which drug to use is often based on factors unrelated to bladder function. If an incontinent patient has dementia or is already taking anticholinergic agents, propantheline is best avoided. If a patient has coexisting hypertension, angina pectoris, or abnormalities of cardiac diastolic relaxation, a calcium channel blocker may be preferred. Imipramine and nifedipine are best avoided in persons with orthostatic hypotension. A tricyclic antidepressant may be preferred for an incontinent patient who needs pharmacotherapy for depression and who does not have orthostatic hypotension. Medications with rapid onset of action, such as oxybutynin, can be used prophylactically if incontinence occurs at predictable times. Occasionally, combining low doses of two agents with complementary actions—such as oxybutynin and imipramine—will maximize benefits and minimize side effects. Some of these agents also can be applied intravesically but only in patients who can catheterize themselves. Vasopressin has only limited efficacy when given by injection in institutionalized patients and by intranasal spray in some care-

TABLE 15–8. DRUGS FOR DETRUSOR OVERACTIVITY

Drug	*Mechanism*	*Dose**
Flavoxate	Smooth muscle relaxant	300–800 mg/day (100–200 mg orally 3 to 4 times per day)†
Diltiazem	Calcium channel blocker	30–270 mg/day (30–90 mg orally 1 to 3 times per day)
Nifedipine	Calcium channel blocker	10–90 mg/day (10–30 mg orally 1 to 3 times per day)
Propantheline	Anticholinergic	22.5–150 mg/day (7.5–30 mg orally 3 to 5 times per day)‡
Oxybutynin	Combination smooth muscle relaxant and anticholinergic	7.5–20 mg/day (2.5–5 mg orally 3 to 4 times per day)
Dicyclomine	Combination smooth muscle relaxant and anticholinergic	30–60 mg/day (10–20 mg orally 3 times per day)
Imipramine	Antidepressant	10–100 mg/day (10–25 mg orally 1 to 4 times per day)
Doxepin	Antidepressant	10–75 mg (10–25 mg orally 1 to 3 times per day)

* Each drug is usually given in divided doses, except for the antidepressants, which may be given as a single daily dose.

† Some reports of uncontrolled studies suggest that doses up to 1200 mg/day may be effective with tolerable side effects; efficacy for *any* dose has not been supported by randomized controlled trials.

‡ Higher doses are occasionally tolerated and effective; should be given in the fasting state.

fully selected nursing home residents. Given the expense of vasopressin and the risk of inducing fluid retention and hyponatremia, general use of the drug should await further studies.

All bladder relaxant medications may cause urinary retention; therefore, the postvoiding residual volume and common indexes of renal function (BUN, serum creatinine, and urine output) should be monitored, especially in patients with detrusor hyperactivity with impaired contractility, in whom the detrusor is already weak. If subclinical urinary retention develops, the associated reduction in functional bladder capacity may attenuate or reverse the drug's efficacy; thus, if incontinence worsens as the dose is increased, the postvoiding residual volume should be measured. Anticholinergic medications can lead to xerostomia and excessive fluid intake, which also may worsen incontinence. Inducing urinary retention and using **intermittent catheterization** may be reasonable for patients whose incontinence defies other remedies (such as those with detrusor hyperactivity with impaired contractility) and for whom intermittent catheterization is feasible. Other remedies for urge incontinence (including **electrical stimulation** and **selective nerve blocks)** have not been studied extensively in the elderly.

Augmentation cystoplasty increases bladder capacity by incorporating a section of intestine or stomach into the bladder. This treatment is reserved for severe cases of intractable detrusor hyperreflexia, especially those associated with a poorly compliant contracted bladder, and is contraindicated in frail patients. Known complications include hyperchloremic metabolic acidosis and secondary osteopenia, urinary tract infection, voiding difficulty, excessive mucus production, potential for secondary neoplasms, and a high likelihood that intermittent catheterization will be needed.

Pads and special undergarments are invaluable if incontinence proves refractory. A wide variety of products are available, so the choice can be tailored to the individual's problem. A launderable bedpad may be preferable for bedridden persons. For those with a stroke, a diaper or pants that can be opened using just the good hand may be preferred. For ambulatory patients with large gushes of leakage, wood pulp pads and diapers are generally preferable to those containing polymer gel. Polymer gel generally cannot absorb the large volume and rapid flow these patients produce, while a wood pulp product can easily be doubled up if necessary. Optimal products for men and women also differ by where on the pad maximal leakage can be absorbed. Finally, whether the patient also has fecal incontinence affects the choice of product.

Condom catheters can be helpful for some men, although they are often associated with skin breakdown and decreased motivation to become dry and may not be feasible for men with a small or retracted penis. **External collection devices** have only recently been devised for women and may be effective for debilitated women in nursing homes. **Indwelling urethral catheters** are *not* recommended for detrusor overactivity because they usually exacerbate contractions. If they must be used (eg, to allow healing of a pressure sore in a patient with refractory detrusor overactivity), a catheter with a small balloon is preferred to minimize irritability and consequent leakage around the catheter. Such leakage almost invariably results from bladder spasm rather than a catheter that is too small. Increasing the size of the catheter and balloon often aggravates the problem and may result in progressive urethral erosion and sphincter incompetence. If bladder spasms persist, oxybutynin can be used. Alternative agents with more potent anticholinergic side effects (eg, belladonna suppositories) should be avoided in the elderly.

Outlet Incompetence

An incompetent outlet is the cause of **stress incontinence.** Outlet incompetence can take one of two forms: urethral hypermobility or intrinsic sphincter deficiency.

Urethral hypermobility: Urethral hypermobility may be improved by weight loss if the patient is obese, by treating precipitating conditions such as atrophic vaginitis or coughing, and (rarely) by insertion of a pessary. **Pelvic muscle exercises** (eg, Kegel's exercises) are often effective, especially if the patient also contracts her pelvic muscles at the time of stress. The pubococcygeal muscle is contracted by interrupting the urine stream, by imagining holding back urine flow, or by having the patient contract her vaginal muscles around an examiner's gloved (or her own) fingers. Simultaneously contracting the abdominal, gluteal, or adductor muscles is counterproductive. Current recommendations are for the patient to sustain a maximal contraction for 3 to 10 sec in sets of 10 contractions and to repeat sets three to five times per day, 3 days per week. Scheduled follow-up visits for encouragement, or biofeedback if available, may be helpful. Experience with weighted vaginal cones to help women perform pelvic muscle exercises is promising but still limited. Cure or improvement can be expected in 60% to 75% of women < 75 yr, especially if the patient is motivated, does the exercises as instructed, and receives written instructions or follow-up visits for encouragement. Whether women > 75 yr can achieve similar success is not known. Efficacy requires continuing the exercises indefinitely.

If stress incontinence is exacerbated by uterine prolapse, a **pessary** may be useful if the patient wishes to defer surgery or is a high operative risk. Pessaries are available in many sizes and shapes (see FIG. 66–4); the cube pessary is easiest to place but requires daily removal and cleaning. Contraceptive diaphragms may ameliorate stress incontinence in younger women, but their efficacy and acceptance in elderly women is unknown.

If not contraindicated, **pharmacotherapy** with an α-adrenergic agonist such as sustained-release phenylpropanolamine 25 to 75 mg bid may be beneficial, especially when given with estrogen. These two agents work for women with intrinsic sphincter deficiency as well. Phenylpropanolamine is inexpensive, available without a prescription, and contained in many diet pills. However, the physician should guide the choice of preparation and prescribe the dose because some capsules contain additional agents such as chlorpheniramine in doses that can be troublesome for elderly patients. Imipramine 10 to 25 mg one to three times daily has beneficial effects on the bladder and the outlet; it is a reasonable choice for patients with both stress and urge incontinence and no evidence of postural hypotension.

If these methods fail or are unacceptable, surgical correction may be warranted for urethral hypermobility. **Anterior colporrhaphy** is less likely to cure stress incontinence than are other bladder neck suspension techniques. Many elderly women will be unable to tolerate a **Marshall-Marchetti-Krantz** procedure, which entails lengthy abdominal surgery and prolonged recovery time. A highly successful alternative suprapubic procedure, the **Burch colposuspension,** requires less extensive surgery and corrects anterior vaginal wall laxity. However, some women lack sufficient vaginal mobility and capacity, and the procedure may exacerbate posterior vaginal wall weakness and cause stranguria and urinary retention. Vaginal bladder neck suspensions (eg, **Pereyra, Stamey, and Raz procedures**) are relatively minor procedures, with brief hospitalizations and easier recovery. When properly performed, these procedures have excellent cure rates in the elderly. The Raz procedure, which is the least obstructive, may be the most appropriate for older women with concomitant bladder weakness.

Intrinsic sphincter deficiency (incompetence): Conservative, nonpharmacologic treatment for sphincter deficiency consists of a toileting and fluid regimen that maintains bladder volume below the leakage threshold. This approach is often appropriate for older women, whose sphincter deficiency is more often the result of atrophy. If this approach fails, surgical correction is effective, but a different approach **(pubovaginal sling)** is often required, morbidity is higher, and chronic urinary retention is more likely to be precipitated than with correction of urethral hypermobility.

New treatments for sphincter deficiency, especially for men who have had a prostatectomy, include implantation of an **artificial sphincter.** With patient selection, about 70% of patients become completely dry, with the remainder using only one or two pads a day; reoperation or revision may be needed in 20%. Another new approach is periurethral injection of **bulking agents.** Short-term success rates with glutaraldehyde cross-linked bovine collagen are 65% to 95% for women but much lower for men. Longer follow-up studies are under way, as are new studies using autologous fat injections. While bulking agents are appealing (injection requires only local anesthesia and little time), success usually involves multiple injections. Experience with persons > 75 yr is limited, and urinary retention (often leading to catheterization) is a risk.

If all other interventions fail, condom catheters or penile clamps may be useful for men. However, most such prostheses require substantial cognitive capacity and manual dexterity and are often poorly tolerated. An alternative product is a penile sheath, such as a McGuire prosthesis (similar to an athletic supporter) or a self-adhesive sheath (especially if it is lined with a polymer gel or cellulose). Some collection devices for women are available. Thin superabsorbent polymer gel pads are often successful because the gel can more readily absorb the smaller amount of leakage associated with stress incontinence. Pads that can be flushed down the toilet are convenient for ambulatory women. Electrical stimulation, a promising alternative for women, is currently under investigation.

Outlet Obstruction

In men: Transurethral resection of the prostate **(TURP)** or even suprapubic or retropubic prostatectomy is feasible for elderly men (see also Ch. 64). Newer approaches, such as **bladder neck incision with bilateral prostatotomy,** have made surgical decompression feasible for even the frailest men. These procedures, as well as TURP in some instances, can be done under local anesthesia and completed in < 30 min of operating time. Unlike TURP and open resections, incision procedures do not fully resolve the problem, since they do not remove the hyperplastic tissue. However, in frail elderly men, relapse of obstruction 2 to 3 yr later may not be an issue.

Administration of α-adrenergic antagonists, such as **prazosin** 1 to 2 mg bid to qid or **terazosin** 2.5 to 10 mg/day, may also help the older man with outlet obstruction. The efficacy of these agents in relieving symptoms is well documented, and postvoiding residual volume, outlet resistance, and urinary flow rate may improve as well. Neither agent is a panacea for outlet obstruction, and trials of these agents have generally excluded men with large residual volumes (ie, > 200 mL), diabetes, heart disease, and hypertension, conditions that are prevalent in the elderly and associated with an increased risk of side effects. However, the physician may be able to treat men symptomatically until more definitive therapy is necessary and feasible.

The 5α-reductase inhibitor **finasteride** 5 mg/day decreases prostate size, but symptom reduction may be modest for 10 to 12 mo. Some investigators have suggested combining therapy with an α-adrenergic antagonist, although this approach has not yet been tested. Clinicians should be aware that finasteride decreases prostate-specific antigen levels by about 50%; therefore, men should be carefully screened for prostate cancer before taking the drug. Also, the prostate eventually grows back to its baseline size when the drug is discontinued.

The use of luteinizing hormone–releasing hormone agonists and antiandrogens to decrease prostate size and relieve symptoms of obstruction in the frail elderly is still investigational; untoward side effects such as hot flashes, erectile dysfunction, gynecomastia, and diarrhea are common.

Urethral stents are a promising nonpharmacologic intervention. Side effects include stent migration and urinary urgency (usually subsiding after a few weeks to months), and long-term follow-up data are lacking. Initial enthusiasm for balloon dilation of the prostate has waned because of the short duration of response. The new transurethral techniques for **microwave hyperthermia** may be more effective than the previous transrectal techniques, but long-term data in the elderly are lacking. While there is increasing experience with **transurethral lasers,** which cause coagulation necrosis and gradual sloughing of prostatic tissue, long-term results and a full safety profile are still lacking.

In women: Surgical correction is usually required for a large **cystocele,** and an outlet suspension procedure should be performed if urethral hypermobility is also present. If the bladder neck is incompetent or the urethral closure pressure is low (< 10 cm H_2O), a different surgical approach may be required to avoid causing sphincter incompetence. Bladder neck obstruction is easily corrected in even the frailest patient. Distal urethral stenosis can be dilated and treated with estrogen. If meatal stenosis is present, more extensive intervention may be necessary; alternatively, dilation can be repeated frequently. However, most women who undergo dilation do not have urethral stenosis but rather an underactive detrusor; for these women, dilation is usually not helpful and may be harmful.

Detrusor Underactivity

The type of incontinence most often associated with an underactive detrusor is **overflow incontinence.** Management of detrusor underactivity is directed at reducing residual volume, eliminating hydronephrosis (if present), and preventing urosepsis. The first step is to decompress the bladder for at least 7 to 14 days with an indwelling catheter. Meanwhile, potential contributors to impaired detrusor function, such as fecal impaction and medication side effects, should be addressed. If decompression does not fully restore bladder function, **augmented voiding techniques** may help if the patient is able to initiate a detrusor contraction or if stress incontinence coexists. Augmented voiding techniques include double voiding or implementing the Credé maneuver (application of suprapubic pressure during voiding—see FIG. 15–3) or the Valsalva maneuver. Bethanechol 40 to 200 mg/day in divided doses is occasionally useful in a patient whose bladder contracts poorly owing to an anticholinergic agent that cannot be discontinued (eg, a tricyclic antidepressant). In other patients, bethanechol may decrease the postvoiding residual volume if sphincter function and local innervation are normal. Because its efficacy is debatable, residual volume should be monitored so that the drug can be discontinued if ineffective.

If the detrusor is acontractile after decompression, any intervention is likely to be futile, and the patient should undergo intermittent catheterization or have an indwelling urethral catheter placed. For persons at home, **intermittent self-catheterization** is usually painless, safe, inexpensive, and effective and does not interfere with activities of daily living. Catheters can be clean rather than sterile. Two or three catheters should be purchased. The catheters are cleaned daily, allowed to air dry at night, sterilized periodically, and may be reused repeatedly. Antibiotic or methenamine mandelate prophylaxis against urinary tract infection is probably warranted if the person gets more than an occasional symptomatic infection or has an abnormal heart valve or an orthopedic

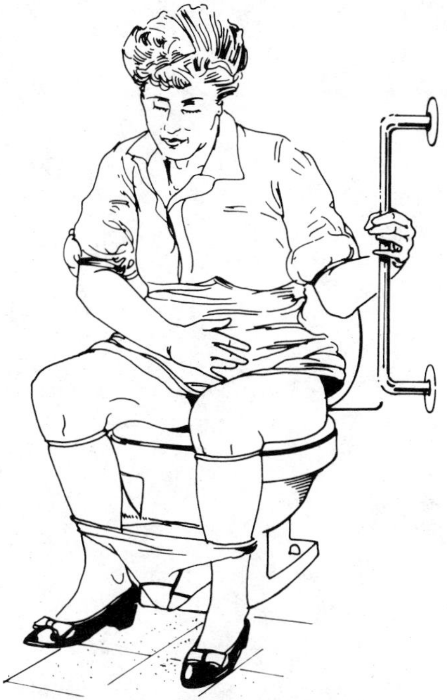

FIG. 15–3. Credé maneuver—application of suprapubic pressure during voiding.

prosthesis. Intermittent catheterization is usually less feasible, although sometimes possible, for debilitated patients who need caregiver assistance. If intermittent catheterization is performed in an institutional setting, sterile rather than clean technique should be used because of the prevalence and virulence of bacteria found in such settings.

Indwelling catheters should be reserved for the acutely ill patient to monitor fluid balance, the patient with a nonhealing pressure sore, the patient with acute urinary retention, the patient who needs temporary bladder decompression, and the patient with overflow incontinence refractory to other measures. Even in long-term care facilities, indwelling catheters are probably indicated for only 1% to 2% of patients. Complications of chronic indwelling catheterization include bladder and urethral erosions, bladder stones, bladder cancer, and urosepsis.

§2. SPECIFIC APPROACHES

SPEC

§2. SPECIFIC APPROACHES

16. HISTORY AND PHYSICAL EXAMINATION

Much of the classic training in obtaining histories and doing physical examinations may need to be modified when assessing a very old or frail elderly patient. The interview may have to be divided into sessions—often one with the patient and the other with the caregiver. Similarly, the physical examination may have to be separated from the interview because of patient fatigue, requiring two sessions. Because a complete history may not be obtainable, the physician may need to make decisions before all data are available, thus placing greater emphasis on the physical examination while attempting to obtain historical data from other sources.

THE HISTORY

Challenges in Obtaining History

Clinicians should be prepared to spend more time interviewing and evaluating elderly patients and should tailor the interview to the individual patient. Aphasia, cognitive dysfunction, or sensory deficits such as hearing or vision loss can interfere with the interview process. Further, terms such as stroke, heart attack, constipation, and dizziness may require interpretation. For example, constipation could mean infrequent bowel movements, hard stool, small stool, or the sensation of incompletely evacuated stool. Standard questions may not apply to patients with functional limitations; eg, a patient whose mobility is severely limited by arthritis will not complain of dyspnea or chest pain with exertion even if he has severe coronary artery disease.

Older patients may present with many nonspecific symptoms, making it difficult to focus the interview. In addition, clinical features of diseases may differ from those seen in younger patients. For example, disease may manifest as functional decline. To determine the duration of symptoms, ask questions pertaining to functional disability (eg, "How long have you been unable to do your own shopping?"). Older patients may underreport symptoms, further complicating history taking, because they consider them part of normal aging; eg, they may not volunteer symptoms of dyspnea, hearing or vision loss, incontinence, gait disturbance, constipation, dizziness, or falls. However, no illness should be attributed to normal aging.

Elderly patients may have difficulty recalling all illnesses, hospitalizations, operations, and drugs used during a lifetime. If the patient's history is incomplete because of memory disturbances, an alternative source for the data (eg, a family member, home health aide, or medical records obtained from another physician or institution) is required. However, the patient's chief complaint may differ from what the family views as the main problem. An extensive **family history** has limited value and should focus on disorders of later life known to have inherited patterns, such as Alzheimer's disease.

Approach to the Interview

Knowledge of the everyday concerns, social circumstances, and psychology of the elderly helps orient and guide the clinician's approach to the older patient, while a thorough knowledge of geriatric medicine provides the framework for the interview.

Traditionally, physicians evaluate patients using the chief complaint to structure the clinical interview. However, older patients often have much to tell that would benefit both doctor and patient and that is often stifled by the chief complaint approach. Asking about a typical day provides the clinician with a snapshot of the patient's quality of life, liveliness of thought, and physical independence. Asking older patients about themselves is especially useful on first meeting, whether in an emergency room, the hospital, or the nursing home. Doctor and patient have a chance to build a bridge, the patient speaking with pride about survival, about accomplishments, and about things that are important to him. The physician allows rapport to develop, which is productive because it promotes the positive side of the expectations of both parties. A good relationship with the patient will also be helpful when meeting the family and later when seeking cooperation and compliance with the health care program.

The doctor must use the power of observation to recognize and interpret the clues suggested during the telling of the history. Clues are often nonverbal, such as the way the story is told, the tempo of speech, the tone of voice, and eye contact. What is omitted or explicitly denied may be important. An elderly person may deny symptoms of anxiety or depression, yet betray them with a lowering of the voice, an enthusiasm that seems subdued, or even a tear. Careful attention to reports about sleep and appetite may unearth information about both physical and mental health. The change in the fit of clothing or of dentures or the reading on a scale provides important information about weight gain or loss. Also important is observing the patient's personal hygiene and dress, who accompanies the patient, and the patient's preference about having that person talk during the interview.

Interview Techniques

To determine historical reliability, you may need to perform a mental status evaluation early in the interview (see Ch. 89); this should be done tactfully so the patient will not be embarrassed or offended or become defensive, especially when a relative is present during such an examination. Anyone accompanying the patient should not answer questions for him, unless the physician asks the person to do so.

Some patients may prefer to have a relative present. However, unless mental status is impaired, interview the patient alone to encourage the discussion of personal matters. Having a relative present without asking the patient's permission implies that the patient is incapable of telling the entire history. Similarly, asking the patient to wait outside while a relative or friend is interviewed can be detrimental to the physician-patient relationship.

To overcome communication problems involving auditory or visual deficits, move close, face the patient directly, and speak clearly and slowly to allow lipreading. If appropriate, the patient should wear his dentures, eyeglasses, or hearing aid to facilitate communication. If the patient has difficulty hearing, examine the auditory canals for cerumen. Shouting at the patient is unnecessary, since age-related increased stiffness of the tympanic membrane and ear ossicles distorts high-volume sound. Using a stethoscope in reverse (speaking into the stethoscope like a microphone while the patient has the ear pieces) may be helpful.

Patients should be interviewed while fully clothed. They may require additional time to respond to questions, undress, and transfer to the examining table for the physical examination (see below) and should not be rushed. An elderly patient may not be able to tolerate a long session; if so, divide the initial evaluation into two sessions.

MEDICAL HISTORY

A review of *past* medical illnesses includes diseases that may have once afflicted patients (eg, rheumatic fever, poliomyelitis), even though they are uncommon today. Younger physicians may not be familiar with past treatment modalities (eg, pneumothorax therapy for tuberculosis and mercury for syphilis). Obtain a history of immunizations (tetanus, influenza, pneumococcus), along with any adverse reactions to them, as well as the results of skin tests for tuberculosis. Although the patient may recall having had surgery, he may not remember the nature of the procedure or the reason for it. If the patient knows where and when he was hospitalized, surgical records can be sought.

A review of *current* medical illnesses and complaints can be conducted systematically (see TABLE 16–1).

DRUG HISTORY

The drug history includes determining which medications—prescribed and over-the-counter (OTC)—are used, at what dose, how often they are taken, who prescribed them, and for what reason. Topical drugs can also cause problems. For example, eye drops used for treating glaucoma are absorbed systemically with effects that may be comparable to intravenous dosing, resulting in cardiovascular, pulmonary, or CNS effects. Systemic absorption and blood levels vary widely.

TABLE 16–1. REVIEW OF SYSTEMS

System	Symptom	Possible Problem
Head	Headaches	Temporal arteritis, depression, anxiety, cervical osteoarthritis, subdural hematoma
Eyes	Loss of near vision (presbyopia)	Common with age
	Loss of peripheral vision	Glaucoma, stroke
	Loss of central vision	Macular degeneration
	Pain	Glaucoma, temporal arteritis
	Glare from lights at night	Cataracts
Ears	Hearing loss	Acoustic neuroma, tumor of the cerebellopontine angle, presbycusis, cerumen, foreign body in the external canal, Paget's disease, trauma from noise, ototoxicity from drugs (eg, aminoglycosides, furosemide, aspirin)
	Loss of high-frequency range (presbycusis)	Common with age
Mouth	Loss of taste	Infection of mouth or nose, adrenal insufficiency, nasopharyngeal neoplasm, drugs (eg, antihistamines, antidepressants), radiation therapy, smoking
	Limited tongue motion	Oral cancer
	Burning mouth	Pernicious anemia
	Pain caused by dentures	Poorly fitting dentures, oral cancer
	Dry mouth	Drugs (eg, diuretics, antihypertensives, tricyclic antidepressants, psychoactives, antihistamines), salivary gland damage (infection, radiation therapy of head and neck neoplasms), autoimmune disorders (rheumatoid arthritis, systemic lupus erythematosus, Sjögren's syndrome), dehydration

(continued)

TABLE 16–1. REVIEW OF SYSTEMS *(Continued)*

System	*Symptom*	*Possible Problem*
Throat	Voice changes	Tumor on vocal cord, hypothyroidism
	Dysphagia	Foreign body, Zenker's diverticulum, esophageal stricture, Schatzki's ring, carcinoma
Neck	Pain	Cervical arthritis, polymyalgia rheumatica
Chest	Pain	Angina pectoris, anxiety, herpes zoster, gastroesophageal reflux, esophageal motility disorders, costochondritis
Cardiovascular	Difficulty in eating or sleeping	Heart failure
	Paroxysmal nocturnal dyspnea	Heart failure, gastroesophageal reflux
Gastrointestinal	One bowel movement q 2–3 days	Normal
	Constipation	Hypothyroidism, hyperparathyroidism, dehydration, hypokalemia, colorectal carcinoma, inadequate exercise, low-fiber diet, drugs (eg, aluminum-containing antacids, opioids, tricyclic antidepressants, anticholinergics), laxative abuse
	Pain, constipation, vomiting, diarrhea	Fecal impaction
	Rectal bleeding	Colon angiodysplasia, ischemic colitis, diverticulosis, colon carcinoma, hemorrhoids
	Fecal incontinence	Cerebral dysfunction, spinal cord lesions, rectal carcinoma, fecal impaction
	Lower abdominal pain (crampy, sudden onset)	Ischemic colitis
	Postprandial abdominal pain (15–30 min after eating, lasting 1–3 h)	Chronic intestinal ischemia

(continued)

TABLE 16–1. REVIEW OF SYSTEMS *(Continued)*

System	*Symptom*	*Possible Problem*
Genitourinary	Urinary frequency	Hyperglycemia
	Frequency, dysuria, hesitancy	Benign prostatic hyperplasia, prostatic carcinoma
	Frequency, dysuria, fever	Urinary tract infection, prostatitis
Musculoskeletal	Proximal muscle pain	Polymyalgia rheumatica
	Back pain	Osteoarthritis, compression fractures, Paget's disease, metastatic cancer, infection (tuberculous spondylitis)
Neurologic	Syncope	Postural hypotension, seizure, cardiac dysrhythmia, aortic stenosis, hypoglycemia
	Fall without loss of consciousness	Transient ischemic attack, drop attack
	Transient interference with speech, muscle strength, or sensation	Transient ischemic attack
	Numbness, tingling in fingers	Spondylotic cervical myelopathy
	Clumsiness in tasks requiring fine motor coordination (eg, buttoning shirt)	Spondylotic cervical myelopathy, arthritis
	Sleep disturbances	Circadian rhythm disturbances, medications, sleep apnea, periodic leg movements, depression, anxiety, parkinsonism
	Change in mental status, fever	Meningitis
	Excessive sweating with meals	Autonomic neuropathy
Extremities	Swollen ankles	Heart failure (bilateral swelling), venous insufficiency, hypoalbuminemia

(continued)

TABLE 16–1. REVIEW OF SYSTEMS *(Continued)*

System	*Symptom*	*Possible Problem*
Extremities *(continued)*	Leg pain	Osteoarthritis, radiculopathy (lumbar stenosis, disk herniation), intermittent claudication, night cramps
Skin	Itching	Dry skin, jaundice, uremia, carcinoma, hyperthyroidism, allergic reaction, lice, scabies

Sometimes it is best to ask the patient or family to bring in all of the pills, ointments, or liquids that are in the medicine cabinet at home. Abuse of OTC drugs can have serious consequences; eg, overuse of laxatives can result in constipation, and aspirin abuse may lead to salicylism.

Simply showing that he has medication vials does not guarantee that a patient is complying with treatment. It may be necessary to count the number of tablets in each vial on the first and subsequent visits. If drugs are administered by someone other than the patient, interview that person as well. Find out how the drugs are stored. Some patients combine all tablets in one vial, making it difficult to differentiate the drugs. A patient may have problems reading the label if the print is small. Some patients have difficulty opening bottles, especially child-resistant containers. Ask patients to demonstrate their ability to read labels, recognize drugs, and open containers. Finally, determine the precise nature of any drug allergies reported.

The clinician should not only review the drug history but also document it. Compiling a medication flow sheet is often useful, and a copy should be given to the patient or caregiver.

NUTRITION HISTORY

Ask what kind of food, how much, and how often the patient eats, including the number of hot meals eaten weekly. Address the patient's *ability* to eat (eg, ask how well he can chew and swallow). Xerostomia (dry mouth) may impair mastication and swallowing. Find out if another physician has prescribed a special diet (eg, a low salt or low carbohydrate diet) or if the patient follows a self-prescribed fad diet. Inquire about the intake of alcohol, dietary fiber, and OTC vitamin preparations, as well as the type of snacks consumed (see also Ch. 2).

The amount of money spent on food and the accessibility of food stores are important issues. A patient may be unable to prepare meals if proper kitchen facilities are unavailable. Others have difficulty preparing meals or feeding themselves because of visual limitations, arthritis, immobility, or tremors. A decreased sense of taste or smell may reduce the pleasure of eating. Patients who are worried about urinary incontinence may reduce their fluid intake, which may lead to poor food intake.

PSYCHIATRIC HISTORY

Psychiatric problems in the elderly may not be detected as easily as those in younger patients. Insomnia or changes in sleep patterns, constipation, changes in cognition, anorexia, weight loss, fatigue, increased preoccupation with bodily functions, increased alcohol consumption, and somatic complaints are common signs (see also Ch. 94). Ask the patient about feelings of sadness, depression, and hopelessness. Episodes of crying may indicate depression. Deafness may contribute to depression. Determine if the patient suffers from delusions or hallucinations. Elicit any history of psychiatric care, including psychotherapy, institutionalization, electroconvulsive therapy, and the use of psychoactive drugs or antidepressants.

Discuss such events as the recent loss of a loved one. Suicide risk is not increased by asking about thoughts of suicide (see Suicide in Ch. 94), and plans (eg, medications, gun) need to be discovered. The sooner suicidal thoughts are discovered, the more likely suicide can be prevented.

FUNCTIONAL STATUS

Evaluate the patient's mobility, continence, self-sufficiency, and mentation. The patient may walk independently or may need a cane, walker, or another person's assistance. Ask about difficulty with stairs. Assess the patient's ability to walk, transfer, toilet, groom, bathe, dress, and feed himself **(activities of daily living)** as well as his ability to cook, use the phone, do laundry, clean, shop, or manage money **(instrumental activities of daily living)**; see also Ch. 17. Input from a caregiver and clinical observation may be necessary to evaluate a very disabled patient.

SOCIAL HISTORY

The social history includes assessment of the patient's living arrangements: number of rooms, plumbing, availability of elevators, heat, and air conditioning. Discuss home features that could lead to falls, such as poor lighting, slippery bathtubs, and unanchored small rugs, and how to remedy them. A home visit is the best way to assess the situation. In addition, valuable information can be gleaned from having the patient describe a typical day, touching upon activities such as reading, television viewing, work, exercise, and hobbies. The patient may also talk about the frequency and nature of meals, social contacts, family visits, and availability of transportation. As the number of older drivers increases, the physician's role in examining patients for impairments that may affect driving ability becomes more important (see Ch. 112).

Identify caregivers and support services available to the patient. Determine the family's ability to assist the patient; a full-time job, traveling time to the patient's home, and the health of family members all play a role (see also SOCIAL SUPPORTS AND FAMILY CAREGIVING in Ch. 110). Probe the patient's attitude toward the family and the family's attitude toward the patient. Note the patient's social network (friends or religious or senior citizens' groups) and status (single, married, widowed, or living in a relationship without marriage). Inquire about sexual practices and satisfaction in order to diagnose sexual problems. Although the questioning must be sensitive and tactful, it should be thorough, exploring the number and sex of sexual partners and the risk of sexually transmitted diseases (see Ch. 68).

An elderly person suffers many losses that may affect health and well-being. The patient may have experienced the loss of a spouse, sibling, child, friend, or pet. Retirement may lead to a loss in income. Economic difficulties brought about by inflation and a fixed income need to be addressed. Financial or health problems may result in loss of a home, social status, or independence. The relationship with a longtime physician may have been lost, either because the physician retired or died or because the patient moved to a new residence.

The social history includes questions about tobacco and alcohol use. Remind the patient about the hazards of smoking; if the patient continues to smoke, be especially careful to warn against smoking in bed. Although alcoholism is a serious problem in the elderly, it is often not diagnosed. Signs of alcoholism may include confusion, anger, hostility, alcohol odor on the breath, and tremors. The CAGE (Cut down, Annoyed, Guilty, Eye-opener) screening questionnaire effectively identifies elderly patients with a history of drinking problems (see also Ch. 99).

Discuss and document the patient's wishes regarding heroic measures for prolonging life in acute or chronic care settings. Determine whether the patient has provided for surrogate decision making in case of incapacity (see Ch. 108).

THE PHYSICAL EXAMINATION

Ask if the patient wants a relative or aide in the room during the examination. Portions of the examination may be more comfortable if the patient is allowed to sit in a chair. Lower the examining table to a height that allows easy access; a footstool facilitates mounting. Be aware of examining gowns that are too long and may cause the patient to trip. Do not leave the patient alone on the table. Maintain his dignity and ensure his privacy; if the examination is conducted in a hospital room and a roommate is present, the curtains must be drawn.

Does the patient appear uncomfortable, restless, malnourished, inattentive, pale, dyspneic, or cyanotic? The patient may look older or younger than the stated age. Preliminarily assess the patient's functioning by, for example, observing his clothing and personal hygiene. If the patient is examined at bedside, note the use of a water mattress, a sheepskin, or restraints, as well as the use of a urinary catheter or adult diaper.

VITAL SIGNS

Measure the patient's **height and weight.** Grab bars near or on the scale are helpful for patients with balance problems. When recording the **temperature,** be aware that hypothermia can be missed if the thermometer does not measure low temperatures. Febrile elderly patients in an ambulatory setting are more likely than younger patients to have a serious disease, but the absence of fever does not exclude infection.

Pulses and **blood pressure** should be checked in both arms. Since many factors can alter blood pressure, take several measurements under resting conditions (see also Ch. 35). Blood pressure may be overestimated in elderly patients because of arterial stiffness. This pseudohypertension is suspected in patients with elevated systolic and diastolic blood pressure but no end-organ damage from hypertension. In patients with pseudohypertension, the brachial or radial artery is still palpable after the blood pressure cuff is inflated to a point greater than the systolic pressure (Osler's sign). However, Osler's maneuver is subject to observer error; its accuracy in predicting pseudohypertension is not known.

Checking for **orthostatic hypotension** is worthwhile, even though it is unclear whether prevalence increases with age in patients who are not hypertensive. Observe the patient for at least 3 min in the standing position, but exercise caution when testing volume-depleted patients. A **postprandial fall in blood pressure** with virtually no compensatory increase in pulse rate has been observed in institutionalized patients (see also Ch. 36).

Respiratory rate in elderly patients is 16 to 25 breaths/min. A rate > 25 breaths/min may signal a lower respiratory tract infection before other clinical signs appear.

ORGAN SYSTEMS

Skin and Nails

The evaluation of skin includes a search for **premalignant and malignant lesions,** as well as for areas of **tissue ischemia** or **pressure ulcers.** The size of an ulceration on the skin surface is less than that of the underlying soft tissue lesion (see also Ch. 14). **Unexplained bruises** may be a clue to abuse of an elderly person. Since the dermis becomes thinner with age, **ecchymoses** may occur easily in traumatized areas of the skin, such as the forearm. An uneven tan after sun exposure may be normal in elderly persons because of a progressive loss of epidermal melanocytes (see also Ch. 101).

With advancing age, longitudinal ridges develop **on the nails,** and the crescent-shaped lunula disappears. The nail plate is thinner and is prone to fracture. In the elderly, black splinter hemorrhages in the middle or distal third of the fingernail are more likely associated with trauma than with bacteremia.

Face

With aging, the eyebrows steadily drop below the superior orbital rim, the chin descends, the angle between the submandibular line and the neck is lost, and the skin wrinkles and becomes drier. Thick terminal hairs develop on the ears, nose, upper lip, and chin. The temporal arteries should be palpated for tenderness and thickening.

Nose

A progressive descent of the nasal tip with age causes the upper and lower lateral cartilages to separate, enlarging and lengthening the nose. Although olfaction acuity diminishes with age, an asymmetric loss is abnormal.

Eyes

A loss of orbital fat with age gradually displaces the eye backward into the orbit **(enophthalmos).** Thus, sunken eyes are not necessarily a sign of dehydration in the elderly. This recession is accompanied by a deepening of the upper lid fold and a slight obstruction of peripheral vision. Pupils and palpebral aperture may get smaller **(pseudoptosis),** and an inversion **(senile entropion)** or an eversion **(senile ectropion)** of the lower lid margins can occur. **Arcus senilis,** a white ring at the limbus, has no pathologic significance. Loss of lens elasticity with age results in reduced ability of the lens to change shape when focusing on close objects **(presbyopia).**

By age 70, many persons are unable to rotate the eye upward > 15° from the horizontal plane because of a decline in extraocular muscle function. The light reflex and accommodation are sluggish, a defect in ocular convergence occurs, and pupil size decreases; however, these findings are not pathologically significant.

A thorough eye examination includes testing of visual acuity and screening for glaucoma and cataracts (see Ch. 102). Before testing visual acuity in the patient who wears glasses, check to see that the glasses are properly centered and the lenses are clean. Tonometry is one important screening tool, but peripheral vision should also be tested. Cataracts are best seen using a positive lens of an ophthalmoscope. Some elderly persons with decreased visual acuity experience visual hallucinations despite normal mental function. The hallucinations are well organized and clearly defined; patients who experience them are rarely frightened and quickly recognize that the hallucinations are not real.

Although signs of hypertension or diabetes may be evident on funduscopic examination, the retina's appearance does not change significantly with age. Because of cortical atrophy, elevated intracranial pressure may not be accompanied by papilledema. Macular degeneration is characterized by areas of black pigment or hemorrhages in and around the macula.

Ears

Tophi may be noted during inspection of the pinna. Examine the external auditory canal for cerumen. If the patient wears a hearing aid, remove and examine it; the ear mold and plastic tubing can become plugged with wax. If the battery is dead, a whistle (feedback) will not be heard when the volume is turned up.

To assess the patient for hearing loss, whisper an easily answered question with your face out of view. Test each ear. Evaluation with a portable audioscope, if available, is recommended. Presbycusis affects the high frequencies. The patient is more likely to complain of difficulty in understanding speech than of an inability to hear (see also Ch. 103).

Temporomandibular Joint

Degeneration of the temporomandibular joint (osteoarthrosis) occurs as teeth are lost and excessive compressive forces occur in the joint. Crepitus may be felt at the head of the condyle as the patient opens and closes his jaw. Jaw movements may be painful (see also Ch. 52).

Mouth

Before examining the mouth, remove any dentures. Denture wearers are at risk for resorption of the alveolar ridges and for oral candidiasis. Improperly fitting dentures can also cause inflammation of the palatal mucosa and ulcers of the alveolar ridges. Edentulous persons who do not wear dentures may have painful, inflamed, fissured lesions at the lip commissures (angular cheilitis); this usually is caused by fungal infections and responds promptly to topical therapy. Inadequate support of the facial musculature accentuates the grooves at lip commissures, creating a moist, protected area conducive to fungal growth.

Look for bleeding or swollen gums, loose and broken teeth, fungal infections, and signs of cancer (leukoplakia, erythroplakia, ulceration, and tumor mass). Patients suffering from xerostomia may have fissuring of the mouth and tongue, and the tongue blade may stick to the buccal mucosa. The teeth may darken with age, as a result of extrinsic stains and less translucent enamel. Erythematous, edematous gingiva that bleeds easily around the teeth can be a sign of gingival and periodontal disease. Bad odor from the mouth may indicate caries, periodontitis, or other oral disease (see also Ch. 52).

Tongue

Examine the dorsal and ventral surfaces of the tongue. Varicose veins on the ventral surface are common. Erythema migrans (geographic tongue) is also considered a normal age-related change. The papillae at the sides of the tongue atrophy with age.

The tongue may be enlarged in an edentulous patient to facilitate mastication; however, enlargement may also be a sign of amyloidosis or hypothyroidism. A smooth, painful tongue may indicate vitamin B_{12} deficiency.

Neck

The thyroid gland in elderly persons lies low in the neck, often beneath the sternum. Examine the gland for enlargement and nodules. In dehydrated elderly patients with parotitis, the parotid gland is swollen, firm, and tender; pus may be expressed from Stensen's duct.

The significance of carotid bruits in asymptomatic patients is unclear. Arterial bruits due to carotid artery stenosis can be distinguished from those due to transmitted heart murmurs by moving the stethoscope up the neck: a transmitted heart murmur gets softer, whereas the bruit of carotid artery stenosis gets louder.

Resistance to passive flexion of the neck is found in patients with either cervical spondylosis or osteoarthritis. Resistance to flexion also occurs in patients with meningitis, but the neck can be rotated passively from side to side. Resistance to lateral rotation, extension, and flexion of the neck occurs with cervical spine disease.

Back and Chest

The back should be examined for **scoliosis** and tenderness. **Spontaneous osteoporotic fractures** of the sacrum (characterized by severe low back, hip, and leg pain and marked sacral tenderness) may occur in elderly patients.

Basilar rales may be heard in the lungs of healthy patients and should disappear after the patient takes a few deep breaths.

Heart

Normally, the size of the heart can be assessed by palpating the apex; however, displacement caused by kyphoscoliosis may make assessment difficult. The most common **systolic murmur** in the elderly is due to aortic sclerosis, which is not hemodynamically significant. **Mitral regurgitation,** significant **aortic stenosis,** and **hypertrophic obstructive cardiomyopathy** also produce systolic murmurs; the murmur of hypertrophic obstructive cardiomyopathy is intensified when the patient performs a Valsalva maneuver. The murmur of **aortic valve sclerosis** peaks early and rarely radiates to the carotid arteries, while the murmur of **aortic valve stenosis** peaks later and is transmitted to the carotid arteries. Narrowed pulse pressure, loud murmur (> grade 2), and a dampened second heart sound are helpful clinical signs of aortic stenosis. However, the classic features of aortic stenosis may not be observed in older patients—the murmur decreases in loudness with advancing age, an audible second heart sound is rare, and narrow pulse pressures are not common. Slowing of the carotid upstroke often does not occur in elderly patients with aortic stenosis because of diminished vascular compliance.

Fourth heart sounds are common in older persons who have no evidence of cardiovascular disease. **Diastolic murmurs** are abnormal in persons of any age. **Heart rates** as low as 40 beats/min may be normal. An unexplained **sinus bradycardia** in apparently healthy persons does not adversely influence long-term cardiovascular morbidity or mortality, although it is associated with abnormalities of atrioventricular or intraventricular conduction (see also Ch. 40).

In patients with **pacemakers** who develop new neurologic or cardiovascular symptoms, physical examination may reveal hypotension, heart failure, cannon waves in the neck veins, or variability of heart sounds, murmurs, or pulses. This complex of symptoms and signs may be related to the loss of atrioventricular synchrony.

Abdomen

The abdominal musculature in elderly persons is often weak. Although most abdominal aortic aneurysms are palpable, only the lateral extent of the aneurysm can be assessed on physical examination. A mass in front of the aorta that is transmitting a pulse does not expand laterally. Check the suprapubic area for evidence of urinary retention.

Rectum

Examine the anorectal area for fissures, hemorrhoids, and strictures, as well as for sensation and anal winks as part of the neurologic examination. A digital examination, performed in both men and women, may reveal a mass or fecal impaction.

Palpate the prostate gland for nodules. Estimating prostate size by digital examination is inaccurate, and size does not correlate with urethral obstruction; however, digital examination allows a qualitative evaluation.

Female Reproductive System

Elderly women should have annual breast examinations by a health professional and should be instructed to perform monthly breast self-examination. Retracted nipples can be everted with pressure around the nipple when retraction is due to age but not when it is secondary to an underlying growth.

Regular pelvic examinations are indicated, and Papanicolaou (Pap) tests should be performed about every 2 to 3 yr until the age of 70 yr (see also CERVICAL CARCINOMA in Ch. 66). Any woman who has not had regular Pap tests should have at least two tests, a year apart, before the screening interval is lengthened. After three consecutive normal results in women > 60 yr old, testing can usually stop. Women who have had a hysterectomy should receive Pap tests if they have any remaining cervical tissue; otherwise no further Pap tests need to be obtained. The pelvic examination may be done in the left lateral position if the patient lacks hip mobility. Postmenopausal reduction of estrogen leads to atrophic changes in the vaginal and urethral mucosa, which appears dry and lacks rugal folds. The ovaries should not be palpable; palpable ovaries suggest malignancy. Check for leakage of urine with coughing.

Musculoskeletal System

Examine the joints for tenderness, swelling, subluxation, crepitus, warmth, and redness (see Ch. 75). **Heberden's nodes** are bony overgrowths at the distal interphalangeal joints, whereas **Bouchard's nodes** are bony overgrowths at the proximal interphalangeal joints. Either can occur in patients with osteoarthritis. Patients with chronic rheumatoid arthritis may have subluxation of the metacarpophalangeal joints with ulnar deviation of the fingers. Hyperextension of the proximal interphalangeal joint and flexion of the distal interphalangeal joint result in a **swan-neck deformity,** whereas hyperextension of the distal interphalangeal joint and flexion of the proximal interphalangeal joint result in a **boutonnière deformity.**

Determine both the active and the passive range of joint motion. Note the presence of contractures. With age, a variable resistance to passive manipulation of the extremities (gegenhalten) sometimes occurs. Test muscle strength and note any atrophy. Wasting of the interosseous and thenar muscles of the hands occurs with age. Test the functional ability of the arms by asking the patient to pick up an eating utensil or to touch the back of the head with both hands.

Feet

Onychomycosis, fungal infection of the toenail, causes the nail to appear thickened and yellow. An ingrown toenail **(onychocryptosis)** has borders that curve in and down. Psoriatic nails are whitish, scale easily, and may have a pitted surface (see also Ch. 77).

The **bunion deformity** consists of a medial prominence of the first metatarsal head and lateral deviation (hallux valgus) and rotation of the big toe. The **bunionette deformity** is a lateral prominence of the fifth metatarsal head. Hyperflexion of the proximal interphalangeal joint results in a **hammer toe.** Hyperflexion of both the proximal and distal interphalangeal toe joints results in a **claw toe.**

Nervous System

The neurologic examination is critically important in the elderly, and reasonable screening can be accomplished in a short time (see also NEUROLOGIC EVALUATION in Ch. 88). Assess **motor function** by noting strength and ability to sit down and get up from a chair or examining table. Compression of the upper arm against the armrest of a wheelchair can injure the radial nerve, resulting in weakness of the extensor muscles of the wrist, fingers, and thumb. Observe **coordination** during walking and transferring. With aging, a woman's gait is described as becoming more waddling, while a man's gait becomes wider-based and smaller-stepped. Check **sensation** when examining the feet and hands. While vibratory sensation in the lower legs decreases with aging, sensation to light touch and pinprick does not change.

Generally, the deep tendon (knee jerk and biceps) **reflexes** do not change with age. Nearly half of older patients have a greatly diminished ankle reflex, but it can be elicited with skillful technique in most of them. Postural reflexes are often impaired with aging, and a loss of postural control may contribute to falls. Postural sway (movement in the anteroposterior plane when the patient remains stationary and upright) also increases in severity with age. Primitive reflexes (eg, the snout and glabella reflexes) may reemerge with aging but are not clinically meaningful.

Evaluation of **tremor** is important and can be done during handshaking and other simple activities. If tremor is detected, note its amplitude, frequency, and whether it occurs at rest, with motion, or with intention.

MENTAL STATUS

Assessment of mental status, a key component of the history and physical examination, is discussed in Ch. 89.

The patient may resent the mental status examination and needs to be reassured that it is routine. The patient must be able to hear the examiner. Pure word deafness, an isolated inability to understand speech, may be mistaken for cognitive dysfunction. Assessing the mental status of a patient who has a speech or language disorder (eg, mutism, dysarthria, aphasia, or speech apraxia—see below) is difficult.

Although the speed with which information is processed and memories are retrieved may decline, abnormalities of consciousness, orientation, judgment, calculations, speech, language, or praxis cannot be attributed simply to age. Questions of orientation alone fail to detect many cases of dementia. Loss of short-term memory is a sensitive indicator of cognitive impairment and can be used as a screening test. Such screening can be followed later by a formal test of mental status.

SPEECH AND LANGUAGE

Evaluation of language function includes assessing spontaneous speech, comprehension of spoken language (performance of verbal commands, yes or no answers to questions, pointing to objects), repetition of words and phrases, word-finding ability, comprehension of written material, and writing. In assessing spontaneous speech, pay attention to the rate of word output, the effort involved in initiating speech, and the length of phrases (see TABLE 16–2). In testing word-finding ability, ask the patient to name objects and parts of objects.

TABLE 16–2. ASSESSMENT OF THE APHASIC PATIENT

Spontaneous speech	Nonfluent aphasia: Lesion is anterior to central sulcus (eg, Broca's aphasia); speaks < 50 words/min; speaks slowly and with effort; pauses between words; often mumbles; experiences naming errors; comprehends well; is unable to repeat sentences verbatim; uses 1- or 2-word phrases Fluent aphasia: Lesion is posterior to central sulcus (eg, Wernicke's aphasia); speaks 100 to 200 words/min; speaks effortlessly but often unintelligibly; experiences naming errors; is unable to comprehend; is unable to repeat sentences correctly; uses incorrect words and grammar
Word-finding ability	Circumlocutory phrase (eg, *what you use to tell time* for *clock*) Nonspecific words (eg, *thing* or *stuff*) Incorrect words (paraphasia) Phonemic paraphasia (eg, *trable* for *table*) Semantic paraphasia (eg, *headman* for *president*) Jargon (eg, *gabbagabbahey* for *pin*)

Adapted from Sherman FT, Meisells SM, Margolis E, Libow LS: "Speech and language disorders," in *The Core of Geriatric Medicine,* edited by LS Libow and FT Sherman. Published 1981 by CV Mosby Company. Copyright 1986 by LS Libow and FT Sherman.

The patient with **dysarthria** may have weakness or poor coordination of the lips, tongue, palate, vocal cords, or respiratory muscles, which interferes with speech production. The patient produces approximate sounds in the correct arrangement. Dysarthria may occur in patients with neurologic diseases (eg, cranial nerve palsies) or lesions that affect the speech mechanism, such as vocal cord tumors. Note speech rhythm and articulation (see TABLE 16–3). Since language function is intact, the dysarthric patient is able to read and write.

The patient with speech **apraxia** is able to move the muscles involved in speech and understands what needs to be done but has difficulty speaking. He can perform overlearned acts (eg, counting) and write sentences without a problem. In contrast, the patient with **aphasia** has difficulty speaking or writing (see TABLE 16–2). Previously acquired language ability is lost. Depressed patients may speak slowly and softly, but language function is intact. Speech arrest may be associated with seizures.

TABLE 16–3. ASSESSMENT OF THE DYSARTHRIC PATIENT

Type of Dysarthria	*Area Damaged*	*Cause*	*Speech Pattern*
Dysarthria of pseudobulbar palsy	Upper motor neurons	Cerebrovascular accident, amyotrophic lateral sclerosis	Slow, great effort required; prolonged, hardly intelligible words
Ataxic dysarthria	Cerebellum	Cerebellar atrophy, multiple sclerosis	Slow, staccato, jerky; irregular separation of syllables; imprecise enunciation; poor coordination of speech and respiration
Hypokinetic dysarthria	Extrapyramidal system	Parkinson's disease	Hesitation, loss of vocal inflection, stoppages and bursts of speed, monotonous tone, poor articulation, diminished voice volume
Paretic dysarthria	Lower motor neurons or neuromuscular transmission	Myasthenia gravis, bulbar palsy, peripheral neuropathies	Difficulty with vibratives (eg, "R"), lingual and labial consonants are not pronounced, nasal quality to voice owing to palatal weakness

Adapted from Sherman FT, Meisells SM, Margolis E, Libow LS: "Speech and language disorders," in *The Core of Geriatric Medicine,* edited by LS Libow and FT Sherman. Published 1981 by CV Mosby Company. Copyright 1986 by LS Libow and FT Sherman.

NUTRITIONAL STATUS

Many of the measurements commonly performed when assessing nutritional status may be unreliable in the elderly. Aging can alter height, weight, and body composition (lean body mass and fat content). Arm span is a reliable estimate of height when calculating body mass index in the elderly. Use of multiple sites instead of only the triceps may provide more reliable skinfold measurements. (See also Ch. 2.)

UNUSUAL PRESENTATIONS OF ILLNESS

Symptoms and signs of **hyperthyroidism** may be subtle in very old patients, and classic eye findings and an enlarged thyroid gland may not be present (see HYPERTHYROIDISM in Ch. 79). Symptoms include weight loss, palpitations, and weakness; clinical signs include fine skin, tremor, atrial fibrillation, and tachycardia. Patients may have an apathetic rather than a hyperkinetic appearance. Those with **hypothyroidism** may present with weight loss rather than weight gain and may have cognitive loss, heart failure, or constipation.

Patients with **hyperparathyroidism** often do not have any of the characteristic symptoms. The clinical picture may be nonspecific: fatigue, decreased intellectual capacity, emotional instability, anorexia, constipation, and hypertension (see HYPERCALCEMIA in Ch. 82).

Instead of presenting with the classic manifestations of headache, jaw claudication, or blindness, patients with **giant cell arteritis** or **polymyalgia rheumatica** may present with respiratory tract symptoms (eg, cough, sore throat, hoarseness) or mental changes (see Ch. 74). They may complain of head pain in the frontal, vertex, or occipital areas rather than in the temporal area.

Elderly patients with **systemic lupus erythematosus** have a lower incidence of Raynaud's phenomenon, malar rash, nephritis, and neuropsychiatric disease than do younger patients (see SYSTEMIC LUPUS ERYTHEMATOSUS in Ch. 75). However, the incidence of pneumonitis, interstitial fibrosis, subcutaneous nodules, and discoid lupus is higher in the elderly. Patients may present with the symptoms of a systemic illness (eg, fever, weight loss, arthritis).

Elderly patients with **fibromyalgia syndrome** are less likely than younger patients to have chronic headaches, anxiety, and symptoms aggravated by weather factors, mental stress, or poor sleep.

The clinical manifestations of **sarcoidosis** in the elderly are variable. Presenting symptoms include shortness of breath, blurred vision, myopathy, adenopathy, and fatigue.

Elderly patients with **bacteremia** may not be febrile, demonstrating instead nonspecific findings such as general malaise or an unexplained change in mental status.

The elderly patient with **urinary tract infection** may be afebrile and may not complain of dysuria, frequency, or urgency (see Ch. 65). Dizziness, confusion, anorexia, fatigue, or weakness may occur.

At initial presentation, the elderly patient with **meningitis** may not have symptoms of meningeal irritation (see Ch. 92). The patient may have fever and a change in mental status without headache or nuchal rigidity.

The older patient with **pneumonia** may present with malaise, anorexia, or confusion. Although tachycardia and tachypnea are common, fever may be absent. Coughing may be mild and without copious, purulent sputum. Coexisting illnesses may alter the presentation of **tuberculosis.** Symptoms may be nonspecific (eg, fever, weakness, confusion, anorexia). Pneumonia and tuberculosis are discussed in Ch. 46.

Older patients with **appendicitis** may complain of diffuse abdominal pain that is not followed by localization to the right lower quadrant (see DISORDERS OF THE APPENDIX in Ch. 62). However, tenderness in this quadrant is a significant early physical sign.

Elderly patients with **biliary disease** may present with nonspecific mental and physical deterioration (malaise, confusion, loss of mobility) without jaundice, fever, or abdominal pain. Abnormal liver function tests may be the only indication that biliary disease is present (see DISORDERS OF THE GALLBLADDER AND BILIARY TREE in Ch. 62).

Patients with **acute bowel infarction** may not have the characteristic abdominal pain and tenderness. These patients may present with acute confusion.

Nonsteroidal anti-inflammatory drugs can mask the pain of **peptic ulcer disease** in elderly patients, who may present with anorexia (see PEPTIC ULCER DISEASE in Ch. 62). Gastrointestinal bleeding may be painless in the elderly.

Patients with **myocardial infarction** may present with dyspnea, syncope, weakness, vomiting, or confusion, rather than with chest pain (see Ch. 37).

Instead of complaining of dyspnea, an elderly patient with **heart failure** may present with confusion, agitation, anorexia, weakness, insomnia, or lethargy (see also Ch. 41). Orthopnea may cause nocturnal agitation in demented patients with heart failure.

Irritability may be the primary affective symptom of **depression** (see Ch. 95). Cognitive loss, often called pseudodementia, is another atypical presentation of depression (see Ch. 90).

17. COMPREHENSIVE GERIATRIC ASSESSMENT

A multidimensional, usually interdisciplinary, diagnostic process intended to determine a frail elderly person's medical, psychosocial, and functional capabilities and problems. Comprehensive geriatric assessment has many immediate and long-term purposes, including achieving a multidimensional diagnostic evaluation, developing an overall plan for treatment and long-term follow-up, arranging for treatment and rehabilitation, facilitating primary care and case management, determining long-term care needs and optimal placement, and making the best use of health care resources.

A comprehensive geriatric assessment differs from a standard medical evaluation in its concentration on frail elderly people with complex problems, its emphasis on functional status and quality of life, and its frequent use of interdisciplinary teams. Although a comprehensive geriatric assessment may be carried out by a primary care physician in an office, generally it is best performed by personnel from several disciplines in a setting organized for their interaction.

The comprehensive geriatric assessment is usually initiated when primary care physicians or community health workers identify functional problems and disabilities. The assessment then continues with more in-depth evaluation of these problems by a physician or interdisciplinary team and the initiation of a therapeutic plan with a goal of maximizing health and functional status, and hence quality of life.

The basic concepts of comprehensive geriatric assessment, which have evolved over the last 60 years, incorporate elements of many disciplines, including the traditional medical history and physical examination, the social services assessment, functional evaluation and treatment methods derived from rehabilitation medicine, and psychometric methods derived from the social sciences. By incorporating all these perspectives into a compact assessment format, geriatricians have created a practical means of viewing the whole patient.

As geriatric care systems have emerged throughout the world, comprehensive geriatric assessment has become a central element. Geared to local needs and populations, geriatric assessment programs vary widely. They differ in comprehensiveness, organization, and structural and functional components. The programs also are based in different settings, including hospital acute care units, hospital rehabilitation units, outpatient and office programs, and home visit outreach programs. Yet despite such diversity, the assessment programs share many common characteristics. Virtually all include multidimensional assessment, using one or more sets of assessment instruments to quantify functional, psychologic, and social parameters. Most use interdisciplinary teams to pool expertise and share enthusiasm in working toward common goals. Moreover, most programs attempt to couple assessment with an intervention, such as rehabilitation, counseling, or placement.

Assessment Settings

A number of factors must be considered when deciding on the setting for a patient's assessment (see TABLE 17–1). A patient with mental or physical impairments may have difficulty complying with recommendations and keeping appointments in several locations. A functionally impaired elder who requires transportation may depend on family members and friends who worry about losing their jobs because of continual demands on their time and energy. Because increased periods of illness cause fatigue, a patient may need bed rest during the assessment process. Also, the interdisciplinary team must allow adequate uninterrupted time to complete the assessment.

TABLE 17–1. FACTORS IN DETERMINING SETTING FOR COMPREHENSIVE GERIATRIC ASSESSMENT

Factor	*Office Setting*	*Outpatient Unit*	*Inpatient Unit*
Level of disability	Low	Intermediate	High
Cognitive dysfunction	Mild	Mild to severe	Moderate to severe
Family support	Good	Good to fair	Good to poor
Acuity of illness	Mild	Mild to moderate	Moderate to severe
Complexity of patient's problems and needs	Low	Intermediate	High
Access to transportation	Good	Good	Good to poor

Most comprehensive geriatric assessments do not require the full range of technology available nor the intense level of monitoring performed by physicians and nurses in acute care inpatient settings. However, hospitalization may be necessary if the assessment cannot be accomplished quickly in an outpatient setting. A specialized geriatric setting outside an acute care hospital (a day hospital or subacute inpatient geriatric evaluation unit) can provide an interdisciplinary team that has the time and expertise to perform services efficiently, an adequate level of monitoring, and beds for patients unable to sit or stand for long periods. Inpatient and day hospital assessment programs can offer intensiveness and speed, and they can care for particularly frail or acutely ill patients. Outpatient programs are usually less costly, and they eliminate the need for an inpatient stay.

Assessment Benefits

More than 25 controlled trials in different settings and a recent meta-analysis have shown that comprehensive geriatric assessment improves patient care and clinical outcomes. The benefits include greater diagnostic accuracy, improved mental and functional status, reduced mortality, decreased use of nursing homes and acute care hospitals, and greater satisfaction with care. Although the degree of benefit varies among the study settings and not all studies document each benefit, virtually all studies show at least some significant benefit. Unfortunately, the cost of these programs has limited their use. Although some cost-effectiveness evaluations indicate that these programs can save money by decreasing hospital readmissions and nursing home stays, few programs are in self-contained care systems that can achieve these subsequent savings. Thus, the growth of these programs has been slow.

Targeting programs to the most appropriate patients is a key issue in demonstrating program impact. Although most elderly people could probably derive some benefit from comprehensive geriatric assessment, frail or ill people derive the most benefit. Programs that include not just consultation but also treatment, rehabilitation, long-term follow-up, and case management also tend to be most beneficial.

ASSESSMENT PROCESS

Patients are referred for comprehensive geriatric assessment when both disease and functional status worsen. If disease alone worsens without affecting functional status, patients can usually be managed in primary care settings by primary care physicians. However, patients who have new, severe, or progressive deficits in functional status should be given a comprehensive geriatric assessment that encompasses the expertise of several disciplines. Also, when new disabilities are detected through periodic screening, comprehensive geriatric assessment may be recommended.

The four principal domains of comprehensive geriatric assessment are **functional ability, physical health, psychologic health,** and **socio-environmental factors.** Assessment of each can be achieved by using certain assessment instruments. Although these instruments are not essential for performing comprehensive geriatric assessment, they make the process more reliable and easier. They also aid communication of clinically relevant quantitative information among health care providers and permit tabulation of clinical data and measurement of change over time.

Several issues need to be considered in selecting an assessment instrument for a specific population: instrument reliability and validity, patient acceptance, time and personnel needed to administer the tests, and relevance and usefulness of the data to be collected. With most (but not all) instruments, these issues are addressed during development, testing, and publication. The instruments described in this chapter are some of the most useful, most widely used, and best validated. However, exclusion of a particular instrument does not imply a negative judgment.

Proper interpretation of the scores of these quantitative tests is based on the original references and clinical experience. TABLE 17–2 summarizes the general features of selected assessment instruments.

TABLE 17–2. GUIDELINES FOR USE OF SELECTED GERIATRIC ASSESSMENT INSTRUMENTS

Instrument	*Who Administers*	*Who Answers*	*Score Range (poor to good)*	*Time Required to Administer (min)*
Katz ADL scale	I	CP,NP	0–6	2–4
Lawton IADL scale	I,SA	S,CP,NP	9–27	3–5
Folstein Mini Mental State Examination	I	S	0–30	5–15
Yesavage Geriatric Depression Scale (short form)	I,SA	S	15–0	3–6
Tinetti Balance and Gait Evaluation	I	S	0–28	5–15

ADL = activities of daily living; IADL = instrumental activities of daily living; I = interviewer; S = subject; SA = self-administer; CP = caregiver proxy; NP = nurse proxy.

Functional Ability

A typical geriatric assessment begins with a review of the major domains of functional ability: **activities of daily living (ADLs)** and **instrumental activities of daily living (IADLs).** The ADLs include self-care activities that people must accomplish to survive without help, such as eating, dressing, bathing, transferring, and toileting. Patients unable to perform these activities usually require caregiver support for 12 to 24 h per day. The IADLs include performing heavy housework, going on errands, managing finances, and telephoning—activities required if the person is to remain independent in a house or apartment. Several reliable instruments have been developed for measuring patients' abilities to perform ADLs and IADLs; perhaps the most widely used are the Katz ADL Scale and the Lawton IADL Scale (see TABLES 17–3 and 17–4). Clinicians use these instruments to detect problems in performing activities and to determine what kind of assistance may be needed. For instance, a top score of six out of six on the Katz ADL Scale indicates that a person has full basic function, usually implying that nursing home care is inappropriate. A score of two usually indicates adequate feeding and continence (since scoring is hierarchical) but impairment of the more advanced activities, implying that a caregiver or nursing home is needed for survival.

TABLE 17–3. ACTIVITIES OF DAILY LIVING SCALE

		Independent	
		Yes	*No*
1. Bathing (sponge bath, tub bath, or shower)	Receives no assistance or assistance in bathing only one part of body		
2. Dressing	Gets clothes and dresses without any assistance except for tying shoes		
3. Toileting	Goes to toilet room, uses toilet, arranges clothes, and returns without any assistance (may use cane or walker for support and may use bedpan or urinal at night)		
4. Transferring	Moves in and out of bed and chair without assistance (may use cane or walker)		
5. Continence	Controls bowel and bladder completely by self (without occasional accidents)		
6. Feeding	Feeds self without assistance (except for help with cutting meat or buttering bread)		
Total ADL score (Number of "yes" answers, out of possible 6)			

A score of 6 indicates full function; a score of 4, moderate impairment; and a score of 2, severe impairment.

Modified from Katz S, Downs TD, Cash HR, et al: "Progress in the development of the index of ADL." *Gerontologist* 10:20-30, 1970. Copyright © The Gerontological Society of America.

When patients have deficits in ADLs and IADLs, physicians usually need additional information about the patient's environment and social situation. For example, the amount and type of caregiver support available, the strength of the patient's social network, and the level of social activities in which the patient participates all influence the approach used to manage the deficits. Such information can readily be obtained by an experienced nurse or social worker.

Besides ADLs and IADLs, this domain includes higher level activities, sometimes called advanced ADLs **(AADLs),** which include exer-

TABLE 17–4. INSTRUMENTAL ACTIVITIES OF DAILY LIVING SCALE

1. Can you use the telephone	without help,	3
	with some help, or	2
	are you completely unable to use the telephone?	1
2. Can you get to places beyond walking distance	without help,	3
	with some help, or	2
	are you completely unable to travel unless special arrangements are made?	1
3. Can you go shopping for groceries	without help,	3
	with some help, or	2
	are you completely unable to do any shopping?	1
4. Can you prepare your own meals	without help,	3
	with some help, or	2
	are you completely unable to prepare any meals?	1
5. Can you do your own housework	without help,	3
	with some help, or	2
	are you completely unable to do any housework?	1
6. Can you do your own handyman work	without help,	3
	with some help, or	2
	are you completely unable to do any handyman work?	1
7. Can you do your own laundry	without help,	3
	with some help, or	2
	are you completely unable to do any laundry at all?	1
8. Do you or could you take medicine	without help (in the right doses at the right time),	3
	with some help (take medicine if someone prepares it for you and/or reminds you to take it, or	2
	are you or would you be completely unable to take your own medicine?	1

(continued)

TABLE 17–4. INSTRUMENTAL ACTIVITIES OF DAILY LIVING SCALE *(Continued)*

9. Can you manage your own money	without help,	3
	with some help, or	2
	are you completely unable to manage money?	1

For each question, the first answer indicates independence; the second, capability with assistance; and the third, dependence. The maximum score is 27, although scores have meaning only for a particular patient, as when declining scores over time reveal deterioration. Questions 4 through 7 tend to be gender-specific; they can be modified by the interviewer.

Adapted with permission from M. Powell Lawton, PhD, Director of Research, Philadelphia Geriatric Center, Philadelphia. For more information, see the review article Lawton MP, et al: "A research and service-oriented multilevel assessment instrument." *Journal of Gerontology* 37:91–99, 1982.

cise and the ability to travel independently on airplanes. However, these AADLs have not been as well quantified and usually are not included in comprehensive geriatric assessment for frail elderly persons.

Physical Health

Most health care professionals quantify physical health by compiling a traditional problem list of defined diagnoses and symptom complexes. Also, most clinicians are aware of a few severity indicators, such as the New York Heart Association four-point functional disability scale (which can help clarify and communicate the degree of disability resulting from a cardiac condition) and the APACHE (Acute Physiology and Chronic Health Evaluation) scale for quantifying the severity of illness among acutely ill persons. Documenting the number of days of hospitalization and disability and the use of related health care services can help to define the severity of health problems, as well.

A number of detailed, disease-specific scales are also available for quantifying levels of function, dysfunction, disability, and handicap attributable to particular diseases; these instruments are similar to the New York Heart Association Scale. Some, such as measurements made in a pulmonary function or physiology laboratory, are purely quantitative; others, such as a quality-of-life scale, are purely qualitative. Still others, such as a dementia-disability scale, include both kinds of information. Well-established disease-related scales exist for dementia, depression, parkinsonism, and multiple sclerosis. One particularly useful scale for the comprehensive geriatric assessment is the Tinetti Balance and Gait Evaluation (see TABLE 17–5). This scale can be used to detect

TABLE 17–5. TINETTI BALANCE AND GAIT EVALUATION

BALANCE

Instructions: Person is seated in hard armless chair. The following maneuvers are tested.

1. Sitting balance	Leans or slides in chair	= 0
	Steady, safe	= 1 ____
2. Rising	Unable without help	= 0
	Able but uses arms to help	= 1
	Able without use of arms	= 2 ____
3. Attempts to rise	Unable without help	= 0
	Able but requires more than one attempt	= 1
	Able to arise with one attempt	= 2 ____
4. Immediate standing balance (first 5 sec)	Unsteady (staggers, moves feet, has marked trunk sway)	= 0
	Steady but uses walker or cane or grabs other objects for support	= 1
	Steady without walker or cane or other support	= 2 ____
5. Standing balance	Unsteady	= 0
	Steady but has wide stance (medial heels more than 4 in. apart) or uses cane, walker, or other support	= 1
	Has narrow stance without support	= 2 ____
6. Nudged (person stands with feet as close together as possible, examiner pushes lightly on person's sternum with palm of hand 3 times)	Begins to fall	= 0
	Staggers, grabs, but catches self	= 1
	Steady	= 2 ____
7. Eyes closed (same position as in #6)	Unsteady	= 0
	Steady	= 1 ____

(continued)

TABLE 17–5. TINETTI BALANCE AND GAIT EVALUATION *(Continued)*

	BALANCE (continued)		
8. Turning 360°	Discontinuous steps	= 0	
	Continuous steps	= 1	_____
	Unsteady (grabs, staggers)	= 0	
	Steady	= 1	_____
9. Sitting down	Unsafe (misjudged distance, falls into chair)	= 0	
	Uses arms or not a smooth motion	= 1	
	Safe, smooth motion	= 2	_____
	Balance score:		_____/16
	GAIT		
Instructions: Person stands with examiner; walks down hallway or across room, first at usual pace, then back at rapid but safe pace (using usual walking aid such as cane, walker).			
10. Initiation of gait (immediately after told to go)	Any hesitancy or multiple attempts to start	= 0	
	No hesitancy	= 1	_____
11. Step length and height	a. Right swing foot Does not pass left stance foot with step	= 0	
	Passes left stance foot	= 1	
	Right foot does *not* clear floor completely with step	= 0	
	Right foot completely clears floor	= 1	_____
	b. Left swing foot Does not pass right stance foot with step	= 0	
	Passes right stance foot	= 1	
	Left foot does *not* clear floor completely with step	= 0	
	Left foot completely clears floor	= 1	_____

(continued)

TABLE 17–5. TINETTI BALANCE AND GAIT EVALUATION *(Continued)*

	GAIT (continued)		
12. Step symmetry	Right and left step length do not appear equal	= 0	
	Right and left step appear equal	= 1	____
13. Step continuity	Stopping or discontinuity between steps	= 0	
	Steps appear continuous	= 1	____
14. Path (estimate in relation to 12-in. floor tiles; observe excursion of one foot over about 10 ft of the course)	Marked deviation	= 0	
	Mild or moderate deviation or uses walking aid	= 1	
	Straight without walking aid	= 2	____
15. Trunk	Has marked sway or uses walking aid	= 0	
	No sway but has flexion of knees or back or spreads arms out while walking	= 1	
	No sway, no flexion, no use of arms, and no use of walking aid	= 2	____
16. Walking stance	Heels apart	= 0	
	Heels almost touch while walking	= 1	____
	Gait score:		____/12
	Total score:		____/28

A score below 26 usually indicates a problem; the lower the score, the greater the problem. A score below 19 indicates a fivefold increased risk of falls.

Modified from Tinetti M: "Performance-oriented assessment of mobility problems in elderly patients." *Journal of the American Geriatrics Society* 34:119-126, 1986; used with permission.

a mobility problem, to quantify the severity of the problem, to identify the aspect of balance or gait most affected for treatment planning, and to establish a quantitative baseline score for monitoring disease progression or treatment effectiveness. Also, the score can predict the risk of falls.

Psychologic Health

Measurement of psychologic health includes the two major quantifiable subdomains of cognition (mental status) and affect (anxiety and depression). Of the several validated screening tests for cognitive function, the Folstein Mini Mental State Examination is one of the best because it efficiently tests the major aspects of cognitive functioning (see FIG. 89–1). Several depression screens are widely used. Among the easiest to use and most widely accepted are the Yesavage Geriatric Depression Scale and the Hamilton Depression Scale (see TABLES 95–2 and 95–3). Sometimes specific psychiatric symptoms (eg, paranoia, delusions, behavior abnormalities) are included in the psychologic assessment, but they are less easily quantified and are rarely included in rating scales.

Socioenvironmental Factors

This domain is complex and currently the least well quantified, probably because of the heterogeneity of its components, which include the social interaction network, available social support resources and special needs, and environmental adequacy. Several instruments are available for documenting this domain, but none are both quantitative and clinically useful. For a checklist that can be used to assess home safety, see TABLE 7–4.

---

18. ESTABLISHING THERAPEUTIC OBJECTIVES: QUALITY OF LIFE ISSUES

In one sense, a discussion of quality of life issues and their influence on establishing therapeutic objectives for the elderly is inappropriate in this book. The chapter title itself reeks of ageism, implying that ill elderly people have distinct quality of life concerns that require a change in traditional therapeutic objectives. But the goals of medical treatment have not changed since the time of Hippocrates, and a patient's age should not affect a consideration of them. Medicine and its practitioners cure when possible, while always caring and relieving suffering.

Although age per se should not become part of the equation for setting treatment goals, several phenomena that are more prevalent with increasing age affect these goals and thus intrude upon this discussion. Chronic disease, physical disability, pain and suffering, cognitive impairment, institutional confinement, diminished life expectancy, heavy health care utilization, accumulated losses, and social isolation, although not unique to old age, are closely associated with it and demand attention when considering ways to enhance quality of life for persons receiving medical care.

Quality of life assessment is a thorny concept, in some ways more suited to philosophy than to medicine. In the context of health care, the focus on quality of life should be narrow, referring to a particular patient's experience. The phrase "quality of life" does not imply any absolute standards; in the absence of disease or medical treatment, quality of life is an intensely personal and thus variable concept. Most people are comfortable talking about their own quality of life, but when asked to determine it for another person, they become appropriately uncertain and reluctant. Frequent and frank discussions with the patient about goals and aspirations for late life allow the physician to act in the most informed and useful way on the patient's behalf.

Concrete, objective parameters may help guide clinicians in treating elderly patients when certain phenomena suggest the need to **modify therapeutic objectives.** Examples of useful indicators include the presence and severity of suffering (either mental or physical) or pain, the likelihood of having previous lifestyle and pleasures restored by treatment, the prognosis for survival, and the prospect that the disease or treatment will cause suffering. Regardless of the patient's age, the adverse impact of a proposed diagnostic test or treatment should always be scrutinized and compared with the potential benefit. Coexisting conditions may influence the net gain or harm, but in principle the need to modify therapy remains unchanged by patient age. These and other ethical issues are discussed more fully in Ch. 109.

Chronic disease accompanied by **chronic functional impairment** is increasingly common with age (see Ch. 17). Some 50% of noninstitutionalized elderly persons have limitations in performing activities of daily living, and more than 80% have at least one chronic disease. More than 33% cannot perform major activities independently; 5% are homebound. About 15% of those over age 75 are homebound; the figure rises to 25% in those over age 80. More than 80% of US health care resources are devoted to chronic illness, and 80% of deaths after age 65 are attributed to chronic disease. Successful treatment of chronic conditions requires a shift in traditional therapeutic emphasis from cure to continuing care. Management that emphasizes improving function, postponing deterioration and disability, and preventing secondary complications characterizes the best of geriatric health care. These principles are merely good common sense applied to therapeutic objectives in the care of older patients.

Cognitive impairment itself does not require a change in therapeutic objectives but does deserve consideration. The severity of loss and its functional impact should be measured and fully evaluated before deciding whether to modify treatment plans. Even a transient iatrogenic discomfort that cannot be explained to an elderly demented patient may require a change in clinical approach and treatment goals. Explanations to demented patients must be made with special care, and obtaining consent is fraught with difficulty.

Diminished life expectancy is another important factor in considering treatment objectives. A patient who has only months of life remaining should not have to spend them enervated, nauseated, and confined by oppressive chemotherapy. When the prognosis for a specific disease indicates a short life span, planning treatment in light of life expectancy is reasonable—regardless of the patient's age. But when life expectancy is based on predictions related to the cohort (eg, 19 yr for a 65-yr-old woman, 14 yr for a man), variability among individuals is so great that calculations based on these data become meaningless. Who is to say that coronary artery bypass surgery with a high probability of improving function should be withheld from an 82-yr-old based on a prediction of "only" 5.3 yr of life remaining? And despite an average of 12 yr of life remaining for a 75-yr-old woman, how can one know if a particular patient will deviate a great deal in either direction from the mean? Finally, it could be argued that older people cherish their last few years, thus increasing the importance of preserving life through medical intervention, whether heroic or ordinary.

Nursing home residents have a disproportionately high prevalence of the characteristics that can affect treatment goals, including reduced life expectancy, poverty, cognitive loss, physical disability, chronic disease, pain and suffering, accumulated losses, and social isolation. Despite these negative characteristics, quality of life is very personal and subjective; therefore, a physician must accurately summarize the treatment issues and present them clearly in terms the patient can understand. Informing the patient and respecting autonomy is crucial, regardless of the patient's age or dwelling. Only when the patient is an informed participant in the decision can the physician be comfortable in modifying treatment objectives. When the patient is unable to participate in such discussions because of cognitive loss, family or friends intimately familiar with the patient's lifestyle and preferences may serve as a proxy for these decisions.

In some cases when life expectancy is diminished and suffering is severe, the patient or proxy may request euthanasia. However, active termination of life has traditionally been forbidden in medicine, and many believe rightly so. Confusing life protection and preservation with purposeful intervention to end life might make physicians and patients uncomfortable and suspicious. Yet in certain clinical situations of hopelessness and suffering, death is the end of pain, not the end of meaningful life. Accordingly, physicians have recently undertaken a reexamination of the bioethical basis for considering assisted suicide. In Holland, legislation has been enacted allowing physicians to end life in carefully specified circumstances of hopeless deterioration (see Ch. 109).

In old age, many phenomena occur that may argue for altering the usual therapeutic objectives. But these phenomena demand individual consideration, and age is largely irrelevant. The quality of human life is, for the most part, a concept that each person must consider; if quality of life becomes a criterion broadly applied to populations when making health care decisions, it will produce more complexities than solutions. Special attention must be given to the personal characteristics of older patients. Including patients in making decisions about treatment usually enhances their quality of life and brings greater satisfaction to the physician.

19. CARE OF THE DYING PATIENT

(See also HOSPICE CARE in Ch. 25)

Helping a patient and family find meaning in the experience of dying is often more important than adhering to medical routines or correcting physiologic abnormalities that are not causing distress or discomfort. The physician has at least two important responsibilities to a dying patient: to allow the patient and family to maintain control whenever possible and to prevent and relieve symptoms as effectively as possible.

People differ in what they consider important, especially when facing death. Some people find spiritual reward in enduring pain or disfigurement; others consider such stressful experiences worse than death. Some find an appropriate time and way to bring life to a satisfying close; others never really make peace with their mortality. The patient's preferences are paramount, and health care providers must take them into account when planning care.

The goal of care should be to achieve the best possible future for a patient, from the patient's perspective. A patient who fears dementia more than death should be treated differently from one who cherishes every moment of life, regardless of its quality. A knowledge of local law and institutional policy governing living wills, durable powers of attorney, and procedures for resuscitation and hospitalization is also important to ensure that patients' wishes are followed when they are no longer able to direct their own care (see also Chs. 108 and 109).

Depending on the patient and the situation, the goal of medical care may include prevention, cure, rehabilitation, or support. For dying patients, supportive care may be the only realistic goal. Yet, to say that a patient's care has changed from curative to supportive care or from treatment to palliation is an oversimplification of a complex decision process. Dying patients may benefit from curative, rehabilitative, or preventive care, just as persons not near death may benefit from supportive care, such as symptom control and psychologic counseling.

All significant medical interventions require careful decision making, regardless of whether a patient appears to be near death. Similarly, access to health care should not be limited because a person is near death. Certain symptoms are more common when death is close, however, and treatment of them should be guided by the patient's life expectancy.

SYMPTOM CONTROL

Both physical and mental distress are common in terminal illnesses. Relieving discomfort allows the patient to live as fully as possible and to focus on the unique issues presented by the approach of death. Patients need symptom control for comfort, and they need reassurance to allay the common fear that suffering will be protracted and that no one will care or control it.

Optimal control of symptoms involves choosing therapy based on etiology. For example, treating vomiting caused by hypercalcemia differs from treating vomiting caused by elevated intracranial pressure. The appropriateness of diagnostic investigations varies, however, depending on how burdensome the test is and how useful the findings may be.

When expected survival is brief, the severity of symptoms frequently dictates initial treatment choices. The fear that a symptom will worsen can be more crippling than the symptom itself, and reassurance that effective treatment is available may be all the patient needs. Other times, a symptom is so severe and the diagnostic alternatives so poor that immediate therapy is required.

Because one symptom can have many causes and may respond differently to therapy as the patient's condition deteriorates, effective treatments must be closely monitored and continuously reevaluated. *Special care must be taken to avoid inadvertent overdosage of medications during periods of altered drug disposition.*

Pain

(See also Ch. 12)

Dying patients with cancer are likely to have severe pain. Although only half of cancer patients have substantial pain, half of those with such pain may never obtain adequate relief. Most often pain persists not because it cannot be well controlled but because both patients and physicians have misconceptions about pain and the drugs, especially narcotics, used to control it. Severe pain in other terminal conditions is less common, but the approach to treatment is virtually the same.

Patients perceive pain differently, depending in part on such factors as fatigue, insomnia, anxiety, depression, and nausea. Thus, treatment must be individualized, taking these factors into account. Often, a supportive environment can help control pain.

The **cause of pain** should be considered when choosing an analgesic because some types of pain respond better to certain treatments. For example, salicylates and nonsteroidal anti-inflammatory drugs (NSAIDs) are helpful for bone pain from metastases, while tricyclic antidepressants, phenytoin, and carbamazepine may be effective for dysesthesias from nerve compression.

The key to pain control is maintaining the analgesic level by scheduled dosing. Controlling pain after it recurs is more difficult than preventing it, partly because pain generates anxiety. Thus, analgesics should be prescribed on a regular schedule, and the patient should be closely monitored for overdosage, underdosage, and adverse effects. As-needed doses may supplement the scheduled doses. In hospice units, nurses or patients become competent at making the necessary dosing or scheduling adjustments.

The choice of analgesic depends largely on the **intensity of the pain.** Assessing pain intensity is subjective and can be done only by talking with and observing the patient. All pain can be relieved with an appropriately potent drug, although sometimes the drug also produces sedation or confusion. Commonly used drugs are aspirin or acetaminophen for mild pain, codeine or oxycodone for moderate pain, and morphine or hydromorphone for severe pain.

Morphine is the most commonly used narcotic in terminal illness. Possible adverse effects include nausea, drowsiness, and confusion. Constipation should be treated prophylactically (see below). The patient usually develops substantial tolerance to the respiratory depressant and sedative effects of morphine but much less tolerance to the analgesic effect.

Morphine can be given by several routes. When it is given orally, a controlled-release form (MS Contin, Roxanol SR) is preferred because of its better absorption and longer duration. However, controlled-release morphine has a slow onset of action. The recommended initial dosage for controlled-release morphine is 90 to 120 mg q 12 h. The usual starting dosage for immediate-release morphine sulfate tablets is 10 to 30 mg q 4 h. A lower dose may be given to elderly and very sick patients to decrease initial drowsiness. In general, the elderly are more sensitive to the analgesic effects of narcotics, but as a population they demonstrate great variability, so doses may need to be increased rapidly if pain persists. The maximum dose is whatever is needed to relieve pain, preferably without unpleasant adverse effects. There is no arbitrary maximum dose. Two rules of thumb are useful in adjusting doses. First, the dose that seriously depresses respiratory function is usually more than twice the stable, tolerated dose. Second, reestablishing pain control when a stable dose becomes inadequate ordinarily requires 1.5 times the previously adequate dose.

When the oral route is not feasible, continuous IV infusions or intermittent IM or subcutaneous injections may be used. Morphine may be administered using a patient-controlled analgesia pump. In addition, morphine is now available in suppositories (5, 10, 20, or 30 mg). Estimated equianalgesic doses for conversion are shown in TABLE 19–1. The actual equianalgesic doses for any one patient vary, so conversions entail close monitoring with prompt correction of overdosage and underdosage.

Because **hydromorphone** is more soluble than morphine, it can be injected in smaller volumes. A pharmacist can prepare hydromorphone for high-dose therapy of up to 100 mg/mL, using commercially available powder for IV use. Hydromorphone is also available as a suppository,

TABLE 19–1. EQUIANALGESIC DOSES OF NARCOTICS USED FOR CHRONIC PAIN

Drug	*Oral Dose (mg)*	*Injectable (Intramuscular or Subcutaneous) Dose (mg)*	*Usual Effective Interval (h)*
Codeine	180–200	75	3–4
Morphine	30	10	3–4
Controlled-release morphine (MS Contin, Roxanol SR)	90–120	Not available	12
Hydromorphone	7.5	1.5	3–4
Methadone	20	10	6–8
Levorphanol	4	2	6–8

Absorption of suppositories is often erratic; doses must be adjusted to the patient's symptoms.

Adapted from information appearing in *The New England Journal of Medicine.* Jacox A, Carr DB, Payne R: "New clinical-practice guidelines for the management of pain in patients with cancer." *The New England Journal of Medicine* 330(9):651–655, 1994; used with permission.

which is especially convenient for patients at home. **Heroin** is more soluble than morphine but has no other proven advantage and cannot be legally prescribed in the USA.

Useful longer-acting alternatives to morphine include **levorphanol** and **methadone.** Pentazocine and other mixed agonist-antagonist drugs are not recommended because of low potency, erratic oral and IM absorption, and a greater incidence of adverse effects, especially psychosis. Furthermore, mixed agonist-antagonist drugs are contraindicated in combination with pure agonist narcotics. Meperidine also is not recommended because it is short acting and produces toxic metabolites that cause psychosis or CNS hyperexcitability at relatively low doses.

A narcotic that produces adverse effects may be effective in a lower dose if potentiated by a tricyclic antidepressant, corticosteroid, or hydroxyzine. **Pain-modification techniques** such as hypnosis, guided mental imagery, counseling for stress and anxiety, and relaxation methods may also help. In extreme cases, the ability to sense pain may need to be eliminated with neurosurgery or anesthesia.

Transdermal patches of **fentanyl** may replace the IM and subcutaneous narcotics discussed above. These patches have a fixed dose, take 12 to 18 h to achieve their effect, and may not have predictable equianalgesic doses. Frequent "rescue" doses of short-acting drugs are needed until the action of the patch becomes stable. **Ketorolac tromethamine,** an NSAID, can also be used to manage pain. For long-term therapy, it may be given orally q 4 to 6 h in 10-mg doses, as needed; however, it is expensive and has not been shown to offer long-term advantages. For short-term management (up to 5 days), ketorolac may be given IM; the recommended loading dose is 30 to 60 mg, followed by 15 to 30 mg q 6 h. Though not approved for IV use, the drug is sometimes given IV; the dosage is the same as for IM administration.

Dyspnea

One of the most feared symptoms and probably the most distressing to a dying patient, dyspnea has several causes. If the cause is identifiable and correctable, the patient and physician may choose to treat it. For example, antibiotics for pneumonia or thoracentesis for a pleural effusion may be appropriate. Oxygen may be psychologically comforting to the patient and family, even when it does not provide a physiologic benefit.

A narcotic can be used to slow respirations and reduce breathlessness when a patient's blood gas levels deteriorate. Often, the body's response to carbon dioxide retention or oxygen decline is severe, although the levels are still physiologically adequate. In this case, blunting the medullary response may obliterate symptoms without producing adverse effects. **Morphine sulfate** 2.5 mg IV q 2 to 4 h as needed or by continuous drip may be used. **Benzodiazepines** may also help relieve anxiety. Useful **nonpharmacologic measures** include providing a cool draft from an open window or a fan at bedside, using relaxation techniques, and maintaining a calming presence.

Anorexia

Common in dying patients, anorexia is usually more distressing to family members than to patients. Counseling may be needed to help them accept anorexia and understand the futility of tube feedings or parenteral nutrition.

If the patient is overwhelmed by a full meal tray, specially prepared foods, small portions, and a flexible meal schedule are recommended. Also, giving a favorite alcoholic beverage a half hour before meals may help. Foods that have strong flavors or smells sometimes stimulate the appetite. Low-dose **corticosteroids** (dexamethasone 1 mg or prednisone 5 mg tid), **megestrol acetate,** or **tricyclic antidepressants** may also improve the appetite and sense of taste. Metoclopramide enhances gastric emptying and may help with anorexia. However, onset may take 1 or 2 wk, which may be too slow for a patient near death. Also, the drug may induce tardive dyskinesia, particularly in elderly patients. Methylphenidate can enhance the patient's interest in food, but it also can cause dysphoric agitation. Thus, it must be introduced only with very careful decision making, and the patient must be monitored closely.

Rarely should a dying patient receive caloric supplementation through tube feeding or IV alimentation. Before starting any artificial feeding, the physician should discuss indications for discontinuance with the patient and family. During discussions with the patient and family, the physician needs to recognize that food and water have a powerful symbolic and psychologic importance. They symbolize our caring for and nurturing of one another, and they can provide comfort and satisfaction to the patient. However, the patient and family need to understand that in certain circumstances, a patient receives more comfort and satisfaction from forgoing nutrition and hydration.

After the decision has been made to forgo nutrition and hydration, supportive care is imperative. Such care includes **good oral hygiene** (brushing the teeth, swabbing the oral cavity, applying lip salve, and providing ice chips for dry mouth). An important physical and psychologic comfort measure, providing oral hygiene can give family members a valuable role in caring for the dying patient.

Nausea and Vomiting

Many seriously ill patients experience nausea, frequently without vomiting. If the cause is easy to treat (eg, hypercalcemia or constipation), specific treatment may be warranted, provided it makes the patient more comfortable. Nonspecific treatment is almost always indicated, however, and **phenothiazine therapy** is the most effective because of its action on the chemoreceptor zone in the medulla. The anticholinergic effects of phenothiazines may be a problem.

Prochlorperazine 10 mg orally before each meal can be given prophylactically. If vomiting precludes using the oral route, the drug can be given as a suppository (25 mg bid) or by IM injection (5 to 10 mg q 3 to 4 h with a maximum of 40 mg/day). **Metoclopramide** is useful for nausea and vomiting caused by decreased gut motility because it increases peristalsis and relaxes the pyloric sphincter. Other helpful antiemetics include corticosteroids (eg, **dexamethasone** and **methylprednisolone)** and antihistamines (eg, **hydroxyzine** and **dimenhydrinate),** which act centrally. Dronabinol, the principal psychoactive substance in marijuana (*Cannabis sativa* L.), is used primarily for the nausea and vomiting associated with chemotherapy. Many elderly persons are not as tolerant of the altered mental state associated with this drug, although experience is limited. As with analgesics for pain control, antiemetics should be given regularly to prevent nausea and improve patient comfort.

If vomiting is caused by obstruction and the patient is near death, consideration should be given to providing conservative treatment without relieving the obstruction. Sometimes, paralyzing the gut with morphine and treating dry mouth with ice chips is better than continuous gastric suction or surgery. Nasogastric suctioning is difficult for a sentient patient to endure except as a short-term measure.

Constipation

(See also Ch. 56)

Most dying patients have constipation because of inactivity, decreased fiber in the diet, dehydration, narcotics, and anticholinergic drugs. Therefore, **laxatives** should be given prophylactically to prevent fecal impaction. Usually, a stool softener (soluble or insoluble fiber or docusate sodium) should be given first. However, if the patient is being given a narcotic, generally a stimulant laxative (eg, casanthranol, senna, cascara sagrada, or bisacodyl) should be given first. Most patients require a stool softener and a stimulant laxative.

Osmotic laxatives stimulate GI function indirectly by increasing the fluid content of feces. **Lactulose,** a semisynthetic disaccharide that is not hydrolyzed by human intestinal enzymes, is an especially effective osmotic laxative for many bedridden patients; however, it is expensive.

If the patient has not had a bowel movement in 3 days and stool is present on rectal examination, a **glycerin or bisacodyl suppository** should be administered. If no bowel movement occurs, a **saline enema** should be administered. The importance of a regular bowel regimen to a dying patient's comfort is often underestimated by physicians.

Pressure Sores

(See also Ch. 14)

Many dying patients are immobile, poorly nourished, cachectic, and therefore at great risk for developing pressure sores. The most important preventive measure is to relieve pressure by rotating the patient q 2 h, by using a specialized mattress, or by using a continuously inflated air-suspension bed. A urinary catheter should be used as a last resort; usually, it is justified only when pain occurs with bedding changes or when the patient or family has a strong preference.

Confusion

The mental changes that can accompany the terminal stage of illness may be distressing to both the patient and family, though many patients are unaware of these changes. Confusion is common and has several causes, including drugs, hypoxia, metabolic disturbances, and intrinsic CNS disease. If the cause can be determined and is easy to treat, treatment may be worthwhile, provided it allows the patient to communicate more meaningfully with family and friends. In other cases, if a patient is comfortable and less aware of the surroundings, it may be better not to provide treatment. The physician should carefully assess the relative merits in each case.

Nonspecific therapy may include tranquilizers (benzodiazepines) if the patient is agitated. Also, low doses of **haloperidol** may help a patient who has disquieting, vivid dreams or threatening hallucinations.

PSYCHOLOGIC INTERVENTIONS

Depression

Most dying patients experience some depression. One patient may have many regrets about his life, while another may be preoccupied with legal, social, or financial problems. Providing **psychologic support** and allowing the patient to express concerns and feelings is the best and simplest course of action. Helping the patient and family settle any unresolved matters may decrease the level of anxiety. A skilled social worker, physician, or nurse can help with conflicts that distance the patient from family members.

Antidepressants should be reserved for patients who have persistent, clinically significant depression. Such patients may be helped by a low dose of an antidepressant once a day at bedtime. For anxiety, a sedating tricyclic should be used and supplemented as needed with another appropriate sedating agent. In the last weeks of life, a sedating antidepressant sometimes provides restful sleep while lifting the patient's depression. Given the circumstance, the usual concerns about possible cardiac and neurologic effects are attenuated. Doxepin and trazodone may provide sedation with milder anticholinergic effects than amitriptyline.

Withdrawn patients and those with vegetative signs may be helped by methylphenidate 5 to 10 mg once a day adjusted to individual response. This drug has a rapid onset and fewer adverse effects than most antidepressants; however, it may precipitate agitation.

Stress

Approaching death is most stressful when it is unexpected or when interpersonal conflicts keep patient and family from sharing their last moments together. Such conflicts can lead to excessive guilt or an inability to grieve among survivors and can cause anguish for the patient. A family member who is taking care of a dying patient at home may also experience physical and emotional stress. The patient may have an altered body image and a loss of self-esteem, fears of abandonment and separation, anxieties, and feelings of hopelessness. Usually, stress in dying patients and families is best treated with compassion, information, counseling, and even time-limited psychotherapy. Sedatives should be used sparingly and only briefly.

When a partner in a marriage dies, the survivor may be overwhelmed by making decisions about legal or financial matters or managing the household. With an elderly couple, the death of one partner may reveal cognitive impairment in the survivor that the deceased spouse had compensated for. Stress is even greater if no support is extended by friends or other family members. Physicians should identify such high-risk situations so they can mobilize the resources needed to prevent undue suffering and dysfunction.

Effective care for the dying usually involves a team because no one caregiver can provide 24-h availability and several disciplines must be consulted to provide all skills and perspectives needed to help the patient. Palliative-care or hospice teams anticipate potential problems and make appropriate arrangements, such as obtaining supplies or narcotics in an emergency. With death impending, an experienced person can comfort the family and may prevent an inappropriate call to the emergency medical system brought on by panic. Dying patients often have spiritual needs that should be recognized, acknowledged, and with the help of one or several team members, addressed as part of the care plan.

Not everyone is at ease with dying patients, but those who choose to work with them find rewards in providing support to the family and comfort to the patient. Nurses who work in a hospice setting do not seem to experience the same degree of burnout that frequently occurs in settings such as oncology or intensive care units. However, staff members may become so involved with the patient or family that they grieve with them. This stressful involvement can be mitigated by a nurturing work environment or a staff support group that meets regularly to share responses to dying patients and their families. Physicians and others who work in less supportive environments may need to form similar support groups and find sources of guidance.

Bereavement

Grieving is a normal process that usually begins before an anticipated death. For the patient, it often starts with denial caused by fears about a loss of control, separation, and an uncertain future, as well as a fear of suffering. The staff can help patients accept the prognosis by listening to their concerns, helping them understand that they can remain in control, explaining what the future probably holds, and assuring them that their pain will be controlled.

The family may also need support in expressing grief. Any member of the health care team who has come to know the patient and family may help them through this process and direct them to professional services if needed. Physicians and others responsible for the care of dying persons need to develop regular procedures that ensure follow-up of grieving family members.

Final Considerations

The last moments of life can have a lasting effect on family, friends, and caregivers. The patient should be in an area that is peaceful and quiet and ensures physical comfort. Some patients close to death may develop noisy bronchial congestion or palatal relaxation, known as the death rattle. If this distresses the family, 0.4 mg of scopolamine or atropine can dry up the patient's secretions and reduce the noise. Also, patients may develop CNS irritability, including agitation and restlessness, which can be relieved with a sedative.

Any stains or tubes on the bed should be covered, and odors should be masked. The family should be encouraged to maintain physical contact, such as holding hands, with the patient. Support personnel such as clergy or friends should be encouraged to be present, if the patient and family desire. If feasible and desired by the patient and family, cultural, spiritual, or ethnic rites of passage should be performed.

SOCIETAL CONCERNS

Financial Concerns

(See also Ch. 114)

Financial coverage for the care of dying persons is problematic. Medicare regulations exclude supportive care except in a hospice setting. However, not all patients qualify for hospice care, and physicians are often reluctant to certify the 6-mo prognosis required for coverage. Even a certified need for a skilled nursing level of care may not gain admission to a nursing home for a short-term, terminally ill patient. Physicians should know the financing options and the financial effects of choices.

Legal and Ethical Concerns

(See also Chs. 108 and 109)

A dying patient should be given appropriate support and symptom relief and vigorous treatment for any reversible aspects of depression and cognitive dysfunction. When the patient or a surrogate proposes an action that seems contrary to the patient's interests, referral to consultants should be available within the institution or agency to ensure that the physician's response is defensible even though it differs from the patient's or surrogate's request.

In some cases, the care of a dying patient may seem to be directed more toward hastening the patient's death than toward prolonging life. Whether such an approach should be construed as good medical care or as the criminal taking of life (homicide or assisting with suicide) is an increasingly debated issue. This problem arises, for example, with patients who request a discontinuance of parenteral hydration and nutrition; with those who choose to forgo treatment expected to yield long, disease-free remissions; and with those who develop suffocating dyspnea that can be relieved only with strong sedation, a treatment that can accelerate death.

Most medical actions that accelerate death are intended to relieve pain or other suffering. In these cases, the forgone life would have been so brief and so anguished that little question remains about whether treatment should have been carried out to prolong life. Once the question is raised, however, the issue of what constitutes wrongful death can be quite difficult.

Criminal law does not differentiate between intentional and unintentional crime, although motivation may extenuate the penalty. Thus, even the patient whose pain is relieved only by doses of narcotics that cause deep sedation and who expectedly dies from the effects of treatment could be construed to be the victim of wrongful death.

There are several reasons why these cases are virtually never brought to court: (1) Most people, including prosecutors, judges, and jurors, do in fact consider motivation in their assessments and usually find no willful destruction, only the pathos of a situation that could have had no better outcome. (2) The means used to bring about the death are those ordinarily used in treatment (analgesics, sedatives, and anesthetics), not those associated with crime (poisons, guns, and knives). (3) The means of death are not as certain to result in death as are those in clearly criminal cases.

Assisting with suicide remains a criminal act in most states, but the laws vary substantially and are rarely invoked. Directly providing a dying patient with lethal drugs and instructions for using them might be grounds for prosecution in some states but not in others. Physicians confronted with such situations should seek legal guidance before acting. Physicians and nurses should recognize that very few cases have been prosecuted. The considerations involved are largely conjectural and are changing rapidly with cultural change.

Charges of homicide rather than of assisting with suicide are more likely to be filed if the patient's interests are not carefully advocated, if the patient lacks capacity or is severely functionally impaired just before death, if documentation is sparse, and if the prosecutor's electoral base is expected to approve. Physicians engaged in vigorous symptom management and forgoing life-sustaining treatment need to document decision making carefully, provide care in a reputable setting, and be willing to discuss these issues honestly and sensitively with patients, other providers, and the public.

Finally, the physician should not use any treatment that is conventionally thought of as a means of homicide (eg, lethal injection), even though the physician may maintain that the treatment was intended to relieve suffering.

Managing Death

When death is expected, families should be prepared for it, and health care professionals should try to ensure that the following issues are addressed:

1. The family should be thoroughly informed about what will happen when the patient dies. If the patient is expected to die at home, the family should be told whom to call (eg, the doctor) and whom not to call (eg, an ambulance service). The family should also be informed about obtaining legal advice and burial services.

2. A physician should make the official determination of death as quickly as possible to reduce the family's anxiety and uncertainty. Families or funeral directors should be provided with a properly com-

pleted death certificate as quickly as possible. Physicians should be aware that on rare occasions, death may be difficult to determine; eg, when severe hypothermia mimics death.

3. Physicians, nurses, and other health care providers should address the family's psychologic needs, providing appropriate counseling, a comfortable environment where family members can grieve together, and adequate time for them to be with the body. Friends, neighbors, and clergy may be available to provide psychologic support to the family. Health care providers should be aware of cultural differences in behavior at the time of death.

4. The health care system should ensure that death did not result from wrongdoing. Even when death was expected, physicians may have a responsibility to report the death to the coroner or police; thus, physicians should know their local laws.

5. A discussion about autopsy can occur either before death or just after. Often, the physician chooses not to raise this issue, but families may have strong feelings, either for or against it. In any case, the discussion of autopsy should not be left to a covering physician or house officer who has not had previous contact with the family. Discussions about organ donation, if appropriate, should take place before death or as soon as possible after death.

6. The body should not present a risk to the public health, which usually means that it must be attended to quickly by persons licensed to do so.

Often, management of death consists of making sure that someone (eg, a nurse or volunteer) is with the body when the family visits after death, offering to help notify clergy or funeral directors, providing reassurance that the patient was comfortable and that family and caregivers did all that could be done, and making follow-up contact a few weeks later with the most closely affected survivor to answer questions and note whether appropriate adjustment is taking place.

20. PREVENTIVE STRATEGIES

Far more people than ever before are living into their 70s and beyond in relatively good health, leading vigorous, independent lives. Recent studies indicate that most body organs function nearly as well in later life as in younger years in those who maintain healthy lifestyles and have no chronic diseases. Of course, chronic diseases and disabilities tend to accumulate with age in many persons, threatening their independence. However, to a large extent, disease and disability in later life are linked to unhealthy behaviors in the earlier years and thus are preventable.

Preventive strategies for older persons have two general objectives: to maintain good health and function through behavioral choices and lifestyles beginning in the early or middle years and continuing through the later years, and to minimize the loss of health and function when chronic disabilities do occur. The latter is the goal of rehabilitation and is addressed in Ch. 29.

Lifestyle

Studies have documented that a lifestyle including regular exercise, good nutrition, moderate (if any) alcohol intake, abstinence from tobacco, involvement in meaningful activities, supportive and satisfying personal relationships, and adequate amounts of sleep (generally 7 to 8 h each night) is associated with a longer, healthier later life.

Exercise: Weight-bearing and aerobic exercise, such as walking or bicycling, 20 to 30 min at least three times a week is associated with improved cardiac capacity, maintenance of muscle strength, and reduction in age-related progressive loss of bone mass. Regular exercise also helps reduce the risk of falls, including those resulting in hip fractures, which often lead to further physical deterioration. Persons in their 60s and 70s who take part in organized fitness programs not only increase their maximum aerobic capacities almost as much as younger persons in these programs but also improve their glucose tolerance and blood lipid levels. Daily stretching exercises are also important for maintaining joint flexibility (see also Ch. 31).

Although organized fitness programs do not appeal to everyone, virtually everyone can make vigorous walking part of an exercise regimen. Maintaining the ability to walk comfortably requires properly fitted, supportive shoes; clean feet; and routine care of nails and skin, including attention to calluses. A podiatrist should be consulted for foot problems that affect comfort or function (see also Ch. 77).

Nutrition: Good nutrition for older persons has not been clearly defined because adequate dietary, metabolic, and longitudinal data are not available. Based on studies of younger adults, however, older persons should have adequate but not excessive amounts of protein (0.6 to 1.0 gm/kg/day, relatively low fat (< 30% of calories) and cholesterol intakes, and the National Research Council's recommended daily allowances of vitamins and minerals in food or as supplements. The importance of including about 1.0 to 1.5 gm of calcium in the daily diet should be stressed, although most older women need to take calcium supplements (see Ch. 73). However, the value of taking more than the recommended daily allowances of food supplements (ie, the megadoses marketed to the general public) has not been proved, and in some cases these doses may be toxic. For example, excessive doses of vitamin A or vitamin D can be toxic. For general use, vitamin D supplements of 400 to 800 IU/day are suggested.

Adequate fiber intake is the simplest means of minimizing constipation and gaining benefits such as reducing the risk of colon cancer and diverticulosis. Such fiber intake can be achieved through a regular nutritious diet that includes grains, fruits, and vegetables. Complex sugars, such as starchy foods, rather than simple sugars are also recommended, although the value of this substitution, like that of fiber intake, has not been proved conclusively. Salt intake should be modest, ie, little or no salt should be added to foods unless more is medically indicated. Data are not available on the impact of adding salt to the food of elderly persons with no history of hypertension or heart failure.

Most important, dietary intake (including alcohol intake) should be tailored to the individual. A person's diet must take into account hereditary tendencies toward hyperlipidemia, a history of alcoholism, evidence of diabetes, a need to achieve weight reduction, activity level, and personal preferences.

Accident Prevention

Accidents, particularly falls, increase markedly with age. Because falls often cause hip fractures and fear of more falls, they are a major cause of a loss of functional independence. Maintaining good physical condition helps prevent such accidents (see also Ch. 7).

The home should have certain safety features, such as handrails on stairways both indoors and outdoors, handrails and nonskid surfaces in showers and bathtubs, good lighting, nonskid rugs, and smoke and fire alarms. The safety of the neighborhood should be assessed, and alternative living arrangements should be considered, if necessary.

Modifying dangerous driving practices, such as avoiding driving at night with impaired night vision, should be strongly encouraged. The need for caution in hazardous situations such as walking or driving in wet or icy conditions should also be emphasized. If a significant decline in mental or physical condition might make driving risky, a decision to stop driving should be considered by the affected person and family members in consultation with the physician. Data indicate that older persons involved in car crashes suffer greater physical damage than younger persons. These injured elderly persons need to be closely evaluated and may require monitoring for a period of time (see also Ch. 112).

Health Issues

The general condition and vigor of the older person should be assessed. Specifically, the physician should assess height and weight, the ability to walk normally, the ability to carry out ordinary daily activities, joint flexibility, and any history or evidence of urinary incontinence. The physician should note any significant changes over time.

Screening: An essential preventive strategy in older persons is routine screening for problems that are likely to develop. Upon early detection, many such problems may be reversed or corrected. Usually part of a general medical examination, the screening procedures are discussed in detail elsewhere in the manual.

Older persons should undergo tests of hearing, vision, blood pressure, and hemoglobin and cholesterol levels, as well as urinalysis. The frequency of such evaluations depends in part on symptoms and findings. For a person with no evidence of abnormalities, these evaluations should be performed every 1 to 3 yr.

The skin, mouth, breasts (male or female), prostate, colorectum, and cervix and uterus should be examined regularly for evidence of early cancer. Colorectal screening should include tests for occult blood. Opinions differ on how often the cervix and uterus should be examined in women over age 65 who have had one normal examination, have no symptoms such as bleeding, and are not receiving estrogen therapy. Some specialists recommend yearly examinations, others recommend one examination every 5 yr (see TABLE 20–1).

Persons of all ages should be advised to avoid extensive sun exposure and to use sunscreen to prevent skin cancer. For dry skin, regular use of lotions is suggested (see also Ch. 101).

Because hypothyroidism can develop unexpectedly in older persons, clinical examinations should include a specific search for even subtle signs and appropriate laboratory follow-up. In patients who are known to be hypothyroid and are taking replacement hormone, thyroxine (T_4) and thyroid-stimulating hormone (TSH) levels should be checked periodically to deal with possible overtreatment and osteoporosis.

Attention should be given to a person's individual profile. If a person has a family history of diabetes or a tendency toward obesity, a glucose tolerance test or a 2-h postprandial glucose test should be considered. A person with a family history of symptomatic osteoporosis, a thin build, or a loss of stature should have radiologic and laboratory examinations for osteoporosis (see also Ch. 73). More frequent pelvic and cytologic

TABLE 20–1. AMERICAN CANCER SOCIETY RECOMMENDATIONS FOR EARLY DETECTION OF CANCER IN ASYMPTOMATIC PEOPLE

Test or Procedure	*Sex*	*Age*	*Frequency*
Sigmoidoscopy, preferably flexible	Men, women	≥ 50 yr	Every 3–5 yr
Fecal occult blood test	Men, women	≥ 50 yr	Every year
Digital rectal examination	Men, women	≥ 40 yr	Every year
Prostate examination*	Men	≥ 50 yr	Every year

(continued)

TABLE 20–1. AMERICAN CANCER SOCIETY RECOMMENDATIONS FOR EARLY DETECTION OF CANCER IN ASYMPTOMATIC PEOPLE *(Continued)*

Test or Procedure	*Sex*	*Age*	*Frequency*
Pap test	Women	All women who are or who have been sexually active or who have reached age 18 should have an annual Pap test and pelvic examination. After a woman has had three or more consecutive satisfactory normal annual examinations, the Pap test may be performed less frequently at the discretion of her physician.	
Pelvic examination	Women	18–40 yr	Every 1–3 yr with Pap test
		> 40 yr	Every year
Endometrial tissue sample	Women	At menopause, if at high risk†	At menopause and thereafter at the discretion of the physician
Breast self-examination	Women	≥ 20 yr	Every month
Breast clinical examination	Women	20–40 yr	Every 3 yr
		> 40 yr	Every year
Mammography‡	Women	40–49 yr	Every 1–2 yr
		≥ 50 yr	Every year
Health counseling and cancer checkup§	Men, women	> 20 yr	Every 3 yr
		> 40 yr	Every year

* Annual digital rectal examination and prostate-specific antigen test should be performed on men ≥ 50 yr. If either is abnormal, further evaluation should be considered.

† History of infertility, obesity, failure to ovulate, abnormal uterine bleeding, or unopposed estrogen or tamoxifen therapy.

‡ Screening mammography should begin by age 40.

§ To include examination for cancers of the thyroid, testicles, prostate, ovaries, lymph nodes, oral region, and skin.

Modified from American Cancer Society: *Cancer Facts & Figures—1993,* revised November 1992.

examinations are indicated if estrogens are being used. Perimenopausal women should be counseled about the benefits and risks of estrogen replacement therapy for preventing osteoporosis, as well as management of menopausal symptoms (see also Ch. 83).

Use of prescription and over-the-counter medications should be reviewed regularly. Such reviews should focus on potential interactions and side effects, and patient compliance. A small daily dose of aspirin is now recommended as prophylaxis for vascular thrombosis, as long as no contraindications exist.

Nosocomial infections can have a major deleterious impact on older persons and require good infection control practices in an institutional setting. With the increased incidence of drug-resistant **tuberculosis,** prevention and monitoring are especially important in older persons whose immune systems are usually less effective. Older persons in chronic care institutions are particularly vulnerable (see also Ch. 46).

Immunizations: Before administering a particular vaccine, the physician should note when the patient last received it. A **tetanus booster** is recommended every 10 yr. The current year's **influenza vaccine** should be given to older persons who have underlying conditions that may reduce immunity or who are prone to pulmonary infections. In fact, many experts recommend yearly influenza immunization for all persons ≥ 65 yr of age.

A once-in-a-lifetime **pneumococcal vaccine** is generally recommended for older persons. Because more local reactions occur with a second vaccination than with the first, revaccination may not be advisable except with overriding indications. More data and further guidance about pneumococcal vaccine use should be forthcoming (see Ch. 85).

Oral health: Because of fluoridated water and frequent regular dental checkups, most older people today still have their own teeth. The physician should stress the importance of continuing good oral health practices, including regular dental prophylactic examinations, early correction of problems, and personal dental care (including use of fluorinated toothpastes) at least twice daily. Keeping the mouth and teeth in good condition is essential for proper nutrition, good appearance, and general enjoyment of life (see also Ch. 52).

Mental and emotional status: Despite recent conclusive evidence, many professionals and laypersons still consider **loss of cognitive function** a normal part of aging. However, any significant decline in memory or other mental function reported by a patient or family member and confirmed by a simple mental status test calls for thorough evaluation because the decline almost certainly results from a disease process, which may be reversible (see Chs. 9, 89, and 90).

Similarly, any evidence of **depression** reported by the patient or family or observed during a routine assessment should be investigated and treated appropriately. Although depression is common in older persons, it is *not* a normal part of aging, and early attention can be beneficial. Depression is frequently associated with physical and social problems that make diagnosis difficult and complicate management. Among depressed elderly persons, the incidence of suicide has increased. The suicide rate increased rapidly between 1980 and 1985 and continues to increase among those > 85 yr; in 1991, the rate for those > 85 yr was twice the national average. Older people who are depressed should be treated with appropriate antidepressants and psychotherapy (see also Ch. 95).

Mental and emotional status can affect **sleep patterns.** Sleep problems are sometimes associated with treatable health conditions and modifiable behavioral and environmental characteristics.

Evidence of **psychosocial stress**—in family relationships, living environments, or marital and sexual relationships—should also be explored with older persons and family members. Significant stresses can interact with and may even affect immune competence and interact with chronic medical conditions. An older person's social and support network of family and friends and involvement in outside activities also help maintain overall health and enjoyment of life. One preventive strategy is to ensure the effectiveness of support networks through counseling and the use of social resources.

21. CLINICAL PHARMACOLOGY

Safe and effective pharmacotherapy remains one of the greatest challenges in clinical geriatrics. The elderly suffer from many chronic illnesses, and consequently, they use more medications than any other age group. An older person's diminished physiologic reserves are further stressed by the effects of drugs and acute or chronic disease, often in an additive manner. Prescribing for the elderly is complicated not only by chronic disease but also by polypharmacy (which is often tolerated less well by older than by younger persons) and by altered pharmacodynamics and pharmacokinetics.

Older patients may respond to drugs differently than do younger patients. Because of age-related pharmacodynamic changes, a drug's effect in older patients may be increased (eg, benzodiazepines) or decreased (eg, β-blockers). Because of age-related pharmacokinetic changes, plasma and tissue concentrations of drugs are usually increased in the elderly, often necessitating a dosage adjustment. In addition, older patients are more susceptible than younger patients to adverse drug reactions, drug-drug interactions, and drug-disease interactions; these reactions may be different in frequency or degree from those in younger patients and less well tolerated. For example, the use of nonsteroidal anti-inflammatory drugs increases the risk of GI hemorrhage, and the use of psychoactive drugs increases the risk of falls and hip fracture, which has serious health and social implications for the elderly.

Because of concern about the ill effects of drugs, the fact that many therapies are of major benefit in the elderly often is forgotten. For example, antibiotics, antiarrhythmics, and thrombolytic therapy can be lifesaving; antihypertensive drugs and pneumonia and influenza vaccines can help prevent or decrease morbidity; analgesics and oral hypoglycemic drugs can improve independence and quality of life. Appropriateness, whether the potential benefits outweigh the potential risks, should guide therapy.

PRESCRIBING PRACTICES

In the USA, recent large-scale surveys indicate that about 66% of people ≥ 65 yr of age use prescription and nonprescription drugs, with < 13% not taking any medications. Women take more medications than men because of their older average age and because they use more psychoactive and antiarthritic drugs. At any given time, the average older person uses 4.5 prescription drugs and 2.1 nonprescription drugs and fills 12 to 17 prescriptions a year.

The frail elderly consume the largest number of medications. Not surprisingly, drug use is greater in hospitals and nursing homes than in the community; a nursing home resident receives an average of seven drugs.

The type of medication used most often by the elderly varies with the setting. For community-dwelling elderly, analgesics, diuretics, cardiovascular drugs, and sedatives are most often prescribed; for nursing home residents, antipsychotics and sedative-hypnotics are the most commonly prescribed drugs, followed by diuretics, antihypertensives, analgesics, cardiac drugs, and antibiotics. Psychoactive drugs are prescribed for 65% of nursing home patients and 55% of residential care patients; 7% of patients in nursing homes receive three or more psychoactive drugs concomitantly.

Polypharmacy refers to the concurrent use of many medications. Although polypharmacy could reflect inappropriate prescribing, it is not by itself an accurate measure of the appropriateness of therapy because older persons often have many conditions that require treatment. However, prescribing practices must be reviewed meticulously. For example, many older hospitalized patients receive drugs that are contraindicated or potentially hazardous or that may adversely interact with other drugs. In nursing homes, physicians overprescribe antipsychotics, benzodiazepines, H_2-receptor antagonists, antibiotics, and laxatives. In most cases, such practices are avoidable. For example, less toxic drugs can often be substituted for those that have anticholinergic side effects. A thorough review of medications can reduce the number of drugs used and, according to limited data, improve patient outcome.

Underuse of some drugs is also a significant problem in elderly patients. For example, nursing homes report a limited use of antidepressants despite a high prevalence of depression. In addition, drugs for incontinence are underused, as are those used for preventive measures (eg, drugs for glaucoma, influenza and pneumococcal vaccines). Thus, many elderly patients miss the potential benefit of therapy that is safe and effective when carefully managed.

DRUG RESPONSE

Aging can alter drug response (see TABLE 21–1) although the variability of age-related differences precludes any attempt at generalization. Many factors affect drug response (see FIG. 21–1), and the effect of aging is often variable. Important factors include those that affect drug concentrations at the site of action (pharmacokinetics), end-organ responsiveness to a given drug concentration (pharmacodynamics), and a host's ability to adapt to the drug's effect (homeostasis). In some cases

TABLE 21–1. EFFECT OF AGING ON DRUG RESPONSE

Drug	*Action*	*Effect of Aging*
Analgesics		
Aspirin	Acute gastroduodenal mucosal damage	↔
Morphine	Acute analgesic effect	↑
Pentazocine	Analgesic effect	↑
Anticoagulants		
Heparin	Activated partial thromboplastin time	↔
Warfarin	Prothrombin time	↑
Bronchodilators		
Albuterol	Bronchodilation	↔
Ipratropium	Bronchodilation	↔

(continued)

TABLE 21–1. EFFECT OF AGING ON DRUG RESPONSE *(Continued)*

Drug	*Action*	*Effect of Aging*
Cardiovascular drugs		
Adenosine	Minute ventilation and heart rate response	↔
Diltiazem	Acute antihypertensive effect	↑
Enalapril	Acute antihypertensive effect	↑
Isoproterenol	Chronotropic effect	↓
Phenylephrine	Acute venoconstriction; acute hypertensive effect	↔
Prazosin	Chronotropic effect	↓
Timolol	Chronotropic effect	↔
Verapamil	Acute antihypertensive effect	↑
Diuretics		
Furosemide	Latency and size of peak diuretic response	↓
Psychoactive drugs		
Diazepam	Acute sedation	↑
Diphenhydramine	Psychomotor function	↔
Haloperidol	Acute sedation	↓
Midazolam	EEG activity	↑
Temazepam	Postural sway, psychomotor effect, sedation	↑
Triazolam	Psychomotor activity	↑
Others		
Levodopa	Dose limitation due to side effects	↑
Tolbutamide	Acute hypoglycemic effect	↓

↑ = increased; ↓ = decreased; ↔ = unchanged.

Adapted from Cusack BJ, Vestal RE: "Clinical pharmacology: Special considerations in the elderly," in *Practice of Geriatric Medicine,* edited by E Calkins, PJ Davis, and AB Ford. Philadelphia, WB Saunders Co, 1986, pp 115–136; used with permission.

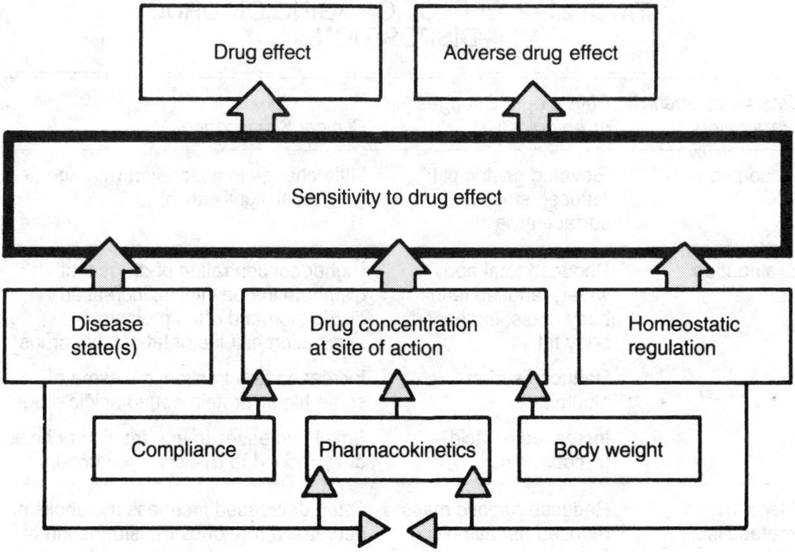

FIG. 21–1. Factors of importance that affect drug response in elderly patients.

(eg, triazolam), a drug's effect may be enhanced by increased plasma concentrations; in others (eg, warfarin), the end-organ effect may be enhanced with no change in concentration.

Some drugs interfere with homeostatic regulation in the elderly. For example, some drugs can cause a drop in blood pressure (eg, tricyclic antidepressants, major tranquilizers, dopaminergic agents, diuretics, many antihypertensives) and precipitate symptomatic orthostatic hypotension. In addition, thiazide diuretics can cause hyponatremia; potassium-sparing diuretics can cause hyperkalemia; and nonsteroidal anti-inflammatory drugs can cause renal impairment. These effects appear more pronounced as age advances.

PHARMACOKINETICS

The physiologic changes of aging can potentially affect pharmacokinetics (see TABLE 21–2). Some of these changes are more important than others.

TABLE 21–2. EFFECT OF AGING ON DRUG DISPOSITION

Pharmacokinetic Parameters	*Physiologic Changes of Aging*	*Clinical Significance*
Absorption	Elevated gastric pH; reduced small-bowel surface area	Little change in absorption with age (ie, no clinical significance)
Distribution	Reduced total body water; reduced lean body mass; increased body fat	Higher concentration of drugs that distribute in body fluids; increased distribution and often prolonged elimination half-life of fat-soluble drugs
	Reduced serum albumin	Increased free fraction in plasma of some highly protein-bound acidic drugs
	Increased α_1-acid glycoprotein	Small decreases in free fraction of basic drugs bound to α_1-acid glycoprotein
Hepatic metabolism	Reduced hepatic mass; reduced hepatic blood flow	Often decreased first-pass metabolism; decreased rate of biotransformation of some drugs; marked interindividual variation in rate of hepatic metabolism
Renal elimination	Reduced renal plasma flow; reduced glomerular filtration rate	Decreased renal elimination of drugs and metabolites; marked interindividual variation

Adapted from Vestal RE: "Aging and pharmacokinetics: Impact of altered physiology in the elderly." *Physiology and Cell Biology of Aging* 8:198, 1979; used with permission of Raven Press.

Absorption

Despite the decrease in small-bowel surface area with aging, changes in drug absorption tend to be trivial and of little clinical consequence.

Distribution

The clinical importance of decreased serum albumin levels and increased α_1-acid glycoprotein with age is not well established. Decreased serum albumin levels in a patient with an acute disease may lead to more problems.

Hepatic Metabolism

The presystemic metabolism of some drugs given orally (eg, propranolol, lidocaine, labetalol, verapamil) is decreased in older persons. As a result, plasma concentration and bioavailability of these drugs are increased, and the drugs' effect may be enhanced in older patients. Consequently, initial doses of these drugs should be reduced by about 30% in elderly patients. The presystemic metabolism of other drugs (eg, imipramine, amitriptyline, morphine, meperidine) is not decreased in the elderly.

Although concentrations of drug-metabolizing enzymes (those related to the cytochrome P-450 systems) do not appear to decline with age, the intrinsic hepatic elimination of many drugs is reduced in older persons. Some experts consider the decline in hepatic clearance to be the result of decreased liver mass. Although liver blood flow decreases with age, this has important effects on hepatic drug elimination only in limited situations when a drug with high clearance (eg, propranolol) is given IV. Since these situations are rare, the clinical significance of decreased liver blood flow is relatively minor.

For drugs subject to reduced liver metabolism (see TABLE 21–3), clearance typically declines 30% to 40%. Theoretically, maintenance drug doses should be reduced by this amount; however, the rate of drug metabolism can vary greatly from person to person. For example, with some drugs, only men have reduced hepatic metabolism (see TABLE 21–3).

Age does not affect the clearance of some drugs, usually those with relatively simple, one-step conjugation metabolism (eg, lorazepam, oxazepam). Older persons are more likely to have reduced clearance of drugs with multistage metabolism (eg, diazepam, chlordiazepoxide). Sometimes, drugs with elimination that is less affected by age can be chosen.

A significant fraction of some drugs is metabolized on the first pass through the liver after absorption. This first-pass extraction effect is reduced in the elderly with certain drugs, including propranolol, labetalol, and verapamil. As a result, more drug reaches the systemic circulation, with potentially decreased dose requirements.

Many drugs produce active metabolites in clinically relevant concentrations. These drugs include older benzodiazepines (eg, diazepam, chlordiazepoxide), tertiary amine antidepressants (eg, amitriptyline, imipramine), major tranquilizers (eg, chlorpromazine and thioridazine but not haloperidol), and opioid analgesics (eg, morphine, meperidine, propoxyphene). Accumulation of active metabolites (eg, N-acetylprocainamide, morphine-6-glucuronide) can produce toxicity in patients with renal insufficiency (ie, many older patients). Thus, knowing the age-related pharmacokinetics of the parent compound alone may be insufficient when calculating the time course of a drug.

Renal Elimination

Renal mass and renal blood flow (mainly in the renal cortex) decrease significantly with age (see Ch. 63). After age 30, **creatinine clearance** declines on average 8 mL/min/1.73 m^2/decade, although about 1/3 of older persons do not show any decline in creatinine clearance. Thus, the decline in glomerular filtration rate is relatively predictable but not

TABLE 21–3. EFFECT OF AGING ON HEPATIC DRUG METABOLISM*

Metabolism Reduced by Age	*Metabolism Unaffected by Age*
Analgesics and anti-inflammatory agents	
Dextropropoxyphene	Acetaminophen
Ibuprofen	
Meperidine	
Morphine	
Naproxen	
Cardiovascular drugs	
Amlodipine	Labetalol
Diltiazem	
Lidocaine†	
Nifedipine	
Propranolol	
Quinidine	
Theophylline	
Verapamil	
Psychoactive drugs	
Alprazolam†	Ethanol
Chlordiazepoxide	Oxazepam
Desipramine†	Lorazepam
Diazepam	Temazepam
Imipramine	Phenytoin
Nortriptyline	Valproic acid
Trazodone	
Triazolam†	
Others	
Levodopa	Erythromycin
	Fluorouracil
	Isoniazid
	Warfarin

* The effect of age on hepatic metabolism is sometimes controversial; in such cases, the effects indicated represent those reported in the majority of studies.

† In men but not in women.

TABLE 21–4. DRUGS THAT HAVE DECREASED RENAL ELIMINATION IN THE ELDERLY

Antibiotics	Amikacin Gentamicin Streptomycin Tobramycin
Cardiovascular drugs	Captopril Digoxin Enalapril Lisinopril N-Acetylprocainamide Procainamide Quinapril
Diuretics	Amiloride Furosemide Hydrochlorothiazide Triamterene
Others	Amantadine Chlorpropamide Cimetidine Lithium Ranitidine

Adapted from Cusack BJ, Vestal RE: "Clinical pharmacology: Special considerations in the elderly," in *Practice of Geriatric Medicine*, edited by E Calkins, PJ Davis, and AB Ford. Philadelphia, WB Saunders Co, 1986, pp 115–134; used with permission.

universal. Decreases in tubular function parallel those in glomerular function. Serum creatinine levels do not increase because older persons have less lean body mass and produce less creatinine.

These physiologic changes have profound effects on renal drug elimination, which is decreased in older persons (see TABLE 21–4). The clinical implications depend on how much renal elimination contributes to total systemic elimination and on the drug's **therapeutic index** (the ratio between therapeutic and toxic doses). Thus, clinical implications are greater for the aminoglycoside gentamicin, a drug that is cleared almost entirely by the kidneys and has a low therapeutic index, than for atenolol, a drug that is eliminated less exclusively by the kidneys and has a higher therapeutic index. Creatinine clearance (measured or estimated) is used to guide drug dose. Computer programs or the Cockcroft-Gault formula (see Ch. 63) helps in making this calculation. This formula predicts creatinine clearance better in ambulatory and hospital patients than in nursing home patients, perhaps because the latter tend to be more frail, with variable nutritional status.

Since renal function is dynamic, maintenance doses of drugs should be adjusted in patients who are acutely ill or dehydrated. Also, in view of the age-related decline in renal function, dose requirements of drugs given long term should be reviewed. The failure to adjust the dose of chronically administered digoxin is one reason why older patients have a high rate of adverse reactions from this drug.

ADVERSE DRUG REACTIONS

The risk of an adverse drug reaction rises exponentially with the number of drugs used (see FIG. 21–2), in part because multiple drug therapy reflects the presence of many diseases and provides opportunity for drug-drug and drug-disease interactions. Aging per se is not an independent risk factor; the risk of adverse drug reactions increases with age primarily because the elderly are sicker and take more drugs. About 1/3 of drug-related hospitalizations and 1/2 of drug-related deaths occur in persons > 60 yr.

Determining the risk associated with specific drugs is a more valid method of assessing the susceptibility of older persons to adverse drug reactions. The elderly are at increased risk with some drugs (eg, flurazepam, nonsteroidal anti-inflammatory drugs, warfarin, heparin, gentamicin, isoniazid, antineoplastic agents, and most antiarrhythmic drugs) but not with others (eg, β-blockers, antihypertensives, lidocaine, propafenone). Increased susceptibility may be the result of age-related changes in pharmacokinetics (eg, gentamicin) or response (eg, warfarin). In other cases, increased susceptibility is attributable to diseases or disorders that are aggravated by drugs; for example, anticholinergic drugs can exacerbate prostatism and diuretics can precipitate postural hypotension. The relationship between aging and the risk of adverse drug reactions is complex. A patient's risk of having an adverse drug reaction must be determined case by case, taking into consideration the possibility of pharmacokinetic changes (because of age or disease), pharmacodynamic differences, the possibility of a drug-drug interaction, and the possible exacerbation of an underlying disorder.

Drug-disease interactions: Exacerbation of a disease by a drug can occur in any age group, but this type of interaction is especially important in older persons because of the increased prevalence of disease and the difficulty in distinguishing often subtle adverse drug reactions from the effects of disease (see TABLE 21–5). Anticholinergic drugs can produce adverse effects that are indistinguishable from the patient's disease (eg, urinary retention in older men with prostatism; increased mental impairment in patients with dementia or parkinsonism; impaired vision in patients with open-angle glaucoma; and exacerbation of chronic gingivitis). Other drug-disease interactions include dyspnea

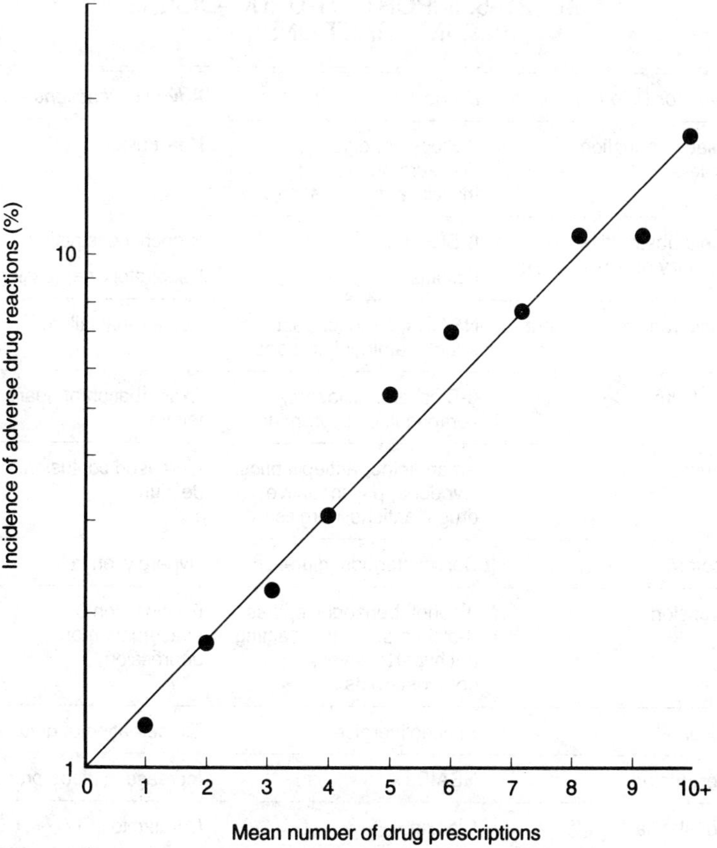

FIG. 21–2. The relationship between the number of drug prescriptions and the incidence of adverse drug reactions in hospitalized medical patients. (From Carbonin P, Pahor M, Bernabei R, Sgadari A: "Is age an independent risk factor of adverse drug reactions in hospitalized medical patients?" *Journal of American Geriatrics Society* 39:1093–1099, 1991; used with permission.)

due to β-blockers in patients with chronic obstructive pulmonary disease; upper GI bleeding due to nonsteroidal anti-inflammatory drugs (NSAIDs) in patients with peptic ulcer disease; azotemia due to NSAIDs in patients with chronic renal failure; heart block due to β-blockers, verapamil, diltiazem, or tricyclic antidepressants in patients with atrioventricular conduction disturbances; and fractures due to corticosteroids in patients with osteoporosis. In all of these cases,

TABLE 21–5. IMPORTANT DRUG–DISEASE INTERACTIONS

Disease or Disorder	*Drugs*	*Adverse Reactions*
Cardiac conduction disorders	β-Blockers, digoxin, diltiazem, verapamil, tricyclic antidepressants	Heart block
Chronic obstructive pulmonary disease	β-Blockers Opioids	Bronchoconstriction Respiratory depression
Chronic renal impairment	NSAIDs, radiocontrast agents, aminoglycosides	Acute renal failure
Heart failure	β-Blockers, diltiazem, verapamil, disopyramide	Exacerbation of heart failure
Dementia	Amantadine, antiepileptics, levodopa, psychoactive drugs, anticholinergics	Increased confusion, delirium
Diabetes	Corticosteroids, diuretics	Hyperglycemia
Depression	Alcohol, benzodiazepines, β-blockers, centrally acting antihypertensives, corticosteroids	Precipitation or exacerbation of depression
Glaucoma	Anticholinergics	Exacerbation of glaucoma
Hypertension	NSAIDs	Increase in blood pressure
Hypokalemia	Digoxin	Cardiac toxicity
Orthostatic hypotension	Antihypertensives, diuretics, neuroleptics, tricyclic antidepressants, L-dopa	Dizziness, falls, syncope
Osteopenia	Corticosteroids	Fracture
Peptic ulcer disease	NSAIDs, anticoagulants	Upper GI bleeding
Peripheral vascular disease	β-Blockers	Intermittent claudication

(continued)

TABLE 21–5. IMPORTANT DRUG–DISEASE INTERACTIONS *(Continued)*

Disease or Disorder	*Drugs*	*Adverse Reactions*
Prostatism	Anticholinergics, α-agonists	Urinary retention

NSAIDs = nonsteroidal anti-inflammatory drugs.
Adapted from Cusack BJ: "Polypharmacy and clinical pharmacology," in *Geriatrics Review Syllabus: A Core Curriculum in Geriatric Medicine*, 1st ed, edited by JC Beck. New York, American Geriatrics Society, 1989, pp 127–136; used with permission.

the clinical exacerbation could be considered disease-related rather than iatrogenic, making diagnosis more difficult. Such problems can often be obviated by choosing safer alternatives when possible.

Drug-drug interactions: Drug-drug interactions are myriad; TABLE 21–6 lists a few interactions of potential clinical importance to illustrate some of the mechanisms whereby they occur. Interactions are basically either pharmacokinetic (causing differences in drug disposition) or pharmacodynamic (causing differences in drug effect). Few prospective studies on drug interactions in older persons have been performed. One study showed that 40% of ambulatory elderly patients were at risk for drug-drug interactions, of which 27% were potentially serious (eg, quinidine-digoxin interaction). Digoxin is frequently prescribed in the elderly; therefore, attention must be paid to drugs, such as quinidine, amiodarone, and verapamil, that decrease digoxin's renal clearance. Older patients are also at increased risk for digitalis toxicity because of the high incidence of heart disease, hypokalemia, and chronic obstructive pulmonary disease.

Inhibition of drug metabolism does not appear to change with age; for example, both cimetidine and ciprofloxacin inhibit theophylline's rate of metabolism by about 30% in young and older healthy persons. Because age has no effect on inhibition of drug metabolism, the risk of drug toxicity is at least the same or increased in older patients when an inhibitor is added to a regimen. Thus, the addition of cimetidine or ciprofloxacin to a theophylline regimen increases the risk of theophylline toxicity, which has serious implications for elderly persons because of their increased sensitivity to chronic theophylline toxicity. Unless concentrations of the index drug are low, its dose should be reduced by about 1/3 to avoid toxicity when a metabolism inhibitor is added.

TABLE 21–6. EXAMPLES OF IMPORTANT DRUG–DRUG INTERACTIONS

Mechanism	*Drug*	*Interacting Drug*	*Effect*
Pharmacokinetic interactions			
Decreased absorption	Digoxin	Antacids, cholestyramine, colestipol	Decreased digoxin effect
	Ciprofloxacin	Sucralfate	Decreased antibiotic response
Altered rate of gastric emptying	Most drugs	Metoclopramide	Increased rate of drug absorption
		Anticholinergic drugs	Decreased rate of drug absorption
Displacement of plasma protein binding	Warfarin	Aspirin, furosemide	Possible increased anticoagulant effect
Inhibition of drug metabolism	Warfarin	Cimetidine, omeprazole, trimethoprim-sulfamethoxazole, metronidazole	Increased anticoagulation, bleeding
	Theophylline	Cimetidine, erythromycin, ciprofloxacin, enoxacin	Theophylline toxicity
Induction of drug metabolism	Warfarin	Barbiturates, rifampin, carbamazepine	Decreased anticoagulation
	Phenytoin	Barbiturates, rifampin	Loss of seizure control
	Theophylline	Phenytoin, rifampin, carbamazepine, smoking	Increase in dyspnea
Decreased active renal tubular secretion	Methotrexate	Salicylate, penicillins, probenecid, other organic acids	Methotrexate toxicity
Decreased renal or nonrenal clearance	Digoxin	Quinidine, verapamil, amiodarone, diltiazem	Digitalis toxicity

(continued)

TABLE 21–6. EXAMPLES OF IMPORTANT DRUG–DRUG INTERACTIONS *(Continued)*

Mechanism	*Drug*	*Interacting Drug*	*Effect*
Pharmacodynamic interactions			
Specific receptor-mediated drug interactions			
Additive effect on cholinergic receptors	Benztropine	Other anticholinergics (eg, tricyclic antidepressants, thioridazine, antihistamines)	Confusion, urinary retention
Competitive blockade of β receptors	Albuterol	β-Blockers	Decreased bronchodilator response
Nonspecific pharmacodynamic interactions			
Effects on cardiac conduction	β-Blockers	Verapamil, diltiazem, digoxin	Bradycardia, heart block
Hypokalemia	Digoxin	Diuretics	Digitalis toxicity
Orthostatic hypotension	Diuretics	ACE inhibitors, tricyclic antidepressants, α-blockers, phenothiazines, vasodilators, levodopa	Falls, weakness, syncope
Reduced renal perfusion	Diuretics	NSAIDs	Renal impairment
Effects on platelet function, coagulation, and mucosal integrity	Aspirin	Warfarin	Gastrointestinal bleeding

ACE = angiotensin converting enzyme; NSAIDs = nonsteroidal anti-inflammatory drugs.

Aging's effect on induction of drug metabolism varies. For example, induction of theophylline metabolism by phenytoin is similar in young and older persons, but induction of drug metabolism by other agents such as dichloralphenazone, glutethimide, and rifampin is unchanged or decreased in older persons. Because induction may be unchanged or decreased in older patients, the potential exists for decreases in drug concentrations and response after an inducing agent is added to a regimen.

Among the most important drug-drug interactions in the elderly are those involving drugs with antimuscarinic activity. Many drug classes have antimuscarinic activity, including anticholinergics used to treat parkinsonism (eg, benztropine), tricyclic antidepressants (eg, amitriptyline, imipramine), antipsychotics (eg, thioridazine), antiarrhythmics (eg, disopyramide), and over-the-counter antihistamines (eg, diphenhydramine). Combinations of antimuscarinics may cause or worsen side effects including dry mouth, blurred vision, constipation, urinary retention, and delirium. The use of more than one antimuscarinic drug should be minimized, and drugs with the least anticholinergic effect should be selected.

Many different classes of agents interact nonspecifically to cause an imbalance between vascular tone and intravascular volume status, putting a patient at risk for orthostatic hypotension and syncope. Combinations of drugs are a common cause of orthostasis, falls, and injury in older persons.

CONSIDERATIONS FOR EFFECTIVE PHARMACOTHERAPY

Therapeutic choices are difficult, especially in frail, very elderly patients who have many diseases and are taking several medications. Because geriatric clinical pharmacology is complex, effective prescribing for the elderly involves special considerations (see TABLE 21–7). The principal clinical concerns include not only efficacy and safety but also the dosage, complexity of regimen, number of medications, costs, and whether the patient can comply with therapy. The goals of prescribing in older patients are to improve compliance, reduce the risk of adverse effects, and improve efficacy. Monitoring for adverse effects and using appropriate doses, simpler regimens, and safer drugs can make prescribing for the elderly effective and relatively safe.

COMPLIANCE

Noncompliance with drug therapy, usually in the form of taking less drug than prescribed (underadherence), is common; about 40% of older patients do not take their medications as directed. Up to 35% of noncompliant older persons may suffer health problems because of their noncompliance; in one study, noncompliance was the cause of 11% of hospital admissions in elderly patients.

TABLE 21–7. GUIDELINES FOR EFFECTIVE PRESCRIBING

1. Ask patients to bring all medicines to the office
2. Restrict prn prescribing to treatment of minor symptoms
3. Select a drug that may treat more than one condition
4. Check for contraindications and potential drug interactions before prescribing a drug
5. Start with low doses, and titrate the dose according to response
6. Monitor patients for adverse reactions
7. Instruct patients about their drug therapy
8. Encourage and routinely check compliance
9. Periodically simplify the therapeutic regimen and stop drugs if possible
10. Place realistic limits on the duration of drug therapy

Adapted from Cusack BJ: "Polypharmacy and clinical pharmacology," in *Geriatrics Review Syllabus: A Core Curriculum in Geriatric Medicine*, 1st ed, edited by JC Beck. New York, American Geriatrics Society, 1989, pp 127–136; used with permission.

Compliance or adherence with drug therapy is affected by many factors (see TABLE 21–8). Poor communication between physician and patient is an important cause of noncompliance. Compliance can be improved by discussing the purpose and benefit of medicines with the patient and by providing written instructions that are clear, simple, informative, and written in large type. Pharmacists and nurses can help teach patients and improve compliance. A standard system for promoting compliance is more effective than an informal, ad hoc approach. A patient's compliance can mean the difference between independent living and institutional placement.

DOSE ADJUSTMENT

Older patients usually require a reduction in drug dose because they are often more sensitive to drugs and are less able to eliminate them. Dose requirements vary considerably from person to person, up to fivefold in some cases. Although generally a starting dose should be reduced in an older patient, the dose should be titrated to the therapeutic response, and the patient should be observed closely for signs of adverse effects, which are usually predictable and dose related.

TABLE 21–8. FACTORS THAT INFLUENCE COMPLIANCE

Increase compliance	Patient's belief that disease is serious Good communication by physician about purpose of medicine Drug calendars and reminder cards Blister-pack packaging of drugs Multicompartment pill boxes Compliance counseling
Decrease compliance	Multiple drug therapy Complicated drug regimen Long duration of therapy Patient's concern that drug will cause toxicity Patient's belief that drug is unnecessary Cognitive impairment Child-proof pill containers
Do not affect compliance	Age Patient's sex Ethnicity Educational level Severity of disease Efficacy or toxicity Drug costs(?)

Adapted from Stewart RB, Caranosos GJ: "Medical compliance in the elderly." *Medical Clinics of North America* 73:1551–1563, 1989; used with permission.

Guidelines for adjusting doses in the elderly are not available for many drugs. However, some important principles help in deciding whether, and by how much, a dose should be adjusted.

In general, conservative initial doses (about 1/3 to 1/2 the usual adult dose) are indicated for **drugs with a low therapeutic index** (the ratio between therapeutic and toxic doses) and with significant adverse effects. Examples include tricyclic antidepressants, benzodiazepines, major tranquilizers, opioid analgesics, antiparkinsonian agents, warfarin, nonsteroidal anti-inflammatory drugs, theophylline, antiarrhythmic drugs, aminoglycosides, digoxin, and some anticonvulsants. In the elderly, the adverse drug reactions of concern (such as hypoglycemia from chlorpropamide, bleeding from warfarin, or confusion from levodopa) are mainly dose related. Conversely, for **drugs with a high therapeutic index,** the dose usually does not need to be reduced significantly compared with that given to younger adults. Examples include acetaminophen, penicillins, and cephalosporins.

Clearance of a drug correlates with **patient size,** which is an often overlooked but important determinant of drug dose. A small woman weighing 40 kg clearly does not need as high a dose as a large man twice her weight.

If a patient has a **clinical problem** that may be exacerbated by a drug, the usual starting dose should be reduced by about 50%, especially if elimination of that drug is reduced with age. As the dose is increased, the patient must be monitored for adverse effects. For example, because of the risk for urinary retention in a patient with mild prostatism, a tricyclic antidepressant (such as nortriptyline, which has anticholinergic properties) should be started at a dose of 10 to 25 mg/day. In such cases, a safer alternative, if available, should be used first.

EFFECTS OF SPECIFIC DRUG CLASSES

Some classes of drugs (including diuretics, antihypertensives, antiarrhythmics, antiparkinsonian drugs, anticoagulants, psychoactive drugs, hypoglycemics, and analgesics) are often associated with adverse reactions in older patients. Pertinent therapeutic principles are reviewed below.

Diuretics

Diuretics are widely used for treating hypertension and heart failure in older patients, who are at increased risk for developing hypokalemia from these drugs. Lower doses of thiazide diuretics (eg, 12.5 to 25 mg hydrochlorothiazide or chlorthalidone) can effectively control hypertension, with reduced risk of hypokalemia and hyperglycemia. The diuretic effect of furosemide is decreased in elderly patients because of reduced secretion of drug to the renal tubules (site of action); however, the clinical relevance is limited because dosing is guided by diuretic response. Doses should be titrated carefully to avoid adverse effects such as azotemia, postural hypotension, and hypokalemia.

Antihypertensives

Although different classes of antihypertensives have comparable efficacy in older white patients, calcium channel blockers and diuretics are the most effective antihypertensives in older black patients. Often the choice of antihypertensive is guided by whether the individual patient is at risk for drug-disease or drug-drug interactions. β-Adrenergic blockers are contraindicated in patients with chronic obstructive pulmonary disease, diuretics in patients with diabetes, clonidine in patients with depression, and vasodilators and α-adrenergic blockers in patients with underlying orthostatic hypotension. Whether certain antihypertensives are preferable because they best preserve quality of life in the elderly is not well established.

Antiarrhythmics

Antiarrhythmics have the same indications and efficacy in older as in younger patients. However, because of altered pharmacokinetics, the dose of some drugs (eg, procainamide, quinidine, lidocaine) should be reduced in the elderly. In addition, the risk for significant adverse reactions to certain drugs (eg, mexiletine and class IC drugs such as encainide and flecainide) increases with age. Because class IC drugs can increase the risk of death, they are not recommended for the treatment of ventricular arrhythmias. Antiarrhythmics should be used cautiously, with close monitoring of the ECG and the therapeutic response.

The clearance of **digoxin** decreases on average 50% in elderly patients with normal serum creatinine levels. Therefore, maintenance doses should be started low (0.125 mg/day) and adjusted according to response and serum digoxin levels. Excessively high doses of digoxin have been one of the most common causes of digitalis toxicity; however, the incidence of digitalis toxicity has decreased in recent years mainly because lower doses are being prescribed. Older patients also develop digitalis toxicity because of factors that increase their sensitivity to digoxin, such as renal failure, advanced heart disease, obstructive airway disease, hypothyroidism, hypokalemia, and acid-base imbalance. Cardiac toxicity is characterized by increased automaticity and conduction defects. Common noncardiac features of toxicity include nausea, vomiting, anorexia, dizziness, and fatigue. Treatment of toxicity includes discontinuing the drug, correcting any potassium deficiency, and administering specific antibody fragments to digoxin if the toxicity is serious. Ventricular arrhythmias are treated with IV lidocaine or phenytoin. Heart block may require a temporary transvenous pacemaker. Although digoxin is frequently prescribed in elderly patients (10% to 20% receive the drug), the indications for treatment are often not clear; in these cases, digoxin may be stopped without risk to the patient.

Antiparkinsonian Drugs

Levodopa clearance is reduced in older patients, who are also more susceptible to postural hypotension and confusion. Therefore, older patients should receive conservative doses of levodopa and should be thoroughly screened for adverse effects, which are usually dose limiting (see Ch. 93). Patients with a diminished response to levodopa may benefit from the newer dopaminergic agents (eg, bromocriptine, pergolide); however, these drugs are not tolerated better in those who become confused while taking levodopa. Because older patients with parkinsonism may be cognitively impaired, anticholinergic agents should be avoided.

Anticoagulants

Warfarin use is common in older patients because of the high incidence of atrial fibrillation. Although aging does not alter the pharmacokinetics of warfarin, sensitivity to the anticoagulation effect may increase with age (recent studies have not confirmed that aging per se increases the risk of bleeding). Thus, older patients may require lower doses (usually < 5 mg/day), but as long as no contraindications exist, old age should not preclude meticulous, low-dose warfarin prophylaxis (the International Normalized Ratio [INR] should be between 2 and 3). Contraindications to warfarin use include uncontrolled hypertension, unsteady gait, history of falls, peptic ulcer disease, previous GI or other mucosal bleeding, syncope, seizures, alcoholism, or history of poor medication compliance.

Psychoactive Drugs

The common practice of prescribing **antipsychotic drugs** for agitated, confused elderly patients is being reevaluated because of concerns about inappropriate use, inadequate supervision, and toxicity. In agitated patients, antipsychotics control symptoms only marginally better than does placebo. Although antipsychotics can reduce agitation and paranoia, they may worsen confusion. In addition, because older patients are at increased risk for tardive dyskinesia, which is irreversible, chronic use of antipsychotics requires informed consent. Patients should be monitored for tardive dyskinesia as well as for other side effects, such as sedation, postural hypotension, anticholinergic effects, akathisia (subjective motor restlessness), and parkinsonism.

Starting doses of antipsychotics should be low (about ¼ the usual adult doses) and increased gradually. Response should be reevaluated regularly, and doses should be reduced and treatment stopped as soon as possible. The risk of falls and hip fracture associated with these drugs (and with other psychoactive drugs such as **long-acting benzodiazepines and antidepressants**) increases with the dose. Anticholinergics (eg, benztropine, trihexyphenidyl) may be used to treat extrapyramidal side effect, although stopping the antipsychotic treatment is usually preferred. Using anticholinergics to prevent extrapyramidal side effects is not recommended.

For a detailed discussion of the pharmacokinetics of psychoactive drugs, see Pharmacotherapy in Ch. 94.

Hypoglycemics

Doses of hypoglycemic drugs, including insulin and the sulfonylureas, should be titrated to prevent symptomatic hyperglycemia without causing hypoglycemia. Because the elderly often have a blunted metabolic response, hypoglycemia is more subtle in presentation.

Aging can reduce insulin clearance, but dose requirements depend on the level of insulin resistance, which varies widely among patients with type II diabetes. Thus, the insulin dosage needed to effectively control diabetes will vary widely. The incidence of hypoglycemia from sulfonylureas may increase with age. For patients with renal impairment, drugs cleared by hepatic metabolism (eg, tolbutamide, glipizide) are preferable. Chlorpropamide is not recommended because older patients are at increased risk of hyponatremia, and the drug's prolonged duration of action is dangerous if toxicity or hypoglycemia occurs. Because serious hypoglycemia occurs predominantly in elderly patients, the initial dose of sulfonylureas should be low and increased slowly. Diet remains a mainstay of treatment provided the patient can comply with it. Dosage recommendations for insulin and sulfonylureas are given in Ch. 80.

Analgesics

Because arthritic conditions are so prevalent in the elderly, nonsteroidal anti-inflammatory drugs **(NSAIDs)** are among the most widely used drugs. The use of NSAIDs is increasing, and over-the-counter preparations are now available. These drugs are well absorbed and highly protein bound; almost all are eliminated by hepatic metabolism. Evaluation of aging's effect on NSAID pharmacokinetics is complicated by the high protein binding, the presence of stereoisomers (mainly propionic acid derivatives), and in patients with renal impairment, the accumulation of metabolites that can be hydrolyzed to re-form the parent drug. Some data indicate that the clearance of salicylate, oxaprozin, and free naproxen is decreased in older patients.

Peptic ulceration and upper GI bleeding are serious consequences of NSAID therapy; the risk is greater when therapy is first begun and when doses are increased. Although aging does not seem to increase the risk for NSAID-induced adverse GI effects, such complications cause considerably more morbidity and mortality in elderly patients.

The risk of NSAID-induced renal impairment may be increased in older patients, but the risk is relatively low. The monitoring of serum creatinine level is a reasonable approach, especially in patients with other risk factors such as heart failure, renal impairment, cirrhosis with ascites, volume depletion, or diuretic use.

22. THE ROLE OF THE PHARMACIST

Advances in health care technology and changes in federal regulations have given increasing importance to the pharmacist's role on the health care team. Besides dispensing drugs, pharmacists collaborate with physicians and counsel patients. Since drug use increases with age (the elderly consume > 30% of all prescription drugs and about 40% of over-the-counter drugs), the pharmacist's expertise is especially important to the elderly.

Pharmacists, as well as physicians, must be aware of the implications of altered pharmacodynamics and pharmacokinetics in elderly patients (see Ch. 21). They should also recognize that the elderly have a high incidence of adverse drug reactions and interactions, poor compliance with drug regimens, and overuse and underuse of drugs. In consultation with the physician, the pharmacist can help avoid or resolve these problems by recommending appropriate or alternative drugs and by advising and monitoring patients, especially concerning compliance.

To meet the need for pharmacists with expertise in handling the special requirements of the elderly, more pharmacy educators are being trained in geriatrics, and pharmacy schools are offering more courses in geriatrics. The American Society of Hospital Pharmacists and the American Society of Consultant Pharmacists recognize and accredit residency programs in geriatric pharmacy, and the number of research-oriented fellowship programs in geriatric pharmacology is growing.

DRUG UTILIZATION REVIEW

The Health Care Financing Administration defines drug utilization review as "a structured, ongoing, quality assurance process to ensure that drugs are prescribed and dispensed appropriately, safely, effectively, and economically."

Drug utilization review (DUR) programs are directed and staffed mainly by pharmacists. The Omnibus Budget Reconciliation Act of 1990 (OBRA 90), which became effective in January 1993, requires that all states establish DUR programs in hospitals and long-term care facilities for drugs reimbursed through Medicaid. Health maintenance organizations and similar organizations, Veterans Administration hospitals, and state programs providing drug services also use DUR programs extensively. A demonstration project was initiated in 1993 to validate the application of DUR at the pharmacy level.

Drug utilization review programs have prospective, concurrent, and retrospective components. **Prospective DUR** is done at the point of sale (ie, the pharmacy) before the patient gets the drug. Pharmacists are required to obtain and record certain information about patients and their drug prescriptions; this information enables the pharmacist to assess the appropriateness of a particular prescription before dispensing it. The pharmacist may collaborate with the prescribing physician to resolve potential problems. Pharmacists must also counsel patients before filling prescriptions covered by Medicaid, with the aim of improving compliance and avoiding medication errors.

Concurrent DUR programs evaluate the use of drugs currently being prescribed. Information on potentially problematic drug use is supplied to prescribers to allow them to adjust therapy before it harms the patient. Concurrent DUR can also be used to control costs.

In **retrospective DUR,** data on aggregate drug use in a health care setting are collected and evaluated to identify trends, overuse and underuse, adverse drug reactions, and drug interactions and to analyze expenditures. In some programs, the appropriateness of prescribing patterns can be assessed by linking drugs to diagnoses. Strategies are developed to correct abuses and inappropriate practices, and corrective actions are transmitted to the prescribers.

SETTINGS FOR PHARMACY SERVICES

The settings in which pharmacy services are provided include community pharmacies, home health care programs, long-term care facilities, and hospitals. Of the nation's 190,000 licensed pharmacists, 112,000 practice in chain store or independent community pharmacies; 40,000 in hospital pharmacies; and 21,000 in consultation, academia, industry, or government.

Community Pharmacies

Traditionally, the community pharmacist has dispensed prescriptions, provided informal advice and counseling (particularly on over-the-counter drugs), referred patients to physicians, and conferred with physicians on drug therapy.

Advances in computer technology have enhanced the counseling role of the community pharmacist (see TABLE 22–1). Most pharmacies use computers to keep patient records, including medication profiles. The medication profile can help identify duplication of drugs, overuse and underuse, allergies, drug interactions, potential adverse reactions, and special counseling needs of individual patients. However, most such programs do not have criteria specific to the elderly. Some computer programs specify when a patient is scheduled for a medication refill or a return visit to the physician. This information enables the pharmacist to identify noncompliance and to counsel the patient more effectively. Because the elderly purchase many over-the-counter drugs (especially analgesics, cough and cold preparations, vitamins, antacids, and laxatives), pharmacist counseling and monitoring of such drug use can decrease the potential for adverse reactions or drug interactions.

Home Health Care Programs

Many disabled elderly persons are cared for at home by family members. In addition, over 9000 agencies are certified to provide services at home to Medicare beneficiaries. Home health care agencies accredited by the Joint Commission on Accreditation of Healthcare Organizations must contract for pharmacy services. The pharmacist is required not only to dispense and deliver medications but also to continually monitor the use of drugs by patients cared for at home. The pharmacist should be able to manage the administration of IV fluids such as total parenteral nutrition and other therapies such as anticoagulation, cancer chemotherapy, and inhalation therapy.

Long-Term Care Facilities

Since 1965, federal regulations have issued specific mandates for pharmacy services in nursing homes and other long-term care facilities. To meet requirements for Medicare and Medicaid reimbursement, pharmacists must conduct monthly **drug regimen reviews,** in which they reevaluate a patient's drug regimen and make appropriate recommen-

TABLE 22–1. COUNSELING RESPONSIBILITIES OF THE PHARMACIST*

Provide name and description of the drug
Discuss special instructions and precautions in preparing, administering, and using the drug
Recommend action to take if a dose is missed
Describe common adverse effects and drug interactions (including interactions with over-the-counter drugs), how to avoid them, and what to do if they occur
Discuss contraindications to the drug
Suggest self-monitoring techniques for drug therapy
Explain how to store the drug properly
Discuss prescription refill procedures

*This is a partial list; pharmacists should provide whatever information they consider important.

dations to the patient's physician. Drug regimen reviews help to decrease polypharmacy, minimize duplication of drugs, prevent significant drug interactions, and reduce the inappropriate or unnecessary use of drugs. The Health Care Financing Administration has established guidelines for use by surveyors in assessing a facility's drug regimen review process (see TABLE 22–2). This list of apparent irregularities reflects problems that have been seen in long-term care facilities.

Other duties of the pharmacist in a long-term care facility include managing the labeling, storage, and security and inventory control of drugs; reporting irregularities in drug regimens to the administration, the director of nursing, and the primary physician for appropriate action; and implementing guidelines for reducing unnecessary drug therapy, particularly psychoactive drugs. The Health Care Financing Administration defines unnecessary drug therapy as the use of any drug in excessive dose, for excessive duration, without adequate monitoring, without adequate indication for its use, or when circumstances indicate that the dose should be reduced or the drug discontinued. One goal of the Omnibus Budget Reconciliation Act of 1987 (OBRA 87) was to reduce the use of antipsychotic drugs as chemical restraints.

Hospital Pharmacies

Hospital pharmacists are responsible for acquiring, storing, and distributing medicines and other pharmaceutical preparations. They also participate in the drug utilization review process, serve on pharmacy

TABLE 22–2. INDICATORS OF APPARENT IRREGULARITIES IN DRUG REGIMEN REVIEWS

General	Multiple orders for the same drug for the same patient by the same route of administration Drugs given without regard for established stop-order policies Orders for drugs that the patient is known to be allergic to Crushing of solid forms of a drug that may cause patient discomfort or undesired blood levels
Drugs given in excess of the recommended maximum dose	Antidepressants Antipsychotics Anxiolytics Hypnotics
Duplication of therapy	Three or more laxatives Two or more hypnotic drugs Two or more antipsychotic drugs Three or more analgesics
Inappropriate duration of therapy	Hypnotic drugs continuously for $>$ 30 days Antibiotic or corticosteroid topical ophthalmic preparations continuously for $>$ 14 days As needed (prn) drugs every day for $>$ 30 days Antipsychotics or antidepressants for $<$ 3 days
Drug use without adequate monitoring	Thyroid drugs without assessment of thyroid function Anticoagulants without assessment of blood clotting function at least every month Antihypertensives without blood pressure checks at least weekly Cardioactive drugs without recording pulse rate daily during first month of therapy and weekly thereafter Diuretics without determining serum potassium levels during first month of therapy Diuretics and cardiotonics (eg, digoxin) without determining serum potassium levels during first month of cardiotonic therapy and every 6 mo thereafter Insulin or oral hypoglycemics without a urine glucose test at least daily or a blood glucose test at least every 60 days Iron preparations, folic acid, or vitamin B_{12} without RBC assessment during first month of therapy Methenamine mandelate, methenamine hippurate, sulfamethoxazole-trimethoprim, or nitrofurantoin in patients with chronic UTIs without at least one urinalysis during first month of therapy

(continued)

TABLE 22–2. INDICATORS OF APPARENT IRREGULARITIES IN DRUG REGIMEN REVIEWS *(Continued)*

Drug use without adequate monitoring *(continued)*	Phenylbutazone or oxyphenbutazone continuously without at least one CBC count during first month of therapy
Drug use without documented indication or with documented contraindication	Anticholinergics with antipsychotic drugs without documented extrapyramidal side effects Aminoglycosides without determining baseline serum creatinine level Nitrofurantoin for conditions other than treatment or prophylaxis of UTIs or without recording BUN or serum creatinine levels Cardiotonics (eg, digoxin) without documentation of heart failure, atrial fibrillation, paroxysmal supraventricular tachycardia, or atrial flutter Cardioactive drugs when pulse is consistently < 60 or > 100 beats/min Methenamine mandelate, methenamine hippurate, sulfamethoxazole-trimethoprim, or nitrofurantoin in patients with chronic UTIs when urine pH is continually > 6
Other	More than two changes in antidepressant therapy within 7 days Repeated loss of seizure control in a patient taking anticonvulsants

Modified from *State Operations Manual, Provider Certification.* Department of Health and Human Services, Health Care Financing Administration, September 1990, Transmittal No. 242.

and therapeutics committees, and often join physicians on clinical rounds. The pharmacist's expertise may be particularly valuable to older patients since age-related changes in pharmacokinetics and tissue sensitivity may be amplified by drugs commonly used to treat acute diseases (eg, antibiotics, antiarrhythmics, anticoagulants, thrombolytic agents).

Many hospital pharmacies provide a number of programs, including comprehensive drug information centers, pharmacokinetic dosing advice to physicians, and nutrition support services. In addition, pharmacists may serve on multidisciplinary teams. For example, as a member of a geriatric assessment unit, the pharmacist obtains a patient's medication history that includes patterns of use for all drug regimens, therapeutic effectiveness, duplication of drugs, adverse drug reactions, and drug interactions. The pharmacist then makes recommendations to optimize drug use (eg, counseling and teaching the patient and family, recommending alternative therapy, or adjusting the current regimen). Similar activities are conducted in hospital-based geriatrics clinics and in community-outreach programs in which patients are seen in satellite clinics, in congregate housing facilities, or at home.

Pharmacists are responsible for dispensing discharge medications and for instructing patients and their caregivers on proper use of these medications. Nurses, who can help establish the most effective means of communicating vital information, should be involved in such instruction. For most elderly patients, instructions for medication use after discharge should be written.

23. GERIATRIC NURSING

In the USA, nurse generalists (often called staff nurses) deliver most nursing care, including geriatric nursing care. Educated in diploma programs, associate degree programs, or baccalaureate degree programs, these registered nurses practice in settings ranging from patients' homes to intensive care units.

Nurse generalists both plan and provide a wide range of geriatric care, dealing with common problems such as skin breakdown, incontinence, eating and feeding problems, falls, confusion, sleep disorders, and discomfort and pain. These nurses also teach elderly patients and their families various self-care and preventive care procedures and provide support (see TABLE 23–1).

Because of their round-the-clock surveillance of patients, nurse generalists also serve as the linchpins of multidisciplinary teams, working closely with physicians. These teams may include attending physicians, house staff, social workers, physical therapists, and other health care professionals. Such teams are useful in hospitals, outpatient clinics, nursing homes, and hospice settings.

GERIATRIC NURSING SPECIALTIES

The first graduate level program in geriatric nursing was introduced in 1966 at Duke University. Today, more than 50 such programs exist in the USA. Nurses graduating from these specialty programs can take a certification examination sponsored by the American Nurses Association to become either a geriatric nurse practitioner or geriatric nurse specialist. Currently, a certification examination is not available for the geropsychiatric clinical nurse specialist.

TABLE 23–1. NURSING ACTIVITIES

Purposes of Nursing	*Giving Care (Examples)*	*Teaching (Examples)*	*Supporting (Examples)*
Promoting health	Providing wound care for pressure sores	Teaching older adults how to maintain healthy bowel patterns	Supporting caregivers of demented elders
Maintaining health	Promoting patient mobility during convalescence	Teaching preoperative patient to turn, cough, and breathe deeply	Encouraging elderly alcoholic to attend Alcoholics Anonymous meetings
Restoring health	Performing range-of-motion exercises with stroke patient	Demonstrating colostomy care to permanent ileostomy patient	Encouraging patient to perform postural drainage care

Modified from Megenity JS, Megenity J: *Patient Teaching: Theories, Techniques and Strategies.* Bowie, Md., Robert J. Brady Co., 1982; used with permission of Appleton & Lange.

Geriatric Nurse Practitioners

As of 1991, more than 60,000 registered nurses had been certified as nurse practitioners, including adult nurse practitioners, family nurse practitioners, and geriatric nurse practitioners. Ideally, elderly patients should receive care from geriatric nurse practitioners; however, only about 4000 have been certified.

Nurse practitioners are usually registered nurses whose formal education and clinical training surpass the basic requirements for licensure. The additional training in the form of a certificate or master's degree program includes from 9 to 24 mo of study and supervised clinical training in direct patient care in a specialty. For a geriatric nurse practitioner, study focuses on normal aging, common problems of old age, management of common problems, and assessment skills in detecting complex problems for referral. Functions include conducting physical assessments; assessing and diagnosing; ordering laboratory and other diagnostic tests; developing and implementing treatment plans for some acute and chronic illnesses; prescribing some medications; monitoring patient status; teaching and counseling patients; and consulting with, collaborating with, and referring patients to other health care professionals. Upon graduation, about 40% of the geriatric nurse practitioners work in nursing homes or for physicians with practices in nursing homes. About 35% work in urban institutions; about 20%, in rural areas.

Today, community health services such as home care agencies, hospices, and clinics are managed primarily by nurse practitioners. These expanded nursing roles have evolved because of the lack of basic health care services in certain areas, especially rural regions and inner cities, and because few physicians make home visits. As medicine has become more and more specialized, access to primary care has become more difficult. Today, nurse practitioners are helping to meet the need for primary care in the community.

Geriatric nurse practitioners may receive third-party reimbursement under the Rural Health Act and, for dependents of military personnel, through CHAMPUS (Civilian Health and Medical Program of the Uniformed Services). Geriatric nurse practitioners are also eligible for Medicare reimbursement in certain long-term care settings.

Geriatric Nurse Specialists

Nurse specialists have substantial clinical experience with individuals, families, and groups; expertise in formulating health and social policies; and demonstrated proficiency in planning, implementing, and evaluating health problems. Unlike nurse practitioners, however, nurse specialists do not have the authority to prescribe medications.

Most geriatric nurse specialists work in hospitals, where they serve on multidisciplinary consultation teams and are available to staff nurses who encounter problems that require their expertise. The specialists provide expert practice protocols for such common problems as skin breakdown, incontinence, sleep disorders, falls, and eating and feeding disorders. The specialists also help staff nurses by serving as liaisons between the hospital and nursing homes and community health agencies. Geriatric nurse specialists also provide continuing education about new research findings to staff nurses.

Geropsychiatric Nurse Specialists

Geropsychiatric nurse specialists are the newest group of nurse specialists caring for the elderly. The number of these specialists currently in practice is not known, partly because the specialty has no certification procedure. In the USA, only a few training programs exist. These nurse specialists often work in hospitals, mental health clinics, and outpatient settings where elderly patients have mental health impairments, especially cognitive changes.

NURSING MANAGEMENT OF COMMON PROBLEMS

Nurses participate in the management of many geriatric problems: pressure sores, urinary and fecal incontinence, eating and feeding problems, falls, confusion, sleep problems, and discomfort and pain.

Pressure Sores

A primary objective of nursing practice is preventing skin breakdown. For elderly patients at special risk for such breakdown, the potential problem should be listed in the nursing care plan. Preventive measures include following a regular observation schedule, turning and massaging the patient as appropriate, and using prophylactic bed surfaces, such as sheepskin, special air mattresses, and air-fluidized beds.

Preventing skin breakdown is paramount. Once a pressure sore progresses to stage 2 (partial-thickness skin loss involving the epidermis and dermis), nursing actions must become more vigorous. These actions may include turning the patient regularly, applying the appropriate dressing, continually monitoring the patient, and documenting all nursing care and observations. If a pressure sore progresses to stage 4 (full-thickness skin loss involving extensive necrosis or damage to muscle, bone, or supporting structure), the nurse should include in the care plan interventions for social isolation, depression, pain, and discomfort (see also Ch. 14).

Urinary and Fecal Incontinence

Preventive nursing measures include instituting a regular toileting schedule using prompted voiding, providing easy and safe access to the bathroom, and planning appropriate timing of diuretics and fluids. When older patients become incontinent, nurse-managed protocols that document patterns of urinary and fecal incontinence and describe therapeutic interventions provide valuable information. For example, information about the bowel patterns of older patients can make a difference between an unwanted outcome (such as a severe impaction or diarrhea from antibiotics and nutritional supplements) and an early, successful resolution.

When **urinary incontinence** occurs, the nurse must understand the cause to develop an appropriate care plan. For example, when incontinence results from an irreversible neurologic cause, the nurse should minimize discomfort and promote appropriate coping responses. If incontinence is acute and reversible, efforts are directed at the underlying problem. When a patient has an episode of delirium, the possibility of incontinence should be anticipated, and the patient should be taken to the bathroom or offered a bedpan or urinal more often than usual. An indwelling catheter should be used only as a last resort and only as long as necessary. When a patient has an indwelling catheter, the nurse should keep the physician apprised of how long it has been in place and may need to advocate its removal.

For any patient with urinary incontinence, the nurse should keep an incontinence chart; every 2 h, the nurse documents the amount of urine voided, the amount lost because of incontinence, any associated symptoms, and any patient comments. Adult urinary incontinence pads and diapers should be used judiciously because they retain urine against the skin. They are inappropriate substitutes for helping the patient get to the bathroom. Every effort should be made to respect patient preferences regarding the management of urinary incontinence (see also Ch. 15).

An embarrassing problem for older patients, **fecal incontinence** may result from IV antibiotics, hyperalimentation, or chemotherapy or from delirium or another neurologic disorder. Nurses should strive to recognize fecal incontinence when possible and prevent its complications. If the patient has diarrhea, the nurse must observe closely for fluid and electrolyte imbalance and for dehydration. The fecal material and the continuous wiping may produce excoriations on the buttocks. Before redness or soreness develops, lotion should be applied to the skin. If the patient cannot exert any bowel control, insertion of a rectal tube should be considered. Because fecal incontinence may be a sign of impaction, this diagnosis should be excluded before therapies are initiated (see also Chs. 53 and 55).

Eating and Feeding Problems

Eating and feeding problems can often be resolved with meticulous nursing assessment and intervention. These nursing activities are distinct from those of the dietitian or nutritionist, but they are just as essential for adequate patient nutrition.

A patient who is unable to swallow, digest, or absorb sufficient food and fluid taken by mouth requires enteral or parenteral feedings. A patient who can ingest nothing by mouth is at particularly high risk for being inadequately nourished. The nurse should carefully document weight loss, decreased skin turgor, changes in bowel habits (especially diarrhea and constipation), and other early signs of declining nutritional status and promptly report this information to the doctor.

When a patient is not eating adequately, the nurse should assess eating and feeding patterns to find out why. Anorexia may result from illness, depression, poorly fitting dentures, dry mouth, or a dislike of the foods provided. In a busy institution with conflicting schedules, inadequate nutrition may result simply because the patient is a slow eater. Eating problems may also result from difficulties in using eating utensils because of paraplegia, muscle weakness, or neuralgia. In such cases, efforts should be made to improve hand strength and muscle coordination so patients can maintain their ability to feed themselves. The nurse may need to work with a physical or occupational therapist to develop a plan for regular muscle strengthening exercises throughout the day.

In many cases of inadequate eating or feeding, nursing interventions solve the problem. Nurses or nursing assistants may place food or nutritional supplements at the patient's bedside, dispense frequent small feedings, instruct dietary services to leave meal trays past the usual time for collection, or consult with dietitians to alter the consistency of the diet. When necessary, nurses should reposition patients to prevent choking and should keep patients from returning to bed too soon after eating to help prevent regurgitation (see also Ch. 2).

Falls

A major cause of morbidity and mortality in the elderly, falls account for most institutional incident reports. Nursing responsibilities include working with other health care team members to prevent falls, document which patients are at high risk, and intervene after falls to determine the extent of injury and to prevent subsequent falls.

Most falls occur during the day when patients are more active and during shift changes. Falls are also common during the night shift when patients who awaken to use the bathroom are confused or disoriented and fewer staff members are available. Nursing care plans should note risk factors for falls, including weakness, altered mentation, proprioceptive problems, and sensory losses. All nursing practice sites should have a plan for preventing or reducing falls; this plan should be part of a quality assurance program.

Specific nursing interventions for preventing falls include using bed rails appropriately, using vest restraints to keep patients in bed, and hiring sitters to observe patients. Sitters can also help ensure that IV lines, nasogastric tubes, and central lines are not pulled out. However, sitters are expensive, and patients may resent having their privacy invaded. An alternative is to place high-risk patients in rooms near the nurses' station or to seat them in comfortable chairs where they can be constantly monitored.

When physical restraints are ordered, the minimum standard for safe nursing practice includes checking the restraints at least hourly and releasing them every 2 h to prevent circulatory impairment and skin breakdown. Probably most important, this regular checking and releasing reassures patients that they have not been tied up and forgotten. Understandably, patients and families resent the use of restraints without appropriate instruction, support, and documentation that all alternatives have been considered and informed consents have been obtained. Documentation should indicate why restraints have been ordered, under what conditions they will be continued, how they will be evaluated, and when they should be discontinued. When appropriate, the nurse should recommend discontinuing the restraints. Restraints should also require new orders every 3 days so that inappropriate use is not continued (see also Ch. 7).

Confusion

Delirious and demented elderly patients are at risk for falls, medication errors, communication problems, and nutritional deficits. They may also become uncooperative, noisy, and violent and may be unable to participate in making medical decisions.

Delirium requires a rapid nursing response. It signals serious medical illness and is a grave prognostic sign. Also, a delirious older person can easily fall and break a hip, thrash out and strike a caregiver or another patient, or become extremely frightened. After evaluating the extent and nature of the problem, the nurse should immediately consult the physician to determine which temporary safety measure should be taken, what clinical information should be gathered to determine the underlying cause, and what, if any, medications are appropriate. Frequently, the delirium is iatrogenic. Therefore, the patient's medications should be reviewed and evidence of hypoxia or other physiologic changes, including cardiac, neurologic, renal, hepatic, or metabolic changes, should be sought. The importance of rapid intervention cannot be overstated. Initially, the most important nursing intervention is to stay with the patient to help alleviate fear and protect the patient from injury (see also Ch. 9 and DELIRIUM in Ch. 90).

In older persons with **dementia,** the cognitive deterioration has evolved over time. Thus, a history obtained from the family or caregiver will reveal behavioral changes and the ways in which the patient and family have adapted. The nurse should document the routines described by the family and other caregivers and incorporate them into the care plan. Most important, the nurse should document what the family says about the patient's usual behavior at home, so the team can try to maintain a similar environment and thus avoid triggering behavioral problems. Regular mental status examinations should be performed and documented. A deterioration of cognition or behavior may indicate superimposed delirium (see also DEMENTIA in Ch. 90).

Sleep Problems

Distinct from chronic sleep disorders, sleep problems in the hospital usually stem from worry related to illness, discomfort with unfamiliar surroundings, pain, and environmental noise. Particularly in the hospital, sleep problems may go unnoticed for several days, leading to sleep deprivation and delirium. Obtaining a sleep history, keeping a sleep flow chart, and documenting the patient's perception of sleeping patterns in the hospital can help in identifying sleep deprivation as the cause of cognitive changes.

Preventing unnecessary noise on the evening and night shifts and unnecessary interruptions, such as those for routine vital signs, may solve the problem. Foods, medications, and therapies should be reviewed for their possible effects on the patient's sleep; if the nurse suspects one of these factors, the suspicion should be reported to the physician and other team members. Caffeine should be avoided, if the patient is willing to give it up. A medication such as theophylline, which may be prescribed to treat lung disease, can severely disturb sleep patterns. Exercise (though highly unlikely in the hospital) should take place early in the day. Even a simple change such as providing a better mattress can be effective. This intervention may be particularly helpful in patients who become disoriented in a flotation bed. Finally, support from the hospital chaplain, volunteers, physician, or the nursing staff may help ease the anxiety related to being sick (see also Ch. 11).

Discomfort and Pain

Providing physical and emotional comfort to an elderly patient may include giving relaxing back rubs; providing favorite pillows, treasured pictures, and personal articles; and giving care with a personal touch. During the rare quiet times in an institution when a nurse can give a bed bath or a back rub or even sit and read with the patient, a great deal of information can be exchanged, both verbally and nonverbally. While cost containment is the rule of the day, the importance of providing comfort measures cannot be overemphasized.

Nurses also play a key role in administering analgesics. When standing orders exist, nurses should give analgesics assiduously. Many narcotics have short half-lives and lose their effectiveness within hours; if they are not given on time, pain recurs. Nurses must also monitor patients for pain and then advise physicians about changing doses or administration times. When analgesics are ordered as needed, nurses must decide when to give them. Waiting for patients to ask for pain medication is usually not the best course. Some patients cannot ask; others wait until the pain becomes severe. Nurses may be able to anticipate the need for analgesics either by time or by upcoming events such as a dressing change, turning, moving, or toileting (see also Ch. 12).

PATIENT TEACHING AND DISCHARGE PLANNING

A large part of geriatric nursing involves teaching patients and families, planning for discharge to ensure that treatments can be carried out safely and effectively, and communicating with the multidisciplinary team.

Patient Teaching

In most patient care settings, the nurse explains tests and procedures to the patient and family. For example, a gastroenterologist may use diagrams in describing an endoscopy to obtain informed consent, but the nurse then elaborates, explaining the procedure based on the patient's ability to understand and retain the information. Nurses also develop patient education pamphlets containing pertinent information and phone numbers in case questions arise. Nurses regularly demonstrate self-care procedures to patients and then have the patients perform the procedures as the nurses observe. Such procedures include irrigating a new colostomy, injecting insulin, and providing wound care for a pressure sore. Ongoing evaluation of the elderly patient's ability to learn new information or behavior should be documented, along with an assessment of the support available in the patient's environment, whether it is the home, a nursing home, or the intensive care unit.

Determining the best teaching method for a particular patient can speed the process dramatically. For instance, some elderly patients learn best when they have written or printed material; others prefer videotaped information. The nurse can tell the multidisciplinary team which methods the patient prefers, so an appropriate unified approach can be tailored to the patient.

Usually, the nurse sees family members more often than other team members do. Continual, open communication with family members lets

TABLE 23–2. DISCHARGE PLANNING STANDARDS*

Discharge planning standards include but are not restricted to the following:

1. All patients have the right to discharge planning, which begins with the initial patient care assessment upon admission and includes consideration of legal and civil rights and the principles of the least restrictive alternatives to care.

2. Discharge planning should be initiated by the primary health care providers. Assessments should be based on skilled nursing care needs and on psychosocial, economic, legal, and environmental factors.

3. Discharge planning must be multidisciplinary.

4. A mechanism for consultation or coordination with a continuing care nurse should be established by the multidisciplinary team. The continuing care nurse is vital to the assessment process in determining the patient's medical and nursing needs after discharge. Based on the nurse's knowledge and community health expertise, the nurse identifies specific levels of nursing care required, while recognizing and using appropriate resources to provide the care.

5. Documentation of the discharge must be consistently maintained on a multidisciplinary sheet in the medical record. The patient care referral form is the vehicle for transfer of patient care information between agencies and must be provided to facilities at the time of discharge.

6. Evaluation is a necessary component of the discharge planning process because it helps identify gaps and inadequacies in the health care services provided by the hospital and the community. This information should be used to generate action in health planning and regulatory activities.

* These standards were developed by the Boston Regional Continuing Care Nurses Association (*Discharge Planning Standards*, 1982) to identify the essential components of the discharge planning process.

them know that their input is valuable. As a result, the nurse is more likely to obtain useful, accurate information about the patient's home. After discharge, the nurse should continue to be available to the patient and family.

Discharge Planning

Nurses play a vital role in discharge planning, which begins at admission and continues through discharge. Nurses help determine when discharge is safe and which setting is most appropriate. Effective discharge planning speeds discharge, decreases the likelihood of readmission, identifies less expensive care alternatives, and helps increase patient satisfaction. One example of discharge planning standards, developed by the Boston Regional Continuing Care Nurses Association, is shown in TABLE 23–2.

Before the patient is discharged or transferred, effective communication between settings helps ensure continuity of care. In most cases, a nurse caring for a hospital patient should call the nurse who will care for the patient after discharge in a nursing home, at home, or through a home care service. The appropriate transfer form should contain complete, accurate information, including resuscitation status, cognitive and physical function, medications, follow-up appointments and studies, and the names and phone numbers of a nurse and physician who can provide additional information. When a patient is transferred to the hospital from a nursing home, the nursing home nurse should inform the admitting nurse about the patient's cognitive and physical status, resuscitation status, medications and medication allergies, and family support.

24. CARE IN NURSING HOMES AND OTHER LONG–TERM CARE FACILITIES

Whether placement in a nursing home or other long-term care facility occurs from a hospital or home setting, the need for institutionalization should be thoroughly assessed. In addition, the services needed must be matched to an institution's ability to provide them.

ASSESSING THE NEED FOR INSTITUTIONALIZATION

Assessing the need for institutional placement must be comprehensive and should include evaluation of medical needs, social support, cognitive or intellectual capacity, and physical function. Because these areas are interrelated, a problem in one area may also cause difficulty in another.

Medical Needs

All medical problems should be evaluated before a patient is institutionalized. The evaluation is done by a physician in collaboration with nurses and social workers to determine the impact of the medical problems on the need for institutionalization, the probability of successful treatment, and most important the nursing home's capability for providing that treatment. While medical problems are rarely the sole factor warranting institutional placement, even modest improvement of a medical condition may forestall the need for a nursing home. For example, if a person who is already dependent on family for care develops urinary incontinence, care at home may become difficult, but evaluating and treating the causes for the incontinence may allow the patient to remain at home. Even when a chronic condition worsens, treatment may delay institutionalization. On the other hand, a nursing home may be the most appropriate place for treating persons with certain medical problems. Many patients with fractures, strokes, or severe physical deconditioning from prolonged illness can benefit from several weeks or months of therapy in a nursing home.

Social Support

Consideration must be given to whether potential caregivers are willing and able to perform the tasks necessary to keep the older person at home. Strongly motivated families usually can perform elaborate and detailed care, but they may be indifferent or become resentful or worn out from assuming such responsibility. Home care often involves a long-term commitment and may prove an unremitting burden to a family. Physicians should watch for and be ready to intervene if elder abuse is suspected (see Ch. 111). The very old may be cared for by equally aged spouses or elderly children whose own frailty or impairment may preclude providing the necessary care, regardless of how much they may wish to do so.

Cognitive Function

Intellectual impairment alone can make institutionalization necessary. Even supportive families may find disruptive behavior, such as nocturnal wandering or paranoia, intolerable. If 24-h care is required, nursing home placement may be appropriate. But mildly to moderately demented patients can often function quite well in their own familiar environment, especially if families have been taught coping strategies for dealing with dementia and periodically get some respite (see RESPITE CARE in Ch. 25). Physicians and other care providers must be supportive not only of the patient but of the family as well.

Physical Function

Evaluating a patient's ability to perform the activities of daily living (ADLs)—bathing, walking, toileting, eating, dressing, and grooming—and instrumental activities of daily living (IADLs)—shopping, cooking, cleaning, managing finances, and using the telephone—is crucial in deciding whether nursing home placement is necessary or appropriate (see also Ch. 17). Although severely impaired mobility may make living at home impossible, other functional impairments may be less of a handicap with adaptive devices. Skillful assessment of patients in their own homes (eg, by an occupational therapist) is extremely useful and may indicate whether the home can be made safer, eliminating the need for institutionalization.

NURSING HOMES

The USA has about 16,000 nursing homes with about 1.9 million beds, which represents about 53 beds for every 1000 people > age 65.

Increased demographic demand indicates that more beds are needed, especially in certain geographic areas. The probability of nursing home placement sometime within a person's lifetime is closely related to age; for those age 65 to 74, the probability is 17%, but for those > 85, it is 60%. Projections indicate that 43% of people who turned 65 in 1990 will spend some time in a nursing home before they die, and more than 50% of those admitted will spend at least a year.

Prospective payment systems, such as those based on diagnosis related groups (DRGs), are often responsible for expedited discharges from hospitals to nursing homes of marginally stable or extremely deconditioned patients. Such patients need considerable amounts of skilled nursing and other therapies to achieve their rehabilitative potential. They will probably be in the nursing home for short stays (< 3 mo) rather than permanently. Medical practitioners must ensure that facilities have the level of staffing and types of personnel necessary to meet the needs of these sick patients.

FINANCIAL ASPECTS

Cost

Nursing home care is expensive both for individuals and for state and federal governments. While the cost is usually far lower than that for acute care hospitalization, lengths of stay average months to years rather than days. In 1990 the average rate per day was about $80. About 60% of nursing home revenue comes from the jointly sponsored federal-state Medicaid programs and about 13% from Medicare. Other sources, such as health insurance plans and individual policies, health maintenance organizations (HMOs), the Veterans Administration, and personal savings, account for the remainder of their revenue.

Patients who pay for their own nursing home stays may find that the fees quickly deplete assets, rendering them indigent and thus eligible for Medicaid. However, **spending down** assets to pay for nursing home care has two consequences for residents: (1) For couples, depletion of joint assets may jeopardize the welfare of the spouse remaining in the community. (2) No assets remain for the patient's return to the community, if that becomes clinically feasible; thus, nursing home placement may become permanent out of financial necessity. (See also FINANCING HEALTH CARE in Ch. 110 and Ch. 114.)

Payment Mechanisms

Payment for nursing home care is changing to reflect the diversity of need in today's long-term care facility. **Case-mix systems,** which tie payment to the care needs of the nursing home population, place patients in hierarchical categories according to the types and amounts of resources their care will consume, such as physical or occupational therapists attending to patients' rehabilitative needs and nurses providing physical care or medical monitoring. Several states (eg, New York, Rhode Island, Texas) have linked Medicaid payments to case mix for many years.

Because this system has been successful, the Health Care Financing Administration (HCFA) is sponsoring a Multi-State Medicare Case-Mix and Quality Demonstration Project to refine and improve the system, based on the experiences of individual states. Called RUG III (Resource Utilization Group, Version III), this federal model is being tested in Kansas, Maine, Mississippi, Nebraska, South Dakota, and Texas. Its category-based classification system uses data from a version of the Minimum Data Set (MDS), the mandated nursing home resident assessment instrument developed as a result of **OBRA 87** (Omnibus Budget Reconciliation Act of 1987, also referred to as the Nursing Home Reform Law). Under this model, nursing home residents are classified hierarchically in one of the three mutually exclusive RUG groups. A distinct category for the cognitively impaired considers not only ability to perform activities of daily living but also decision-making ability, orientation, and short-term memory.

There are concerns that case-mix systems put a premium on physical care but pay little attention to psychosocial and quality-of-life–enhancing services, especially for residents with dementia. Because these systems offer financial incentives to provide care for the neediest patients, they may create an environment in which nursing homes foster dependence or maintain high-level care needs to maximize reimbursement. Performance evaluations based on review and audit of relevant care plans are needed to ensure that this does not happen. The Minimum Data Set and a required interdisciplinary care planning process, developed under OBRA 87, should make this evaluation easier.

Level of Care

In 1986, the Department of Health and Human Services in association with the Institute of Medicine issued a report entitled "Improving the Quality of Care in Nursing Homes," which contained a number of provisions that were incorporated into OBRA 87. One of the most significant changes that occurred under OBRA 87 was the consolidation of two levels of care—the Skilled Nursing Facility level for Medicare beneficiaries and the Intermediate Care Facility level for Medicaid recipients. This change to a so-called single level of care was motivated not by a belief that all nursing home residents have the same care needs but by an attempt to redress program inequities that had gradually developed because of payment differentials between Medicare and Medicaid.

When initially established, these two care level designations were intended to take into account how much skilled care was needed, but gradually they came to represent only payment indicators. Patients qualifying for payment by Medicare were admitted to skilled nursing facilities; after exhausting that benefit, they were transferred to a designated intermediate care facility, which was paid for by Medicaid. This shift in location was usually triggered by a change in payer status and

TABLE 24–1. NURSING HOME SERVICES REQUIRED FOR FEDERAL CERTIFICATION

Licensed charge nurse on site 24 h/day
Registered nurses 8 h/day, 7 days/wk
Certified nurses aides
Full-time social worker if facility has > 120 beds
Medical director
Licensed nursing home administrator
Qualified therapeutic recreational therapist*
Licensed pharmacist†
Rehabilitative therapists†
Dentists†
Qualified dietitian‡
Pastoral services†
Physician services†

* Federal requirements give several alternatives for this position.

† Nursing home *must* employ or obtain the services of these persons as needed for resident care.

‡ If not employed by the facility, the food services manager must have frequently scheduled consultations with a dietitian.

rarely reflected an actual change in the resident's underlying care needs. Because Medicaid reimbursement rates often provided for little more than room and board and were kept artificially low in many states, scandalous incidents of patient neglect occurred, which OBRA 87 sought to rectify. Through the Nursing Home Reform Law, OBRA 87 stipulated that a Medicare- or Medicaid-certified nursing home must provide all the services needed to enable each resident to attain and maintain the highest practicable level of physical, mental, and psychosocial functioning, regardless of the source of payment (see TABLE 24–1). Nursing home associations in some states have resorted to litigation against the state's Medicaid agency, an action permitted under the Boren amendment, to raise reimbursement rates to a level that at a minimum covers a resident's assessed care needs.

PATIENT CARE ASPECTS

Although nursing homes are part of the medical continuum of care, they should not be considered hospitals for the chronically ill. Rather, they should be considered places where people live and where health care and many other services are provided. Many people fear nursing home placement and regard it as a life sentence of mental and physical imprisonment. Too often, nursing home residents are deprived of their rights because institutional regimentation and routines take priority over personal choices and preferences. To protect residents, the federal Nursing Home Requirements for Participation in Medicare or Medicaid give equal weight to residents' rights, quality of life, and quality of care.

Because the typical nursing home resident has complex problems, OBRA 87 emphasizes comprehensive assessment by a **multidisciplinary team.** Whether the team consists solely of such core members as the physician, nurse, and social worker or also includes a nutritionist, pharmacist, physical and occupational therapists, and others, each member has a responsibility to ensure that four activities are carried out. (1) The resident is thoroughly assessed; (2) a comprehensive care plan is developed; (3) the care plan is implemented; and (4) the success of the care plan is evaluated, and appropriate modifications are made.

Medical Services

Physicians providing care to nursing home residents assume a complex responsibility that requires time, energy, and commitment if it is to succeed. They must assess and advocate appropriate interventions. Assessing the need for rehabilitative therapy is especially important but not well understood by most physicians and, therefore, is almost routinely delegated to therapists (see Ch. 29).

Physicians must see patients as often as medically necessary but not less than every 60 days. Regulations require that certain patients, such as those with dementia and delirium, undergo further evaluation using standardized Resident Assessment Protocols. These guidelines were established by the Health Care Financing Administration (HCFA) to help identify the causes of common problems and ensure that interventions are specific and appropriate. Visits, even if routine, should not be perfunctory; patients should be examined, medication status assessed, and laboratory tests ordered as needed. Findings should be documented in the patient's chart to keep other staff members informed about any problems. If possible, the physician who cares for the resident in the nursing home should also treat the person's acute illness if hospitalization becomes necessary.

Caring for a nursing home patient often involves considerable interaction with the family. Rapport can be established at the outset if the patient and family are made to feel that someone in authority is listening and trying to address their concerns. Physicians can alleviate fears of abandonment by engaging in positive discussions of what can be done, even if it is only palliative, rather than stressing the withholding or stopping of treatment (which relatives may perceive as subtle instances of abuse and neglect—see Ethical Considerations, below). An interdisciplinary team can more easily address problems and advocate good geriatric care, particularly if residents and families are included in the decision-making process. Organized family meetings, in which the physician, social worker, and nurse participate, can be particularly helpful.

Two trends may help solve some of the problems identified in medical care in nursing homes. One is that some physicians are limiting their practice to long-term care facilities. If physicians spend enough time in the nursing home to participate in team activities and be readily available for consultation with other staff members when clinical changes in patients presage the onset of serious illness, the quality of care may improve markedly over that given in hurried bimonthly visits. The appeal to physicians of practicing full time in long-term care facilities is enhanced when physicians can combine the practice with teaching medical students and house staff and when they can monitor their patients' hospital care should they wish to. Such activities can help the nursing home physician remain current with patient care practices and maintain interest in caring for the chronically ill.

The second trend is that many nursing homes are hiring nurse practitioners or physician assistants, who likewise improve care by seeing patients when needed, alerting the physician to serious problems, reviewing old medical records, interviewing families, and performing other important tasks. However, not all tasks can be delegated, and federal requirements continue to mandate periodic physician visits and close involvement in patient care.

Similarly, medical students and house staff can provide valuable services in long-term care facilities while learning skills not taught elsewhere (eg, how to conduct a functional assessment, use a cognitive-screening instrument, and care for the chronically ill). This exposure also makes them aware that not all nursing home residents are obtunded, dehydrated, and febrile, a misconception often held when the only contact with such patients is in a hospital emergency department.

In 1974 the position of **medical director** was required as part of the federal conditions for participation in Medicare. With OBRA 87, the medical director's responsibilities for coordinating the medical care in the facility and for implementing resident care policies were specified.

The medical director's role varies with the type of nursing home and the degree of authority granted by the administrator. Nine tasks and functions help define the medical director's role: (1) participate in administrative decision making, (2) assist in the development of educational programs, (3) organize and supervise medical services, (4) participate in quality assurance programs, (5) serve as a spokesman for the nursing home's mission to the community, (6) assist in establishing employees' health programs, (7) maintain knowledge of regulatory, social, political, and economic factors affecting patient care services, (8) provide leadership for research and development, and (9) participate in developing the policies and procedures that ensure the rights of residents and staff.

Hospitalization of Nursing Home Residents

The issue of when to transfer nursing home residents to a hospital requires several considerations. In some nursing homes, physicians, nurse practitioners, or physician assistants are present for several hours every day, and a highly skilled nursing staff is available to manage IV lines, suctioning equipment, and sometimes ventilators. In other nursing homes, physician visits are sporadic, and few experienced nurses are on staff; therefore, a patient may need to be transferred to a hospital for technical or highly skilled care.

Nursing home staff often try to avoid hospitalizing patients, because all too often patients return from a hospitalization with urinary catheters and pressure sores. Patients are often confused, severely deconditioned, and receiving psychoactive medications. Many families and residents also prefer to avoid hospitalization not only for these reasons but because treatment in hospitals can be dehumanizing and impersonal.

When transfer to a hospital does occur, medical records should accompany the patient. A phone call from a nursing home nurse to a hospital nurse is useful to explain the patient's diagnosis and reason for transfer, the patient's baseline functional and mental status, the patient's medications, and care directives as expressed in a living will.

Ethical Considerations

Because many nursing home residents are cognitively impaired, they are rarely consulted about their preferences for daily routines, diagnostic tests, or treatments. Decision-making capacity is usually assumed to be lacking, and even when choices are expressed, they may be overridden by staff or family. In many institutions, sensitive or empathetic discussions about advance medical directives rarely take place. As a result, the resident's fears and concerns about illness and dying are not addressed, and his wishes about resuscitation, hospitalization, and aggressive treatment are not established. Informed consent, the process by which patient and family members are fully informed of the potential risks and benefits of testing and treatment options, may be similarly neglected.

Medications may be given surreptitiously when patients refuse them. In fact, mixing medications in food to hide them is a fairly common practice, with both psychoactive drugs and essential cardiac and pulmonary medications, and should be discouraged. Except in emergencies, such abuse of residents' rights is proscribed. Regulations prohibiting this practice are enforced in mental health facilities but usually not in nursing homes.

Other forms of abuse, neglect, and mistreatment are also of concern. The typical resident is physically and cognitively vulnerable and can be easily abused. Residents are unable to leave the facility, they may have infrequent visitors, and their complaints, when voiced, are often not believed. Despite federal regulations that attempt to safeguard residents, better protection is needed.

How much physical and psychologic abuse exists is unknown. Subtle types of abuse—eg, using drugs and physical restraints (disingenuously labeled "safety devices") to manage disruptive behavior—are difficult to monitor. Evidence of pinching, slapping, or yanking may be hard to prove, because ecchymosis and skin tears occur easily in the elderly, even without abuse.

While some residents manage to protect their own rights, often family members serve as an advocate. However, not all residents have families who are concerned enough to participate in their care, and residents and family members may fear reprisals. Although a public advocacy system exists and nursing homes can be cited by regulatory agencies, instances of abuse and mistreatment rarely come to the attention of authorities. In addition, residents or families who insist on transfer to another institution may have difficulty finding one that will accept a patient and family labeled as "troublemakers."

QUALITY-OF-CARE ASSESSMENT

Methods for evaluating quality of care in nursing homes are under scrutiny. The 10th Federal Circuit Court of Appeals ruled in Smith vs. Heckler that the government is responsible for ensuring that a facility is actually *providing* good care, not merely *capable* of doing so. Thus, outcome measures have replaced many of the more structural aspects of quality assessment.

Through the Health Care Financing Administration, the federal government requires states to maintain surveillance agencies. These agencies inspect nursing homes to make sure they are complying with state regulations and adhering to specific requirements for participation in Medicare and Medicaid programs. The inspection report for a particular facility, including any deficiencies cited, must be provided to the nursing home's attending physicians and may be useful to families or physicians when selecting a nursing home. However, no report can substitute for a personal visit when choosing a nursing home.

Through actual observations of care, interview of residents and staff, and review of the clinical records, surveyors attempt to assess a facility's performance. Physical findings or events that are objective and easily measured (such as falls, contractures, use of nasogastric feeding tubes, development of urinary tract infections or pressure sores) help indicate the quality of care, particularly nursing care. However, quality-of-life factors are difficult to assess. If a surveyor observes that residents' rights are being violated, examples of the violations can be submitted along with evidence of poor care. A statement of deficiencies can show that the facility has systemic problems.

In the past, nursing homes were divided conceptually into those offering skilled services for "sicker" people who required more care from licensed nurses or rehabilitative services and those offering custodial services (a euphemism for warehousing) for the vast majority of demented, disabled nursing home residents. Today, facilities that receive any federal funding, whether Medicare or Medicaid, must be able to provide all services to its residents if and when they need them (see TABLE 24–1). Nursing home operators and staff are beginning to realize that they must take a new approach to caring for demented, frail, or debilitated residents if they wish to preserve the residents' independence and function. Maintenance and rehabilitation must be pursued with equal vigor. Practitioners can demand that their nursing home patients receive all the services necessary to attain and maintain the highest level of functioning, although coverage of these services by Medicaid varies by state.

The level of services can also vary considerably. Some nursing homes provide IV therapies, enteral nutrition through gastrostomy or jejunostomy tubes, hyperalimentation, and chronic oxygen treatment or ventilator support; others do not. Some homes have a full-time activities staff; in others, activities are minimal. Activity programs of high quality often include scheduled group events as well as leisure time and self-selected diversional choices for residents, especially those who are cognitively impaired or bedridden. Some homes provide personal services such as hairdressing and makeup, which are psychologically important to some residents but are usually paid for by residents' personal funds (out-of-pocket expenses).

Some homes have programs for persons with special needs. For example, a special unit for patients with dementia may provide a supportive physical environment where trained staff and creative programming diminish the use of physical and pharmacologic restraints and focus on preserving the patient's residual skills. Some facilities specialize in providing intensive rehabilitation for patients with hip fractures or head injuries. In fact, many homes segregate patients who need acute rehabilitation and skilled services after hospitalization (usually those patients with Medicare coverage) from patients whose needs may be similar although theoretically of lesser intensity (usually those with Medicaid coverage). Medicaid units often have fewer staff members and may not provide any rehabilitative services. However, a federally certified nursing home must provide care to meet a resident's assessed needs, whether the resident's care is covered by Medicare, Medicaid, or private payment. Some nursing homes are not federally certified and are licensed only by the state. Unless state regulations are comprehensive and well enforced, the lack of federal certification may indicate poor quality of care.

Social services vary as well. Usually, social workers provide minimal assistance to patients and families; however, in better facilities they help alleviate transfer trauma, identify social withdrawal and isolation, and actively assist in maintaining the residents' psychosocial well-being. Good social workers also help ensure that families are given timely information and assistance when applying for Medicare or Medicaid coverage, planning appropriate discharge, or learning about other services.

Although some states set minimum nurse:resident ratios, staffing ratios vary considerably. In homes that have only a minimal staff, the staff rarely has time to adequately care for sicker or needier patients, particularly those with dementia; such situations place unrealistic burdens on the nursing staff. Social workers, nurses, and physicians, as well as patients and their families, should be aware that some residents require more nursing care and should demand appropriate staffing levels on all shifts in all parts of the facility. If health care professionals refuse to accept substandard care for their patients, then perhaps nursing homes can shed their generally unsavory reputation.

BOARD–AND–CARE FACILITIES

Known variously as adult care homes, domiciliaries, or rest homes, board-and-care facilities offer an alternative for elderly persons who can no longer live independently but who function well enough to not need the constant supervision provided in nursing homes. These facilities typically provide shelter, meals, minimal assistance with personal care, and sometimes supervision of medication administration.

While many elderly persons are able to pay their own expenses in board-and-care facilities, a large number are funded through the federal Supplemental Security Income (SSI) program at a cost of more than $8 billion annually. More than 70,000 board-and-care homes in the USA provide services to more than one million frail, disabled people. The number of homes is increasing, sometimes at the instigation of the state, since they offer an economic, federally funded means of accommodating the rising number of elderly persons who would otherwise require nursing home care paid for with state Medicaid funds.

Minimally regulated and sometimes unlicensed, the facilities serve a dual population, about 50% elderly and about 50% deinstitutionalized mentally ill, often mixed or cared for together. While some excellent homes exist, many facilities tend to warehouse the disabled in substandard buildings with few skilled staff members. Investigation by the House of Representatives Subcommittee on Health and Long-Term Care has uncovered widespread misuse of medications in adult care homes.

Physicians who have patients in board-and-care facilities should make every effort to ensure that they are safe and are receiving appropriate care. This may necessitate making a personal visit or sending a nurse or social worker to ascertain that the facility complies with fire and safety regulations, keeps and stores proper medication records, and attends to health care needs.

ASSISTED–LIVING PROGRAMS

Concern over the lack of services and quality of care in the existing board-and-care system has led to a new movement to provide housing with health care. While assisted living (or supportive housing, enriched housing, congregative care) has not yet been precisely defined, it attempts to steer long-term care away from the almost exclusively medically oriented direction traditionally taken by nursing homes. One such program developed in Oregon, a leader in exploring alternatives to nursing homes, is modeled on facilities in Denmark and Sweden.

Assisted-living programs appear to be more cost-effective than nursing homes. Residents maintain their independence in a more humane, personalized setting where housekeeping services, meals, social support, and supervision of personal care (assistance with activities of daily living) and medication administration are available as needed. In some states (eg, New York), assisted-living programs are carried out in existing board-and-care facilities with supplemental care provided by a home health agency, since the cost of supplying services to a group of residents in one location is lower than that of serving individuals scattered throughout the community.

Many variations of these programs are being tried and are attracting the attention of some large corporations, who view them as potentially lucrative. The nursing home industry, which stands to lose in this trend toward deinstitutionalization, has not been enthusiastic about assisted-living programs and has sought, at least in one state (Florida), to block their development.

Health care practitioners should keep informed about these programs as they become established so they can help their patients select one that is well run and safe and that offers high-quality services.

LIFE–CARE COMMUNITIES

During the 1970s and 1980s, life-care or continuing care retirement communities grew in number to meet the needs of older people who wanted to remain active in their communities and involved with other elderly people. Those who choose to live in life-care communities also want to ensure that their assets will provide supportive services when and as those services become necessary.

The American Association of Homes for the Aging defines a continuing care retirement community as an organization that offers a contract intended to remain in effect for the resident's lifetime. At a minimum, this contract guarantees shelter and access to various health care services; however, it may include much more. An entrance fee, paid when moving to the community, and monthly payments thereafter are typically required to purchase a continuing care contract.

Continuing care retirement communities are found all across the country. Unfortunately, in some communities, because of unscrupulous real estate dealers or well-intentioned but inept management, the assets of the residents have been wiped out. If well financed and managed, these communities provide a broad range of housing, social, supportive, and health services that enable their residents to live comfortably.

Three types of continuing care retirement communities are generally recognized: those covered by an all-inclusive contract, those covered by a modified contract that limits the amount of long-term care that will be provided before the monthly fee is increased, and those covered by a fee-for-service contract that bills for health services as they are used.

Communities may be housed in a single building, or they may be spread out across multi-acre campuses that provide a variety of housing options (ranging from efficiency apartments to cottages with several rooms). Many have community buildings where organized social events take place, dining rooms, sports facilities, clubs, planned outings, and vacation options. In addition to residential and recreational programs, continuing care retirement communities usually offer a variety of home care, adult homes, day programs, and nursing homes. Access to physicians is usually provided, and most programs are affiliated with local acute care facilities.

25. HOME HEALTH CARE

The home care industry represents several aspects of care delivered to persons in their own homes. The largest component of the industry is home health care, usually defined as the Medicare-certified component of home care; it includes home health agencies that provide nursing, skilled care, attendant care, and hospice services; medical equipment companies; and infusion service companies. Nonmedical components of the industry include those that provide such services as emergency alarm device monitoring and security surveillance, non–Medicare-covered home attendant care, homemaker services, and Meals-on-Wheels. Patients may need several services, or their needs may change from one type of service to another.

Home care is a desirable option for older people who wish to remain in their own homes but, because of frailty or disability, require some form of health services, either temporary or ongoing, to do so. Home health care received its biggest boost in 1965 with the advent of Medicare and Medicaid, which fund many home care services. Although Medicare covers only intermittent and short-term services, it provides about 60% of home health care agency revenue. Medicaid and private insurance (including HMOs) provide 11% and 15%, respectively, and private payments account for the remaining 14% of home health care revenue.

Several factors contribute to the growth and desirability of home health care programs: (1) Given the increase in life expectancy and the burdens of chronic illness, many more older people need health care services. (2) Most people *prefer* to be cared for at home, especially if this is an alternative to or delays the need for nursing home care. (3) Technologic advances make treatments possible in the home that were once available only in hospitals (eg, IV therapy, dialysis, parenteral and enteral nutrition, and ventilator support). In addition, mobile laboratories can provide such services as x-rays, ECGs, and blood testing, further diminishing the need for institutional care. (4) Changes in government and private reimbursement methods for medical care, particularly those based on diagnosis related groups (DRGs), are aimed at shortening hospital stays and place a greater demand on services for recovery and rehabilitation. (5) In general, home care may be no more expensive than institutional care if home health aide hours and skilled service visits are kept to a minimum.

As of 1991, home health care agencies in the USA numbered about 9300. Some of them are proprietary (for profit), others are voluntary (not for profit); some are privately sponsored, others are publicly (government) sponsored; some are freestanding (community based), others are associated with a hospital or nursing home. About 25% of the nation's home health care agencies are affiliated with larger organizations (chains).

Home care agencies can be as simple or complex as any other health care organization. Most agencies have an administrator or director who is responsible for the business and managerial aspects of the agency. Often this person is a doctor, nurse, or social worker who has moved to an administrative position. The director of patient services is responsible for the recruitment, scheduling, performance, and supervision of the caregiver staff. In small agencies, the administrator may also serve as the director of patient services; in large agencies, the administrative infrastructure may include a medical director, in-service educators and trainers, quality assurance–utilization review coordinators, invoice processors, and data systems analysts.

Some home care providers have both professional staff (eg, nurses, therapists, social workers) and nonprofessional staff (eg, home health aides or home attendants). Both types of workers spend most of their time in patients' homes, where their visits range from < 1 h to 24 h/day, depending on patient needs.

Persons needing home care are often referred for services after hospitalization, although prior hospitalization is not a requirement. Typically, a social worker, nurse, discharge planner, case manager, or physician decides that home care services will speed discharge, facilitate recuperation, or prevent nursing home admission or hospitalization. Evaluation for home care should be comprehensive, encompassing an assessment of functional ability, mental status, psychosocial needs, nutritional status, and medication use and compliance (see also ASSESSING THE NEED FOR INSTITUTIONALIZATION in Ch. 24). In addition, the patient's home environment and community resources must be considered.

The home health agency develops a preliminary care plan from information provided by hospital staff or obtained during a visit with the patient. This plan and orders for care are then given to the physician for signature. Without a physician's signed order, the agency cannot provide services. The agency reports to the physician at least every 62 days, at which time orders must be rewritten. Physicians who do not get involved in home care deprive their patients of educational services, close medical monitoring, early warning signs of changes in medical status, and the benefit of medical therapies provided in the home.

Most home health agencies arrange for vendors to deliver supplies or durable medical equipment (eg, commodes, wheelchairs, walkers) to the patient's home. Medications are usually purchased through pharmacies. Companies specializing in devices and solutions for enteral and parenteral nutrition, IV solutions and equipment, ventilators, or other high-technology devices may serve as a vendor to an agency or as an independent home care service. Third-party payers are usually billed directly by vendors, although other arrangements do exist.

THE PHYSICIAN'S ROLE

Medicare legislation for home health care is based on the premise that the physician acts as the gatekeeper, ordering services when appropriate and referring patients to programs of more intensive care when reasonable and necessary. Physician orders are required for all services except attendant care. To guard against fraud and abuse, physicians are precluded from referring patients to or writing orders for any home health program in which they have a financial interest of more than 5%.

Reimbursement for physician services in home care has long been considered inadequate and has recently undergone revision, although reimbursement rates remain low. In an effort to encourage home care, policy makers have adopted a Medicare Fee Schedule with a new billing code system using Current Procedural Terminology (CPT). The system includes six codes for home services, allowing flexibility in billing. However, no mechanism as yet exists by which a physician can be reimbursed for such tasks as supervising visiting nurse services, reviewing care plans and writing orders, taking telephone calls from patients or family, or coordinating care, unless a home visit is made. Most physicians continue to sign orders for home care services, although they tend to be minimally involved with agency staff because of the financial disincentives to active participation in the home care plan. However, the agency's skilled on-site clinicians can act as the physician's eyes and ears by monitoring the patient's medical condition.

TABLE 25–1. MEDICARE REQUIREMENTS FOR HOME HEALTH CARE BENEFITS

Beneficiary requirements	Must be homebound Must need one or more of the following qualifying services: Skilled nursing care Physical therapy Speech therapy
Service requirements	Must be reasonable and necessary Must be offered in the patient's residence Must be ordered by the physician Must be provided on an intermittent basis

TYPES OF HOME HEALTH CARE PROGRAMS

Whatever their organization or affiliation, home health care agencies can be classified into three major types of programs: certified home health agency, long-term home health care, and hospice care.

CERTIFIED HOME HEALTH AGENCY

The Certified Home Health Agency (CHHA), reflecting the influence of Medicare, provides skilled services under the direction of licensed physicians. To be certified, an agency must meet state licensing requirements as well as federal conditions for participation in the Medicare program. Agencies so designated may then be reimbursed by Medicare, Medicaid, or private third-party insurers.

Several requirements must be met for patients to be considered eligible for home health care benefits under Medicare (see TABLE 25–1). One is that the patient must be **homebound**—to leave home would require considerable effort or put the patient's health at risk. However, periodic visits to a physician's office or clinic are expected. Another requirement is that the patient need **skilled care** from at least one qualifying service: nursing, physical therapy, or speech therapy (see TABLE 25–2). Occupational therapy can be given only if another qualifying service is also needed, but once begun, occupational therapy can be continued even if it remains the sole service. Once a patient qualifies for Medicare-covered home care benefits, he is also eligible for ancillary services (see TABLE 25–3).

Although nursing assistants are an important element of home health care programs, their services are being increasingly limited by third-party payers to control costs. For example, the use of nursing assistants

TABLE 25–2. PARTIAL LIST OF SKILLED–CARE SERVICES

Nursing	Teaching: Teach patient how to use medications, select a proper diet, use prosthetic or other devices, follow safe practices and prevent accidents, control bowel and bladder, modify behavior Assessment: Perform physical examination; assess environment, functional support systems, health knowledge, nutritional status Monitoring: Monitor patient's self-care, wound status, fluid status, medication use and side effects, coping ability Case management: Arrange for referrals, order supplies and equipment, make appointments, obtain transportation, confer with and coordinate services of other care providers, supervise nursing assistants Treatment: Provide chronic wound care; parenteral feeding; tracheostomy, ostomy, and catheter care; range-of-motion exercises; pain management; venipuncture; IV drug administration; injections; fecal disimpaction
Physical therapy	Evaluation and functional assessment, including customizing a wheelchair Exercises: Passive, active, resistive, therapeutic, stretching Training: Gait, prosthetic device, transfers Therapy: Chest physical therapy, ultrasound, hot or cold pack application, whirlpool
Occupational therapy	Evaluation and assessment: Activities of daily living (ADLs) Training: Adaptive devices, ADLs Teaching: Retrain muscles, adapt therapy or disability to home environment, make splints and braces
Speech therapy	Evaluation and assessment: Speech, language, hearing, swallowing disorders Training: Alaryngeal speech, language processing, speech and voice use, aural rehabilitation
Medical social work	Assessment: Social support, emotional factors Counseling Assistance: Placement (eg, in day-care, social programs), housing, financial services

TABLE 25–3. ANCILLARY SERVICES*

Occupational therapy
Medical social services
Home health aide services
Medical intern or resident services†
Medical supplies
Durable medical equipment
Prosthetic devices

* Available to patient when general Medicare eligibility criteria are met, and need for one or more of the qualifying services is determined.

† Home health agencies affiliated with an approved medical training program can bill for the services of interns or residents making home visits, or physicians must bill Medicare using a CPT code.

primarily to watch a demented patient while family members are at work can be very expensive. The number of hours of reimbursable nursing assistant services is usually < 2 h/day, 5 days/wk, but the actual number of visit-hours is usually less. Patients typically stay in CHHA programs for several weeks to months and are often discharged abruptly when reimbursement benefits cease.

LONG–TERM HOME HEALTH CARE

Long-term home health care programs, paid for either by Medicaid or privately by the patient or family (or in some states funded by Medicaid under a 2176 waiver program), may differ substantially from the CHHA model. Eligibility criteria and services vary by state; information on available programs can usually be obtained from either the state office or agency for the aging, the department of social service, or the health department.

A prototype for such programs is New York's Nursing Home Without Walls, a capitated long-term home care program. Designed primarily for patients who might otherwise require institutionalization, this program provides home health aides, case management, and limited skilled services in the home. Patients receive services as long as they meet state criteria for nursing home placement and the cost does not exceed a percentage of what would be paid for comparable care in a nursing home. Attaining a therapeutic goal or continuing to need skilled services is not required as it is for Medicare patients in a CHHA program.

Although long-term home health care programs are widely accepted by patients and families, they have not proved effective in forestalling institutionalization. Accordingly, many policy makers consider the programs supplementary rather than substitutive and are eager to restrict their growth. However, because these programs are capitated, costs can be limited to an agreed-upon maximum level.

HOSPICE CARE

Hospice services are offered by more than 22% of home health agencies to care for terminally ill patients and provide support to their families. Initially philanthropic, they are now covered by Medicare, and some states (eg, Florida, Kentucky, Michigan, and New York) include them under Medicaid.

While most hospice programs are home based, and Medicare and Medicaid regulations stipulate that at least 80% of the agency's care be provided to patients in their homes, states are now required to offer hospice services to nursing home residents. To receive reimbursement for hospice care, patients must be eligible for Medicaid or Medicare. In addition, a physician must certify at the beginning of each certification period that the illness is terminal and that the patient has less than 6 mo to live if the disease runs its normal course (although physicians no longer have to guarantee life span). Patients who elect the Medicare hospice benefit must indicate their willingness to waive Medicare benefits for services outside the hospice program for conditions related to their terminal illness. The eligibility to receive care for other intercurrent problems is not affected (eg, a hospice patient with lung cancer can be treated for injuries sustained in an automobile accident).

The hospice employs multidisciplinary teams consisting of a physician, a registered nurse, a social worker, and a counselor. This is the only home health care program in which Medicare specifies that a physician must be a salaried member of the team. **Core services** that must be provided in a federally funded hospice program are nursing, medical, and social services and bereavement counseling. **Additional services** include physical and occupational therapy, home health aide services, medical supplies, general counseling, and short inpatient stays.

The reimbursement formula has both prospective and retrospective features; although a cap is specified ($11,600 in 1992), intensity of services can fluctuate depending on the patient's needs. Physicians are often unsure of their ability to predict remaining life expectancy, and hospices continue to be unwilling to accept the financial risk of having patients outlive benefits, since the programs may not discharge patients. Therefore, the average length of hospice care is still only about 6 wk, often too short a time to help the patient and family prepare for death by improving the physical, mental, and spiritual quality of the remaining life, which is the aim of hospice programs.

A patient's own physician need not relinquish primary medical responsibility to the hospice physician. However, many primary care physicians have neither the expertise in pain management and symptom control nor the accessibility to other team members for home visits and problem solving; therefore, they often willingly turn over the case. (See also Chs. 19 and 110.)

OTHER NONINSTITUTIONAL SERVICES

Many community-based elderly persons benefit from other types of services, such as the outpatient programs offered at adult day-care centers. Spouses or relatives providing care to a homebound person may find respite care programs helpful.

CONGREGATE OUTPATIENT SERVICES

(See also Ch. 110)

Congregate services are referred to as adult day care, adult day health care, day hospital, aftercare, and medical day-care programs, as well as by other names. Regardless of the term, all of these outpatient programs tend to share certain features. Therefore, in this discussion, the generic term **day care** is used.

Although recognized as a necessary and cost-effective component of the long-term care system, day-care programs are still relatively uncommon, with only about 2000 programs in the USA compared with more than 16,000 nursing homes. The National Institute on Adult Day Care expends much time and effort getting practitioners and policy leaders to recognize the importance of day care and is a resource for information about programs.

Most day-care programs tend to be small, averaging 20 clients. Persons with medical, physical, or cognitive disabilities or those who need socialization are brought to a center for several hours a day, several days a week, for group activities designed to delay institutionalization and improve well-being.

Medicare does not cover the costs associated with travel to and from day-care centers. Unless a patient is entitled to Medicaid benefits, which cover transportation costs in some states, or is able to pay privately for travel costs, a program may be inaccessible. Some centers use donated funds to subsidize transportation and match financial means with a sliding-fee scale to accommodate patients.

While programs vary, they usually conform to one of three models (see TABLE 25–4). The **day hospital model** emphasizes rehabilitation or intensive medical-nursing care, along with recreational and social activities to improve functional independence or recuperation. It is designed for persons recovering from acute events such as stroke, amputation, or

TABLE 25–4. MODELS OF CONGREGATE OUTPATIENT PROGRAMS

	Restorative or Rehabilitative Model (Day Hospital)	*Maintenance or General Model*	*Psychosocial or Mental Health Model*
Duration of program	Time limited	Long term	May be time limited
Target population	Patients with major disabilities or serious illnesses (strokes, fractures, etc)	Frail, chronically ill, or disabled elderly	Patients with fewer physical disabilities, cognitive impairment, affective disorders, social impairment
Services	Core services* plus: Rehabilitation (physical therapy, occupational therapy, speech therapy) Nursing Medical social work	Core services plus: Screening or monitoring chronic illnesses Social, recreational, educational activities (health promotion, disease prevention) Physical exercises	Core services plus: Counseling Group therapy Cognitive retraining
Goals	Rehabilitate Restore function Improve clinical status	Delay or prevent institutionalization Improve self-image Prevent loneliness, isolation, and withdrawal Eliminate monotony of daily existence Prevent exacerbation of chronic disease	Improve mental health Manage medication Modify behavior Encourage self-expression Develop coping techniques

* Transportation, nutrition, activity programs.

fractures. These programs are usually time-limited, ranging from 6 wk to 6 mo. The ratio of professional staff to patients is high, making the programs costly.

The **maintenance model** of day care combines social and recreational services with limited skilled services often aimed at preventing deterioration. The program is designed to help patients maintain or enhance an existing level of functioning for as long as possible. Because the ratio of professional staff to patients is lower, this type of program is less costly to operate. Although benefits are realized with prolonged involvement, demand often exceeds available resources, limiting the duration of care that can be provided. In addition, because of transportation difficulties and lack of third-party payment, access to the programs may be quite limited.

The **social model** may resemble either a typical senior citizens' center, providing care to ambulatory persons with varied psychosocial needs, or a mental health center, providing care to older persons with dementing or mental illnesses. Care may be ongoing or limited in duration. In almost all cases, patients must be ambulatory or able to enter and get around in a wheelchair, must be continent, and must not be socially disruptive within the controlled environment of the center. Unfortunately, these criteria may discriminate against some of those with dementia, who might benefit a great deal from participation and whose caregivers would get a few hours of respite.

Some day-care centers specialize in serving those with dementia. Services include family support activities; recreational activities designed to maintain stability and orientation; and attempts to modify disruptive behavior by providing positive, consistent reinforcement for efforts at self-control and socially appropriate behavior. Although these services cannot halt the inexorable progression of dementia, quality-of-life–enhancing improvements in functional capacity, even if temporary, and relief of caregiver burden are often accomplished.

Formulating discharge criteria is one of the most difficult issues faced by time-limited day-care programs, which are usually those with a rehabilitation orientation. Once a patient has reached his maximum potential, discharge is required. Patients may come to depend on the support provided by the program and resist discharge, or they may become depressed, feeling that their condition will regress or that they could improve if allowed to remain in the program. Therefore, **discharge planning** needs to begin even before admission, with the potential for ultimate discharge a part of enrollment criteria. The staff, as a team, needs to define goals and track progress. Unfortunately, follow-up programs usually do not exist to ease the transition.

Because many patients require some formal support after leaving a day-care program, assessing posttreatment needs is important. Discussing needs with patients and families to identify community resources helps to ensure continuity of care and prevent families from feeling abandoned. Gradually decreasing the number of days per week spent at the day-care center, periodically evaluating patient readiness for discharge, and emphasizing that discharge represents an achievement and a sign of readiness for independence, not punishment, may help alleviate some of the anxiety patients experience when leaving a program.

RESPITE CARE

Some 60% to 80% of the care for disabled elderly persons living in their own homes is provided by a spouse, child, other family member, or friend. Many caregivers find the constant responsibility of caring for someone who is physically or cognitively dependent on them to be physically, emotionally, and financially draining. Respite care is often sought by caregivers to relieve the strain of caregiving or because of personal illness.

Respite care is a generic term applied to the temporary supportive care of an elder by a substitute caregiver. The elder normally lives in the community with a caregiver, and respite care serves to maintain and strengthen the regular caregiver's well-being and ability to sustain care at home. Individual programs may be more specifically defined and may be further restricted by law (eg, respite care may be limited to 28 days in a calendar year).

Respite care assists the patient indirectly by assisting the usual caregiver directly. Just because day care or other long-term care programs provide a measure of relief to the caregiver does not make them respite care programs.

Over half the states have some sort of respite care program. Several states (eg, Florida, Texas, Wisconsin, South Carolina, Delaware, and New York) have legislated programs. Medicaid supports slightly less than half the programs, various grants support another quarter of the programs, and private funds pay for the rest.

Programs can be divided into four major types: (1) in-home programs provided by special respite agencies or by home care agencies with a respite program; (2) community programs provided by adult day-care providers, respite care cooperatives, or freestanding respite facilities; (3) programs offered by long-term care institutions such as board-and-care facilities or nursing homes that accept people for limited stays; and (4) hospital programs that take people into hospital beds.

Respite services need to be carefully planned. A home visit should be made to interview the elderly person and the caregiver and to learn about the patient's home environment and routines. A medical and psychosocial assessment should be undertaken to ascertain if the person has any special requirements. In case of medical or other emergencies, a detailed emergency plan should be worked out with the caregiver. A discharge plan can address continued support services for the returning caregiver.

Several states have respite associations, and organizations such as the Alzheimer's Association or Area Agencies on Aging can act as a referral source for practitioners trying to assist patients and families. A respite report is available from the Bowman Gray School of Medicine in Winston-Salem, North Carolina.

26. HOSPITALIZATION

Almost half of all adult hospital beds are filled by patients > 65 yr, and often hospitalization for these patients is followed by an irreversible decline in functional status and changes in lifestyle and quality of life. About 75% of those ≥ 75 yr who are functionally independent when admitted from their homes are not functionally independent when discharged; 15% are discharged to nursing homes.

In many cases, the decline cannot be attributed to the problem that led to hospitalization. Even when an acute disease, such as pneumonia, is cured in a few days or a hip fracture repair is technically perfect and uncomplicated, the patient may never return to prehospitalization functional status. In one large group of patients who had hip fracture repairs, only 20% returned to their preoperative functional level.

A high percentage of hospitalized elders discharged to nursing homes never return to their homes or community. About 55% of patients > 65 yr who enter nursing homes remain for more than a year. Many others are discharged to hospitals or other long-term care facilities, or they die. Even when the nursing home stay is supposed to be short (eg, until the patient is rehabilitated or until arrangements can be made for home care), circumstances frequently dictate otherwise. The family may discover the advantages of institutionalization. Home caregivers may not be available. The rent on the patient's apartment may have lapsed. The patient's need to spend down financially to obtain nursing home care may have left insufficient funds for getting started again. Or the patient may not recover sufficiently to return home.

Some of the decline in hospitalized elders can be attributed to iatrogenic complications and nosocomial infections. Adverse drug reactions occur at rates as high as 36% in hospitalized patients, and most of these problems occur in older persons. In some cases, the cause may be age-associated changes in pharmacokinetics, but more important is the number of prescription drugs commonly given to elderly patients: 6 to 12 different drugs during a single hospitalization is not unusual. Many medications have the potential to contribute to the adverse effects of hospitalization described below. Nosocomial infections also occur more commonly in older patients. Part of the increased risk can be attributed to longer hospital stays, more serious illnesses, and the interventions commonly used for the elderly. Urinary tract infection, particularly after catheterization, is the most common nosocomial infection. Pneumonia, soft tissue infection, and *Clostridium difficile* colitis are also common.

However, much of the functional decline in hospitalized elders is not related directly to iatrogenic complications or nosocomial infections. Instead, the decline results from the interaction between the effects of aging and the stresses of hospitalization.

EFFECTS OF AGING AND HOSPITALIZATION

Several factors associated with hospitalization and bed rest interact with changes of usual aging, decreasing the ability to function independently and initiating a cascade of events that often culminates in diminished quality of life. These changes of usual aging include decreased vasomotor stability; reduced muscle strength and aerobic capacity; decreased respiratory function; demineralization; impaired skin integrity; a tendency toward incontinence; decreased taste, smell, thirst, and dentition; and a tendency toward confusion (see TABLE 26–1).

Decreased Vasomotor Stability

With increasing age, autonomic function changes, and one of the most clinically important manifestations is baroreceptor insensitivity. This insensitivity combined with age-associated decreases in body water and plasma volume, which can be exacerbated by disease- or drug-associated dehydration, results in a tendency toward orthostatic hypotension that can lead to syncope. Bed rest in the supine position results in decreased plasma volume and peripheral vascular resistance, which further increase the risks of orthostatic hypotension and syncope. Sedative drugs and the intense hypotensive effects of some antihypertensive medications can further contribute to the possibility of syncope.

Syncope under any circumstances can result in injury. In the hospital, the possibility of injury is increased because patients often faint while getting out of a high hospital bed, sometimes while climbing over the bed rails. Patients also faint in the bathroom, where they often strike hard objects.

Reduced Muscle Strength and Aerobic Capacity

With aging, muscle mass, muscle strength, and aerobic capacity (maximum oxygen uptake, $\dot{V}O_2max$) decrease, leading to a progressive loss of reserve capacity for physical activity. Aerobic capacity decreases as the result of reduced peripheral oxygen use related to the diminished muscle mass and strength.

With complete inactivity, muscle strength decreases by 5% per day. Even young men on bed rest lose muscle strength at a rate of 1.0% to 1.5% per day (10% per week). Inactivity rapidly contributes to muscle shortening and changes in periarticular and cartilaginous joint structure, both of which contribute to limitation of motion and development of contractures. The most rapid changes take place in the legs. Bed rest also markedly diminishes aerobic capacity, causing substantial reductions in $\dot{V}O_2max$. Loss of muscle strength is also a major cause of falls in the elderly and may contribute to the inordinate number of falls that take place in the hospital.

TABLE 26–1. INTERACTION OF AGING WITH HOSPITALIZATION

Changes of Usual Aging	*Effects of Hospitalization*	*Potential Primary Effects*	*Potential Secondary Consequences*
Vasomotor instability (baroreceptor insensitivity and reduced total body water)	Reduced plasma volume, inaccessibility of fluids	Syncope, dizziness	Fall, fracture
Reduced muscle strength and aerobic capacity	Immobilization, high bed and rails	Deconditioning, fall	Dependency
Decreased ventilation	Increased closing volume	Reduced Pa_{O_2}	Syncope, delirium
Reduced bone density	Accelerated bone loss	Increased fracture risk	Fracture
Fragile skin	Immobilization, shearing forces	Pressure sore	Infection
Tendency toward urinary incontinence	Barriers, tethers (eg, IV lines, catheters)	Functional incontinence	Catheter, family rejection
Altered taste, smell, thirst, and dentition	Barriers, tethers (eg, IV lines, catheters), therapeutic diets	Dehydration, malnutrition	Reduced plasma volume, tube feeding
Tendency toward confusion	Isolation, lost glasses, lost hearing aid, additional sensory deprivation	Delirium	False labeling, physical restraint, chemical restraint

Modified from Creditor MC: "Hazards of hospitalization of the elderly." *Annals of Internal Medicine* 118(3):219–223, 1993; used with permission.

For an older person who has diminished physiologic reserves but still can perform daily activities, such as walking, toileting, and bathing, the accelerated losses of muscle strength and aerobic capacity after even a few days of bed rest may result in a prolonged loss of independent function. Even if the loss is reversible, rehabilitation requires extensive and expensive intervention because reconditioning takes longer than deconditioning.

Decreased Respiratory Function

The mechanics of respiration are also altered with aging (see Ch. 45). Costochondral calcification and reduced muscle strength, especially of the diaphragm, diminishes rib cage expansion; residual capacity and closing volume increase; and more dependent alveoli fail to ventilate as a result of airway closure. This combination reduces arterial oxygen tension (PaO_2), so that a value of 70 to 75 mm Hg is not uncommon in a 75-yr-old.

The supine position further reduces ventilation by increasing the closing volume enough to cause an additional fall in PaO_2, which may produce symptoms, such as confusion, somnolence, or dyspnea. This fall in PaO_2 may also contribute to syncope and predispose the patient to pneumonia.

Demineralization

In healthy young men on bed rest, vertebral bone loss accelerates to 50 times the involutional rate. The loss incurred from 10 days of bed rest takes 4 mo to restore. Some of the loss is caused by lack of weight bearing, but the general negative nitrogen balance associated with immobilization probably contributes. Many elderly persons, particularly thin white women, are osteoporotic on admission, and the hospital stay may accelerate the condition.

Impaired Skin Integrity

Age-associated skin changes include thinning of the epidermis and dermis, reduced vascularity, decreased epidermal turnover, and a loss of subcutaneous fat. Direct pressure on the skin greater than the capillary perfusion pressure of 32 mm Hg for as little as 2 h can result in skin necrosis. After short periods of immobilization, sacral pressures reach 70 mm Hg and pressure under the unsupported heel averages 45 mm Hg. Unusual shearing forces result from movement by patients sitting in wheelchairs or propped up in beds. Not surprisingly, pressure sores frequently develop in the hospitalized elder. The rate may be accelerated by incontinence and poor nutrition.

Urinary Incontinence

Many hospitalized patients have difficulty implementing their usual strategies for avoiding urinary incontinence. The environment is unfamiliar, and the path to the toilet may not be clear. Illness or injury may impair ambulation. The high bed may be intimidating, and bed rails may pose a barrier. Various pieces of equipment—such as IV lines, nasal oxygen lines, and catheters—act as restraints. Psychoactive agents may diminish the perception of a need to void, inhibit bladder function, and further impair ambulation. Anticholinergics, narcotics, and constipation may lead to overflow incontinence, and diuretics may precipitate urge incontinence.

More than 40% of hospitalized patients > 65 yr become incontinent, many within a day of being hospitalized. The functional incontinence that occurs in the hospital explains the discrepancy between incontinence rates in community-dwelling persons and newly hospitalized patients. Unfortunately, many health care personnel and families do not understand that continence is likely to be reestablished when the illness resolves and the patient returns home; thus, some patients are sent to nursing homes because of what would be reversible incontinence.

Decreased Taste, Smell, Thirst, and Dentition

Malnutrition and dehydration can develop rapidly in a hospitalized elder. Because thirst perception is diminished, dehydration may need to be severe before thirst drives a sick elder to reach for a glass of water. Dehydration, in turn, can lead to sedation, inanition, and confusion, further reducing the ability to eat and drink.

Anorexia is a common feature of many illnesses. Age-associated decreases in taste and smell make changes in dietary habits less tolerable, and under the best of circumstances, hospital food is unfamiliar; more often, it is unappetizing. Therapeutic diets, such as low-salt diets, are apt to make food even less appealing. Eating in bed with trays, utensils, and water out of easy reach is difficult, particularly when bed rails and restraints limit movement. Commonly, by the time someone arrives to help feed a patient, the food cools and is even less appetizing. If, as is so often the case, dentures have been left at home or misplaced, all the other problems are compounded by an inability to chew.

Confusion

Age and illness produce a tendency toward confusion that may be exacerbated by reduced visual and auditory input. The reduction in sensory input that occurs with immobilization can produce intellectual and perceptual disorders. Not surprisingly, an elderly person whose eyeglasses and hearing aid are left at home may become confused when placed in a hospital bed in a quiet room with subdued lighting. Besides the sensory deprivation, frequent awakenings in a strange bed, the effects of psychoactive drugs, and the stress of surgery or illness may affect the elderly patient's mental status and may lead to delirium.

PREVENTIVE STRATEGIES

The negative effects of hospitalization often begin immediately and progress rapidly. In theory, formal geriatric assessment of hospitalized elderly patients should help identify risk factors. Unfortunately, in practice, by the time consultation and intervention occur, the problems have evolved. Although the formal assessment is useful for long-term management and for evaluating the effects of intervention, the time it takes may actually delay care that could prevent decline.

The hospital environment should be designed to prevent significant functional decline among elderly patients. Physicians should exert as much influence as possible to ensure that necessary changes are made throughout the hospital because elderly patients use almost all services. Acute care geriatric units may provide safer environments than general hospital units.

Hospitalization

Geriatric patients should be kept active during hospitalization. There is little evidence of the therapeutic value of bed rest, so patients should be out of bed, unless activity is prohibited for a specific reason. Written orders should emphasize the need for activity except for specific purposes or designated periods of recumbency.

High beds are for the staff's convenience, not the patient's. Patients do not *fall* out of bed in the hospital any more than they *fall* out of bed at home. They are injured as they *climb* in and out of high beds. If the hospital does not provide the modified, less hazardous beds that are available, written orders should direct that the patient's bed be in the lowest position. In most circumstances, bed rails should be removed or kept down; bed rails produce injury much more often than they prevent injury.

Not every patient needs an IV line. Nor is nasal oxygen required as often as it is ordered. Oral fluid orders should be explicit, and when making rounds, the physician should check that the fluids are fresh and accessible. Family, friends, and staff should be urged to regularly offer something to drink. Having dentures available and using them may preclude the need for enteral or parenteral nutrition.

Family members should be encouraged to bring eyeglasses and hearing aids that have been left at home as well as daily newspapers, books, and magazines. Also, the family should bring a clock and wall calendar, if the hospital does not provide them. If possible, family members should join the patient at mealtimes, making sure the patient sits up in a chair while eating. Patients should be encouraged to dress in comfortable street clothes (a sweat suit, for example) in the morning and in pajamas at bedtime. If hospital regulations forbid this, physicians and families should lobby to change the restrictions.

Carpeting provides safe footing and is easy to maintain. Yet only a few hospitals have it, so patients should be reminded to be careful about their footing and to wear shoes or slippers.

Only essential medications should be ordered. Nonessential drugs, such as those for evening sedation, should be avoided. Many drugs, including antihistamines, may have adverse anticholinergic effects on bladder and bowel function, cognition, and blood pressure; therefore, they should be used only when essential. Environmental modification, such as moving the patient to a site that provides greater sensory stimulation, should be tried before ordering psychoactive drugs.

Most important, relationships among physicians, nurses, and other health professionals need to reflect the interdisciplinary care required by the elderly, even on acute care units. Mutual objectives require communication beyond the simple writing of an order by a physician and its execution by a nurse. Some hospitals have implemented primary care nursing or a variation of it, in which one nurse has around-the-clock responsibility for a particular patient, just as an attending physician does. In any case, physicians and nurses must work in partnership. Because few physicians and nurses make regular rounds together anymore, a physician caring for an older hospitalized patient must seek out the responsible nurse and discuss shared objectives for the patient.

All personnel assigned to units where elderly patients reside must understand the unique requirements for their care and share in implementing care. Patients should be encouraged to walk and should be assisted with ambulation by doctors, nurses, and family members throughout the day, not just by the physical therapist during the 15-min formal session once or twice a day. To be beneficial, high-tech medicine requires high-touch care.

Discharge Planning

Hospital discharge must be carefully planned and appropriately instituted. A social worker or discharge planning coordinator should be involved in discharge planning, and the consultation should begin soon after admission. Such early involvement by social services personnel may shorten the length of stay and prevent the need for nursing home placement. Early planning is also needed so that equipment, such as a hospital bed or oxygen, can be delivered to the patient's home and arrangements for home nursing care can be made. When nursing home admission is considered, a geriatrician should perform a thorough evaluation.

Patients being discharged to their homes need detailed instructions about follow-up care, and family members or other caregivers must be trained to provide it. Failure to teach them how to use medications, implement treatment, and monitor recovery increases the likelihood of adverse outcomes and readmission. Follow-up appointments and medication schedules should be written down for the patient and family. A copy of a brief discharge summary plan should be given to the patient or family in case questions arise about care before the official summary plan is sent to the primary care physician.

When patients are discharged to a nursing home or another hospital, communication is especially important. A written summary should be sent with the patient. This summary should include not only the standard medical information but also a summary of mental and functional status, the times the patient last received medications, known drug allergies, advance medical directives, and family contacts. Optimally, a nurse should call the receiving institution to review such information shortly before the patient is transferred.

27. SURGERY: PREOPERATIVE EVALUATION AND INTRAOPERATIVE AND POSTOPERATIVE CARE

Indications for surgery in older persons often differ from those in younger persons. Since life expectancy in the elderly is measured in months or years rather than in decades, prophylactic surgery is less important. However, treatment of serious illness is essential whenever cure or alleviation of pain or disability is possible. Because elective procedures for older patients are given more consideration as to whether they should be performed, emergency procedures are more common.

Emergency operations commonly performed on elderly patients include those for a fractured hip, strangulated hernia, complications of gallbladder disease, intestinal obstruction, and intra-abdominal catastrophes, such as ruptured aortic aneurysm or mesenteric thrombosis. Elective operations likely to be performed include those for cancer (chiefly involving the colorectal area, breast, and uterus), cataract, inguinal hernia, urinary incontinence, rectal prolapse, aortic aneurysm, and diseases of the peripheral arteries (particularly the internal carotid arteries and the arteries of the legs).

Other operations that might be justified in younger patients are not indicated in the very old except in unusual circumstances. Such procedures include cosmetic surgery, extensive reconstructive dental procedures, renal transplantation, joint replacement when severe pain is absent, and cholecystectomy for asymptomatic gallstones. *However, chronologic and physiologic ages are not necessarily equivalent.* The indications for surgery in an older patient who is fit and "younger than his years" are essentially the same as those in a younger patient. This is especially true of heart surgery, which may be beneficial and may carry a low risk in carefully chosen elderly patients. Thus, each person should be assessed individually, and judgments should be based on an individual's problem and physiologic status, not on age alone.

In the USA in 1990, 36% of all hospitalized patients ≥ 65 yr underwent a surgical procedure. Some 6,569,000 operations (or 28% of all procedures) were performed on patients in this age group. Since the geriatric population is expected to increase in future decades, the implications for hospitals and physicians are significant.

In the elderly, postoperative complications are more common, and mortality is higher. An initial complication is much more likely to lead to other complications; failure of one organ to function adequately is more likely to lead to failure of other organs. In one study, the mortality rate for patients ≥ 70 yr undergoing elective cholecystectomy was nearly 10 times that for younger patients. In a study of abdominal operations, the mortality rate for those 80 to 84 yr was 3%; for those 85 to 89 yr, 9%; and for those ≥ 90 yr, 25%.

Emergency operations carry a greater risk than elective ones in all age groups, particularly the elderly. For example, from 1974 to 1986, in operations for peptic ulcer with massive bleeding at Massachusetts General Hospital, the mortality rate was 10.6% for patients $\leq$ 70 yr and 41.9% for patients $\geq$ 70 yr. A corollary observation is that certain indicated surgical procedures should be treated electively; eg, inguinal hernia and abdominal aortic aneurysms are associated with a low mortality rate when handled as elective procedures and a high mortality rate when handled as emergency procedures because of strangulation or rupture.

PREOPERATIVE EVALUATION

A preoperative evaluation for elective surgery should include a history, physical examination, laboratory examinations, and an assessment of the surgical risks, including those related to age. Such risks result from compromised physiologic systems (eg, cardiovascular, respiratory, renal, immunologic), which may not necessarily be related to the primary diagnosis. Before elective surgery, such system deficits can be identified, and attempts can be made to correct them. Before emergency surgery, complete evaluation or correction is impossible; therefore, system failure is much more common.

Before surgery, the surgeon tells the patient about the procedure and any possible complications or disabilities. The surgeon then obtains informed consent (see also Chs. 108 and 109).

History

The history can furnish important clues, but many older patients suffer from deafness, memory deficits, or confusion and are unable to identify symptoms. Also, they tend to deny having any disabilities. Thus, obtaining a history can require a great deal of time and patience. Many patients have multiple disabilities. For example, one study of patients > 65 yr found an average of more than three disabilities; a study of more than 2000 autopsies found an average of seven significant lesions.

A complete history of drug use is especially important. A study of 178 chronically ill patients, for instance, showed that 59% made medication errors; 26% of the errors were potentially serious. Therefore, patients should be instructed to bring all their medications to the doctor's office or hospital and to describe exactly how they use them.

Because nutritional deficiencies are common in the elderly and not limited to the poor, nutritional status should be determined. Low levels of serum potassium or albumin are fairly common and potentially serious.

Physical Examination and Laboratory Tests

The skin, oral mucosa, and tongue can provide information about hydration and nutrition. The neck should be examined for lymph nodes, thyroid masses, carotid pulsations, and bruits. Blood pressure should be measured, and the heart, lungs, and breasts should be examined. The abdomen should be examined for asymptomatic lesions such as hernias, aortic aneurysms, and masses. Rectal examinations are mandatory, as are pelvic examinations in women. Femoral, popliteal, and pedal pulses should be noted, and any evidence of venous disease, such as varicose veins, postphlebitic ulcers, or edema, should be identified.

Urinalysis, peripheral blood count, a limited blood chemistry profile, and measurement of coagulation factors are necessary. Perioperative serum electrolyte studies are useful for patients who take diuretics. Also, a chest x-ray and an ECG are obtained before patients undergo surgery.

Risk Assessment

The physician must estimate the patient's ability to withstand an operation. The prognosis may be good for those who have survived the ages at which ischemic heart disease and strokes have claimed the lives of peers. Other prognostic factors are the patient's general mood and mental status.

The operative risk is increased by coexisting conditions such as coronary artery occlusive disease, carotid artery occlusive disease, chronic obstructive or bronchospastic lung disease, chronic renal insufficiency, cirrhosis, arterial or venous disease of the legs, and severe malnutrition.

Cardiac problems: The presence of certain cardiac conditions contraindicates elective noncardiac procedures. Recent myocardial infarction dramatically increases the risk of surgery. One study reported a mortality rate of 40% for those who had surgery within 3 mo of an acute myocardial infarction, compared with 14% for those who had a healed infarction. A series from the Mayo Clinic indicated that patients who had surgery within 3 mo of a myocardial infarction had a 37% reinfarction rate. This rate decreased to 16% between 3 and 6 mo after a myocardial infarction and to 4% to 5% > 6 mo after a myocardial infarction.

A patient who has heart failure is not a candidate for elective surgery. Patients whose heart failure is still evident preoperatively are more likely to develop frank postoperative failure and pulmonary edema than those who are no longer in failure or who have no history of failure. Patients with jugular venous distention and a third heart sound are at increased risk.

Consideration should be given to using digitalis, diuretics, and vasodilators to improve cardiac performance preoperatively and reduce the risks of surgery. Digitalis is recommended for patients who have a history of previous heart failure or cardiac dysfunction as evidenced by signs of impaired ventricular response, nocturnal angina, atrial fibrillation or flutter with rapid ventricular response, or frequent episodes of paroxysmal atrial or junctional tachycardia. Patients receiving digitalis should be closely monitored for digitalis toxicity during the perioperative period.

The exercise tolerance of patients with cardiac disease should be assessed by asking them about usual daily activity and how easily they tire. Nonspecific T wave and ST segment changes in a stable ECG are relatively unimportant when the history is unremarkable and a thorough physical examination has been performed. New ischemic patterns, however, should be assessed with serial tracings, and a cardiology consultation should be requested before an elective procedure.

Premature atrial contractions are a benign finding unless they occur frequently, which may indicate impending atrial fibrillation or supraventricular tachycardia. Preoperative ECG abnormalities that correlate with postoperative cardiac death include five or more premature ventricular contractions per minute and a rhythm other than sinus. Occasional solitary premature ventricular contractions do not require preoperative treatment.

In general, no drug commonly used to treat heart disease should be withdrawn before surgery, including β-blockers. In fact, withdrawing these drugs suddenly could be dangerous. If the patient has been stabilized on a regimen of calcium channel blockers preoperatively, administration should be continued. However, if a β-blocker is used concomitantly with verapamil or nifedipine, myocardial depression may be enhanced, increasing the risk of heart failure. The anesthesiologist should be informed of the use of these drugs because they alter the body's response to anesthetics and other vasoactive drugs. Use of an antiarrhythmic such as lidocaine, procainamide, phenytoin, or quinidine is a concern for the anesthesiologist primarily because it indicates an underlying organic lesion.

Hypertension should be controlled before surgery, and antihypertensive drugs should not be withdrawn. Patients with untreated or inadequately controlled hypertension have greater absolute reductions in blood pressure during anesthesia than those with adequately controlled hypertension. If a patient is taking a thiazide diuretic, the anesthesiologist should be informed, and the patient's serum potassium level should be checked. If the level is < 3.5 mEq/L, surgery should be postponed until adequate potassium supplementation has been provided.

Carotid artery occlusive disease: The influence of this disease on perioperative mortality and stroke is more controversial. Carotid artery occlusive disease in patients undergoing myocardial revascularization does appear to increase the perioperative stroke rate. In other types of operations, however, an increased rate of perioperative strokes may be limited to patients who have had transient ischemic attacks or to those who have severe occlusive disease of both internal carotid and vertebral arteries.

Pulmonary disease: Chronic obstructive or bronchospastic lung disease also increases the risk of surgery, mainly for patients with severe disease who have a forced expiratory volume of < 1 L at 1 sec (FEV_1). Preoperatively, the bronchospastic component may improve with bronchodilator therapy. The patient should not smoke preoperatively and would likely benefit from a few days of active physical therapy, including the use of broncholytic agents and percussion.

Liver disease: Evidence of impaired liver function before surgery is especially ominous. Attempts to improve liver function preoperatively are limited to correcting coagulation abnormalities with vitamin K or protein blood products such as fresh frozen plasma or coagulation concentrates.

Renal disease: Renal function is assessed by measuring BUN and creatinine levels. Dehydration may lead to prerenal azotemia, which can be corrected by administering fluids. If BUN and creatinine levels remain high, peritoneal dialysis or hemodialysis may reverse the uremia and reduce the high surgical risk.

Malnutrition: Preoperatively, the patient should be evaluated for symptoms and signs of malnutrition, a common problem in the elderly. According to one study, about half the patients > 65 yr who require surgery for serious disease have had a recent weight loss ranging from 5 to 50 lb. Since weight loss may lead to complications such as delayed wound healing, preoperative nutritional supplements should be provided when possible. This supplementation can include high-caloric foods, vitamins, enteral feedings (continuous or intermittent), or if necessary, total parenteral nutrition.

Anesthetics: Most anesthesiologists use the following classification recommended by the American Society of Anesthesiologists to assess a patient's anesthetic risk: **class 1** indicates a normally healthy patient; **class 2**, a patient who has mild systemic disease; **class 3**, a patient who has severe systemic disease that is not incapacitating; **class 4**, a patient who has incapacitating systemic disease that is a constant threat to life; and **class 5**, a moribund patient who is not expected to survive for 24 h with or without surgery.

Although age is not a factor in this classification, a greater proportion of older patients falls into the higher risk classes. One study demonstrates that although patients > 50 yr accounted for only 35% of the surgical population, they had a disproportionately high rate (45%) of deaths from anesthetics.

Drugs: Responses to drugs are often altered in the elderly as a result of differences in pharmacokinetics and tissue responses. The use of several drugs leads to the risk of drug interactions as discussed in Ch. 21.

Trauma: Assessing and managing trauma is similar in young and older patients. The initial assessment consists of identifying immediate life-threatening conditions by following the ABCs of trauma management: **A**irway, **B**reathing, and **C**irculation. An adequate airway is maintained with neck extension, an oropharyngeal airway (if the patient is unconscious but breathing), or an endotracheal or a nasotracheal tube (if the patient has an obstructed airway or inadequate ventilation). Once airway and ventilation are ensured, attention should be given to maintaining an adequate blood pressure. Hypotension from hemorrhage can usually be controlled by applying pressure directly to the bleeding site and replacing blood volume. Exploring wounds and placing clamps are inadvisable except for thoracic vascular injuries. Intra-abdominal hemorrhage is best managed in the operating room after a brief evaluation in the trauma area.

Adequate blood pressure generally can be achieved by vigorous blood volume replacement, usually with crystalloids such as lactated Ringer's solution or 0.9% sodium chloride solution, followed as soon as possible by appropriate replacement blood products. Vasopressors rarely are needed to maintain blood pressure in the trauma patient. The goals of blood pressure management include achieving a normal mental status when possible and maintaining normal coronary artery and renal perfusion. A urine output of at least 1 mL/kg/h is a reasonable goal; output should not drop below 0.5 mL/kg/h.

Once the ABCs are addressed, other life-threatening conditions are evaluated by physical examination. A chest examination and x-ray can identify a penetrating injury as well as pneumothorax, hemothorax, or a widened mediastinum—all of which require further evaluation. Abdominal examination can identify a penetrating abdominal injury as well as tenderness in the conscious patient. A rectal examination can identify intestinal bleeding from contusion or perforation injuries and prostatic injuries. Pelvic instability should be examined to identify pelvic fractures, which can be lethal. Examining the urinary meatus for blood is important before placing a urinary catheter. The presence of blood requires cystourethrography to rule out urethral injuries. If the patient has a urethral injury, catheterization should be suprapubic rather than transurethral. The extremities should be examined for fractures and dislocations of long bones.

The unconscious patient in whom significant blunt abdominal trauma is suspected and the conscious patient in whom intraperitoneal hemorrhage is suspected should undergo diagnostic infraumbilical peritoneal lavage. The lavage fluid should be examined for RBC and WBC counts and measured for bilirubin content and amylase activity. An RBC count of $> 100,000/\mu L$ strongly suggests intraperitoneal hemorrhage; an RBC count of 50,000 to $100,000/\mu L$ is borderline and indicates the need for further abdominal examination, peritoneal lavage, computed tomography imaging, or other diagnostic procedures. A WBC count $> 500/\mu L$ suggests an injury to a viscus. The presence of bile or amylase suggests injury to the pancreas, intestine, or biliary system.

Additional imaging procedures may be carried out in a stable patient. In a patient who has hematuria, an IV urogram should be obtained to identify urinary tract injuries. When necessary, renal trauma may be evaluated with abdominal computed tomography and vascular contrast. Abdominal or chest computed tomography imaging and arteriography can be carried out in a stable patient to evaluate a widened mediastinum or to identify intraperitoneal hemorrhage. The diagnostic accuracy of computed tomography in this setting has not yet been fully evaluated. Ultrasonography is undergoing clinical investigation and appears to be diagnostically useful in the trauma patient.

INTRAOPERATIVE CARE

Selecting the proper operative procedure depends on a number of factors, including the patient's ability to withstand an operation, the surgeon's skill, and the operating conditions. Generally, the simpler the operation that will produce the desired result, the better. Separate procedures for purely prophylactic purposes rarely should be performed. Thus, a routine appendectomy is seldom indicated during the course of an operation for acute cholecystitis in an elderly patient. If, however, a large gallstone is found during a right colectomy for cancer and adequate exposure has been achieved, the stone should be removed by either cholecystectomy or cholecystostomy to reduce the risk of early postoperative acute cholecystitis.

Anesthetic Agents and Techniques

Regional anesthesia should be used when feasible in elderly patients who are fair to poor risks. For example, a brachial block using the axillary approach is excellent for operations on the arm. Most inguinal hernia operations can be performed with local anesthesia. **Spinal anesthesia** is usually preferred to peridural anesthesia or individual nerve block for extraperitoneal operations below the umbilicus; it is frequently used for inguinal hernia repairs, anorectal operations, prostatic resections, hip pinnings, and leg amputations.

General anesthesia in an elderly patient nearly always requires intratracheal intubation to maintain an adequate airway. This anesthesia is preferred for abdominal operations because extensive exploration is usually necessary, and spinal anesthesia is rarely satisfactory. Induction requires an agent such as thiobarbiturate. Anesthesia is usually maintained by gases that are eliminated mainly through the lungs. In many cases, preliminary insertion of a nasogastric tube may be necessary to prevent aspiration of gastric contents. Patients with clinically significant heart disease or advanced respiratory disease should receive oxygen by mouth before and during barbiturate induction.

The usual inhalation agents are nitrous oxide, halothane, enflurane, isoflurane, and methoxyflurane. These agents may be supplemented by

IV morphine or meperidine. Some anesthesiologists prefer fentanyl because of its short duration of action, which allows the dosage to be closely controlled.

The **dissociative agent** ketamine, a potent analgesic that can be administered IV or IM, is useful in geriatric patients. Ketamine may be the sole anesthetic used for burn debridements and dressing changes or for positioning the patient for hip pinning before induction of spinal anesthesia. Relatively small doses provide analgesia while maintaining adequate blood pressure. The IV dosage is 1 to 2 mg/kg at a rate of 0.5 mg/kg/min. Hallucination upon emergence from ketamine anesthesia is unusual in elderly patients.

When used judiciously, **muscle relaxants,** such as succinylcholine, tubocurarine, and pancuronium, are well tolerated by older patients. Overdosage occurs, however, if the anesthesiologist uses the dosage appropriate for younger patients because the size and vigor of skeletal muscle is usually decreased in the elderly. A peripheral nerve stimulator may be used to determine the proper dosage.

Intraoperative Monitoring

Pulse, cuff blood pressure, and ECG should be monitored in all patients undergoing surgery. For a lengthy procedure, a urinary catheter is usually needed to monitor urine output. If the operative field involves the pelvis, draining the bladder often aids operative exposure.

Temperature should be measured and recorded during all major operations because significant hypothermia is a common sequela of a long procedure, particularly when the viscera are exposed. After a complicated operation, a rectal temperature of 32.2° to 35° C (90° to 95° F) or lower is common. Even this degree of hypothermia can lead to death secondary to ventricular fibrillation, which is thought to occur at 31.6° C (89° F). Thus, measures should be taken to maintain a reasonable body temperature, including warming all fluids, maintaining a reasonable operating room temperature, keeping the abdominal viscera in the abdominal cavity as long as possible, and using warm 0.9% sodium chloride solution for lavage.

Central venous pressures should be monitored with the catheter tip in an intrathoracic vein such as the superior vena cava. These pressures reflect intravascular volume and are particularly valuable when blood loss has occurred. The normal pressure is 8 to 10 mm Hg. Lower pressures generally indicate the need for blood or fluid replacement; elevated pressures may occur with right ventricular or biventricular heart failure. Pulmonary arterial hypertension secondary to pulmonary disease, high bronchial airway pressure, and right ventricular failure may elevate central venous pressure out of proportion to the left ventricular end-diastolic pressure. Such an elevation suggests adequate blood volume when, in fact, blood volume is inadequate.

To monitor left ventricular filling pressure, **a balloon-tipped pulmonary artery (Swan-Ganz) catheter** must be passed through the right ventricle into the pulmonary artery, and pulmonary capillary wedge pressures must be obtained. Normally, 4 to 12 mm Hg indicates adequate blood volume. In left ventricular failure, wedge pressures may rise to ≥ 40 mm Hg. These measurements arc particularly valuable guides to intraoperative management of fluid replacement therapy and management of cardiac inotropic activity and peripheral vascular resistance when vasopressor support is used in patients with cardiac dysfunction.

Continuous peripheral arterial blood pressure measurement is essential for complicated operative procedures, particularly vascular surgery. Continuous measurements may be taken by placing an intra-arterial catheter in the radial artery and connecting it to a transducer. This is especially useful during carotid artery surgery, in which brief periods of hypotension are poorly tolerated and may result in intraoperative cerebral infarction.

Intraoperative fluid replacement by the anesthesiologist should be conservative, providing maintenance fluids and replacing lost blood and fluids. Excessive fluid replacement is a common mistake that can be dangerous in the elderly, who may have difficulty eliminating additional fluid because of exaggerated or prolonged aldosterone and antidiuretic hormone (ADH) responses postoperatively. Also, because of underlying pulmonary, cardiac, hepatic, and renal deficiencies, compensating for excess fluids takes longer in the elderly than in younger patients.

Complications can follow any of these invasive procedures. For example, pulmonary artery catheters can cause pulmonary hemorrhage, and although rare, intra-arterial catheters can produce thrombosis and gangrene of fingers. Such complications have led to the recent development of methods such as **transcutaneous monitoring of tissue oxygen tension,** which is safe and beneficial for elderly patients with pulmonary disorders.

Abdominal Incision

Exposure of the operative field is the foremost consideration in choosing an incision. Generally, when wide exposure is needed, as for resection of an abdominal aortic aneurysm, a long vertical midline incision is best. However, the patient's body habitus should also be considered. For example, a cholecystectomy in a patient with a narrow costal margin usually can be undertaken more readily through a vertical incision than through the usual subcostal incision. In a very obese patient with a pendulous omentum, a supraumbilical transverse incision usually can be substituted for a vertical one; this may avoid the deep-fat omentum and prevent a subsequent wound seroma. Because chronic obstructive GI disease is common in geriatric patients, upper abdominal incisions should be selected carefully. Generally, vertical incisions in the epigastrium are less painful postoperatively and allow for more effective clearing of pulmonary secretions.

Although laparoscopic cholecystectomy is indicated for many patients, open cholecystectomy is preferable for many elderly patients. Compared with younger patients, elderly patients pose more difficult technical problems and are more likely to have acute cholecystitis and common bile duct stones. Also, older patients who are poor cardiac or pulmonary risks may not tolerate the elevation of the diaphragm required for laparoscopy.

POSTOPERATIVE CARE

After high-risk operations, most patients are treated in intensive care units overnight or for up to 72 h before being returned to the surgical floor. Geriatric patients are especially likely to require this pattern of care.

Certain preventive considerations are important in the care of older patients, even when convalescence is uncomplicated. Ambulation should begin soon after surgery; for several days this may require two assistants. Patients who do not ambulate soon after surgery are more likely to develop thromboembolism. One study showed that after repair of a fractured hip, 10% of elderly patients developed pulmonary embolism, compared with only 0.2% of the general surgical population > 40 yr. Elderly patients are also at risk for acute confusion, particularly at night ("sundowning"). Thus, they must be protected, especially at night, from such dangers as dislodging their catheters and tubes and falling from bed. Using constant nighttime attendants, eg, a family member or special aide, is preferable to using physical or chemical restraints. Several measures help prevent decubitus ulcers on the sacrum, trochanters, and heels—thoroughly washing and lubricating the skin, frequently changing position, and when necessary, applying alternating air-pressure mattresses, sheepskins, and foam pads.

Feeding tubes, nasogastric tubes, IV lines, and drains are all essential for postoperative care but are potential sources of sepsis unless handled properly. Sterile technique must be used in handling surgical drains. Profuse drainage (eg, from the biliary tree or an intestinal fistula) requires sterile adherent collection bags.

Intestinal stomas require meticulous skin care and attention to intestinal output. Usually skin sutures are removed after a week, but if the patient is malnourished or being treated with corticosteroids, they must be left in place longer.

INTENSIVE CARE

Monitoring all physiologic functions is essential during the patient's stay in the intensive care unit. Pulse, blood pressure, temperature, respiratory rate and depth, and state of consciousness must be measured and recorded on flow charts. Hourly urine output should also be noted. Central venous pressure must be monitored when oligemia or fluid depletion requires that large volumes of fluid be administered, particularly when cardiac or pulmonary reserve is limited. Also, a postoperative ECG should be recorded; if necessary, another ECG may be recorded later. Chest x-rays should be taken immediately after the operation and then daily. If cardiorespiratory problems are present, the usual laboratory studies of blood and blood chemistry must be supplemented with arterial blood gas determinations.

At times, additional monitoring may be required. For example, arterial catheters may remain in place for days or weeks to obtain direct blood pressure measurements. Such a catheter must be observed frequently to make sure that it has not been dislodged and that circulation to the fingers has not been compromised. When the right ventricular pressure reading obtained by central venous pressure monitoring does not adequately reflect left ventricular pressure, a pulmonary artery (Swan-Ganz) catheter may be inserted in the operating room or the intensive care unit. Such a situation may occur with severe pulmonary artery disease, severe left ventricular failure related to ischemia, or other diseases associated with significant pulmonary hypertension. The data obtained by the pulmonary artery catheter help maintain adequate blood volume and determine physiologic treatment of the patient's cardiac inotropic state and peripheral vascular resistance.

Early Postoperative Complications

Many postoperative problems occur in the first 2 or 3 days following surgery. Some of the most common ones include hypotension, hypothermia, respiratory problems, delirium, pain, fluid and electrolyte imbalance, acid-base abnormalities, and nutritional deficiencies.

Hypotension: **Hypovolemia,** the most common cause of hypotension in the early postoperative period, results from inadequate replacement of intraoperative fluid losses, inordinate bleeding, or internal losses of fluid such as reaccumulation of ascites or third-space losses. Third-space losses represent intravascular fluid losses caused by tissue edema, especially in the operative site. After abdominal surgery, considerable intraperitoneal hemorrhage can occur, although it may produce relatively few physical findings. The usual test for such occult hemorrhage is to administer large amounts of blood or fluids; if blood pressure immediately rises to normal levels, followed by a rapid recurrence of hypotension, abdominal reexploration for bleeding is usually indicated.

The patient's course during the operation must be reviewed, noting the anesthetics used, the estimated fluid loss, and the fluid replacement. The patient's **respiratory status** must be assessed as well. If the endotracheal tube is still in place, the chest is examined to make sure the tube has not blocked a main stem bronchus or a pneumothorax has not developed. If the tube has been removed, the rate and depth of respirations must be determined because reintubation may be necessary.

Drains and catheters should be examined for escaping blood. Laboratory tests, including arterial blood gas determinations, ECG, peripheral hematocrit, and if necessary, a chest x-ray, should be performed.

Vasopressors should not be given unless severe hypotension is thought to be compromising coronary or cerebral blood flow or is found to be caused by cardiogenic or neurogenic shock.

Postoperative hypotension caused by shock from heart failure is a major concern. This may be either left ventricular failure resulting from **myocardial ischemia or infarction** in coronary artery disease or right ventricular failure related to pulmonary arterial hypertension secondary to an acute **pulmonary embolus.** These causes of failure are rare, however, in the immediate postoperative period. If myocardial ischemia is suspected, an ECG tracing should be compared with the preoperative tracing. If the patient has myocardial ischemia, hypovolemia must be avoided. Even if blood volume is adequate, the ischemia may be exacerbated by tachycardias. Management also includes using vasodilators, such as transdermal or IV nitrates, and obtaining serial ECGs to assess the drugs' efficacy. Also, β-blockers and calcium channel blockers can diminish cardiac ischemia, if they are used with care and their negative inotropic properties are considered. Blood should be drawn to measure cardiac isoenzyme levels, which can be used subsequently to distinguish between myocardial ischemia and infarction.

Other causes of hypotension are unusual in the early postoperative period. Septic shock can develop in a patient who had preoperative signs of **sepsis,** eg, a patient with severe intra-abdominal sepsis or massive burns. Because **arteriosclerotic peripheral vascular disease** is common in the elderly, blood pressure should be checked in both the right and left brachial arteries. A discrepancy could indicate obstructive lesions in the brachiocephalic or subclavian arterial system. **Factitious causes** should also be considered, especially if the history and physical examination do not correlate with the severity of hypotension. Pressure monitors must be inspected to be certain they are functioning properly.

Hypothermia: Immediately after a prolonged operation, the patient's temperature may be in the 32.2° to 34.4° C (90° to 94° F) range. Any further reduction should be prevented because bradycardia, cardiac irregularity, and cardiac arrest could occur in the 31.1° to 31.6° C (88° to 89° F) range. Hypothermia can be treated by warming all IV and other fluids and by using blankets and covers to raise the patient's core temperature.

Respiratory problems: In the early postoperative period, respiratory problems are particularly important. Because the usual signs of shallow, ineffective respirations and cyanosis are not always present, other signs such as extreme restlessness or hypotension should be noted. Arterial blood gas determinations can confirm respiratory problems.

Treatment depends on the underlying cause and may include relatively simple measures such as reintubation, repositioning an endotracheal tube, or applying positive end-expiratory pressure **(PEEP).** If inadequate reversal of muscle relaxants or narcotics may be the cause, oxygen should be given immediately, and arterial blood gas determinations should be obtained.

Respiratory difficulty in the immediate postoperative period is usually treated successfully over a few days; sometimes, however, protracted ventilatory support is needed. Mechanical ventilation may, in turn, introduce other complications.

When prolonged **ventilatory assistance** is required, volume-controlled ventilators usually ensure adequate tidal volume despite changes in pulmonary compliance. Oxygen should be delivered at the lowest concentration that maintains an acceptable PaO_2. Inspired oxygen concentrations of $\leq 40\%$ are usually well tolerated indefinitely; higher concentrations, however, may cause oxygen toxicity with alveolar collapse, interstitial edema, and hyaline membrane formation.

When increased PaO_2 is needed, PEEP may be used to maintain positive airway pressure throughout the ventilatory cycle. This does not allow airway pressure to return to the level of atmospheric pressure, but it does allow a minimum of the designated PEEP to be maintained. Use of PEEP is believed to open collapsed alveoli, thus permitting ventilation of perfused alveoli, and to provide adequate ventilation at a higher functional residual capacity. If PEEP is used in a hypovolemic patient, however, it may produce hypotension by blocking blood return to the left side of the heart. In this case, volume replacement must be carried out before significant PEEP is instituted.

Mechanical ventilation usually requires an **endotracheal tube,** which may be left in place for at least 5 days with few complications. If longer intubation is needed, a low-pressure cuff-type tube should be used to prevent tracheal erosion, which could result in such complications as late tracheal stenosis or fatal hemorrhage. Meticulous care of the endotracheal tube is essential for preventing lung contamination. For instance, sterile gloves should be worn when the trachea and bronchi are suctioned. Tracheal specimens for culture should be drawn periodically. Severe tracheobronchial bacterial infection or pneumonia requires appropriate antibiotic therapy. Sufficient humidity should be delivered by the ventilator to prevent inspissation of bronchial secretions. Highly viscous, thick bronchial secretions and bronchospasm are treated with mucolytic and bronchodilating agents, respectively.

When a patient is extubated, good pulmonary cleansing should be maintained. Deep breathing and coughing at regular intervals should be encouraged. Nasogastric suctioning may be necessary to stimulate coughing. Occasionally, bedside bronchoscopy is necessary to remove secretions from specific lobes or from the peripheral bronchial tree. Early ambulation helps stimulate breathing, and an upright position increases lung capacity by 15% to 25%.

Other supportive measures include preventing abdominal distention by using a nasogastric tube and avoiding tight abdominal binders and dressings. Narcotics should be used cautiously to avoid narcosis, which would prevent adequate pulmonary cleansing.

Elderly patients who have a marginal pulmonary reserve are likely to develop major areas of collapse, atelectasis, or heart failure. Death is likely if the exact cause of the pulmonary failure is not determined and corrected immediately. The most common causes include pneumonia, pulmonary edema, pulmonary embolus, fat embolus, and adult respiratory distress syndrome (ARDS).

Adult respiratory distress syndrome is *a respiratory failure with life-threatening respiratory distress and hypoxemia, associated with various acute pulmonary injuries*. In the early phase, this syndrome is difficult to recognize because the chest x-ray is normal. The patient is in obvious respiratory distress, however, exhibiting agitation, cyanosis, and grunting with respiratory effort. Frequently, arterial blood gas determinations show surprisingly low PaO_2 values, often in the 30 or 40 mm Hg range, and respiratory alkalosis with a low $PaCO_2$. The latter eventually begins to rise as respiratory acidosis and further respiratory failure develop. On x-ray, perihilar and diffuse parenchymal infiltrates appear.

The treatment of adult respiratory distress syndrome includes fluid restriction (usually to 1000 to 1500 mL/day), diuresis (induced with drugs such as furosemide or ethacrynic acid), and mechanical ventilation. Relatively high tidal volumes (12 to 15 mL/kg) are used along with PEEP, and appropriate antibiotics are administered based on sputum culture results.

Postoperative delirium: Many geriatric patients in an intensive care unit develop delirium, ranging from mild confusion to total psychotic disorientation. Many factors, including environmental and physiologic derangements, are responsible. Preexisting dementia, fluid and electrolyte imbalance, drugs, loss of sleep, frequent interruptions for nursing care, and loss of ability to keep track of time all contribute to disorientation. As recovery progresses, the condition should clear (see also Ch. 9).

Postoperative pain: The elderly are more tolerant of and philosophical about pain than younger adults (see Ch. 12). Because of changes in neural pathways, the elderly may actually be less aware of pain. As a result, patient-controlled analgesia, in which patients control their own IV narcotic delivery, may be less effective. Patient-controlled analgesia should be monitored closely because an elderly patient may become confused and disoriented from the narcotic.

Many elderly patients have a compromised response to drugs, particularly narcotics, that can lead to prolonged or exaggerated effects (see Ch. 21). Because of their sensitivity to narcotic side effects, the elderly also tend to experience hallucinations and disorientation, making postoperative management more difficult. Thus, when it comes to managing postoperative pain with narcotics, the adage "a little goes a long way" is apropos.

Fluid and electrolyte imbalance: Managing fluids and electrolytes is difficult because the capacity to maintain homeostasis is reduced in the elderly. A relatively narrow margin exists between too little and too much fluid in the treatment of these patients. Proper **fluid replacement** can be determined only by close monitoring. Initially, a rough estimate can be made, but it should be followed by a definitive plan, which can then be modified to optimize blood pressure, pulse, and urine output.

For several days after an operation, the body normally retains water and sodium in response to increased aldosterone and antidiuretic hormone. Therefore, *excessive fluid administration should be avoided in an elderly patient whose cardiovascular function is reduced.* Enough fluid should be given to provide for urine output of 0.5 mL/kg/h or about 30 mL/h to replace insensible fluid losses and to replace other measured or estimated external losses. In the early postoperative period, all this fluid is usually given IV.

When external losses are not great, fluid requirements for 24 h usually range from 1500 to 2500 mL. Considerably more fluid may be needed, however, if excessive third-space sequestration of fluids occurs—eg, as happens with distended bowel or inflamed subcutaneous tissues from burns. Precautions should be observed in these cases because the sequestered fluid usually is mobilized on the third to fifth postoperative days. Central venous pressure, pulmonary wedge pressure, and urine output provide further guidance for fluid management.

The amount of insensible fluid loss is relatively constant, usually averaging 600 to 900 mL daily. This amount may rise to 1500 mL daily with hypermetabolism, hyperventilation, or fever. Insensible loss usually is replaced with 5% D/W.

After a few postoperative days, fluid overload is no longer a danger, and about 1 L of fluid daily is needed to replace the urine volume required to excrete the catabolic end products of metabolism. The urine volume usually is *not* replaced on a milliliter-for-milliliter basis because an output of 2 to 3 L on a given day could represent fluids given during the surgical procedure or excessive fluid administration. Gastrointestinal losses, which are usually isotonic or slightly hypotonic, are replaced with 0.9% sodium chloride solution. When the estimated loss is slightly above or below isotonicity, appropriate adjustments can be made in the daily water intake. Maintenance fluids should be administered at a steady rate over 24 h.

Electrolyte replacement must include 40 mEq/L/day of potassium to replace urine losses and about 20 mEq/L to replace gastrointestinal losses. Inadequate potassium replacement may prolong postoperative ileus; if hypokalemia is not corrected, resistant metabolic alkalosis may develop. Calcium and magnesium also may be replaced if serum values warrant.

Excessive administration of isotonic solutions results in overexpansion of the extracellular compartment. This is well tolerated in younger adults but may be dangerous in geriatric patients because of their limited cardiopulmonary reserves. Theoretically, sodium and chloride requirements in the immediate postoperative period are minimal. If little or no sodium chloride is given at this time, however, a prolonged hyponatremia and hypochloremia will persist after normal salt retention. Therefore, 50 to 90 mEq/day of sodium usually maintains a normal serum osmolality and serum sodium level. If external losses occur—for instance, from nasogastric suction or diarrhea—additional salt should be given.

Hyponatremia, *a serum sodium concentration below the normal range of 136 to 145 mEq/L,* is a particularly perplexing but relatively common problem in geriatric patients. It may present as confusion or a seizure a few days after surgery. The sodium level may drop from 140 mEq/L to as low as 115 mEq/L, with symptoms appearing when it falls below 130 mEq/L.

The physician must determine whether the patient's total body sodium content is increased, normal, or diminished. Pulmonary edema, excessive peripheral edema, or evidence of major third-space losses suggests increased total body sodium content. The relationship between total body water and total body sodium content must also be determined. Total body free water content may be elevated because of excessive 5% D/W administration postoperatively or because the body's response to surgery is altered, resulting in excessive antidiuretic hormone. After evaluating the patient's total body water and total body sodium content, the physician should decide whether to administer or withhold free water or sodium in subsequent fluids.

If hyponatremia results from water overload, 0.9% sodium chloride solution and a diuretic should be given cautiously; if hyponatremia results from inadequate sodium intake, 0.9% sodium chloride solution should be given cautiously. In either case, electrolyte levels should be monitored frequently; 3% or 5% sodium chloride solution is rarely indicated and can result in excessive and dangerous hypernatremia.

Acid-base derangements: Acid-base abnormalities often occur postoperatively. The major abnormalities are respiratory acidosis, respiratory alkalosis, metabolic acidosis, and metabolic alkalosis. Diagnosis may be suspected on clinical grounds, but confirmation requires arterial blood gas determinations and nomogram interpretation.

Respiratory acidosis is *a primary increase in* Pa_{CO_2}*; pH is decreased and carbon dioxide content increased if renal function is intact.* This abnormality is produced by many factors that reduce pulmonary function, including inadequate ventilation with airway obstruction, atelectasis, pneumonia, pleural effusion, hypoventilation, and abdominal distention. It is particularly serious in patients who have chronic obstructive pulmonary disease and chronic compensated respiratory acidosis because it may be markedly accentuated postoperatively. Although restlessness, hypertension, and tachycardia may indicate inadequate ventilation with hypercapnia, they may also result from pain.

Respiratory alkalosis is *a primary decrease in* Pa_{CO_2}*; pH is increased and carbon dioxide content decreased.* This abnormality is caused by excessive carbon dioxide elimination, which may result from hyperventilation induced by apprehension or pain or from excessive mechanical ventilation. Mild respiratory alkalosis is of little consequence, and most patients require no therapy. Moderate respiratory alkalosis, however, may result in cerebral vasoconstriction. In those with extracranial arterial disease, this vasoconstriction further compromises cerebral blood flow and may result in irreparable cerebral damage.

Metabolic acidosis is *a primary decrease in ECF HCO_3^-; pH and carbon dioxide content are decreased.* This abnormality has many potential causes, but in the postoperative patient the cause is usually renal dysfunction. The kidneys normally maintain acid-base balance by excreting nitrogenous waste products and acid metabolites and by reabsorbing sodium bicarbonate in the renal tubule. When renal damage impairs these functions, or when an excessive loss of alkaline gastrointestinal fluids from the pancreas or the lower gastrointestinal tract occurs, metabolic acidosis may result. Therapy consists of administering IV fluids with an appropriate chloride-to-bicarbonate ratio (such as lactated Ringer's injection).

Other disorders that can lead to metabolic acidosis include diabetic acidosis, which is treated with insulin, and cardiac arrest, which requires large amounts of IV sodium bicarbonate. This lactic acidosis also occurs with poor tissue perfusion resulting from severe soft tissue damage or any state of diminished oxygen delivery to tissues.

Severe acidosis further impairs the circulation by decreasing smooth muscle responsiveness to vasopressors such as epinephrine. Attempts to correct the acidosis by giving large amounts of sodium bicarbonate are futile, unless blood volume or circulation is restored. When adequate tissue perfusion is restored, lactic acid is quickly metabolized, and the pH returns to normal. Using lactated Ringer's injection for the ECF deficit accompanying hemorrhagic shock concomitant with whole blood administration does not aggravate lactic acidosis. Instead, lactate rapidly decreases, and pH returns to normal.

Metabolic alkalosis is *a primary increase in blood HCO_3^-; pH and carbon dioxide content are increased.* This abnormality results from uncompensated losses of acid and retention of bases. Usually, the patient has some degree of hypokalemia. Cellular potassium depletion results in a corresponding entry of hydrogen and sodium ions. Thus, intracellular pH is lowered, and extracellular alkalosis develops.

Metabolic alkalosis may follow an aldosterone-stimulated exchange of sodium and hydrogen ions for potassium, resulting in a **paradoxic aciduria.** This syndrome may occur with prolonged nasogastric suctioning or repeated vomiting. The dangers of metabolic alkalosis are related to potassium depletion and include cardiac arrhythmias, tetany, digitalis sensitivity, and paralytic ileus. Less serious symptoms include irritability and neuromuscular excitation.

Nutritional deficiencies: With a geriatric surgical patient, three questions regarding nutritional management must be addressed.

1. *Should the patient receive postoperative nutritional support?* Patients who should receive early, aggressive nutritional support include

those with primary malnutrition, those with complications such as sepsis or associated injuries, and those admitted late in the course of their disease who have lost > 10% of their premorbid weight. This support may be supplemental oral feedings, tube feedings, or total parenteral nutrition, depending on the patient's condition. If anorexia or dysphagia makes oral feeding difficult or impossible but gastric motility and absorption are normal, enteral feedings may be given by continuous drip. If intestinal motility and absorption are adequate, the enteral route is preferable to the parenteral route because it involves fewer complications, costs less, and may have a trophic effect on the intestine itself. Total parenteral nutrition is used when normal intestinal motility or absorption is absent.

2. *What level of caloric intake will enable the patient to respond adequately to the operation?* A brief increase in metabolism as measured by oxygen consumption occurs postoperatively, unless a complication such as sepsis develops. The metabolic rate in the early postoperative period, however, does not exceed twice the normal basal metabolic rate (BMR) and is usually only 20% to 40% above it. The Harris-Benedict equation for determining BMR in men is as follows:

$$BMR = 66 + (13.7 \times W) + (5.0 \times H) - (6.8 \times A)$$

The equation for women is as follows:

$$BMR = 665 + (9.6 \times W) + (1.7 \times H) - (4.7 \times A)$$

In these equations, the BMR is expressed in kilocalories; W is the ideal body weight in kilograms; H is the height in centimeters; and A is the age in years. Although age, sex, height, and weight are considered in determining basal caloric requirement, body temperature, protein losses through wounds, and muscular work related to physical activity such as ambulation are ignored. Thus, an adequate estimate for total daily caloric requirement is 1.2 to 2 times the BMR as determined above.

3. *What mixture of substrates, proteins, carbohydrates, and fats will adequately meet the patient's metabolic needs without producing a negative nitrogen balance?* Determining the appropriate mixture is more complex. The total caloric requirement is met with carbohydrate, protein, and fat. Carbohydrate (glucose) infused at a rate of 5 mg/kg/min provides enough calories to prevent amino acid breakdown as an energy source and suppresses endogenous glucose production via hepatic gluconeogenesis, which requires mobilization of amino acids as gluconeogenic precursors.

This glucose infusion rate also approximates the maximum rate of glucose oxidation for a patient on strict bed rest. Any additional glucose in such a patient is not used for adenosine triphosphate production but is simply converted to fat. At this infusion rate, the respiratory quotient is just below unity, indicating that the glucose is oxidized to carbon dioxide, water, and energy and is not being stored as fat.

In most patients, protein is infused at 0.5 to 1.0 gm/kg/day; in some patients, the rate can be carefully increased to 1.5 to 2.5 gm/kg/day. In most geriatric patients, the lower rate may be used. Nitrogen balance analysis and kinetic amino acid turnover studies show that this rate maintains a positive nitrogen balance in adults and injured children. Although the effectiveness of this protein infusion rate has not been studied in the elderly patient, it represents a reasonable first approximation.

Glucose given at 5 mg/kg/min and protein at 1.5 gm/kg/day do not meet the patient's total caloric requirement. Therefore, fats must be given either parenterally or enterally. Fats supply essential fatty acids and furnish enough calories to minimize the need for mobilization of endogenous proteins for energy and gluconeogenesis.

Other Postoperative Complications

Certain complications can occur either in the intensive care unit or later during convalescence. These include cardiorespiratory arrest, thromboembolism, acute renal failure, stress ulcers, antibiotic-associated pseudomembranous colitis, hemorrhage, wound infections, intra-abdominal abscesses, anastomotic suture leakage, dehiscence, and urinary tract infection.

Cardiorespiratory arrest: **Respiratory arrest** may result from airway obstruction or respiratory depression, or it may be secondary to cardiac arrest. **Airway obstruction** may be caused by mucus, blood, or a foreign body in the endotracheal tube or tracheobronchial tree, an aspirated food bolus in the larynx, or vocal cord spasm. **Respiratory depression** may result from primary pulmonary disease (such as bacterial pneumonia), pneumonia from aspiration of vomited gastric contents, or pulmonary embolus; it may also occur as a narcotic side effect. In the postoperative patient, **cardiac arrest** is associated with ventricular fibrillation or asystole; initial treatment for either is the same.

Cardiac or respiratory arrest requires immediate treatment. An absence of ventilation for 3 min can be fatal. If the patient does not die, brain damage may occur. Treatment is based on the ABCD mnemonic of resuscitation: **A**irway, **B**reathing, **C**irculation, and **D**efinitive treatment. Establishing an airway and adequate breathing or ventilation are achieved by performing mouth-to-mouth resuscitation, using a bag-valve-mask device, or using an endotracheal tube and manual or mechanical ventilation. A reasonable breathing rate for adults is 12 breaths per minute while using 100% oxygen.

Primary cardiac arrest also leads immediately to cerebral anoxia and loss of respiratory exchange. Thus, circulation must be reestablished. In the postoperative period, the arrest usually occurs when the patient is not being monitored and after the endotracheal tube has been removed. A few chest compressions can be used to determine whether the airway is open. Then ventilation must be maintained either by intermittent chest compression or by intubation and mechanical ventilation, if necessary. A hard blow with the fist to the sternum sometimes produces a return of cardiac rhythm, but if it does not, external cardiac compression is necessary. Rarely, thoracotomy and cardiac massage may be needed.

For further treatment of the cardiac arrest, drugs and an ECG are necessary. In 85% of cases, sudden cardiac arrest is caused by ventricular fibrillation. Further treatment depends on whether asystole, fibrillation, or bradycardia (or idioventricular rhythm) appears on the ECG. **Bradycardia** is treated with atropine sulfate 0.5 to 1.0 mg IV or isoproterenol 1 to ≥ 5 μg/min IV to obtain a reasonable ventricular rate.

Fibrillation is treated by cardioversion (defibrillation), initially with 200 to 300 joules. If this is unsuccessful, epinephrine (5 to 10 mL of a 1:10,000 solution) should be administered IV or transtracheally; if these routes are not available, intracardiac injection may be used. Epinephrine administration is then followed by cardioversion. If these measures fail, other factors such as arterial oxygenation or acidosis should be considered. Oxygenation may be quickly identified by obtaining arterial blood gas values and should be treated accordingly. During CPR, acidosis occurs rapidly. Sodium bicarbonate, 1 or 2 ampules (7.5%, 44.6 mEq), may be injected rapidly IV and repeated every 5 to 10 min. (If possible, calcium or catecholamine preparations should not be given at the same injection site.) Arterial pH should be monitored frequently to avoid paradoxical acidosis.

If fibrillation persists, repeated cardioversion, IV epinephrine, and possibly antiarrhythmics such as lidocaine, procainamide, or bretylium tosylate may be used. In critical situations, when cardiac inotropism is weak and digitalis toxicity is not suspected, calcium chloride 10 mL in a 10% solution may be given IV to increase inotropic activity.

For **asystole,** cardioversion alone may be attempted. But usually, asystole must be converted to fibrillation using epinephrine before cardioversion can be performed.

Preventive measures may be taken to avoid cardiac arrest. Patients at increased risk include those who have anemia, infection, or a history of heart disease, which increases the heart's work load; serious electrolyte or acid-base abnormalities; severe hypovolemia; hypervolemia and severe pulmonary edema; arrhythmias; or excessive digitalization. From a practical point of view, patients at risk should be placed on cardiac monitors. If the monitor shows a recent onset of more than three premature ventricular contractions per minute, particularly if they are multifocal or appear early in the diastolic phase (near the T wave), lidocaine should be given IV 50 to 100 mg (ie, 1 to 2 mg/kg) at a rate of 25 to 50 mg/min; if no response occurs, a second dose may be given after 5 min. This is generally followed by a continuous infusion of 1 to 4 mg/min (ie, 20 to 50 μg/kg/min). The dosage should be reduced in patients > 70 yr, those with heart failure or liver disease, and those taking drugs that either reduce hepatic blood flow or reduce lidocaine metabolism.

Older patients in cardiac arrest, especially those with a terminal illness, present serious ethical and social considerations. Resuscitation may not be in the patient's best interest if expectations for his health are not as good as they were before the arrest (see also Chs. 41, 108, and 109).

Thromboembolism: A thromboembolism may present as peripheral thrombophlebitis, pulmonary embolism, or both. Patients who have had previous thromboembolism, prolonged operations, or prolonged postoperative immobilization, as well as those who are obese, are at increased risk for developing thromboembolism. Most fatal pulmonary emboli originate from peripheral thrombophlebitis in the legs.

Many prophylactic measures can reduce the incidence of thrombophlebitis; the most important ones are appropriate anesthesia, expeditious operations, and early ambulation. Other measures include postoperative use of elastic stockings, pneumatic compression devices, and anticoagulants. Disagreement exists about the choice and amount of anticoagulant that should be used. Because prophylactic heparin, even in small doses, can lead to hemorrhage, many surgeons restrict its use to high-risk patients. Heparin can be replaced by oral warfarin sodium within a few days. The antiplatelet drug aspirin is also used prophylactically for thromboembolism but does not appear to be as effective as heparin.

Anticoagulation is generally considered the therapy of choice for established thromboembolism. In adults, a loading dose of IV heparin (5,000 to 10,000 u.) is given, followed by a continuous IV infusion for 7 days. The initial dosage of 1,000 u./h is adjusted to increase partial thromboplastin time to twice normal. On the first or second day of therapy, warfarin is started. Usually, the warfarin dose is adjusted to elevate prothrombin time to 1.5 times normal. This treatment is generally successful.

If anticoagulation is contraindicated or if embolization recurs despite anticoagulation, a vena cava filter may be inserted either directly or percutaneously through the right internal jugular vein. When inserted accurately and expeditiously, this filter substantially eliminates recurrent embolization.

Today venous interruptions of the superficial femoral vein are rarely necessary, although ligation of this vein and vena cava ligation were common in the past. The latter procedure was discontinued because of a lack of competent anastomotic veins about the ligature, immediate hyperdistention of distal veins, and subsequent excessive edema of the legs. Vena cava clips, which allowed blood to pass but strained out nearly all emboli, were also used previously but have been replaced by the vena cava filter. Pulmonary embolectomy is still used successfully in selected cases of life-threatening cardiogenic shock resulting from massive pulmonary emboli.

Acute renal failure: After surgery, acute renal failure is more common in older patients than in younger ones because of the compromised renal reserve resulting from coexisting diseases, such as atherosclerosis and diabetes. Acute renal failure is associated with a rapidly increasing azotemia and usually oliguria (< 500 mL/day).

Causes of postoperative acute renal failure fall into three diagnostic categories: prerenal, renal, and postrenal. The most common **prerenal causes** are severe dehydration and a severely diminished blood volume, cardiac failure, hepatorenal syndrome, and septicemia. The most common **renal causes** result from a direct injury to the kidneys and include acute tubular necrosis, which follows episodes of renal ischemia resulting from hypotension during or after an operation, or which is associated with renal injury from toxins such as hemoglobin or myoglobin; acute renal artery or vein occlusion resulting from the operation; and acute nephritis, which is associated with potentially nephrotoxic drugs such as the aminoglycosides, contrast dyes for arteriography, and papillary necrosis in diabetes. The most common **postrenal causes** are related to blockage of the ureters or the prostatic urethra.

A progressive rise in serum creatinine is diagnostic of acute renal failure, but the urinary sediment also should be examined. Red cell casts and red cells suggest a vascular, neoplastic, or glomerulonephritic cause. Eosinophils in urine suggest nephrotoxic drugs as the cause. Renal ultrasonography is useful in detecting postrenal obstructive causes of acute renal failure.

Prophylaxis chiefly involves preventing hypotension and maintaining adequate urinary flow during the postoperative period. Because renal injury from nephrotoxic drugs may be dose-related, levels of drugs such as aminoglycosides should be monitored closely. Potential renal injury from myoglobin should be anticipated in clinical circumstances such as extremity crush injuries in trauma or acute severe arterial occlusive disease and profound extremity ischemia. Maintaining a high glomerular filtration rate and alkalinizing urine with sodium bicarbonate are helpful.

Treatment of a patient with failing kidneys is difficult. In the early stages, an adequate blood volume must be maintained. Meticulous measurements of intake and output and daily weights are needed to monitor fluid and electrolyte therapy. Dosages of drugs excreted by the kidney, such as digoxin and many antibiotics, must be adjusted. Acid-base balance and nutrition must be closely monitored.

Dialysis may be needed for patients with concomitant oliguria, increasing acidosis, and heart failure. The indications for dialysis (either hemodialysis or peritoneal dialysis) are retention of nitrogenous solutes (urea and creatinine) and uremic encephalopathy or serositis (evidence of pericarditis, pleuritis, or inflammation of other serous membranes), overexpansion of the blood volume and heart failure, hyperkalemia (serum potassium > 6 mEq/L), and metabolic acidosis (pH < 7.2).

Stress ulcers: *Superficial mucosal erosions of the stomach occurring after stressful conditions, eg, trauma, burns, sepsis, or operations.* Stress ulcers produce upper GI bleeding that can vary from minimal to life-threatening. The patient may vomit bright red blood, or a coffee-ground vomit may appear in nasogastric tube aspirates. Stress ulcers may develop at any time during the postoperative period but usually occur before oral intake has resumed and when the abdomen is distended and concomitant pulmonary complications are present. Diagnosis is best made by upper gastrointestinal endoscopy.

Prophylaxis, which involves treating pulmonary complications, preventing gastric distention by decompression via a nasogastric tube or gastrostomy, and maintaining a neutral or alkaline pH in the stomach, is very successful. Gastric acidity may be controlled by giving antacids via a nasogastric tube to maintain gastric pH above 5.5 or by giving histamine H_2-receptor antagonists (eg, cimetidine) IV. The first method requires additional nursing time to monitor pH and to deliver antacids hourly, making it more expensive. Thus, most institutions currently use H_2-receptor antagonists for prophylaxis. Care must be taken, however, to avoid the dose-related CNS side effects of cimetidine, which are thought to occur more frequently in elderly patients. These effects include confusion, delirium, slurred speech, and hallucinations.

If stress bleeding does occur, conservative **treatment** by endoscopic coagulation or angiographic embolization may be effective. Severe hemorrhage may require surgery—either a high gastrectomy plus vagotomy or a total gastrectomy. Because these operations are associated with a high perioperative mortality, prevention of stress ulcers is extremely important (see also Ch. 62).

Antibiotic-associated pseudomembranous colitis: When diarrhea, which is common after abdominal operations, occurs in a postoperative patient who has received antibiotics, antibiotic-associated pseudomembranous colitis should be considered. Generally limited to the colon, this inflammatory disorder is characterized by membrane-like plaques of exudate that replace necrotic colonic mucosa. The pseudomembranous plaques consist of fibrin, mucin, leukocytes, and sloughed necrotic cells. The underlying mucosa shows varying degrees of superficial necrosis, edema, and inflammation.

Exposure to antibiotics is thought to alter the balance in normal gut flora, allowing overgrowth of *Clostridium difficile*. The diarrhea usually develops within 3 to 4 wk after antibiotic exposure. Clindamycin and lincomycin are the antibiotics most frequently associated with pseudomembranous colitis, although ampicillin, cephalosporins, penicillin, amoxicillin, tetracycline, chloramphenicol, and trimethoprim-sulfamethoxazole have also been implicated. Diagnosis is usually made by bacterial stool culture, stool examination for *C. difficile* toxin, and sigmoidoscopy. Both oral vancomycin 500 mg q 6 h and metronidazole 7.5 mg/kg q 6 h or 500 mg q 6 h are generally safe and effective treatments. This disease is usually self-limiting, but in extreme cases, treatment with IV corticosteroids and emergency colectomy may be necessary. Food sources containing *Lactobacillus*—eg, yogurt or buttermilk—help restore more normal flora.

If diarrhea does occur in a postoperative geriatric patient, stool specimens for bacterial culture and toxin analysis should be obtained immediately. In one study, *C. difficile* assays were performed on specimens from 691 postoperative patients with watery diarrhea; 75 of them had confirmed *C. difficile* infections. The average age of the involved patients was 68 yr. The average time from the initial administration of antibiotics to the onset of diarrhea was 2.7 days. Many of these patients were immunosuppressed because of cancer, sepsis, or diabetes. In 30% of them, the diarrhea disappeared after the antibiotics were discontinued; the others required specific therapy with vancomycin, bacitracin, or metronidazole. Two deaths occurred as a direct result of this type of colitis.

Hemorrhage: Massive bleeding during long operations in which large amounts of blood are transfused and hypothermia and coagulopathy are present may result in hemorrhagic complications. These complications also may occur during convalescence when a secondary operation is required for a complication. The standard treatment includes discontinuing anticoagulant therapy, reversing the effects of heparin with protamine, and transfusing fresh frozen plasma, cryoprecipitate, and platelets.

If bleeding is intolerable during surgery, the surgeon may have to stop the procedure, insert large packs, and close the abdomen. During the next 48 h, the coagulopathy should be vigorously corrected, using fresh frozen plasma, cryoprecipitate, fresh whole blood, and platelets, as necessary. After 48 h, the capillary bleeding usually stops, and the packs can be removed and the surgery completed.

Wound infections: The incidence of wound infections increases with age, possibly because elderly patients are more likely to undergo operations with a high potential for such infections. These procedures include cholecystectomy, herniorrhaphy, colon or other bowel resection, amputations, hysterectomy, total hip replacement, and total knee replacement. For these operations, prophylactic antibiotics should be given.

Wound infections are usually suggested by fever that appears 3 to 5 days after an operation. Physical examination of the wound may elicit more tenderness than is usually expected. Warmth and redness near the wound suggest an infection or early cellulitis. Any superficial wound fullness or swelling, which suggests fluid collection, should be closely examined and may be drained. Fluid obtained should be gram-stained and cultured for aerobic and anaerobic bacteria. The wound does not have to be opened extensively to allow drainage. Rather, complete drainage can usually be achieved by opening a small portion of the incision and inserting a rubber or cloth drain to ensure an opening or tract.

Intra-abdominal abscesses: These abscesses, which are not within the wound but are deep to the fascia, are also suggested by persistent fever and, in many cases, by localized abdominal or flank tenderness. Intra-abdominal abscesses include subphrenic, subhepatic, pelvic, and intraloop abscesses, all of which may be difficult to localize. The computed tomography scan is useful in diagnosing and localizing these abscesses, and ultrasonography is a valuable adjunctive imaging modality. Percutaneous placement of catheters for drainage, using these imaging techniques, has been successful in many cases. Surgery (including operative drainage of the abscess), however, remains the final method of therapy.

Anastomotic suture leakage: Such leakage may occur during healing if the anastomosis dehisces. When this happens, GI contents, feces, bile, pancreatic secretions, or urine may leak into the peritoneal or retroperitoneal spaces. These rare complications are very dangerous if not treated promptly. They occur in the first 10 days postoperatively and are marked by acute onset of an unusual degree of abdominal pain and tenderness.

Treatment consists of immediate reexploration. When possible, the suture line is exteriorized from the abdomen. In cases such as perforation of a duodenal stump, the only possible course is to place drains close to the perforation. In perforations of low colonic anastomoses, drainage and a proximal colostomy are necessary.

Dehiscence: *Disruption of either the skin or fascial closure.* **Skin dehiscence** delays complete skin healing but has little significance otherwise. **Fascial dehiscence,** however, is usually associated with evisceration or herniation of intraperitoneal organs and is a life-threatening condition.

Dehiscence of an abdominal incision often is heralded by profuse discharge of clear fluid from the incision. In nearly all cases of fascial dehiscence, resuture of the incision is necessary. The only treatment for evisceration is placing sterile towels over the exposed bowel and immediately returning the patient to the operating room for fascial closure. In fascial dehiscence, late hernia formation is common.

Urinary tract infection: The risk of urinary tract infection is higher in geriatric surgical patients and is particularly associated with catheterization of the lower genitourinary tract during surgery. The usual symptoms and signs of a urinary tract infection may appear days later, especially in older men with bladder outlet obstruction from benign prostatic hyperplasia.

28. ANESTHESIA CONSIDERATIONS

When an elderly patient is brought to the operating room for a surgical procedure, the anesthesiologist faces a complex physiologic and pharmacologic situation. For the elderly, the risk of anesthesia is greater, the recovery is longer, and the possible complications are more ominous.

Physiologic Considerations

With aging, both functional and structural changes account for the reduced ability to adapt to change in the environment. Height, weight, and body surface area decrease; metabolically active cell mass decreases; body fat increases; muscles shrink; and the liver and kidneys lose about one third of their weight. Commonly used measures of organ function such as cardiac index, oxygen consumption, and glomerular filtration rate tend to underestimate function in the elderly. Many physiologic changes associated with normal aging affect anesthesiologic care (see TABLE 28–1).

Pharmacokinetics

Pharmacokinetics deals with the relationship between the dose of drug administered and the concentration of drug delivered at the site of action. Although age does not affect the absorption of most orally administered drugs, age-related changes in body composition do affect drug distribution. In the elderly, the volume of distribution for water-soluble drugs is decreased, so that a smaller loading dose is required to achieve a given plasma concentration. In practice, therefore, the dose of most water-soluble drugs should be reduced to avoid an overdose. Conversely, the volume of distribution for lipid-soluble drugs in proportion to total body weight may be increased in the elderly.

Most drugs are metabolized by the liver and excreted by the kidneys. In the elderly, drug clearance is decreased because of age-related effects on these organs. TABLE 28–2 lists a number of drugs commonly used during anesthesia and summarizes several pharmacokinetic parameters.

PREOPERATIVE CONSIDERATIONS

Before surgery, the anesthesiologist must evaluate the elderly patient and consider whether preoperative medications or special monitoring or interventions are necessary.

TABLE 28–1. ANESTHETIC IMPLICATIONS OF AGE–RELATED CHANGES

Organ System	*Physiologic Change*	*Functional Change*	*Anesthetic Implications*
Connective tissue	↑ Fibrous tissue ↓ Elasticity	↑ Stiffness	Difficulty positioning patients for intubation and surgery
Bones	↓ Calcium	↑ Fragility	
Joints	Calcium deposition	↓ Mobility	
Skin	↓ Subcutaneous tissue	↑ Fragility ↓ Thermal insulation ↓ Protection of bony surfaces	Predisposition to: Injury from adhesives, monitoring devices, and tape Heat loss (hypothermia) Pressure sores
Pulmonary system	↑ Airway space ↓ Alveolar space ↓ Diffusing capacity	↓ Ability to acquire and deliver oxygen Ventilation-perfusion mismatch ↓ Alveolar ventilation	Tracheal intubation, positive pressure ventilation, and general anesthesia lead to increased ventilation-perfusion mismatch ↓ Alveolar ventilation slows uptake of inhaled anesthetics
	↓ Compliance of lung–chest wall unit	↑ Work of breathing	Regional anesthesia can impair function of accessory muscles of respiration, causing predisposition to respiratory insufficiency
	↓ Chemoreceptor responsiveness	↓ Ventilatory response to hypoxia and hypercapnia	Sedative and narcotic administration cause further predisposition to respiratory insufficiency

(continued)

TABLE 28–1. ANESTHETIC IMPLICATIONS OF AGE–RELATED CHANGES *(Continued)*

Organ System	*Physiologic Change*	*Functional Change*	*Anesthetic Implications*
Cardiovascular system			
Heart	Left ventricular hypertrophy ↓ Distensibility	↓ Maximal cardiac output ↓ Contractility	↓ Maximal cardiac output, ↑ uptake of inhaled anesthetics Most anesthetic agents are negative inotropic agents and vasodilators; hemodynamic response to anesthetic drugs is greater than expected ↑ Sensitivity to changes in intravascular volume
Vessels	Calcium deposition ↓ Compliance ↓ Diffusing capacity	↑ Peripheral resistance ↓ Peripheral perfusion	
Kidney	↓ Number of nephrons ↓ Renal perfusion ↓ Creatinine clearance	Altered water and sodium homeostasis ↓ Elimination of some drugs and their metabolites	Predisposition to fluid and electrolyte abnormalities ↓ Elimination of drugs causes predisposition to relative overdosing and drug toxicity
Liver	↓ Activity of some hepatic enzymes ↓ Number of hepatocytes ↓ Perfusion	↓ Metabolism of some drugs	Predisposition to relative overdosing and drug toxicity

↑ = increased; ↓ = decreased.

TABLE 28–2. PHARMACOKINETICS OF DRUGS USED DURING ANESTHESIA

Drugs	*Clearance*	*% Excretion**	
		Renal	*Biliary*
Lipid-soluble drugs			
Induction agents			
Thiopental	Liver	—	—
Diazepam	Liver	—	—
Lorazepam	Liver	—	—
Midazolam	Liver	—	—
Ketamine	Liver	—	—
Etomidate	Liver, plasma esterase	—	—
Propofol	Liver	—	—
Narcotics			
Meperidine	Liver	—	—
Fentanyl	Liver	—	—
Sufentanil	Liver	—	—
Water-soluble drugs			
Narcotics			
Morphine sulfate	Hepatic, renal metabolism	—	—
Alfentanil	Hepatic, renal metabolism	—	—
Neuromuscular blockers			
Metocurine	—	43	< 2
Pipecuronium	—	70	20
Pancuronium	—	80	10
Tubocurarine	—	45	10–40
Vecuronium	—	15–25	40–75
Atracurium	Hoffman elimination, ester hydrolysis	0	0
Succinylcholine	Plasma cholinesterase	0	0

(continued)

TABLE 28–2. PHARMACOKINETICS OF DRUGS USED DURING ANESTHESIA *(Continued)*

		% Excretion*	
Drugs	*Clearance*	*Renal*	*Biliary*
Water-soluble drugs *(continued)*			
Anticholinesterases			
Neostigmine	Renal excretion, hepatic metabolism	50	—
Pyridostigmine	Renal excretion, hepatic metabolism	75	—
Edrophonium	Renal excretion, hepatic metabolism	75	—

*Data are not available for lipid-soluble drugs.

Preoperative Evaluation

Most elderly patients have existing medical problems, which are superimposed on age-related physiologic changes, complicating management for the anesthesiologist. A thorough history and physical examination is an integral part of formulating an anesthesia plan for the elderly patient. A review of previous hospital records or an interview with family members or friends can help define the patient's medical history. A list of the patient's medications can also provide important information about disease processes. The conditions of particular importance to the anesthesiologist are described in TABLE 28–3.

One of the best sources of information is the elderly patient's primary care physician, who may have records of past medical history, functional status, medications, and allergies. Frequently, test results obtained to prepare a patient for anesthesia can be compared with earlier results available from the primary care physician.

The most important question the anesthesiologist has to answer is not whether the patient is in perfect condition but whether the patient is in optimal condition for the anticipated surgery. Several authorities have tried to identify predictors of adverse outcome. In 1977, Goldman retrospectively identified a number of variables associated with cardiac risk and assigned each a relative weight. He found that not only cardiac problems but also a patient's age and the type of surgery affected cardiac outcome (see TABLE 28–4). Several investigators have since applied the Goldman Cardiac Risk Index prospectively and found that it is not useful in predicting adverse outcome; however, it remains a com-

Table 28–3. ANESTHETIC IMPLICATIONS OF CERTAIN DISORDERS

Disorder	*Physiologic Changes*	*Anesthetic Implications*
Cardiovascular system		
Hypertension	Diastolic dysfunction Left ventricular hypertrophy Impaired coronary blood flow Ventricular ectopy, sudden death End organ damage (heart, brain, kidney)	Poorly controlled hypertension predisposes patient to intraoperative blood pressure lability, which contributes to myocardial ischemia and to CNS and renal complications Postpone elective surgery Consider invasive monitoring for emergent surgery
Coronary artery disease (especially recent myocardial infarction) Heart failure Arrhythmias Aortic stenosis	↑ Incidence of perioperative morbidity (myocardial infarction, pulmonary edema) and mortality	Postpone elective surgery Consider coronary artery surgery or angioplasty in patients with coronary artery disease Perioperative invasive monitoring may ↓ risk of complications
Pulmonary system		
Reactive airways disease Asthma COPD	Predisposition to: ↓ Airflow Arterial desaturation ↑ Pulmonary vascular resistance Right-sided heart failure Ventilation-perfusion mismatch	Optimize preoperative pulmonary function: Treat infection Administer bronchodilators Advise patient to stop smoking Avoid drugs associated with histamine release Consider regional anesthesia to avoid tracheal intubation Perioperative monitoring and respiratory care require: Ventilation Arterial line Pulse oximetry
Endocrine system		
Diabetes mellitus	Poor perioperative glucose control	Avoid oral hypoglycemic agents in perioperative period

(continued)

TABLE 28–3. ANESTHETIC IMPLICATIONS OF CERTAIN DISORDERS *(Continued)*

Disorder	*Physiologic Changes*	*Anesthetic Implications*
Endocrine system *(continued)*		
Diabetes mellitus *(continued)*	Autonomic dysfunction Silent myocardial ischemia Gastroparesis Renal dysfunction Neuropathy	Check blood glucose level frequently Consider invasive monitoring Patient is at risk for aspiration Patient may have fluid and electrolyte abnormalities Blood pressure may be labile
Musculoskeletal system		
Degenerative joint disease	Limited mobility	Problems positioning patients for surgery, regional anesthesia, intubation
	Use of NSAIDs	Impaired platelet function
Rheumatoid arthritis	Use of corticosteroids	Need for stress dose corticosteroid coverage
	High prevalence of atlanto-occipital subluxation and arytenoid involvement	Intubation is hazardous

↑ = increased; ↓ = decreased; COPD = chronic obstructive pulmonary disease; NSAIDs = nonsteroidal anti-inflammatory drugs.

monly used index. Nearly all of the studies agree that a prior myocardial infarction (especially a recent one) or a reduced cardiac functional capacity greatly increases the risk of a postoperative adverse cardiac event. Perioperative optimization of medical problems does improve outcome, and the patient's own physician, by virtue of an established relationship, can best determine that cardiovascular status and respiratory function are optimized, that blood pressure and blood glucose level are well controlled, and that the doses of medication are appropriate for the patient's current condition.

The anesthesiologist may request specific studies to better evaluate a patient's ability to undergo anesthesia and the surgical procedure.

TABLE 28–4. GOLDMAN CARDIAC RISK INDEX

Variable	*Point Value*
Third heart sound or jugular venous distention	11
Recent myocardial infarction	10
Nonsinus rhythm or premature atrial contractions on ECG	7
> 5 Premature ventricular contractions	7
Age > 70 yr	5
Emergency surgery	4
Poor general medical condition	3
Intraperitoneal, intrathoracic, or aortic surgery	3
Important valvular aortic stenosis	3

Predictive Class	*Point Range*	*Cardiac Complication Rate*
I	0–5	1%
II	6–12	7%
III	13–25	14%
IV	> 26	78%

Adapted from information appearing in Goldman L, Caldera DL, Nussbaum SR, et al: "Multifactorial index of cardiac risk in noncardiac surgical procedures." *New England Journal of Medicine* 297:845, 1977; used with permission.

These studies may include an exercise stress test or cardiac catheterization. When the requested data are available, the anesthesiologist can formulate an anesthesia plan that best fits the patient's needs.

Preoperative Medication

Many anesthesiologists avoid preoperative sedation for elderly patients because it further reduces the already compromised ventilatory response to hypoxia and hypercapnia. The muscarinic anticholinergics, such as atropine and scopolamine, are generally not needed to decrease oral secretions because newer anesthetics cause fewer secretion problems in the airways. Besides producing an unpleasantly dry mouth, atropine and scopolamine can cause CNS side effects. Atropine, usually considered stimulatory, may produce excitement and delirium; scopolamine, a sedative amnestic, can cause agitation, restlessness, and hallucinations in elderly patients. If an anticholinergic is necessary, glycopyrrolate, which is poorly lipid soluble and does not cross the blood brain barrier, is the drug of choice.

INTRAOPERATIVE CONSIDERATIONS

Anesthesia

Depending on the circumstances, the anesthesiologist may provide monitored anesthesia care, regional anesthesia, or general anesthesia.

Monitored anesthesia care: When patients do not need analgesia for a procedure or when the surgeon administers it, the anesthesiologist provides monitored anesthesia care, which consists of monitoring the patient's vital signs and providing sedation as needed. Procedures such as cataract surgery, pacemaker placement, inguinal hernia repair, and extracorporeal shock wave lithotripsy are often done with monitored anesthesia care.

Regional anesthesia: This type of anesthesia includes spinal anesthesia, epidural anesthesia, and blockade of other major nerves such as the cervical or brachial plexus. Procedures of the lower abdomen, pelvis, and legs can be done with spinal or epidural anesthesia in certain patients. Spinal or epidural blockade produces profound sympathetic block, which can precipitate hypotension in patients with inadequate volume status. In the elderly, epidural anesthetics have a faster onset and a greater spread; the duration of action can be prolonged because of reduced clearance. Whenever possible, adjuvant therapy with anticholinergics should be avoided because of the high risk of inducing delirium and other complications.

General anesthesia: General anesthesia provides loss of consciousness, amnesia, analgesia, and a variable degree of muscle relaxation. Generally, the patient's airway is secured with an endotracheal tube, and ventilation is controlled. Most of the general anesthetics are potent myocardial depressants and vasodilators. The metabolism of these drugs is governed by the pharmacokinetic factors described above.

The dosage requirements for the induction agents propofol, midazolam, and thiopental are significantly reduced in the elderly. Ketamine and etomidate have been suggested as induction agents of choice for geriatric patients because of their minimal effects on the cardiovascular system, but little information is available about the effect of age on exact dose requirement. The volatile anesthetics halothane, enflurane, and isoflurane impair the already attenuated chemoreceptor response in the elderly. Also, the minimal alveolar concentration of these agents decreases linearly with age.

The muscle relaxants pancuronium and tubocurarine have an increased duration of action in the elderly because the termination of their activity depends largely on renal and hepatic clearance. This is not true of the shorter-acting neuromuscular blockers atracurium and vecuronium. Few data are available on the effects of aging on succinylcholine activity, but it is commonly held that the longer circulatory time in the elderly allows more time for hydrolysis of the drug, so that a larger initial dose may be necessary.

The duration of action of opioids is also prolonged in the elderly because clearance is decreased and sensitivity to these drugs is increased. The sedative and respiratory depressant effects of opioids may contribute to the postoperative pulmonary complications frequently observed in this age group.

In hip fracture surgery, both regional and general anesthesia are used, and considerable debate exists over which is the best technique with respect to early and late survival and the incidence of postoperative thromboembolic disease and confusion. Investigators have found no difference in the incidence of postoperative confusion between elderly patients who had regional anesthesia and those who had general anesthesia for hip fracture repair. The current consensus is that spinal anesthesia has no advantage over general anesthesia in improving either short-term or long-term outcomes in elderly patients undergoing surgical hip repair. Regional anesthesia does provide some protection against deep venous thrombophlebitis, but it is not associated with a sustained improvement in outcome.

Other Considerations

Obtaining vascular access to use monitoring devices and to administer drugs, fluids, and blood can be a challenge in the elderly. Arthritic changes can make intubation and positioning for surgery difficult. Also, increased skin fragility makes the elderly person prone to injury from restraining devices, tape, Bovie pads, and adhesive monitoring devices such as ECG electrodes. Extra padding should be placed on operating tables, and care should be exercised in positioning extremities to avoid injury.

The elderly also have significant problems with perioperative temperature regulation. Heat production is reduced as a result of their lower basal metabolic rate. Thinning of the skin and loss of subcutaneous fat make the skin a less effective insulator, so that body heat conservation is also impaired. The relative increase in body surface area with respect to body mass and the impaired vasomotor response in older persons predispose them to heat loss. During anesthesia, the thermoregulatory center in the hypothalamus is anesthetized; patients are pharmacologically paralyzed and given sympathetic blocking agents. Thus, heat production is prevented, and heat loss is promoted. A major sequela of hypothermia is the surge in oxygen consumption that occurs with shivering during the rewarming period. If oxygen demand exceeds supply, hypoxemia, acidosis, and circulatory changes occur, and the elderly patient may be unable to compensate. To minimize the risk of hypothermia and its sequelae, the operating room, inspired gases, IV solutions, and antibacterial solutions used to prepare the surgical site should be warmed. Forced-air warming blankets help prevent heat loss and should be used, especially when patients are hypothermic.

POSTOPERATIVE ANALGESIA

Controlling postoperative pain in the elderly can be difficult. The major goal of such control is patient comfort; a secondary goal is decreased morbidity and mortality. Adequate analgesia may improve cardiovascular and pulmonary function. By preventing the stress response to postoperative pain, adequate analgesia may also lower the incidence of postoperative myocardial events.

Much of the decrease in ventilatory function after thoracic and abdominal surgeries results from surgical trauma and splinting from postoperative pain. Postoperative analgesia cannot undo the decrease in ventilatory function produced by surgical trauma or lung resection. However, anesthesiologists and surgeons can help prevent splinting by providing adequate analgesia, thus helping patients breathe deeply and cough, improving mucous removal and avoiding atelectasis. By avoiding atelectasis, patients also reduce the risk of postoperative pneumonia and hypoxia.

Patients who receive adequate postoperative pain relief generally walk earlier and are discharged sooner than those who do not. Thus, adequate analgesia helps in achieving the overall goal of most surgical procedures: to return the patient to an improved functional state in the community, which benefits both the patient and society. Also, by shortening the hospital stay, adequate analgesia reduces the cost of medical care.

To achieve postoperative analgesia, an anesthesiologist may use a narcotic, a nonsteroidal anti-inflammatory drug, or a regional anesthetic method. Each choice has its advantages and disadvantages as a modality for analgesia in the elderly (see also Ch. 12).

Narcotic Analgesics

Narcotic analgesics have been the traditional mainstay of postoperative pain control. However, before ordering a narcotic, the physician should consider its effect and side effects. The same dose given to a young adult and an older adult will have a stronger effect on the older one. In older patients, important clinical side effects are usually dose related and include sedation, confusion, respiratory depression, and constipation. Despite these concerns, by far *the most common error in narcotic use is undermedication.*

Intramuscular injections produce initially high plasma drug levels that can cause undesirable side effects; then the levels rapidly decline, leading to a recurrence of pain. Thus, patients are alternately overdosed and uncomfortable. In an alert older person, meticulous titration of narcotic in the recovery room followed by **patient-controlled analgesia** provides excellent pain relief. Patient-controlled analgesia provides a more stable blood level of medication, avoiding the roller-coaster effects of IM dosing.

Unfortunately, not every elderly patient is a candidate for patient-controlled analgesia. A confused or demented patient cannot safely or effectively use this method. If regional techniques and nonsteroidal anti-inflammatory drugs are ineffective or inappropriate, a **continuous narcotic infusion** may be useful. Fentanyl is an appropriate choice because of its relative lack of hemodynamic side effects. However, hepatic clearance of the drug is decreased in the elderly. Also, the drug is lipophilic, and the increased proportion of body fat in the elderly leads to an increased volume of distribution. These factors increase the elimination time in the elderly. Because the volume of distribution and clearance of a drug cannot be precisely determined for an individual patient, the proper loading dose and infusion rate must be estimated. In the recovery room, patients can be given fentanyl 15 to 25 μg IV q 5 min until the desired analgesic effect is reached. The goal is to avoid excessive sedation or respiratory depression while maintaining blood pressure and pulse within acceptable limits. Once a patient is made comfortable with a loading dose of fentanyl in the recovery room, an infusion can be started at 1 μg/kg/h. The patient should then be monitored in the recovery room for at least 2 h, so that the infusion can be adjusted. On the surgical unit, hourly nursing assessments of vital signs, respirations, mental status, and arousability should be performed. Often, such intense monitoring is available only in a step-down or intensive care unit.

Nonsteroidal Anti-Inflammatory Drugs

Nonsteroidal anti-inflammatory drugs (NSAIDs) are very useful for controlling pain in the elderly. For minor procedures, oral doses of NSAIDs often provide excellent pain relief. For more painful procedures, NSAIDs can supplement other methods of analgesia. Ketorolac can be administered IV or IM, and indomethacin can be given rectally in patients unable to tolerate oral preparations.

The advantage of these drugs is their relative lack of sedative or respiratory depressant effects. When an NSAID is combined with a narcotic, less narcotic is needed, so undesirable side effects decrease. Ketorolac should be given cautiously to a patient who has received large narcotic doses. The added pain relief from the NSAID can unmask the respiratory depressant effects of the narcotic.

The potential benefits of NSAID therapy must be weighed against the possible complications. Use of NSAIDs can irritate the GI tract, predispose patients to ulcers and bleeding, cause sodium retention, and impair renal function. These drugs also interfere with platelet function.

If a patient has a bleeding diathesis or has undergone a craniotomy where even a small amount of postoperative bleeding could be disastrous, NSAIDs should not be used. For these persons, acetaminophen q 4 h may provide some relief.

Regional Techniques

Regional analgesia can often be extremely beneficial for elderly patients. One advantage of regional techniques is the reduced amount of narcotic needed. The disadvantages include the hemodynamic changes associated with epidural local anesthetics and the potential for intravascular injection, infection, bleeding, and nerve damage. When a regional anesthetic block is performed before a painful stimulus (ie, surgery) is initiated, pain relief lasts longer than would be expected from the pharmacokinetics of the local anesthetic. When the pain does recur, it is less intense, and lower doses of narcotic can be used. The mechanism for this phenomenon appears to occur at the spinal cord level and involves modulation of the impulses eventually received in the brain.

Regional analgesic techniques range in complexity from instillation of local anesthetic into the surgical incision to specific nerve blocks to continuous epidural infusions of local anesthetic, a narcotic, or a combination of the two. The choice of technique depends on the surgical site and the relative complexity and potential advantages or disadvantages of a particular technique.

Pain relief after limb surgery is often accomplished with a single-dose nerve block or a continuous infusion. For hand and elbow procedures, the axillary approach is used to block the brachial plexus because this approach can be used with relative ease and it has a lower incidence of complications than the other approaches to this plexus have. If a need for prolonged analgesia is anticipated, a catheter is inserted and an infusion of local anesthetic is begun postoperatively. Often an infusion of bupivacaine 0.125% is sufficient for complete pain relief. The infusion rate is usually started at 8 to 10 mL/h and titrated to desired effectiveness.

After knee procedures, a continuous femoral sheath catheter technique can be used. Although the sciatic nerve is not blocked with this approach, patients still receive adequate analgesia. The femoral catheter infusion may be supplemented by low-dose narcotics or ketorolac. For both the axillary and femoral sheath blocks, a blunt tip needle may be used. The same needle may be used for both single-dose and continuous infusion techniques. The distinct pop felt when the needle enters the sheath signals an excellent end point for proper needle placement. This pop is much more evident with the blunt needles than with the traditional B-bevel needles. Also, with the blunt needles, entering the adjacent artery is more difficult, and the incidence of nerve damage is decreased.

Epidural analgesia: After hip, abdominal, or thoracic procedures, a continuous epidural technique is often used for analgesia. An infusion of bupivacaine 0.125% to 0.0625% solution containing fentanyl 4 to 5 μg/mL usually provides excellent analgesia. When the epidural catheter is placed at the dermatome level where discomfort is perceived, the amount of local anesthetic and narcotic can be reduced, minimizing the possibility of toxicity. For hip procedures, a lumbar, epidural catheter placement is used; for abdominal procedures, a low-thoracic, epidural catheter placement is used; and for thoracotomies, a midthoracic, epidural catheter placement is used. Fentanyl is lipophilic and does not spread widely in the epidural space, so the catheter must be placed close to the segmental area of the lesion. The need for precise catheter placement can be circumvented by using epidural morphine, which spreads more readily in the epidural space. However, the rostral spread of morphine may result in late respiratory depression.

The most common complication is inadvertent removal of the catheter during routine nursing care. Meticulous taping of the catheter and nursing education can reduce this problem. Urinary retention secondary to the local anesthetic and the narcotic occurs and is more prevalent in elderly men. Migration of the catheter to the subcutaneous tissues or the spinal space can also occur. The former results in a lack of pain relief; the latter can result in disastrously high spinal anesthesia. Fortunately, the latter rarely occurs.

In an elderly patient, an epidural infusion must be titrated precisely, and intravascular volume must be maintained by close monitoring of fluid status. Blood loss of 300 to 500 mL from a hip wound drain can result in severe hypotension in an elderly patient with a sympathetic blockade if volume resuscitation is not promptly instituted.

Postoperative pain control in the elderly patient is best accomplished by a dedicated, functioning pain control service. Strict attention to the patient's hemodynamic parameters and mental status along with a thorough understanding of the altered effects of various medications in the elderly are essential. Cooperation between the surgical, nursing, and pain service staffs can provide safe and effective analgesia for even the most frail elderly patient.

29. REHABILITATION

Rehabilitation refers to a combination of physiatrics; physical, occupational, and speech therapy; psychiatric counseling; and social work directed toward helping persons maintain or recover their physical capacities. Often, rehabilitation is needed after stroke and hip fracture. It is also commonly needed after serious cardiac events or illnesses associated with prolonged bed rest that results in deconditioning.

In geriatric rehabilitation, the goal is usually to help the person regain functional independence after a loss caused by a medical or surgical event. For some younger persons, the goal is to achieve full, unrestricted function, but for older persons, the challenge is to restore the ability to perform as many activities of daily living **(ADLs)** as possible.

Progress may be slow for elderly patients. Even for those who regain their premorbid functional status, the rehabilitation process is very slow and may take months. Many factors common among the elderly (eg, lack of endurance because of cardiovascular complications, suboptimal nutritional status, lack of motivation, depression, dementia, diminished muscle strength, and reduced joint mobility, coordination, and agility) contribute to a pessimistic functional prognosis and a long restorative process. Any of these factors may have an adverse effect on regaining function. Also, a lengthy rehabilitation may place a great financial burden on an elderly person.

Despite these problems, age alone is not a reason to postpone or avoid rehabilitation. With modifications, even impaired older persons can benefit greatly from rehabilitation programs.

REHABILITATION PROGRAMS

Rehabilitation may require only one discipline, but usually it draws on the coordinated efforts of more than one. When a complex problem requires expertise from several disciplines, a rehabilitation team can develop a program to coordinate therapy.

Usually, rehabilitation programs are organized around a particular type or set of problems. For example, a program may be designed to help patients recover from hip fracture, stroke, myocardial infarction, or heart surgery. The program can coordinate the needed services in an environment designed to facilitate recovery. Also, persons with similar conditions can work together toward a common goal, encouraging each other and reinforcing the rehabilitation training.

Rehabilitation programs for geriatric patients include medical care that would not be needed for younger adults. Nurses and therapists can more easily adjust goals and the intensity of care to older patients when they are not integrated with younger ones, who usually can handle more intensive, demanding therapy. Also, in segregated programs, older patients will not compare their progress with that of younger patients and thus become discouraged. Moreover, the social work needed to provide postdischarge care can be more readily integrated into the program.

Many different settings have geriatric rehabilitation programs, and the extent, aggressiveness, and duration of treatment varies from program to program. Although rehabilitation may begin in the hospital, organized rehabilitation programs rarely exist there. Rehabilitation hospitals usually provide the most extensive and aggressive care and should be considered for patients who have the most potential and who can participate in aggressive intervention. Patients in rehabilitation hospitals must receive and be able to tolerate at least 3 h of therapy daily. Many nursing homes have programs as well, but they are far less intensive. Generally, these programs are limited to 1 h daily and fewer than 5 days a week. Services may be delivered in outpatient settings or at home, but these alternatives cannot deliver the two or three daily treatments and the variety of services supplied in institutions. Providing care to a disabled elderly person at home is most desirable, but it can be physically and emotionally taxing to a caregiver. The spouse may not be physically able to help, and the children may be too busy with their own families. Home health aides are available in some communities but usually cannot provide round-the-clock care. Thus, when the disability is severe, institutionalization may be necessary. Nonetheless, creative home care may be possible, especially for those with substantial financial resources.

At the start of treatment, the duration of therapy must be considered and discussed with patients and their families because not all persons can invest the time needed for optimal results. For example, after a hip fracture, complete rehabilitation may take 6 or 8 wk; after a stroke, it may take several months. For patients unable or unwilling to remain in a rehabilitation facility that long, the goals must be altered. Determining the goal of rehabilitation helps determine how and where to accomplish it.

Rehabilitation is initiated by a physician who writes a referral containing instructions to an allied health professional. Like any prescription, this referral is a legal document. Without it, the allied health professional cannot treat the patient.

Because the allied health professional is carrying out the physician's orders, the physician establishes the goal of therapy and is responsible for the efficacy and side effects of treatment. Therefore, referrals should be appropriately detailed, including all relevant information and some initial directions. An appropriate referral would be: "Independent in ambulation 1 mo poststroke. Please evaluate and treat for stability and strength" or "3 wk post–hip fracture. Please continue therapy for independent transfer and gait." Although many therapists accept vague orders such as, "Physical therapy to evaluate and treat," this type of order is not adequate. Physicians who are unfamiliar with writing orders to therapists should consult with senior therapists, physiatrists, or orthopedic surgeons.

Before prescribing any exercise program, the physician should determine that the patient is medically stable and advise the therapist about any chronic cardiac, pulmonary, neurologic, or musculoskeletal limitations. Older patients may have several problems, and treatment must often be prioritized. Physicians should work closely with therapists to decide which problems to work on first and when to move on to others.

A **physiatrist,** a physician who specializes in rehabilitation medicine, treats patients with disabilities, coordinating a team of physicians and allied health professionals, and helps patients develop and implement a comprehensive treatment plan. This plan is not limited to the hospital but extends to the patient's community, family, friends, occupation, and lifestyle.

After performing an evaluation, the therapist creates a treatment plan. The therapist then implements and monitors the plan, adjusting goals and interventions.

Often, leisure or recreational therapy is part of the care plan for demented or institutionalized patients who need physical activity but who do not need the specialized resources of physical therapy. Social workers and discharge planners are responsible for plans for discharge and postdischarge care. Nurses are responsible for augmenting formal therapy and reinforcing the lessons taught during therapy sessions.

THERAPEUTIC MODALITIES

Persons undergoing rehabilitation may require therapeutic exercises, training in ADLs, transfer training, and treatment for pain and inflammation.

THERAPEUTIC EXERCISES

Depending on the patient's needs, the following therapies may be used: range-of-motion exercises, muscle strengthening exercises, proprioceptive neuromuscular facilitation, coordination exercises, use of a tilt table, general conditioning exercises, and ambulation exercises.

Restricted motion is a common problem after a stroke or prolonged bed rest. It can cause pain, reduce functional abilities, and predispose patients to pressure sores.

Range-of-Motion Exercises

Goniometric range-of-motion evaluation should be recorded before therapy and regularly thereafter. Normal range-of-motion values are shown in TABLE 29–1. Typically, the values for certain joints are lower in fully functional elderly persons than they are in younger persons. Still, persons with this age-related reduction in range of motion should be able to perform ADLs without assistance.

Moving a joint frequently within its full range maintains the range of motion. **Active range-of-motion exercise** is used when a patient is able to exercise without assistance. **Active assistive range-of-motion exercise** is used when the muscles are too weak (requiring additional strengthening exercises) or when joint movement causes discomfort. **Passive range-of-motion exercise** is used when a patient cannot actively participate (see FIG. 29–1).

Assistive or passive exercise must be carried out *very gently*. Restricted joints can easily be damaged by aggressive movements, and

TABLE 29–1. NORMAL VALUES FOR RANGE OF MOTION OF JOINTS*

Joint	*Motion*	*Range*
Hip	Flexion	0° to 115°–125°
	Extension	115°–125° to 0°
	Hyperextension†	0° to 10°–15°
	Abduction	0° to 45°
	Adduction	45° to 0°
	Lateral rotation	0° to 45°
	Medial rotation	0° to 45°
Knee	Flexion	0° to 120°–130°
	Extension	120°–130° to 0°
Ankle	Plantar flexion	0° to 40°–50°
	Dorsiflexion	0° to 20°
Foot	Inversion	0° to 35°
	Eversion	0° to 25°
Toes		
Metatarsophalangeal joints	Flexion	0° to 20°–30°
	Extension	0° to 80°
Interphalangeal joints	Flexion	0° to 50°
	Extension	50° to 0°
Shoulder	Flexion to 90°	0° to 90°
	Extension	0° to 50°
	Abduction to 90°	0° to 90°
	Adduction	90° to 0°
	Lateral rotation	0° to 90°
	Medial rotation	0° to 90°
Elbow	Flexion	0° to 145°–160°
	Extension	145°–160° to 0°
	Pronation	0° to 90°
	Supination	0° to 90°

(continued)

TABLE 29–1. NORMAL VALUES FOR RANGE OF MOTION OF JOINTS* *(Continued)*

Joint	*Motion*	*Range*
Wrist	Flexion	0° to 90°
	Extension	0° to 70°
	Abduction	0° to 25°
	Adduction	0° to 55°–65°
Fingers		
Metacarpophalangeal joints	Flexion	0° to 90°
	Extension	0° to 20°–30°
Interphalangeal joints	Flexion	0° to 120°
	Extension	120° to 0°
Interphalangeal distal joints	Flexion	0° to 80°
	Extension	80° to 0°
Finger	Abduction	0° to 20°–25°
	Adduction	20°–25° to 0°
Thumb		
Metacarpophalangeal joints	Flexion	0° to 60°–70°
	Extension	60°–70° to 0°
Interphalangeal joints	Flexion	0° to 90°
	Extension	90° to 0°
Thumb	Abduction	0° to 40°–50°
	Adduction	40°–60° to 0°

* Ranges are for persons of all ages; age-specific ranges have not been established.
† Extension beyond midline.

bones made fragile by osteoporosis can break with minimal stress. Movements producing severe pain should be avoided, although some discomfort may be unavoidable. Passive exercise should never be applied to joints adjacent to an unfixed fracture.

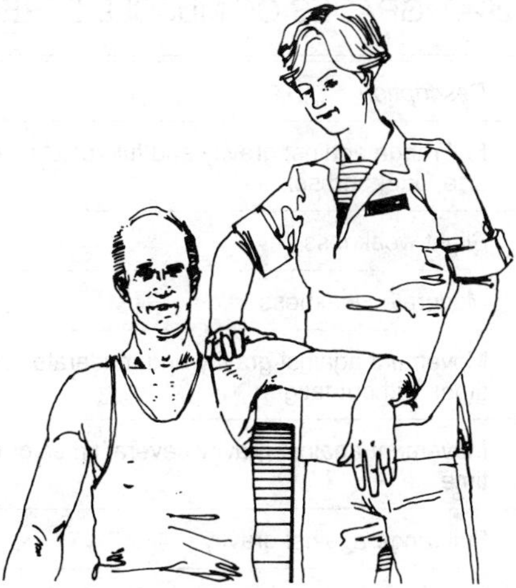

FIG. 29–1. Passive range of motion at the shoulder joint.

Tight muscles can be stretched more vigorously than a tight joint. Thus, before beginning treatment of a restricted joint, the therapist must determine if the problem involves muscles or ligaments and tendons. The joint must be moved beyond the point of pain but without causing residual pain. Momentary forceful stretching is not as effective as sustained moderate stretching. Sustained stretching may be accomplished by applying 5- to 50-lb weights with pulleys for 20 min a day. Manual stretching is both time-consuming and fatiguing for therapists. When tissue temperature is raised to about 43° C (109° F), stretching exercise is usually more effective and less painful (see HEAT AND COLD, below).

Muscle Strengthening Exercises

Many techniques can be used to increase muscle strength, but all involve two basic principles: **resistance** (applied manually or mechanically) and **progression,** eg, progressive resistive exercise. Resistance may be applied with just gravity or may be increased with weights or mechanical resistance. When the exercise becomes easy, the resistance is increased. In this way, exercise builds muscle mass, increases strength, and helps improve endurance. Muscle strength can be graded as described in TABLE 29–2.

TABLE 29–2. GRADES OF MUSCLE STRENGTH

Grade	*Description*
5 or N (Normal)	Full range against gravity and full resistance for the patient's size, age, and sex
N − (Normal minus)	Slight weakness
G + (Good plus)	Moderate weakness
4 or G (Good)	Movement against gravity and moderate resistance at least 10 times without fatigue
F + (Fair plus)	Movement against gravity several times or mild resistance one time
3 or F (Fair)	Full range against gravity
F − (Fair minus)	Movement against gravity and complete range one time
P + (Poor plus)	Full range with gravity eliminated but some resistance applied
2 or P (Poor)	Full range with gravity eliminated
P − (Poor minus)	Incomplete range of motion with gravity eliminated
1 or T (Trace)	Evidence of contracture (visible or palpable) but no joint movement
0 (Zero)	No palpable or visible contracture and no joint movement

Proprioceptive Neuromuscular Facilitation

Proprioceptive neuromuscular facilitation helps promote useful neuromuscular activity in patients who have upper motor neuron damage with resulting spasticity. For example, applying strong resistance to the left elbow flexor (biceps) of a patient with a right hemiplegia causes the right elbow to flex through contraction of the hemiplegic biceps. The exact mechanism is not clearly understood, but it is thought that reflex-related proprioception results in movement of the extremity. The patient can gain feelings of muscle contraction, further helping maintain the joint's range of motion. Various techniques (eg, Brunnstrom, Rood, and Bobath) are widely used.

Coordination Exercises

These task-oriented exercises involve the repetition of a meaningful movement. Unlike range-of-motion and muscle strengthening exercises, coordination exercises involve more than one joint and one muscle. No matter how simple the movement, a meaningful movement such as picking up an object or touching a body part requires various muscles to contract and relax in a coordinated manner. Coordination exercises provide a simple way to improve skills, but they require repetition.

Use of a Tilt Table

In persons with orthostatic hypotension from paraplegia or quadriplegia, prolonged bed rest, or immobilization, a tilt table may be used to help reestablish hemodynamic balance. The supine patient is strapped to a padded table fitted with a footboard, and the table is tilted manually or electrically. The angle is increased very slowly to 85° in an upright position, as tolerated by the patient. Initially, the duration of each treatment depends on the patient's tolerance but should not exceed 45 min. Treatments are given once or twice daily. The success rate depends on the disability and the duration of immobilization.

General Conditioning Exercises

These exercises are used to treat the effects of debilitation, prolonged bed rest, or immobilization. The exercises combine various interventions to reestablish hemodynamic balance, increase cardiorespiratory capacity, and maintain range of motion and muscle strength.

Ambulation Exercises

These exercises aim to improve walking on level surfaces either independently or with the assistance of a person or device. Before starting ambulation exercises, a patient may need range-of-motion and muscle strengthening exercises. If individual muscles remain weak or spastic, an orthotic device, such as a brace, may be used. Training may begin on parallel bars, especially if the patient's balance is impaired, and progress to walking with aids, such as a walker, crutches, or cane. With some patients, an assistive belt helps the therapist prevent falls. Anyone assisting patients should know how to properly support them (see FIG. 29–2).

If the patient will need to use stairs after rehabilitative therapy, training should start as soon as the patient can walk safely on level surfaces. Ascent starts with the better leg, and descent with the affected leg (ie, "good is up and bad is down"). A patient who will be walking outdoors should be taught how to step over a curb. Patients who use walkers must learn special techniques for traversing curbs or using stairs. Before discharge, the social worker or therapist should arrange to have secure handrails installed along all stairs in the patient's home.

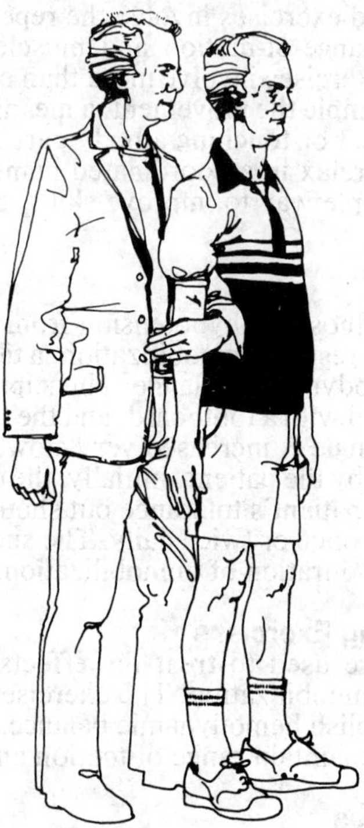

Fig. 29–2. Supporting a patient during ambulation. If the patient is wearing a waist belt, the left hand is used to grasp it in the back.

ACTIVITIES OF DAILY LIVING TRAINING

Activities of daily living (ADLs) include personal hygiene, grooming, bathing, dressing, feeding, toileting, and transferring. Instrumental activities of daily living (IADLs) include cooking, cleaning, shopping, managing medications, managing finances, using the telephone, and traveling. Not everyone needs to accomplish all these activities to remain independent, and with assistance from the patient and family, the social worker and therapist can determine which ones are essential. The patient's physical and social responsibilities at home determine training needs. Even in an institution, training in ADLs is crucial for maintaining dignity and physical independence (see Ch. 30).

Before training begins, the therapist must assess the patient's functional status. Ideally, this assessment takes place in the patient's home; however, assessment in that setting is rarely feasible, and a simulated environment is typically used. The evaluation may indicate a need for self-help devices or training.

TRANSFERRING

The inability to transfer safely is one reason elderly patients become or remain institutionalized. When patients cannot transfer independently from bed to chair, chair to commode, or chair to a standing position, they generally require 24-h attendants. Thus, transfer capability is an essential part of evaluation and treatment in rehabilitation programs.

Transfer training is particularly important after a hip fracture or stroke. The techniques used depend on whether the patient can bear weight on one or both legs, has sound balance, or has hemiplegia. Assistive devices can sometimes help, and for persons who have difficulty going from a seated to a standing position, raising the level of the chair or using a self-lifting chair may be beneficial.

TREATMENT OF PAIN AND INFLAMMATION

Therapies for pain and inflammation include heat, cold, electric stimulation, traction, massage, and acupuncture.

Heat and Cold

Heat increases blood flow and the extensibility of connective tissue; decreases joint stiffness, pain, and muscle spasm; and helps resolve inflammation, edema, and exudates. Heat application may be superficial or deep. The intensity and duration of the physiologic effects are determined mainly by tissue temperature, the rate of temperature elevation, and the area treated.

Indications for heat are acute and chronic traumatic and inflammatory conditions such as sprains, strains, fibrositis, tenosynovitis, muscle spasm, myositis, painful back, whiplash injuries, various forms of arthritis, arthralgia, and neuralgia.

Superficial Heat

Infrared heat: Applied with a lamp, an infrared heat treatment usually lasts 20 min and is repeated daily. Contraindications include advanced heart disease, peripheral vascular disease, impaired skin sensation (particularly of temperature and pain), and significant hepatic or renal insufficiency. Precautions must be taken to avoid burns.

Hot packs: Use of hot packs is the most common method of applying heat. Commercially available hot packs consist of cotton cloth containers filled with silicate gel. They are placed in boiling water, left to cool, and applied when they reach a temperature that will not burn the skin. Wrapping the packs in several layers of towels helps protect the skin from burns. Contraindications are the same as for infrared heat.

Paraffin wax: Heat can also be applied by melting paraffin wax to 49° C (120° F). Wax above 54.4° C (130° F) should not be used. Since the heating effect is relatively short-lived, radiant heat may be applied immediately afterward.

Paraffin can be applied by dipping, immersing, painting, or wrapping; a hand is easy to dip or immerse, whereas a knee or elbow is best treated by painting. Paraffin wax is usually used to apply heat to small joints; it should not be used on open wounds or on persons allergic to paraffin.

Hydrotherapy: Hydrotherapy may be used to enhance wound healing or to apply heat. Agitated warm water stimulates blood flow and debrides wounds. This treatment is often done in a Hubbard tank (a large, industrial Jacuzzi) at 35.5° C to 37.7° C (96° F to 100° F).

Total immersion at temperatures of 37.7° C to 40° C (100° F to 104° F) may also be used to help relax muscles and relieve pain. Warm baths, especially whirlpools, are particularly useful in conjunction with range-of-motion exercise. For localized areas, the whirlpool and lowboy are used. Hydrotherapy has no contraindications. However, patients may become fatigued during treatment, and blood pressure may fall.

Deep Heat

Shortwave diathermy: Though it appears to be less efficacious than previously thought, shortwave diathermy is still used sometimes to treat inflammation, the pain of urinary calculi, pelvic infections, and acute and chronic sinusitis. Contraindications include malignancy, hemorrhagic conditions, peripheral vascular disease, loss of sensation, and nonremovable prostheses, pacemakers, or electrophysiologic braces.

CAUTION: *Shortwave diathermy cannot be used in people with metallic implants (eg, bars, screws, plates) because the heated metal may cause a burn. Implanted devices may also malfunction or be destroyed. No metallic substance should be in contact with the skin.*

Microwave diathermy: Simpler to apply than shortwave diathermy, microwave diathermy has more accurate output measurement and better deep heating without undue heating of the skin. It is also more comfortable. Microwaves are selectively absorbed into tissues with high water content (eg, muscles), producing deeper heat and less superficial damage. Despite its advantages, microwave diathermy is not used as widely as shortwave diathermy or ultrasound. Indications and contraindications are the same as for shortwave diathermy.

Ultrasound: Ultrasound is the use of high-frequency sound waves to penetrate deep into the tissue (4 to 10 cm), providing thermal, mechanical, chemical, and biological effects. This therapy may be used to treat limited range of motion caused by muscle shortening and fibrosis, skin or subcutaneous tissue scarring, calcific bursitis and tendinitis, pain from postoperative neurofibromas (especially when embedded in scar tissue), phantom pain, bursitis, myositis, tenosynovitis, epicondylitis, spondylitis, contusions, neuritis, and reflex dystrophies such as Sudeck's atrophy, causalgia, and shoulder-hand syndrome. Other possible indications are sciatica and other forms of radiculitis, myofascial pain syndrome, and chronic skin ulceration.

Ultrasound should not be used to treat ischemic tissue, hemorrhagic diathesis, malignancies, anesthetized areas, or areas of acute infection. Also, it should not be used over the eyes, brain, spinal cord, ears, heart, reproductive organs, brachial plexus, or healing bone.

Cryotherapy

Cold application may be beneficial in treating muscle spasm, myofascial or traumatic pain, acute low back pain, and acute inflammatory lesions as well as in inducing local anesthesia. The choice between heat and cold therapies is often empiric. When heat does not work, cold is applied. However, for acute low back pain, cryotherapy seems to be better than heat therapy.

Cold may be applied locally using an ice bag or cold pack. Local cooling may also be produced by evaporation of volatile fluids, such as ethyl chloride. The spread of cold on the skin depends on the thickness of the epidermis, its underlying fat and muscle, the water content of the tissue, and the rate of blood flow. Care must be taken to avoid tissue damage (ie, frostbite) and general hypothermia.

Electric Stimulation

Electric stimulation of denervated skeletal muscle and innervated muscle that cannot be contracted voluntarily may help treat or prevent disuse atrophy and muscle spasticity—especially in those with hemiplegia from cerebrovascular accident, traumatic paraplegia and quadriplegia, and peripheral nerve injuries. The unipolar technique uses a large dispersive electrode at a distant part of the body and a smaller active electrode on the muscle being treated. This technique uses a lower current than the bipolar method and is the method of choice when it produces the desired contractile response. The bipolar technique uses two small electrodes over the ends of the muscle. This technique is useful for severely degenerated muscles caused by gross anatomic or physiologic interruption of the nerve supply and for unusually high skin impedance (eg, when edema exists in the area being treated).

Usually, 10 to 20 muscle contractions per session are sufficient. Overstimulation may cause muscle fatigue, which may eventually result in damage. Electrode burns may result from inadequate skin contact or too much current. This technique should not be used in persons with advanced cardiac disease or a pacemaker. It also should not be used over the eyes.

Transcutaneous electric nerve stimulation (TENS) is a low-frequency variation of electric therapy used for pain relief. Stimulation may be applied several times daily, each session ranging from 20 min to several hours, depending on the severity of pain. Often, patients are taught to use the TENS device and decide when to apply the treatment. The patient feels a gentle tingling sensation without an increase in muscle tension.

This technique is particularly useful for chronic back pain, rheumatoid arthritis, sprained ankle, contusion, postherpetic neuralgia, causalgia, phantom limb syndrome, and trigger points. It may also aid callus formation of a nonunited fracture. When the electrodes are improperly placed on the skin, erythema may develop. This treatment should not be used by a person with advanced cardiac disease or a pacemaker because it may precipitate an arrhythmia. It also should not be applied over the eyes.

This therapy varies from highly effective to virtually ineffective. But TENS is harmless, and the unit's small size and portability as well as the low cost of operation make it attractive.

TRACTION

Spinal traction is used to overcome extrinsic muscle spasm and to keep bony surfaces aligned while fractures heal. A weight and pulley system, the patient's body weight, and manual or motorized force can be used. The force may be applied continuously or intermittently.

Cervical traction is often used for chronic neck pain from cervical spondylosis, disk prolapse, whiplash, or torticollis. A moderate weight (5 to 10 lb) is used for safety and patient comfort. Some advocate using a much greater weight. Sustained traction with > 20 lb is poorly tolerated for more than a few minutes, but motorized intermittent rhythmic traction is generally well tolerated.

Lumbar traction is rarely used today, although it is sometimes recommended for treating painful lumbar osteoarthritis or spondylolisthesis. The value of lumbar traction in treating acute discogenic pain is debatable, and because it requires prolonged bed rest, it always poses a risk for elderly persons.

MASSAGE

Massage may be used to relieve pain, reduce swelling and induration associated with trauma (eg, fracture, joint injury, sprain, strain, bruise, or peripheral nerve injury), and mobilize contracted tissues. Massage should be relaxing and pleasurable and should be considered for low back pain, arthritis, periarthritis, bursitis, neuritis, fibrositis, hemiplegia, paraplegia, quadriplegia, multiple sclerosis, and cerebral palsy. Massage should not be used to treat infections or thrombophlebitis.

ACUPUNCTURE

Acupuncture involves penetrating the skin with needles at specific body sites, frequently far from the site of pain. The needles, made of stainless steel, gold, or platinum, are very thin. A needle is twirled rapidly and intermittently for a few minutes, or a low electric current is applied. Although the mechanism of action is not fully understood and not everyone believes that the technique is helpful, many believe that it stimulates endorphin production, generating powerful analgesic and anti-inflammatory effects.

Acupuncture should be performed only by trained persons. Sterilized or new needles are needed to prevent infection.

THERAPEUTIC AND ASSISTIVE DEVICES

During rehabilitation, a patient may require an orthotic device, such as special shoes, a walker, crutches, a cane, leg brace, neck brace, corset, splint, or wheelchair. A person may also need self-help devices to perform ADLs.

ORTHOTIC DEVICES

Orthotic devices provide support for damaged joints, ligaments, tendons, and muscles. Although some orthotic devices are standard items, most are made to fit the needs and anatomy of individual patients.

Shoes

For safe ambulation, a physically disabled person needs well-constructed orthopedic shoes, which may have steel shanks and low rubber heels shaped to increase ankle or foot stability. The height of the shoes (oxford or high top) and closing system (shoelace, strap, buckle, or Velcro) may be modified to meet the patient's needs. If one leg is shorter than the other, a lift made of light material, such as cork, may be needed.

Walkers, Crutches, and Canes

These devices can aid ambulation in persons with chronic disability and those who have suffered an injury or undergone surgery. Walkers provide a movable, stable platform that protects the patient from falls, but they are not constructed to support weight. Walkers also slow gait and make climbing stairs and crossing thresholds difficult.

FIG. 29–3. Proper cane height. The patient's elbow should be bent at slightly less than a 45° angle when maximum force is applied.

Ordinary crutches are usually inappropriate for the elderly, who often lack the upper-body strength and motor coordination to use them. Canadian crutches, which have forearm supports and hand grips, require less upper-body strength and are useful for the chronically disabled.

Canes help with balance and reduce the weight-bearing forces across the hip. Several types of canes are available, including some with four legs (called quad canes) that offer considerably more stability but, like

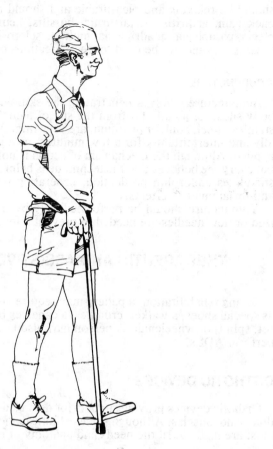

walkers, slow gait. The height of a cane must be adjusted so that the patient's elbow is bent at slightly less than 45° when maximum force is applied. The head of the cane should provide a secure grip (see FIG. 29–3).

Leg Braces

A short leg brace, which stops just below the knee, is used for ankle disabilities. A knee brace, which extends from midthigh to midcalf, may be used for disabilities confined to the knee (eg, an inability to lock the knee caused by extensor weakness). A long leg brace, which reaches midthigh, is indicated for disabilities in both the ankle and knee. A long leg brace with a pelvic band and hip joint is used for disabilities of the ankle, knee, and hip. However, such a brace is seldom practical for a geriatric patient because it greatly increases the energy demands of walking.

A weight-bearing brace, with which the weight is borne at the tibial condyle or ischial tuberosity, may be prescribed for a patient with a nonunited fracture who cannot bear body weight on the affected leg.

Neck Braces

A neck brace is used to immobilize the head or to minimize weight bearing of the head. It can be attached to a rigid corset; usually it is not worn in bed. Soft neck braces are generally preferred because they are more comfortable and are less likely to injure the skin. Fitting a neck brace properly is essential to obtaining benefit.

Corsets

A corset is used to immobilize the thoracic or lumbar spine. Prolonged use may result in weakening of the abdominal and spinal muscles; corsets should not be used for vague reasons or in an attempt to improve a person's figure.

Arm Splints

The static splint maintains the range of motion of wrist and finger joints and prevents contractures. It should be ordered whenever contracture is likely, such as after a stroke. The dynamic splint allows wrist and fingers to perform such tasks as pinching and grasping and is often used with quadriplegic patients.

Wheelchairs

Two types of wheelchairs are available: indoor (large wheels in the rear) and outdoor (large wheels in the front). Most geriatric patients use the indoor model. Persons maneuvering in tight quarters may find a smaller model useful. A **one-arm-drive wheelchair** may be suitable for a hemiplegic patient with good coordination. A **motorized wheelchair,** which requires little strength, is prescribed for a patient who has little or no arm function. Because the wheelchair can go up to 5 mph, the user should have good coordination, vision, and judgment.

SELF–HELP DEVICES

Kitchen and Bathroom Aids

Many kitchen activities require considerable strength, coordination, and stamina, and certain devices can help impaired elders prepare meals. A high stool with a backrest provides comfort while a person works on a countertop. A rolling cart can transport heavy or cumbersome articles and decrease the number of trips between the kitchen and dining table. If the oven is too low to use comfortably, a tabletop electric broiler oven may be used. Heavy pots can be replaced with lighter aluminum ones, and unbreakable plastic dishes can be used rather than breakable china.

Tools with long handles such as a dustpan and duster can help avoid the need to stoop. Using a long-handled reacher for retrieving items from high shelves can avoid the need to climb on a ladder or step stool. Other useful items include an electric can opener, a jar opener installed on the wall, and a rubber cover that can be slipped over the door knob to provide a better grip. Occupational therapists can evaluate cooking skills and often can recommend creative and useful devices to improve a person's ability to function in the kitchen.

The bathroom is a particularly dangerous place for impaired elders. Space is tight, and surfaces are often slippery. Blood pressure may fall after micturition, defecation, or showering, causing a person to feel faint or lose balance. Assistive devices are often needed in the bathroom to ensure safety and improve function. Again, an occupational therapist can evaluate the person's needs. A hand-held shower head with an extension hose may be easier to use than a regular shower, particularly with a shower chair. Guardrails enable a person to get in and out of the tub more easily and safely. A bar of soap on a piece of rope can be hung from the neck to prevent losing the soap or slipping on it while bathing or showering. Instead of buying such soap, a person can place a regular bar of soap in a small bag made from a dishcloth with a loop of soft string attached, or a person can use a mitten with a pocket for soap. A shower caddy may be used to store necessary articles for bathing. Alternatively, a child's pool raft or a small air mattress can be floated in the tub with the necessary items on it. A raised toilet seat, available in medical and surgical supply stores, can make standing easier after using the toilet. Bathroom storage shelves should be adjusted to a convenient height.

Dressing Aids

Devices such as a long-handled shoehorn, hairbrush, comb, and toothbrush can help an impaired elder dress independently. A ring or an 18-in. cord with a metal hook at the end can be attached to a zipper, enabling women to close zippers in the back of their dresses. Other useful items for patients with limited range of motion of the hand or arm joints include a bootjack, elastic shoelaces, front-closure brassieres, and button hooks.

Aids for Low Vision
(See also Ch. 102)

Many devices can help persons with poor eyesight. In addition, a number of support groups are available to offer advice and recommendations.

Hand-held magnifiers, with or without a light attachment, are often used by persons whose vision is mildly or moderately impaired. A concave magnifying mirror may help with grooming. Eyeglasses and telescopic lenses that can be permanently attached to the upper part of eyeglasses are available to supplement poor vision. Large-print editions of newspapers, magazines, and books are also available. Public libraries and bookstores have books available on audiotapes, and radio reading services are available.

Although moderate illumination is helpful for low vision, too much causes a whiteout effect, and too little causes a blackout effect. Reflected lighting is often better than direct lighting. A strong contrast of light and dark on a flat floor, as in a hospital corridor, may create the illusion of a step. Colors of hospital or other institutional interiors should be selected with the low-vision population in mind; pastels may please the medical staff but may be invisible to those with low vision. A door or the protruding corner of a wall should be painted with a high-contrast color.

THERAPY FOR SPECIFIC PROBLEMS

Therapies for specific problems include therapy for blind persons, speech therapy, and cardiovascular, stroke, hip fracture, and leg amputation rehabilitations.

THERAPY FOR BLIND PERSONS

Rehabilitation for blind persons includes training them to rely more on the other senses, training in specific skills and the use of devices for the blind, restoring psychologic security, and assisting them in dealing with and influencing the attitudes of others. When older persons become blind, the goals of rehabilitation are often more limited than those for younger adults. Establishing realistic goals is essential to success.

The patient must learn to develop skill and confidence in walking and traveling, learn a new means of spatial orientation, and develop conversational skills to overcome the lack of eye contact. Some elders may also want to learn to read and write in braille. During rehabilitation training, group discussions are useful for sharing experiences, difficulties, frustrations, fears, and other feelings.

SPEECH THERAPY

Speech patterns change with age. Healthy elders tend to speak in lower frequencies and have slightly increased voice tremor, laryngeal tension, and air loss. Also, consonant enunciation becomes imprecise, and the rate of articulation slows. Some healthy elderly persons have a limited vocabulary, disturbed prosody, and a tendency to make semantic errors.

Aphasia

An impairment in interpretation and formulation of language. In about 93% of people, speech and language functions are mediated by the left hemisphere of the brain. Aphasia occurs in about 40% of patients with strokes in the left hemisphere. Aphasia may be fluent, nonfluent, or global. **Fluent aphasia** is a deficit in comprehension. People with this condition can usually produce speech easily, but often they use jargon and word substitution. In **nonfluent aphasia,** comprehension is better than expression. People with this condition have extreme difficulty with speech production. In **global aphasia,** severe impairments in comprehension and expression coexist.

Recovery from aphasia generally continues for 1 to 2 yr after a stroke. The goal of speech therapy is to establish the most effective means of communication for the patient. For severely impaired patients, direct treatment with drills and repetitive practice is not effective, but a communication book with photographs and pictures can be useful. Less severely impaired patients may benefit from the stimulation approach (repetitive presentation of linguistic stimuli) and the programmed approach (a learning process for reacquiring language behavior). For mildly aphasic patients, a context-centered approach that emphasizes ideas and thoughts rather than words is effective.

The patient's family and close friends can provide essential therapy at home, but they may experience enormous stress, frustration, and even anger. The physician and speech pathologist should provide extensive guidance to help family and friends understand that the patient is not mentally ill so that they can be extremely patient at all times, use simple sentences but not baby language, take safety precautions since the patient may not be able to call for help, use gestures and point to objects to supplement speech, phrase questions so the patient can answer yes or no by nodding or shaking the head, and avoid interrupting no matter how long the patient takes to say something.

Dysarthria

A group of speech abnormalities resulting from disturbances in muscular control caused by damage to the central or peripheral nervous system and resulting in weakness, slowness in response, or incoordination of the speech mechanism. The second most common communication disorder in elderly patients, dysarthria may be flaccid, spastic, ataxic, hypokinetic, hyperkinetic, or mixed and may involve several or all of the basic mechanical processes of speech: respiration, phonation, resonance, articulation, and prosody.

Treatment depends on whether dysarthria results from an acute neurologic episode (eg, stroke, head trauma, or surgery) or a chronic progressive disease. After an acute illness, the goal of therapy is to restore and preserve speech. With a progressive disease, the patient is encouraged to maintain premorbid function for as long as possible. However, the patient eventually will begin to experience various dysarthric speech patterns and will have to modify his speech to control rate, consonant emphasis, and articulation. Some patients may be able to adjust without practice. In very advanced cases, an augmentative communication system may be required.

Verbal Apraxia

A motor speech disorder caused by an impairment in initiation, coordination, or sequencing of muscle movements for volitional production of phonemes. Apraxia may occur in patients with brain damage caused by stroke, head injury, or surgery. Although no significant muscle weakness, slowness, or incoordination in reflex and automatic response is apparent, prosodic alterations may occur.

When a patient has a nonfluent aphasia with apraxia, melodic intonation therapy (the use of natural melody patterns to facilitate speech) may be used. However, if the patient has poor auditory comprehension, this type of therapy is not helpful. Intensive practice of sound patterns and speech is an alternative approach.

Laryngectomy

A partial laryngectomy alters voice quality; a total laryngectomy results in nearly total loss of the ability to speak. A patient with a total laryngectomy has three options: reconstructive surgery (neoglottis or shunt), esophageal speech, or electrolarynx. Esophageal speech requires the patient to take air into the esophagus and expel it forcefully, causing a vibration in the upper narrow portion of the esophagus. The articulation techniques are the same as those for normal speech. However, not every patient can master esophageal speech. Tissue elasticity is essential for esophageal speech, and radiation therapy often makes tissues lose elasticity. An artificial larynx, such as an electrolarynx, can restore speech by producing external vibrations that result in sound. A number of support groups are available for persons who cannot speak.

CARDIOVASCULAR REHABILITATION

(See also Ch. 31)

Cardiovascular rehabilitation may be useful for some elderly persons who have suffered a myocardial infarction and some who have severe heart failure. The goal of cardiac rehabilitation is to help the patient maintain or regain independence, given his physical capability.

For those in poor physical condition because of cardiac disease or physical inactivity, the heart's maximum working capacity is greatly reduced. Restoring cardiac reserve is especially important after an acute myocardial infarction, whether the patient is young or old (see also Ch. 37). Activity should be minimized immediately after a myocardial infarction, then increased gradually. Although morbidity and mortality rates are higher in older patients, most can eventually resume their previous level of physical activity.

Each patient responds differently to the stress of severe illness, so the rehabilitation program must be individualized. Typical programs begin with light activities and progress to moderate activities under the supervision of a physical therapist or nurse. The level of physical activity can be expressed in metabolic equivalents (METs). Light to moderate housework is about 2 to 4 METs; heavy housework or yard work is about 5 to 6 METs. Under normal working and living conditions (excluding recreational activities), a person rarely exceeds 6 METs. About 1 wk after an uncomplicated myocardial infarction, a 2-MET exercise test may be performed to evaluate progress. Before discharge, an exercise test of 4 to 5 METs helps guide physical activity at home.

The New York Heart Association's maximum allowable workloads for functional classes of cardiac patients appears in TABLE 29–3. During hospitalization, all physical activities should be controlled to keep the heart rate below 60% of the maximum for the patient's age; during the home recovery period, the heart rate should be kept below 70% of the maximum. (At age 60, the maximum heart rate is about 160 beats per minute.)

Patients with unstable angina should not exercise at all. Other conditions—including heart failure, arrhythmias, and valvular disease—may increase the risk from even gentle exercise. Persons at high risk should exercise only under the supervision of a trained attendant in a well-equipped cardiac rehabilitation facility.

Patients who can tolerate a 5-MET exercise test for 6 min can safely perform at least sedentary activities at home but must have sufficient rest between them. Upon discharge, the patient should be given a detailed home activity program.

Common problems during the home recovery period include emotional stress and unnecessary restrictions of activity. The result may be inactivity, which is detrimental to recovery. Therefore, the physician and allied health professionals should provide sufficient psychologic support and explain which activities can be undertaken and which cannot be undertaken.

Although geriatric patients may not ask about sexual activity, the physician should give appropriate advice. As a guide, young couples expend 5 to 6 METs during intercourse. Whether older couples expend more or less is not known; however, most can be advised to resume sexual activity but to avoid overexertion and to stop and rest as necessary (see also Ch. 68).

TABLE 29–3. NEW YORK HEART ASSOCIATION CLASSIFICATION OF SUSTAINED AND INTERMITTENT WORKLOADS

Functional Classification of Cardiac Patients	*Physiologic Symptoms*	*Maximum Workload (Calories per minute)*		*Maximum METs*
		Sustained	*Intermittent*	
I	Cardiac disease but without resulting limitations of physical activity: ordinary physical activity does not cause undue fatigue, palpitation, dyspnea, or anginal pain	5.0	6.5	6.5
II	Cardiac disease resulting in slight limitation of physical activity: comfortable at rest; ordinary physical activity results in fatigue, palpitation, dyspnea, or anginal pain	2.5	4.0	4.5
III	Cardiac disease resulting in marked limitation of physical activity: comfortable at rest; less than ordinary physical activity causes fatigue, palpitation, dyspnea, or anginal pain	2.0	2.7	3.0
IV	Cardiac disease resulting in inability to carry on any physical activity without discomfort; symptoms of cardiac insufficiency or of the anginal syndrome may be present even at rest; if any physical activity is undertaken, discomfort increases	1.5	2.0	1.5

Modified from Karwal SS: "Cardiac rehabilitation," in *Current Therapy in Physiatry, Physical Medicine and Rehabilitation,* edited by AP Ruskin. Philadelphia, WB Saunders Company, 1984, p 328; used with permission.

STROKE REHABILITATION

After a stroke, two distinct recovery processes occur. The neurologic recovery occurs to varying degrees, depending on the mechanism, location, and size of the lesion. In general, the smaller the lesion, the better the recovery. About 90% of this recovery usually occurs within 3 mo. The remaining 10% occurs much more slowly. Recovery from a hemorrhagic stroke is particularly slow. The second type of recovery, improvement in functional performance can be enhanced by rehabilitation.

Rehabilitation potential refers to the likelihood of recovery and depends on general condition, the range of motion of joints, muscle strength of the affected and unaffected sides of the body, bowel and bladder function, premorbid functional and cognitive ability, social situation (including prospects of returning to the community), ability to participate in a rehabilitation regimen under the supervision of nurses and therapists, learning ability, motivation, and coping skills.

After an assessment, the rehabilitation team formulates goals and sets target completion dates. The team must communicate these goals and dates to the patient and family to avoid unrealistic expectations. The physician should not raise false hope but should explain the patient's prospects as positively as possible.

Early Rehabilitation

The rehabilitation program should be started as soon as the stroke victim is medically stable. Such an early start may prevent secondary disabilities, such as contractures and pressure sores, and help avoid depression.

Patients can safely begin sitting up once they are fully conscious and their neurologic deficits are no longer progressing, usually within 48 h of the stroke. Early in the rehabilitation period when the involved extremities are still flaccid, passive range of motion through the normal range three to four times daily for each joint should be provided at bedside. For patients with hemiplegia, one or two pillows should be placed under the affected arm to prevent dislocation of the shoulder. A well-constructed sling should be used for arm flaccidity, so that the weight of the arm and hand does not overstretch the deltoid muscle and cause subluxation of the shoulder. A posterior foot splint should be applied with the ankle in a 90° position to prevent equinus deformity (talipes equinus) and foot drop.

Regaining the ability to get out of bed and transfer to a chair or wheelchair independently has a positive psychologic effect and is important for all other aspects of rehabilitation. Patience and close supervision by the therapist are necessary until the patient can transfer safely. Besides motor and sensory paralysis, the patient may have incoordination, dyspraxia, visual field defects, and impaired judgment.

Reeducation and coordination exercises of the affected extremities should be added as soon as tolerated, often within a week. Active exercise of the unaffected extremities without fatigue must also be encouraged. Various ADLs, such as moving in bed, turning, changing position, and sitting up, can be performed.

Active and assistive exercise of the affected extremities should be started shortly afterward to maintain range of motion and, if indicated, to increase muscle strength. In hemiplegic patients, the most important muscle for ambulation is the unaffected quadriceps. If weak, this muscle should be strengthened to assist the hemiplegic side.

Resistive exercise for hemiplegic extremities is controversial because it may increase spasticity. If resistive exercise is used, the therapist should observe muscle activity closely because spasticity is insidious; if spasticity occurs, resistive exercise should not be used.

Ambulation

Standing exercise is safest using the parallel bars. First, the patient works on standing from the sitting position. The height of the seat may need to be adjusted. When the patient walks, the distance between the feet should be 6 in. or more while holding onto the bar with the sound hand. If the hemiplegic arm is flaccid, a sling should be worn, as described above. The patient must stand with the hips and knees fully extended, leaning slightly forward and toward the sound side. A hemiplegic patient is subject to vertigo and must change body position slowly when standing up or turning. After standing, the patient should take a moment to establish equilibrium before walking.

The patient should be reminded to take a shorter step with the hemiplegic leg and a longer step with the sound leg. When the patient first begins walking without the parallel bars, the therapist may need to physically assist and later supervise. Generally, a patient uses a cane or walker when first walking without the parallel bars. The diameter of the cane handle should be large enough to accommodate an osteoarthritic hand.

Most hemiplegic patients have a gait abnormality, but if a patient can walk safely, the therapist should not attempt to fully correct the abnormality. The goal is not to restore a normal gait but to establish and maintain a safe gait.

Spasticity may or may not help ambulation. Slightly spastic knee extensors can lock the knee during the stance phase. However, spastic knee extensors cause hyperextension, or genu recurvatum, and a knee brace with an extension stop may be necessary. When resistance is applied to spastic plantar flexors, ankle clonus occurs; a short leg brace without a spring mechanism minimizes this problem.

The basic principle of the stair climbing exercise, good is up and bad is down, can be used by the stroke patient. Ideally, when the patient ascends the stairs, the railing should be on the unaffected side, so the patient can grasp it. The patient should not look up the staircase; doing so may cause vertigo. When the patient descends, the affected side should be against the railing, and a cane should be used. When a hemiplegic person falls, he almost always falls on the hemiplegic side. With the affected side against the railing, the patient can lean against it and help prevent a fall.

Preventing Falls

One goal of rehabilitation is to prevent falls, which are the most common accidents among stroke victims. Usually, the patient explains the fall by saying, "The knees gave way." If muscles are weak, particularly in the trunk and leg, initial strengthening exercises should be performed. The patient should be assessed for orthostatic hypotension; if it is present and symptomatic, it should be treated with support stockings, medication, or tilt table training. Stroke victims should take special care to wear comfortable, supportive shoes with rubber soles and heels. Women's heels should be no higher than 3/4 in.

Other Problems

Patients with **hemianopia** should be made aware of it and taught to move their heads toward the hemiplegic side when scanning. Family members should be advised to place important objects on the patient's good side and to approach the patient on that side.

Many activities require **fine coordination** of the arms and hands. After a stroke, that coordination may be absent, leading the patient to become frustrated. Therefore, a patient may need to modify activities and use assistive devices.

Some stroke patients develop intermittent **spasticity,** which may be painful and debilitating. Heat or cold therapy can temporarily decrease spasticity and allow muscle stretching. Drugs such as diazepam and methocarbamol have limited value and cause sedation.

Most hemiplegic hands and wrists exhibit flexor spasticity. Unless the patient performs range-of-motion exercises several times a day, flexion contracture may develop rapidly, resulting in pain and difficulty maintaining personal hygiene. Patients and families should be taught and strongly encouraged to perform range-of-motion exercises to prevent contractures. A hand or wrist splint may also be useful, particularly at night. The splint should be easy to apply and to clean.

HIP FRACTURE REHABILITATION

(See also Ch. 8)

Rehabilitation After Surgery

Rehabilitation should be started as soon as possible after surgery. At first, therapy may be directed at increasing strength and preventing atrophy on the unaffected side. Initially, only isometric exercise should be used on the affected limb, while keeping it fully extended. A pillow should never be placed under the knee because flexion contracture of the hip and knee may result.

Gradual mobilization of the affected limb should lead to full ambulation. The speed of rehabilitation depends in part on the type of surgery performed. After prosthetic replacement, therapy usually progresses more rapidly; less rehabilitation is needed, and the functional outcome is better than for nail-and-plate or pin-and-plate fixation. Ideally, full weight-bearing ambulation may start on the second postoperative day. Ambulatory exercises should begin between 4 and 8 days postoperatively, and stair climbing should start about 11 days postoperatively.

The patient should be taught to perform daily exercises to strengthen the trunk muscles and quadriceps of the affected leg. Any prolonged lifting or pushing of heavy items, stooping, reaching, or jumping can be harmful. Sitting on a chair, particularly a low one, for a long period should be avoided, and the patient should use the chair arm for support when standing up. While sitting, the patient should keep the legs uncrossed. The amount of mechanical stress does not differ greatly whether the patient uses one or two canes, and using two may interfere with certain ADLs.

Before discharge, a therapist should evaluate the patient's home to determine if additional training or assistive devices are needed.

Rehabilitation Without Surgery

Nonsurgical treatment is generally associated with a poor functional prognosis. During immobilization, which usually lasts at least 6 to 8 wk, preventing secondary disabilities (pressure sores, muscle atrophy, joint contractures, and general deconditioning) is important.

After the immobilization period, the patient should undergo a rehabilitation program similar to the one for postoperative patients; however, it should be preceded by general conditioning exercises and should progress more slowly.

Some physicians believe that weight bearing should not be permitted unless x-rays demonstrate union of the bone. However, union is rarely detected in 8 wk and usually not for at least 10 to 12 wk after injury. Others suggest comparing x-rays under non–weight-bearing and weight-bearing conditions to establish healing. If no change is found, weight bearing can proceed. The patient often begins weight bearing, even if told not to, as soon as no discomfort is felt. Relying on the patient's perception seems more reasonable than basing a decision solely on x-ray findings.

LEG AMPUTATION REHABILITATION

Before surgery, the physician should explain the extensive rehabilitation program that will be needed after surgery. Psychologic counseling may be indicated. The team of health care professionals should discuss with the patient whether rehabilitation should include the use of a prosthesis or a wheelchair.

Immediately after surgery, prevention of secondary disabilities, especially contractures, must be begun. Flexion contracture of the hip or knee may develop rapidly after surgery and make prosthetic fitting and use difficult. Exercises for general conditioning, stretching of the hip and knee, and strengthening of all extremities should be started as soon as the patient is medically stable. Endurance exercises may also be prescribed. The elderly amputee should begin standing and balancing exercises with parallel bars as early as possible.

The functional prognoses for above-the-knee amputees and below-the-knee amputees differ greatly. The weight of the above-the-knee prosthesis and the control of the knee joint require energy and skills that some elderly patients may not have. On the other hand, elderly below-the-knee amputees are usually fitted with prostheses and become functionally ambulatory.

Stump Conditioning

Conditioning assists the natural process of shrinking that must occur before a prosthesis can be used. All stumps must be tapered, so an elastic stump shrinker or elastic bandages are applied and maintained on a 24-h basis. Continuous use of an elastic stump shrinker or elastic bandages also helps prevent edema, and such prevention is essential. Though an elastic stump shrinker is easy to apply, the bandages may be preferred because the amount and location of pressure can be better controlled with bandages. The disadvantage of elastic bandages is the need to reapply them whenever they become loose. After a few days of stump conditioning, rapid shrinkage may occur.

Prosthesis

Early ambulation with a pylon or temporary prosthesis not only makes the amputee active but also accelerates stump shrinkage, prevents flexion contracture, and reduces phantom limb pain. The socket of the pylon is made of plaster of paris and should fit the stump snugly. Various temporary prostheses with adjustable sockets are available. Ambulation can start on the parallel bars, and the patient can progress to walking with crutches or canes until a permanent prosthesis is made.

The prosthesis should be lightweight and should meet the needs and safety requirements of the patient. Providing a perfect prosthetic fit is an art. If the prosthesis is made before the stump stops shrinking, adjustments may be needed to satisfy the patient and produce a good gait pattern. For most geriatric patients with a below-the-knee amputation, the patellar-tendon-bearing prosthesis with a solid ankle, cushion heel foot, and suprapatellar cuff suspension is best. Unless a special need exists, a standard below-the-knee prosthesis with thigh corset and waist belt is not prescribed because of its weight and bulkiness.

The most common complaint is pain in the stump. When phantom limb pain and other conditions can be ruled out, an ill-fitting socket is usually the cause. The socket may be too small, the stump may be edematous, or the patient may have gained weight.

Care of the Stump and Prosthesis

The patient should be instructed in stump hygiene. Because a leg prosthesis is intended only for ambulation, a patient should not wear it while sleeping. At bedtime, the stump should be inspected thoroughly (with a mirror if the patient is inspecting it), washed with mild soap and warm water, and dried thoroughly. Then talcum powder should be applied. If the skin of the stump is too dry, lanolin or petrolatum may be applied. If the stump sweats excessively, an antiperspirant may be applied. Any skin inflammation must be treated immediately by removing the irritant and applying talc or a low-potency corticosteroid cream or ointment. If a break occurs in the skin, the prosthesis should not be used until the wound has healed.

The stump sock should be changed daily, and mild soap may be used to clean the inside of the socket. A prosthesis is neither waterproof nor water-resistant. Therefore, if even part of it becomes wet, it must be dried immediately and thoroughly; heat should not be used.

Wheelchair Use

Whether or not elderly patients use a prosthesis, they should have an **amputee wheelchair.** These wheelchairs have a longer span between the wheel axles to compensate for the absence of leg weight and prevent tilting. With proper maintenance, a wheelchair lasts 5 to 10 yr. The wheelchair can be used in several circumstances. For instance, it can be used during the night when putting on a prosthesis is bothersome and using crutches without a prosthesis is unsafe. At other times, perhaps because of the condition of the stump, the patient may not be able to use the prosthesis. Moreover, even if a patient can walk independently to perform ADLs, walking long distances may be difficult or inadvisable.

Bilateral Amputation

An elderly person with bilateral below-the-knee amputations usually can manage two prostheses fairly well. However, most elderly persons with bilateral above-the-knee amputations are unable to walk with prostheses because they do not have the necessary energy and strength. The functional prognosis for those with a combination of above-the-knee and below-the-knee amputation varies greatly. When the person walks with prostheses, the below-the-knee side becomes the functional leg and a manual knee lock may sometimes be required on the above-the-knee prosthesis. A bilateral amputee needs a pair of canes or crutches to walk, and even with two prostheses, the walking distance is limited. A wheelchair must be used outdoors and for long distances.

Phantom Limb, Phantom Limb Pain, and Painful Stump

Phantom limb, a painless awareness of the amputated part possibly accompanied by mild tingling, is experienced by almost every new amputee. The sensation can be so vivid that some amputees can describe the position of the foot, which is often very closely related to its position at the time of amputation. This sensation may last from several months to several years but usually disappears without treatment. Frequently, patients sense only part of the missing limb; many patients sense only the foot, which is the last phantom sensation to disappear. The phantom limb sensation is not harmful unless an amputee, without thinking, attempts to stand with both legs and falls.

Phantom limb pain in the amputated part is more likely to occur if the patient had a painful condition before amputation. Various treatments such as simultaneous exercise of the affected limb and the contralateral limb, massage of the stump, percussion of the stump with fingers, use of mechanical devices (eg, a vibrator), and ultrasound have been reported to be effective. Medications (including tricyclic antidepressants and carbamazepine) may be helpful.

A **painful stump** involves mild to severe pain on palpation or when a pylon or prosthesis is used. This stump pain is localized and different from phantom limb pain. The most common causes of stump pain are a painful amputation neuroma or a spur formation at the amputated end of the bone. An amputation neuroma is usually palpable. Spur formation may be diagnosed by palpation and x-ray examination. Treatments include injection of corticosteroids or analgesics in the neuroma or the surrounding area, use of cryotherapy, or continuous tight bandaging of the stump. The most effective modality is daily ultrasound treatment for 5 to 10 sessions. Surgical resection of the neuroma often has disappointing results. The only effective treatment of a spur formation is surgical resection.

Follow-up Care

A patient who successfully completes the program of prosthetic rehabilitation and returns to the community should be followed up every 3 to 6 mo for the first 2 yr. The stump usually continues to shrink with use. Eventually (usually within the first 2 yr), the stump may become too small and a new socket will be needed. Because of continuous use, various components of the prosthesis may deteriorate, possibly resulting in an altered gait. The circulatory status of the sound leg should be examined at follow-up. Unfortunately, many persons with a below-the-knee amputation eventually require an above-the-knee amputation.

30. OCCUPATIONAL THERAPY

In geriatrics, the goal of occupational therapy is to enhance the older adult's ability to function. Because of disease, trauma, disuse atrophy, environmental deprivation, and age-related changes in biologic, psychologic, and social functions, older adults often have difficulty performing routine tasks of daily living, such as climbing stairs to get to the bathroom or opening food containers to prepare meals. Such functional disabilities critically alter well-being and quality of life. In occupational therapy, these disabilities are assessed and managed to optimize function or slow decline.

ASSESSMENT OF TASK PERFORMANCE

Occupational therapy classifies life tasks (ie, occupations) as functional mobility, personal self-care, home management, leisure, and work. **Functional mobility** involves gross body movements needed for more skilled tasks, such as maintaining standing balance while dressing. **Personal self-care** includes feeding, bathing, maintaining hygiene, grooming, toileting, dressing, and communicating basic needs. **Home management** involves indoor and outdoor tasks for maintaining independent living, such as preparing meals, taking medications, managing finances, mowing the lawn, and using public transportation. **Leisure** involves tasks performed for enjoyment, relaxation, and socialization; **work** involves tasks performed for pay as well as those done to contribute to family and society, such as caregiving and volunteer jobs.

Functional mobility and personal self-care tasks are referred to as basic **activities of daily living (ADLs). Instrumental activities of daily living (IADLs)** apply only to home management and work tasks. Assessments of functional mobility and personal self-care have become standardized; assessments of home management, leisure, and work are often individualized, covering only the tasks that a particular person must perform.

Occupational therapists evaluate the following dimensions of task performance: skill, habit, and the personal and environmental factors that might affect performance.

Skill Assessment

Skill is the ability to initiate, perform, and complete tasks efficiently. Skill assessment involves observing older adults carry out tasks. Because task performance is influenced by the physical environment (eg, a walk-in shower stall that allows a person with impaired mobility to shower) and the social environment (eg, a solicitous spouse), skill assessment should be done in the setting where the task is actually performed. If this is not possible, a simulated home, leisure, or work environment in the occupational therapy clinic may be used.

The results of skill assessment are summarized in a listing of tasks. A rating of **competence** signifies that the person can do a task independently, adequately, safely, and within a reasonable time. A rating of **disability** signifies that the person cannot meet these criteria. The degree of assistance needed should be classified as minimal (up to 25%), moderate (up to 50%), maximum (up to 75%), or total (100%), and the type of assistance should be specified. A hierarchy of types of assistance might be (1) preparation of materials (arranging clothing on the bed before a person dresses); (2) encouragement (telling the person, "Good try!"); (3) instruction (directing the person, "Put your right arm into the sleeve"); (4) manual guidance (therapist putting own hand over patient's hand and guiding it into a shirt sleeve); and (5) physical assistance (therapist dressing a patient).

Habit Assessment

Having the competence to perform a task is not the same as using that competence in daily life. A depressed patient, for example, may be capable of preparing meals but may fail to do so because of a lack of interest; a patient with cardiopulmonary disease may perform adequately in the morning but become so fatigued by the afternoon that preparing dinner is not feasible. Usually, repeated observation of a person's daily living habits is not practical. Therefore, habit assessment relies on an interview with the patient and reports from caregivers. Observation during the skill assessment can also provide valuable information. Dentures caked with food particles, dirty clothes scattered on the bedroom floor, and a rancid odor emanating from the refrigerator are telltale signs of a deficit.

No uniform system exists for describing habit deficits. Certain behaviors seen in older patients, sometimes called **maladaptive patterns,** are marked by inconsistency, imbalance, disorganization, inflexibility, and social inappropriateness. Patients who feed themselves at one meal but refuse to do so at the next exemplify **inconsistency.** Activity **imbalance** refers to a person performing too few tasks, tasks that lack diversity, or tasks that are poorly paced. Patients who spend all day watching television and neglect household chores illustrate this type of deficit. The salient feature of **disorganization** is an inability to anticipate, plan, and carry out a plan; hence, patients delay starting tasks, gather task materials haphazardly, proceed in a way that is not consistently goal-directed, and participate in activity that leads to fatigue, frustration, and feelings of incompetence. **Inflexibility** is characterized by an inability to vary routines to accommodate unforeseen or changing circumstances and an inability to adjust emotionally when routines are changed. This pattern is apparent in a patient who tries to maintain a lifelong housecleaning schedule even though it now causes exhaustion. **Socially inappropriate behaviors** disregard standards of behavior, particularly those involving promptness, sociability, independence, cleanliness, and neatness.

Determining whether a task performance dysfunction results from a skill deficit or habit deficit is a key decision for the occupational therapist. Intervention for a person who lacks the skill to perform a task differs from that for a person who lacks the will to perform a task or the ability to manage time effectively.

Assessment of Personal and Environmental Factors

Successful task performance requires that the older adult coordinate and integrate many abilities. Performing even a simple task such as dressing requires the **sensorimotor ability** to perform the task, the **cognitive ability** to plan it and execute the plan, and the **affective ability** to want to do the task and to persevere until it is completed. Furthermore, the physical and social environments must facilitate task performance.

Impairments of sensorimotor abilities include aberrations in sensation, perception, range of motion, muscle strength, muscle tone, endurance, balance, dexterity, and coordination. Cognitive impairments include inattention, distractibility, loss of concentration, impaired judgment, indecision, memory deficit, apraxia, cognitive rigidity, and poor problem-solving skills. Affective impairments include apathy, depression, anxiety, perceived incompetence, frustration, a lack of persistence, and decreased coping skills. If the cause of the task dysfunction is correctly identified, the impairment can often be compensated for or remediated.

Impairments may be evaluated during the skill or habit assessment or independently. For example, an occupational therapist may observe instability as a patient stands and undresses, gets into the bathtub, and reaches overhead to get a towel. Later, a standardized test, such as the Performance Oriented Assessment of Balance, may be administered to obtain more information about the extent and nature of the balance disorder. Similarly, an occupational therapist may note that regardless of the ADL or IADL, a patient drops objects soon after grasping them. Additional tests of static and dynamic grip strength (eg, pinch meter, manual muscle test) may be performed to further define the hand impairment. Also, data collected by other health care professionals, such as physical therapists, neuropsychologists, and speech pathologists, may be used to help understand impairments.

Impairments do not inevitably result in disability. An impairment may not be severe enough to adversely affect performance, or adaptive techniques may compensate for an impairment. Nonetheless, identifying an impairment can enable the start of preventive interventions before task performance deteriorates. For instance, progressive resistive exercises may be started at the first sign of deteriorating manual strength.

Task performance dysfunctions may also result from environmental factors. The **physical environment** includes lighting (focused light on work areas, light switches placed so that lights can be turned on before entering a room), walking surfaces (intact carpeting, no electrical cords in walkways), resting surfaces (stable chairs), and the condition and placement of objects in the environment (unfrayed electrical cords, no clutter). The environment should be free of barriers, especially for people using wheelchairs or walkers. For the cognitively impaired, cues that orient (eg, a picture of a toilet on the bathroom door) may enhance safety or function. Objects in the environment, namely furniture, appliances, and tools, should support task performance. For example, many older patients have difficulty rising from chairs that are too low—a problem that can often be resolved by raising the chair height with chair leg extenders or seat cushions. Finally, the environment should elicit an appropriate level of stimulation and positive emotion.

Features of the **social environment** that directly affect task performance are the attitudes of caregivers toward functional independence and caregiving and the competence of caregivers in providing rehabilitative care. The more disabled elderly patients are, the more dependent they are on their caregivers and the more important an assessment of the patient-caregiver interaction becomes. Although standardized protocols are available for assessing physical environmental factors (eg, architectural barriers and safety features in the home), assessment of social environmental factors involves individualized observation and clinical judgment.

Functional Diagnosis

The occupational therapy assessment yields a descriptive summary of task performance in terms of competence and disability, habit adaptation and maladaptation, abilities and impairments, and environmental influences. The functional diagnosis indicates the tasks that a patient cannot perform or has difficulty performing and the impairments or environmental factors that appear to be responsible for this dysfunction.

Although the primary purpose of assessing task performance is to plan occupational therapy interventions, assessment data may also be used for other purposes. An inability to perform tasks necessary for survival or independent living indicates the need for services from family members, neighbors, friends, or health and social services. When the care needed cannot be provided in the home, the occupational therapist alerts the physician. Assessment data may also be useful when competence is being determined for legal purposes. Repeated assessments of task performance are valuable for monitoring the effects of medical interventions on function. For example, extrapyramidal reactions, agitation, and confusion are potential side effects of psychoactive medications. Periodic reassessment of task performance can detect deterioration and signal the need for adjusting the dosage of the medication.

INTERVENTION

Interventions include therapeutic activity to reduce impairments, acquire skills, and acquire habits; the use of splints and assistive devices; and environmental and social adaptations.

THERAPEUTIC ACTIVITY

Activity is inherently therapeutic, and function improves by engaging in purposeful activity. Using purposeful activity as therapy requires the following: The patient and the occupational therapist must be partners in determining and prioritizing intervention goals and in selecting therapeutic tasks; tasks used as therapy must be meaningful to the patient; tasks used as therapy must be commensurate with the patient's ability; and as performance improves, tasks of increasing difficulty must be introduced to stimulate further improvement.

Impairment Reduction

Remediation is accomplished through **therapeutic exercise** for the specific type of impairment. For example, fine motor exercises may be used to alleviate incoordination; visual-perceptual exercises, to correct problems in scanning the visual field; memory retraining, to enhance recognition and recall; and assertiveness exercises, to develop skill in expressing needs. Such exercises simply provide a means to an end; thus, developing an interest or proficiency in the activity is not as important as reducing the impairment. For example, because weaving or sewing is a good activity for relearning fine motor skills, patients may weave or sew, even though they have no particular interest in pursuing it as a hobby.

Interventions to reduce an impairment should be used only if a patient's prognosis indicates that improvement can be expected. Memory retraining might be attempted for patients recovering from a stroke but not for those with dementia.

Skill Acquisition

With this type of intervention, a particular activity is pursued for its own sake. Skills may be developed in functional mobility, personal self-care, home management, leisure, or work tasks, as appropriate. The essence of skill acquisition is practicing tasks under controlled, supervised conditions with the task materials and the movement patterns being selected to promote success. For many patients, putting on a pullover is easier than putting on a cardigan, so training in dressing may begin with the former and progress to the latter. Assistance is given only when needed and only to the extent needed as determined by the skill assessment. As the patient improves, assistance is reduced. Skills learned in occupational therapy must be adapted to the home, leisure, or work situation. Thus, patients practice using a variety of training materials, and they continue practicing until they can comfortably integrate the tasks into their daily routines. During therapy, the therapist reinforces the patient's sense of competence.

Skill acquisition is used when a patient needs adaptive techniques, healthier movement or behavior patterns, or new skills. When impairments cannot be corrected, patients are taught adaptive techniques, which compensate by using the patients' strengths. Thus, patients with paralyzed extremities resulting from a stroke learn to dress the paralyzed extremities before the nonparalyzed ones and learn to complete bilateral dressing tasks (tying shoes, buttoning buttons) using only one hand. Programs designed to acquire skill in protecting arthritic joints, promoting proper body mechanics, and developing more effective interpersonal techniques are examples of interventions involving healthier movement or behavior patterns.

Habit Acquisition

The goal of habit training is to provide the incentive, structure, and endurance needed to develop and sustain an ordered, yet flexible, pattern of daily living. The patient learns to organize tasks from beginning to end, link tasks into effective routines, and understand the social norms or expectations regarding task performance. Routines provide efficiency, and because they are almost automatic, they minimize the need for continuous planning. Key elements of habit training in occupational therapy include clarifying values to determine task priorities, examining how time is spent, acknowledging maladaptive patterns, exploring and practicing alternative routines, and consolidating new habit structures.

The patient learns to conserve physical and mental energies through training in time management, ergonomic techniques, and stress management. Tasks are spaced so that labor-intensive ones are distributed over a day or week. Schedules are arranged to provide the best balance of personal self-care, home management, leisure, and work tasks, approximating the schedule used in the discharge setting. Opportunity is then provided within occupational therapy to try out new routines.

Group activities allow patients to experience many leadership and helper roles and to practice social behaviors. The groups are task oriented and are similar to groups that older patients are likely to encounter in senior centers, day-care centers, nursing homes, and religious and fraternal organizations; they may engage in cooking, discussions of current events, card playing, exercises, music groups, and religious activities. In essence, for patients with habit deficits, the occupational therapist designs a socialization experience in which real-life expectations for life tasks are conveyed.

USE OF SPLINTS AND ASSISTIVE DEVICES

Splints

Splints are fabricated to prevent deformity or promote function. Static hand splints are applied to maintain the wrist in a neutral position, the fingers in extension, and the thumb in opposition to prevent flexion deformities. A wrist cock-up splint holds the wrist in extension but leaves the fingers free. A foot drop splint helps maintain 90° ankle flexion.

Assistive Devices

Self-help aids are typically used to promote safety or compensate for specific impairments. Some of the safety aids most commonly used by older patients are canes, rails on the side and back of the bathtub, non-skid mats on the bottom of the bathtub or shower, shower chairs or benches, reachers, and bedside commodes. Extended handles on tools (eg, eating utensils, combs and brushes, and shoehorns) compensate for range-of-motion restrictions. Raised toilet seats and chair leg extenders compensate for diminished leg strength; while tools with built-up handles, spring-loaded or electric controls, or grippers accommodate reduced manual strength. Tremors may lessen with the use of weighted tools, and spills may be prevented by using cups with lids and rocker spoons.

For those with sensory impairments, stimuli can be enhanced; for instance, enlarged dials can be added to telephones for those with decreased vision. Or the type of sensory input can be changed; for instance, a telephone ring (auditory signal) can be replaced with a flashing light (visual signal) for the hearing impaired. Memory aids include automatic dialing telephones, medication organizers and reminders, and pocket devices that cue people by beeping or talking at the appropriate time. These examples are only some of the self-help aids that occupational therapists prescribe for older patients.

PHYSICAL AND SOCIAL ENVIRONMENTAL ADAPTATIONS

Physical Environmental Interventions

These interventions aim to change the physical environment so that it supports task performance needs. Safety needs may be met by removing risks or installing new elements. Also, since both understimulation and overstimulation adversely affect task performance, the amount of auditory, visual, tactile, olfactory, gustatory, vestibular, or social stimulation may be changed as appropriate.

Accessibility may be improved by removing or modifying architectural barriers (such as doors, doorjambs, and thresholds), adding ramps, and lowering work surfaces and storage areas. Accommodating a walker may require rearranging furniture. For some patients with mental impairments, signs and pictures indicating the location of rooms and objects may help.

Social Environmental Interventions

The social environment supports the patient's task performance needs when caregivers value functional independence and know how to promote it. Older patients often depend on caregivers to schedule life tasks, provide needed materials, and give appropriate assistance. Thus, caregivers should be involved in the older adult's program.

If a caregiver is unable to provide care safely and adequately, alternative resources need to be identified. Many caregivers are elderly themselves and lack the energy or strength to cope with a high level of task dysfunction.

INTERVENTION CONSIDERATIONS

A distinguishing characteristic of geriatric medicine is the simultaneous management of several clinical problems. Often, these problems translate into functional deficits that have many causes. Older patients with hip fracture may need to use a walker to reduce stress on the hip joint, but at the same time they may not be able to learn to use it effectively because of cognitive impairment secondary to dementia. Engaging depressed patients in activity may be complicated by their decreased vision secondary to macular degeneration or reduced grip strength secondary to osteoarthritis.

Learning is at the core of occupational therapy interventions, and learning may take longer as people age, largely because of the reduced efficiency of the mechanisms that receive, process, and act on information. The extent of these changes is variable, however, and many elderly persons remain highly efficient learners. These normal age-related changes may be compounded by disease-related changes that compromise attention, concentration, memory, problem solving, judgment, and the ability to respond motorically. Therefore, training programs designed to manage task performance dysfunctions must take into account changes in learning capability. In general, older adults learn best when they are involved in tasks that have personal meaning and they can control the pace of learning. The environment should have adequate ambient and focused lighting and should be free of distracting stimuli. Some elderly persons may have difficulty distinguishing relevant cues from irrelevant ones (eg, distinguishing the start button on a microwave oven from other buttons), so relevant cues should be emphasized orally, visually, or manually. A supportive social environment helps reduce the frustration associated with the struggle to relearn basic skills.

The traditional outcome of rehabilitation is independent functioning; however, in geriatric practice, functional independence may not be feasible. When independence is not possible, patients may be able to achieve a measure of independence that benefits them and their caregivers. For example, physical stress on a caregiver is reduced when patients learn to bear some weight during transfers. Even when patients remain totally dependent, occupational therapy may result in their becoming more cooperative with caregivers, particularly during ADLs. For example, violent reactions during dressing may be avoided in a patient with dementia if the caregiver provides breakfast beforehand and shows each garment to the patient before putting it on.

31. EXERCISE

About 35% of noninstitutionalized persons > 65 yr of age describe themselves as being limited in some type of activity. Some limitation results from chronic disabling conditions or from normal aging, but much results from disuse of muscles and joints. Yet the physiologic changes associated with exercise translate into practical benefits.

BENEFITS OF EXERCISE

Improvements in Functional Capacity

Only 29% of those > 65 yr report doing any regular exercise, including walking. Aerobic capacity (usually limited more by cardiovascular than respiratory decline) is so low that even in healthy seniors (≥ 65 yr), carrying out activities such as making beds, doing light shopping, or dressing and undressing may use ≥ 50% of the average person's maximal capacity. Raising the maximal capacity by even 10% to 15% greatly improves functional ability and quality of life and prolongs independence. The very sedentary (ie, those who do not walk outside the house or exercise) achieve even greater benefit from a small increment in physical activity.

Exercise goals differ among subgroups of the older population and from those of younger persons. In those > 75 yr, the emphasis is on maintaining flexibility, strength, coordination, and balance, as well as aerobic conditioning. Aerobic or cardiovascular conditioning improves the ability of the heart and lungs to supply muscles with oxygen and is best accomplished by walking, jogging, cycling, or swimming. To be effective, aerobic conditioning exercise must be sustained for at least 15 to 20 min at a time. Walking and range-of-motion exercises are appropriate for previously sedentary persons. In those 65 through 74 yr and those ≥ 75 who have remained physically active, exercise may also include moderate aerobic conditioning. Physicians should prescribe activity based on a patient's previous exercise experience, current activity, general physical condition, and medical history.

Other Benefits

Aging, especially in sedentary persons, is associated with an increase in body fat and a decrease in lean body mass. (The loss of muscle mass is sometimes called sarcopenia.) Exercise enhances weight control by expending more calories and suppressing appetite, but it is not a substitute for decreasing caloric intake in those who are overweight. When exercise accompanies negative caloric balance, fat is lost and lean body mass is preserved as long as daily protein intake exceeds 1.2 gm/kg. Blood pressure declines independently of weight reduction. HDL cholesterol rises and LDL cholesterol falls. Persons with diabetes, particularly type II (non–insulin-dependent), may benefit from increased insulin sensitivity associated with exercise-facilitated uptake of glucose by muscle.

Physical activity retards osteoporosis by slowing the rate of bone loss, but adequate dietary calcium (1 to 1.5 gm/day) is needed for healthy bone remodeling. Other treatments for osteoporosis may also be required (see Ch. 73). Increased muscle strength may protect vulnerable joints (eg, quadriceps exercises improve knee function) and the lower back, thus enhancing overall physical ability. A strength-training program for the biceps, triceps, and quadriceps muscles in nonagenarians has resulted in increased muscle size and strength. Thus, age is not a contraindication to strength training.

Although the appropriate use of growth hormones and anabolic steroids has not yet been defined, they have been shown to increase muscle mass. These drugs are most beneficial to persons whose plasma growth hormone or testosterone levels are low. However, studies that show a possible improvement in function (ie, strength) are inadequate, and no conclusions have been reached about their effectiveness beyond increasing plasma growth hormone or testosterone levels.

Studies suggest that perceived well-being and self-image improve with regular exercise, probably as a result of both social interaction and physical conditioning. Symptomatic improvement of depression and certain aspects of cognitive function, including reaction time, has also been reported. Anxiety (particularly its somatic manifestations) decreases, and sleep patterns and bowel function may improve. Ultimately, drug therapy may be reduced in dosage or need.

RISKS OF EXERCISE

The most serious adverse effects of exercise are cardiovascular, including sudden death. Although such sequelae are rare, they usually occur in persons with decreased left ventricular function and myocardial ischemia. A survey of cardiac arrests occurring in cardiac rehabilitation centers showed a nonfatal arrest rate of 1/34,673 patient-exercise hours and a fatal arrest rate of 1/116,402 patient-exercise hours. No comparable data exist for cardiac arrests among community-dwelling elderly exercising in unsupervised settings. The risk of sudden death increases severalfold during vigorous exercise; however, at comparable exertion levels, those who exercise regularly are at lower risk than those who are sedentary. Since inactivity is an independent risk factor for ischemic heart disease, the relative risks and benefits of exercise in addition to loss of bone mass and muscle strength must be assessed individually.

Possible injury from falls and other musculoskeletal complications should be considered. All active older persons should wear shock-absorbing shoes with traction soles (eg, running or walking shoes).

Proper warm-up, gentle stretching, and gradual onset of activity help prevent injuries. Most community-dwelling elderly are able to walk; walking, coupled with stretching exercises, is an excellent way to maintain function and reduce the risks of extreme inactivity.

EVALUATION OF EXERCISE ABILITY

Preexercise screening facilitates choosing an appropriate activity program for all except those for whom any physical exertion is an unwarranted risk. Some 10% to 43% of community-dwelling persons who volunteer to participate in unsupervised moderate exercise programs (ie, achieving 70% to 85% of maximal heart rate) are medically excluded and thus require a lower level of exercise. Reasons for exclusion include active coronary artery disease or clear risk factors, severe arthritis or other musculoskeletal disability, and uncontrolled hypertension or diabetes. Of these exclusions, 70% to 80% occur *before* stress testing.

Aerobic conditioning should not be an automatic exercise goal but is appropriate for many young-old and for those > 75 yr who have always been physically active.

Assessment should include previous and current activity; cardiovascular, mental, and metabolic status; balance; and gait stability. Subtle cognitive decline might limit a person's ability to follow an exercise prescription, and sensory impairment or balance problems could predispose to falls.

The pertinent **history** should include the above areas, as well as respiratory symptoms, musculoskeletal complaints, and drug history (all medications as well as alcohol and tobacco use). **Physical examination** should focus on visual and mental status and on the cardiovascular, respiratory, and musculoskeletal systems, including range of motion. The patient's walk should be observed, and functional capacity should be assessed by observing how far the patient can walk and whether the patient can climb stairs. If the history suggests a high-risk patient or if abnormalities occur with moderate exertion, then **noninvasive tests** such as exercise thallium scintigraphy, rest adenosine-thallium scintigraphy, or exercise echocardiography may help determine an appropriate exercise program. Nutritional status and weight should also be evaluated. Although individual health status and the availability of recent test results determine which tests are needed, in general **laboratory tests** should include a resting ECG, hematocrit and blood glucose studies, urinalysis, and any tests indicated by the history and physical examination. For many, an exercise stress test is *not* required.

TABLE 31–1 lists common drugs that may affect ability to exercise. Patients taking drugs that can cause volume depletion or orthostatic hypotension should have blood pressure and pulse checked while both reclining and standing. Patients taking diuretics should have potassium levels measured. β-Adrenergic blockers do not preclude regular exer-

TABLE 31–1. COMMON DRUGS THAT MAY AFFECT ABILITY TO EXERCISE

Drugs	*Side Effects*
Antihypertensives Hypnotics Tranquilizers	Orthostasis, falls, sedation
Diuretics	Hypokalemia → arrhythmias, muscle cramps Dehydration → orthostasis, falls, thermoregulatory disturbance
Antidepressants	Orthostasis, falls, arrhythmias, sedation
Insulin, oral hypoglycemics	Hypoglycemia
β-Adrenergic blockers	Decreased heart rate, fatigue, masking of hypoglycemic symptoms except sweating

cise, but the blunting of exercise-induced tachycardia must be considered. Patients taking these drugs must rely on their own sense of perceived exertion—see under EXERCISE STRESS TESTING, below.

Persons with diabetes need to be evaluated for metabolic control, particularly risk of hypoglycemia; as exercise increases, those taking insulin or oral hypoglycemics should be monitored for need to reduce dosage. Insulin must not be injected directly into muscle groups used in exercise; the increased blood flow may speed insulin uptake and precipitate hypoglycemia. For example, a walker or tennis player should inject the insulin subcutaneously into the abdominal tissue.

EXERCISE STRESS TESTING

Graded exercise testing identifies a safe range for heart rate and blood pressure during exercise, whether or not the person has coronary artery disease. Patients without evidence of coronary artery or other cardiovascular disease do *not* require stress testing *if the planned exercise program consists of only walking.* Stress testing is recommended for those who plan to do more intense exercise or those with a history of significant cardiovascular disease.

Maximal stress testing is not required, although patients should reach at least 85% of age-predicted maximal heart rate (see THE EXERCISE PRESCRIPTION, below, for calculation of maximal heart rate). Either a treadmill or a bicycle ergometer provides a satisfactorily graded stress

TABLE 31–2. BORG RATING OF PERCEIVED EXERTION SCALE

6	
7	Very, very light
8	
9	Very light
10	
11	Fairly light
12	
13	Somewhat hard
14	
15	Hard
16	
17	Very hard
18	
19	Very, very hard

Adapted from Borg G: "Perceived exertion as an indicator of somatic stress." *Scandinavian Journal of Rehabilitation Medicine* 2:92–98, 1970; used with permission.

under continuous ECG monitoring. Although treadmills use walking, which is a familiar activity, many older persons have problems with balance, particularly as speed and grade increase. The modified Balke or Naughton protocols are tolerated better than the Bruce protocol. Because bicycle ergometers allow the patient to sit and hold on to handlebars, they are appropriate for persons with gait or visual disorders. However, since cycling is less common than walking, local muscle fatigue may impede performance before an adequate heart rate is reached.

Patients should continue taking their usual medications, including digitalis or β-adrenergic blockers, when testing. If heart rate and blood pressure are suppressed by medication, the rating of perceived exertion **(RPE)** is used to gauge the patient's graded exercise testing responses. The Borg RPE is one such scale (see TABLE 31–2). The patient rates his perception of overall effort according to the scale. Perceived exertion and heart rate together predict maximal capacity more accurately than heart rate alone, aiding fitness evaluation and the subsequent exercise prescription.

Submaximal values (eg, heart rate, blood pressure) achieved at a given work load can also be used to assess fitness and monitor the effect of exercise. As fitness improves, the heart rate required to reach a given level of exertion falls. Some researchers have used RPEs to regulate exercise intensity; however, these ratings have not proved accurate in guiding heart rate range at the lower work levels appropriate for older persons. One practical guideline: If a person is unable to talk comfort-

TABLE 31–3. CRITERIA FOR STRESS TEST TERMINATION

Premature ventricular contractions Multifocal In pairs, with increasing frequency Ventricular tachycardia ($\geq$ 3 in a row) Blood pressure abnormalities Fall in systolic $\geq$ 10 mm Hg Systolic > 250 mm Hg Diastolic > 115 mm Hg New-onset atrial tachycardia, fibrillation, or flutter Second- or third-degree heart block Angina, faintness, marked fatigue, dyspnea, nausea, pallor, confusion	Claudication or significant musculoskeletal pain Significant ST segment depression (> 1 mm of horizontal or down-sloping ST segment depression at 80 msec from J point, or > 2 mm or up-sloping ST segment depression at 80 msec from J point) ST segment elevation Achievement of 85% of age-predicted maximal heart rate

Adapted from Posner JD, et al: "Exercise capacity in the elderly." *American Journal of Cardiology* 57:56c, 1986; used with permission.

ably while exercising, he is probably exceeding the anaerobic threshold (about 50% of VO_2max), ie, building an oxygen debt. The pulse should be checked promptly to ascertain that it is within the training range (see THE EXERCISE PRESCRIPTION, below).

Problems With Testing the Elderly

True **maximal stress testing** is defined as *reaching a plateau of oxygen consumption*. Predictions from submaximal treadmill tests systematically underestimate (by 15% to 25%) maximal capacity in elderly patients, partly because of reduced mechanical efficiency in sedentary persons. Patients must adapt to the treadmill or bicycle ergometer before testing, and their ability to understand and perform the test should be assessed. Maximal heart rates in North American elderly populations may exceed those assumed in common VO_2max prediction nomograms, possibly because these populations are in poorer condition than the European populations for whom the nomograms were developed.

Precise assessment of maximal capacity increases the accuracy of an exercise prescription. However, $\geq$ ⅓ of elderly patients do not meet the criteria for maximal stress testing. Furthermore, maximal tests increase the risks of testing, particularly in those with impaired cardiovascular or musculoskeletal function. Testing to 85% of age-predicted maximal heart rate equals or exceeds the level of exertion recommended in exercise programs for the elderly. ECG abnormalities oc-

TABLE 31–4. CARDIOVASCULAR RESPONSES TO AEROBIC EXERCISE

	Submaximal	*Maximal*
In the elderly		
Heart rate	↓	± ↓
Stroke volume	↑	↑
Cardiac output	± ↓	slight ↑
Systolic blood pressure	↓	↓
Diastolic blood pressure	↓	↓
Oxygen uptake ($\dot{V}O_2$)	± ↓	↑
In patients with cardiovascular disease		
Heart rate	↓	±
Stroke volume	↑	± ↑ especially with high intensity
Cardiac output	±	± ↑ especially with high intensity
Systolic blood pressure	↓	± variable
Diastolic blood pressure	↓	± variable
Oxygen uptake ($\dot{V}O_2$)	± ↓	↑

↓ = decrease, ↑ = increase.
Adapted from Lowenthal DT, Pollock ML: "Cardiac response to exercise in health and disease." *Seminars in Respiratory Medicine* 14(2):97, 1993; used with permission from Thieme Medical Publishers, Inc.

curring at less than 85% of age-predicted maximal heart rate identify those who should not exercise or who require medically supervised exercise. Indications for terminating an exercise stress test are listed in TABLE 31–3.

Results of Stress Tests

Symptoms and ECG changes occurring near maximal exertion are relative contraindications to an exercise program. Unless the medical and family history suggests a high risk of coronary artery disease, activity may still be prescribed at a lower heart rate, generally 75% of that at which abnormalities occurred, although initially the activity should be medically supervised.

ST segment abnormalities are most indicative of coronary disease when they occur with angina, arrhythmias, or an abnormal blood

TABLE 31–5. CAUSES OF FALSE–POSITIVE ST SEGMENT CHANGES DURING EXERCISE STRESS TESTING

Hyperventilation	Other cardiac abnormalities (valvular disease, asymmetric septal hypertrophy)
Abnormal ventricular depolarization-repolarization	Vasoregulatory abnormalities
Left ventricular hypertrophy	Use of cardiac glycosides
Left-sided intraventricular conduction delays	Hypokalemia
Wolff-Parkinson-White syndrome	ST segment depression at rest

Adapted from Shepard RJ: "Prognostic value of exercise testing for ischemic heart disease." *British Journal of Sports Medicine* 16:220–229, 1982; used with permission.

pressure response or at very low exertion. A pretest high likelihood of disease (history of symptoms or risk factors) also increases the test's positive predictive value. Patients who develop hypotension or significant ST segment depression during the first 3 min of exercise have a substantial risk of high-level (triple-vessel or left main artery) coronary disease and require prompt diagnostic follow-up. Exercise is contraindicated until a definitive diagnosis is made and symptoms are appropriately treated.

TABLE 31–4 compares the cardiovascular responses to aerobic exercise in the elderly with responses in patients who have ischemic heart disease. Notably, neither group experiences a change or fall in oxygen uptake with submaximal exercise. However, training can bring about a rise in oxygen uptake during maximal stress. Submaximal stress testing is insufficient for assessing cardiovascular capacity.

Elderly persons who develop significant ST segment depression *without* chest pain or other symptoms, particularly at higher levels of exertion, are difficult to assess. For instance, 25% to 50% of abnormal exercise stress tests occur in asymptomatic older persons, particularly women; however, 25% to 45% of these abnormal test results are normal when the test is repeated, or the ST segment depression resolves with conditioning. TABLE 31–5 lists causes of false-positive test results.

THE EXERCISE PRESCRIPTION

Warm Up and Cool Down

Exercise sessions should begin with 5 to 10 min of gentle stretching and flexibility exercises for the neck, trunk, and limbs (eg, sitting stretches to reach the toes; neck rotation; and hamstring, quadriceps, and lateral trunk stretches). The person should hold the stretch for 10 sec (just beyond what is comfortable) and *refrain from bouncing* (ballistic maneuvers); bouncing increases muscle tension by stimulating antagonist muscles. Light limb exercises should follow. Such warm-up periods decrease musculoskeletal complications and reduce myocardial ischemia during exercise.

Cool-down and flexibility exercises should be repeated at the end of the session; muscles tend to shorten during more vigorous exertion, and stretching after the workout decreases the risk of muscle cramps. When aerobic conditioning is contraindicated, stretching and range-of-motion activities can be prescribed either alone or before and after walking.

Target Heart Rate

For aerobic conditioning, a program that produces a training benefit in sedentary elderly persons is based on **heart rate reserve,** which is calculated as **maximal heart rate (MHR:** 220 minus age in years) minus **resting heart rate (RHR).** A training benefit occurs when 30% to 45% of the heart rate reserve is added to the RHR. This is the **target heart rate range,** about 65% to 80% of predicted MHR, somewhat lower than the 70% to 85% of MHR recommended by the American Heart Association for aerobic conditioning in younger persons.

The target heart rate range for a 70-yr-old with an RHR of 84 is calculated as follows:

$$220 - \text{age} = \text{MHR}$$
$$220 - 70 = 150$$

$$\text{MHR} - \text{RHR} = \text{heart rate reserve}$$
$$150 - 84 = 66$$

Figure 30% and 45% of heart rate reserve

$$30\% \times 66 = 20 \qquad 45\% \times 66 = 30$$

Add to RHR

$$84 + 20 = 104 \qquad 84 + 30 = 114$$

$$\text{Target heart rate range} = 104 \text{ to } 114$$

This method allows for variability in RHR. Persons who are not physically fit, who generally have a higher RHR and thus smaller heart rate reserve, require a smaller increment to achieve training benefit. This calculation may underestimate the true range, but taking a conservative approach and reassessing the increase in range after a period of sustained training is better than overestimating the range.

To calculate an exercise heart rate, the radial pulse is palpated in the first 10 sec after ceasing activity (exercise heart rates fall off very rapidly). The result is multiplied by 6, which should yield a rate within the calculated target range. Each person should be taught to adjust, or titrate, the intensity of exercise. If the heart rate is below the target range, intensity should be increased; eg, a person who is walking should adopt a brisker pace. Conversely, if the heart rate is above the target range, intensity should be reduced.

Initially, participants' calculations of heart rate should be checked by a monitor or by a person skilled in performing such measurements. Because the pulse is measured for only a fraction of a minute, an error of a single beat is multiplied sixfold.

Most studies show that an optimal training benefit results from a 30-min period of increased heart rate three to four times a week. Lower-intensity exercise (50% to 60% of MHR) may produce a training benefit if duration is extended. However, less frequent exercise is unlikely to improve fitness. Exercising more than five times a week increases the risk of musculoskeletal injury; high-intensity exercise increases both musculoskeletal and cardiovascular risk, especially if the target range is exceeded. *Participants should not exercise beyond the stress test intensity.*

Initially, most sedentary persons are unable to sustain a target heart rate for 30 min. A program should begin gradually, eg, by alternating 2 to 3 min of exercise with 2 to 3 min of rest over 15 min. Activity should be increased by 2 to 3 min/wk until a total of 30 min is reached. Then the exercise interval should be increased by 1 to 2 min/wk until the target heart rate can be sustained for 30 min. For previously inactive persons > 75 yr, lower-intensity and more frequent but shorter periods of activity are advised. An appropriate goal would be 15 to 20 min of walking six times a week.

The previously inactive or frail patient > 75 yr should use shorter intervals to build endurance (eg, alternate 30 sec of activity with 30 sec of rest) and increase the activity intervals by 30 to 60 sec/wk as endurance improves. In those who are physically unfit, work capacity may be so low that aerobic conditioning occurs as the by-product of a program that otherwise would produce no training benefit. Clinical signs of improved aerobic capacity include a lower RHR and decreased perceived exertion. The distance walked in 6 min can also be used to assess fitness: The patient is asked to walk a measured course (eg, up and down a 100-ft hall) for 6 min. As fitness improves, the patient is able to walk farther during the 6-min period. Fitness also means strength. The frail elderly may benefit from very low-level, repetitive weight training, especially when it involves the lower extremities. Falls may be reduced or even prevented by incorporating strengthening exercises (ie, *resistance* or *static* exercise) into the routine (see TABLE 31–6). Examples of strengthening exercise include the use of free weights (eg, 5 to 10 lb) and frequent repetition on Medex, Nautilus, or Universal types of equipment.

Activity intensity is often expressed in metabolic equivalents, or **METs** (*one MET is the oxygen expenditure at rest, about 3.5 mL/kg of*

TABLE 31–6. EXERCISE STANDARDS FOR HEALTHY ELDERLY ADULTS

	AHA	*ACSM*
Frequency	3 days/wk*	3–5 days/wk
Intensity	50–60%*	50–85% $\mathring{V}O_2max$
Duration	20–30 min*	20–60 min
Mode	Walk, run, swim, cross-country ski, cycle	Same plus dance, skip rope, row, climb stairs, and participate in endurance sports
Resistance	Important but not specific; 1 set, 8–10 repetitions; moderate intensity	2 days/wk; same but moderate to high intensity*

AHA = American Heart Association, ACSM = American College of Sports Medicine.
* Minimum standard.
Adapted from Lowenthal DT, Pollock ML: "Cardiac response to exercise in health and disease." *Seminars in Respiratory Medicine* 14(2):98, 1993; reprinted with permission from Thieme Medical Publishers, Inc.

body weight per minute). Maximal oxygen uptake **(MET capacity)** can be derived from stress test data. When the heart rate response is normal, 80% of MHR corresponds to 70% of MET capacity. TABLE 31–7 shows the MET level of some common activities.

Specific Exercise Programs

Exercise programs should always be individualized. A *written* exercise prescription should detail the recommended activity, including initial intensity, duration, frequency, and ways to increase activity as fitness improves. The prescription should include instructions to stop exercising promptly and see a physician if ischemia-related symptoms develop (eg, chest pain, marked dyspnea, dizziness, claudication, or extreme fatigue). Patients should also be told to drink ample amounts of fluid and to refrain from vigorous activity in extreme heat and cold. Physicians should consult exercise physiologists or physicians or nurses in cardiac rehabilitation units if they are uncertain about the details of an exercise prescription.

Generally, jogging is inappropriate for older persons not already accustomed to it. Walking, cycling, dancing, and swimming all provide excellent conditioning (aerobic or otherwise), with less stress on the lower back, hips, knees, and ankles. Swimming is particularly benefi-

TABLE 31–7. METABOLIC REQUIREMENT OF COMMON ACTIVITIES

Activity	*METs*	*Kcal/h*
Walking at 2–3 mph Cycling (level) at 6 mph Light stretching exercises Swimming (with float board) Light to moderate housework	2–4	180–300
Walking at 4 mph Cycling at 8 mph Golf (walking, pulling cart) Light calisthenics Swimming (treading water) Heavy housework or yard work	5–6	300–360
Walking-jogging at 5 mph Swimming (1/2 mile in 30 min) Cycling at 11–12 mph Recreational tennis Hiking	7–8	420–480

MET = metabolic equivalent.

Adapted from Hanson PG, et al: "Clinical guidelines for exercise training." *Postgraduate Medicine* 67(1):120–138, 1980. Copyright © McGraw-Hill, Inc.; used with permission.

cial in persons with painful joints. Physical activity should also be incorporated into a person's daily routine. For example, using a shopping cart may enable a person to walk to stores rather than drive or ride, and taking stairs may be preferred to using an elevator.

Men and high-risk women should begin exercising in a supervised setting; low- or average-risk women may not require supervision. Medically supervised exercise programs can be found through hospital or cardiac rehabilitation programs, the American Heart Association, or senior citizen groups. Persons with a history of heart disease and those with abnormal stress test results who are allowed to exercise should begin programs more vigorous than walking only under supervision. If no adverse effects occur after 3 to 6 mo, such persons may continue independently at the same intensity level.

Very frail elderly persons, those who cannot walk several blocks without difficulty, and those with cognitive impairment precluding reliable self-monitoring also should increase activity only under supervision. If musculoskeletal symptoms of overuse occur, the activity should be stopped or changed (eg, swimming instead of jogging) until the person is pain free. If injury or illness causes exercise to cease for > 1 wk, activity should be resumed at a lower intensity.

Exercise may be performed alone or with a group. Except for those who require supervision (generally provided in a group setting), either is appropriate. The social interaction of a group may provide psychologic support and facilitate adherence to the program. Selecting an activity the person likes, setting attainable goals, and providing encouragement and reinforcement during training and at follow-up visits also foster adherence.

With appropriate screening and individualized exercise prescriptions, regular physical activity can and should be incorporated into the lifestyles of older persons. Increased activity can bring major benefits in functional capacity, sense of well-being, and other improvements in health.

§3. ORGAN SYSTEMS

INTRODUCTION

CARDIOVASCULAR DISORDERS

PULMONARY DISORDERS

GASTROINTESTINAL DISORDERS

GENITOURINARY AND GYNECOLOGIC DISORDERS

HEMATOLOGIC DISORDERS

HEMATOLOGIC DISORDERS *(Continued)*

MUSCULOSKELETAL DISORDERS

METABOLIC AND ENDOCRINE DISORDERS

INFECTIOUS DISEASE

NEUROLOGIC DISORDERS

NEUROLOGIC DISORDERS *(Continued)*

PSYCHIATRIC DISORDERS

SKIN DISORDERS

EYE DISORDERS

EAR, NOSE, AND THROAT DISORDERS

§3. ORGAN SYSTEMS: INTRODUCTION

CARDIOVASCULAR DISORDERS

§3. ORGAN SYSTEMS: INTRODUCTION

32. AGING PROCESSES

The large number of theories on aging can be attributed in part to the newness of biologic gerontology, a discipline that has received intensive research support only in the past 15 yr. But it can also be attributed to the fact that no single theory could possibly explain all the aging processes. Just as ongoing research in oncology uncovers many mechanisms for the origin of cancers, further research in biologic gerontology will find many aging mechanisms at the molecular, cellular, organ, and organism levels.

The major current theories of aging can be divided into two types: those that suppose aging events occur randomly and accumulate with time (stochastic theories) and those that suppose aging is predetermined (nonstochastic theories).

STOCHASTIC THEORIES

Error Catastrophe Theory

This theory proposes that over time an accumulation of errors in protein synthesis results in impaired cellular function. No biologic process is 100% accurate, and errors in transcription and translation could lead to protein abnormalities. However, most research indicates that transcription and translation continue to function well with advancing age; if this theory were correct, aging would occur at an unchanged pace from birth. Other findings that do *not* support this theory include evidence that there is (1) no change in amino acid sequence in proteins from young and old animals, (2) no increase in defective tRNAs with age, and (3) no age-related differences in the accuracy of poly(U)-directed protein synthesis. In fact, most alterations of protein found with aging are posttranslational.

Cross-Linking Theory

This theory proposes that the cross-linking of proteins and other cellular macromolecules leads to age-dependent diseases and disorders. Although this theory cannot explain all the changes associated with aging, it may account for some. Extracellular collagen becomes increasingly cross-linked in humans and animals. Although this cross-linking decreases mobility of certain tissues, it does not appear to have a major clinical impact. However, the cross-linking of glycosylated proteins may play an important role in age-dependent opacification in crystalline lens protein and eventual cataract development. Cross-linking between glycosylated immunoglobulins and glomerular basement membrane proteins and between glycosylated lipoproteins and arterial wall proteins has also been proposed as important in the development of age-dependent glomerular and arterial diseases in humans and in animals.

Wear and Tear Theory

This theory proposes that the cumulative damage to vital irreplaceable body parts leads to the death of cells, tissues, organs, and finally the organism. For example, DNA is constantly damaged throughout life, and recent studies indicate the loss of DNA at the ends of chromosomes (telomeres) in certain organisms with aging. If DNA repair is incomplete or age-related impairments in repair mechanisms occur, cellular function might progressively decline. In fact, DNA repair capacity positively correlates with species life span, suggesting a role of efficient DNA repair in the evolution of longevity. However, studies of DNA repair during the aging of experimental animals do not show a consistent decline with aging. (Some studies show a decline; others show no change.) Such studies are complicated by multiple DNA repair mechanisms and uncertainty about which mechanisms are most critical to aging. Further refinement of the techniques for detecting DNA damage may help clarify whether it does accumulate with aging.

Free Radical Theory

Free radicals are highly reactive molecules that can damage membrane proteins, enzymes, and DNA. The most important source of free radicals is oxygen metabolism, which yields the superoxide radical O_2^-. Proponents of this theory believe that low-level free-radical damage accumulates over time, resulting in the findings associated with aging. Studies in which various antioxidants were fed to animals found an increase in life expectancy, but in many of these studies antioxidant administration was accompanied by weight loss—a potential confounder because it independently produces a significant increase in life expectancy. However, levels of the naturally occurring cellular antioxidant superoxide dismutase correlate well with life span in primates, supporting this theory. Finally, in some lower forms of life, mutations leading to defects in the production of free-radical–quenching enzymes are also associated with shorter life span.

NONSTOCHASTIC THEORIES

Pacemaker Theories

Certain organs or organ systems (eg, the immune and neuroendocrine systems, notably the hypothalamus) are thought to be intrinsic pacemakers of the aging process, genetically programmed to involute at specific times during an organism's life span. This programmed senescence is hypothesized to affect the aging of the entire organism.

With aging, both B- and T-cell functions decline, controlled largely by the major histocompatibility complex (MHC). T-cell functions are more impaired, the decline paralleling the involution of the thymus gland, which begins in adolescence. In studies of mice that are identical except for MHC, B- and T-cell functions closely correlate with life span. Also, the age-related increase in malignancies may be related to the age-dependent decline in cellular immune surveillance.

As another example, adrenergic activity increases with age and β-mediated vasodilation decreases. These changes may be linked to age-related increases in blood pressure, impaired carbohydrate tolerance, and altered sleep patterns.

Studies of hypophysectomized animals receiving hormone replacement therapy suggested that aging was slowed and prompted a search for a death hormone, whose level increases with age, or a Methuselah hormone, whose level decreases with age. However, no data support these notions.

All of these theories fail to explain the origin of the changes in the pacemaker system itself. Also, they fail to take into account that not all organisms have well-developed immune or neuroendocrine systems.

Genetic Theories

Genetic factors are important determinants of aging, although most mechanisms involved are unknown. Life span is remarkably specific for each species, yet even within species genetic factors are important. In humans, the life expectancy of identical twins is more similar than that of siblings, and some families demonstrate a strong predisposition for longevity. Mutant varieties of *Caenorhabditis elegans,* a nematode, have been produced with life spans increased by 50%; the increase appears to result from a single gene in some strains. Researchers are now attempting to clone and examine this gerontogene.

VARIABILITY

Some biologic changes in the elderly are related to aging alone, while others result from disease. In evaluating and managing health and disease in the elderly, it is important, although not always possible, to understand and recognize the difference.

The rate of age-related decline in organ function varies greatly; thus, people become less alike as they age. Also, within any individual, the functions of different organs decline at different rates, so that kidney function may decline more quickly than heart or lung function.

Age-adjusted criteria have been established for several clinically important functions; eg, spirometric measures are commonly expressed as "percent of expected" for age and body size, and cardiac exercise tolerance tests use age-adjusted criteria for maximum heart rate. With aging, glomerular filtration rate (GFR) declines, and creatinine clearance falls about 10 mL/min for each decade. Because endogenous creatinine production also falls, however, normal serum creatinine levels remain unchanged. Thus, in the elderly, serum creatinine levels reflect a substantially lower GFR. Understanding these changes is important in prescribing drugs for the elderly. However, these are *average* changes for age, and the variability in function makes applying averages to each individual difficult.

USUAL (AVERAGE) VS. SUCCESSFUL (PURE) AGING

Many factors modify the effects of the intrinsic aging process. The observed changes produced by these factors have been classified as either usual aging or successful aging.

Usual aging refers to *changes due to the combined effects of the aging process and of disease and adverse environmental and lifestyle factors*. **Successful aging** refers to *the changes due solely to the aging process, uncomplicated by damage from environment, lifestyle, or disease*.

For example, oxygen consumption declines in most sedentary elderly people (usual aging), but it increases in elderly people who begin to regularly perform aerobic exercise after a long period of sedentary living in which oxygen consumption has declined (successful aging). Thus, persons who age successfully can achieve levels of oxygen consumption equal to those of sedentary young adults. Therefore, it should not be assumed that the differences in clinical status between elderly patients and younger persons represent only the effects of aging. These differences depend on varying mixtures of age-dependent and disease-related effects.

A disability or abnormal finding often results from a disease rather than normal aging. For example, elderly people with low hematocrits are often incorrectly diagnosed as having an "anemia of old age" without further diagnostic evaluation or treatment. However, since studies have shown that no age-dependent change in hematocrit occurs in healthy community-dwelling elderly people, a low hematocrit always indicates an abnormality. In fact, most common clinical laboratory measures are not significantly influenced by normal aging (see Ch. 113). There are a few exceptions; eg, oral glucose tolerance diminishes, but fasting blood glucose levels remain in the normal range.

Many normal age-dependent reductions in biologic functions reduce compensatory reserve. With successful aging, these changes may never produce clinical symptoms and illness, but when other factors affect an older person, the reduced reserve may cause problems. For example, the normal age-related decline in cerebral blood flow may not cause symptoms until an antihypertensive agent aggravates orthostatic hypotension, producing syncope. The average nonagenarian has only about

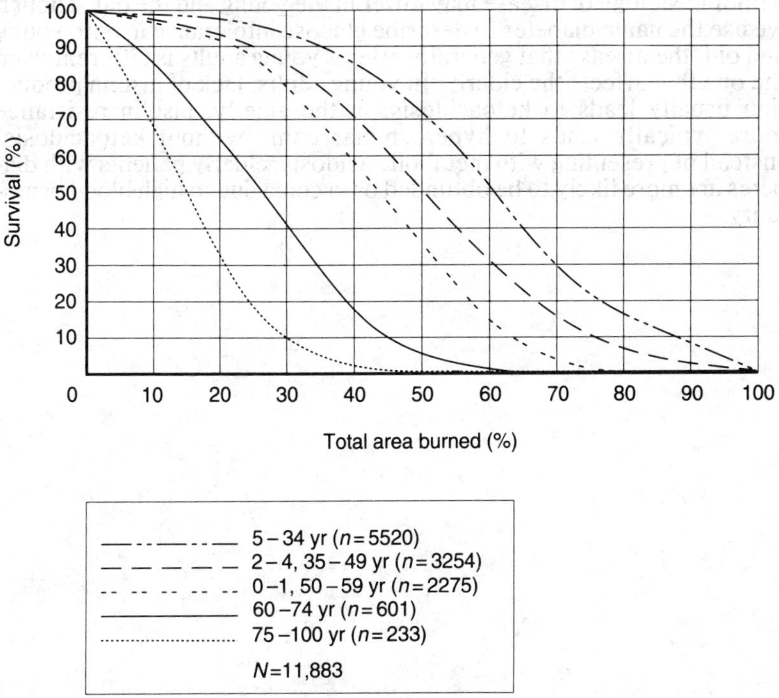

FIG. 32–1. Survival of patients as a function of the total percentage of body surface burned and age. (Modified from Rowe JW: *Cecil Textbook of Medicine*, ed. 18, edited by RL Cecil, JB Wyngaarden, LH Smith. Philadelphia, WB Saunders Company, 1988, p 25; used with permission.)

half the pulmonary function of a normal 30-yr-old, so that acute bacterial pneumonia may lead to serious hypoxemia. With renal function normally reduced by 40% in later life, any further loss may result in inadequate function. Major systemic stress, such as burns, is more likely to cause death in the elderly, probably reflecting reductions in the physiologic function and the reduced reserve of several organ systems (see FIG. 32–1).

Aside from increasing vulnerability to disease, age also affects the way some diseases present in the elderly. Typically in the young, hyperthyroidism presents with hyperactivity and tremor, but in the elderly, it may present as lethargy, heart failure, and confusion. Also, pathophysiology of disease may differ in the young and the old. Though we use the name diabetes to describe glucose intolerance in both young and old, the disease that generally affects young adults is different from the one that affects the elderly. In young adults, lack of insulin production usually leads to ketoacidosis; in the elderly, insulin resistance more typically leads to hyperosmolar coma without ketoacidosis. Instead of presenting with metabolic acidosis, elderly patients with diabetes are more likely to be obtunded or in coma due to high blood osmolality.

§3. ORGAN SYSTEMS: CARDIOVASCULAR DISORDERS

33. NORMAL CHANGES OF AGING

Age-related changes in cardiovascular structure and function increase the probability of disease, modify the threshold at which symptoms and signs arise, and affect the clinical course and prognosis. The widespread prevalence of disease in elderly persons complicates gerontologic study. In particular, occult forms of disease (eg, occult coronary artery disease) can exaggerate functional declines often attributed to aging.

The impact that lifestyle and other variables—such as level of physical activity, diet, smoking and alcohol use, educational and socioeconomic status, and even personality traits—have on cardiovascular function is difficult to assess at a single point in time (eg, as in a cross-sectional study) or over a longer period (eg, as in a longitudinal study). Such variables probably account for the diversity of results and opinions in the scientific literature.

Evidence is mounting that lifestyle and diet can modify age-associated increases in arterial stiffness and pressure. For example, dietary sodium has a greater effect on arterial pressure with age. The rate at which the aorta stiffens with age, as manifested by increased pulse wave velocity, depends on exercise and dietary habits, particularly the amount of sodium ingested. In a Chinese study population whose participants were on a low-sodium diet (44 mmol/24 h) for about 2 yr, the expected age-associated increase in aortic, arm, and leg pulse velocities did not occur.

The sedentary lifestyle of many community-dwelling older persons has led to erroneous conclusions regarding the impact of aging on cardiac functional reserve capacity. In a healthy sedentary population encompassing all ages, arterial stiffness varied inversely with aerobic capacity. This inverse relationship occurred above and beyond the effects of age. Compared with older persons who are sedentary, those who remain physically fit can have up to twice the maximal work capacity and their percentage of body fat does not increase. Indeed, recent studies indicate that, in some instances, the impact of lifestyle on cardiovascular function may be far greater than that of aging.

CARDIOVASCULAR STRUCTURE

The Heart

An aging heart can atrophy, remain unchanged, or show moderate or marked hypertrophy. Atrophy usually coincides with various wasting diseases and is not part of normal aging. This is also true of the extreme ventricular thickening found in some (usually hypertensive) women. A modest increase in left ventricular wall thickness with age is normal in normotensive persons, and an exaggerated increase occurs in hypertensive patients (see Ch. 35).

Left atrial dimension increases with age, even in otherwise healthy persons. A slight increase in left ventricular cavity size may occur, but in studies this has not usually been statistically significant. The cardiac silhouette on chest x-ray enlarges slightly with age when patients are followed up by serial examinations; however, this increase is also clinically normal.

The amount of fibrous tissue increases with age but does not contribute appreciably to cardiac mass. Rather, an increase in myocyte size underlies heart wall thickening. While some myocytes enlarge, others are replaced by fibrous tissue.

Nearly 50% of patients > 70 yr have detectable amyloid in the cardiovascular system, and the incidence rises sharply thereafter. About 50% of the involved hearts have only small amounts of amyloid confined to the atria. Whether cardiac amyloidosis is part of normal aging is debatable; it is not an invariable finding, even in centenarians.

Senile cardiac amyloidosis has two immunologically distinct forms: one is limited to atrial deposits and the other is characterized by ventricular deposits and often minor extracardiac deposits as well. Cardiomegaly is not characteristic, as it is in the much rarer primary amyloidosis that may occur in the elderly. In the senile form, amyloid accumulation is associated with atrophied myocardial fibers, and the heart is not firm, large, or waxy.

The Vasculature

Arterial walls stiffen with age, and the aorta becomes dilated and elongated. This appears to result not from atherosclerosis but from changes in the amount and nature of elastin and collagen as well as from calcium deposition. In particular, changes in the cross-linking of collagen may render it less elastic. With aging, glycoprotein eventually disappears from elastin fibrils, elastin becomes frayed, and its calcium content increases. The higher mineral (calcium, phosphorus) content of elastin is associated with an increase in more polar amino acids. While the total mucopolysaccharide content (ground substance) of the interstitial matrix is unaltered with aging, the amount of dermatan sulfate and heparan sulfate increases and that of hyaluronate and chondroitin decreases. Arterial stiffness may also be due in part to increased arterial tonus. The incidence and severity of subintimal thickening and atherosclerosis also rise markedly. Whether age-related changes occur in vascular permeability, smooth muscle function, gene expression, or the inflammatory response to injury is not known.

CARDIOVASCULAR FUNCTION

Cardiovascular function and cardiac output are determined by the interaction of several variables, each of which is ultimately dependent on biophysical mechanisms that regulate cardiac muscle and ventricular function (see FIG. 33–1).

Cardiac Filling and Preload

Factors that determine ventricular volume (ie, fiber stretch, end-diastolic blood volume, and filling pressure) are sometimes referred to

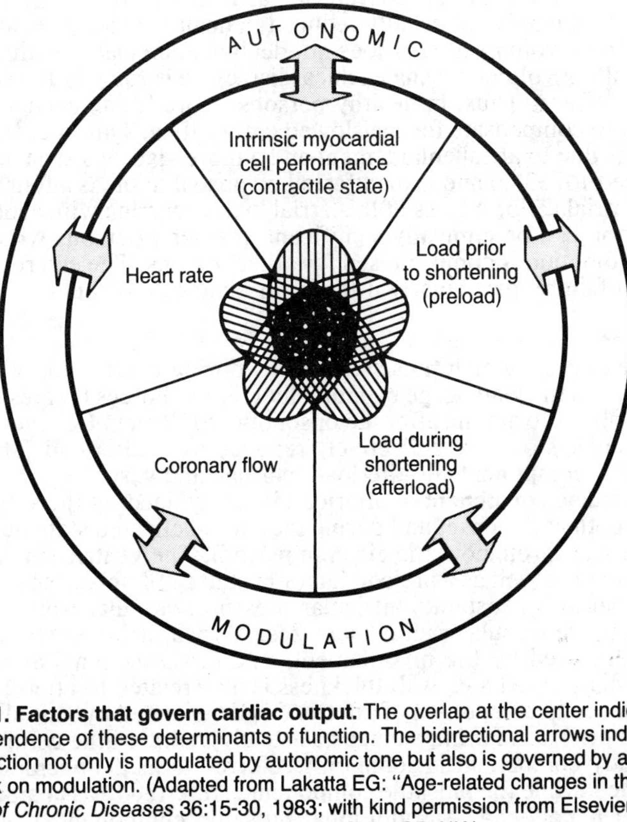

FIG. 33–1. Factors that govern cardiac output. The overlap at the center indicates the interdependence of these determinants of function. The bidirectional arrows indicate that each function not only is modulated by autonomic tone but also is governed by a negative feedback on modulation. (Adapted from Lakatta EG: "Age-related changes in the heart." *Journal of Chronic Diseases* 36:15-30, 1983; with kind permission from Elsevier Science Ltd, The Boulevard, Langford Lane, Kidlington OX5 1GB, UK.)

as preload. Preload is related to the filling volume and degree of myocardial stretch before excitation; hence, it is one determinant of myocardial function and pump performance. Left ventricular compliance (inverse of stiffness) affects the atrioventricular pressure gradient, which determines left ventricular filling rate. A reduction in ventricular compliance with age remains unproved because its measurement requires the simultaneous determination of pressure and volume.

The **early diastolic filling rate** progressively slows after the age of 20 yr, so that by 80 yr, the rate is reduced up to 50% (see FIG. 33–2). This reduction in filling rate (demonstrated by echocardiography, radionuclide angiography, and Doppler ultrasonography) is attributed either to structural (fibrous) changes within the left ventricular myocardium or to residual myofilament Ca^{++} activation from the preceding systole (ie, prolonged isometric relaxation), which is discussed in greater detail below.

Despite the slowing of left ventricular filling early in diastole, end-diastolic volume is not usually reduced in healthy elderly persons. Because stroke volume at rest does not decline appreciably with age, the at-rest filling volume during each cardiac cycle is roughly the same regardless of age. Thus, in healthy persons, more filling occurs later in diastole to compensate for the slowed early filling. This later filling response is due to atrial enlargement and a more vigorous atrial contraction (see FIG. 33–2) and is manifested on auscultation as a fourth heart sound (atrial gallop). Loss of this atrial kick occurring with acute atrial fibrillation can be clinically significant in elderly persons whose ventricular function is compromised for other reasons. The end result may be heart failure, particularly if the ventricular rate is rapid.

Afterload

The extent to which muscle shortens during contraction varies inversely with the load borne by individual fibers. Forces that resist myocardial fiber shortening after the onset of myofilament Ca^{++} activation (ie, during systole) are collectively referred to as afterload. There are two major components of afterload: cardiac and vascular.

The cardiac component of afterload is determined by the ventricular radius, both at the onset and during the Ca^{++}-activated state (ie, at end diastole and throughout the ejection period). The ventricular radius is an afterload as well as a preload factor because of Laplace's law, which states that at a constant ventricular pressure, vascular wall stress increases as ventricular radius increases. Myocardial wall stress is the force generated by the myofilaments and cross-sectional area of the myocardial wall. Thus, wall thickness is also related to afterload.

The vascular component of afterload is determined by vascular input impedance. Vascular impedance has steady and pulsatile components: the steady component is commonly referred to as **peripheral vascular resistance,** while the pulsatile component is referred to as **characteristic vascular impedance.** An additional pulsatile component of vascular afterload is the **reflected pulse wave.** Thus, the total arterial load placed upon the left ventricle can be characterized by peripheral vascular re-

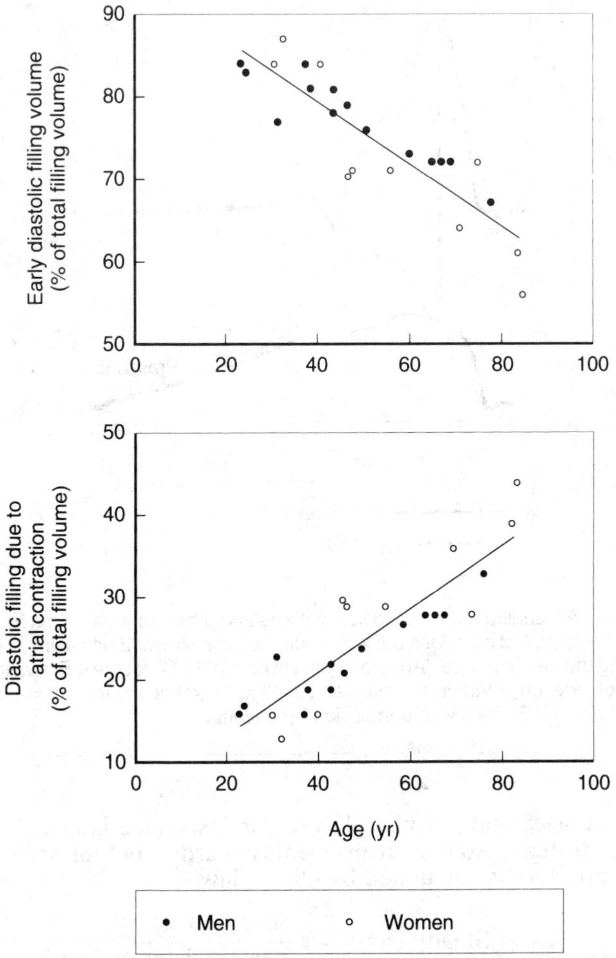

FIG. 33–2. Age-associated decrease in early diastolic filling rate is compensated for by an increase in filling due to the atrial contraction. (Based on data from Swinne CJ, Shapiro EP, Lima SD, Fleg JL: "Age-associated changes in left venticular diastolic performance during isometric exercise in normal subjects." *American Journal of Cardiology* 69:823–826, 1992.)

sistance, characteristic vascular impedance, and pulse wave reflection. The extent to which each of these factors changes with age varies dramatically among individuals.

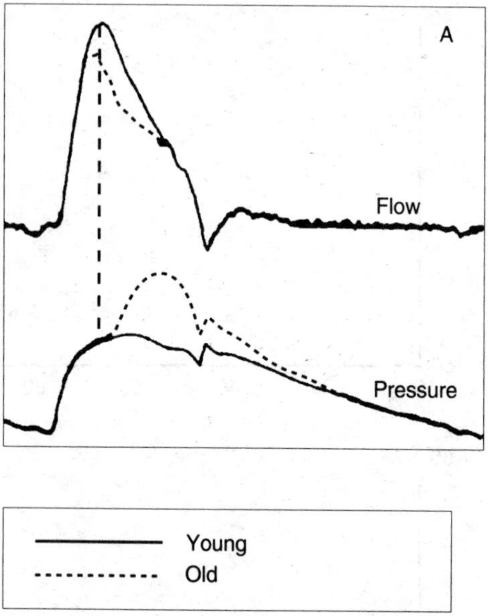

FIG. 33–3. *A,* Ascending aortic blood flow velocity and pressure wave forms from a young and an old person. Not only does peak pressure become elevated with aging, it also peaks later during the cardiac cycle. (Adapted from Nichols WW, O'Rourke MF, Avolio AP, et al: "Effects of age on ventricular-vascular coupling." *American Journal of Cardiology* 55:1179-1184, 1985; used with permission.) *(continued)*

The average total peripheral vascular resistance is calculated indirectly from steady-state measurements of cardiac output or flow. Mean arterial pressure is calculated by Ohm's law:

$$\text{Steady flow} = \frac{\text{mean pressure}}{\text{mean resistance}}$$

Some studies report that basal peripheral vascular resistance increases with age; others have not found this to be so.

Characteristic aortic impedance is usually < 10% of total vascular impedance. Calculated from instantaneous measurements of pressure and flow harmonics, it is determined in part by aortic stiffness, aortic wall thickness and diameter, and aortic pressure.

One index of vascular stiffness is **pulse wave velocity,** which increases with age, owing to the changes in arterial structure noted above. Age-associated increases in pulse wave velocity and late aug-

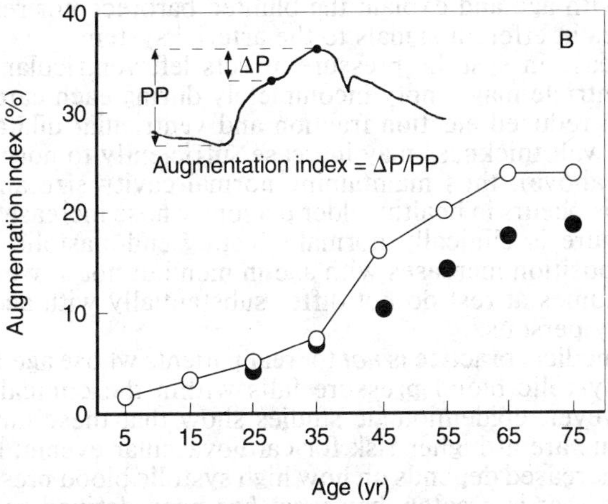

FIG. 33–3 *(Continued). B,* Augmentation index of the carotid artery pressure pulse in healthy persons, measured by applanation tonometry. The augmentation index is defined as the ratio of Δ P:PP; Δ P is the pressure difference from the shoulder to peak; PP is pulse pressure. The ○ population included mild hypertensives. (Based on data from Kelly R, et al: "Noninvasive determination of age-related changes in the human arterial pulse." *Circulation* 80:1652-1659, 1989). The ● population excluded clinical hypertensives (blood pressure > 140/90 mm Hg). (Based on data from Vaitkevicius P, et al: "The age-associated increase in arterial stiffness is attenuated by chronic exercise." *Circulation* 84:II-29, 1991.)

mentation of carotid pressure pulse are blunted in older athletes. Although aortic stiffness is a well-known concomitant of aging, an increase in characteristic aortic impedance has recently been demonstrated via probes that simultaneously measure blood flow and pressure.

Because of increased aortic pulse wave velocity, pressure waves from peripheral sites are returned to the heart sooner in older persons. Pressure in the aortic root continues to rise and peaks later in systole, thereby altering the pressure pulse contour (see FIG. 33–3). Arterial stiffening and the associated increase in pulse wave velocity appear to cause the increase in systolic blood pressure within the clinically normal range that is associated with aging. Some physiologists suggest that this increase in systolic blood pressure reflects a resetting of the baroreceptor reflex to a higher level in the elderly. The same structural changes that render the aorta stiffer and cause pulse wave velocity to increase could be responsible for less baroreceptor stimulation for a given change in aortic pressure. Alternatively, afferent nerve impulses may vary with age and explain the blunted baroreceptor response, as may changes in efferent signals to the arterial system.

The increase in systolic pressure affects left ventricular afterload. The left ventricle may empty incompletely during each cardiac cycle, leading to a reduced ejection fraction and ventricular dilatation. Left ventricular wall thickness may increase sufficiently to normalize wall stress (see above), thus maintaining normal cavity size and ejection fraction; this occurs in healthy older persons whose increase in systolic blood pressure is clinically normal. Resting end-diastolic volume in the seated position increases with age in men but not in women. End-systolic volumes at rest do not differ substantially with age in otherwise healthy persons.

Current medical practice is *not* to treat patients whose age-associated increased systolic blood pressure falls within the clinically normal range. However, epidemiologic studies show that these untreated elderly persons are at higher risk for cardiovascular events; how much the risk is increased depends on how high systolic blood pressure rises. An increase that is greater than what has been defined as normal is referred to as **isolated systolic hypertension** (see Ch. 35).

How the heart and vasculature adapt to age-associated changes is summarized in FIG. 33–4. Strikingly similar changes occur in patients in whom the heart has adapted to hypertension by an increase in mass. In addition, in patients with systolic plus diastolic hypertension, peripheral vascular resistance also increases substantially.

Myocardial Contractility

In addition to preload and afterload, myocardial and left ventricular pump performance depends on the myocardial contractile state (also referred to as intrinsic myocardial cell performance, contractility, inotropic state, or excitation-contraction coupling). The extent to which myofilaments become Ca^{++} activated during systole is determined by the extent of diastolic stretch (preload). Myofilament shortening during contraction (afterload) affects how long Ca^{++} remains bound to the myofilaments throughout systole. Myocardial fiber length both before and during shortening is a modulatory factor of the strength of the heartbeat. The effects of preload and afterload in altering myofilament Ca^{++} activation mimic those of inotropic stimulants, which also alter Ca^{++} activation before or during contraction.

Because many factors interact to regulate cardiac performance (see FIG. 33–1), the intrinsic contractile behavior of myocardial fibers cannot be determined in situ. One index of myocardial contractility that is generally considered superior to others is the trajectory of end-systolic volume vs. mean arterial pressure (sometimes referred to as **Emax**) derived from a series of pressure-volume loops measured over a range of cardiac volumes. In noninvasive studies, a crude index of this trajectory (ie, the ratio of end-systolic arterial pressure to end-systolic volume) is not reduced at rest with age in either healthy men or women.

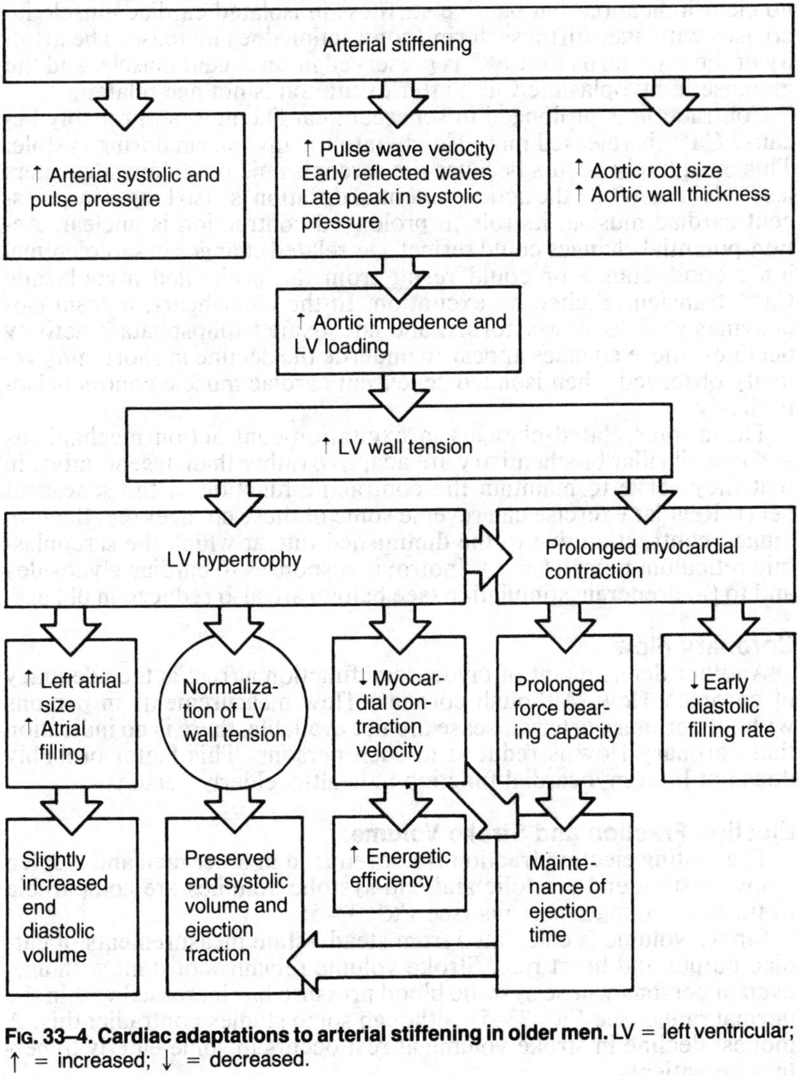

FIG. 33–4. Cardiac adaptations to arterial stiffening in older men. LV = left ventricular; ↑ = increased; ↓ = decreased.

Age-associated changes in the mechanisms that govern excitation-contraction coupling in cardiac muscle have been demonstrated in animal models. Some of these changes are related in part to alterations in gene expression. Studies in rats show that contractile force production, at least at low stimulation, is preserved in old age. While there is no clear indication that passive stiffness in isolated cardiac muscle increases with age, stiffness during contraction does increase. The affinity of the myofibrils for Ca^{++} is preserved in senescent muscle, and the increase in myoplasmic Ca^{++} after excitation is not age related.

Contraction is prolonged in senescent cardiac muscle, probably because Ca^{++} is released more slowly into the myoplasm during systole. This most likely occurs because the sarcoplasmic reticulum sequesters less calcium. While the action-potential duration is also longer in senescent cardiac muscle, its role in prolonged contraction is unclear. Action-potential changes could reflect age-related changes in sarcolemmal ionic conductance or could result from the prolonged myoplasmic Ca^{++} transient elicited by excitation. In the older heart, myosin isoenzymes shift to slower forms, and adenosine triphosphatase activity declines; these changes appear to underlie the decline in shortening velocity observed when isolated senescent cardiac muscle contracts isotonically.

These interrelated changes in excitation-contraction mechanisms and myofibrillar biochemistry are adaptive rather than degenerative, in that they serve to maintain the contractile function of the senescent heart. Regular exercise can reverse some of these changes (eg, the prolonged contraction due to the diminished rate at which the sarcoplasmic reticulum pumps Ca^{++}). Inotropic responses to cardiac glycosides and to β-adrenergic stimulation (see below) are also reduced in old age.

Coronary Flow

Another determinant of myocardial function at rest is the adequacy of coronary flow. Although coronary flow measurements in persons without coronary artery disease are not available, there is no indication that coronary flow is reduced in such persons. This factor probably does not limit myocardial function in healthy elderly persons.

Ejection Fraction and Stroke Volume

The resting ejection fraction is not reduced in older men and women whose resting end-diastolic and end-systolic volumes are comparable to those of younger persons (see FIG. 33–5).

Stroke volume is calculated from steady-state measurements of cardiac output and heart rate. Stroke volume remains constant with age, even in persons whose systolic blood pressure has increased within the normal range (see FIG. 33–5), although some studies contradict this. A modest decline in stroke volume at rest occurs in some elderly hypertensive patients.

Heart Rate

The heart rate at rest is modulated by relative sympathetic and, more important, parasympathetic tone. In healthy men, the supine basal heart rate does not change with aging; in the sitting position, the heart rate decreases slightly. Spontaneous variations in heart rate over a 24-h period occur less often with age in men without coronary artery dis-

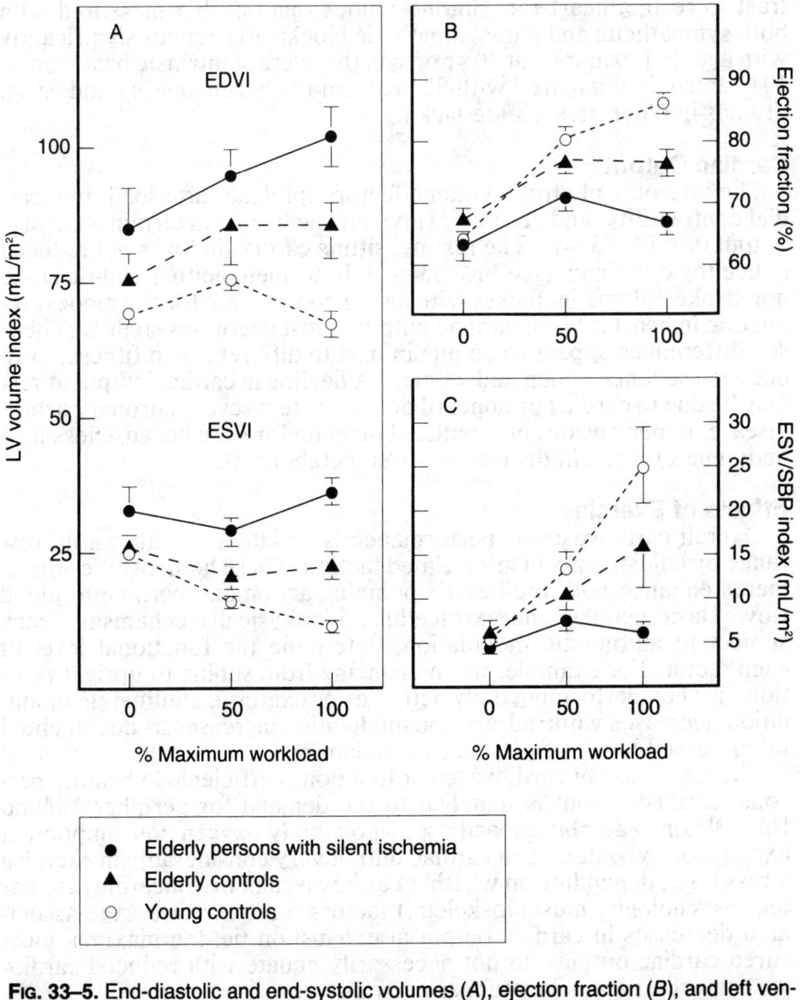

Fig. 33–5. End-diastolic and end-systolic volumes (*A*), ejection fraction (*B*), and left ventricular contractility index, ESV/SBP (*C*) at rest and during vigorous cycle exercise in the seated position in healthy younger and older men and in older men with silent myocardial ischemia. EDVI = end-diastolic volume index; ESVI = end-systolic volume index; LV = left ventricle; SBP = systolic blood pressure. (From Fleg JL, Schulman SP, Gerstenblith G, et al: "Additive effects of age and silent myocardial ischemia on the left ventricular response to upright cycle exercise." *Journal of Applied Physiology* 75:499–504, 1993; used with permission.)

ease. Variations in the sinus rate with respiration also diminish. In contrast to resting heart rate, **intrinsic sinus rate** (ie, that measured with both sympathetic and parasympathetic blockade) declines significantly with age. For example, at 20 yr of age, the average intrinsic heart rate is 104 beats/min compared with 92 beats/min between ages 45 and 55 yr. Studies in older persons are lacking.

Cardiac Output

The interplay of stroke volume factors (preload, afterload, myocardial contractility, and coronary flow) and heart rate determines cardiac output (see FIG. 33–1). The resting, sitting cardiac index is not reduced in healthy older men (see FIG. 33–6*C*). In women, neither end-diastolic nor stroke volume increases with age to compensate for the modest reduction in heart rate, so cardiac output at rest decreases slightly. These sex differences appear to be due in part to differences in fitness, even between sedentary men and women. A decline in cardiac output at rest may be due to cardiac or noncardiac factors (eg, severe coronary artery disease, hypertension, or a reduced demand for flow because less lean body mass results in decreased basal metabolism).

Effects of Exercise

Overall cardiovascular performance is maintained within a narrow range by adjustments in interrelated factors. These homeostatic adjustments enhance both the heart's pumping action and peripheral blood flow. Basic cellular and extracellular biophysical mechanisms, each subject to autonomic modulation, determine the functional level of each factor. For example, when changing from supine to upright position or when performing daily activities or exercise, cholinergic modulation decreases while adrenergic modulation increases as documented by increased levels of plasma catecholamines.

The regulation of cardiovascular function is efficient. In healthy persons, cardiac output is matched to the demand for peripheral blood flow. **Maximal aerobic capacity,** ie, whole-body oxygen consumption at exhaustion ($V\text{O}_2$max), and cardiac output vary considerably in exercise stress tests, depending on whether cardiovascular or noncardiovascular (eg, psychologic, musculoskeletal) factors limit exercise. Age-associated decreases in cardiac output at exhaustion (ie, the maximal measured cardiac output) do not necessarily equate with reduced cardiovascular reserve, as in younger persons.

The maximum exercise capacity and maximal oxygen consumption decline with age but to a variable extent among individuals. Elderly persons in good physical condition can match or exceed the aerobic capacity of unconditioned younger persons. This indicates either that physical deconditioning causes the decline in some older persons or that physical conditioning can retard aging's effect on cardiorespiratory function.

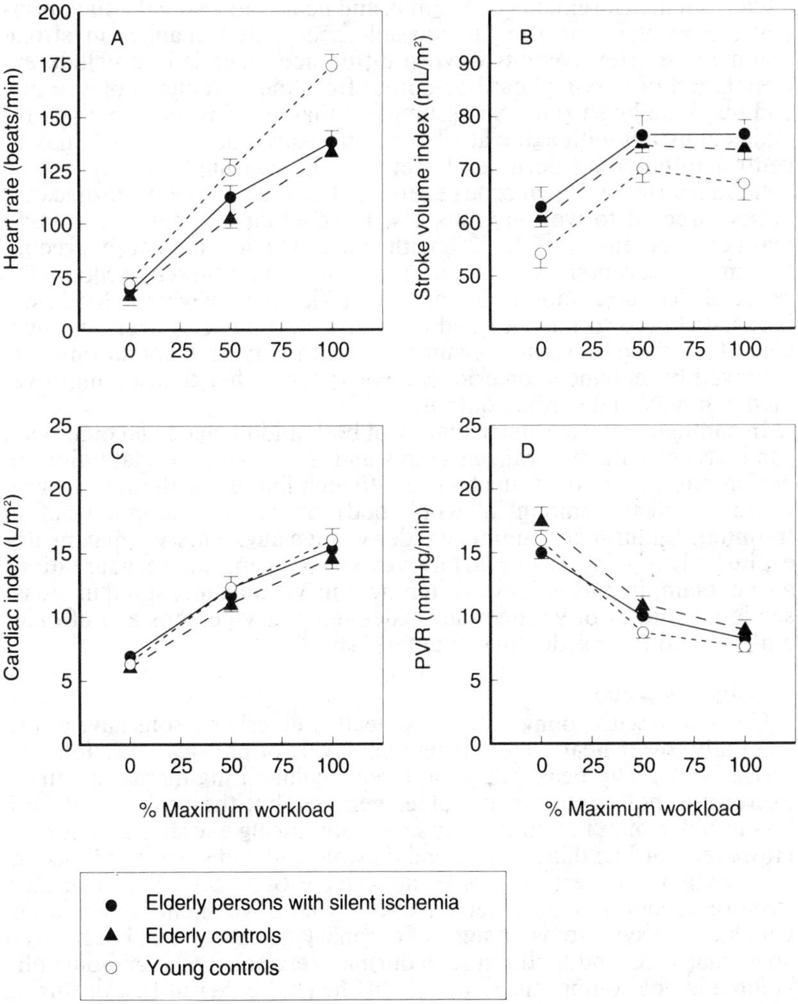

FIG. 33–6. Heart rate (*A*), stroke volume (*B*), cardiac index (*C*), and peripheral vascular resistance (*D*) at rest and during exercise in subjects studied in FIG. 33–5. (Based on data from Fleg JL, Schulman SP, Gerstenblith G, et al: "Additive effects of age and silent myocardial ischemia on the left ventricular response to upright cycle exercise." *Journal of Applied Physiology* 75:499–504, 1993.)

Maximal cardiac output and stroke performance are often extrapolated from measurements of VO_2max and heart rate using the Fick principle. However, specific but variable age-related changes in stroke volume and arteriovenous oxygen difference essentially preclude extrapolation of maximal cardiac output from measurements of VO_2max and maximal heart rate. An assumption that arteriovenous oxygen remains constant with aging attributes a measured decline in VO_2max to central rather than peripheral factors. This assumption may not be valid, because during vigorous exercise stress tests, 90% of cardiac output is directed to working muscles. In sedentary persons, lean body mass can decrease 10% to 12% with aging, which could cause a reduction in arteriovenous oxygen difference that could thereby account for reduced VO_2max. Another factor is the efficiency by which blood flow is redistributed to muscles and oxygen is extracted by working muscles. Improved oxygen consumption with physical conditioning is achieved by enhanced arteriovenous oxygen rather than by improvements in maximal cardiac output.

In summary, the aerobic capacity of both middle-aged and older men can increase with endurance training and is mediated by adaptations in peripheral and cardiac mechanisms (depending upon the intensity of exercise and the amount of whole-body oxygen consumption before training). Endurance training in older women augments VO_2max nearly exclusively by increasing arteriovenous oxygen. These adaptations also explain, in part at least, differences in VO_2max measured in cross-sectional studies of younger and older sedentary persons and of older athletes and their sedentary counterparts.

Cardiac Reserve

Compared with younger persons, healthy elderly persons have a substantially lower heart rate during high levels of physical exertion (see FIG. 33–6*A*). The peak rate of left ventricular filling increases during exercise in both younger and older persons, but the peak rate is 50% less in older than in younger persons both during exercise and at rest. However, cardiac dilatation at end diastole and end systole still occurs during vigorous exercise in older men (see FIG. 33–5*A*). This dilatation is more pronounced in elderly persons who have silent ischemia (ie, who have no symptoms or signs of coronary disease at rest but have an abnormal ECG and thallium scan during exercise). Thus, end-diastolic volume is not compromised by a "stiff heart," either at rest or during exercise. However, end-diastolic pressure, which has not been measured in healthy older and younger persons during exercise, may be expected to increase with age. During vigorous exercise, the left ventricular stroke volume, which depends upon the end-diastolic and end-systolic volumes, is *not* reduced in healthy elderly persons (see FIG. 33–6*B*). Thus, the cardiac dilatation at end diastole outweighs the concomitant age-associated deficiency in end-systolic volume (see FIG. 33–5*A*).

The maximum cardiac index is only slightly decreased with age in healthy men (see FIG. 33–6*C*). Stroke volume in older women is not as well maintained because women have a relatively smaller end-diastolic volume during exercise. Thus, the maximum cardiac output during vigorous cycle exercise decreases more in older women than in men because older women have a reduced heart rate and stroke volume.

Because neither men nor women can reduce left ventricular end-systolic volume sufficiently during vigorous exercise, ejection fraction increases less compared with that in younger persons (see FIG. 33–5*B*). The failure to increase the left ventricular ejection fraction during exercise is more severe in older persons who have silent ischemia. An age-associated decrease in myocardial contractile reserve or a failure of ventricular afterload to sufficiently decrease can cause left ventricular end-systolic volume to be insufficiently reduced during exercise in healthy older persons. The peripheral vascular resistance declines to about the same extent during vigorous exercise in healthy older and younger persons (see FIG. 33–6*D*). The ratio of systolic blood pressure to end-systolic volume, an index of myocardial contractility, decreases with age during vigorous exercise but not at rest. The apparent decrease in left ventricular contractility is more severe in older persons with silent ischemia than in those who are healthy (see FIG. 33–5*C*).

β-Adrenergic Modulation

β-Adrenergic stimulation has two effects on myocardial contraction: The strength is enhanced and the duration is decreased. Because heart rate increases dramatically in response to β-adrenergic stimulation, the contraction must be briefer to permit myocardial relaxation and proper filling of the ventricle during a shorter diastole.

β-Adrenergic modulation of pacemaker cells accounts in part for an increased heart rate during exercise. Rapid infusions of β-adrenergic agonists (eg, isoproterenol) have been used to demonstrate a diminished heart rate response with age (see FIG. 33–7*A*). Ejection fraction is increased to a lesser extent in older than in younger men (see FIG. 33–7*B*). Forearm vascular dilatation in response to intra-arterial infusion of isoproterenol is less in older than younger men (see FIG. 33–7*C*). Catecholamines also modulate venous tone and thus its capacitance during stress. α-Adrenergic–mediated venoconstriction during exercise is not impaired with aging and is a major factor facilitating the return of blood to the heart. The effect of β-adrenergic stimulation in relaxing veins decreases with age (see FIG. 33–7*D*).

The hemodynamic pattern observed in many healthy older persons during exercise (ie, reduced heart rate and greater cardiac dilatation at end diastole and end systole with maintenance or augmentation of stroke volume) occurs in younger persons who exercise while receiving β-blocker therapy. β-Adrenergic blockade also abolishes the age-associated decrease in the peak left ventricular filling rate in the sitting position, both at rest and during vigorous exercise.

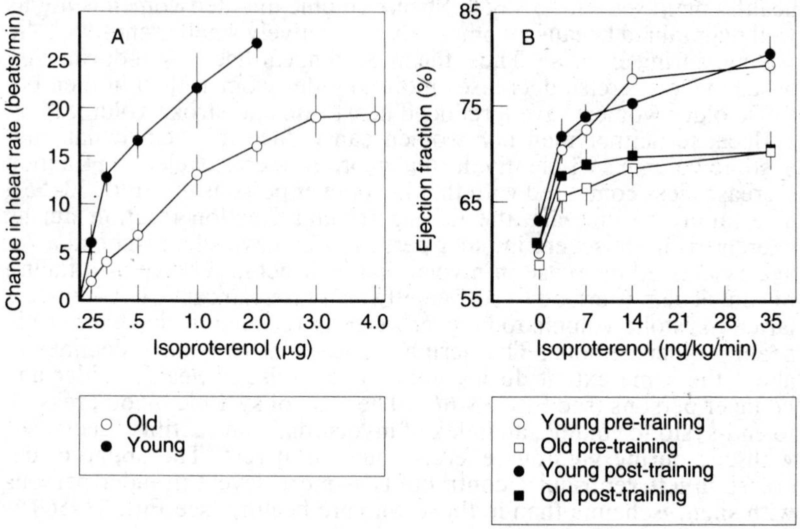

FIG. 33–7. *A,* The effect of rapid infusions of IV isoproterenol in increasing heart rate in healthy young and older men at rest.

B, The effect of isoproterenol in increasing the left ventricular ejection fraction in younger and older healthy men in the supine position before and after chronic endurance training. Endurance training had no effect on this index of cardiac pump function or on its response to isoproterenol. *(continued)*

SUMMARY

Overall cardiovascular function in most healthy elderly persons is sufficient to meet the body's needs for pressure and flow at rest. The resting heart rate is unchanged with aging. Heart size is essentially similar in younger and older adults, although heart-wall thickness increases modestly with age mainly because of an increase in myocyte size. While early diastolic filling rate is reduced, an enhanced atrial contribution to ventricular filling maintains filling at a normal volume. Although systolic blood pressure at rest increases with age, the end-systolic volume and ejection fraction are not altered, partly because of increased left ventricular thickness.

Physical work capacity declines with age, but how much this can be attributed to reduced cardiac reserve is not certain. Part of the age-related decline in maximal oxygen consumption appears to be caused by peripheral rather than central circulatory factors (eg, a decrease in lean muscle mass rather than loss of cardiac function). Some elderly

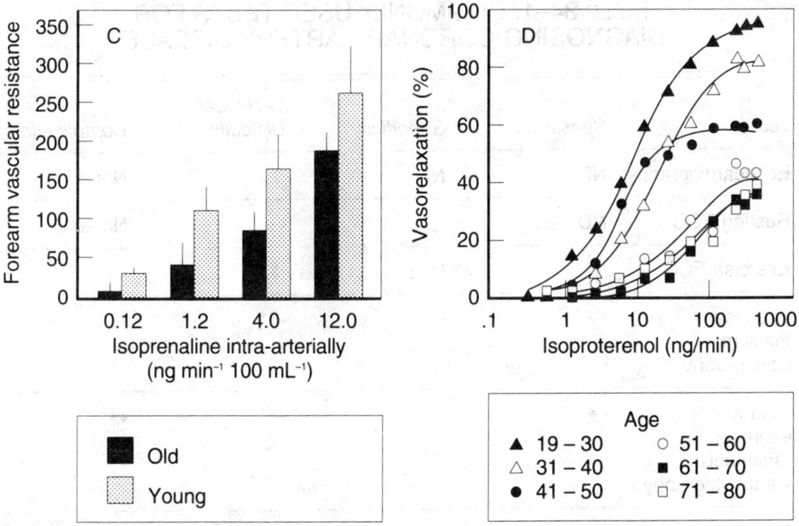

FIG. 33–7 *(Continued). C,* The effect of intra-arterial isoproterenol (isoprenaline) infusions in decreasing the forearm vascular resistance in healthy younger and older men.

D, The effect of IV arterial infusion of isoproterenol in relaxing dorsal hand veins, previously constricted by phenylephrine, in men of varying ages.

(From Lakatta EG: "Cardiovascular regulatory mechanisms in advanced age." *Physiological Reviews* 73:413–465, 1993; used with permission.)

persons experience cardiac dilatation, which increases stroke volume sufficiently to counter the well-known age-related decrease in exercise heart rate; as a result, a high cardiac output can be maintained during exercise. A diminished responsiveness to β-adrenergic modulation is among the most notable changes that occur in the aging cardiovascular system. In contrast, α-adrenergic responsiveness appears to remain intact.

34. DIAGNOSTIC EVALUATION

While new technology is enhancing the accuracy of cardiologic diagnosis, clinicians may be relying on it excessively. For example, an evaluation for coronary artery disease could include any of the following tests: chest x-ray, standard exercise ECG, ambulatory ECG monitoring, an invasive electrophysiologic study, exercise thallium scin-

TABLE 34–1. COMMONLY USED TESTS FOR DIAGNOSING CORONARY ARTERY DISEASE

Test	*Sensitivity*	*Specificity*	*Technical Difficulty*	*Complications*
Echocardiography	ND	ND	↑	None
Resting ECG	ND	↓	↔	None
Exercise ECG	↑	Mild	↑	↔
Exercise thallium scintigraphy	↔	↔	↔*	↔
Rest and exercise radionuclide ventriculography	↔	↓	↔*	↔
Catheterization	NM	NM	↑	↑

ND = no data available; NM = not meaningful.
Arrows denote whether parameter is increased (↑), decreased (↓), or no different (↔) in older persons compared with younger ones.
* Although thallium scintigraphy and radionuclide ventriculography are not more difficult to perform in the elderly, they are subject to age-related difficulties in performing maximal aerobic exercise tests when they are combined with exercise testing.

tigraphy, M-mode and two-dimensional echocardiography, radionuclide ventriculography at rest and during exercise, CT scan, and cardiac catheterization. Many of the commonly used tests for diagnosing coronary artery disease are compared in TABLE 34–1. To determine which tests are necessary, clinicians need to consider the patient's history and physical examination findings.

THE HISTORY

The patient's overall health and level of functioning help determine a realistic diagnostic approach and therapeutic goal. The elderly patient is generally more concerned with quality than with quantity of remaining years. The benefits of an aggressive cardiac workup may be lost if the patient has other health problems that interfere with quality of life.

For example, an 80-yr-old with severe osteoarthritis and occasional episodes of exertional angina is unlikely to benefit significantly from extensive evaluation for coronary artery disease unless the arthritic symptoms are ameliorated.

Age-related lifestyle changes often mask important symptoms (eg, exertional angina pectoris and dyspnea may be denied because the patient no longer walks far or fast enough to experience them). Furthermore, the symptom may be atypical and therefore misleading. For example, the age-associated decrease in left ventricular compliance may produce exertional dyspnea rather than angina. Multisystem disease often reduces the specificity of cardiac symptoms (eg, orthopnea may result from gastroesophageal reflux, and syncope may be due to orthostatic hypotension, carotid sinus hypersensitivity, vertebral artery compression, or inner ear disorders). Memory or attention deficits may prevent the patient from accurately recalling or describing the cardiac symptom in question.

The drug history may explain sudden cardiac decompensation. For example, a nonsteroidal anti-inflammatory drug may exacerbate heart failure as a result of sodium retention. Adding a diuretic and quinidine to a stable regimen of digitalis may precipitate digitalis toxicity in the elderly; smaller body size and diminished renal function increase susceptibility. Conversely, noncompliance or inaccurate compliance with a prescribed drug regimen is common and may result in the need for hospitalization. In a study of 220 ambulatory patients $\geq$ 60 yr of age, 60% made medication errors, averaging 2.6 mistakes per patient; 40% of these were potentially serious.

THE PHYSICAL EXAMINATION

Given the limitations of the cardiac history in many older patients, the physical examination often assumes greater importance.

Blood Pressure

Blood pressure measurement is essential because hypertension is the most common treatable cardiovascular risk factor in the elderly. Blood pressure is measured in the supine or sitting position and after 2 min of quiet standing. About 20% of persons > 65 yr of age have an orthostatic decline > 20 mm Hg; if the pulse rate does not increase to compensate for the loss in blood pressure, then autonomic insufficiency, sinus node dysfunction, or a drug side effect is suggested.

Arterial blood pressure is measured in both arms to exclude significant stenosis distal to the origin of the subclavian artery. Systolic blood pressure is first estimated by palpation, because an auscultatory gap (disappearance and later reappearance of the Korotkoff sounds) is more prevalent in older persons and may lead to systolic pressure being greatly underestimated. Measurements of systolic blood pressure in the peripheral arteries are inaccurate for estimating central systolic blood pressure because such measurements do not take into account the characteristic exaggeration of late systolic peak pressure seen in aging central arteries. A sclerotic noncompressible brachial or radial arterial wall that remains palpable at suprasystolic cuff pressure suggests generalized arteriosclerosis. This may result in a falsely high measurement of systolic blood pressure (ie, pseudohypertension, which is suspected when very high cuff pressure is seen without apparent target-organ damage). Measuring intra-arterial pressure confirms the diagnosis.

Central venous pressure is best estimated from the right internal jugular vein because the left brachiocephalic (innominate) vein is often compressed by both the aortic arch and the left external jugular vein, the latter often being kinked near its junction with the left subclavian vein. A bruit in the neck, abdomen, or groin indicates a high probability of carotid, aortorenal, or peripheral vascular disease. A prominent midline abdominal pulse with bruit suggests an abdominal aortic aneurysm.

Heart Sounds

Heart sounds are usually softer in older persons, probably because the volume of lung tissue between the heart and the chest wall increases with age. Audible splitting of the second heart sound (S_2) occurs in only about 30% to 40% of elderly patients. Easily audible splitting that increases with inspiration suggests right bundle branch block. Because the elderly heart relies on atrial contraction to compensate for diminished early left ventricular filling, a fourth heart sound (S_4) is normal whereas a third heart sound (S_3) is always abnormal. This situation is reversed in younger persons. Kyphoscoliosis and other chest-wall deformities complicate interpretation of the apical impulse and other precordial movements.

Systolic ejection murmurs (most often aortic) are found in $\leq$ 55% of elderly patients. These benign murmurs are distinguished from those of significant aortic valvular stenosis or hypertrophic obstructive cardiomyopathy by their short duration, low intensity (usually grade 1 or 2), and failure to radiate (see also Ch. 38). Age-related stiffening of the arterial tree may result in a brisk upstroke of the carotid artery pulse tracing, even when severe aortic stenosis is present. Pulmonary valve murmurs are much less common in the elderly.

Other Findings

Pulmonary rales are more likely to represent atelectasis, pulmonary fibrosis, or an acute inflammatory process in an older person than in a younger one. Emphysematous lungs can produce factitious hepatomegaly by displacing the liver inferiorly. Peripheral edema may be secondary to venous varicosities, lymphatic obstruction, or low serum albumin, rather than right-sided heart failure.

LABORATORY TESTS

Standard Electrocardiography

(See also Ch. 40)

Although the heart size tends to increase with age (see Ch. 33), limb lead and precordial QRS voltages decrease with age. No *age-specific* criteria for ECG diagnosis of left ventricular hypertrophy have been developed. In a study of more than 500 institutionalized elderly patients in sinus rhythm, a terminal P-wave deflection of > 0.04 mm in lead V_1 had a sensitivity of 32%, a specificity of 94%, and a positive predictive value of 31% for left atrial enlargement. The well-documented age-related increases in ectopic beats, PR and QT intervals, left axis deviation, and right bundle branch block have no prognostic significance in older persons who have no clinical heart disease.

An ECG pattern of myocardial infarction may be the initial manifestation of significant coronary artery disease. In the Framingham study, > 25% of all patients with myocardial infarctions presented silently and had a prognosis similar to those with clinical manifestations. However, an ECG pattern of poor R-wave progression in leads V_1 to V_4 has low specificity or predictive value for anterior myocardial infarction in the elderly, probably because of age-related increases in resting lung volume and anteroposterior chest diameter. The most common ECG abnormality in the elderly is nonspecific change in ST segments or T waves, often secondary to digitalis, diuretic, antiarrhythmic, or psychoactive drug use, with little independent prognostic significance. However, in the absence of the drugs listed above, and when voltage criteria for left ventricular hypertrophy are met, these ST–T-wave changes presage increased cardiovascular morbidity and mortality.

Ambulatory Electrocardiographic Monitoring

Given that complex arrhythmias on ambulatory ECG monitoring in healthy elderly persons are relatively common, finding such an arrhythmia does not necessarily explain a patient's complaints. An accurate diary allows correlation of symptoms with ECG rhythm disturbances. When symptoms are infrequent and nondisabling, an ECG event recorder is economical and allows up to 2 wk of intermittent monitoring. Alternatively, a small device can transmit an ECG via telephone to a central recording facility when symptoms occur. Ambulatory ECG monitoring is useful for detecting asymptomatic episodes of myocardial ischemia (usually defined as ≥ 60 sec of flat or down-sloping ST-segment depression ≥ 0.1 mV). The number of asymptomatic ischemic episodes can be used to identify patients at increased risk for future coronary events.

Electrophysiologic Testing

Electrophysiologic testing includes recording of His bundle activity, atrial pacing, programmed atrial or ventricular stimulation, and map-

TABLE 34–2. DIAGNOSTIC VALUE OF EXERCISE ELECTROCARDIOGRAPHY FOR DETECTING CORONARY ARTERY DISEASE

Age (yr)	*Sensitivity (%)*	*Specificity (%)*
< 40	56	84
40–49	65	85
50–59	74	88
≥ 60	84	70

Adapted from Hlatky MA, Pryor DC, Harrell FE, et al: "Factors affecting sensitivity and specificity of exercise electrocardiography: Multivariable analysis." *The American Journal of Medicine* 77:64–71, 1984; used with permission.

ping of tachyarrhythmias. However, ambulatory ECG recording is generally more sensitive than atrial pacing–determined sinus node recovery time for detecting the sick sinus syndrome. Similarly, the HV interval (*conduction time from the His deflection to ventricular activation*) has little independent prognostic significance unless extremely prolonged. Programmed ventricular stimulation is used predominantly in older persons with life-threatening ventricular arrhythmias; the low morbidity rate and overall favorable results are the same as in younger persons (see also Ch. 40).

Exercise Testing

Exercise testing has a similar safety profile and diagnostic yield in elderly and in younger patients. Test sensitivity increases with age, consistent with the higher prevalence and severity of coronary artery disease in the elderly, whereas specificity decreases modestly with age, probably because of the higher prevalence of left ventricular hypertrophy, nonspecific resting ST-segment abnormalities, and valvular heart disease in older patients (see TABLE 34–2). Several investigators have shown that exercise-induced ST-segment depression has significant diagnostic and prognostic value in older patients with chest pain. Furthermore, in postinfarction patients age 65 to 70 yr, a blunted increase in the heart rate–blood pressure product and the occurrence of major ventricular arrhythmias identify patient subsets at high risk for cardiac death.

Several physiologic and nonphysiologic factors must be considered in applying diagnostic exercise testing to the elderly:

1. The lower maximal aerobic capacity requires a protocol that begins at low energy expenditures and advances in small increments (eg, the Naughton, Sheffield, or modified Balke protocols).
2. Maximal heart rate declines progressively by about one beat per minute yearly through at least the 80s.
3. Systolic blood pressure at rest and at any given external work load is higher in older persons, although age-related differences are less prominent at maximal effort.
4. The ability to exercise is often limited by noncardiac factors (eg, arthritis, neurologic disorders, or peripheral vascular disease).
5. Older persons may fail to exercise maximally because of psychologic factors (eg, unfamiliarity with vigorous exercise, fear, or insufficient motivation).

The following are alternatives to treadmill exercise testing: (1) bicycle ergometry for persons with gait disturbances but good lower-extremity strength; (2) arm ergometry with a hand-cranked ergometer for those incapable of leg exercise; (3) atrial or esophageal pacing to increase heart rate in those incapable of exercise but without atrioventricular conduction disease; and (4) use of IV dipyridamole or adenosine to maximize coronary flow heterogeneity. Widespread experience with pharmacologic stress tests and their demonstrated safety and efficacy in older patients make them the preferred alternative for patients unable to perform treadmill or bicycle exercise.

Phonocardiography and Pulse-Wave Recording

Phonocardiography and pulse-wave recording are used primarily for research and for teaching cardiac physical diagnosis. The phonocardiogram can differentiate between a fourth heart sound (S_4) and a split first heart sound (S_1) or ejection click and between a delayed pulmonary valve closure sound, an opening snap, and a third heart sound (S_3). In contrast to younger patients, older persons with severe aortic valvular stenosis may misleadingly show a rapidly rising carotid arterial pulse.

IMAGING TECHNIQUES

Chest X-ray

Cardiomegaly may be simulated by kyphoscoliosis, other chest-wall deformities, or age-related aortic elongation and unfolding. Even without such changes, the cardiothoracic ratio normally increases modestly with age but rarely exceeds 50%.

Aortic knob calcification is visible in about 30% of the elderly but has no pathologic significance. In contrast, intracardiac calcification—most commonly on the aortic valve (signifying valvular stenosis) and the mitral anulus—is almost always pathologic. Calcification of the pericardium (constrictive pericarditis) or the left ventricular wall (old myocardial infarction) is seen occasionally. Coronary artery calcification, best seen on fluoroscopy, does not necessarily signify a major stenosis, as it does in younger patients.

Echocardiography

Accurate echocardiograms cannot be obtained in about 25% of elderly patients, partly because of chest-wall abnormalities and pulmonary hyperinflation. M-mode studies, although less useful than two-dimensional (2-D) studies for detailed assessment of cardiac anatomy (eg, segmental left ventricular wall motion abnormalities, severity of mitral stenosis, and detection of intracardiac masses), are easier to quantify. Age-related changes seen on M-mode echocardiograms include modest increases in aortic root and left atrial dimensions, an increase in left ventricular wall thickness with unchanged cavity size, and a diminution of mitral valve E-F closure slope—the rate of mitral valve closure in early diastole (see TABLE 34–3 and FIG. 34–1). These changes rarely fall outside normal limits for any parameter except perhaps E-F slope. Age does not significantly affect fractional shortening and velocity of circumferential fiber shortening (measures of global left ventricular function).

Echocardiography can detect thickened aortic or mitral valve leaflets or a calcified mitral anulus, the most common sources of systolic murmurs in the elderly. Pericardial effusions, atrial myxomas, left ventricular thrombi, and valvular vegetations are also best detected by echocardiography, particularly two-dimensional.

Transesophageal echocardiography should be considered in older patients with suspected heart disease and suboptimal transthoracic echocardiograms. The transesophageal technique is particularly useful for detecting thrombi in the left atrium or left atrial appendage, aortic dissection, valvular vegetations, and prosthetic valve dysfunction. Recently, an increased risk for thromboembolic events associated with cardiac surgery has been shown in older patients with intra-aortic atherosclerotic debris detected by transesophageal echocardiography.

Cardiac Doppler testing, combined with echocardiography, is used to quantify aortic valvular stenosis. The transvalvular pressure gradient (roughly 4 × [Doppler blood flow velocity]^2) correlates closely ($r > 0.9$) with the catheter-measured gradient. Similar correlations are found for mitral stenosis, which is now increasingly recognized in the elderly. A more widespread application involves assessment of diastolic dysfunction. The rate of early diastolic left ventricular filling, as determined by the Doppler E-wave velocity, declines with age (analogous to the decrease in E-F slope seen on M-mode echocardiograms). To compensate, the atrial contribution to ventricular filling in late diastole, the A-wave velocity, increases with age (see Ch. 33). Thus, an E/A-wave velocity ratio ≤ 1.0 is normal for elderly persons, but it is pathologic in younger persons. Doppler color flow mapping is useful

TABLE 34–3. M-MODE ECHOCARDIOGRAPHIC PARAMETERS IN HEALTHY PERSONS

	Group 1 (Age 25–44 yr)	*Group 2 (Age 45–64 yr)*	*Group 3 (Age 65–84 yr)*
Mitral valve E-F slope (mm/sec)	102.3 ± 3.7	79.0 ± 3.8*	67.1 ± 5.2†
Aortic root dimension (mm)	30.9 ± 0.6	32.0 ± 0.6	32.9 ± 0.8‡
Left ventricular wall thickness (mm)			
Systolic	15.4 ± 0.5	17.6 ± 0.7	18.8 ± 0.6*
Diastolic	8.7 ± 0.3	9.8 ± 0.5	10.7 ± 0.5*
Systolic/m^2	7.6 ± 0.3	9.2 ± 0.3	10.0 ± 0.4†
Diastolic/m^2	4.3 ± 0.1	5.0 ± 0.2*	5.7 ± 0.2†§
Left ventricular dimension (mm)			
Systolic	34.4 ± 1.1	32.1 ± 0.9	32.1 ± 1.4
Diastolic	51.8 ± 1.0	50.8 ± 1.3	51.2 ± 1.4
Systolic/m^2	17.3 ± 0.5	16.7 ± 0.5	16.8 ± 0.6
Diastolic/m^2	26.0 ± 0.5	26.4 ± 0.6	27.0 ± 0.7
Fractional shortening of minor semiaxis	0.34 ± 0.01	0.36 ± 0.01	0.37 ± 0.02
Velocity of circumferential fiber shortening (circ/sec)	1.17 ± 0.04	1.23 ± 0.04	1.30 ± 0.08

± = mean standard error; circ = circumference.
* $P < 0.01$
† $P < 0.0001$
‡ $P < 0.05$ vs. Group 1
§ $P < 0.05$ vs. Group 2
Adapted from Gerstenblith G, Fredericksen J, Yin FCP, et al: "Echocardiographic assessment of a normal adult aging population." *Circulation* 56:273–278, 1977; reproduced with permission of *Circulation*. Copyright 1977 American Heart Association.

for detecting and estimating the severity of valvular regurgitation. However, the high prevalence of mild multivalvular regurgitation in apparently healthy older persons must be considered when interpreting test results.

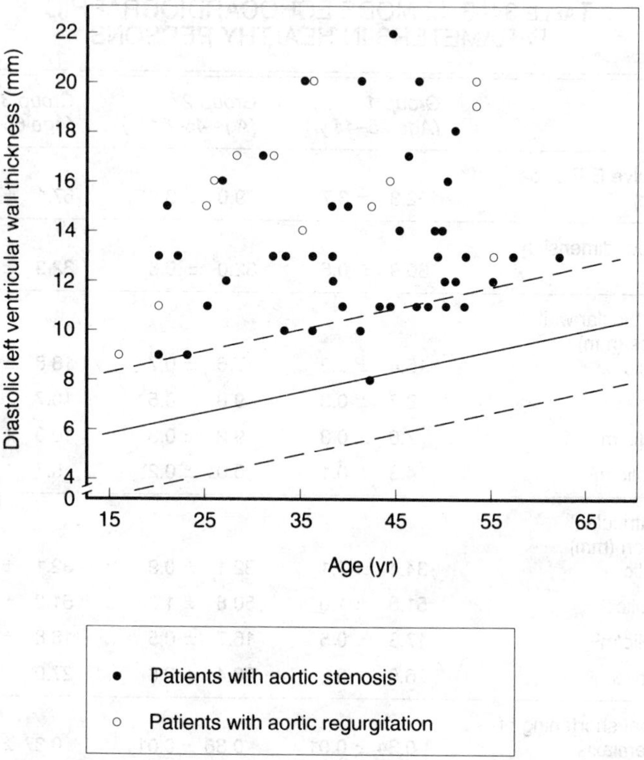

FIG. 34–1. Comparison of the increase in diastolic left ventricular wall thickness with aging vs. that induced by aortic valvular disease. The solid line represents the age regression in normal persons, and the dashed lines indicate the 95% tolerance limits. The wall thickness in most of the patient group lies well above the age-adjusted normal limit. (Adapted from Sjögren AL: "Left ventricular wall thickness in patients with circulatory overload of the left ventricle." *Annals of Clinical Research* 4:310–318, 1972; used with permission.)

Intravascular ultrasound is an exciting new technique that allows detailed morphologic assessment of coronary artery disease. This procedure will probably be used increasingly in patients of all ages with coronary artery disease to determine the suitability of a specific intervention, such as balloon angioplasty, laser therapy, or stent placement.

Radioisotope Studies

Although radioisotope techniques lack the high spatial resolution of echocardiography, they are particularly well suited for quantifying ventricular function and for detecting heterogeneities in myocardial perfusion.

Radionuclide ventriculography is the most accurate technique for assessing global left and right ventricular function, especially in the elderly (given the limitations of echocardiography). Two methods are used: (1) After peripheral injection of technetium-99m, the **first-pass technique** records the initial passage of the radioisotope through the cardiac chambers, usually with a highly sensitive multicrystal camera. (2) The more common **equilibrium-gated blood-pool technique** allows the tracer to equilibrate within the blood and then the intracardiac counts gated to the ECG are determined over many cardiac cycles. Gated imaging allows many measurements of left ventricular function up to several hours after injection of a radioisotope. Both techniques can accurately measure global and regional left ventricular systolic performance as well as changes in the left ventricular volumes. Several studies using radionuclide ventriculography show no age-related changes in left ventricular ejection fraction at rest. First-pass studies afford the most accurate assessment of right ventricular ejection fraction, since they avoid the problem of chamber overlap intrinsic to the equilibrium technique.

Both first-pass and gated radionuclide techniques can be used to measure left ventricular ejection fraction during bicycle exercise. Although the ejection fraction in younger persons is normally increased by ≥ 5 points on exercise, about 25% of normal men and 40% of normal women > 60 yr of age have a blunted response. Thus, a normal exercise response in elderly persons is probably best defined as *any increase in ejection fraction from the resting value*.

In a large study of patients with chest pain who underwent exercise radionuclide ventriculography, the sensitivity of the test for coronary artery disease was unaffected by age or sex, although specificity was decreased in women, particularly those > 60 yr of age (see TABLE 34–4). For unknown reasons, normal older women have a blunted increase in ejection fraction compared with men. Thus, if the criteria for men are applied, many women will have a falsely abnormal ejection fraction response, resulting in a fall in specificity. Older men appear to use the Frank-Starling mechanism (ie, increased end-diastolic volume) to enhance stroke volume more than do older women, both at rest and during upright cycle exercise; women rely more on increases in heart rate to augment cardiac output during exercise.

Myocardial perfusion imaging with thallium 201 at rest and particularly during exercise is generally considered the most accurate noninvasive test for detecting coronary artery disease in all age groups. Thallium

TABLE 34–4. DIAGNOSTIC VALUE OF RADIONUCLIDE VENTRICULOGRAPHY IN DETECTING CORONARY ARTERY DISEASE

Group (age)	*Sensitivity (%)**	*Specificity (%)**	*Disease Prevalence (%)*
Men (< 60 yr)	88 (449)	53 (94)	82
Women (< 60 yr)	91 (82)	27 (107)	43
Men (> 60 yr)	96 (101)	46 (13)	88
Women (> 60 yr)	92 (38)	7 (14)	70

* Figures in parentheses are numbers of patients studied.

From Cobb FR, Higgenbotham M, Mark D: "Diagnosis of coronary disease in the elderly," in *Coronary Heart Disease in the Elderly,* edited by NK Wenger, CD Furberg, E Pitt. New York, Elsevier Science Inc., 1986; used with permission.

201 concentrates in normally perfused cardiac muscle and substitutes itself for potassium during sodium-potassium exchange. Perfusion defects at rest generally indicate a previous myocardial infarction. Segmental defects on exercise that resolve or improve within 3 to 4 h signify exercise-induced ischemia. Specificity of the exercise ECG declines with age, probably because of the higher prevalence of resting ST-segment abnormalities (see above). Thus, a large percentage of older patients who have left ventricular hypertrophy or bundle branch block, or who are receiving digitalis, are optimal candidates for thallium exercise studies if a noninvasive test for coronary artery disease is desired.

In a series of patients undergoing exercise thallium scintigraphy, test sensitivity for detection of coronary artery disease was nearly identical (90% vs. 86%) for persons > 60 yr of age and those younger. Specificity was also similar, although the number of older persons without coronary artery disease was small. The extent of exercise-induced thallium defect is a useful prognostic indicator in elderly patients with known or suspected coronary artery disease. In a recent study, the combination of ST-segment depression on the exercise ECG and a thallium perfusion defect identified a group of apparently healthy older persons who had a 48% incidence of coronary events during the subsequent 5 yr.

Positron emission tomography (PET) assesses both myocardial blood flow and metabolism after IV injection of a radiolabeled fatty acid. The test is very sensitive, but minimal data are available on its use in the elderly. The high cost of the tomographic camera and the need for an on-site cyclotron for radioisotope generation have thus far limited its application.

Other Noninvasive Imaging Modalities

Computed tomography (CT) of the heart is useful in diagnosing cardiac masses and pericardial effusions, although echocardiography is the initial procedure of choice. Cardiac CT may be particularly helpful in distinguishing pericardial fat from effusion, a distinction that is often impossible with echocardiography. Echo-free pericardial spaces, indicating either fat or effusion, increase in prevalence with age and are demonstrable in about 10% of women > 80 yr.

Computed tomography is the procedure of choice for defining pericardial thickening, a necessary component of constrictive pericarditis. It is also highly effective in detecting lipomatous hypertrophy of the intra-atrial septum, an abnormality limited to the elderly, which has been associated with supraventricular arrhythmias and sudden death. The patency of coronary artery bypass grafts can be assessed using recent refinements to fast CT, thus avoiding routine postbypass cardiac catheterization. A drawback of this technique is the need for IV injection of iodinated contrast media.

Magnetic resonance imaging (MRI) can characterize both cardiac anatomy and metabolism without ionizing radiation. It can assess myocardial viability in patients who have suffered an infarction, in those with chronic heart failure, and in numerous other conditions. It provides an alternative to echocardiography for measuring chamber size and thickness. Gating image acquisition to the ECG allows ventricular function assessment. However, high cost and substantial overlap with echocardiography are major restrictions to its use.

Cardiac Catheterization

Cardiac catheterization with **coronary angiography** remains the gold standard for diagnosis. No other procedure measures intracardiac pressures or defines the coronary artery anatomy. In addition, percutaneous balloon dilatation of the coronary arteries and cardiac valves has broadened the use of catheterization beyond that of selecting candidates for cardiac surgery.

In the multicenter Coronary Artery Surgery Study (CASS), the incidence of death and major complications associated with coronary angiography in patients ≥ 65 yr was low but still significantly higher than that in younger patients (see TABLE 34–5). This may be partly explained by the higher prevalence of cardiomegaly and left ventricular dysfunction in the elderly and the greater difficulty encountered in obtaining vascular access. Nonetheless, coronary angiography is appropriate for many older patients with heart disease.

Digital subtraction angiography (a computer-enhanced imaging technique) may offer greater safety by allowing a 75% reduction in the amount of contrast medium.

TABLE 34–5. COMPLICATIONS OF CORONARY ANGIOGRAPHY

Complication	Incidence (per 1000 cases) Age < 65 yr (n = 17,165)	Age ≥ 65 yr (n = 2144)	P
Death	0.6	1.9	0.038
Nonfatal myocardial infarction	2.9	7.9	0.001
Vascular events	8.4	8.4	NS
Arterial embolism	0.5	1.9	0.025
Neurologic events	1.0	3.7	0.001
Ventricular fibrillation	3.8	4.2	NS

NS = not significant

Adapted from Gersh BJ, Kronmal RA, Frye RL, et al: "Coronary arteriography and coronary artery bypass surgery: Morbidity and mortality in patients ages 65 years or older. A report from the Coronary Artery Surgery Study." *Circulation* 67:483–490, 1983; reproduced with permission of *Circulation.* Copyright 1983 American Heart Association.

35. HYPERTENSION

A persistent elevation of systolic and/or diastolic arterial pressure of primary or secondary origin that may impair heart, brain, or kidney function.

In industrialized societies, both systolic and diastolic blood pressure tend to rise until about age 60. After that, systolic pressure may continue to rise, but diastolic pressure tends to stabilize or decline. More than 50% of Americans ≥ 65 yr have abnormally elevated systolic or diastolic pressures. In some primitive societies, however, neither systolic nor diastolic pressure increases with age, and hypertension is practically nonexistent. This difference is attributed to less dietary sodium (< 60 mEq/day) in these populations.

According to the Fifth Report of the Joint National Committee on Detection, Evaluation, and Treatment of High Blood Pressure, systolic pressure elevation is defined as ≥ 140 mm Hg and diastolic pressure elevation as ≥ 90 mm Hg (see TABLE 35–1). **Isolated systolic hyperten-**

TABLE 35–1. CLASSIFICATION OF HYPERTENSION BY ARTERIAL PRESSURE LEVELS

Classification	*Systolic Pressure (mm Hg)*	*Diastolic Pressure (mm Hg)*
Normal blood pressure	< 130	< 85
High normal blood pressure	130–139	85–89
Hypertension		
Stage 1 (mild)	140–159	90–99
Stage 2 (moderate)	160–179	100–109
Stage 3 (severe)	180–209	110–119
Stage 4 (very severe)	≥ 210	≥ 120

From "The Fifth Report of the Joint National Committee on Detection, Evaluation, and Treatment of High Blood Pressure." *Archives of Internal Medicine* 153(2):154–183, 1993.

sion is defined as a systolic pressure of ≥ 140 mm Hg and a diastolic pressure of < 90 mm Hg. Formerly, it was defined as a systolic pressure of ≥ 160 mm Hg; this revision reflects the importance of systolic pressure as a risk factor for cardiovascular disease.

The prevalence of elevated arterial pressure in the USA has led many to believe that a rising arterial pressure associated with aging is normal and innocuous. To the contrary, several multicenter prospective studies have shown that the higher the systolic or diastolic pressure, the greater the cardiovascular and total morbidity and mortality rates. Moreover, these studies have shown that an elevated systolic pressure is a better predictor of cardiovascular complications than an elevated diastolic pressure. In fact, isolated systolic hypertension increases the risk of cardiovascular death by 2 to 5 times and the risk of stroke by 2.5 times; it also increases overall mortality by 51% compared with age-, race-, and sex-matched normotensive people.

In general, hypertension predisposes a person to heart failure, stroke, renal failure, coronary heart disease, and peripheral vascular disease. Antihypertensive therapy reduces the risk of developing many of these catastrophic complications. For example, treating hypertension has helped reduce the incidence of fatal stroke in the USA by almost 60% and fatal myocardial infarction by almost 50%. Similar treatment benefits have been reported by researchers in Europe; for instance, the European Working Party on Hypertension in the Elderly demonstrated a 60% reduction in fatal myocardial infarction. The Systolic Hypertension in the Elderly Program **(SHEP)** in the USA also demonstrated a reduction in fatal and nonfatal stroke and nonfatal myocardial infarction.

Etiology

The causes of arterial hypertension are no different in elderly patients than in younger patients (see TABLE 35–2). **Primary (essential) hypertension,** afflicting at least 90% of the 50 million hypertensive Americans, may develop from changes in any or all of the pressor and depressor mechanisms responsible for maintaining normal arterial pressure levels.

Many different mechanisms may underlie hypertension. Among the more important **pressor** mechanisms are increased participation of the adrenergic nervous system and/or catecholamines; increased activity of the renopressor (renin-angiotensin) system (systemically or in autocrine systems of arteries, heart, brain, or other organs); reduced distensibility of the great vessels (eg, from atherosclerosis) with augmented left ventricular impedance; excessive production of pressor hormones; occlusive diseases of the renal arteries or aortic coarctation; and altered regulation of fluid and electrolyte balance. The last mechanism may be associated with either subclinical renal parenchymal disease or the hormonal and humoral factors that directly affect fluid and electrolyte balance. Underactivity of various **depressor** systems including the kallikrein-kinin system, the prostaglandins, atrial natriuretic peptide, and others may also play a role.

Each of these pressor and depressor mechanisms helps control arterial pressure in normotensive and hypertensive people of all ages. Catecholamine (particularly norepinephrine) levels increase with age, which suggests reduced β-adrenergic receptor responsiveness (down regulation). However, α-adrenergic receptor responsiveness seems to be unchanged. Plasma renin activity and angiotensin II levels are suppressed in elderly people with hypertension, but this has not been associated with intravascular volume expansion. Thus, participation of the pressor and depressor mechanisms seems to be as variable and unresolved in elderly hypertensive patients as it is in younger patients.

Because atherosclerosis is common in the elderly, the presence of an atherosclerotic renal arterial lesion is a major secondary etiologic consideration. Such a lesion may elevate arterial pressure de novo or aggravate essential hypertension. Underlying endocrine disorders (eg, thyroid diseases, hypercalcemic diseases, release of humoral agents from malignant tumors, primary aldosteronism, and pheochromocytoma) also may account for a recent onset of hypertension in the elderly.

Because elderly patients frequently have many diseases, medications (including over-the-counter drugs) should be considered when identifying the cause of recent onset, aggravation, or complication of hypertension. Some medications and diseases may predispose hypertensive patients to complications. For example, use of digitalis and a diuretic may cause hypokalemia-related cardiac arrhythmias; chronic diarrhea and

TABLE 35–2. CLASSIFICATION OF SYSTEMIC ARTERIAL HYPERTENSION BASED ON ETIOLOGY

Primary (essential) hypertension	Borderline (labile) essential hypertension Established essential hypertension Isolated systolic hypertension

Secondary hypertension	Renovascular hypertension
	  Atherosclerotic renal arterial disease
	  Nonatherosclerotic (fibrosing) renal arterial disease
	  Renal arterial aneurysm
	  Embolic renal arterial disease
	  Extravascular compression (eg, tumors, fibrosis)
	Renal parenchymal diseases
	  Chronic pyelonephritis
	  Chronic glomerulonephritis
	  Polycystic disease
	  Diabetic glomerulosclerosis
	  Others: amyloidosis, obstructive disease, etc
	Hormonal diseases
	  Thyroid diseases
	    Hyperthyroidism
	    Hypothyroidism
	  Adrenal diseases
	    Cushing's disease and syndrome
	    Primary hyperaldosteronism
	      Adenoma, bilateral hyperplasia
	    Adrenal enzyme abnormalities
	  Pheochromocytoma
	  Others: ectopic production of pressor hormones in metastatic tumors, growth hormone, hypercalcemic diseases, and hyperparathyroidism
	Coarctation of the aorta
	Drugs, chemicals, and foods
	  Antidepressants (tricyclics, monoamine oxidase inhibitors)
	  Steroidal compounds (corticosteroids, estrogens)
	  β-Adrenergic receptor agonists
	  Cyclosporine (immunosuppressive therapy)
	  Over-the-counter cold preparations (nasal decongestants, phenylpropanolamine)
	  Milk-alkali syndrome, hypervitaminosis D
	  Excessive dietary sodium intake
	  Excessive alcohol intake
	  Others: licorice, snuff, etc
	Radiation nephritis or arteritis
	Erythropoietin renal lithotripsy

Modified from "The Fifth Report of the Joint National Committee on Detection, Evaluation, and Treatment of High Blood Pressure." *Archives of Internal Medicine* 153(2):154–183, 1993.

laxative abuse may also predispose a patient to hypokalemia; corticosteroids may produce a hypokalemic form of hypertension; cyclosporine, tricyclic antidepressants, monoamine oxidase (MAO) inhibitors, and phenylpropanolamine and other vasoconstrictors in over-the-counter cold preparations may also elevate arterial pressure.

Pathogenesis and Pathophysiology

The hemodynamic characteristics of elderly hypertensive patients are similar to those of younger hypertensive patients. However, in the elderly, calculated total peripheral resistance may be higher and compliance of the large arteries may be lower. Arterial pressure is the product of two hemodynamic variables: cardiac output and vascular resistance to blood flow through systemic circulation (total peripheral resistance). Cardiac output, in turn, is the product of two variables: heart rate and stroke volume. Enhanced myocardial contractility or venous return may increase stroke volume. Vascular resistance may be increased by adrenergic stimulation, increased renopressor activity, and many circulating hormonal or humoral substances. The many factors that can increase arteriolar smooth muscle tone and total peripheral resistance are presented in TABLE 35–3. All these factors act interdependently in normal and hypertensive persons.

TABLE 35–3. MECHANISMS THAT ALTER VASCULAR RESISTANCE

Constriction	*Dilation*
Active	Active
Adrenergic stimulation	Certain prostaglandins
Catecholamines: norepinephrine, epinephrine	Kinins: bradykinin, kallidin
Renopressor: angiotensin II	Histamines
Cations: calcium, potassium (high levels)	Peptides: atrial natriuretic factor, insulin, vasoactive intestinal polypeptide, calcitonin gene-related peptide, parathormone, endorphins, enkephalins, renal medullary neutral lipid substance, phospholipid
Hormonal and humoral substances: vasopressin, serotonin, certain prostaglandins	Cations: potassium (low levels), magnesium
Passive	Passive
Extravascular edema	Reduced blood or plasma viscosity
Vessel wall water-logging	Increased tonicity
Increased blood or plasma viscosity	Heat
Proximal obstruction: thrombosis, embolus	
Cold	

TABLE 35–4. FACTORS LEADING TO CARDIAC ENLARGEMENT IN ELDERLY PERSONS WITH HYPERTENSION

Increasing afterload associated with hypertensive vascular disease
Increased coronary vascular resistance
Reduced coronary blood flow and flow response
Increased blood viscosity
Collagen tissue deposition
Reduced number of adrenergic receptor sites

Recent studies strongly indicate a local renin-angiotensin system within the vascular myocyte and suggest that this system may also contribute to the tone of vascular smooth muscle. This may explain the effectiveness of the angiotensin converting enzyme (ACE) inhibitors in patients with low plasma renin activity, including the elderly.

Atherosclerotic disease, so common in the elderly, reduces large artery distensibility, resulting in elevated systolic pressure as the left ventricle ejects its stroke volume into a more rigid and less compliant aorta. This **reduced distensibility of the aorta** and other large arteries is a major factor in the pathophysiology of isolated systolic hypertension and augments left ventricular impedance. Other pathologic conditions that can contribute to systolic hypertension in the elderly are hyperthyroidism, aortic insufficiency, malnutrition (with clinical or subclinical beriberi), diseases with arteriovenous fistulas, and fever.

As **vascular resistance increases,** so do systolic and diastolic pressures. The heart adapts to this progressively increasing afterload by a process of concentric hypertrophy (see TABLE 35–4). Because of the frequent coexistence of myocardial ischemia, blood supply to the myocardium may be insufficient—even if arterial pressure is not dramatically elevated. These changes are compounded by cardiac enlargement; reduced β-adrenergic responsiveness; and possible deposition of collagen, amyloid, and other substances in the aging myocardium, even if hypertension is not present.

Each of the above factors may cause **reduced myocardial contractility of the left ventricle** that may eventually predispose it to heart failure. This process may be aggravated further by exogenous obesity. Obesity is associated with expanded intravascular volume, increased venous return to the heart, and elevated cardiac output. This volume overload provides an eccentric component to the left ventricular hypertrophy and may explain the facilitated heart failure observed in obesity-associated hypertension.

In contrast to the plasma volume expansion that occurs with obesity, **intravascular volume contracts** as arterial pressure and total peripheral resistance rise in most patients with essential hypertension. Because

renopressor system activity seems to be reduced and less sensitive in elderly patients with primary hypertension, an attenuated relationship between intravascular volume and the renopressor system results. This may explain the enhanced responsiveness to diuretics and calcium antagonists in some elderly hypertensive patients (particularly those with isolated systolic hypertension). The superiority of calcium antagonists over other agents, however, has not yet been proved.

Laplace's law is another important hemodynamic consideration in elderly hypertensive patients. Myocardial oxygen demand is directly related to left ventricular wall tension, which in turn is directly related to the product of the left ventricular diameter and the systolic pressure generated within this chamber during contraction.

In hypertensive patients (and even in elderly normotensive people), left ventricular and systolic vascular pressures are increased. Both of these tension-dependent factors further increase left ventricular demand for oxygen, which explains the development of coronary artery insufficiency and angina pectoris and provides a rationale for reducing arterial pressure in patients who have only mild diastolic hypertension or isolated systolic hypertension.

Hypertension may also impair **brain and kidney function.** Transient ischemic attacks and strokes may impair brain function, which results in reduced sensory, motor, and intellectual function. Hypertension diminishes **renal parenchymal function** in a manner similar to the aging process. Histologic evidence of nephrosclerosis in hypertensive and aging patients demonstrates the altered structure associated with impaired parenchymal function. Thus, renal blood flow decreases in proportion to cardiac output reduction. Consequently, intrarenal vascular resistance increases, and the glomerular filtration rate and the ability to concentrate urine decrease. Hypertension and aging synergistically exacerbate these changes. In patients with untreated essential hypertension, the lower the renal blood flow, the higher the serum uric acid concentration, explaining the high incidence of hyperuricemia in these patients.

Symptoms and Signs

Hypertension, when uncomplicated and not associated with target organ involvement, is usually a **silent disease.** The medical literature suggests that hypertension is associated with headaches, epistaxis, and tinnitus, but these complaints are nonspecific. Young patients with borderline or mild **essential hypertension** and no target organ involvement may have symptoms of cardiac awareness (rapid heart rate, palpitations, or ectopic beats) associated with physiologic findings that confirm a hyperdynamic circulation. These changes may also occur in older patients and in those with severe hypertension.

Symptoms and signs occur more often in **secondary hypertension. Pheochromocytoma** may be associated with headache, flushing, blood pressure lability, and hypermetabolism. **Occlusive renal arterial disease** may produce a sudden onset or worsening of hypertension, headaches, and renal arterial bruits that are systolic and (more significantly) diastolic in timing. Patients with **renal parenchymal disease** may experience recurrent urinary tract infection and urinary frequency, nocturia, impaired ability to concentrate urine, microscopic or gross hematuria, and (with advanced disease) anemia. In younger patients, the coexistence of hypertension and anemia suggests renal parenchymal disease (if hemoglobinopathy is excluded); in the elderly, it may suggest a **neoplasm.**

Elderly patients with **thyroid disease** may not have the characteristic symptoms of hyperthyroidism or hypothyroidism; therefore, a recent onset of hypertension without renal arterial disease or other evident cause indicates the need to rule out thyroid disease (see Ch. 79). Those with **primary aldosteronism** exhibit muscle weakness, nocturia, isosthenuria, altered carbohydrate metabolism, and hypokalemic alkalosis. **Cushing's disease** is suggested by hypokalemic alkalosis and the typical facies, hirsutism, purplish abdominal striae, buffalo hump, and new appearance of acneiform lesions.

In patients with essential hypertension, the presence of symptoms or signs suggests **target organ involvement.** With **cardiac involvement,** the earliest complaints are easy fatigability, palpitations, and atrial or ventricular ectopy. Chest pain in patients without occlusive coronary artery disease reflects increased myocardial oxygen demand with persistently elevated arterial pressures and cardiomegaly (left ventricular hypertrophy). More advanced stages of cardiac involvement are marked by symptoms and signs of heart failure: exertional dyspnea, orthopnea, peripheral edema, and increased ventricular irritability. Edema without heart failure suggests secondary hypertension. A third heart sound (ventricular gallop rhythm) may develop, usually in association with a fourth heart sound (atrial gallop), which reflects the reduced distensibility and compliance of the hypertrophic left ventricle. A sudden onset of back pain and hypertension suggests aortic dissection.

The earliest symptom of **renal involvement** is nocturia; later symptoms and signs result from functional renal impairment: frequency, proteinuria, anemia, and edema. Sensory or motor deficits signal **brain involvement;** subtle symptoms of transient ischemic attacks include transient speech impediments, numbness of fingers and extremities, and unusual weakness. Sudden onset of a severe vertical headache and hypertension suggests a subarachnoid hemorrhage.

All patients should be examined for hypertensive retinopathy. In elderly patients, this should not be confused with the sclerotic changes of increased arteriolar light striping, arteriovenous nicking, and tortuosity. Arteriolar (and venular) constriction and the appearance of hemorrhages, exudates, and papilledema suggest advancing and more severe degrees of hypertensive vascular disease.

The physician should listen for renal, carotid, aortic, brachial, and femoral arterial bruits. A carotid bruit with symptoms of a transient ischemic attack suggests embolic phenomena from that vessel. *Occlusive disease is more likely when a renal arterial bruit has a diastolic component than when it has only a systolic component.*

Laboratory Data

Laboratory studies in patients with hypertension should include a **blood count** (with hemoglobin, hematocrit, and white blood cell count); an **ECG** (to identify early evidence of left ventricular hypertrophy, left atrial abnormality, and arrhythmias); selected **blood chemistries** such as fasting blood glucose and serum levels of creatinine, uric acid, potassium, and lipids including high-density and low-density cholesterol fractions; and a **urinalysis.** A slightly elevated hemoglobin or hematocrit suggests hypertension-induced hemoconcentration, which may be confirmed by a proportionately higher plasma protein concentration. Hyperuricemia may indicate that the patient is taking a diuretic or is predisposed to gout; in an untreated hypertensive patient, hyperuricemia may indicate reduced renal blood flow.

The **chest x-ray** is less sensitive than the **ECG** for detecting cardiac enlargement. Electrocardiographic evidence of left atrial enlargement provides an early clue to left ventricular hypertrophy before it can be detected by the usual criteria of increased voltage, delayed intrinsicoid deflection of the QRS complex, or left ventricular hypertrophy and strain pattern. The enlarged left atrium does not indicate atrial disease per se. Rather, it indicates reduced left ventricular distensibility associated with the development of left ventricular hypertrophy.

Even more sensitive than the ECG, the **echocardiogram** clearly demonstrates ventricular hypertrophy in a patient whose ECG shows only a left atrial abnormality. Moreover, before systolic functional changes are apparent, diastolic functional changes are revealed by echocardiographic or radionuclide studies showing a reduced left atrial filling rate. Echocardiographic evidence of left ventricular hypertrophy usually precedes early evidence of **renal functional impairment,** which includes renal blood flow slightly reduced in proportion to the height of serum uric acid concentration. Later evidence of renal impairment includes rising serum creatinine or BUN concentrations, as well as reduced creatinine clearance (glomerular filtration rate) and ability to concentrate urine.

Hypercalcemia is frequently associated with hypertension. When hypercalcemia occurs in younger patients, the clinician should first rule out hyperparathyroidism; in older patients, the clinician should first rule out metastatic bone disease. Because hypercalcemia is frequently associated with diuretic therapy, this possibility should be explored when taking the patient's history.

Proteinuria occurs infrequently in patients with uncomplicated essential hypertension. When daily urinary protein excretion exceeds 400 mg, nephrosclerosis (associated with essential hypertension or aging) is not likely to be the cause; the entire differential diagnosis of renal parenchymal disease should be considered. A fresh urine sample with an alkaline pH suggests hypokalemia or primary aldosteronism.

Diagnosis

The diagnosis of hypertension depends on finding elevated arterial pressure as defined in TABLE 35–1. The elevated pressure should be documented on at least three separate occasions with at least two separate blood pressure measurements on each occasion.

Proper measurement technique is especially important in the elderly patient. Blood pressure should be measured in both arms during the initial examination and periodically thereafter. Frequently, occlusive atherosclerotic disease of the subclavian or brachial artery reduces systolic pressure in one arm, producing an abrupt, unexplained decline. Measurements should be obtained while the patient is supine or sitting and immediately after the patient stands because postural (orthostatic) hypotension is common in elderly patients, particularly after meals.

If pressures are persistently and strikingly elevated but chest x-ray and ECG indicate that cardiac size is normal, the physician should suspect **pseudohypertension.** This finding occurs when the sphygmomanometer cuff cannot compress a sclerotic brachial artery. A direct arterial pressure measurement may be needed to verify this phenomenon. Once true hypertension has been diagnosed, the physician must determine whether it is primary or secondary.

Treatment

Nonpharmacologic measures include maintaining an ideal body weight, moderating alcohol intake (≤ 1 oz of ethanol equivalent per day), controlling dietary sodium (≤ 100 mEq/day), exercising regularly, and avoiding smoking. (Smokers who take certain antihypertensive drugs such as propranolol have more hypertensive complications, eg, stroke, and myocardial infarction, than smokers who take other drugs such as thiazide diuretics.) These measures may not control arterial pressure completely, but they may control it adequately in some patients and reduce the number and doses of antihypertensive drugs needed in others.

Isolated systolic hypertension: The efficacy of reducing systolic arterial pressure in elderly patients with isolated systolic hypertension has been demonstrated in several clinical studies. These patients are at greater risk for stroke, myocardial infarction, and premature death than normotensive people; the elevated pressure and larger heart increase myocardial oxygen demand. The multicenter SHEP study strongly demonstrated that elevated systolic pressure can be controlled with diuretics (eg, hydrochlorothiazide or chlorthalidone, starting at 12.5 or 25 mg and increasing, if necessary, to 50 mg). Alternatively, β-blockers alone and in combination with a diuretic were also effective in the SHEP study. Also, angiotensin converting enzyme **(ACE)** inhibitors or calcium antagonists may be effective.

Stages 1 and 2 hypertension: Patients whose diastolic pressure ranges between 90 and 109 mm Hg and whose blood pressure is not controlled by nonpharmacologic means may respond to a diuretic, β-blocker, ACE inhibitor, calcium antagonist, α_1-blocker, or α/β-blocker in submaximal doses (see TABLE 35–5). The Fifth Report of the Joint National Committee on Detection, Evaluation, and Treatment of High

Blood Pressure indicates that diuretics and β-blockers are preferred because placebo-controlled multicenter studies have demonstrated reduced total and cardiovascular morbidity and mortality with these drugs. Similarly controlled studies have not been conducted with the other drugs.

The α_1-blockers and α/β-blockers are particularly pertinent for men already taking an α_1-blocker for benign prostatic hyperplasia. How-

TABLE 35–5. ANTIHYPERTENSIVE AGENTS

Agent	*Average Daily Dose*	*Maximum Daily Dose*
Diuretics (selected agents are compiled in equivalent dosage forms)		
Chlorothiazide	125–500 mg once a day	500 mg
Hydrochlorothiazide	12.5–50 mg once a day	100 mg
Furosemide	20–320 mg once a day	2.0 gm
Spironolactone	25–100 mg once a day	200 mg
Ganglionic blocker		
Trimethaphan	1 mg/mL IV	——
Adrenergic inhibitors		
Centrally acting α-agonists		
Clonidine	0.1 mg bid	1.2 mg
Guanabenz	4.0 mg bid	32 mg
Methyldopa	250 mg bid	3.0 gm
Peripheral-acting adrenergic antagonists		
Guanadrel	10 mg once a day	100 mg
Guanethidine	10 mg once a day	150 mg
Reserpine (typical of rauwolfia alkaloids)	0.05 mg once a day	0.25 mg
α_1-Adrenergic antagonists		
Doxazosin	1.0–16 mg once a day	16 mg
Prazosin	1.0 mg bid–tid	20 mg
Terazosin	1.0–20 mg once a day	20 mg

(continued)

TABLE 35–5. ANTIHYPERTENSIVE AGENTS *(Continued)*

Agent	*Average Daily Dose*	*Maximum Daily Dose*
Adrenergic inhibitors *(continued)*		
β-Adrenergic antagonists		
Acebutolol	100–800 mg once a day	800 mg
Atenolol	25–100 mg once a day	100 mg
Betaxolol	5–40 mg once a day	40 mg
Bisoprolol	5–20 mg once a day	20 mg
Carteolol	2.5–10 mg once a day	10 mg
Metoprolol	50–200 mg once a day	200 mg
Nadolol	20–40 mg once a day	240 mg
Pindolol	10–60 mg once a day	60 mg
Propranolol	40–240 mg once a day	480 mg
Timolol	10–20 mg bid	80 mg
Combined α/β-inhibitor		
Labetalol	100–600 mg bid	1200 mg
Vasodilator		
Hydralazine	10 mg bid	200 mg
Calcium antagonists		
Amlodipine	2.5–10 mg once a day	10 mg
Diltiazem	30 mg tid	360 mg
Felodipine	5–10 mg once a day	20 mg
Isradipine	2.5–10 mg once a day	10 mg
Nicardipine	60–120 mg once a day	120 mg
Nifedipine	10 mg tid	180 mg
Verapamil	80 mg tid	480 mg

(continued)

TABLE 35–5. ANTIHYPERTENSIVE AGENTS
(Continued)

Agent	*Average Daily Dose*	*Maximum Daily Dose*
Angiotensin converting enzyme inhibitors		
Benazepril	10–40 mg once a day	40 mg
Captopril	12.5 mg once a day	150 mg
Cilazapril*	2.5–5 mg once a day	5 mg
Enalapril	5 mg once a day	40 mg
Fosinopril	10–40 mg once a day	80 mg
Lisinopril	10 mg once a day	40 mg
Perindopril*	1–16 mg once a day	16 mg
Quinapril	5–80 mg once a day	80 mg
Ramipril	1.25–20 mg once a day	20 mg
Spirapril*	12.5–50 mg once a day	50 mg

* Not available in the USA.

Modified from "The Fifth Report of the Joint National Committee on Detection, Evaluation, and Treatment of High Blood Pressure." *Archives of Internal Medicine* 153(2): 154–183, 1993.

ever, adding another α-blocker for hypertension may provoke postural hypotension—a potentially dangerous symptom in a patient who arises from bed frequently with nocturia.

If the initial dose of any of these drugs fails to control blood pressure, the dose may be increased. This action is consistent with the currently advocated individualized stepped-care approach to treatment (see TABLE 35–6).

As an alternative to increasing the dose, a second drug may be added; this approach prevents side effects from maximum doses of the first drug. Thus, adding a β-blocker to hydrochlorothiazide 25 mg/day may prevent hypokalemia and hyperuricemia. In general, elderly patients respond to diuretics. Calcium antagonists and ACE inhibitors are also effective with elderly patients, including blacks and those who have not responded to lower doses of β-blockers prescribed for coexisting angina pectoris.

TABLE 35–6. INDIVIDUALIZED STEPPED–CARE APPROACH TO DRUG THERAPY

Step 1	Begin with submaximal dose of one of the following: Thiazide diuretic β-blocker Angiotensin converting enzyme inhibitor Calcium antagonist α_1-blocker α/β-blocker
Step 2	Take one of the following measures: Give up to the maximum dose of the step 1 choice Add a second drug from the step 1 choices Use an alternative step 1 drug
Step 3	Take one of the following measures: Give up to the maximum doses of both step 2 choices Add a third drug from the step 1 choices Use an alternative step 1 drug

Stages 3 and 4 hypertension: In patients with severe hypertension, any of the first-step drugs may be prescribed. If this does not control blood pressure adequately, however, a second or third drug may be necessary. These can be added sequentially, using lower doses first, then increasing doses or adding different drugs.

Tailoring therapy by selecting drugs most appropriate to the pressor mechanisms of specific patients is possible. For example, the black or obese patient, who is more volume-dependent and has lower plasma renin activity, may respond well to a diuretic or calcium antagonist. The patient with renal arterial disease (unilateral but not in a solitary kidney) may be more responsive to an ACE inhibitor.

Therapy with β-blockers may be appropriate for patients with a previous myocardial infarction, angina pectoris, migraine headaches, or glaucoma. An oral β-blocker prescribed for hypertension usually does not adequately treat glaucoma as well. If the patient has not had side effects from prolonged therapy with a topical β-blocker, he probably will not have adverse effects from the addition of an oral agent.

The ACE inhibitors may be particularly valuable in hypertensive patients with heart failure. These drugs have been shown to improve left ventricular function, reduce hospital admissions for left ventricular dysfunction, prevent heart failure after a myocardial infarction, and prevent a second myocardial infarction. These findings have been demonstrated in the recent controlled, multicenter studies SOLVD (Studies of Left Ventricular Dysfunction) and SAVE (Study Against Ventricular Enlargement).

If the patient is already taking digitalis, a diuretic should be prescribed with care. Serum potassium levels should be closely monitored to prevent cardiac arrhythmias associated with hypokalemia. Impotence may result in patients treated with diuretics, adrenergic inhibitors, and β-blockers; the ACE inhibitors and calcium antagonists have been reported to produce fewer side effects.

Although elderly hypertensive patients have no more side effects from prolonged treatment than younger patients, they are more likely to have postural (orthostatic) hypotension from agents that inhibit adrenergic function. Also, centrally acting agents may be more likely to cause depression, forgetfulness, vivid dreams or hallucinations, and sleep problems.

Patients with chronic obstructive lung disease, asthma, or heart block greater than first degree should not be treated with β-blockers; calcium antagonists may be more appropriate. Patients with low heart rates may be good candidates for calcium antagonists that do not markedly reduce heart rate.

All hypertensive patients should continue therapy after blood pressure is controlled because it is likely to rise if therapy is discontinued. Therapy can be "stepped down," but this should be done slowly, one drug at a time. If blood pressure rises, therapy must be "stepped up" again.

36. HYPOTENSION

Subnormal arterial blood pressure.

Many age-related physiologic changes affect blood pressure. Numerous studies in Western countries have shown an association between age and blood pressure elevation. But paradoxically, age-related elevations in blood pressure also increase the risk of hypotension.

Baroreflex mechanisms regulate systemic blood pressure by resisting transient decreases and damping transient increases in arterial pressure. With age, baroreflex response to both hypertensive and hypotensive stimuli progressively declines. Also, hypertension reduces baroreflex response. Thus, baroreflex function is most impaired in elderly, hypertensive patients. Signs of such impairment include increased lability in blood pressure in response to daily activities and an increased response to hypotensive stimuli, particularly medications.

The diminished baroreflex response may be caused partly by arterial stiffening, which results in damping of baroreceptor stretch and relaxation during changes in arterial pressure. Reduced adrenergic responsiveness by the aged heart may diminish baroreflex-mediated cardioacceleration during hypotensive stimuli. These changes become clinically significant when common hypotensive stresses, such as postural changes, can no longer be offset by compensatory increases in heart rate or vascular resistance.

With age, cerebral blood flow declines. Risk factors for cerebrovascular disease (eg, hypertension, heart disease, diabetes mellitus, and hyperlipidemia) further decrease cerebral blood flow. Thus, elderly patients who have such risk factors may develop cerebral ischemia from even a fairly small drop in blood pressure.

Cerebral autoregulatory mechanisms usually compensate for acute reductions in blood pressure. Current data suggest that autoregulation of cerebral blood flow is generally maintained with age, except in certain persons who have symptomatic orthostatic hypotension. Chronic hypertension, however, raises the lowest blood pressure at which autoregulation can maintain cerebral blood flow. Below this level, blood flow may decline, increasing the risk of cerebral ischemia. Although an *acute* reduction in blood pressure may not be tolerated well by a hypertensive elderly patient, a *gradual* reduction, using a variety of agents, can be accomplished without compromising cerebral blood flow.

ORTHOSTATIC HYPOTENSION

A reduction ≥ 20 mm Hg in systolic blood pressure upon standing upright.

Orthostatic hypotension, a common clinical manifestation of impaired blood pressure homeostasis, occurs in 15% to 20% of noninstitutionalized elderly persons. Its prevalence increases with age, cardiovascular disease, and basal blood pressure elevation. Many elderly people have wide variations in postural blood pressure, which is closely associated with basal supine systolic blood pressure; ie, when basal supine systolic blood pressure is highest, the decline in postural systolic blood pressure is greatest.

Orthostatic hypotension is a significant risk factor for syncope and falls in elderly persons, even those without other evidence of autonomic nervous system dysfunction.

Etiology

Orthostatic hypotension in the elderly has two distinct clinical presentations: physiologic (attributable to normal aging) and pathologic (attributable to disease).

Physiologic orthostatic hypotension: In healthy elderly persons, this type of hypotension varies dramatically from day to day, is related to blood pressure elevation, and is associated with the exaggerated plasma norepinephrine response to postural change that is characteristic of aging. It often is provoked by common hypotensive stresses, such as volume depletion, ingestion of hypotensive drugs, or Valsalva's maneuver during voiding. Although generally asymptomatic and labile, physiologic orthostatic hypotension may be sufficient to compromise cerebral blood flow and cause dizziness or syncope. Prolonged bed rest may further compromise blood pressure homeostasis, resulting in severe postural hypotension.

Pathologic orthostatic hypotension: Usually symptomatic, this type of hypotension often is associated with postural dizziness or syncope. Acute orthostatic hypotension most commonly results from dehydration during an acute illness. In young patients, excessive cardioacceleration upon standing suggests hypovolemia rather than autonomic dysfunction as the cause of orthostatic hypotension. But in normal elderly persons, cardioacceleration is often blunted, so it may not occur in patients whose orthostatic hypotension results from hypovolemia. A much less common cause of acute orthostatic hypotension is adrenocortical insufficiency accompanied by hyponatremia and hyperkalemia (see TABLE 36–1).

Chronic orthostatic hypotension is usually associated with symptoms of autonomic nervous system dysfunction such as a fixed heart rate, incontinence, constipation, inability to sweat, heat intolerance, impotence, and fatigability.

If no cause is evident, orthostatic hypotension may be primary or idiopathic. **Pure autonomic failure** (previously called **idiopathic orthostatic hypotension**) is characterized by lower basal plasma norepinephrine levels in the supine position, no increase in norepinephrine levels upon standing, a lower threshold for the pressor response to infused norepinephrine, and an increased pressor response to tyramine despite the release of less norepinephrine at sympathetic nerve endings. These findings suggest that norepinephrine is depleted from sympathetic nerve endings, resulting in postsynaptic denervation supersensitivity.

Patients with **Shy-Drager syndrome** have normal levels of circulating norepinephrine and a normal response to infused norepinephrine and tyramine, but their plasma norepinephrine levels do not increase upon standing. This syndrome is associated with neuron degeneration in several areas of the central nervous system, including the corticobulbar, corticospinal, extrapyramidal, and cerebellar systems of the brain, as well as the intermediolateral columns of the spinal cord. Thus, Shy-Drager syndrome is a central nervous system disorder of sympathetic blood pressure control, usually associated with extrapyramidal and cerebellar symptoms.

Disorders of the **peripheral autonomic nervous system** also cause pathologic orthostatic hypotension. They include insulin-dependent diabetes mellitus, in which severe peripheral neuropathy and other end-organ damage occur, and less common disorders such as amyloidosis, vitamin deficiencies, and neuropathies associated with malignancies, particularly cancers of the lung and the pancreas.

TABLE 36–1. CAUSES OF ORTHOSTATIC HYPOTENSION

Systemic disorders	Dehydration Adrenocortical insufficiency
Pure autonomic failure	
Central nervous system disorders	Shy-Drager syndrome Brain stem lesions Parkinson's disease Myelopathy Multiple cerebral infarcts
Peripheral and autonomic neuropathies	Diabetes mellitus Amyloidosis Tabes dorsalis Paraneoplastic syndromes Alcoholic and nutritional diseases
Drugs	Phenothiazines and other antipsychotics Monoamine oxidase inhibitors Tricyclic antidepressants Antihypertensives Levodopa Vasodilators β-Blockers Calcium channel blockers

Modified from Lipsitz LA: "Syncope in the elderly." *Annals of Internal Medicine* 99(1):92–105, 1983; used with permission.

Perhaps the most common cause of orthostatic hypotension is the use of **medications,** such as phenothiazines, tricyclic antidepressants, antianxiety agents, and antihypertensives, including those with central effects (such as methyldopa and clonidine) and those with peripheral effects (such as prazosin, hydralazine, and guanethidine). Because of age-related impairments in ventricular diastolic filling, elderly people depend on adequate venous return to generate a normal cardiac output. Medications that reduce venous return, particularly nitrates and diuretics, commonly produce orthostatic hypotension. With many medications, orthostatic hypotension may result even from usual therapeutic doses.

Diagnosis

The clinician should not assume that an elderly person who complains of postural dizziness and light-headedness is suffering from orthostatic hypotension. Rather, blood pressure and pulse rate should be measured after the patient has been recumbent for at least 5 min and after the patient has been standing quietly for 1 min and then for 3 min. A hypotensive response may be immediate or delayed. Prolonged standing or a tilt test may be needed to detect a delayed hypotensive response. Before therapy is initiated, blood pressure should be measured on several occasions to confirm that orthostatic hypotension persists.

Treatment

The goal of therapy is to reduce or eliminate symptoms; often this can be achieved without completely correcting orthostatic hypotension. Regardless of the cause, orthostatic hypotension should be treated in the stepwise fashion described below.

Initial therapy: The first therapeutic considerations include correcting hypovolemia and evaluating the patient's prescription and over-the-counter (OTC) medications to identify a possible cause. A patient with chronic orthostatic hypotension should be instructed to rise slowly after lying in bed or sitting in a chair for a long time. Dorsiflexing the feet before standing often promotes venous return to the heart, accelerates the pulse, and increases blood pressure. Crossing the legs while standing may also help increase blood pressure. A high salt diet aimed at producing a modest weight gain may blunt the symptoms of orthostatic hypotension in many patients. Elastic stockings that cover the calf and thigh and, in some cases, abdominal binders may be effective. Elevating the head of the bed 5° to 20° prevents the diuresis and supine hypertension caused by nocturnal shifts of interstitial fluid from the legs to the rest of the circulation.

Medications: If despite these measures, the patient remains symptomatic, medication may be needed. Various drug regimens have been tried, but most have been ineffective or require further study. However, **fludrocortisone acetate** appears to be effective for most types of orthostatic hypotension. Given in daily doses of 0.1 to 1.0 mg orally until mild peripheral edema develops, this mineralocorticoid increases extracellular fluid and plasma volume and sensitizes blood vessels to the vasoconstrictive effect of norepinephrine. These physiologic changes compensate for the homeostatic impairment that occurs upon rising in most persons with mild to moderately severe orthostatic hypotension. Complications of fludrocortisone therapy include supine hypertension and heart failure. Because hypokalemia can develop with mineralocorticoids, serum potassium should be measured every few months during treatment.

Drugs under study include nonsteroidal anti-inflammatory drugs such as indomethacin, the central α_2-antagonist yohimbine, the α_2-agonist clonidine, and β-adrenergic antagonists that block β_2-vasodilator receptors or have intrinsic sympathomimetic activity, such as pindolol. The central α_2-antagonist yohimbine can increase central sympathetic nervous system outflow. When such outflow is reduced (as in Shy-Drager syndrome), α_2-agonists, which inhibit central sympathetic outflow in normal persons, can act on peripheral α_2-receptors in the veins. This action promotes venoconstriction, thereby increasing venous return. Midodrine, a direct α_1-agonist, is helpful in some patients with Shy-Drager syndrome or pure autonomic failure.

Various sympathomimetic agents such as ephedrine and phenylephrine have yielded inconsistent results. On the other hand, 250 mg caffeine each morning attenuates orthostatic hypotension in younger patients and can be used safely in the elderly. Ergot alkaloids, including oral ergotamine tartrate and dihydroergotamine given subcutaneously with caffeine, have also been helpful in some patients. In severe cases of orthostatic hypotension that resist traditional approaches, erythropoietin may be useful.

POSTPRANDIAL HYPOTENSION

A decline in arterial blood pressure that occurs after a meal.

Postprandial hypotension is a clinical abnormality of blood pressure homeostasis in the elderly. Studies of clinically stable, unmedicated elderly patients, both institutionalized and noninstitutionalized, show significant decreases in blood pressure after morning and noon meals; such decreases do not occur in younger persons or in elderly persons who have not just eaten a meal. Up to one third of institutionalized and noninstitutionalized elderly persons have a postprandial blood pressure decline $\geq$ 20 mm Hg within 75 min of eating a meal. This decline can be even greater when hypotensive medications are taken before a meal. The incidence of postprandial hypotension is greatest among hypertensive elderly persons and those who have postprandial syncope or autonomic nervous system dysfunction. Postprandial hypotension is probably a common cause of syncope and falls in the elderly. In one study of institutionalized elderly persons, it accounted for 8% of syncopal episodes.

Etiology, Symptoms, Signs, and Diagnosis

The mechanism of postprandial hypotension is thought to be related to impaired baroreflex compensation for splanchnic blood pooling during digestion. Dysautonomic patients with postprandial hypotension have impaired forearm vasoconstriction, reduced systemic vascular resistance, and abnormal sympathetic nervous system control of heart rate after a meal. Thus, alterations in autonomic control of heart rate and vascular resistance are probably underlying causes of this syndrome.

Postprandial hypotension has two clinical presentations: (1) a physiologic, age-related phenomenon that is rarely symptomatic unless exacerbated by other hypotensive stresses and (2) a more severe pathologic syndrome related to autonomic insufficiency in which more profound hypotension is accompanied by syncope.

Blood pressure should be measured before and after meals in geriatric patients who experience postprandial dizziness, falls, syncope, or other cerebral or cardiac ischemic symptoms.

Treatment

Without clinical trials to evaluate treatments for postprandial hypotension, management is based on common sense. Symptomatic patients should not take hypotensive drugs before meals and should lie down after meals. Reducing dosages of hypotensive drugs and eating small, frequent meals may also help. Recent data suggest that walking after a meal may help restore normal circulation in some patients. This should be attempted only when the patient is under close observation.

Studies of patients with autonomic insufficiency suggest that indomethacin 50 mg q 6 h, caffeine 250 mg with or without dihydroergotamine 6 to 10 μg/kg s.c., or somatostatin 12 to 16 μg s.c. before a meal may ameliorate postprandial hypotension. Caffeine should be given only in the morning so the effect wears off by evening, allowing sleep and avoiding drug tolerance.

37. CORONARY ARTERY DISEASE

A condition in which one or more of the coronary arteries is narrowed by atherosclerotic plaque or vascular spasm.

Coronary artery disease reflects an imbalance between myocardial oxygen supply and demand. This imbalance, which represents myocardial ischemia, is expressed clinically as angina or myocardial infarction. Most sudden cardiac deaths are arrhythmic secondary to coronary artery disease.

Prevalence

The prevalence and severity of coronary artery disease increase dramatically with age. The increase is greater in men than in women and reaches a peak between the sixth and seventh decade, at which point it declines slightly. The increase in women continues steadily until the eighth decade. The prevalence is about 60% in both sexes at the eighth decade and thereafter. Despite the high prevalence of coronary artery disease in the elderly, symptomatic disease is noted in only 10% to 20% of this population. This discrepancy may be due to (1) decreased activity levels (work loads that would ordinarily trigger ischemic symptoms may be encountered less frequently in the elderly), (2) increased likelihood of a neuropathy that alters pain sensation, or (3) age-associated myocardial and possibly pericardial changes, making dyspnea more likely to occur than chest pain when ischemia is present. The prevalence of disease detected on thallium stress testing also increases, from 2% in the fifth and sixth decades to > 25% in the ninth decade.

Diagnosis

(See also Ch. 34)

Coronary artery disease should be strongly suspected in persons with known coronary risk factors (see Prevention, below) and in those with signs of noncoronary atherosclerosis, such as cerebrovascular or peripheral vascular disease. The probability of disease (which is higher in an elderly person), as well as the sensitivity and specificity of a test (see TABLE 34–1), determine a test's accuracy. Thus, a positive test result is more predictive, and a negative result less so, in an older person.

Exercise stress testing is useful for diagnosing coronary artery disease and for predicting subsequent coronary death in middle-aged persons with two or more risk factors. It is probably equally useful in the elderly (see TABLE 34–2). Exercise stress testing is also used to evaluate the severity of coronary artery disease. Left main artery or triple-vessel obstructions typically produce systolic hypotension (a fall in systolic blood pressure of > 15 mm Hg from one exercise level to the next) as well as several types of ECG changes. These include global changes (ie, those occurring in both the anterior and inferior leads), marked changes (> 2 mm of ST-segment shift), prolonged changes (those persisting > 8 min after exercise), early changes (those occurring during stage 1 or stage 2 of the standard Bruce treadmill test), and the appearance of malignant ventricular arrhythmias.

Two points should be considered when evaluating a stress ECG. First, ST and T changes cannot be interpreted if a person has left bundle branch block or left ventricular hypertrophy or is taking digoxin, all of which are more likely in older than in younger persons. Under these circumstances, thallium stress testing is a better alternative. Second, older patients often cannot exercise to 90% of predicted maximum heart rate because of respiratory or musculoskeletal disease. In older persons who cannot exercise to the desired heart rate or work load, **thallium scan or ECG testing** after the administration of a pharmacologic stress such as dipyridamole or adenosine may be used to diagnose significant coronary artery disease. Adenosine probably has a greater incidence of side effects, such as impulse formation or conduction system disturbances. Pacing may also be used to increase the heart rate and so induce ischemia in appropriate patients. However, not only is insertion of a pacemaker an invasive procedure, but the stress provoked by pacing is often not comparable to that induced by exercise.

In addition to scintigraphic and ECG evidence of ischemia, functional evidence may be provided by **echocardiography.** Echocardiography performed during dobutamine infusion and then during or immediately after exercise can help diagnose, localize, and assess the severity of ischemia-induced left ventricular dysfunction. The diagnostic sensitivity and specificity are similar to those of other imaging modalities. Advantages include using less expensive technology and avoiding radiation exposure.

Prevention

The principles of coronary artery disease management are similar for all patients, and **risk factor modification** may be as important in older patients as in younger ones. Measures should be taken to decrease the progression of coronary atherosclerosis in both symptomatic and asymptomatic elderly persons.

Data from the Framingham Heart Study indicate that **systolic blood pressure** is the strongest discriminator of coronary artery disease risk in men $>$ 45 yr old. A study of persons $>$ 60 yr of age with isolated systolic hypertension (systolic pressure $\geq$ 160 mm Hg without diastolic hypertension) has shown that treatment decreases the risk of major cardiovascular outcomes.

Total cholesterol levels have been related to unfavorable cardiovascular outcomes in the elderly, although not in the Framingham data. High levels of **low-density lipoprotein (LDL)** cholesterol represent a significant risk factor for cardiovascular disease; conversely, high levels of **high-density lipoprotein (HDL)** cholesterol are associated with reduced risk. Drug and dietary interventions to lower LDL levels have been shown to reduce cardiovascular risk in middle-aged populations. Although similar data are not available for the elderly, recommending dietary changes and pharmacotherapy for older persons with coronary artery disease and abnormal lipid levels is probably prudent (see also Ch. 81).

Many studies correlate **cigarette smoking** with increased cardiovascular risk in the elderly. Studies also show that cessation of smoking for as little as 1 to 5 yr markedly reduces risk.

Physical inactivity is an additional risk factor for the development of coronary artery disease. The benefits of exercise may be related to maintenance of normal blood pressure, a favorable influence on the lipid profile, decreased neurohumoral activation, and improved glucose tolerance. However, since asymptomatic disease is so prevalent in the elderly, older persons should undergo a supervised exercise test before initiating, and at regular intervals while participating in, a regular exercise program (see Ch. 31).

ANGINA PECTORIS

A clinical syndrome due to myocardial ischemia characterized by episodes of precordial discomfort and pressure, typically precipitated by exertion and relieved by rest or sublingual nitroglycerin.

Angina pectoris is a clinical manifestation of coronary artery disease. The discomfort of angina, which is highly variable, is most commonly felt beneath the sternum. It may be a vague, barely troublesome ache, or it may rapidly become a severe, intense, precordial crushing sensation. Some patients do not perceive the discomfort as pain.

Angina is usually triggered by physical activity and typically persists for no more than a few minutes, subsiding with rest. Angina is worsened when exertion follows a meal. It is also exaggerated in cold weather. Walking into the wind or first contact with cold air on leaving a warm room may also precipitate an attack. Angina may occur at night **(nocturnal angina),** which may be a sign of recurrent left ventricular failure, an equivalent of nocturnal dyspnea.

Attacks may vary in frequency from several a day to occasional episodes separated by symptom-free intervals of weeks or months. They may increase in frequency **(crescendo angina)** to a fatal outcome or may gradually decrease or disappear if an adequate collateral circulation develops, if the ischemic area becomes infarcted, or if heart failure supervenes and limits activity.

Any change in the pattern of symptoms—increased intensity of attacks, decreased threshold of stimulus, longer duration, or occurrence when the patient is sedentary or awakening from sleep—should be viewed as serious. Such changes are termed **unstable angina,** which may be prodromal to acute myocardial infarction.

Treatment

The treatment of elderly persons with angina should begin with an attempt to identify other superimposed and treatable illnesses that may increase myocardial oxygen demand and decrease its supply, such as anemia, infection, hyperthyroidism, and arrhythmias. If any of these conditions are present and treated, the angina may possibly be eliminated.

Pharmacotherapy: The primary drug options are the same for elderly as for younger patients: nitrates, β-blockers, and calcium antagonists. Age-associated changes in pharmacokinetics and pharmacodynamics (eg, decreases in serum albumin and lean body mass and increases in α_1-acid glycoproteins and body fat) may influence the choice and dose of these drugs. Aging is also associated with a change in the cardiovascular response to certain medications including β-agonists and digitalis. Older persons are also more likely to be taking other medications that may alter the pharmacokinetics of cardiovascular agents.

Nitrates act primarily by lowering preload through venous dilation, which decreases venous return and hence ventricular cavity size, and to a lesser extent by reducing afterload through arteriolar dilation. They may also produce coronary vasodilation. Nitroglycerin given sublingually 0.3 to 0.6 mg or as a lingual aerosol spray 0.4 mg provides relief during an acute ischemic episode and is useful for prophylaxis. Unfortunately, the anti-ischemic effect of both oral (20 to 40 mg qid) and topical (5 to 20 mg/24 h) nitrate preparations is significantly attenuated if the drug is given continuously. This can be avoided by intermittent dosing. Removing the transdermal patch overnight or using oral preparations bid or tid may prevent the development of nitrate tolerance. However, this may leave the patient insufficiently protected between doses.

Preexisting diminished intravascular volume, impaired venous valves, and a diminished baroreceptor reflex make older patients more susceptible to the hypotensive effects of nitrates. Thus, it is important to begin with a low dose, increase the dose slowly, and instruct patients to lie down when they first take any nitrate preparation.

β-Blockers work primarily by reducing myocardial oxygen demand; they decrease heart rate, myocardial contractility, and blood pressure. Secondarily, they increase myocardial oxygen supply through the reduction in heart rate (since most of the coronary flow occurs during diastole). In addition, propranolol has been shown to produce a rightward shift of the oxyhemoglobin dissociation curve, thus increasing release of oxygen to ischemic tissues.

The choice of β-blocker should be based on the drug's associated properties. Low doses of relatively cardioselective drugs (atenolol 50 mg/day or metoprolol 100 mg/day) may be used when blockade of β_2-receptors is undesirable. However, the selectivity is only relative because blockade of β_2-receptors occurs at moderate to high doses. Hydrophilic β-blockers (atenolol 50 to 200 mg/day or nadolol 40 to 80 mg/day) should be considered when treating patients with hepatic disease or when CNS side effects need to be minimized. Lipophilic β-blockers (propranolol 80 to 240 mg/day, metoprolol 50 to 100 mg bid, or timolol 10 to 20 mg bid) may be preferable in patients with coexisting renal disease.

Secondary prevention is an important additional benefit of some β-blockers. Studies have shown that timolol (20 mg/day), propranolol (160 to 240 mg/day), and metoprolol (100 to 200 mg/day) decrease the risk of subsequent infarction and death when given after myocardial infarction.

Because of pharmacodynamic and pharmacokinetic changes (described in Ch. 21), the β-blocking properties of these drugs are diminished in the elderly. The age-related reduction in cardiovascular responsiveness to β-agonist stimulation results in less reliance on catecholamines and more dependence on the Frank-Starling mechanism to increase cardiac work during times of stress (see Chs. 33 and 41). This suggests that β-blockers as anti-ischemic agents may be less effective in elderly than in younger patients.

Preexisting disease, such as bronchospastic pulmonary disease, claudication, insulin-dependent diabetes mellitus, impaired ventricular function, and conduction system disease, may render the elderly more sensitive to the side effects of β-blockers. Prolonged therapy may result in up-regulation of cardiac β-receptors and hence produce an increased sensitivity to endogenous catecholamines if β-blockers are abruptly withdrawn. Thus, *β-blockers should be withdrawn slowly, if possible,* when therapy is discontinued in angina patients.

Calcium antagonists are useful for treating stable and unstable angina. This group of drugs includes nifedipine 30 to 120 mg/day, diltiazem 90 to 360 mg/day, verapamil 120 to 480 mg/day, and the newer dihydropyridines, amlodipine 5 to 10 mg/day and felodipine 5 to 10 mg/day.

Calcium antagonists act primarily by decreasing coronary and peripheral vascular resistance, although verapamil (and to a considerably less extent, diltiazem) has negative inotropic and chronotropic effects. These agents exert an anti-ischemic effect (1) by decreasing coronary artery resistance and preventing spasm, which increases myocardial oxygen supply, and (2) by inducing peripheral vasodilation, which decreases myocardial oxygen demand. They also have antiplatelet properties and an antihypertensive effect, which makes them useful in patients with coexisting hypertension.

Because calcium antagonists have a peripheral vasodilating effect, they should be given cautiously to elderly patients. Hypotension can occur with peripheral vasodilation, especially in patients who are volume depleted. A sympathetic reflex-induced increase in cardiac work may also occur, which can be prevented by the concomitant administration of a relatively small dose of β-blocker. Some calcium antagonists also have negative inotropic, chronotropic, and dromotropic effects, which affect primarily persons with preexisting impaired ventricular function or conduction system disease or those taking fairly high doses of β-blockers. No significant rebound phenomenon appears to occur on withdrawal of calcium antagonists.

Aspirin (325 mg/day) has been shown to reduce by 50% the rate of myocardial infarction and death in patients with unstable angina, to provide secondary prevention after myocardial infarction, and to improve patency of saphenous vein grafts after bypass surgery.

Surgical treatments: If pharmacotherapy fails to control symptoms, or if noninvasive studies (eg, the treadmill test) or the clinical setting (eg, recurrent ischemia in the postinfarction period) indicates that the patient is at high risk despite medical therapy, **cardiac catheterization** should be considered to evaluate the suitability of angioplasty or coronary artery bypass surgery. The risks of cardiac catheterization, including cerebral and peripheral embolization, renal failure, and death, are higher in the elderly. This increased risk may be because older patients are more likely to have preexisting coronary and peripheral vascular disease, renal insufficiency, and left ventricular dysfunction.

Some reports indicate that **angioplasty** is associated with a lower success rate and an increased rate of acute complications in the elderly. However, more recent studies indicate that the success rate (83%) is comparable to that in younger patients (86%) and that the complication rate (9%) is only slightly higher than that in younger patients (6%).

If a patient's coronary artery anatomy is not suitable for angioplasty, **bypass surgery** should be considered. Although the mortality rate may be two to three times higher in older than in younger persons, this is primarily because the elderly are more likely to have hypertension, impaired ventricular function, and extensive coronary artery disease. The overall mortality rate of 5% to 6% in the elderly is low enough for surgery to be recommended if indicated. Although morbidity and hospitalization time and costs are greater in the elderly, the risk of complications is declining. In addition, the long-term pain relief and survival rates of bypass surgery compare favorably with those of drug therapy.

MYOCARDIAL INFARCTION

Necrosis of myocardial tissue resulting from obstruction of a coronary artery.

In the USA, most patients hospitalized with acute myocardial infarction are > 65 yr of age. The elderly are less likely to have precordial pain and more likely to have dyspnea, fatigue, weakness, or CNS symptoms such as confusion and dizziness. The different symptomatology may reflect the greater likelihood that an older person has preexisting cerebrovascular disease or heart failure.

The incidence of infarct complications, including heart failure, pulmonary edema, ventricular rupture, and death, is significantly higher in older patients. Again, these changes may result from preexisting left ventricular dysfunction and possibly from lower contractile reserve in noninfarcted regions related to diminished β-agonist responsiveness. Older patients are also more likely to have smaller and non–Q-wave infarcts than are younger persons. This may be because the elderly are more likely to have hypotension and superimposed illnesses, such as pneumonia or anemia, which may induce a small, non–Q-wave infarction in the absence of associated coronary thrombus. Important topographic changes—regional dilation and thinning in the infarcted area and compensatory hypertrophy in noninfarcted tissue—that occur after Q-wave infarction are also related to advancing age.

Treatment

Because of a high complication rate, elderly persons benefit from close monitoring in a coronary care unit.

Early **thrombolysis** (within 6 h of a transmural infarction) decreases mortality and improves left ventricular function. The addition of aspirin 160 mg/day provides more benefit than that achieved with thrombolysis alone. However, thrombolytic therapy is not used as often in older patients with acute infarctions. This may be related in part to the increased likelihood of coexisting illnesses, delayed presentation, and atypical symptoms and ECG changes. Although the elderly are at increased risk for intracerebral hemorrhage, the risk may be attenuated if the dose of thrombolytic agent is weight-adjusted. When assessing the benefit-to-risk ratio, the physician should remember that the benefit of thrombolytic therapy is increased in those who are treated early and in those who have extensive anterior infarctions.

Drug therapy is otherwise the same as that used in younger patients. However, because the elderly have a markedly heterogeneous response, with no strict age-related rules, *therapy must be individualized.* **Anticoagulants** are given cautiously for two major reasons: (1) heparin is associated with an increased risk of bleeding in older women, and (2) the hazards of chronic warfarin therapy are compounded by the increased risk of falls. **Aspirin** is approved for prevention of reinfarction after myocardial infarction. Although studies have focused on middle-aged populations, it is reasonable and prudent to give aspirin to the elderly as well. As in younger patients, **β-blockers** may be used for their secondary prevention effects (see above). Such therapy is particularly beneficial for those who are at increased risk for recurrent myocardial infarction.

Medically supervised rehabilitation after myocardial infarction results in improved conditioning similar to that observed in younger patients. Target heart rates are best assessed on a Bruce treadmill test performed 3 to 6 wk after the infarction. If no evidence of exercise-induced ischemia, arrhythmia, or deterioration of left ventricular function exists, an exercise program sufficient to raise the heart rate to 70% of the maximum achieved heart rate can then be recommended (see Ch. 31). Sexual activity can usually be resumed 8 to 14 wk after myocardial infarction (see Heart Disease under EFFECTS OF MEDICAL PROBLEMS ON SEXUALITY in Ch. 68).

38. VALVULAR HEART DISEASE

In elderly patients, the predominant causes of valvular heart disease are degenerative calcification, myxomatous degeneration, papillary muscle dysfunction, and infective endocarditis; rheumatic and syphilitic diseases are less common causes. These disorders are superimposed on the normal changes of aging, which include fibrotic thickening and increasing opacity of the mitral and aortic valves. Noninvasive imaging techniques are important in establishing a diagnosis. Although medical management is appropriate for most older patients, surgery is indicated when symptoms interfere with daily activities or when hemodynamically important valvular disease occurs acutely and surgery can be accomplished with acceptable risk.

AORTIC VALVE DISEASE

Diseases of the aortic valve that occur in the elderly include aortic stenosis and aortic regurgitation, both acute and chronic.

AORTIC STENOSIS

An abnormal narrowing of the aortic valve orifice.

Aortic stenosis, the most clinically significant valvular lesion in the elderly, increases in frequency with age. The severity of the stenosis is often underestimated because its progression is so gradual. Aortic stenosis with calcification predominates. Calcification of a congenital bicuspid valve occurs in the younger elderly, whereas calcification on the aortic aspect of a tricuspid aortic valve is typical in patients > 75 yr of age. The 20% of elderly patients with rheumatic aortic stenosis often have associated mitral valve disease.

Symptoms and Signs

The majority of patients with aortic stenosis are asymptomatic. For those who experience symptoms, the prognosis is extremely poor. Chest pain is an early symptom. Presyncope (transient alteration of consciousness) progresses to effort syncope, which occurs in about ⅓ of symptomatic patients. Activity-precipitated symptoms may not occur in sedentary patients. Exertional dyspnea may progress to pulmonary edema. About ½ of elderly patients with severe aortic stenosis have heart failure, often heralded by atrial fibrillation. The loss of late diastolic filling of the poorly compliant ventricle due to a loss of atrial contraction may precipitate heart failure.

Physical findings include a narrow pulse pressure and a slowly rising, small-volume carotid pulse, with a systolic thrill in some patients. However, the poorly compliant arterial wall may mask these abnormalities, rendering the carotid pulse relatively normal. The cardiac apex impulse is forceful and sustained, but this finding may be masked by kyphosis. The first heart sound is soft. The aortic component of the second heart sound is also soft; it may be inaudible when stenosis is severe and life-threatening. Reverse splitting of the second sound may occur with left ventricular failure. A fourth heart sound is common, but this sound disappears in the ¼ of elderly patients who develop atrial fibrillation. Ejection sounds are rare because the valve cusps are immobile.

A harsh, loud crescendo-decrescendo systolic murmur, often associated with a thrill, is maximal at the upper right sternal border. The murmur peaks in mid to late systole and often radiates throughout the precordium and into the neck. This late peaking is often the best clue to severe aortic stenosis. The murmur's high-frequency components are often transmitted to the lower left sternal border and toward the cardiac apex during most of systole and may mimic the murmur of mitral regurgitation. The murmur's intensity does *not* correlate with the severity of the obstruction. With the decreased cardiac output of critical stenosis, the basal systolic murmur may soften or may be absent. Basal diastolic murmurs of aortic regurgitation are heard in more than ½ of patients with aortic stenosis. Because of vascular stiffening, hypertension can coexist with severe aortic stenosis in elderly patients.

Laboratory Findings

The ECG shows evidence of left ventricular hypertrophy, although hyperinflated lungs may mask increased left ventricular voltage. Cardiac enlargement on chest x-ray is evident when heart failure supervenes, although heart size often remains normal before its onset. Poststenotic aortic dilatation is a frequent finding. Dense calcification of the aortic valve is best seen on the lateral chest x-ray. Lack of calcification on chest x-ray and echocardiogram virtually excludes the diagnosis of critical aortic stenosis.

Two-dimensional echocardiography is used to assess cardiac chamber size, wall thickness, wall motion, valve leaflet motion, valve orifice size, and valvular calcification. Doppler measurement of intracardiac blood velocity permits calculation of the severity of valvular regurgitation or obstruction, and serial measurements can determine progression of hemodynamic severity. Such studies are helpful in identifying appropriate candidates for cardiac catheterization. When severe stenosis is suspected, exercise testing is *contraindicated* because of the high risk of exercise-related syncope and death.

Diagnosis

Echocardiography and Doppler studies help differentiate aortic stenosis from the benign aortic sclerosis found in ⅓ to ½ of elderly persons. The latter is typically asymptomatic and without hemodynamic significance; the basal systolic murmur is short and peaks early, and the carotid pulse is normal.

The chest pain of aortic stenosis must be differentiated from that of coronary disease. Likewise, the syncope must be distinguished from that due to atrioventricular block or tachyarrhythmias—two conditions that often occur in older patients. The dyspnea must be differentiated from that of chronic obstructive pulmonary disease or cardiomyopathy, and the murmur from that of hypertrophic cardiomyopathy, mitral annular calcification, papillary muscle dysfunction, and aortic sclerosis. Cardiac catheterization, which is sometimes required to make these differential determinations, is warranted in patients with severe aortic stenosis to identify coexisting coronary atherosclerotic obstruction that may require simultaneous coronary artery bypass graft surgery. Unrecognized or uncorrected significant concomitant coronary disease increases the risk of early postoperative mortality. Recognizing severe aortic stenosis is important because it has an adverse prognosis if untreated and a high operative success rate when identified.

Treatment

Aortic valve replacement is indicated for hemodynamically significant symptomatic aortic stenosis (see VALVE REPLACEMENT in Ch. 44), because only ½ of medically treated elderly patients survive > 5 yr after onset of angina, heart failure, or syncope. Patients often die suddenly. Symptomatic patients with severe aortic stenosis have a mortality rate of up to 50% at 1 yr and 65% at 2 yr.

Even in octogenarians and nonagenarians, aortic valve replacement improves survival and quality of life. The procedure can be performed in patients who meet the New York Heart Association's class 3 and class 4 criteria. Recent reports cite a perioperative mortality rate as low as 4% to 5% in elderly patients, with a surgical mortality rate of 5% to 10% even after the onset of heart failure. Improved surgical techniques have decreased the incidence of perioperative stroke caused by calcified valvular debris. The 5-yr survival rate is 70%, and long-term improvement is reported in symptom relief and hemodynamic status. Concurrent coronary bypass surgery may increase the risk of postoperative complications and death, primarily because it requires increased time on cardiopulmonary bypass.

Operative mortality is increased when clinical deterioration mandates emergency surgery. A high rate of *emergency* valve replacement surgery in elderly women compared to that in men raises concern that aortic stenosis is being diagnosed and treated less aggressively in women.

Porcine heterograft valves have an advantage over mechanical valves in that anticoagulation is not needed, but they may be less durable and may require reoperation when the patient is even older.

The role and efficacy of **catheter balloon valvuloplasty** for aortic stenosis have been delineated in recent years; the high rates of restenosis and posthospital mortality warrant its use only for symptomatic palliation of severely ill patients who are not candidates for surgery (see PERCUTANEOUS BALLOON VALVULOPLASTY in Ch. 44). Ultrasonic debridement of calcium from a stenotic aortic valve is no longer used because progressively severe aortic regurgitation often occurs.

Elderly patients with noncritical aortic stenosis require serial surveillance because the stenosis often progresses in severity, although at an unpredictable pace.

ACUTE AORTIC REGURGITATION

Sudden development of retrograde blood flow through an incompetent aortic valve into the left ventricle during ventricular diastole.

Trauma, infective endocarditis, or aortic dissection may cause acute aortic regurgitation. Acute severe heart failure is precipitated by abrupt ventricular volume overload without compensatory hypertrophy or dilatation.

Symptoms, Signs, and Laboratory Findings

Sudden, severe heart failure or acute pulmonary edema occurs with tachycardia and often with hypotension. The heart failure may mask the anticipated brisk arterial upstroke, wide pulse pressure, and collapsing pulse contour. The pulse pressure may be narrowed because of elevated left ventricular diastolic pressure. The first heart sound is soft, and the left sternal border decrescendo diastolic murmur is harsh and shortened by the raised ventricular filling pressure.

The ECG may be normal initially. Echocardiography helps confirm the diagnosis and often shows early mitral valve closure.

Diagnosis and Treatment

Acute aortic regurgitation must be differentiated from other causes of sudden severe heart failure (eg, papillary muscle, chordal, or septal rupture). The pulmonary edema may be erroneously attributed to myocardial infarction because the heart is not enlarged, the wide pulse pressure may be absent, and the murmur may not be appreciated. Urgent valve replacement is generally indicated for acute severe heart failure.

CHRONIC AORTIC REGURGITATION

Long-standing retrograde blood flow through an incompetent aortic valve into the left ventricle during ventricular diastole.

Chronic aortic regurgitation may be caused by valve leaflet disease (congenital or rheumatic disease, myxomatous degeneration, or secondary to endocarditis) or by aortic annular root dilatation (eg, as in syphilis, rheumatoid spondylitis, Marfan's syndrome).

Symptoms and Signs

Mild to moderate aortic regurgitation is often asymptomatic for many years, with preserved exercise tolerance, because of the sizable stroke volume of the dilated, hypertrophied ventricle and the lowered peripheral vascular resistance.

Rheumatic aortic regurgitation occurs predominantly in men and often remains asymptomatic, even in old age. A short, soft basal diastolic murmur is characteristic and may be accentuated by hypertension.

Syphilitic aortic regurgitation is more severe and has a worse prognosis, often because of an associated aortic aneurysm. A long, loud, decrescendo basal diastolic murmur, often with a short basal systolic murmur, is characteristic.

In symptomatic patients, effort intolerance and dyspnea may progress to heart failure. Chest pain is often attributable to associated coronary atherosclerosis. Palpitations usually do not reflect arrhythmias but rather are due to the forceful ejection of blood.

The findings of severe regurgitation include bounding peripheral arterial pulses, a wide pulse pressure, occasionally a bisferious pulse (pulsus bisferiens), and a hyperactive precordium with a rocking motion. The high-pitched diastolic murmur is best heard at the cardiac base. It is louder at the upper right sternal border in aortic root disease and more prominent along the left sternal border in aortic leaflet disease. There may be an associated diastolic thrill and a spindle-shaped systolic murmur of increased aortic outflow. Both third and fourth heart sounds are common, as is an apical diastolic rumble **(Austin Flint murmur).**

Laboratory Findings

Cardiac enlargement with a dilated aorta and occasionally an aortic aneurysm is characteristic on chest x-ray. Linear calcification of the ascending aorta is typical in syphilitic aortic regurgitation. This contrasts with the x-ray findings of benign aortic calcification. The ECG shows left ventricular hypertrophy. On echocardiography, the left ventricular cavity is enlarged, often with early diastolic fluttering of the anterior mitral valve leaflet. Enlarging ventricular dimensions and evidence of ventricular dysfunction in the symptomatic patient are indications for surgery.

Treatment

Medical management is the same as that for heart failure and includes sodium restriction, diuretic and vasodilator therapy, and at times, digitalis. Drugs that cause bradycardia should be avoided, because relative diastolic prolongation can increase the regurgitation and accentuate symptoms. Patients who remain symptomatic after receiving optimal medical therapy should be considered for valve replacement; the results are less satisfactory than in patients with aortic stenosis because of frequent severe underlying ventricular dysfunction. Bioprosthetic valves are favored because they do not require anticoagulant therapy, which may be associated with higher risk of bleeding in the elderly.

MITRAL VALVE DISEASE

Diseases of the mitral valve include mitral stenosis and mitral regurgitation, both acute and chronic, and that due to a calcified mitral annulus or to mitral valve prolapse.

MITRAL STENOSIS

An abnormal narrowing of the mitral valve orifice.

Mitral stenosis, due predominantly to rheumatic heart disease, is usually identified before old age and accounts for about 1/3 of mitral valve disease in the elderly. Its severity is usually such that an adequate response to medical therapy was obtained. However, this incidence may decrease because of the reduced incidence of rheumatic fever in developed countries. Commissural fusion and fibrosis occur, as does calcification of the leaflets and chordae. Some degree of mitral regurgitation often coexists. Less often, progressive extension of mitral annular calcification causes moderately severe mitral stenosis. One third of patients > 70 yr have calcium deposition in the aortic or mitral valve.

Symptoms, Signs, and Diagnosis

The clinical features are comparable to those in younger persons and include a loud first heart sound, an apical diastolic rumble with presystolic accentuation, and an opening snap. The latter may soften or disappear with valvular calcification, and the diastolic murmur may become softer. A right ventricular parasternal impulse is often palpable, and venous pressure may be elevated. Atrial fibrillation is more common in elderly patients, as is complicating arterial embolism.

Left atrial enlargement is often seen on chest x-ray. Electrocardiographic evidence of right ventricular hypertrophy is uncommon. Echocardiography with Doppler flow studies can document mitral stenosis and help estimate its severity. Left atrial myxoma may mimic mitral stenosis and can be differentiated by echocardiography.

Treatment

Most elderly patients with mild to moderate mitral stenosis are in sinus rhythm with few or no symptoms and respond well to medical therapy. Although atrial fibrillation often precipitates clinical deterioration and sometimes pulmonary edema, digitalis, verapamil, or β-blocker therapy can slow the ventricular response rate. The onset of atrial fibrillation may also cause peripheral arterial embolism. Pharmacologic or electrical cardioversion to sinus rhythm may restore compensation.

Although elderly patients with mitral valve disease and atrial fibrillation are at increased risk for bleeding, **anticoagulation** is recommended because of the high risk of valve thrombosis and peripheral arterial embolism. Brain hemorrhage occurs in 1% of anticoagulant-treated patients annually—an eightfold increase in risk compared with that in patients who have not received anticoagulant therapy—and major hemorrhage is reported in 3%. Some recent reports have challenged the excess bleeding risk in elderly patients. Lower levels of anticoagulation are currently recommended, with prolongation of the international normalized ratio (INR) to 2 to 3; this may lessen the risk of bleeding complications.

Valve replacement is warranted for progressively severe symptomatic mitral stenosis, because the calcified valve is rarely amenable to commissurotomy. Embolization per se is not an indication for valve surgery. The high risk of thrombosis associated with prosthetic valves mandates anticoagulant therapy. Evidence demonstrating the efficacy of catheter balloon valvuloplasty remains inconclusive, particularly in elderly patients.

ACUTE MITRAL REGURGITATION

Sudden development of retrograde blood flow, during systole, from the left ventricle into the left atrium through an incompetent mitral valve.

Acute, often massive, mitral regurgitation in elderly patients is commonly due to chordal rupture or the development of a flail mitral leaflet. The underlying disorder may be myocardial infarction, papillary muscle rupture, infective endocarditis, or mucoid degeneration of the valve cusps. Idiopathic chordal rupture also occurs.

Symptoms, Signs, and Laboratory Findings

The characteristic findings include sinus tachycardia and a new, harsh, early systolic apical murmur, often with a thrill. The murmur ends early, when the noncompliant left atrium can no longer accept additional volume. The first heart sound is soft, and the accentuated pulmonic component of the second heart sound reflects the acute pulmonary hypertension. A ventricular diastolic sound (S_3) is characteristic, and an atrial gallop may be present. Pulmonary venous congestion and often pulmonary edema develop rapidly, as evidence of hemodynamic significance.

Both the ECG and the chest x-ray may be normal initially, but pulmonary venous congestion soon supervenes. Echocardiography confirms the diagnosis and often suggests the cause; hyperkinetic left ventricular function is usually seen.

Diagnosis and Treatment

Echocardiography can differentiate acute mitral regurgitation from septal rupture. Valvular vegetations of infective endocarditis may also be demonstrated. Transesophageal echocardiography has been performed safely in selected elderly patients, providing decision-making information for surgery.

Acute mitral regurgitation is treated in the same way as acute pulmonary edema of other cardiac cause. Hemodynamic instability, characterized by hypotension with pulmonary edema, often requires intra-aortic balloon counterpulsation to permit cardiac catheterization and the subsequent induction of anesthesia for surgery. Acute massive mitral regurgitation typically requires urgent valve replacement. Clinical deterioration is an urgent indication for valve replacement, although the mortality risk increases with emergency surgery. The mortality risk also increases when myocardial infarction causes acute mitral regurgitation, since concomitant coronary bypass surgery, which increases pump time, may be required.

CHRONIC MITRAL REGURGITATION

Long-standing retrograde blood flow, during ventricular systole, from the left ventricle into the left atrium through an incompetent mitral valve.

Chronic mitral regurgitation accounts for 2/3 of mitral valve disease in the elderly. About 1/2 of affected patients have a history of rheumatic fever and about 1/2 have associated aortic valve disease, usually aortic regurgitation. Isolated mitral regurgitation often results from papillary muscle dysfunction following myocardial infarction. Calcification of the mitral annulus and myxomatous valve degeneration leading to mitral valve prolapse also cause chronic mitral regurgitation and are discussed separately below.

Symptoms, Signs, and Laboratory Findings

The usual presentation includes atrial fibrillation, which may precipitate hemodynamic deterioration; an apical holosystolic murmur, often with a soft first heart sound; and heart failure. Complicating systemic embolism may occur, as a result of either rheumatic disease or myocardial infarction. When mitral regurgitation is due to papillary muscle dysfunction, a spindle-shaped apical murmur is heard during midsystole. Electrocardiographic abnormalities and echocardiographic evidence of regional wall motion abnormalities may suggest coexisting coronary disease. Echocardiography can also delineate overall ventricular function.

Treatment

Atrial fibrillation in mitral regurgitation is managed the same as that in mitral stenosis, and heart failure is treated in the usual manner. Most elderly patients with chronic mitral regurgitation either are asymptomatic or respond readily to medical therapy for heart failure. Surgery is indicated when medical therapy fails to control the heart failure and ventricular function deteriorates. Because papillary muscle integrity may be more important in older than in younger persons, mitral valve reconstruction may be preferable to valve replacement for older patients. Surgical plication or valvuloplasty may be effective for myxomatous degeneration, but case series of mitral valve repair in the elderly are not yet available. When valve replacement is needed, mechanical valves are typically chosen; they are more durable, and the left atrial enlargement, atrial fibrillation, or both already indicate a need for anticoagulation.

Mitral valve replacement is associated with less satisfactory results and a higher mortality rate than aortic valve replacement. This is because ventricular dysfunction is significantly greater in patients with mitral valve disease in whom surgery is indicated, and until recently little attention has been given to preserving the mitral apparatus (mitral valvuloplasty). A large percentage of deaths are due to embolic cerebrovascular accident, particularly when atrial fibrillation is present.

MITRAL REGURGITATION FROM MITRAL ANNULAR CALCIFICATION

Mitral regurgitation due to calcification of the mitral valve ring.

About 6% of persons > 60 yr, predominantly women, have mitral annular calcification. Calcification prevents annular systolic contraction and may limit valve leaflet closure. Although the mitral regurgitation is rarely hemodynamically significant, conduction disturbances may result from extension of the calcification. Recent data suggest that such calcification doubles the risk for stroke, independent of other risk factors.

Patients are often asymptomatic. An apical systolic murmur that radiates widely, occasionally to the back, is associated with a soft first heart sound. Characteristic findings on chest x-ray and dense horseshoe-shaped calcifications on echocardiography define the condition. Patients rarely require therapy other than that needed to control the ventricular response rate to atrial fibrillation.

MITRAL REGURGITATION FROM MITRAL VALVE PROLAPSE

Mitral regurgitation associated with bulging of one or both mitral valve leaflets into the left atrium during ventricular systole.

Myxomatous valvular degeneration, which increases in frequency with aging, is the major cause of mitral valve prolapse in the elderly. Mitral valve prolapse, severe enough to require surgical intervention, is more common in elderly men than in elderly women. The associated dissolution of collagen in the elongated chordae tendineae may explain the high incidence of chordal rupture that often produces life-threatening heart failure in these patients. Myxomatous degeneration of the aortic valve often coexists.

Symptoms, Signs, and Laboratory Findings

Presenting symptoms may include disabling chest pain inconsistent with the pain of myocardial ischemia, palpitations or syncope due to arrhythmia, and heart failure secondary to mitral regurgitation. Heart failure appears to be more common in men. Arrhythmias are common, even in patients with normal ventricular function. The onset of atrial fibrillation may accentuate both mitral and tricuspid valve prolapse and often precipitates hemodynamic deterioration.

The clinical picture includes a midsystolic click or clicks and a late systolic or holosystolic murmur, with characteristic postural variations such as an earlier, louder murmur and earlier and more clicks on assuming the upright position. In contrast to the prominent clicks in younger persons, the mitral regurgitant murmur predominates in elderly patients. Although patients often have a long history of cardiac murmur, the mitral regurgitation may progressively worsen. Systemic embolization and sudden death may occur.

The ECG often shows abnormalities. The left ventricle may be enlarged, although the ejection fraction remains normal.

Diagnosis

When chest pain is the predominant finding in mitral valve prolapse, ventricular function is often preserved. Even so, coronary arteriography is often needed to differentiate the chest pain of mitral valve prolapse from that of coronary atherosclerosis. Palpitations may be due to both ventricular and supraventricular arrhythmias, and an ambulatory ECG is helpful in documenting the cause. Echocardiography may differentiate mitral valve prolapse from other causes of mitral regurgitation and can help assess ventricular chamber size and function.

Treatment

Anticoagulants are given to prevent systemic emboli, which occur predominantly with atrial fibrillation and heart failure. Digitalis is used to control the ventricular response to atrial fibrillation. Heart failure is managed with digitalis, diuretics, and vasodilators. Mitral valve replacement may be indicated for progressive ventricular dilation, which occurs predominantly in men; the surgical risk is acceptable because ventricular function is usually preserved.

TRICUSPID VALVE DISEASE

Diseases of the tricuspid valve include tricuspid regurgitation and tricuspid stenosis.

TRICUSPID REGURGITATION

Retrograde blood flow from the right ventricle into the right atrium caused by inadequate closure of the tricuspid valve orifice during ventricular systole.

Tricuspid regurgitation is most often caused by a dilated valve ring secondary to right ventricular failure. Infective endocarditis is a less common cause (see Ch. 39). The holosystolic murmur (maximal along the lower left sternal border) is accentuated on inspiration. A large positive systolic wave in the jugular venous pulse is also present. Medical treatment of heart failure lessens the regurgitation.

TRICUSPID STENOSIS

An abnormal narrowing of the tricuspid valve orifice.

Tricuspid stenosis is rare except in patients with multivalvular rheumatic heart disease or with the carcinoid syndrome. The lower left sternal border diastolic rumble increases on inspiration. A diastolic elevation of the jugular venous pulse occurs (with poor or absent Y descent) and hepatomegaly is present, without other evidence of heart failure. Medical therapy is indicated for mild disease. Surgical repair is rarely required.

PULMONARY VALVE DISEASE

Pulmonary valve disease is extremely rare in the elderly. When present, it is characterized by the murmur of pulmonary insufficiency, usually due to pulmonary hypertension secondary to chronic pulmonary disease or left ventricular failure. Treatment of underlying disorders is appropriate.

IDIOPATHIC HYPERTROPHIC SUBAORTIC STENOSIS

The form of hypertrophic cardiomyopathy associated with a left ventricular outflow gradient.

Prevalence and Pathophysiology

Idiopathic hypertrophic subaortic stenosis (**IHSS**) is relatively common in the elderly. A disproportionate septal thickening narrows the left ventricular outflow tract. Hypertrophic cardiomyopathy may also occur without asymmetric septal hypertrophy; mitral annular calcification may displace the mitral valve anteriorly, producing an outflow gradient. Abnormal ventricular compliance elevates the ventricular diastolic pressure, with a resultant increase in left atrial volume and pressure and pulmonary venous congestion. Hypertrophic cardiomyopathy occurs more often in women and has a more favorable prognosis in older patients than in younger ones, with less likelihood of sudden cardiac death (see also HYPERTROPHIC CARDIOMYOPATHY in Ch. 41).

Symptoms and Signs

Patients may present with chest pain, dyspnea, dizziness, palpitations, and syncope (caused by tachyarrhythmias or decreased cardiac output from outflow obstruction). Ventricular tachycardia is common and increases the likelihood of sudden death. Supraventricular tachyarrhythmias, more likely to occur as atrial dimensions increase, are also common. Because the atrial contribution to ventricular filling is important for maintaining stroke volume in the elderly, atrial fibrillation may cause rapid hemodynamic deterioration.

A characteristic late systolic murmur from the lower left sternal border to the apex terminates before the second heart sound. The characteristic bisferious carotid pulse has a rapid upstroke and a subsequent percussion wave. A prominent fourth heart sound is typical, but it disappears at the onset of atrial fibrillation. The apex impulse is double in character. Provocative maneuvers (eg, Valsalva) accentuate the systolic murmur, which decreases or disappears on squatting; however, many elderly patients cannot adequately perform these maneuvers. The murmur may also disappear as systolic dysfunction and cavity dilatation occur. An aortic regurgitant murmur may be due to coexisting calcific aortic valvular disease.

Laboratory Findings

The ECG is rarely normal. It shows left atrial abnormality and left ventricular hypertrophy, with left anterior fascicular block in about 20% of patients. Septal hypertrophy may also produce nonspecific inferior and apical Q waves mimicking myocardial infarction. The cardiac silhouette enlarges when ventricular systolic function deteriorates. Two-dimensional echocardiography is diagnostic, although systolic cavity obliteration and the outflow gradient may lessen with aging, rendering the systolic anterior motion of the mitral valve more important. An ambulatory ECG to document arrhythmias should probably be obtained annually, because serious arrhythmias are often asymptomatic.

Diagnosis

Often IHSS is not suspected because brisk carotid pulses, basal systolic murmurs, and fourth heart sounds are common in elderly persons without heart disease. Differentiating IHSS from valvular aortic stenosis or coronary heart disease with papillary muscle dysfunction is important because the therapies differ. Nitroglycerin, diuretics, vasodilators, digitalis, and other positive inotropic agents often exacerbate outflow obstruction and symptoms, which are best treated with β-blockers or verapamil. The murmur must also be differentiated from murmurs due to aortic sclerosis, mitral regurgitation, and mitral valve prolapse, all of which are common in the elderly. The chest pain of IHSS does not necessarily reflect coronary disease, although ischemic infarction may occur even in patients with normal coronary arteries.

Treatment

Amiodarone 200 to 300 mg/day orally has been reported to reduce the risk of sudden death from ventricular tachycardia. This effect has not been shown with β-blockers or verapamil. Supraventricular tachyarrhythmias also respond to amiodarone. Anticoagulation is indicated to prevent embolization in patients with atrial fibrillation or frequent supraventricular tachyarrhythmias. Propranolol provides the best relief for both the dyspnea and the chest pain, because of the predominant diastolic dysfunction. Nifedipine may be given with propranolol, or verapamil may be given alone. Amiodarone has little effect on chest pain or dyspnea.

In the late stage of IHSS, when systolic function deteriorates, digitalis and diuretics may be used safely to improve function. When digitalis and warfarin are given concomitantly with amiodarone, their doses should be reduced because amiodarone potentiates their effects. Myomectomy is rarely indicated, except in symptomatic patients with a significant ventricular outflow gradient refractory to medical therapy. If mitral valve replacement is indicated for mitral regurgitation, a low-profile valve should be used because of the small ventricular cavity present in IHSS. Prophylaxis against infective endocarditis is indicated for invasive and surgical procedures.

39. INFECTIVE ENDOCARDITIS

Infective endocarditis has become more prevalent in the elderly despite the development of modern antibiotics. More than half of all cases of infective endocarditis occur in persons > 60 yr of age. Several factors account for the high prevalence in the elderly: increases in the total number of elderly persons and in the number with prosthetic valves, a higher prevalence of hospital-acquired bacteremia, longer survival of persons with rheumatic valvular lesions, and fewer new cases of rheumatic heart disease.

Etiology

The underlying cardiac lesions that predispose the elderly to endocarditis tend to differ from those in younger patients. The increased incidence of atherosclerosis in the elderly may be a factor, since atheromatous deposits can cause turbulence and, hence, thrombus formation. All forms of valvular disease increase the risk of endocarditis, although about 40% of elderly patients with endocarditis have either no valvular lesions or undetermined ones. Of the 60% who do have valvular disease, about 30% have rheumatic lesions, about 25% have calcified valves, and about 5% have mitral valve prolapse (see Ch. 38).

The aortic valve is involved in 20% to 40% of cases. The high incidence of aortic valve involvement probably reflects the increased prevalence of aortic stenosis with calcification in the elderly. Until age 60, aortic stenosis with calcification is most commonly caused by rheumatic heart disease; from age 60 to 75, a calcified congenital bicuspid valve is most often implicated; and after age 75, degeneration of a normal valve is the leading cause. The mitral valve is involved in 25% to 70% of endocarditis cases, and both the aortic and mitral valves are involved in about 10% to 25%. Infections involving congenital heart defects other than those of the bicuspid valve occur infrequently in the elderly.

The development of infective endocarditis involves two events. First is an alteration in the endocardial surface, which then permits the deposition of platelets and fibrin. The resulting thrombus or vegetation most often arises in areas of increased turbulence. Second is transient bacteremia, which allows the thrombus to be colonized. **The source of bacteremia** is usually unknown. Sites of primary infection include the mouth, the GU tract (particularly after procedures involving instrumentation), the GI tract, skin and decubitus ulcers, surgical wounds, and IV catheters.

Bacterial properties—eg, the increased adherence of certain streptococcal and staphylococcal species—make some organisms more likely than others to cause infective endocarditis. *Streptococcus* spp are the most common, accounting for 25% to 70% of endocarditis cases, although the viridans streptococci are less prevalent in older than in younger populations. Enterococci, which often inhabit the GU and lower GI tracts, can account for up to 25% of endocarditis cases in elderly men. Frequent urinary tract infections and procedures involving instrumentation (especially in men with prostate disease) explain the increased frequency of enterococcal bacteremia and endocarditis. *S. bovis*, a nonenterococcal group D streptococcus, can be isolated in up to 25% of endocarditis cases in persons > 55 yr. Many such cases are associated with underlying and often asymptomatic malignant or premalignant GI lesions, especially colon carcinoma.

Staphylococci account for 20% to 30% of all endocarditis cases in the elderly. The predominant species, *Staphylococcus aureus*, often causes nosocomial endocarditis, and many cases are discovered only incidentally at autopsy. *S. epidermidis* is isolated in < 5% of cases of native valve endocarditis, but in elderly as in younger patients, it is the most common single cause of cases involving prosthetic valves.

Gram-negative aerobic bacilli remain a rare cause of endocarditis (only 2% to 3% of cases), often involving a prosthetic valve. *Bacteroides* spp are rare isolates in older patients, as in younger ones. Mixed infections are rare in the elderly. Fungal endocarditis occurs in < 5% of cases; it is usually due to *Candida* spp or is secondary to fungemia from an indwelling intravascular catheter and often affects a prosthetic valve.

Culture-negative endocarditis, *a suggestive clinical syndrome without an isolated organism,* accounts for 10% to 20% of cases. The inability to isolate an organism from blood cultures may be due to prior antibiotic administration, fastidious pathogens, or inadequate laboratory techniques. Right-sided endocarditis and uremia are also associated with culture-negative endocarditis. More often, endocarditis is missed in the elderly because the diagnosis is not considered.

Symptoms and Signs

The clinical manifestations of infective endocarditis are diverse and may involve almost any organ system. Symptoms of endocarditis usually occur within 2 wk of the inciting bacteremia, although diagnosis may take much longer. **Fever** is the single most common finding. Nonspecific generalized complaints of anorexia, fatigue, confusion, weight loss, and night sweats are also common. Because the presentation is sometimes atypical (eg, without fever), infective endocarditis in the elderly may not be recognized and treated until it has progressed to a late stage. In these cases, it has an extremely poor prognosis.

On physical examination, **cardiac murmurs** are found in > 90% of patients, due to a predisposing valvular abnormality or to the infection itself. Murmurs are not found in most patients with tricuspid valve endocarditis. New or changing cardiac murmurs are described in 36% to 52% of infective endocarditis cases diagnosed by strict clinical criteria, although these murmurs are heard less frequently in the elderly. The symptoms and signs of **heart failure** may also be present, occurring secondary to underlying heart disease or valvular destruction. **Splenic enlargement** occurs in 25% to 60% of patients, correlating with longer durations of infection.

About 50% of patients with infective endocarditis have cutaneous or peripheral manifestations. **Petechiae** are most common, arising in crops and found on the conjunctivae, palate, buccal mucosa, extremities, and skin above the clavicles. Splinter hemorrhages appear as linear, dark streaks beneath the fingernails or toenails; however, these lesions are also common in noninfected elderly persons and in those with occupation-related trauma. **Osler's nodes**—small, tender subcutaneous nodules that develop in the pulp of the digits or on the thenar eminences—contrast with **Janeway lesions**—small, hemorrhagic, or erythematous nontender macules on the palms or soles. Janeway lesions are due to septic emboli and are associated more often with acute endocarditis, especially that caused by *S. aureus*. Ophthalmologic examination may reveal pale-centered, oval hemorrhages **(Roth spots)** on the retina. Although Roth spots are highly suggestive of infective endocarditis, they are also seen in patients with collagen-vascular and hematologic disorders.

Other clinical manifestations may involve other organ systems as a result of thromboembolic phenomena. Emboli to the spleen may cause left upper quadrant abdominal pain radiating to the shoulder, a splenic friction rub, or signs of a left pleural effusion. Emboli to the kidney may cause flank or back pain, suggesting renal infarction. Patients with tricuspid valve endocarditis may develop pulmonary emboli and present with dyspnea, cough, pleuritic chest pain, and hemoptysis, especially if pulmonary infarction has occurred.

Cerebral embolism and rupture of an intracranial **mycotic aneurysm** are devastating complications, and the patient may present with the signs of a cerebrovascular accident; this may distract the clinician from the infectious cause of the disease. Fever and a stroke syndrome in any patient should warrant consideration of the possibility of infective endocarditis. Most cerebral emboli involve the distribution of the middle cerebral artery or one of its branches. Clinical signs of emboli include hemiparesis, cranial nerve palsies, corticosensory loss, aphasia, ataxia, alterations in mental status, or a combination thereof. Persistent headache may be the only symptom signifying an intracranial mycotic aneurysm before rupture.

Diagnosis

The single most important laboratory finding in the diagnosis of infective endocarditis is **bacteremia** or **fungemia.** The bacteremia of endocarditis is usually continuous, and with few exceptions, blood cultures are positive. In patients who have not previously received antimicrobial therapy (the major reason for culture-negative endocarditis—see Etiology, above), negative blood cultures probably account for < 5% of endocarditis cases on native valves when blood cultures are handled by experienced laboratory personnel.

Laboratory analysis may show several nonspecific abnormalities. Anemia occurs in 70% to 90% of cases, worsens with duration of illness, and is usually characterized by normochromic-normocytic indices. However, patients with acute endocarditis often do not present with anemia. The ESR is elevated in 90% to 100% of patients. Urine cultures may reveal proteinuria (50% to 65% of cases) and microscopic hematuria (30% to 50% of cases). Bacteriuria may occur when endocarditis is caused by enterococci or *S. aureus*. Up to 50% of patients with subacute bacterial endocarditis who have the infection for 6 wk have a positive rheumatoid factor, but this is also seen in 24% of cases of acute *S. aureus* endocarditis in injection drug abusers. A positive rheumatoid factor must be interpreted cautiously in an aged patient because a significant titer is detected in 5% to 10% of healthy elderly people.

Echocardiography with Doppler ultrasonography has become the most accurate and widely used imaging modality in patients with suspected or proven endocarditis. Echocardiography is a sensitive and accurate method for detecting valvular vegetations, valvular destruction, and the hemodynamic sequelae of regurgitation. The overall sensitivity of two-dimensional transthoracic echocardiography for detecting vegetations is about 80%. Because some older persons with valvular sclerosis have focal thickening on one or more valvular structures, valve masses are not synonymous with vegetations.

Transesophageal echocardiography is more sensitive than the transthoracic approach for detecting vegetations; it is particularly helpful in patients in whom the standard transthoracic approach to imaging is difficult (eg, those with emphysema, prosthetic valves, or poor transthoracic windows, or those on mechanical ventilators). Transesophageal echocardiography can also demonstrate multiple vegetations, satellite lesions, fistulas, ring abscesses, valvular perforations, and aneurysms when transthoracic echocardiography shows only the vegetation.

Prophylaxis

Antibiotic prophylaxis is indicated in older patients with valvular disease, particularly those with calcified and prosthetic heart valves, who are at especially high risk for developing endocarditis. Preventing infective endocarditis will assume even greater importance as the percentage of elderly persons in the population increases and as more persons have prosthetic valves implanted, undergo invasive diagnostic and therapeutic procedures with a potential for bacteremia, and retain their native dentition.

Treatment

Choosing an appropriate antimicrobial agent is of primary importance in the successful management of infective endocarditis. Bactericidal agents must be given for optimal therapy. In acutely ill patients, empiric therapy should be started immediately after obtaining blood cultures to limit valvular damage.

Treatment is based on the likely infecting microorganism in the specific clinical setting. A subacute presentation in a non–injection drug abuser with native valves suggests infection with streptococci or enterococci, and the standard empiric regimen should consist of high-dose IV penicillin G (or ampicillin) combined with gentamicin. In acute-onset disease or in an injection drug abuser, therapy should target *S. aureus*. In non–drug abusers with native valves, a penicillinase-resistant penicillin (eg, nafcillin) or a cephalosporin (eg, cefazolin) is appropriate initial therapy. However, in injection drug abusers, many strains of *S. aureus* are resistant to all β-lactam antibiotics, and vancomycin is the empiric agent of choice. If the patient has a prosthetic valve, therapy is initially directed at *S. aureus* and *S. epidermidis*. Because many strains of *S. epidermidis* are resistant to β-lactam antibiotics, vancomycin is the agent of choice.

Once the infecting microorganism is isolated from blood cultures and susceptibility testing is performed, the antimicrobial regimen should be altered to provide the therapy that is most effective with the least toxicity and cost (see TABLE 39–1). Peak and trough antibiotic concentrations should be ascertained to ensure that blood concentrations are appropriate for elderly patients, since excretory and metabolic functions are often impaired. Therapy is continued for at least 2 wk longer in patients with prosthetic valves.

Some patients with infective endocarditis may need valve replacement (see VALVE REPLACEMENT in Ch. 44). Indications for surgery are hemodynamic deterioration from valve dysfunction, fungal endocarditis, persistent infection despite appropriate antimicrobial therapy, repeated relapses after completion of therapy, early postoperative prosthetic valve endocarditis, intracardiac extension of the infection, "complicated" prosthetic valve endocarditis, and recurrent emboli. With appropriate preoperative assessment and preparation, valve replacement can be safely performed in the elderly patient.

TABLE 39–1. ANTIMICROBIAL THERAPY FOR INFECTIVE ENDOCARDITIS*

Organism	*Regimen*
Streptococci (penicillin MIC ≤ 0.1 μg/mL)	Aqueous penicillin G 10–20 mU/day for 4 wk† or Aqueous penicillin G 10–20 mU/day plus gentamicin‡ 1 mg/kg (maximum 80 mg) q 8 h for 2 wk or Aqueous penicillin G 10–20 mU/day for 4 wk plus gentamicin‡ 1 mg/kg (maximum 80 mg) q 8 h for first 2 wk
Streptococci (penicillin MIC > 0.1 and < 0.5 μg/mL)	Aqueous penicillin G 20 mU/day for 4 wk plus gentamicin†,§ 1 mg/kg (maximum 80 mg) q 8 h for first 2 wk
Enterococci or other streptococci (penicillin MIC ≥ 0.5 μg/mL)	Aqueous penicillin G 20–30 mU/day or ampicillin 2 gm q 4 h plus gentamicin‡ 1 mg/kg (maximum 80 mg) q 8 h for 4–6 wk
Staphylococci (methicillin-susceptible) on native valve	Nafcillin 2 gm q 4 h or oxacillin 2 gm q 4 h for 4–6 wk with or without gentamicin‡ 1 mg/kg (maximum 80 mg) q 8 h for first 3–5 days

(continued)

Table 39–1. ANTIMICROBIAL THERAPY FOR INFECTIVE ENDOCARDITIS* *(Continued)*

Organism	*Regimen*
Staphylococci (methicillin-resistant) on native valve	Vancomycin** 30 mg/kg/day (maximum 2 gm) divided q 6 or 12 h for 4–6 wk
Staphylococci (methicillin-resistant) on prosthetic valve	Vancomycin** 30 mg/kg/day (maximum 2 gm) divided q 6 or 12 h plus rifampin†† 300 mg orally q 8 h for 6 wk or longer plus gentamicin‡ 1 mg/kg (maximum 80 mg) q 8 h for first 2 wk
HACEK organisms	Ampicillin 2 gm q 4 h or ceftriaxone 1 gm q 12 h plus gentamicin 1.7 mg/kg q 8 h for 4 wk
Enterobacteriaceae	Cefotaxime 2 gm q 4 h or imipenem 0.5 gm q 6 h or aztreonam 2 gm q 6 h plus gentamicin 1.7 mg/kg q 8 h for 4–6 wk
Pseudomonas aeruginosa	Piperacillin 3 gm q 4 h or ceftazidime 2 gm q 8 h or imipenem 0.5 gm q 6 h or aztreonam 2 gm q 6 h plus gentamicin 1.7 mg/kg q 8 h
Fungi	Amphotericin B 1 mg/kg/day plus flucytosine‡‡ 150 mg/kg/day orally in 4 divided doses

HACEK = *Hemophilus, Actinobacillus, Cardiobacterium, Eikenella,* and *Kingella;* MIC = minimal inhibitory concentration.

* Patients with normal renal and hepatic function. Unless indicated, all antimicrobial agents are given IV. Regimen should be continued for at least 2 wk longer if patient has a prosthetic valve.

† Preferred in elderly because aminoglycosides are likely to result in toxicity.

‡ Maintain peak serum concentrations at 3 μg/mL.

§ Use if the patient has a prosthetic valve, but continue the penicillin for a total of 6 wk.

** Maintain peak serum concentrations at 30–45 μg/mL if given q 12 h and 20–35 μg/mL if given q 6 h.

†† Use for coagulase-negative staphylococci; value for coagulase-positive staphylococci is controversial.

‡‡ Maintain serum concentrations at 50–100 μg/mL.

Adapted from Baldassarre JS, Kaye D: "Principles and overview of antibiotic therapy," in *Infective Endocarditis,* ed. 2, edited by D Kaye. New York, Raven Press, 1992, pp. 169–190; as based on material appearing in Bisno AL, Dismukes WE, Durack DT, et al: "Antimicrobial treatment of infective endocarditis due to viridans streptococci, enterococci, and staphylococci." *JAMA* 261:1471–1477, 1989.

40. ARRHYTHMIAS AND CONDUCTION DISORDERS

The normal changes with aging that affect the heart and cardiovascular system (see Ch. 33) influence the incidence, significance, and treatment of cardiac arrhythmias in elderly persons.

TACHYARRHYTHMIAS AND ECTOPIC BEATS

Incidence

Ectopic beats—whether supraventricular or ventricular, simple or complex, detected at rest or during routine activity or exercise—increase in frequency with age, even in persons carefully screened to exclude latent coronary artery disease. A study of randomly selected patients > 70 yr of age revealed supraventricular ectopic beats in 10% and ventricular ectopic beats in 8%. Those with supraventricular ectopic beats had no increased risk of sudden death over follow-up periods of 6 to 18 yr. The prognostic significance of ventricular ectopic beats on resting ECG is not as clear-cut. Some studies found no increase in age-adjusted risk of sudden death, while other studies found cardiac mortality increased two- to threefold.

On 24-h ambulatory ECG monitoring, isolated ventricular ectopic beats were found in 80% of healthy persons aged 60 to 85 yr who were screened to exclude coronary artery disease. Frequent supraventricular and ventricular ectopic beats (> 100 in 24 h) were noted in 26% and 17%, respectively. Over a mean follow-up period of 10 yr, neither supraventricular nor ventricular ectopic beats were associated with a higher incidence of coronary events. Short asymptomatic episodes of paroxysmal supraventricular tachycardia occurred in 13%, ventricular couplets in 11%, and unsustained ventricular tachycardia in 4%. Younger healthy persons have a much lower incidence of these arrhythmias. In contrast, atrial flutter and fibrillation, sinus bradycardia < 40 beats/min, sinus pauses > 1.6 sec, and high-degree atrioventricular block were rare or nonexistent in the older healthy persons.

In another study of patients aged 65 to 100 yr, ventricular tachycardia was detected in 4% of women and 10% of men using 24-h ambulatory ECG monitoring. Ventricular tachycardia was associated with increased left ventricular mass and a higher incidence of left ventricular dysfunction and heart failure. Even when persons with known coronary artery disease were excluded, those with ventricular tachycardia more often had abnormal left ventricular function. Although data are not yet available, the prognosis will probably be shown to depend on the presence and severity of underlying heart disease.

In apparently healthy adults undergoing treadmill exercise testing (those with no overt heart disease but in some cases having abnormal exercise ECGs), both supraventricular and ventricular ectopic beats increased in incidence with age: in one study, that of isolated supraventricular ectopic beats increased from 8% to 76% and that of isolated ventricular ectopic beats from 11% to 57% between the third and ninth decades. Asymptomatic runs of ventricular tachycardia, none longer than six beats, were seen in nearly 4% of apparently healthy persons ≥ 65 yr, a prevalence 25 times that in younger persons. Over a mean follow-up period of 2 yr, none of these elderly persons with unsustained exercise-induced ventricular tachycardia experienced angina, myocardial infarction, syncope, or cardiac death.

In another study, 80 apparently healthy persons aged 51 to 77 yr with frequent or repetitive exercise-induced ventricular ectopic beats were evaluated. Only three cardiac deaths occurred over a 5.6-yr mean follow-up period, an incidence identical to that in age-matched controls. Therefore, the mere presence of supraventricular or ventricular ectopic beats, even if frequent or complex, is not an accurate marker for organic heart disease or increased cardiac mortality in older patients. Such ectopic activity may not require specific therapy.

Histologic Changes With Aging

The reasons for the increased incidence in ectopic beats in the elderly are not fully understood. Age-associated increases in left atrial size and pressure may partially account for the increase in supraventricular ectopic beats. The increase in ventricular ectopic beats may be related to age-associated increases in left ventricular mass and catecholamines. Both supraventricular and ventricular ectopic beats occur more often and are more complex in patients with structural heart disease, which increases dramatically with age.

Animal studies suggest that overload of ionized calcium (Ca^{++}) in the senescent myocardium may play an important role in arrhythmogenesis. Under conditions that enhance cell Ca^{++} loading, senescent myocardium is more likely to spontaneously release Ca^{++} from the sarcoplasmic reticulum, ie, to undergo diastolic after-depolarization. This greater likelihood for Ca^{++} overload may render the older heart more susceptible to arrhythmias when calcium homeostasis is disturbed, as in response to inotropic drugs or during postischemic reflow. Furthermore, the threshold for Ca^{++}-dependent ventricular fibrillation is lower.

SPECIFIC ARRHYTHMIAS

As outlined in TABLE 40–1, specific arrhythmias include supraventricular ectopic beats, supraventricular tachycardias (eg, paroxysmal supraventricular tachycardia, atrial fibrillation), ventricular ectopic beats, and ventricular tachycardia.

TABLE 40–1. RELATIONSHIP OF ARRHYTHMIAS TO AGE AND MORTALITY

Arrhythmia	*Effect of Age on Prevalence*	*Effect on Mortality in Otherwise Healthy Patients*	*Therapy*
Supraventricular ectopic beats	Increased	None	None
Paroxysmal supraventricular tachycardia	Increased	Probably none	Digoxin, β-blocker, or calcium antagonist
Atrial fibrillation (chronic)	Increased	Increased	Above drugs; attempt at cardioversion; ? anticoagulation
Ventricular ectopic beats	Increased	Probably none	None in healthy patients; ? antiarrhythmic drugs if heart disease is present
Ventricular tachycardia	Increased	Probably none	? Antiarrhythmic drugs in healthy patients; antiarrhythmic drugs, AICD, or endocardial resection if the patient has coronary artery disease

AICD = automatic implantable cardioverter-defibrillator.

The seemingly benign nature of both supraventricular and ventricular arrhythmias in healthy elderly persons does not mean that these arrhythmias are similarly benign in patients with heart disease. *Regardless of age, the nature and severity of underlying heart disease are of much greater prognostic significance than the arrhythmia itself.* Because few data exist regarding the significance of specific arrhythmias in old age, the following discussion focuses on standard diagnostic and therapeutic measures.

SUPRAVENTRICULAR ECTOPIC BEATS

Isolated supraventricular ectopic beats, common in the elderly, are probably related in part to the increase in atrial pressure or volume associated with aging and with the development of organic heart disease.

Even frequent supraventricular ectopic beats rarely require specific treatment. However, they may indicate a propensity for sustained supraventricular tachyarrhythmia.

ATRIAL (SUPRAVENTRICULAR) TACHYCARDIAS
(Narrow QRS Tachycardias)

Paroxysmal supraventricular tachycardia is characterized by a regular narrow QRS complex at 150 to 200 beats/min. Usually due to a reentrant mechanism, it can often be terminated by vagal maneuvers (eg, Valsalva's maneuver, gagging, or carotid sinus massage). NOTE: *Carotid sinus massage should not be performed on elderly patients until significant carotid stenosis has been excluded by physical examination.* It should also not be performed on any patient with a bruit. If vagal maneuvers are unsuccessful and hypotension is absent, verapamil 5 to 10 mg IV should be given over 2.5 to 5 min. With its rapid onset of action and low risk of hypotension, IV adenosine is an alternative to verapamil. If the arrhythmia precipitates hypotension, cerebral ischemic symptoms, angina pectoris, or heart failure, immediate cardioversion is indicated, starting at 25 to 50 joules. Digoxin is the preferred prophylaxis for paroxysmal supraventricular tachycardia because of its documented efficacy and once-daily dosing. β-Adrenergic blockers or calcium antagonists are alternatives.

Atrial tachycardia with block is usually caused by digitalis toxicity. Treatment consists of withholding digitalis and correcting hypokalemia.

Multifocal atrial tachycardia is common in elderly patients with chronic obstructive pulmonary disease. Here, the P-wave morphology, PR interval, and cycle length vary from beat to beat. Although treatment is directed at correcting the underlying condition, verapamil is usually effective as short-term therapy.

Although not usually a cause of hemodynamic impairment, **accelerated junctional rhythm** may be a sign of a serious underlying disorder. It is characterized by a heart rate of 70 to 130 beats/min; the P wave is usually inverted and may precede, follow, or fall within the QRS complex. In the elderly, digitalis toxicity and acute inferior myocardial infarction are the most common causes. Sudden regularization of the ventricular rate in an elderly patient receiving digoxin for chronic atrial fibrillation suggests this diagnosis. Treatment is directed at the underlying disorder, such as digitalis toxicity, myocardial infarction, or heart failure.

Atrial flutter should be suspected if a patient has a regular tachycardia at a ventricular rate close to 150 beats/min. Carotid massage (see warning, above) should cause an abrupt slowing of the ventricular response and the emergence of "sawtooth" flutter waves at about 300/min, which confirms the diagnosis. Coronary artery disease and chronic obstructive pulmonary disease are common causes of atrial flutter in the elderly. Digoxin is the drug of choice if the patient is hemodynamically stable. Otherwise, low-level DC cardioversion (25 to 50 joules) almost always converts flutter to sinus rhythm.

Atrial fibrillation is recognized by a lack of organized atrial activity and the totally irregular timing of the QRS complexes. In contrast to the other atrial tachyarrhythmias, atrial fibrillation is much more likely to be chronic than acute. Hypertension, coronary artery disease, and mitral valve disease are the most common predisposing conditions in elderly and middle-aged patients. Additional considerations include amyloidosis, sick sinus syndrome, and thyrotoxicosis.

In contrast to isolated supraventricular or ventricular ectopic beats, atrial flutter or fibrillation usually signifies organic heart disease. Established atrial fibrillation in otherwise healthy persons **(lone atrial fibrillation)** appears to substantially increase the risk of cardiovascular morbidity and mortality. In studies, such mortality was increased two- to thirteenfold and stroke more than fivefold in men aged 40 to 65 yr. Thus, *even if no organic heart disease is apparent, atrial fibrillation should never be considered benign.*

As in younger patients, initial treatment of atrial fibrillation is directed toward slowing the ventricular response to 60 to 100 beats/min with digoxin, verapamil, or propranolol given IV. Long-term control of ventricular rate is also achieved with these agents, which are sometimes given in combination. Digoxin and verapamil are contraindicated in the Wolff-Parkinson-White syndrome, which is rare in the elderly. Because of the associated atrioventricular nodal disease, about 1/3 of older patients with atrial fibrillation have a controlled ventricular response and require no specific therapy. Before electrical cardioversion is attempted for chronic atrial fibrillation, the cause and duration of atrial fibrillation, atrial size, and the risks of alternative therapy with anticoagulants should be considered. Because chronic (and even lone) atrial fibrillation has a substantially increased risk of cerebral embolism, anticoagulation should be strongly considered in any elderly patient with this arrhythmia (see also MITRAL STENOSIS in Ch. 38). However, given the increased risk of thromboembolic events in patients with chronic atrial fibrillation, an early attempt at cardioversion (generally within a few weeks of diagnosis) is probably warranted in most elderly patients. Chemical cardioversion with quinidine or other class I drugs may be considered in older patients with atrial fibrillation, although a recent meta-analysis suggests that patients receiving long-term quinidine therapy have an increased mortality rate. The multicenter AFASAK (Atrial Fibrillation, Aspirin, and Anticoagulation [Kopenhagen]) and SPAF (Stroke Prevention in Atrial Fibrillation) studies showed that warfarin reduced the incidence of thromboembolic events in elderly patients with nonrheumatic atrial fibrillation. In the SPAF study, low-dose aspirin also reduced such events, though only in patients $\leq$ 75 yr old.

Ventricular Ectopic Beats

Although ventricular ectopic beats, whether isolated or frequent and complex, do not appear to adversely affect the long-term risk of cardiovascular mortality in clinically healthy elderly persons, even simple ventricular ectopic beats increase the risk in patients with documented coronary artery disease. Nevertheless, it has yet to be shown that treating isolated ventricular ectopic beats in these patients reduces the long-term risk of death. Furthermore, the Cardiac Arrhythmia Suppression Trial (CAST) recently demonstrated that the powerful class IC antiarrhythmic drugs flecainide and encainide actually *increased* the mortality rate in patients with asymptomatic or mildly symptomatic frequent ventricular ectopic beats after acute myocardial infarction. This finding challenges the belief that suppression of ventricular ectopic beats in such patients necessarily translates into improved survival. These drugs had a similar adverse effect on survival in patients younger than 60 yr.

The generally higher risk of reactions to antiarrhythmic drugs in the elderly dictates a conservative approach, starting with low doses and titrating cautiously until density of ventricular ectopic beats is reduced by 75% and ventricular tachycardia is eliminated. The combination of low-dose quinidine and tocainide was generally effective and well tolerated in a pilot study of elderly patients with coronary artery disease and frequent ventricular ectopic beats. Low-dose combination therapy with various agents probably warrants investigation to minimize the risks of adverse effects from any single drug. As with supraventricular ectopic beats, treatment should be directed at resolving underlying or exacerbating factors, such as electrolyte disturbances, hypoxia, or heart failure.

Ventricular Tachycardia

Ventricular tachycardia is usually a regular tachycardia with broad QRS complexes and a rate of 100 to 200 beats/min. Although a distinction from paroxysmal supraventricular tachycardia is often difficult when the QRS complex is widened, a diagnosis of ventricular tachycardia is strongly suggested by atrioventricular dissociation, fusion beats, and QRS duration > 0.14 sec or a QRS axis between $-90°$ and $-180°$. Severe myocardial ischemia, acute myocardial infarction, digitalis toxicity, or heart failure commonly precipitates ventricular tachycardia in the elderly.

Sustained ventricular tachycardia requires immediate attention. If ventricular tachycardia is well tolerated hemodynamically, a rapid IV infusion (bolus) of lidocaine 50 to 75 mg, followed by another 50 mg 2 min later, may be given initially. Recurrent ventricular tachycardia or lidocaine-resistant ventricular tachycardia may be treated with IV procainamide or β-blocking drugs. Current data, derived largely from studies of younger patients, suggest that bretylium is the most effective drug for ventricular tachycardia that is refractory to lidocaine. In the elderly, as in younger patients, *ventricular tachycardia associated with hypotension or syncope requires immediate electrical cardioversion.*

Ventricular tachycardia precipitated by an acute event, such as myocardial infarction or digitalis toxicity, has a low recurrence and does not require chronic prophylaxis. However, ventricular tachycardia without an obvious precipitant is known as **primary ventricular tachycardia;** it has a 1-yr recurrence of about 35% and requires aggressive prophylaxis. In one study, the mean age of patients who had an out-of-hospital cardiac arrest caused by a primary arrhythmia was 68.5 yr, and these patients had a 1-yr mortality rate of 29%.

The most promising approach to patients with primary recurrent symptomatic ventricular tachycardia appears to be intracardiac programmed electrophysiologic stimulation, a technique in which the malignant arrhythmia is induced and the efficacy of various antiarrhythmic agents in preventing it is assessed in a special catheterization laboratory. In a randomized trial of 57 patients (86% men, mean age 59 yr), antiarrhythmic therapy determined by this method resulted in a lower rate of symptomatic ventricular tachyarrhythmia than did an empiric approach. Other studies show a marked reduction in the 1- to 2-yr mortality rate when drug therapy for recurrent ventricular tachycardia is determined by this technique. A less-invasive but similarly labor-intensive approach using ambulatory ECG monitoring with or without exercise testing has also been successful, as demonstrated by the preliminary results of the multicenter ESVEM (Electrophysiology Study Versus Electrocardiographic Monitoring) trial.

The availability of amiodarone and several other new antiarrhythmic drugs increases the likelihood that a successful medical regimen can be found. Patients in whom neither of the above approaches is successful are possible candidates for an automatic implantable cardioverter-defibrillator or endocardial resection guided by intraoperative mapping. In a large series of patients with recurrent ventricular tachycardia or ventricular fibrillation, about ½ were treated with these invasive approaches. Long-term survival was similar in elderly and younger patients, although surgical mortality was higher in the elderly.

GENERAL TREATMENT CONSIDERATIONS

Many new antiarrhythmic drugs and several pacemaker innovations have expanded the therapeutic options for arrhythmias. Although the roles of these newer agents and devices for the older cardiac patient have not been completely defined, their benefits and limitations have begun to be determined. Cardiac pacemakers are discussed under BRADYARRHYTHMIAS, below.

Antiarrhythmic Drugs

The half-life of **digoxin** is prolonged because elderly persons have a reduced glomerular filtration rate; this reduction and a generally smaller body size result in a higher serum digoxin level in older persons. Despite the widespread availability of serum drug-level testing, digitalis toxicity continues to be relatively common in the elderly, primarily because digoxin is often used to treat heart failure and atrial arrhythmias. (For a more detailed discussion of digoxin and digitalis toxicity, see Antiarrhythmics in Ch. 21.) **Quinidine** clearance is reduced by 34% and elimination half-life is prolonged from 7.3 h to 9.7 h in persons 60 to 69 yr of age compared with those 23 to 29 yr of age. Evidence that quinidine therapy increases serum digoxin levels by about 100% may be particularly significant in the elderly, in whom these two drugs are often co-prescribed.

Because hepatic flow decreases with age, the infusion rate of **lidocaine** should be reduced to avoid CNS toxicity, which is common in the elderly. Similar dosage adjustments are necessary with **propranolol** and other **β-blockers** that undergo first-pass hepatic metabolism. The clinical significance of age-related decreases in the binding of propranolol to β-adrenergic receptors is unknown.

BRADYARRHYTHMIAS

Because intrinsic conduction system disease and acute processes such as myocardial infarction and digitalis toxicity are more prevalent, bradyarrhythmias are more common in the elderly. However, sinus bradycardia < 40 beats/min, sinus pauses > 1.6 sec, and high-degree atrioventricular block are rare in healthy persons > 60 yr old. These conduction disturbances are often associated with ischemic, hypertensive, or amyloid heart disease.

Histologic Changes in the Conduction System

Widespread histologic changes that occur in the conduction system with age may help account for the striking age-related increase in the incidence of bradyarrhythmias and conduction disturbances. The number of pacemaker cells in the sinoatrial node progressively declines beginning by age 60 yr; only about 10% of the cells are still present at age 75 yr. The sinoatrial node becomes enveloped by fat, which may partially or completely separate the node from the atrial musculature.

Age-associated changes in the His bundle include loss of cells, more fibrous and adipose tissue, and amyloid infiltration. The left side of the cardiac skeleton, which includes the central fibrous body, the mitral and aortic annuli, and the proximal interventricular septum, undergoes some degree of fibrosis. The atrioventricular node, His bundle, and proximal left and right bundle branches may be involved because of their proximity to these structures. In extreme cases, the resultant "idiopathic" fibrosis may cause atrioventricular block; it is the most common cause of chronic atrioventricular block in the elderly.

Age-Related Changes in the Electrocardiogram

Some age-related histologic changes in the conduction system are apparent on the standard 12-lead ECG. Although resting heart rate does not change with age, the respiratory variation in resting sinus rate (known as sinus arrhythmia) decreases. In addition, measurements of heart rate variability by time or frequency domain analyses demonstrate reduced heart rate variability in the elderly. The PR and QT intervals are somewhat prolonged with age, but QRS duration is unchanged. High-resolution surface electrocardiography in healthy volunteers has localized the increase in PR interval to a delay that is proximal to the His bundle; conduction time from the His bundle to the ventricle appears to be unrelated to age.

The QRS frontal plane axis shifts leftward over time, probably reflecting the combined effects of fibrosis in the anterior fascicle of the left bundle branch and mild age-related left ventricular hypertrophy. In a review of ECGs from elderly persons, such left axis deviation was the most common abnormality, occurring in 51%. In patients with no organic heart disease, neither first-degree atrioventricular block nor axis deviation leftward of −30° is associated with increased cardiac morbidity or mortality.

SPECIFIC BRADYARRHYTHMIAS

Specific bradyarrhythmias include sinus bradycardia, sinoatrial block, atrioventricular block, sick sinus syndrome, and left and right bundle branch block. The prevalence and effect on mortality for some of these bradyarrhythmias are shown in TABLE 40–2.

Sinus bradycardia, *a sinus rate of < 60 beats/min,* may indicate excellent physical conditioning; however, in the elderly it often indicates intrinsic sinus node disease. Inferior myocardial infarction, hypothermia, myxedema, or increased intracranial pressure may cause this arrhythmia. A longitudinal study of apparently healthy persons between 40 and 80 yr of age with sinus rates < 50 beats/min found no increase in cardiovascular morbidity or mortality over a 5-yr mean follow-up period.

Sinoatrial block occurs when sinus node impulses fail to depolarize the atria. Such block is often 2:1, resulting in a ventricular rate that is exactly one half the sinus rate. Common causes in the elderly are intrinsic conduction system disease, ischemia, and digitalis toxicity.

First-degree atrioventricular block, *prolongation of the PR interval ≥ 0.22 sec,* may be seen in healthy persons with high vagal tone. It also may be caused by intrinsic conduction system disease or by various medications (eg, digoxin, β-blockers, calcium antagonists, and class IA antiarrhythmic drugs). No therapy is required.

TABLE 40–2. RELATIONSHIP OF BRADYARRHYTHMIAS AND CONDUCTION DISTURBANCES TO AGE AND MORTALITY

Arrhythmia	*Effect of Age on Prevalence*	*Effect on Mortality in Otherwise Healthy Patients*	*Therapy*
Sinus bradycardia	Probably none	None	None
First-degree atrioventricular block	Increased	None	None
Second-degree atrioventricular block			
Mobitz type I	Probably none	Probably none	None*
Mobitz type II	Increased	Increased	Pacemaker
High-grade	Increased	Increased	Pacemaker
Third-degree (complete) atrioventricular block	Increased	Increased	Pacemaker
Sick sinus syndrome	Increased	None	Pacemaker for *symptomatic* bradycardia only
Left bundle branch block	Increased	Increased	None known
Right bundle branch block	Increased	None	None

* Withdraw digoxin, β-blocker, or calcium blocker if given.

Second-degree atrioventricular block has three different patterns. **Mobitz type I (Wenckebach) block** is recognized by prolongation of the PR interval that progresses until a ventricular complex is dropped. Because this type of block is usually proximal to the His-Purkinje system, the QRS complex typically appears normal. Digitalis toxicity and acute inferior myocardial infarction are common precipitating factors. This conduction disturbance is usually transient and rarely requires specific therapy. In **Mobitz type II block,** the PR interval is fixed but QRS complexes are dropped. Because the site of block is at or below the His bundle, the QRS complex is often wide. Mobitz type II block is most often associated with acute anterior myocardial infarction, myocarditis, or advanced sclerodegenerative conduction system disease. Patients with this arrhythmia are usually symptomatic and often present with syncope due to inadequate cerebral perfusion **(Stokes-Adams attack).** Because of its symptomatic presentation and frequent progression to complete heart block, Mobitz type II block is usually treated with a permanent pacemaker. Similarly, **high-grade block** is often symptomatic, may progress to complete heart block, and is usually treated with permanent pacing.

Third-degree (complete) atrioventricular block is characterized by the inability of any atrial depolarizations to activate the ventricle. Block within the atrioventricular node is usually associated with normal QRS complexes and an escape rate close to 60 beats/min. Common causes are acute inferior myocardial infarction and digitalis toxicity. In most instances, block within the atrioventricular node is transient. However, block within the ventricles is accompanied by wide QRS complexes and a slow escape rate, often < 40 beats/min. Such block may occur in patients with severe sclerodegenerative conduction system disease or extensive acute anterior myocardial infarction. Because these patients usually respond poorly to atropine and isoproterenol, pacemaker insertion is necessary.

Sick sinus syndrome encompasses a variety of rhythm disturbances that reflect sinoatrial node dysfunction and are often associated with dysfunction elsewhere in the conduction system. Although sick sinus syndrome is associated with many different cardiac diseases, coronary artery disease or a primary sclerodegenerative process is most often responsible. Patients may present with bradyarrhythmias (sinus bradycardia, sinus pauses or arrest, sinoatrial exit block, or atrial fibrillation with a slow ventricular response) or with the so-called **bradycardia-tachycardia syndrome,** in which a supraventricular tachycardia terminates in a long period of asystole. Therefore, symptoms may consist of palpitations or chest pain during tachycardia, and dizziness or syncope during bradycardia. The tachycardia—paroxysmal supraventricular tachycardia, atrial flutter, or atrial fibrillation—is treated with digoxin, other antiarrhythmic agents, or cardioversion (as outlined above); bradycardia associated with syncope should be treated by permanent pacing.

The prevalence of **bundle branch block** increases with age. Although left bundle branch block is usually associated with ischemic or hypertensive cardiac disease, complete right bundle branch block is often seen in apparently healthy older men, who appear to have a satisfactory prognosis. An analysis of the predominantly male, multicenter Coronary Artery Surgery Study population confirmed an independent adverse effect of left, but not right, bundle branch block on mortality over the subsequent 5 yr. *In women, however, right and left bundle branch block are highly—and equally—indicative of underlying cardiac disease.*

GENERAL TREATMENT CONSIDERATIONS

Acute Therapy

Acute therapy for bradyarrhythmias is required if the patient has hypotension, cerebral or cardiac ischemia, heart failure, and in the case of acute myocardial infarction, frequent ventricular ectopic beats. Placing the patient in the supine position with the legs elevated often ameliorates hypotensive sequelae acutely. Atropine given rapidly IV in a 0.5-mg bolus may be repeated at 3- to 5-min intervals until a total dose of 0.04 mg/kg has been given. If atropine is ineffective or causes intolerable side effects, an isoproterenol drip can be started at 1 to 4 μg/min and then titrated to produce a ventricular rate of 60 beats/min. When neither drug is successful, or if isoproterenol is *contraindicated* because of ischemia or infarction, temporary transvenous pacing should be used.

Cardiac Pacemakers

In one series, ⅔ of pacemakers were implanted in patients > 70 yr old; about half of these were implanted for high-degree atrioventricular block and the other half for sick sinus syndrome. Recent studies show that sick sinus syndrome now accounts for 48% of all pacemaker implants. Permanent ventricular pacing has eliminated the accelerated mortality rate formerly associated with complete heart block. However, the long-term prognosis for patients with sick sinus syndrome is determined primarily by the presence and severity of underlying heart disease. Permanent pacing for sick sinus syndrome should therefore be based on ECG documentation of symptomatic bradyarrhythmia. Pacemakers are not warranted in asymptomatic elderly patients with chronic bifascicular block, with or without a prolonged PR interval, because complete heart block rarely occurs.

Newer types of pacemakers, such as dual-chamber atrioventricular synchronous pacemakers, improve maximal exercise cardiac output and work capacity compared with traditional fixed-rate ventricular pacemakers. Therefore, such pacing modes may be extremely beneficial to active elderly patients. Although not conclusively documented, the greater dependence on the atrial contribution to ventricular filling with age means that atrioventricular synchronous pacing should have an enhanced benefit in the elderly.

In addition, a higher incidence of atrial fibrillation and a higher mortality rate have been demonstrated in patients treated with ventricular pacemakers compared with atrial or dual-chamber atrioventricular synchronous pacemakers. In a study involving 950 patients, the benefits of dual-chamber pacing were particularly prominent in patients > 70 yr old with sick sinus syndrome. At 7 yr postimplantation, atrial fibrillation developed in 47% of patients with ventricular pacemakers compared with only 9% of those with dual-chamber units; corresponding mortality rates were 72% vs. 51%. Thus, otherwise healthy elderly patients in sinus rhythm who require pacing for sick sinus syndrome should probably be given units that preserve atrioventricular synchrony.

A permanent pacemaker has a low but significant rate of **complications.** Abrupt loss of pacing—due to battery failure, fibrosis around the catheter site, myocardial perforation, lead fracture, or electrode dislodgment—may result in marked bradycardia or asystole. Catheter perforation of the right ventricle may cause a pericardial friction rub or, rarely, tamponade. In patients with little overlying subcutaneous tissue, the pulse generator may extrude or the pacing wire may erode through the skin. Occasionally, a patient has difficulty adjusting psychologically to pacemaker implantation. All pacemaker patients should have regular follow-up physical and ECG examinations.

41. HEART FAILURE AND CARDIOMYOPATHY

HEART FAILURE

Heart failure occurs when cardiac output is unable to meet metabolic demands. It cannot be defined numerically in terms of cardiac output or ejection fraction, because metabolic demands vary from patient to patient. Compromised systolic or diastolic ventricular function, or both, resulting in elevated ventricular end-diastolic pressure, may lead to heart failure. While isolated left- or right-sided heart failure is not rare, combined left- and right-sided heart failure is more common.

Heart failure is common in patients > 65 yr of age; its prevalence rises exponentially from the 6th decade. It has become more widespread over the past two decades and is now the most common diagnosis in elderly hospitalized patients. Heart failure is usually eminently treatable, in older as in younger patients.

Etiology

The principal causes of heart failure are divided into four categories: impediments to forward ejection, impaired cardiac filling, volume overload, and myocardial failure (see TABLE 41–1). About 75% of cases in older persons occur in association with systemic arterial hypertension, which impedes forward ejection, and with coronary artery disease, which leads to primary myocardial failure. Despite the high prevalence of clinical coronary artery disease in older persons (about 20%), about 1/3 to 1/2 of elderly hospitalized patients who died of heart failure had no postmortem evidence of myocardial infarction or of significant coronary artery disease. Valvular disease may contribute to impaired car-

TABLE 41–1. PRINCIPAL CAUSES OF HEART FAILURE

Impediments to forward ejection	Systemic arterial hypertension or elevated systemic vascular resistance Aortic valve stenosis Supravalvular stenosis (coarctation) Subaortic stenosis (left ventricular outflow tract membrane) Obstructive hypertrophic cardiomyopathy Pulmonary hypertension
Impaired cardiac filling	Ventricular hypertrophy (symmetric or asymmetric) Myocardial diastolic dysfunction Pericardial disease (constriction or tamponade) Restrictive heart disease (endocardial or myocardial) Ventricular aneurysm
Volume overload	Valvular regurgitation Increased intravascular volume Increased metabolic demands (thyrotoxicosis, anemia, certain skin disorders) Arteriovenous shunts or fistulas
Myocardial failure	Primary Loss of functioning cardiac muscle (myocardial infarction or myocardial ischemia) Cardiomyopathy Myocarditis Secondary Drug-induced Systemic disease (hypothyroidism) Chronic overload

diac filling or volume overload. Dilated cardiomyopathy and high output failure (due to conditions such as thyrotoxicosis, anemia, arteriovenous fistulas, fever, and some skin diseases, such as Kaposi's sarcoma and psoriasis) are less common in elderly patients.

Pathophysiology

Typical age-related changes, such as increased interstitial fibrosis, prolonged myocardial relaxation, and increased collagen cross-linking (see also Ch. 33), make the older patient's cardiovascular system more vulnerable to a number of systemic illnesses. Exacerbating factors include noncompliance with medication regimens, use of nonsteroidal anti-inflammatory drugs, infection, hypo- or hyperthyroidism, anemia, ischemia, hypoxia, and hypo- or hyperthermia.

The heart adapts to increased work load through one or more of the following mechanisms: increased sympathetic stimulation, myocardial hypertrophy, or the Frank-Starling mechanism. With the Frank-Starling mechanism, the degree of end-diastolic fiber stretch within a physiologic range is proportional to the systolic mechanical work expended in the ensuing contraction. Because myocardial and vascular responsiveness to β-adrenergic stimulation is reduced with age, and because recent data suggest that the myocardial hypertrophic response to a given increase in afterload is impaired, the elderly depend more on the Frank-Starling mechanism.

Diastolic dysfunction: A prolonged myocardial relaxation time with an increase in myocardial stiffness, which decreases filling rate or volume, causes elevated left ventricular diastolic pressure at rest and during exercise. Thus, pulmonary and systemic venous congestion may occur and produce symptoms of heart failure even if systolic function is normal or nearly normal. The high prevalence of diastolic dysfunction with preserved systolic function in elderly patients with heart failure is well documented. Between 50% and 60% of older patients with heart failure have adequate ventricular contractile function, with normal or only slightly reduced ejection fractions.

Symptoms, Signs, and Diagnosis

Symptoms and signs of heart failure (eg, edema) are similar in all patients, but atypical presentations are more common in the elderly. Patients may present with nonspecific signs of illness (eg, somnolence, confusion, disorientation, weakness, fatigue, and failure to thrive). A reliable history may be more difficult to obtain in patients who are cognitively impaired. Elderly patients may have no history of dyspnea.

Patients with **diastolic dysfunction** often have acute onset of symptoms and abrupt clinical deterioration. Underlying hypertension or coronary artery disease is common, and patients often present in acute decompensation related to acute ischemia or hypertension. However, systemic congestion with a normal ejection fraction does not necessarily indicate diastolic dysfunction. Other pathologic entities that should be considered include volume overload, valvular regurgitation, hypertrophic cardiomyopathy, pericardial constriction (acute tamponade or chronic pericarditis), restrictive cardiomyopathy, and high-output states. In contrast, the course of heart failure in patients with **systolic dysfunction** tends to be a gradual, progressive decline.

Signs of right-sided heart failure may accompany systolic dysfunction but are less frequently observed in patients with predominantly diastolic dysfunction. A big, baggy heart (laterally displaced point of maximal impulse) is compatible with systolic dysfunction; a forceful, minimally displaced apical impulse with an S_4 and no S_3 gallop is compatible with diastolic dysfunction.

Differentiating impaired systolic function from impaired diastolic function is important when selecting treatment. However, the clinical distinction between heart failure due mainly to systolic dysfunction and that due to diastolic dysfunction usually *cannot* be made at the bedside. An objective measure of left ventricular systolic function is often needed.

Noninvasive studies of left ventricular diastolic motion and studies of ventricular diastolic filling using Doppler echocardiographic and radionuclide scintigraphic techniques are useful in distinguishing diastolic from systolic dysfunction, as well as in diagnosing other diseases mentioned above. Patients with diastolic dysfunction typically have good or preserved systolic function (ejection fraction or fractional shortening) but impaired diastolic filling or ventricular relaxation. Those with systolic dysfunction generally have good ventricular filling but decreased ejection fraction and impaired systolic wall motion.

Unlike jugular venous distention and hepatojugular reflux, peripheral edema is *not* a reliable sign of heart failure in the elderly. While an S_4 gallop does not necessarily indicate clinically significant heart disease, an S_3 or early diastolic gallop usually does. Inspiratory rales may be heard in the lower half of the lung fields.

Prognosis

The prognosis for patients with heart failure depends on the underlying cause and whether associated diseases are present. While treatment may not prolong long-term survival in patients with chronic severe heart failure, it may enhance short-term survival. Improved quality of life, rather than prolonged survival, may have to be the ultimate goal in the elderly.

Treatment

The management of heart failure in older patients includes nonpharmacologic as well as pharmacologic therapies.

Nonpharmacologic therapies: Correcting underlying contributing factors, modifying the diet, reducing weight if needed, and engaging in physical exercise are some nonpharmacologic approaches to treating heart failure. Acute contributing factors include fever, hypoxia, myocardial ischemia, blood loss, infection, malignant hypertension, and pulmonary emboli. Chronic contributing factors include valvular disease (aortic stenosis being the most common), ventricular hypertrophy, hypertension, metabolic disease (eg, hyper- or hypothyroidism), and cardiomyopathy.

Dietary modifications to reduce fat and cholesterol, increase fruit and vegetable intake, and decrease caloric intake (if needed) are advisable. A low salt diet may benefit older patients with severely reduced systolic function (ejection fraction $< 20\%$) and renal insufficiency.

However, salt restriction is probably not indicated in those with fairly good systolic function (ejection fraction ≥ 35%), especially if they are hyponatremic (serum sodium level ≤ 135 mEq/L). A progressive loss in the kidney's sodium concentrating ability occurs with age, and salt restriction may cause or exacerbate hyponatremia.

Physical exercise can help reverse a number of age-associated cardiac changes that probably result from the sedentary lifestyle that is typical in older persons. Normal walking for ≥ 30 min every other day may help not only to improve cardiovascular function but also to enhance balance, gait, and muscle strength and to protect against falls and injuries.

Pharmacologic therapies: Although systolic and diastolic dysfunction are discussed separately, usually they coexist, at least some of the time, and may need to be treated together.

Elderly patients with **impaired diastolic function** are often erroneously treated for systolic heart failure with large doses of potent diuretics, digitalis, and vasodilators that may exacerbate the condition. Thus, therapy should be appropriate for the pathophysiology (see TABLE 41–2).

When systolic function is preserved, therapy is aimed at improving ventricular filling and relaxation rather than at reducing preload, which may exacerbate the already impaired ventricular filling. Agents that may enhance ventricular diastolic filling include calcium channel blockers and β-blockers. If the patient's left ventricular end-diastolic pressure is on the steep portion of the pressure-volume curve, a small dose of an angiotensin converting enzyme **(ACE)** inhibitor or a mild diuretic may be helpful. Therapy, however, must be individualized.

Emphasis should be on avoiding preload reduction and digitalis, if possible. The primary goals are to optimize ventricular early diastolic filling and reduce ventricular end-diastolic pressure. The atrial contribution to ventricular filling should be restored or augmented in patients with atrial arrhythmias by converting to and maintaining normal sinus rhythm (either pharmacologically or electrically). Elderly persons in particular depend on the atrial kick to attain adequate ventricular filling.

The mainstays of therapy for **impaired systolic function** are bed rest, digitalis, diuretics, and vasodilators (including ACE inhibitors), with reduction of preload and afterload. However, prolonged bed rest should be avoided because it may result in physical deconditioning, muscle wasting, and thromboembolic events. The patient should sit in a chair with the legs elevated. Bed or chair rest enhances diuresis, as does supplemental oxygen. Improved oxygenation of peripheral tissues increases renal perfusion, decreases vascular tone, and consequently reduces preload and afterload. Leg and toe exercises as well as elastic stockings may reduce the risk of thromboembolism. The use of low-dose anticoagulants is also advisable.

TABLE 41–2. DRUGS USED TO TREAT HEART FAILURE IN THE ELDERLY

Drug Group	*Agent*	*Dosage*	*Adverse Effects or Problems*	*Indications*
Digitalis	Digoxin	0.125–0.250 mg/day	Arrhythmia	SD
	Digitoxin	0.05–0.10 mg/day	Arrhythmia	SD
Diuretics	Chlorthalidone	25–100 mg/day	Hypotension	SD
	Furosemide	20-1000 mg/day	Hypokalemia	SD
Vasodilators	Nitroglycerin (oral)	6.5–19.5 mg q 6 h	Headache, drug tolerance	SD
	Nitroglycerin (ointment)	0.5–2 in. q 6 h	Headache, drug tolerance	SD
	Nitroglycerin (transdermal patch)	5–30 mg q 12–24 h	Headache, drug tolerance	SD
	Isosorbide dinitrate	10–60 mg q 4–6 h	Headache, drug tolerance	SD
	Nitroprusside	0.5–10 µg/kg/min IV	Hypotension, thiocyanate toxicity	SD
	Hydralazine	25–75 mg q 6–8 h	Fluid retention	SD
	Minoxidil	5–100 mg/day	Fluid retention, tachycardia, hirsutism	SD
	Prazosin	1–7 mg q 8 h	Postural hypotension, drug tolerance	SD
ACE inhibitors	Captopril	6.25–100 mg q 8 h	Hypotension, azotemia, reduced regional blood flow	SD
	Enalapril	10–40 mg/day		SD

(continued)

TABLE 41–2. DRUGS USED TO TREAT HEART FAILURE IN THE ELDERLY *(Continued)*

Drug Group	*Agent*	*Dosage*	*Adverse Effects or Problems*	*Indications*
Calcium channel blockers	Verapamil	40–120 mg q 12 h	Negative inotropy, heart block	DD
	Nifedipine	10–40 mg q 8 h	Negative inotropy, hypotension, reflex tachycardia	DD
	Diltiazem	30–90 mg q 8 h	Negative inotropy, heart block	DD
β-Blocker	Metoprolol	6.25–100 mg/day	Negative inotropy, bradycardia	DD and SD
Nonglycoside inotropic agents				
Sympatho-mimetic amines	Dopamine	1–5 μg/kg/min IV	Tachycardia	SD
	Dobutamine	1–10 μg/kg/min IV	Tachycardia	SD
Phosphodi-esterase inhibitor	Amrinone	1–10 μg/kg/min IV	Fever, GI intolerance, thrombocytopenia	SD

SD = systolic dysfunction; DD = diastolic dysfunction.

The value of long-term **digitalis therapy** in elderly patients has recently been questioned. Digitalis is useful for acute and chronic severe heart failure in patients with sinus rhythm or atrial fibrillation. It may be less useful in patients with *mild* chronic heart failure and sinus rhythm. While the inotropic response to cardiac glycosides may be diminished, the toxic effects, usually due to elevated plasma levels, are not reduced with age. Higher steady-state plasma levels and the prolonged plasma half-life of digoxin are due in part to the age-related decline in renal excretory capacity. Variability in distribution and extrarenal clearance further affects the predictability of serum digoxin levels in the elderly.

Fortunately, diuretics, vasodilators, antihypertensive agents, and new inotropic agents are effective in treating the symptoms and signs of acute and chronic severe heart failure. **Vasodilator therapy** reduces afterload, thereby enhancing myocardial shortening and increasing stroke volume. The most frequently used vasodilators and perhaps the most effective agents for heart failure are the ACE inhibitors (eg, captopril and enalapril). They work predominantly on the peripheral vasculature. ACE inhibitors are very effective in patients who are refractory to digitalis, diuretics, and other vasodilators. Alone or in combination with nitrates, hydralazine, and diuretics, the **ACE inhibitors** may be effective in reducing filling pressures, increasing cardiac output and renal blood flow, and improving exercise tolerance.

Several recent multicenter studies, including the V-HeFT (Vasodilator–Heart Failure Trial), the CONSENSUS I (The Cooperative North Scandinavian Enalapril Survival Study), and the SOLVD (Studies of Left Ventricular Dysfunction) trials, have shown that certain vasodilators improve survival among patients with chronic heart failure. The V-HeFT I trial demonstrated this benefit with hydralazine and nitrates (isosorbide dinitrate). In the CONSENSUS I trial, enalapril decreased mortality and improved function in patients with severe heart failure and poor ejection fraction. In the V-HeFT II study, enalapril had an added benefit on survival compared with the combination therapy of hydralazine plus isosorbide dinitrate. The SOLVD trials showed similarly positive effects of enalapril on survival in patients with heart failure and poor ejection fraction.

Although smaller doses of diuretics or vasodilators are effective in some elderly persons, other patients require doses equal to those for younger persons. Caution should be exercised when administering any diuretic or vasodilator to an elderly person for the first time. Initial doses should be lower, with smaller increments over longer intervals. Adverse effects of nitrates or hydralazine, such as tachycardia, may occur (rarely) in the elderly because of an age-related reduction in cardioacceleratory capacity.

In patients who do not respond adequately to therapy with digitalis, diuretics, and vasodilators, **inotropic agents** such as amrinone (available only for IV use) and its analog, milrinone, may be effective. These two agents improve the stroke-work index and reduce pulmonary artery pressure. Milrinone has direct inotropic effects on cardiac muscle and, at high doses, has a direct vasodilatory effect.

Prazosin, an arterial and venous system vasodilator, may reduce systemic and pulmonary venous pressure and may increase cardiac output. However, its effectiveness and its propensity for tachyphylaxis in elderly patients have not been extensively studied.

A combination of newer drugs and the more traditional agents will likely have synergistic effects. ACE inhibitors, nitrates, hydralazine, and diuretics all appear to be quite effective in the elderly at doses that cause relatively few adverse effects.

CARDIOMYOPATHY

Cardiomyopathy generally refers to a diffuse or generalized myocardial disorder often without a known underlying cause; patients have idiopathic or primary involvement of the myocardium. However, valvular, hypertensive, or coronary artery disease may coexist with primary cardiomyopathy. The three main types of primary ventricular dysfunction (which may overlap) are dilated or congestive cardiomyopathy, hypertrophic cardiomyopathy, and restrictive or infiltrative cardiomyopathy.

DILATED CARDIOMYOPATHY

Dilated cardiomyopathy is characterized by impaired systolic function with dilation of chambers and increased muscle mass without full compensatory increase in wall thickness. About 10% of patients with this condition are > 65 yr old.

This disorder is usually chronic; patients present with effort dyspnea and fatigability because of elevated left ventricular diastolic pressure and low cardiac output. Less often, the onset is acute and associated with fever if an infective agent is responsible, in which case it is called **myocarditis.** Acute myocarditis appears rarely in the elderly and may be difficult to diagnose clinically. The common causes are viruses, especially coxsackievirus, and rickettsiae.

Diagnosis is made by excluding specific factors that may result in diffuse myocardial dysfunction (eg, doxorubicin toxicity, radiation damage, and chronic alcoholism). Echocardiographic evidence of four-chamber dilation with depressed systolic ventricular function confirms the diagnosis. Dilated or congestive cardiomyopathy may be misdiagnosed as heart failure that is caused by coronary artery disease.

Treatment should be aimed at managing heart failure due to systolic dysfunction, treating arrhythmias, and preventing thromboembolic events. Vasodilator drugs, especially ACE inhibitors and diuretics, in addition to antiarrhythmic agents, digitalis, and anticoagulants, are emphasized. Immunosuppressive therapy has been proposed for the treatment of subacute and chronic myocarditis, but the therapeutic efficacy and side effects of immunosuppressive agents in elderly patients is not established.

HYPERTROPHIC CARDIOMYOPATHY

(See also Idiopathic Hypertrophic Subaortic Stenosis in Ch. 38)

Hypertrophic cardiomyopathy is characterized by normal or small chamber size, increased wall thickness, hyperdynamic systolic ejection, and impaired diastolic filling. The disorder occurs not infrequently in older persons. The symptoms—dizziness, syncope, dyspnea, chest discomfort, and palpitations—are similar in older and younger patients. Left ventricular outflow tract obstruction, mitral annular calcification, aortic regurgitation, and aortic valve calcification may be seen on Doppler echocardiography. The ventricular hypertrophy may be substantial and it may be concentric, especially in elderly patients with a history of hypertension.

Treatment for older patients with hypertrophic cardiomyopathy is similar to that for younger patients. β-Blockers, calcium channel blockers, and possibly low doses of ACE inhibitors may be helpful. Antibiotic prophylaxis to prevent infective endocarditis may be indicated for certain procedures (eg, dental procedures).

RESTRICTIVE CARDIOMYOPATHY

Restrictive cardiomyopathy, often caused by amyloid heart disease, is characterized by increased myocardial stiffness secondary to infiltrative pathology (diastolic dysfunction). Other causes of restrictive cardiomyopathy include postradiation damage and postoperative pericarditis. The atria are often dilated and systolic function is also impaired. In addition to enlarged atria, other findings include small ventricles, thick walls (both ventricles and the interatrial septum), a "sparkling" of the thickened myocardium on echocardiography, low QRS voltage and arrhythmias or conduction defects on the ECG, and elevated ventricular filling pressures.

The term restrictive cardiomyopathy does not apply to all old hearts that contain amyloid. **Senile cardiac amyloidosis** is a separate pathologic entity that is common in the very old. Its prevalence rises to 80% in those > 95 yr. The heart's macroscopic appearance is normal, but amyloid deposition, usually in the atria, is evident microscopically.

Treatment, directed at optimizing ventricular filling and enhancing diastolic function, is the same for younger and older patients.

42. PERIPHERAL VASCULAR DISEASES

There are two distinct systems of small blood vessels—one supplying skin and subcutaneous tissue and the other supplying skeletal muscle. Blood flow to the skin is under α-adrenergic control, and vasodilation is mostly due to reduction of α-adrenergic stimulation. Skin generally requires little blood flow for adequate nutrition. Blood flow to muscle is under relatively little α-adrenergic control; β-adrenergic receptors play a role in increasing blood flow during exercise. Muscle requires little blood flow at rest but needs 500 to 1000 times as much for ordinary walking.

Peripheral circulatory problems, both arterial and venous, increase in frequency with age and deleteriously affect functional capacity and lifestyle. Because the function of the peripheral circulation is accessible to direct scrutiny, thorough physical examination is the key to proper evaluation and treatment. Laboratory tests help confirm the diagnosis and quantify the extent of disease.

ARTERIAL DISEASES

Arterial diseases include peripheral atherosclerosis, small-vessel syndrome, and Raynaud's phenomenon. Giant cell arteritis and polymyalgia rheumatica are discussed in Ch. 74.

PERIPHERAL ATHEROSCLEROSIS

(Arteriosclerosis Obliterans)

Occlusion of blood supply to the extremities by atherosclerotic plaques (atheroma).

Progressive atherosclerosis in the extremities is a very common, age-related disease that parallels the development of atherosclerosis in the coronary and cerebral vessels. The pathologic process, beginning many years before clinical findings are apparent, is slow and insidious. Almost 70% of a vessel's lumen must be occluded before the disease can be clinically recognized. Atherosclerosis involves the legs much more extensively than the arms, and symptoms are usually confined to the former.

Etiology and Pathophysiology

The **risk factors** for peripheral atherosclerosis, similar to those for atherosclerosis elsewhere, include cigarette smoking, diabetes mellitus, hyperlipidemia, hypertension, polycythemia, family history, homocystinuria, and in women, early hysterectomy or ovariectomy. Diabetes and smoking are particularly important.

Since the chief determinant of blood viscosity is the hematocrit, any condition (eg, polycythemia) that increases the hematocrit increases the resistance to blood flow and shearing force against vessel walls. This causes injuries to the intima into which platelets and lipids move and thus form atheromas. Poorly controlled diabetes mellitus also leads to intimal injury and the buildup of atheromas. Low estrogen levels, whether from ovariectomy or menopause, hasten atheroma formation. The lipid-lowering effects of estrogen are one important reason why postmenopausal women who have no contraindications should receive estrogen replacement therapy.

How smoking damages the arteries is still unclear, but carbon monoxide and the metabolites of smoke components probably have a toxic effect on the intima. Because nicotine is a direct arterial vasoconstrictor, damage may be heightened when distal blood flow is restricted. Even after peripheral atherosclerosis becomes clinically evident, continuing to smoke accelerates arterial deterioration. In fact, the incidence of limb amputation is 10 times higher in those who continue to smoke after developing arterial occlusion than in those who quit.

Symptoms and Signs

The cardinal and most specific symptom of peripheral atherosclerosis is **intermittent claudication:** *pain, tightness, or weakness in an exercising muscle that occurs on walking and is relieved promptly (in < 5 min) by rest*. The pain is most often described as "squeezing." It results from muscle hypoxia, its coronary counterpart being angina pectoris. If the femoropopliteal artery is occluded, pain almost always occurs in the calf; if the aortoiliac artery is occluded, pain usually occurs in the hip and buttocks. By definition, claudication never occurs while sitting or standing still. Most important, claudication forces the person to halt; walking either is too painful or results in loss of muscle function and a fall.

The distance at which claudication occurs may change over time but tends to be remarkably constant from day to day if external conditions are unchanged. Cold and windy weather, inclines, and rapid walking shorten the distance at which claudication occurs. Using canes or crutches does not improve walking distance, since muscle function is normal until hypoxia occurs. With mild claudication, a person may walk up to six blocks without stopping, but the usual distance is less than three blocks and, in severe cases, may be only a few yards.

Less specific symptoms of peripheral atherosclerosis—numbness, paresthesias, coldness, and pain on rest—relate to the foot's cutaneous circulation. **Numbness and paresthesias** may also be caused by concomitant diabetic neuropathy. However, foot or toe numbness that occurs on walking suggests arterial disease and can be likened to claudication. It results from maximal vasodilation of muscle arterioles, with stealing of blood flow from the skin.

A **sense of coldness** may be secondary to vasoconstriction rather than to arterial occlusion and is very common in the elderly. A recent increase in coldness, coldness in only one limb, or coldness that persists after a night's sleep suggests arterial insufficiency. **Foot pain at rest** is a dire symptom, indicating that blood flow capacity is reduced to < 10% of normal; it *must be evaluated and treated immediately*. The pain is paresthetic and burning, most severe distally, and typically worse at night, preventing sleep. Partial relief is often possible with the foot in the dependent position (ie, below heart level). Pain from ischemia must be distinguished from other causes; for example, the pain of diabetic neuropathy may be similar but is generally bilateral and extends above the feet.

Claudication is the earliest symptom in a patient accustomed to walking. However, some elderly people are relatively sedentary and rarely walk far enough to have claudication; therefore, they present later with foot pain at rest or even gangrene. Gangrene represents necrosis of tissue. It first appears as nonblanching cyanosis (ecchymosis), followed by blackening and mummification of the involved part. In diabetic or other patients with peripheral neuropathy, dependent rubor and subsequent gangrene may occur without pain.

Because older people usually have many areas of occlusion, they are unlikely to have **Leriche's syndrome** (*localized aortoiliac occlusion*), in which the distal vessels are usually patent and the feet are healthy. Patients with Leriche's syndrome have hip claudication and impotence secondary to hypotension in the internal iliac arteries. Elderly patients with aortoiliac disease generally also have femoropopliteal and tibial occlusions, so distal flow may be seriously impaired. Leriche's syndrome should be considered in the differential diagnosis of impotence in the elderly; however, older patients with Leriche's syndrome may be bothered more by claudication.

Diagnosis

Examination of the peripheral pulses is key to confirming the diagnosis of peripheral atherosclerosis. The posterior tibial pulse is always present in healthy persons, although it may be difficult to feel if the patient has edema or prominent malleoli. It is best palpated with the patient supine and the examiner on the same side as the pulse. Meticulous palpation under the medial malleolus is necessary; dorsiflexing and everting the foot slightly may help move the artery into a more superficial position.

The dorsalis pedis artery extends along the dorsomedial aspect of the foot and is frequently subject to vasoconstriction; its pulse is absent in about 5% of healthy persons. The lateral tarsal pulse can occasionally be felt lateral to this artery.

The popliteal artery is generally the most difficult to palpate; the patient should be supine and relaxed, with the knee slightly flexed. The artery may be located posteriorly, laterally, or medially in the popliteal space. Very deep palpation may be necessary in obese persons.

Measurement of pulse strength is subjective and depends on the pulse pressure, girth of the extremity, and patient age, as well as on the sensitivity of the examiner. If an artery remains patent, its pulse tends to become more prominent with aging because the media loses smooth muscle and elastic tissue, predisposing to ectasia. The upstroke of the pulse wave is more important than the amplitude. Bruits heard over the femoral arteries indicate aortoiliac disease.

When the presence or strength of a peripheral pulse cannot be determined clinically, **Doppler ultrasonography** can be used to assess arterial patency. However, a Doppler signal does not prove that pulsatile flow is adequate; a signal may be perceived when the vessel's systolic blood pressure is as low as 30 mm Hg. For a Doppler study to be satisfactory, a blood pressure cuff must be used to measure systolic pressure (pressure above which the signal cannot be detected). For this purpose, a normal-sized arm cuff can be placed just above the ankle. Wide cuffs can be used to measure thigh pressures, which may be falsely elevated because of difficulty in occluding the femoral artery. The Doppler instrument is placed over the artery to be tested (usually the posterior tibial or dorsalis pedis artery). The clinician must search carefully for a Doppler signal before assuming a zero blood pressure.

The Doppler measurement is also useful in evaluating arterial insufficiency in a pulseless limb (eg, by determining the **ankle-brachial index**). In healthy limbs, this index should not be < 1, although an index > 0.6 indicates but does not prove adequate resting blood flow to the foot. In some cases of mild arterial disease, the ankle-brachial index may be about 1 because of cuff artifact or peripheral vasoconstriction in the involved leg. Rechecking the blood pressure at the ankle after exercise is helpful. Because vasodilation occurs after exercise, blood pressure will fall if the proximal artery is occluded; the magnitude and duration of the fall after exercise correlate with the degree of arterial insufficiency. In addition, many elderly and diabetic patients have heavily calcified arteries that are difficult to compress, thereby making ankle pressure appear falsely high. Thus, foot viability must never be based solely on a Doppler measurement; *examination of the foot is essential.* Other techniques for assessing the degree of ischemia (eg, plethysmography or percutaneous oxygen electrode measurements after transient arterial occlusion) require a great deal of expertise.

Temperature differences between the toes of each foot and color changes are particularly important. The foot should be elevated above heart level for 20 sec to determine whether pallor develops. A severely ischemic foot may appear pale even when horizontal. With the foot in the dependent position, **pallor** lasting for > 30 sec or **rubor** (a homogeneous, violaceous color, which may require 1 to 2 min to reach its maximum) appearing after 20 sec indicates < 10% of normal blood flow capacity. Rubor is more pronounced in the toes and extends proximally for various distances. Both prolonged pallor and rubor, well correlated with pain on resting, are grim signs. More extensive obliterative disease may compromise tissue viability and lead to skin ulceration or frank gangrene, particularly of the toes, heels, and lateral malleoli.

In evaluating persons with atherosclerosis, serum lipid levels should be measured. A full lipid profile, including total cholesterol, HDL, LDL, and triglyceride levels, should be obtained in the fasting state. Measuring the total cholesterol level alone is inadequate because some persons will have normal levels of total cholesterol but abnormal levels of the other lipid parameters (see Ch. 81).

Treatment

Treatment is based on disease severity as determined from history, physical examination, and the patient's general condition. Patients can be categorized into three broad groups: (1) those who are asymptomatic, (2) those who have only intermittent claudication, and (3) those who have significant foot ischemia, with or without claudication.

Asymptomatic patients: Most patients with peripheral atherosclerosis, including the elderly, have no symptoms; collateral vessels adequately perfuse their feet. Many patients > 70 yr have weak or missing pedal pulses but have no difficulty with their extremities unless they experience an infection, trauma, or thermal injury, which may cause serious problems because a marginal circulation cannot meet the increased metabolic demands of the tissue. Therapy consists primarily of preventive measures (see TABLE 42–1).

Patients with intermittent claudication: Medical therapy is somewhat limited in patients who have intermittent claudication. They should be given foot care instructions (see TABLE 42–1) and advised to avoid smoking, to lose weight if necessary, and to walk as much as possible. As soon as they experience claudication, they should rest and then continue walking. In a small but significant number of patients who follow these instructions, symptoms ameliorate within the first 3 mo.

Results of **drug therapy** for claudication are mixed. Vasodilators have been ineffective. Pentoxifylline, the first of a new class of drugs approved for treating claudication, decreases blood viscosity and improves red blood cell flexibility, leading to improved blood flow through arterioles and capillaries. In a double-blind, controlled study, subjects increased mean walking distance by about 50 m. However, clinical results have been disappointing. The recommended dose is 400 mg orally tid.

Questions have been raised about using β-adrenergic blocking agents in patients who have **both coronary and peripheral atherosclerosis.** Except for β-blockers that have intrinsic sympathomimetic activity, these drugs are mild peripheral vasoconstrictors and could aggravate intermittent claudication. Because this rarely happens, however, these drugs should not be withheld from a patient who has both heart disease and claudication. β-Blockers have been shown to increase the longevity of patients with atherosclerotic coronary artery disease, and this advantage clearly outweighs a possible slight decrease in the distance at which claudication occurs.

The only clearly effective treatment for intermittent claudication is **surgery,** either arterial bypass or, in less severe cases, percutaneous transluminal angioplasty. The decision for or against surgery must be based on, among other factors, the patient's age, general health, and lifestyle; whether the patient has heart disease; and the location of the lesions.

Angiography, an invasive procedure that determines the feasibility of surgery, should be performed *only* if surgery is being seriously considered. It allows visualization of the entire peripheral tree from the distal aorta through the tibial vessels. For surgery to be successful, a major vessel beyond the obstruction must be patent, with good distal flow beyond this patent area.

TABLE 42–1. PREVENTIVE AND THERAPEUTIC MEASURES FOR PATIENTS WITH PERIPHERAL ATHEROSCLEROSIS

Stressor or Contributing Factor	*Preventive or Therapeutic Measure*
Cold	Avoid extreme cold; dress warmly in winter; avoid bathing or swimming in cold water
Heat	Never apply heat to the feet; avoid sun exposure to feet and legs
Exercise	Walk regularly to improve circulation
Position	Keep legs level with the bed during sleep; avoid crossing them while sitting
Cleanliness	Wash feet with mild soap and lukewarm water and dry them thoroughly, especially between the toes to avoid skin breakdown and infection
Dry scaly skin	Apply lanolin or cold cream to the feet and gently massage it into dry scaly areas
Toes and toenails	Have a podiatrist or family member cut toenails straight across, being careful to avoid cutting in at the corners or too close to the skin
Corns and calluses	Consult a podiatrist; avoid corn remedies and plasters
Local medication	Avoid strong antiseptics and tincture of iodine because they may damage the skin; use only medications ordered by the physician
Shoes and socks	Do not walk barefoot; wear clean socks every day and comfortable, properly fitting shoes, preferably with square or round toes with adequate room in the toe boxes; avoid garters or hose with elastic tops
Injuries	Avoid foot injuries, even minor ones, by following the suggestions above; examine feet weekly for cracks, cuts, or color changes; consult a physician if any of these occur, with or without pain

The more proximal the lesion, the better the clinical results of **bypass surgery** and the longer the graft remains patent. With localized aortoiliac disease, the graft patency rate at 5 yr is > 90%. In femoropopliteal disease, 5-yr patency rates are probably 60% to 70%. Femorotibial grafts have a 5-yr patency rate well below 50%, and patency rates are even lower with generalized disease. In bilateral arterial occlusion, a femoropopliteal bypass may unmask claudication in the contralateral limb, resulting in only slight clinical improvement. A second operation would then be necessary to increase claudication-free walking distance significantly.

Percutaneous transluminal angioplasty offers an alternative to bypass surgery for short stenoses in the aortoiliac and proximal-femoral areas. Although it is a relatively simple procedure that can be performed under local anesthesia, complications (eg, arterial rupture and distal embolization of ruptured atheromatous plaques) may require emergency surgery. Therefore, a patient undergoing percutaneous transluminal angioplasty must be capable of withstanding a full surgical procedure.

Significant coronary artery disease is a contraindication to peripheral arterial surgery for two reasons: (1) heart disease increases operative mortality, (2) angina, the limiting factor after a successful bypass, may prevent or mitigate any improvement in walking distance.

Patients with significant foot ischemia: Evidence of severe cutaneous ischemia (eg, pain on resting, dependent rubor, and tissue loss) is a much stronger indication for surgery. Greater risks are justified to relieve disabling pain or prevent amputation, although conservative care is often indicated if the patient is a poor surgical risk. Patches of dry gangrene, particularly on the toes, should be allowed to demarcate because autoamputation of toes may result in proximal healing. Ischemic ulcers can heal if the surrounding blood flow is adequate; they may respond to pressure relief, debriding agents (eg, collagenase), and local antiseptic solutions (eg, povidone-iodine applied bid). Soaking the foot in body-temperature water also helps treat infected lesions. Pentoxifylline is of uncertain benefit, but it has few side effects and can be tried. β-Blockers should be avoided.

Elderly patients who have no tissue loss or pain at rest should not undergo surgery, even if they have florid dependent rubor. However, if tissue breakdown begins in a foot, arteriography and surgery are generally indicated. In patients with severe heart disease, amputation is sometimes preferable to the risk of bypass surgery.

Two relatively low-risk surgical procedures can be considered in elderly patients who have severe aortoiliac disease and whose feet are threatened with tissue loss or amputation. A **femorofemoral bypass** subcutaneously across the lower pelvic area may help save a limb if the disease is unilateral. The graft patency rate with this procedure is almost as good as that with aortofemoral bypass. A subcutaneous **bypass from an axillary to a femoral artery** may be helpful if the disease is bilateral. These grafts often clot but may be reopened by performing a local thrombectomy within a few days of closure. The 5-yr graft patency rate is about 50%.

When a limb is threatened, the presence of stenoses in many areas is not a contraindication to surgery. Bypass of the most proximal occlusion often increases collateral flow around more distal occlusions sufficiently to salvage the limb. Angioplasty for a short iliac stenosis may precede femoropopliteal or femorotibial bypass surgery.

SMALL–VESSEL SYNDROME

Cutaneous ischemia or local areas of cyanosis or necrosis in a hand or foot with generally adequate circulation.

Ischemia in a foot or hand with palpable pulses suggests a number of diagnostic possibilities in the elderly: cryoglobulinemia, cryofibrinogenemia, disseminated intravascular coagulation, essential thrombocytosis, polycythemia, vasculitis secondary to drug-induced systemic lupus erythematosus, presence of the lupus anticoagulant, scleroderma, or emboli from an arterial aneurysm, the heart, or atheromatous plaques.

Symptoms, Signs, and Diagnosis

Patients usually present with a cyanotic or gangrenous digit and may have many small lesions on several extremities. Occasionally, an entire foot or hand is cyanotic or exhibits dependent rubor. Patients with peripheral atherosclerosis and pulseless limbs must also be evaluated for small-vessel syndrome if cutaneous ischemia suddenly and inexplicably worsens or if they develop local areas of cyanosis or necrosis but the rest of the foot or hand is adequately perfused. This evaluation is particularly important when a hand is involved because severe ischemia is uncommon in the upper extremities, even if atherosclerosis is advanced.

A thorough **history** is important. Drug use (eg, procainamide, hydralazine, and phenytoin) may induce systemic lupus erythematosus; other findings may include arthralgias and pleural effusion. Weight loss and other symptoms of anorexia may suggest a malignancy responsible for cryofibrinogenemia or disseminated intravascular coagulation. Back pain may point to multiple myeloma responsible for cryoglobulinemia. Acute gangrene with fever may suggest septicemia, leading to cryofibrinogenemia or disseminated intravascular coagulation. Splenomegaly may point to essential thrombocytosis, a megakaryocytic myeloproliferative disease generally characterized by digital or cerebral ischemia but sometimes involving abnormal bleeding. A history of myocardial infarction should prompt suspicion of a ventricular aneurysm.

Physical examination should include a search for abdominal, femoropopliteal, and subclavian aneurysms (see Ch. 43). Popliteal aneurysms are most notorious for shedding small emboli and should be considered if ischemia is confined to one foot. Atrial fibrillation and a dyskinetic left ventricular impulse suggest the heart as a possible source of emboli.

Laboratory evaluation should include a CBC with platelet count, a coagulation screen, and tests for cryoproteins, antinuclear antibodies, and the lupus inhibitor. Lupus inhibitor is a misnomer; most patients with this protein do not have systemic lupus erythematosus, although the **lupus inhibitor** is found in about 10% of patients with the disease. The protein, *an immunoglobulin that interferes with phospholipid-dependent coagulation tests,* binds to phospholipids that accelerate the activation of prothrombin to thrombin by factor Xa. Administering normal plasma does not correct the defect. Venous and small arterial thrombi occur in 27% of patients with the lupus inhibitor. The mechanism of thrombosis is unknown, but inhibition of prostacyclin synthesis is a possible factor.

An echocardiogram should be performed if mitral valve disease or ventricular aneurysm is suspected, and a sonogram of the aorta and popliteal arteries may be necessary to rule out a pulsatile mass. The diagnosis of **atheromatous emboli** (fracturing of plaques) is reached by exclusion. Occasionally, this entity presents with the appearance of **livedo reticularis** (a lacy network of cyanotic-looking superficial vessels on the anterior side of the leg), but a lupus syndrome must still be ruled out.

Treatment

Aneurysms must be surgically repaired. Cardiac embolism is an indication for chronic anticoagulation therapy with warfarin. Atheromatous emboli are treated with antiplatelet drugs, including aspirin.

Appropriate therapy for patients with the lupus inhibitor has not been established, although both antiplatelet drugs and anticoagulation therapy have been advocated. Recent evidence suggests that only warfarin, at the level used for treating cardiac embolism, is effective.

RAYNAUD'S PHENOMENON

A syndrome of peripheral vasospasm with intermittent cutaneous pallor or cyanosis.

Symptoms and Signs

Exposure to cold typically causes blanching and then cyanosis of the hands, feet, and sometimes the ears and nose. An erythematous phase follows upon entering a warm environment. These episodes can be painless or associated with varying degrees of pain, numbness, and sense of coldness. Many older persons experience only a blanching or cyanotic phase, which may develop even when the ambient temperature is not very cool. Patients tend to have cool hands and feet even in a warm environment. If the problem is severe or of long duration, sclerodactyly may occur.

Diagnosis

Symptoms are usually unilateral if Raynaud's phenomenon is the result of previous frostbite or a thoracic outlet syndrome; otherwise Raynaud's phenomenon after age 40 is almost always a harbinger of internal disease. Secondary causes include hypothyroidism, drug-induced systemic lupus erythematosus, cryoglobulinemia, cryofibrinogenemia, cold agglutinin disease, scleroderma, and **CREST syndrome** (*c*alcinosis, *R*aynaud's phenomenon, *e*sophageal dysfunction, *s*clerodactyly, *t*elangiectasia).

Raynaud's phenomenon is a helpful clue to the diagnosis of **hypothyroidism,** which must be considered even if other symptoms are lacking. Patients with scleroderma, systemic lupus erythematosus, and cryoproteinemia may present with infarcted digits. A **cryoprotein** mandates evaluation for occult malignancy. Patients with cold agglutinin disease often have a low-grade lymphoma.

Almost all patients with **scleroderma** have Raynaud's phenomenon, which can precede all other manifestations by many years. Sclerodactyly is not diagnostic of scleroderma; diagnosis requires skin tightening in areas other than the hands and feet or visceral involvement (see SCLERODERMA in Ch. 75).

Treatment

In general, treatment of Raynaud's phenomenon per se should be conservative in the elderly. Cardiovascular reflexes are often impaired, and subclinical coronary and cerebrovascular disease may be present. Therefore, patients respond intensely to vasodilators and can develop orthostatic hypotension with serious consequences. Yet, nifedipine 10 mg orally tid is usually safe and effective. Griseofulvin 250 mg orally bid may also be helpful. Ketanserin, a selective 5-hydroxytryptamine$_2$ receptor antagonist, was reported to be beneficial in one large study, but the drug is not yet available in the USA. However, most patients do well enough by wearing warm clothing, avoiding extreme cold, and not smoking.

Patients with scleroderma should usually be treated more vigorously because attacks of Raynaud's phenomenon are associated with reversible decreases in renal and cardiac blood flow and with echocardiographic evidence of impaired myocardial contractility. If the patient is also hypertensive, an angiotensin converting enzyme inhibitor, which promotes renal as well as peripheral blood flow, is an excellent choice for therapy.

VENOUS DISEASES

Venous diseases include deep venous thrombosis, chronic deep venous insufficiency, superficial thrombophlebitis, and varicose veins.

DEEP VENOUS THROMBOSIS

The presence of a thrombus in a deep vein.

Etiology

The mechanisms behind venous clotting can be classified under **Virchow's triad:** factors involving the movement of blood, the blood itself, and the vessel wall. Since no propelling cardiac force moves venous blood, the emptying of veins in the extremities depends entirely on skeletal muscles that pump and on one-way valves in the lumen that inhibit retrograde flow. Thus, immobilization or even a relatively sedentary existence favors venous stasis and predisposes to thrombosis. Since incompetent venous valves lead to deep venous thrombosis, which itself damages the valves, deep venous thrombosis tends to be a recurring phenomenon. Any factor that increases hematocrit leads to greater blood viscosity and a higher incidence of clotting.

Symptoms and Signs

The hallmark of deep venous thrombosis is the rapid onset of unilateral leg swelling with dependent edema. Generally, swelling is first noted upon awakening. An ambulatory patient has maximal swelling at the ankle and lower leg, usually occurring over 1 or 2 days. Pain may be present but is usually not severe. Physical examination often reveals pitting edema and a mild to moderate increase in skin temperature over the calf or thigh. In patients with heart failure and deep venous thrombosis, *both* legs are swollen but the phlebitic one more so.

A gap always occurs between the level of thrombosis and the location of edema. With popliteal and lower femoral venous occlusion, edema involves only the lower leg and ankle. With the clot at the midfemoral vein area, most or all of the leg is swollen. With upper femoral and external iliac vein involvement, the thigh is also swollen. If present, tenderness occurs in the calf for femoropopliteal and in the medial thigh for iliofemoral venous thrombosis.

Calf vein thrombosis may be asymptomatic or may involve mild tenderness and little or no edema. There are four to six deep calf veins (anterior tibial, posterior tibial, and peroneal); because all of them drain into the popliteal vein, occlusion of one or two is unlikely to impair venous drainage.

Phlegmasia cerulea dolens, a serious form of iliofemoral venous thrombosis, is characterized by massive thigh and calf edema and a cold, mottled foot. Pedal pulses are usually absent, and the leg is quite tender. Findings are secondary to proximal iliac vein thrombosis and associated arteriospasm. The danger of massive pulmonary embolism is great, even if the patient is receiving anticoagulation therapy. Foot gangrene also occurs but less often. Phlegmasia cerulea dolens may be mistaken for arterial embolism, but misdiagnosis can be avoided by keeping in mind that acute arterial occlusion does *not* cause edema. Phlegmasia cerulea dolens often indicates occult malignancy.

Diagnosis

The sudden onset of lower leg swelling in a gravitational distribution without trauma and a precipitating factor suggests a diagnosis of deep venous thrombosis. However, laboratory confirmation is needed if the onset of swelling is not clearly acute and the findings are not entirely typical.

Risk factors: In a patient with deep venous thrombosis, risk factors should be identified; the major ones are immobilization and decreased physical activity, venous damage, obesity, heart failure, polycythemia, thrombocytosis, dehydration, malignancy, fractured hip, and estrogen use (see TABLE 42–2).

If a risk factor is obvious (eg, bed confinement or heart failure), no further evaluation is necessary for femoropopliteal and tibial vein thromboses. However, all patients with iliofemoral venous thrombosis should have an abdominal diagnostic study (ultrasonography is usually adequate) to rule out extrinsic compression by tumor and clot in the inferior vena cava. Right iliofemoral venous thrombosis is of particular concern if no local problem exists in the right lower extremity. Because the inferior vena cava is located on the right, iliofemoral venous compression related to an abdominal tumor must be suspected when thrombosis occurs on that side. The left common iliac vein, on the other hand, is normally compressed by the right iliac artery and is more likely to become thrombosed from reasons other than tumor compression.

If a risk factor is not obvious, especially in patients with recurrent and migratory deep venous thrombosis, other tests are indicated to look for hypercoagulable states and tumors. These generally include stool tests for occult blood; platelet count; tests for antinuclear antibody, cryoproteins, lupus inhibitor, antithrombin III deficiency, and occasionally, protein C and protein S deficiency; abdominal ultrasonography or CT scanning; and rectal, pelvic, and breast examinations.

One clue to antithrombin III deficiency is relative resistance to heparin. Heparin acts primarily as an antithrombin by forming complexes with antithrombin III. When levels of antithrombin III are reduced, heparin's prolongation of the partial thromboplastin time is also reduced.

Protein C is a vitamin K–dependent anticoagulant; patients with protein C deficiency typically develop venous thromboembolism if warfarin therapy is initiated without heparin. Vitamin K procoagulant factors need time to be reduced.

Diagnostic tests: If no swelling is present and the patient is ambulatory, deep venous thrombosis can usually be ruled out by using a tape measure to compare the circumference of the legs at several levels. The most important measurement is just above the ankles. Calf vein thrombosis without swelling is common only in sedentary or bedridden patients and is, therefore, an important consideration in the nonambulatory elderly. This diagnosis can be made only through laboratory evaluation.

TABLE 42–2. RISK FACTORS FOR DEEP VENOUS THROMBOSIS

Risk Factor	*Comment*
Immobilization and decreased activity	Bed rest during acute illness increases risk; cardiovascular and chronic pulmonary disease, chronic arthritis, or dementia often limit walking
Obesity	Weight gain leads to less activity; obesity is associated with decreased production of plasminogen activator by venous endothelium (essential for normal thrombolysis of early clots)
Hip fracture	Factors include immobilization and injury to femoral vein and its tributaries
Estrogen	Decreases blood levels of antithrombin III; can lead to venous dilatation and stasis
Malignancy	Patients with early lesions may have venous clotting as a paraneoplastic effect; hypercoagulability often occurs because of thrombocytosis, circulating cryoproteins, or disseminated intravascular coagulation; those with advanced cancer may become immobile
Others	Previous deep venous thrombosis and other causes of venous damage, heart failure, polycythemia, thrombocytosis, dehydration

Although **radiocontrast venography** is rarely needed, it is the gold standard for confirmation of deep venous thrombosis. It provides an anatomic map of the deep venous system, from tibial veins to the common iliac vein. To ensure that the contrast material is directed into the deep rather than superficial veins, this material is injected through a dorsal foot vein with the leg in the dependent position or with a tourniquet above the ankle. Venous occlusion can be seen as a cutoff of flow or as a filling defect in the vessel, with contrast material streaming around it. In the tibial area, a sparsity of visible veins is diagnostic. Radiocontrast venography should be *avoided in patients with significant renal failure* (creatinine level > 3 mg/dL) and used with caution in those with mild azotemia. Passage of contrast material through the renal tubules can exacerbate preexisting renal disease. It is important to maintain good hydration, both before and 6 to 8 h after the dye study.

Impedance plethysmography can indirectly demonstrate venous thrombi by detecting changes in venous volume when a thigh tourniquet is applied and removed. If a proximal vein is occluded, the usual rapid and large increase in venous volume is likely to be dampened when occlusive pressure is applied. Changes in venous volume are detected by applying a very low amperage current to the calf. Since blood is a good conductor, an increase in venous volume should decrease electrical impedance and, therefore, the voltage necessary to sustain it. Failure to decrease impedance with pressure applied by a tourniquet indicates venous thrombosis.

Plethysmography is reliable only for occlusions above the knee and those of recent onset. If a week or more has elapsed, venous return through collateral circulation leads to a false-negative result. Although controversial, the sensitivity and specificity of impedance plethysmography are probably about 75% for thrombi above the knee.

Real-time ultrasonography with color Doppler is now the technique of choice for diagnosing deep venous thrombosis above the knee. The femoral vein in the inguinal area and the popliteal vein can easily be imaged. The major signs of acute thrombosis are lack of venous compressibility and a visible filling defect in the lumen. If the clot is chronic, the vein is usually compressible and flow is seen around a partially lysed clot. This method has sensitivity and specificity rates of 95%. In general, if ultrasonography fails to reveal any clot, venous thrombosis above the knee is very unlikely.

Radionuclide venography can be performed even in patients with severe azotemia or allergy to contrast material. Macroaggregated albumin tagged with technetium is injected into a dorsal foot vein to outline the venous tree, and special equipment can detect filling defects. Although the tibial veins are not visualized, thrombi in the inferior vena cava can be detected. False-negative results are common, but positive results are generally accurate. Although they do not provide as much detail as conventional venography, radionuclide studies have the advantage of allowing for perfusion lung scanning and venography with one injection.

Isotopes injected IV for diagnosis of small vein thrombi, used mainly in research, have greatly increased understanding of venous thrombosis. Fibrinogen tagged with iodine 125 accumulates in areas of active clotting, indicating a hot spot in the calf. Its long half-life allows for scanning a week after a single injection. The test is accurate only in nonedematous limbs, where the fibrinogen can follow a small clot in the soleal sinusoids until it reaches the upper tibial area. The test is cumbersome and expensive because it requires tagging the patient's own fibrinogen to eliminate risk of viral hepatitis. It is also overly sensitive, detecting thrombi that will never become clinically significant. More recently, platelets labeled with indium 111 have been similarly used.

Differential Diagnosis

Other conditions, such as trauma, can mimic deep venous thrombosis. Traumatic edema should be suspected if the patient noted its onset during or shortly after walking. Forcefully dorsiflexing the foot on sudden downward movement can **rupture the plantar tendon** or injure the gastrocnemius muscle. The swelling tends to be asymmetric and confined, occurs above the ankle, is very tender, and is often associated with visible ecchymosis.

Palpation of the popliteal fossa is also important. A **popliteal cyst,** by extension into the calf, can cause upper leg swelling and later can compress the popliteal vein. Again, this diagnosis should be suspected if the edema develops initially during physical activity. A sonogram can easily confirm or eliminate this possibility.

Treatment

The objective is to prevent pulmonary embolism and chronic venous insufficiency.

Anticoagulation therapy: The mainstay of treatment is anticoagulation therapy, beginning with heparin and continuing with warfarin. **Heparin** is given s.c. q 6 h, IV q 4 h, or by continuous IV infusion. If the continuous IV route is used, the patient must first receive a rapid infusion (bolus) of 5,000 to 10,000 u. The initial infusion rate is usually 1000 u./h; thereafter, the rate is adjusted according to the partial thromboplastin time, which should be kept between 1.5 and 2.0 times the normal control value. The partial thromboplastin time must be measured daily, since the necessary flow rate may change.

Continuous IV infusion offers the most flexibility in adjusting dose. Accurate infusion is critical; inadvertent increases in rate can lead to severe bleeding, and temporary interruptions of the infusion can lead to inadequate anticoagulation within 1 h. When an IV infusion is restarted, a rapid infusion (bolus) of 5000 u. must generally be given. Recently, IV heparin 10,000 to 12,000 u. q 12 h has been found to be as effective as continuous IV. The duration of heparinization is debatable, but one recommendation is 4 days for femoropopliteal thrombosis and 5 to 7 days for iliofemoral thrombosis.

Periodic platelet counts should be obtained in patients receiving heparin therapy, usually after 5 days of therapy. *Heparin therapy should be discontinued if the patient develops thrombocytopenia,* which occurs in about 1% of patients. A small proportion of them develop arterial and venous thrombi called the **syndrome of paradoxical thrombosis.** Although the exact mechanism of this syndrome is not clear, heparin-dependent platelet antibodies and abnormal amounts of immunoglobulin may deposit on endothelial cells. In the laboratory, the rate at which normal platelets release serotonin increases when they are exposed to heparinized plasma from these patients.

To avoid discontinuity in anticoagulation therapy, **warfarin** should be started 4 days before heparin is stopped. Factor VII, which is not involved in the intrinsic clotting pathway, is the only clotting factor significantly depressed during the first 2 days of warfarin administration. The prothrombin time should be adjusted to a level 1.2 to 1.4 times the normal control value (INR of 1.6 to 2.4). For uncomplicated venous thrombosis, at least 3 mo of therapy is usually recommended, but patients at high risk for recurrent thrombosis may need extended therapy.

Patients > 70 yr (especially women) receiving warfarin therapy are at high risk for severe hemorrhage and its consequences. Vascular integrity is impaired, and even a small head injury can lead to intracranial bleeding. A small GI hemorrhage in a patient with atherosclerosis can trigger a myocardial infarction or a stroke. Since many older people with arthritic and neurologic problems fall frequently, warfarin should generally be *avoided* in patients > 80 yr and frail persons > 70 yr.

Because many drugs either potentiate or inhibit warfarin, the known effects of all drugs should be reviewed before any drugs are prescribed. Patients should be advised to clear use of all new drugs, including OTCs, with their primary care doctor.

Inferior vena cava filter (umbrella): Patients who need an alternative to warfarin either could receive short-term heparin treatment only or after heparin therapy could have a filter (umbrella) inserted into the inferior vena cava. Umbrella insertion provides long-term protection against pulmonary emboli. Other reasons for umbrella insertion include (1) hemorrhage while receiving anticoagulation therapy, (2) bleeding diatheses that prevent anticoagulation, (3) phlegmasia cerulea dolens, (4) survival after massive pulmonary embolism, and (5) recurrent pulmonary embolism in an adequately anticoagulated patient.

The umbrella is usually inserted through the external jugular vein, passed through the right atrium, and placed in the inferior vena cava just below the renal veins. If this is technically difficult or the patient already has a transvenous cardiac pacemaker, the umbrella can be inserted through a femoral vein. The umbrella acts as a plication device, preventing large pulmonary emboli. The complication rate is low, although occasionally an umbrella can loosen and migrate into another vein or even into a pulmonary artery. Although pulmonary embolism from thrombi in the legs after umbrella insertion is uncommon, it can occur after a few months when emboli travel through collateral veins.

The decision to use an umbrella depends on the likelihood of recurrence of deep venous thrombosis, the presence of pulmonary emboli, and the location of the venous clot. Tibial vein thromboses rarely embolize and can remain untreated in patients at high risk for hemorrhage. Iliofemoral thrombi embolize often, and an umbrella is strongly indicated if the patient cannot be placed on warfarin.

Thrombolytic therapy: Extensive clotting leads to permanent venous valvular damage and residual venous occlusion. Patients with severe iliofemoral venous thrombosis and massive edema are at particularly high risk for chronic venous insufficiency and should be considered for thrombolytic therapy (eg, streptokinase, urokinase, or tissue plasminogen activator). Although heparin prevents further clotting, it does not lyse preformed thrombi.

Since the risk of bleeding is higher with these agents, contraindications to their use (eg, a coagulopathy, recent GI bleeding, recent stroke, history of cerebral hemorrhage, uremia, or surgical procedures within the preceding 7 days) must be considered. The older the patient, the greater the risk of hemorrhage. The risks of severe bleeding must be weighed against the morbidity of chronic, severe leg edema. Thrombolytic therapy is advisable in a small number of elderly patients. It is unlikely to be effective for clots more than 3 days old.

Streptokinase and urokinase differ. Streptokinase forms a complex with plasminogen activator, whereas urokinase directly lyses the clot. Streptokinase is occasionally associated with allergic reactions. Although urokinase can be given repeatedly, streptokinase cannot be repeated for 6 mo because it induces antibodies that cause drug resistance and increase the chance of a serious allergic reaction. Streptokinase may be ineffective following streptococcal infections.

Before starting thrombolytic therapy, heparin's effect must be allowed to abate. The average dose of streptokinase is 100,000 u./h administered for 12 h, after a loading dose of 250,000 u. in the first hour. The patient should be monitored closely during infusion, and a hematocrit value should be obtained q 3 to 4 h. Urokinase is also administered for 12 h, whereas tissue plasminogen activator is given for 2 h.

Serial thrombin times are used to monitor the drug's action. *Elevation of the thrombin time to at least twice normal is necessary with streptokinase or urokinase.* On the other hand, tissue plasminogen activator acts only within the clot and does not raise thrombin time. If the thrombin time cannot be raised, thrombolytic therapy should be stopped and heparin restarted for two reasons: (1) No rise in thrombin time means that no fibrin split products are being formed, which means that no clot lysis is occurring. (2) Without an elevation in thrombin time, the patient is not anticoagulated and is at high risk for pulmonary embolism.

Prophylaxis

Because of the high incidence of deep venous thrombosis (usually asymptomatic) in certain clinical situations, prophylaxis is of considerable interest. Studies with fibrinogen I 125 show a 20% to 25% rate of deep venous thrombosis in routine postoperative patients > 40 yr. Similar rates are found in immobilized patients with myocardial infarction or heart failure. After hip surgery, the incidence of deep venous thrombosis approaches 50%. Several methods of prophylaxis are available for high-risk patients.

Low-dose heparin is the most widely used. The usual dose is 5000 u. s.c. q 8 to 12 h. Significant bleeding is rare at this dosage. Controlled studies show the risk of both deep venous thrombosis and pulmonary embolism is significantly decreased in surgical patients > 40 yr. Heparin is *contraindicated* in patients who undergo ophthalmologic or neurosurgical procedures. Low-dose heparin is of limited prophylactic value in patients who undergo orthopedic procedures involving the extremities. **Full-dose heparin or warfarin** is effective in these cases, although each carries a significant risk of hemorrhage.

Oscillating boots applied to the calves are another, even safer, method of prophylaxis. A pump rhythmically inflates the boot to between 30 and 40 mm Hg and then deflates it, thus keeping the peripheral veins drained. Results are comparable to those of low-dose heparin but without risk of bleeding. **Galvanic stimulation** of calf muscles, begun intraoperatively and continued until the patient is ambulatory, is also quite effective.

Low-molecular-weight dextran may be used in some high-risk patients to prevent venous thrombosis. Its strong antiplatelet effects decrease both aggregation and adhesiveness. However, it is also a volume expander, and expansion can lead to fluid overload in patients with borderline cardiac or renal status. Dextran is also associated with acute renal failure and allergic reactions. Thus, it does not seem suitable for general use.

Even when other prophylactic measures are taken, appropriate **mobilization** must be accomplished. Patients should be mobilized as quickly as possible and encouraged to move their legs frequently while in bed. Prolonged bed rest poses many risks in addition to deep venous thrombosis and pulmonary embolism.

CHRONIC DEEP VENOUS INSUFFICIENCY
(Postphlebitic Syndrome)

A syndrome occurring after thrombosis, involving destruction of the deep and communicating venous valves of the leg and obliteration of the thrombosed veins.

Chronic deep venous insufficiency is almost always the result of previous symptomatic or asymptomatic deep venous thrombosis, although most patients cannot recall having had episodes consistent with that disorder. Rarely, arteriovenous fistula in the leg causes chronic venous stasis, leading to chronic venous hypertension and eventual valvular incompetence. The fistula is usually caused by trauma in the inguinal area, which may be accidental or iatrogenic (eg, after cardiac catheterization or angioplasty via the femoral vein). Since fistulas are associated with continuous bruits, the inguinal and upper femoral areas should be auscultated in patients with chronic venous insufficiency, especially if the findings are unilateral.

Symptoms and Signs
Chronic venous insufficiency rarely causes pain. The symptoms and signs of stasis are chronic edema, which is generally worse at the end of the day; hyperpigmentation around the medial malleolus and just above it; stasis dermatitis (scaling and pruritus) and hyperemic ulcers in the same area; and varicose veins.

If edema is severe and persistent, fibrosis leads to secondary lymphedema and trapped fluid. The calf becomes permanently enlarged and hard. Ulcers then occur more often and are more difficult to heal.

Prevention and Treatment

The vicious circle of increasing edema and ulceration can be prevented by elastic support. Since elderly people often find it difficult to bandage their legs each day, elastic stockings should be prescribed. A stocking that exerts 30 mm Hg pressure from the toes to just below the knee is usually sufficient, especially since significant edema of the thighs is rare. Patients should elevate their legs intermittently during the day and avoid standing still for extended periods. Ambulation should *not* be limited. If significant swelling persists overnight, patients should sleep with their legs elevated 3 to 4 inches above heart level.

For severe edema, pumps can reduce swelling. Older models exert a uniform pressure in rhythmic fashion to the edematous leg through an encircling sheath. More advanced models exert the pressure in a distal-to-proximal direction, providing more efficient venous return.

Ulcerations are also treated by elastic support and leg elevation. Topical antimicrobial therapy (eg, povidone-iodine) and warm soaks are indicated for infected lesions. A plaster boot often aids healing of large, clear ulcers. Although the boot has to be changed every 1 to 2 wk, this is preferable to limiting ambulation, especially in the elderly. A boot should not be applied if the ulcer shows signs of infection.

SUPERFICIAL THROMBOPHLEBITIS

Inflammation associated with a thrombosed superficial vein.

Etiology

In > 90% of cases, superficial thrombophlebitis occurs in varicose veins (see VARICOSE VEINS, below). Stasis within these incompetent veins leads to clotting, which can be prevented with elastic bandages or stockings.

In some cases, phlebitis occurs without varicose veins or is recurrent and migratory. A potential harbinger of internal disease, this occurrence should prompt assessment for occult neoplasm, especially pancreatic cancer; thrombocytosis or polycythemia; antithrombin III deficiency; collagen-vascular disease; presence of cryoprotein or lupus inhibitor; and protein C or S deficiency.

Symptoms, Signs, and Diagnosis

Superficial phlebitis is a more inflammatory process than is deep venous thrombosis. The usual presenting symptom is pain. Physical examination reveals an area of erythema, warmth, and tenderness overlying a palpable venous cord. The cord represents the thrombosed vein and is easily felt superficially. Often, many areas of thrombosis occur along the course of a superficial vein, usually along a segment of the great saphenous vein at the medial aspect of the leg or at the small saphenous vein in the posterior calf.

Superficial phlebitis rarely leads to pulmonary embolism. However, pulmonary embolism can occur when a clot propagates into the femoral vein, as a result of phlebitis of the great saphenous vein propagating up the thigh toward the inguinal area.

Treatment

For superficial phlebitis below the knee, treatment consists of warm soaks, decreased ambulation, and a nonsteroidal anti-inflammatory drug. The process is self-limited, and signs of inflammation usually fade within 5 to 10 days. There may be no residual findings, or the patient may have a nontender cord, which represents a permanently thrombosed vein. The cord may calcify months or even years later.

For superficial phlebitis in the lower thigh, a short course of heparin is advisable. Treatment can be discontinued as soon as signs of inflammation are gone, if further propagation is not evident. If the cord reaches the upper thigh, the great saphenous vein should be ligated at its most proximal point. This minor procedure can be performed under local anesthesia.

VARICOSE VEINS

Dilated, tortuous superficial veins associated with incompetent venous valves.

Many elderly people have moderate to large varicose veins. Often the varicosities involve only superficial veins, dilated because of incompetent valves. Valvular incompetence can be secondary to chronic venous insufficiency but typically results from primary valvular degeneration, which has a strong hereditary predisposition.

Diagnosis

Primary varicose veins must be distinguished from **secondary varicose veins** so that the secondary causes (eg, chronic venous insufficiency of the deep veins) can be addressed. Primary varicose veins lack signs of stasis and have evidence of deep and communicating vein incompetence on a tourniquet test. In this test, venous filling time is recorded when the patient rises from Trendelenburg's to a standing position. The measurement is then repeated with a tourniquet placed at various levels on the leg. *All* varicose veins fill rapidly in retrograde fashion. However, when the deep and communicating veins are competent (as occurs with secondary varicose veins), compression of the superficial veins impedes retrograde filling. If the deep veins are totally competent, complete venous filling after tourniquet application requires at least 45 sec.

Treatment

Primary varicose veins represent no danger, although they may lead to superficial phlebitis and may bleed easily if traumatized. Venous ligation and stripping procedures have almost no role in the care of the elderly. Surgery for primary varicose veins is only cosmetic, and recurrence is common. Elastic support is the only treatment necessary.

In secondary varicose veins, the cause rather than the varicose veins must be treated. For example, for varicose veins secondary to chronic venous insufficiency, stripping is useless because the pathogenesis of the venous insufficiency is related to hypertension in the deep venous system.

43. ANEURYSMS

A localized dilatation of an artery secondary to loss of smooth muscle and elastic tissue in the media.

In the elderly, aneurysms are most likely to occur at branching points (eg, the terminal aorta) or at areas of stress (eg, the popliteal artery) and are almost always of atherosclerotic origin. Systemic hypertension is a major risk factor. When a local dilatation develops, blood flow velocity decreases, leading to increased pressure against the arterial wall. This in turn results in more dilatation and perpetuates a vicious circle that often terminates in rupture of the artery. Saccular aneurysms are more likely to rupture than fusiform aneurysms because the total wall pressure is applied to a smaller area. Clinical findings and prognosis vary with the aneurysm's location and size.

THORACIC AORTIC ANEURYSM

About 80% of thoracic aortic aneurysms are secondary to atherosclerosis associated with hypertension. Tertiary syphilis remains responsible for about 14%, and these are always located in the ascending aorta. Other causes include congenital factors, Marfan's syndrome, and blunt trauma to the chest (1%).

Symptoms and Signs

Symptoms and signs are related to the site of the lesion. Dilatation of the **ascending thoracic aorta** rarely causes pain until the aneurysm ruptures. Examination may reveal a loud aortic closing sound and an early decrescendo diastolic murmur of aortic regurgitation secondary to dilatation of the aortic ring. The murmur, usually heard best in the aortic area, may be accompanied by a louder systolic murmur. Palpating the chest of a thin person who is leaning forward may reveal a pulse along the right sternal border.

Although asymptomatic when small, aneurysms of the **transverse thoracic aorta** may cause symptoms and signs of mediastinal compression—hoarseness secondary to compression of the recurrent laryngeal nerve, dysphagia, wheezing, and superior vena cava syndrome—as they enlarge. Since these aneurysms may resemble mass lesions on chest x-rays, they can easily be confused with bronchogenic carcinomas and mediastinal neoplasms.

Aneurysms of the **descending thoracic aorta** are generally asymptomatic until very large, and they can even penetrate the spine without causing pain.

Diagnosis

Diagnosis is usually made coincidentally upon review of routine chest x-rays. Generally, good posteroanterior and lateral views can distinguish the aorta from other mediastinal structures, and CT can confirm the diagnosis. If an aneurysm seems likely on chest x-ray, contrast CT is recommended to verify its size and location and to distinguish it from a silent aortic dissection. Angiography should be performed only if surgical repair is considered.

Treatment

The decision to perform surgery is based on the aneurysm's size and location, the presence of symptoms, and the patient's general condition. Aneurysms < 5 cm in transverse diameter rarely rupture, but those > 10 cm often do. Pain or compression symptoms suggest an increased likelihood of rupture.

The transverse thoracic aorta is the most critical site for surgery because it requires not only total cardiopulmonary bypass but also reanastomosis of the extracranial arteries into the graft. The descending thoracic aorta is less critical because only partial cardiopulmonary bypass is required to protect the kidneys and spinal cord. Lesions of the ascending thoracic aorta are of intermediate risk.

Surgery should not be considered for most older patients. Rather, they should have chest x-rays every 4 to 6 mo. Asymptomatic thoracic aortic aneurysms < 8 cm in size that are not expanding call for a conservative approach. Hypertension should be treated with drugs that do not increase cardiac stroke volume (which can stress the aortic wall). β-Blockers (nonvasodilator type) and calcium channel-blockers are the drugs of choice; methyldopa, clonidine, and diuretics can also be used. Vasodilators (eg, hydralazine, prazosin, and angiotensin converting enzyme inhibitors) should be avoided.

ABDOMINAL AORTIC ANEURYSM

The distal aorta is the site of the most common and most dangerous atherosclerotic aneurysms. They often involve the proximal common iliac arteries and rarely (< 2%) extend above the level of the renal arteries. These lesions almost always remain silent until they reach, or are close to, the point of rupture. An estimated 1 of 250 people > 50 yr die of a ruptured abdominal aortic aneurysm.

Symptoms, Signs, and Diagnosis

Most abdominal aneurysms can be detected by palpation. *Thorough palpation of the abdominal aorta in the elderly is unquestionably one of the most important components of the physical examination.* Typically, an aneurysm appears as an expansile mass that has both lateral and anterior pulsations. However, often only a strong pulse is felt, making it difficult to distinguish the aneurysm from generalized ectasia and tortuosity. In persons of normal girth, the aortic pulse is generally palpable in the epigastrium. A strong pulse is normal in thin patients, whereas any pulse may signal an aneurysm in obese patients. About 50% of aneurysms are associated with a bruit.

Too often, the lesion is missed or is suspected only after an abdominal x-ray is taken for another reason. An anteroposterior view may indicate curvilinear aortic calcification near the midline, whereas a lateral film may outline the aneurysm's calcified anterior and posterior walls.

Ultrasonography is the method of choice for confirming the diagnosis. It is virtually 100% accurate, providing precise information on the aneurysm's size, shape, and location. The likelihood of rupture is directly related to the aneurysm's transverse and anteroposterior diameters and inversely related to its length. Rupture is not likely with diameters < 5 cm; thereafter, the rupture rate rises quickly. Abdominal aortic aneurysms have a much faster expansion rate than thoracic aortic aneurysms.

Initially, the rupture is usually a small perforation, blocked from leaking for hours or even days by pressure from a retroperitoneal blood clot. If it is diagnosed rapidly, lifesaving surgical repair may be possible. Unexplained abdominal or lower back pain with a prominent pulsation should suggest a ruptured aneurysm until proved otherwise. In an older obese patient, sudden pain suggests the diagnosis, even if a pulsation is undetectable.

In some cases, immediate exploratory laparotomy is indicated. However, if the index of suspicion is low and the onset of pain is recent, contrast CT of the abdomen can be performed. If the aneurysm has already ruptured, retroperitoneal swelling can usually be seen. Diagnosis of rupture is the only advantage a CT scan has over ultrasonography.

Prognosis

Many studies confirm the high mortality rate associated with unrepaired abdominal aortic aneurysms. The 5-yr survival rate varies from 14% to 37%. Complications of abdominal aortic aneurysms other than rupture occur infrequently. Mural thrombi may embolize to the legs. Rarely, consumption coagulopathy occurs, resulting in thrombocytopenia, elevated thrombin time, fibrin split products in the blood, and a bleeding diathesis. An infection in the aneurysm is even more rare, but if it occurs *Salmonella* is most often implicated. Patients with a recurrent *Salmonella* septicemia of unknown origin should be evaluated for an arterial aneurysm.

Surgical repair prolongs life. With an experienced surgical team, elective repair has an operative mortality rate of < 3%, even though most patients have other manifestations of atherosclerotic disease. Contraindications to surgery include recent transient ischemic attacks and unstable angina.

Treatment

Abdominal aortic aneurysms > 5 cm in diameter usually should be repaired. Repair of slightly smaller lesions might be considered, particularly if serial sonograms show progressive enlargement and if the patient is otherwise healthy. Patients with small aneurysms can be followed up clinically and with ultrasonography every 6 mo.

Treatment of patients who have both coronary artery disease and an abdominal aneurysm is controversial. Some authorities advocate coronary angiography and bypass surgery as the first intervention, but most reserve this approach for patients with severe heart disease. Most surgeons forgo coronary angiography in patients with little or no angina and a good ejection fraction (as determined by radionuclide left ventricular cineangiography).

The management of patients with significant stable angina is open to question. One promising technique is the use of thallium scanning of the heart before and after IV injections of dipyridamole. Evidence of blood flow redistribution after dipyridamole administration is well correlated with postoperative myocardial infarction. Conventional submaximal stress tests and 48-h ambulatory ECG monitoring also can help to assess the need for coronary bypass before aneurysm repair.

POPLITEAL ARTERIAL ANEURYSM

The popliteal artery is the second most common site of aneurysm formation. Knee movements subject the artery to trauma. In addition, compression of the artery as it leaves Hunter's canal in the lower thigh leads to poststenotic dilatation, which is then exacerbated by the development of atherosclerosis. Most lesions are asymptomatic. Patients with patent aneurysms have pulsatile masses in the popliteal fossa, but an occluded aneurysm may be mistaken for a cyst. Ultrasonography is diagnostic.

Thromboembolism—either acute or as a series of small emboli to the foot—is the most common complication (16% of cases) and often necessitates amputation. Occasionally, the popliteal pulse disappears and reappears as the thrombus changes position in the aneurysmal sac. Other complications include rupture (about 10% of cases), popliteal vein compression and thrombosis, and posterior tibial nerve compression with radiating pain or sensory loss in the calf.

Treatment

Occluded aneurysms do not require specific treatment; patients should be managed as for peripheral arterial occlusion (see PERIPHERAL ATHEROSCLEROSIS in Ch. 42). Patent aneurysms, however, are quite dangerous because of the high risk of rupture and thromboembolism. Surgery is required unless the patient is very debilitated or is expected to die shortly of another cause. Spinal or even local anesthesia can be used, if necessary. The aneurysm is not resected but is bypassed and separated from the circulation by proximal ligation. Other aneurysms should be sought; 50% of patients with popliteal aneurysms also have popliteal aneurysms in the other leg, and 35% have abdominal aortic aneurysms.

FEMORAL ARTERIAL ANEURYSM

Femoral aneurysms have a course similar to that of popliteal aneurysms, can be confirmed by ultrasonography, and require surgical repair.

CAROTID ARTERIAL ANEURYSM

Carotid aneurysms are rare, occur in the midneck area, and present as pulsatile masses. Rupture is rare, but they are a source of cerebral emboli. A carotid aneurysm must be distinguished from the much more common tortuosity and bending of a carotid artery, which lacks clinical consequence. **Kinking,** usually with a strong pulse just above the clavicle, more often on the right side, is common in the elderly. Ultrasonography is useful in distinguishing kinking from aneurysmal dilatation. Surgical repair is usually indicated for carotid arterial aneurysm.

AORTIC DISSECTION

(Dissecting Aneurysm; Dissecting Hematoma)

A hemorrhage into the media after an initial intimal tear.

Aortic dissection is often inappropriately called a dissecting aneurysm. The tear occurs because of medial necrosis or severe atrophy, often as a result of chronic, sustained hypertension. Dissection secondary to Marfan's syndrome is rare after age 55.

The initial intimal tear is almost always just distal to the aortic valve **(proximal type)** or just beyond the left subclavian artery **(distal type).** Proximal dissections are reported more often, but the prevalence of distal dissections may be underestimated because clinical findings can be more subtle.

Symptoms and Signs

Symptoms are variable. Pain may be excruciating, radiating throughout the chest and back; mild and limited to one small area of the back or chest; or totally absent. The clinical findings reflect what happens to the hematoma that forms in the media, which may do any of the following: (1) extend distally along the aorta; (2) clot at any point along the aorta; (3) extend distally into any major aortic branch and compress the lumen; (4) become the major blood-flow channel in any aortic branch; (5) reenter the aorta or a branch through a second, more distal intimal tear; or (6) perforate through the adventitia at any point.

Distal dissection: The dissection may cause mild back pain, but pain is often absent. The presenting complaint is often related to regional ischemia. Patients may have abdominal pain due to mesenteric ischemia, flank pain and hematuria secondary to renal infarction, paraplegia from anterior spinal artery involvement, or leg pain because of iliac artery occlusion. Ischemia may be promptly and spontaneously reversed if the dissecting hematoma reenters the normal lumen; for example, femoral pulses that were missing may suddenly reappear. *Many areas of acute ischemia should always suggest a possible aortic dissection.*

Spontaneous healing of a dissection usually involves clotting of the hematoma followed by fibrosis around it. However, the aortic wall remains weak, and a true saccular aneurysm can develop. Because there is little support to the wall, the aneurysm usually expands and soon thereafter ruptures. During acute dissection, rapid expansion of a saccular aneurysm portends imminent rupture. Expansion occurring weeks or months later is generally less dire, although the aneurysm may rupture within days. A patient with a thoracic aortic dissection may present with the symptoms of a sudden abdominal aortic aneurysm.

A distal dissection usually perforates near the initial tear, with blood tracking into the left pleural cavity. Frequently, an initial small perforation is sealed off by a clot. A small left pleural effusion on chest x-ray may be the only clue.

Proximal dissection: Because proximal dissections often involve the aortic valve ring, the extracranial arteries, and the pericardium, they are more dangerous than distal dissections. A regurgitation murmur and a loud sound on aortic closure can usually be heard. Less frequently, hemodynamically significant acute aortic regurgitation results in low cardiac output, with pulmonary edema and hypotension. Rarely, silent dissection produces chronic aortic regurgitation, and the physician discovers either an asymptomatic diastolic murmur or a murmur and left ventricular failure.

Neurologic symptoms (eg, hemiplegia and aphasia) are common presenting complaints. The dissection may occlude both the innominate and left carotid arteries. If focal neurologic signs are present, the corresponding carotid pulse should be either diminished or absent. A lower blood pressure in the right arm is expected with left hemiplegia, as compression of the innominate artery should affect both the subclavian and carotid arteries.

If the false channel is prominent in the transverse aortic wall, findings of **mediastinal compression**—hoarseness, unilateral external jugular venous distention, and a unilateral Horner's syndrome—can occur. Death often results from rupture of the dissection into the pericardial space.

Diagnosis

Aortic dissection can be a great masquerader, with an onset that can be acute or insidious. Since the diagnosis is easily missed, certain constellations of findings should always trigger consideration of this entity (see TABLE 43–1).

Initially, **chest x-ray** is important for evaluation of the aortic shadow. The aorta almost always is somewhat prominent, especially in the elderly, but this finding is not specific to dissection. The aortic shadow is usually tortuous and uncoiled owing to long-standing hypertension, and sometimes it is very dilated. Aortic calcification not extending to the shadow's borders suggests a false channel and is specific for dissection only if a lateral view demonstrates a lack of calcium in the anterior or posterior wall.

If, after clinical evaluation and review of chest x-rays, the index of suspicion is *not* very high, echocardiography or contrast CT is indicated. Transthoracic two-dimensional **echocardiography** is useful only for proximal dissection. It can usually demonstrate the false channel and detect even subclinical degrees of aortic regurgitation. It may also demonstrate early mitral valve closure, which indicates acute aortic regurgitation. **CT scanning** can demonstrate the false channel and also

TABLE 43–1. CONSTELLATIONS OF FINDINGS IN AORTIC DISSECTION

Chest pain, hypertension, and aortic regurgitation
Chest pain radiating to the back
Chest pain with either a normal ECG or one showing left ventricular hypertrophy
Chest pain and no femoral or subclavian pulses
Chest pain and the sudden appearance of a pulsatile abdominal mass
Neurologic symptoms, with a contralateral weak carotid pulse
Left hemiplegia and hypotension in the right arm
Unilateral jugular venous distention
Many areas of ischemia
Limb embolectomy that fails to recover a thrombus
Sudden pericardial effusion

accurately delineate the aortic calcification. It appears to be as sensitive as arteriography. If both echocardiography and CT scanning results are unequivocally negative, dissection has not occurred.

Transesophageal echocardiography is now the most sensitive and specific method of diagnosing aortic dissection. In fact, it detects very small intimal flaps from very limited dissections, many of which are asymptomatic.

Aortography, usually performed in retrograde fashion through a femoral artery, can be used to assess the extent of damage and to plan a surgical approach. The aortogram typically shows the false channel, the compression of major branches, and the site of intimal tear. If the false channel contains unclotted blood, it fills with contrast material. A false channel containing clotted blood does not opacify. This finding has prognostic value, since clotting is the first step in the healing process. However, if the catheter enters the false channel, pressure from the injected contrast material can cause perforation.

Treatment

Uncomplicated **distal dissections** can be treated medically. Systemic blood pressure must be treated to decrease the rising pressure against the aortic wall: *immediate control should be obtained with a titratable agent administered by continuous IV infusion.* Either a sympathetic ganglionic blocking agent such as trimethaphan camsylate or an α- and β-adrenergic blocking agent such as labetalol can be used. At the same time, oral therapy is begun with a β-blocker and a diuretic. The dosage of oral agents is increased until the IV infusion is no longer needed. Pure vasodilators (eg, prazosin, nitroprusside, and hydralazine) and angiotensin converting enzyme inhibitors (eg, captopril and enalapril) should be *avoided* because they lead to increased left ventricular contraction—producing increased pressure against the aortic wall—and may do more harm than good. Centrally acting vasodilators (methyldopa and clonidine) have little or no effect on cardiac output and can be used if necessary. If β-blockers are contraindicated, verapamil can be used.

Surgery must be considered if pain is not reduced within the first few hours of medical therapy and eliminated within the first 2 days. After discharge, patients should be followed up weekly for the first month and at least every 3 mo afterwards. Chest x-rays should be obtained after 1 mo and every 3 to 4 mo for the first 2 yr to look for development of a saccular aneurysm. Mortality rates after 3 and 5 yr for patients with uncomplicated distal dissections are about the same, whether they are treated medically or surgically.

Proximal dissections are much more dangerous and tend to cause severe complications if treated only medically. Perforation rates are high, with pericardial tamponade being the most common cause of death. Hypertension should first be controlled with IV drugs if the patient is stable, and then surgery should be performed. Synthetic grafts that can be placed inside the thoracic aorta have simplified surgery and reduced mortality. A graft with an attached aortic valve is also available for patients with severe aortic regurgitation. After graft insertion, the false channel can be obliterated into the true lumen. A distal saccular aneurysm or interference with blood flow through any major distal aortic branch mandates repair at the local site. Thus, a combined thoracoabdominal approach is often necessary.

The small, atypical intimal tears found only by transesophageal echocardiography should be treated medically.

---

44. CARDIOVASCULAR SURGERY AND PERCUTANEOUS INTERVENTIONAL TECHNIQUES

The growing number of elderly but active patients with symptomatic heart disease has had a major impact on cardiovascular medicine in the USA. Treatments such as cardiovascular surgery, percutaneous transluminal coronary angioplasty, other percutaneous revascularization techniques, and balloon valvuloplasty are performed increasingly on elderly patients. For example, the number of patients undergoing coronary artery bypass surgery increased fivefold between 1975 and 1980, and in 1990 over 40% of these procedures were performed on patients ≥ 65 yr.

Indications for these procedures are different in older patients than in younger ones. The results of medical therapy, the coexistence of other disorders, and the short-term and long-term morbidity and mortality rates for surgery also differ in the elderly. Much of the data on percutaneous transluminal coronary angioplasty and percutaneous balloon valvuloplasty comes from a younger patient population and should not be extrapolated directly to elderly patients, especially very elderly patients. The application of these procedures to the elderly is likely to be altered substantially in the next decade.

The results of cardiovascular surgery and percutaneous interventional techniques in the elderly have improved substantially, but realistically, they will probably never be as good as those in younger patients. Recognition of the increased risk mandates meticulous patient selection and an awareness of potential intraoperative and postoperative complications. The increased risk must be weighed against the potential benefit. In selected elderly patients, excellent survival and functional improvement can be achieved.

CORONARY ARTERY BYPASS SURGERY

Clinical Profile

Direct comparisons between older and younger patients undergoing coronary artery bypass surgery or angiography alone are scanty, but the National Heart, Lung, and Blood Institute's Coronary Artery Surgery Study **(CASS)** Registry, limited to patients undergoing angiography between 1974 and 1979, is a valuable resource. Analyses of clinical and angiographic variables suggest that older patients were sicker than younger ones—a difference that could reflect the longer duration of disease in the elderly or referral patterns that lead to the selection of older patients with more severe disease or symptoms.

Older CASS patients more often had unstable angina and a history of heart failure and had a greater number of associated medical diseases than did younger patients. High-risk coronary artery disease, as evidenced by left main coronary artery stenosis of ≥ 70% and triple vessel disease, was more common in older patients undergoing coronary artery bypass surgery and receiving medical treatment. Similarly, indexes of left ventricular dysfunction, including an impaired left ventricular ejection fraction, abnormal left ventricular wall motion, cardiomegaly, and an elevated left ventricular end-diastolic pressure, were noted more frequently in elderly patients.

More recent studies of older patients undergoing coronary artery bypass surgery, such as large data bank registries from the Cleveland Clinic and Emory University, support the CASS data, particularly in regard to the greater number of coexisting conditions such as diabetes mellitus, hypertension, cerebrovascular disease, peripheral vascular disease, chronic obstructive pulmonary disease, severe and unstable angina, triple vessel disease, and left ventricular dysfunction in the elderly surgical population. These studies also show that more elderly women than elderly men undergo coronary artery bypass surgery. These variations in preoperative status are important and appear to partially account for differences between older and younger patients in length of hospital stay, short-term mortality, and long-term mortality after coronary artery bypass procedures.

Perioperative Mortality and Morbidity Rates

Analysis of 35 series of coronary artery bypass surgery performed in patients ≥ 65 yr from 1969 to 1990 reveals a perioperative mortality rate ranging from 0% to 21.1%. This wide range reflects different patient selection criteria, the relatively small size of some series, changing results over the first two decades of coronary artery bypass surgery, and age differences within the elderly population.

In the CASS Registry, the early mortality rates for isolated coronary artery bypass surgery were 5.2% in elderly patients and 1.9% in those < 65 yr. Mortality increased with age even within the elderly group: 4.6% in patients 65 to 69 yr, 6.6% in those 70 to 74 yr, and 9.5% in those ≥ 75 yr.

More recent large surgical series show improved overall operative mortality rates but a continuing trend of higher mortality with increasing age. In a large Cleveland Clinic series, the operative mortality for patients < 65 yr was < 1%; for patients 65 to 74 yr, 2%; and for those > 75, 4.3%. In six series of coronary artery bypass surgery in octogenarians performed during the 1980s, predominantly after 1985, the operative mortality ranged from 0% to 12%. Octogenarians without other significant medical illnesses who underwent elective coronary artery bypass surgery had a much lower operative mortality rate than patients with one or more coexisting illnesses or those needing urgent or emergency surgery.

The reasons for increased perioperative mortality in the elderly are not clear. In part, the increased mortality is expected in a patient population considered at high risk on the basis of many clinical and angiographic features. Elderly CASS patients considered at lower risk because of stable angina, good left ventricular function, few or no associated medical conditions, and no heart failure or left main coronary artery disease had a significantly lower perioperative mortality (see TABLE 44–1).

For the most part, the technical details of coronary artery bypass surgery are unaltered in elderly patients, although their tissues may be more friable. Abnormalities of the ascending aorta resulting from aging or severe calcific atherosclerosis or both may complicate arterial cannulation or proximal anastomoses in older patients. Intraoperative epicardial or transesophageal echocardiography appears to help minimize these difficulties and to facilitate diagnosis and modification of surgical technique. Increased use of intraoperative echocardiography may help reduce the risk of atheroembolism, but more data are needed.

Nonetheless, analysis of the CASS and other data suggests that other unmeasured or as yet unidentified variables intrinsically associated with aging adversely influence the outcome of coronary artery bypass surgery (see TABLE 44–2). In an analysis of 7658 patients undergoing isolated coronary artery bypass surgery, age ≥ 65 yr was an independent adverse predictor of survival, although not the most powerful. This emphasizes that the greater the risk of a procedure, the more stringent the criteria for its implementation should be.

TABLE 44–1. INDEPENDENT PREDICTORS OF MORTALITY AFTER CORONARY ARTERY BYPASS SURGERY IN ELDERLY PATIENTS

Predictors of Perioperative Mortality	*Predictors of Late Mortality (in perioperative survivors)*
Left ventricular dysfunction	Left ventricular dysfunction
Ejection fraction < 50%	Functional impairment caused by heart failure
Pulmonary rales	Abnormal left ventricular wall motion
Prior myocardial infarction	Increased left ventricular end-diastolic pressure
Heart failure	Associated medical conditions
Increased left ventricular end-diastolic pressure	Peripheral vascular disease
Emergency surgery	
Prior coronary artery bypass surgery	
Class IV angina (angina with minimal activity)	
Unstable angina	
Current cigarette smoking	
Left main coronary artery stenosis	
Associated medical illnesses	
Hypertension	

Perioperative morbidity is also higher in the elderly, in whom stroke, supraventricular arrhythmias, transient psychoses, heart block, pulmonary embolism, postoperative bleeding, respiratory distress, and renal failure occur more frequently than in younger persons. This increased morbidity results in longer hospital stays, and as age increases, so does length of stay. For example, among CASS patients, the mean length of hospital stay was 11.4 days in those < 65 yr, 12.9 days in those 65 to 69 yr, 14.0 days in those 70 to 74 yr, and 16.5 days in those ≥ 75 yr. Since that study, the absolute duration of hospitalization has declined in all age groups, although the elderly, particularly the oldest age groups, continue to require longer hospitalization.

Long-term Results

Survival rates: In a large series from the Cleveland Clinic, the 10-yr survival rate was 78.8% for those < 65 yr and 64.2% for those 65 to 74 yr. The 8-yr survival rate was 53.3% for patients ≥ 75 yr. Preoperative left ventricular dysfunction and associated medical diseases strongly affect long-term survival. The 10-yr survival rate was 68% in patients ≥ 65 yr with normal left ventricular function but only 58% in those with left ventricular dysfunction.

The overall 5-yr survival (including perioperative mortality) rate for CASS patients was 83% in elderly patients with normal left ventricular wall motion, 89% in those who had no associated medical conditions,

TABLE 44–2. INDEPENDENT PREDICTORS OF MORTALITY AFTER CORONARY ARTERY BYPASS SURGERY IN PATIENTS OF ALL AGES

Severity of heart failure
Left main coronary artery stenosis of ≥ 70%
Age ≥ 65 yr
Severity of abnormal left ventricular wall motion
Female sex
Unstable angina pectoris

and only 37% in those with left ventricular dysfunction. Thus, key elements in the preoperative assessment of the elderly are analyses of clinical and angiographic characteristics together with the operative risk at the physician's institution.

Functional outcome: Several studies note that angina is relieved as effectively or possibly more effectively in older patients than in younger ones after surgery, although reduced activity in the elderly may also relieve angina. Nevertheless, older patients who successfully undergo coronary artery bypass surgery report good outcomes, and mental health function appears better in patients ≥ 65 yr than in those < 65 yr. In older patients, as in younger ones, the symptomatic benefits of coronary artery bypass surgery tend to be better in men, with angina having a higher recurrence in women.

Surgery vs. medical therapy: No data from randomized controlled studies are available on the elderly. Information from large, multicenter randomized trials of coronary artery bypass surgery and medical therapy cannot be extrapolated directly to the elderly because these trials, conducted when perioperative mortality in the elderly was high, excluded patients > 65 yr.

A comparison of surgical and medical therapy in 1491 CASS patients with symptomatic angina pectoris shows a cumulative survival rate at 6 yr (after adjustment for major differences in baseline characteristics) of 79% in the surgical group and 64% in the medical group. Relief of chest pain was also significantly greater in surgical patients. A small, nonrandomized series comparing surgical and medical therapy in octogenarians showed that the 3-yr survival rates were 77.4% for the surgical group and 55.2% for the medical group. Also, function improved significantly in the surgical group but not the medical group. However, nonrandomized studies are subject to bias and cannot supplant a randomized trial. No amount of statistical adjustment can eliminate all bias, and such bias could significantly influence conclusions.

TABLE 44–3. CONSIDERATIONS IN ASSESSING THE ELDERLY FOR CORONARY ARTERY BYPASS SURGERY

Severity of symptoms and their effect on quality of life
Pharmacologic therapy of angina pectoris and heart failure
Efficacy
Toxicity
Psychosocial factors
Patient's desires, motivation, and lifestyle
Physiologic age (as opposed to chronologic age)
Associated medical diseases
Coexisting cardiac conditions
Severity and extent of coronary artery and valvular heart disease
Potential for adequate revascularization
Left ventricular function

Very likely, the improved survival among the surgical groups in both studies reflects the high-risk preoperative status of elderly patients. In the CASS Registry a subset of lower-risk older patients who had mild stable angina, well-preserved left ventricular function, and no left main coronary artery disease showed a survival pattern that mirrored those in randomized trials of younger patients with similar characteristics; ie, there was no difference in survival between those treated surgically and those treated medically.

Assessment

A preoperative assessment that focuses on the whole patient, not just a specific organ or system, is crucial to a successful outcome (see TABLE 44–3). Certain factors specific to the elderly should be considered when deciding whether to perform coronary artery bypass surgery.

In older patients, an assessment of the severity of angina pectoris and its effect on quality of life may be complicated by vagaries of memory, the masking of symptoms by reduced physical activity, the frequency of anginal equivalents such as dyspnea, and coexisting medical conditions simulating angina, such as cervical spine disease and diaphragmatic hernias.

Even when elderly patients change their lifestyles to reduce activity levels, medical control of angina pectoris often is hampered by the severity of symptoms and coronary pathology. *Attaining maximum medical therapy is more difficult in the elderly* for these reasons:

1. Alterations in pharmacokinetics, eg, from decreased renal function and hepatic perfusion, may result in higher plasma levels of some drugs.

2. The elderly are more likely to experience adverse effects secondary to age-related changes in cerebral blood flow, impaired reflexes leading to orthostatic hypotension, and associated diseases.

3. Social factors leading to reduced compliance and comprehension may limit the efficacy of medical therapy.

An understanding of the patient's desires, motivation, and lifestyle is also important in determining therapy. In this regard, an evaluation of physiologic age as opposed to chronologic age may be helpful. Close attention to coexisting medical conditions is essential. A clinical and social history, physical examination, and routine laboratory investigations should provide most of the necessary information.

The clinical data must be reviewed along with angiographic assessment of the severity and extent of disease, the potential for adequate revascularization, and the presence and severity of left ventricular dysfunction and other cardiac conditions (eg, aortic stenosis and conduction disease).

Postoperative Treatment

In the postoperative intensive care unit, where physiologic monitoring and respiratory support may be prolonged, preventing sepsis is a major goal. The higher incidence of postoperative psychoses and a tendency toward reduced mobility in the elderly require that attention also be given to chest physiotherapy and wound care. This is particularly true in the very old, ie, those > 80 yr. Gradual but steady resumption of normal activity, mobility, and independence are the major objectives of postoperative treatment.

PERCUTANEOUS TRANSLUMINAL CORONARY ANGIOPLASTY

Percutaneous transluminal coronary angioplasty (PTCA) is a less invasive procedure and has a shorter recovery time than coronary artery bypass surgery, both of which are advantages in elderly patients, particularly those with coexisting diseases that could adversely affect short-term and long-term outcomes. In 1990, nearly 50% of PTCAs in the USA were performed in people > 65 yr.

Further study is needed to compare the risk-vs.-benefit ratio of PTCA with that of coronary artery bypass surgery and to determine whether PTCA is an equally effective approach to revascularization. Several randomized tests are under way. Meanwhile, a critical review of published data on PTCA in the elderly provides the best information for decision making.

Clinical Profile

Elderly patients undergoing PTCA are sicker than younger ones, as is the case with patients undergoing coronary artery bypass surgery. Analysis of the National Heart, Lung, and Blood Institute's PTCA Registry and other large registries from individual medical institutions confirms that older PTCA patients have more extensive coronary artery disease and are more symptomatic with a higher frequency of class III angina (angina with light exercise), class IV angina (angina with minimal activity), and unstable angina. Unstable angina occurs in up to 80% of those > 75 yr, compared with about 50% of patients < 65 yr. Diabetes mellitus, hypertension, and a history of heart failure are more frequently seen in the elderly. In the National Heart, Lung, and Blood Institute's PTCA Registry, the incidence of prior heart failure was 4% in persons < 65 yr and > 9% in those > 65 yr. In a large series from the Mayo Clinic, the incidence of prior heart failure was 24% in persons > 75 yr.

Results

The technical feasibility of PTCA in the elderly is well established. In more recent series of elderly patients, the initial success rate ranges from 82% to 96%, which approximates the success rate in younger patients. The technical success rate is high even for very old patients. As with coronary artery bypass surgery, however, the mortality and morbidity rates for PTCA are higher in the oldest patients. In a large series from the Mayo Clinic, the mortality rate associated with PTCA was 1.2% in those 65 to 70 yr and 6% in those > 75 yr. Similarly, in a large registry series of multivessel PTCA in the elderly from the Mid-American Heart Institute, the mortality rate was 0.8% for patients 65 to 69 yr and 6.3% for those > 80 yr.

The increase in procedure-related mortality in the oldest patients appears to be largely attributable to advanced disease in frail persons. The most powerful predictor of procedural mortality is diffuse coronary artery disease. Age per se, even among patients > 65 yr, has been found to be an independent predictor of procedural mortality in some series but not in others. The same is true of poor left ventricular function.

Overall, long-term survival after PTCA is good in elderly patients, even in the very old. For example, a series from the Mayo Clinic reported a 4-yr survival rate of 86% in those > 75 yr, a percentage comparable with those for younger subgroups (see also TABLE 44–4).

Most elderly patients with angina who undergo successful coronary artery bypass surgery obtain excellent long-term relief. On the other hand, patients > 75 yr who undergo PTCA appear to have more recurrent angina than do younger patients. Older patients have more extensive coronary artery disease, and limited procedures are often performed in frail elderly persons. Restenosis occurs in 30% to 40% of successful PTCA cases; a higher restenosis rate has not been found in the elderly. However, predisposing factors for restenosis such as unstable angina and diabetes mellitus are more common in older patients.

Thus, the increased recurrence of angina may be related largely to more severe coronary artery disease. The extent of coronary artery disease appears to be the strongest independent predictor of late adverse

TABLE 44–4. INDEPENDENT PREDICTORS OF MORTALITY AFTER PERCUTANEOUS TRANSLUMINAL CORONARY ANGIOPLASTY IN ELDERLY PATIENTS

Predictors of Periprocedural Mortality	*Predictors of Late Mortality (in periprocedural survivors)*
Extensive coronary artery disease	Extensive coronary artery disease
Ejection fraction < 40%	Coexisting medical problems
	Left ventricular dysfunction

outcome in older patients. The number of coexisting medical conditions and left ventricular dysfunction are also independent predictors of late adverse outcome.

Assessment

Treatment for coronary artery disease must be individualized. The decision to perform revascularization and the choice of coronary artery bypass surgery or PTCA should be based on a realistic appraisal of the likelihood of success. Age should not be the sole criterion, but the patient's physiologic age and general physical condition are important considerations. The physician must also consider the significance of other medical conditions, the patient's ability to tolerate medications, the patient's activity level and expectations, and the technical feasibility of the particular revascularization procedure. Enhancing independence and quality of life are important goals in treating elderly patients with symptomatic angina.

VALVE REPLACEMENT

(See also Ch. 38)

Clinical Profile

Since the 1980s, patients undergoing valve replacement surgery have been older than those undergoing it in the 1960s and early 1970s. In Olmstead County, Minnesota, between 1980 and 1983, the peak incidence of valve replacements in men was in the 75-yr to 79-yr age group, and in women, in the 65-yr to 74-yr age group. At the Mayo Clinic between 1981 and 1985, 50% of aortic valve replacements for stenosis were in patients ≥ 70 yr; between 1965 and 1980, only 21% of these replacements were in patients ≥ 70 yr.

In patients undergoing aortic valve replacement at the Mayo Clinic, degenerative (senile) calcification is the most common cause of aortic stenosis. The incidence of congenital bicuspid aortic valves has declined slightly, and the incidence of postinflammatory (primarily rheumatic) disease has declined markedly. This pattern may relate to the increasing age of patients undergoing aortic valve replacement and to other factors such as referral patterns, changing life expectancy, and the impact of newer noninvasive diagnostic techniques. In patients undergoing mitral valve replacement, the incidence of postinflammatory disease has similarly declined, whereas that of degenerative mitral valve disease has increased.

Results

The results of valve replacement in elderly patients have improved because of refinements in surgical and myocardial preservation techniques and advances in preoperative and postoperative care. Although comparable results have been reported in older and younger patients, advanced age is generally considered a significant risk factor for early morbidity and mortality, partly because of an association with coexisting diseases.

A review of 14 recent series that included 1947 patients > 70 yr who underwent aortic valve replacement during the 1970s and 1980s revealed an overall operative mortality rate of 12.7% (range, 5.9% to 28%), which is higher than that in younger patients. Operative mortality is higher for those with aortic valve insufficiency than for those with aortic stenosis; it is also higher for emergency and urgent operations. Operative mortality is higher for combined aortic valve replacement and coronary artery bypass surgery than for aortic valve replacement alone. With isolated elective aortic valve replacement for stenosis in patients in their mid-70s, the expected operative mortality rate is 5% to 6%, based on the largest recent surgical series.

A review of six recent series of 315 octogenarians undergoing aortic valve replacement for stenosis primarily during the 1980s shows an overall operative mortality rate of 15.5%.

Mortality for multiple valve replacements is considerably higher. The wide range of reported results reflects the nature and cause of the lesions, the acuity of clinical presentations, differences in patient selection criteria, changing surgical techniques, and the valves replaced.

As expected, postoperative morbidity is generally higher in the elderly, with an increased frequency of respiratory distress, bleeding, supraventricular arrhythmias, conduction disturbances, delayed wound healing, psychoses, and stroke. Whether advanced age alone is associated with a poorer long-term functional result is not clearly established. However, judiciously timed valve replacement in the symptomatic elderly patient with severe valvular heart disease usually results in long-term survival and symptomatic improvement. Long-term (5 to 10 yr) survival with valve replacement appears far superior to that attainable with medical therapy alone.

Assessment

An assessment of the severity of symptoms, coexisting medical diseases, associated cardiac conditions, and psychosocial factors is as important for the patient with valvular heart disease as it is for the patient with primary coronary artery disease.

Age alone does not contraindicate valve replacement or repair. The indications for the procedure in the elderly are similar to those in younger patients: the severity of symptoms, the nature of the valve lesion (whether regurgitant or stenotic), the cause of the disorder, and left ventricular function.

Using **coronary angiography** to identify lesions that are caused by significant stenosis but can be bypassed is a generally accepted part of the preoperative assessment in the elderly. In **aortic stenosis,** poor left ventricular function apparently does not contraindicate surgery, provided the mechanical effects of the valve lesion are the primary cause of the patient's clinical status. In **valvular insufficiency,** prolonged delay in referring an elderly patient for surgery may result in irreversible left ventricular dysfunction, with a markedly adverse impact on early and late results.

The **choice of a valve substitute** in the elderly warrants a comprehensive preoperative assessment and discussion with the patient. In patients who have sinus rhythm, a **biologic prosthesis** (especially an aortic one) is associated with a lower incidence of thromboembolism. A biologic prosthesis is particularly valuable in patients $\geq$ 70 yr because long-term durability of the prosthesis is less important and the risks of chronic anticoagulant therapy are higher. In this age group, biologic prostheses (eg, Carpentier-Edwards, Hancock) are generally recommended. The favorable hemodynamic characteristics of certain low-profile mechanical valves (eg, St. Jude Medical, Medtronic-Hall, Starr-Edwards) may warrant their use in specific situations; often this decision can be made with confidence only during the operation.

Aortic valve decalcification for senile degenerative calcific valve disease on a tricuspid aortic valve is no longer recommended because of a high incidence of subsequent acute valve insufficiency. On the other hand, elderly patients with mitral regurgitation may benefit from **mitral valve repair,** thus avoiding the need for valve replacement.

The prevalence of coronary artery disease in elderly patients with valvular disease raises the question of whether **coronary revascularization** should be performed at the same time as valvular surgery, particularly in patients who do not have angina or prior myocardial infarction. The increased operative mortality entailed by performing concomitant coronary artery bypass surgery has diminished in recent years, but no randomized controlled studies comparing the merits of the two approaches are available.

Generally, severely obstructed but operable coronary arteries should be bypassed at the time of valve surgery, even when angina is absent.

However, the decision to perform coronary artery bypass surgery should be based on the clinical and hemodynamic status of the patient both preoperatively and intraoperatively.

PERCUTANEOUS BALLOON VALVULOPLASTY

For frail elderly patients with aortic stenosis who are not surgical candidates or who are high-risk surgical candidates, balloon valvuloplasty offers palliation of symptoms. The major limitation of balloon aortic valvuloplasty is a high rate of restenosis. Within 2 yr, about 80% of patients have recurrent symptoms leading to a second balloon valvuloplasty, aortic valve replacement, or death. Therefore, patients who are surgical candidates are better treated with surgery.

Results

For frail persons who are not considered surgical candidates, balloon aortic valvuloplasty has a relatively low mortality rate. In the National Heart, Lung, and Blood Institute's Balloon Valvuloplasty Registry, 83% of the patients were > 70 yr, and 80% were not surgical candidates. During the procedure, 3% died; the 30-day mortality rate was 14%. However, morbidity was relatively high; 31% experienced significant complications before discharge, the most common being a need for blood transfusion.

Series reporting acute hemodynamic results in balloon aortic valvuloplasty are remarkably consistent. The average aortic valve area typically increases by 0.3 cm^2 (from 0.5 cm^2 to 0.8 cm^2) with significant reduction in symptoms. Thus, the procedure offers considerable relief and acceptable mortality risk in very ill patients.

Percutaneous balloon mitral valvotomy is comparable to surgical commissurotomy, providing similar hemodynamic improvement, symptomatic improvement, and intermediate-term symptom-free survival. In patients > 65 yr, the procedure-related mortality is usually ≤ 3%. The success of balloon valvuloplasty depends heavily on the characteristics of the diseased mitral valve. Pliable, noncalcified, and less severely stenotic mitral valves are associated with the best results. However, elderly patients with mitral stenosis most often have thickened, nonpliable, and calcified mitral valves because of long-term rheumatic disease. In the largest series of elderly patients undergoing balloon mitral valvotomy at Massachusetts General Hospital, the procedure was an unqualified success in 46% of cases, and the mitral valve area was increased to > 1 cm^2 in 86%. Performed by experienced clinicians, balloon valvuloplasty is a very good option for patients with pliable, noncalcified mitral valves or for those in whom cardiac surgery offers an increased risk.

SURGERY FOR COMPLICATIONS OF MYOCARDIAL INFARCTION

When the left ventricular free wall, papillary muscle, or interventricular septum ruptures following an acute myocardial infarction, mortality is very high unless surgical repair is promptly undertaken.

Left-Ventricular Free-Wall Rupture

This type of rupture occurs in 1% to 3% of all patients with a myocardial infarction and is more common in the elderly. Such ruptures are also more common in women and in those with first infarcts. Usually, the rupture occurs abruptly and unexpectedly so that emergency surgery is not feasible. Rarely, a subacute rupture occurs, causing cardiovascular collapse; the patient presents with signs of cardiac tamponade. In such a patient, emergency cardiac surgery, perhaps after rapid stabilization with pericardiocentesis, volume expansion, intra-aortic balloon pump placement, and other medical therapy, offers hope of survival.

Papillary Muscle Rupture

Postinfarction rupture of a papillary muscle with resulting severe mitral regurgitation is more common in the elderly. At the Mayo Clinic, the average age of 22 patients undergoing surgery for this condition was 68 yr. In all but three cases, surgery was performed within 3 wk of the myocardial infarction and the overall operative mortality rate was 27%. Short-term and long-term mortality was slightly higher in patients with ejection fractions $< 45\%$, but age was not a predictor of survival. Patients with papillary muscle rupture and severe mitral regurgitation should undergo surgery promptly because they may deteriorate rapidly, and surgery generally has good results. Age should not be a major consideration.

Ventricular Septum Rupture

The results of surgery for rupture of the ventricular septum are somewhat less encouraging. A Mayo Clinic series of 77 patients with postinfarction septal rupture seen between 1965 and 1991 had an average age of 68 yr. Among patients with cardiogenic shock, only the group that underwent prompt surgical repair included survivors, and even in this group the mortality rate was 62%. Among patients with heart failure, about 50% of those undergoing surgery survived, but none of the patients treated medically lived longer than 30 days. Age was found to be an independent predictor of survival. Prompt surgery is advised for most patients with postinfarction rupture of the ventricular septum.

§3. ORGAN SYSTEMS: PULMONARY DISORDERS

GASTROINTESTINAL DISORDERS

§3. ORGAN SYSTEMS: PULMONARY DISORDERS

45. THE EFFECTS OF AGE ON THE LUNG

Aging affects not only the physiologic functions of the lungs (ventilation and gas exchange) but also the ability of the lungs to defend themselves. The specific biologic mechanisms responsible for these changes are unknown. For example, it is not known whether the progressive decline in pulmonary function results from exposure to environmental toxins or from progressive subclinical exhaustion of internal respiratory reserve and repair caused by aging itself.

The association of airway obstruction with age may be partially explained by an accumulation of inflammatory injuries. Repeated disruption of the balance of inflammatory mediators and humoral protection (elastase and antielastase, oxidant and antioxidant), neutrophil recruitment, and tissue repair that culminates in inflammatory lung destruction and airway obstruction has been well documented in cigarette smokers. Accumulated environmental oxidant injuries could result in similar, although usually less extensive, lung destruction in nonsmokers.

Airway obstruction (but not chronic bronchitis) is associated with increased age-specific death rates from all causes (most of which result from cardiovascular disease). In fact, survival parallels preservation of ventilatory function. The Baltimore Longitudinal Study of Aging showed that persons with the greatest loss of ventilatory function had a fourfold to sixfold risk of death from coronary artery disease. Besides increasing the risk of death from chronic obstructive pulmonary disease and heart disease, airway obstruction increases the risk of lung cancer. *Thus, an increased risk for three of the five leading causes of death in men and for three of the seven leading causes of death in women can be identified by impaired pulmonary function on spirometric testing.*

Pulmonary Compliance

Age-related changes in ventilation and gas distribution result primarily from changes in compliance of the lungs and the chest wall. Lung volumes at rest are determined by the equilibrium between inward elastic tissue forces of the lung and outward forces of the chest wall and muscles of respiration. During the developmental years, growth of the lungs and chest wall parallels the growth of the body and correlates closely with height. At about age 55, respiratory muscle strength begins to weaken. This weakened outward muscular force and the increased stiffness of the chest wall (decreased compliance) are counterbalanced by a loss of elastic recoil of the lungs (increased compliance).

Lung recoil results from the combined effects of parenchymal elastic fibers and inward-directed surface forces from the air-fluid interface of the terminal respiratory units. There is no evidence that the surface forces or the opposing surfactant effect is altered with age. Therefore, the age-related loss of elastic recoil probably results from a change in the elastic fibers. Yet, after the early 20s, age has no effect on the length or diameter of individual elastic fibers, and no evidence suggests that the overall elastin or collagen content of the lung changes with age. Thus, the age-related increase in lung compliance may result from lost alveolar attachments or damage to the elastic fibers. An exaggerated increase in alveolar dilatation without loss of alveolar attachments, described as "senile lung," has been found in a small number of autopsies of patients > 60 yr. This architectural disruption in the older lung increases the proportion of collapsible small airways.

With age, the chest wall gradually becomes stiffer, probably as a result of ossification of cartilage-rib articulations and progressive dorsal kyphosis. The increased outward pull of the stiffer chest wall combined with the reduced ability of the lung to pull inward results in a small, age-related increase in total lung capacity and a larger increase in functional residual capacity (the volume at which the lung comes to rest at the end of a quiet expiration) and residual volume (the volume that remains in the lung after a maximal expiration).

Rates of Airflow

During forced expiration, increasing contraction of the voluntary muscles of the chest wall and the elastic recoil of the lungs increase expiratory airflow until dynamic compression of the airways limits further expiratory flow (usually after about 25% of the vital capacity has been exhaled). Collapse of the airways occurs at the equal pressure point; it is prevented by intra-alveolar (upstream) pressure generated by the elastic recoil of the lung. Age-related loss of this elastic recoil results in early collapse of poorly supported peripheral airways. Therefore, dynamic compression of the smaller airways in older lungs may lead to decreased flow at low lung volumes, similar to the small airway obstruction produced by chronic cigarette smoking.

Forced expiratory airflows peak at age 20 in women and age 22 in men as a result of the patterns of growth and muscle development of the chest wall. The decreases in forced vital capacity (FVC) and maximal expiratory flow rate that occur until age 40 are thought to result from changes in body weight and strength rather than tissue attrition. Cross-sectional studies of pulmonary function have identified a constant (linear) decline of 24 mL of forced expiratory volume in the first sec (FEV_1) and 21 mL in the FVC with each increasing year of age in men. These observations are based on single examinations of persons of various ages in the general population. However, when participants are followed, the annual decline in FEV_1 is small at first and increases more rapidly with age.

Distribution of Ventilation

The elastic fibers within alveolar walls are tethered to the respiratory and terminal bronchioles, helping to maintain the patency of these small conducting airways at low lung volumes. The loss of these elastic attachments leads to increased compliance, collapse of small conducting airways, nonuniformity of alveolar ventilation, and air trapping. One consequence is an increase in physiologic dead space with increasing age.

Arterial Oxygen Tension

The linear deterioration of arterial oxygen tension (PaO_2) associated with aging (about 0.3%/yr) has long been recognized. This gradual decline in PaO_2 with advancing age parallels the loss of elastic recoil and the increase in physiologic dead space. As described earlier, the progressive loss of elastic recoil leads to a reduction in airway caliber, early airway closure, and maldistribution of ventilation. Although collapse of peripheral airways decreases ventilation to distal gas exchange units, perfusion remains unaffected. Thus, a ventilation-perfusion imbalance is created that accounts for most of the reduction in PaO_2. The ventilation-perfusion imbalance is particularly treacherous in older persons because the PaO_2 (and thus oxygen delivery) may be further compromised by age-associated reductions in cardiac output. When ventilation and perfusion are evenly matched, changing cardiac output has little effect on PaO_2. As ventilation-perfusion inequalities worsen, the PaO_2 decreases at any given cardiac output; further loss of cardiac output magnifies the reduction in oxygen delivery.

Diffusing Capacity

The single-breath carbon monoxide diffusing capacity (DL_{CO}) peaks in the early 20s, then gradually declines because of both morphologic changes (loss of alveolar-capillary surface area) and increasing heterogeneities in ventilation or blood flow. The loss of surface area for gas exchange results from the destruction of alveoli with an accompanying loss of capillary bed. The reduction in DL_{CO} is estimated at 0.5% (0.2 mL/min/mm Hg)/yr; women have 10% lower diffusing capacity values than men of the same age and height. The age-related decline in DL_{CO} is not linear.

Pulmonary resistance to gas diffusion comes from two sources: the area and thickness of the alveolar-capillary membrane and the ability of the gas to combine with elements of the blood. Age-related decreases in total pulmonary diffusing capacity result primarily from a loss of membrane diffusing capacity, which becomes more prominent after age 40.

Control of Breathing

Heart rate and ventilatory responses to hypoxia and hypercapnia diminish with age; thus, otherwise healthy elders may be more vulnerable to poor outcomes from diseases producing lower oxygen levels (eg, pneumonia, chronic obstructive pulmonary disease). Age appears to attenuate chemoreceptor function, either at peripheral or central chemoreceptors or in the integrating CNS pathways. The ventilatory response to hypoxia is reduced by 51% in healthy men ages 64 to 73 compared with healthy men ages 22 to 30; the ventilatory response to hypercapnia is reduced by 41%.

The reduced ventilatory responses to hypoxia and hypercapnia in the elderly are independent of the changes in mechanical properties of the lung. These ventilatory responses are accompanied by decreased inspiratory occlusive pressure—a measure of total neuromuscular drive to breathe, which is unaffected by mechanics of the respiratory system. Thus the elderly, who are most likely to be afflicted with chronic pulmonary diseases, are least able to defend against acute hypoxia or hypercapnia because of reductions in both their mechanical ability to ventilate and their diminished neural drive to breathe.

Exercise Capacity

The ability to deliver oxygen to the tissues (maximal oxygen consumption, or $V_{O_2}max$) is the standard measurement of physical work (exercise) capacity. The $V_{O_2}max$ measures the integrated performance of the three components of the system transporting oxygen from outside air to working muscles: pulmonary ventilation, blood circulation, and muscle tissue. At any age, the $V_{O_2}max$ is related to the physical dimensions of these components: pulmonary (vital capacity, diffusing capacity), cardiovascular (heart volume, blood volume, RBC mass), and skeletal (muscle mass). Because body size is such an important component of $V_{O_2}max$, this measure of fitness often takes weight into consideration and is expressed as maximal oxygen uptake per kilogram of body weight, or $V_{O_2}max/kg$. Measurement of lean body mass is a more reliable predictor of cardiorespiratory performance than weight, especially in obese persons. Lean body mass may be obtained from body weight by correcting for body fat, an estimate made from skin fold measurements or underwater weighing.

Work capacity (as measured by $V_{O_2}max$) increases during childhood, peaks in the late teens, plateaus until the mid-20s, then gradually declines. The increase results from the growth of muscle, heart, and lungs, and the decline results in part from gradual reductions in maximal heart rate and muscle mass with advancing years. The gradual decline in oxygen delivery (32 mL/min/yr in men and 14 mL/min/yr in women) can be approximated by an equation, although only body size and age are considered in the regression.

Decreases in cardiac output may result from specific changes in cardiac biochemistry and metabolism, such as age-related declines in maximal myocardial oxygen consumption and substrate oxidation rates. Although pulmonary function measurements such as FEV_1 decline with age, reduced ventilation seldom limits exercise in healthy persons. However, in patients with a ventilatory capacity reduced sufficiently to limit exercise, the FEV_1 is a reasonably accurate indicator of maximal ventilation in exercise. Typically, the reduced $V_{O_2}max$ in elderly persons with mild to moderate airway obstruction results from cardiovascular deconditioning associated with lower levels of habitual physical activity. Regular training can substantially slow the decline in maximal oxygen delivery from age-related cardiovascular deconditioning.

The differences in work capacity between similarly aged men and women largely disappear when other factors, such as size (lean body mass), hemoglobin level, and levels of structured activity (training) are taken into account. The same is true for differences among races.

Finally, total muscle mass gradually declines with increasing age because of a reduction in the number of muscle fibers. Because the metabolic capacity, enzymatic profile, and capillary density of the muscle fibers in elderly persons appear to be the same as those in younger persons, the age-related decrease in aerobic exercise capacity is quantitatively linked to attrition of lean muscle mass, not to functional impairment of the muscles or pulmonary changes. This decline, too, may be slowed by exercise training.

Defense Mechanisms

The defense mechanisms of the lungs include clearance mechanisms, humoral immunity, and cellular immunity.

Clearance mechanisms: An inverse relationship exists between age and the rate of mucociliary transport. However, the importance of mucociliary transport as a pulmonary defense mechanism has not been clearly demonstrated, even though it removes inhaled particulate matter from the ciliated airways. Nevertheless, clinical observation of patients with Kartagener's syndrome (situs inversus, chronic sinusitis, and bronchiectasis) who also have immotile spermatozoa and lack pulmonary ciliary function suggests that primary ciliary immotility leads to recurrent respiratory tract infections and, eventually, chronic bronchitis and bronchiectasis. If these observations are correct, the diminished mucociliary clearance associated with increasing age may have clinical significance.

The loss of an effective cough reflex (and subsequent aspiration) contributes to an increased susceptibility to pneumonia in the elderly. The elderly are subject to many conditions associated with reduced consciousness, including sedative use and neurologic diseases, which may result in the loss of an effective cough reflex. When other clearance mechanisms are intact, the cough reflex is not essential for respiratory tract clearance, though it is a powerful adjunct. However, when a patient has dysphagia or impaired esophageal motility, conditions that occur more often in old age, an intact cough reflex is a necessary defense.

Humoral immunity: Blood immunoglobulin levels are only a rough guide to humoral immune competence. Despite the lack of age-related changes in IgA and IgG levels, the acute antibody response to extrinsic antigens, such as pneumococcal and influenza vaccines, is considerably reduced in old age. Possibly, the circulating immunoglobulin levels reflect an increased production of antibodies to various intrinsic antigens (ie, autoantibodies), which replaces the production of antibodies to extrinsic antigens. Interestingly, serum values of IgM decrease with age, although the significance of this observation remains unknown (see also Ch. 84).

The ability to generate an effective humoral response depends on the interaction among helper T cells, suppressor T cells, macrophages, and B cells. Age-related reductions in helper T cell activity, increases in suppressor T cell activity, and the reduced ability of B cells to produce normal heterogeneous high-affinity antibodies in response to an antigen have all been seen. In contrast, the mucosa-associated IgA secretory antibody production shows no age-related decline in functional capabilities.

Cellular immunity: With age, cell-mediated immunity decreases. One manifestation of cell-mediated immunity, delayed hypersensitivity, is demonstrated clinically by the number of positive skin reactions to five common antigens. The number of positive skin tests declines in those $>$ 60 yr; in one study, this skin test hyporesponsiveness correlated with increased mortality over 2 yr. A functional depression in lymphocytes in those ages 75 to 96 compared with those ages 25 to 50 has been demonstrated experimentally by a reduced blastogenic response to plant mitogens (phytohemagglutinin and concanavalin A mitogens).

The decline in cell-mediated immunity with increasing age correlates with an increasing frequency of secondary tuberculosis (reactivation tuberculosis). However, even though a reduction in thymic hormone levels is clearly age related, the association of thymic involution to increased susceptibility to infection in the elderly remains speculative.

46. PNEUMONIA AND TUBERCULOSIS

PNEUMONIA

An inflammatory reaction to microbes or microbial products involving the pulmonary parenchyma.

Pneumonias are the most common fatal infections; they are the sixth leading cause of death by disease in the USA, and the fourth leading cause of death in the elderly. Sir William Osler referred to pneumonia as "a special enemy of old age" in the first edition of his famous textbook, but he referred to it as "the friend of the aged" in the third edition. It is perhaps befitting that he eventually died of a lingering case of pneumonia, during which his major regret was that he "would not be able to witness the autopsy."

A review of 44,684 cases of pneumonia in Massachusetts between 1921 and 1930 showed that the incidence of pneumonia increased about fivefold for patients in their 80s compared with those in their 20s. Far more striking was the nearly hundredfold increase in the mortality rate for those > 70 yr, a rate that increased about 10% for each decade after age 20. Pneumonia is found in 25% to 60% of elderly patients at autopsy, often a late complication of another fatal condition.

The hospitalized elderly have a threefold greater incidence of nosocomial pneumonia than do younger patients. It is the most common fatal nosocomial infection in acute-care facilities and also a major problem in chronic-care facilities, where its prevalence may be as high as 50 times that in age-matched, home-based patients. The yearly incidence varies from 20/1000 to 40/1000 for community-acquired pneumonias to 100/1000 to 250/1000 for pneumonias acquired in chronic-care facilities. At any given time, as many as 2.1% of nursing home residents may have lower respiratory tract infections.

Etiology

Because expectorated sputum is contaminated during passage through the upper airways, valid information concerning the distribution of specific pathogens is limited. In addition, no specific pathogen is detected in 30% to 50% of cases. More reliable diagnostic specimen sources—transtracheal aspirate culture, blood culture, and specific serologic tests—implicate the following microorganisms as the most common causes of pneumonia in the elderly: *Streptococcus pneumoniae*, gram-negative bacilli, anaerobic bacteria, *Legionella pneumophila*, and viruses, especially the influenza virus. Other well-established but less common pulmonary pathogens in all populations are *Staphylococcus aureus* and *Hemophilus influenzae*.

The pneumococcus: *S. pneumoniae*, also known as the pneumococcus, is the most common bacterial cause of community-acquired pneumonia in both older and younger persons. In most studies, *S. pneumoniae* accounts for 15% to 50% of all pneumonias in adults. The attack rate of pneumococcal pneumonia is estimated to be 46/1000 persons ≥ 65 yr old. Studies based on expectorated sputum samples in community-acquired pneumonia indicate that the recovery rate of *H. influenzae* is second only to that of *S. pneumoniae*; however, interpretation is difficult because either organism may be simply an oropharyngeal contaminant. Strains of *H. influenzae* account for 8% to 20% of pneumonias. These organisms are frequently recovered from the oropharynx of patients with chronic bronchitis.

Gram-negative bacilli: These pathogens are found relatively infrequently in patients with community-acquired infection. They are far more common in institutional settings, where *Klebsiella, Pseudomonas aeruginosa, Enterobacter* spp, *Proteus* spp, *Escherichia coli*, and other gram-negative bacilli appear to account for 40% to 60% of all pneumonias.

Gram-negative bacilli have a propensity for colonizing the posterior pharynx in debilitated and seriously ill patients. Throat cultures show that the colonization rate correlates directly with the severity of associated disease and the degree of functional impairment. Therefore, the high incidence of gram-negative bacillary pneumonia in institutions occurs simply because severely ill or impaired persons are more likely to be found there. Nevertheless, the epidemiology of organisms *within a particular institution* dictates patterns of colonization and antibiotic sensitivity.

Anaerobic bacteria: Anaerobes appear to play an important role in both community-acquired and nosocomial pneumonia in the elderly. Elderly patients have a tendency to aspirate because they often use sedatives and have associated conditions (such as neurologic disorders) and other illnesses that alter consciousness. Anaerobes are estimated to account for up to 20% of community-acquired pneumonia; these common oropharyngeal commensal organisms probably play a role in almost *all* aspiration pneumonias. The more common anaerobes include *Fusobacterium nucleatum, Bacteroides melaninogenicus*, peptostreptococci, peptococci, and occasionally *B. fragilis*.

Obtaining a specimen for anaerobic culture and etiologic identification is difficult. Expectorated sputum becomes contaminated by the normal flora of the upper airways. Specimens obtained by transtracheal aspiration yield a high number of anaerobes.

Legionella species: Older persons are more susceptible to legionellae. A review of 182 cases in the 1976 Philadelphia outbreak indicated that 75% of patients infected with *L. pneumophila* were > 40 yr old; the risk of infection among those > 60 yr was about twice that for younger persons. Subsequent studies continue to show a direct correlation between attack rate and patient age.

Of the pneumonias caused by the 23 recognized *Legionella* spp, *L. pneumophila* accounts for about 85%, and *L. micdadei* accounts for most of the remaining 15%. Although the pulmonary infection referred to as **legionnaires' disease** occurs sporadically, epidemics can occur and usually are associated with hotels or hospitals. The diagnosis can be missed unless special tests—using respiratory secretions for direct fluorescent antibody stain and culture on special media and examining urine for *L. pneumophila* antigen—are used to make the diagnosis.

Viruses: Viral causes of pneumonia in elderly patients include influenza and parainfluenza viruses, respiratory syncytial virus, and possibly adenoviruses. The most important viral agent of pulmonary infections in adults, especially in the elderly, is **influenza** (see Ch. 47). Attack rates are age-related, with the incidence in persons > 70 yr about four times that in those < 40 yr. The increased morbidity and mortality rates in the elderly are far more impressive; persons > 65 yr account for about 90% of influenza-associated deaths in the USA. Epidemics, sometimes with high mortality rates, are especially problematic in chronic-care facilities; thus, annual influenza vaccination is recommended for staff and residents (see Ch. 85).

Influenza A virus is the most common cause of severe and even fatal illness, in part because of its propensity for antigenic shift. Influenza B, usually relatively benign in younger persons, also may be associated with serious infection and high mortality rates in the elderly. While parainfluenza viruses and respiratory syncytial virus are important pulmonary pathogens in children, they infrequently invade healthy adults; however, the relative frequency of their occurrence in the elderly presumably reflects waning immunity.

Pathogenesis

Microorganisms reach the tracheobronchial tree via four routes: (1) inhalation, (2) aspiration, (3) direct inoculation from contiguous sites, and (4) hematogenous spread. Inhalation and aspiration are much more frequently involved than the other two routes. Pneumonitis occurs when the normal defense mechanisms of the lungs are overwhelmed or impaired.

Two major factors predisposing to pneumonia are oropharyngeal colonization and silent aspiration. **Colonization of the oropharynx** with various gram-negative bacilli occurs often, especially in patients whose underlying illness requires treatment in an intensive care unit. Predisposing factors include poor oral hygiene; abnormal swallowing; increased adherence of gram-negative bacilli to mucosal cells; debility from cardiac, respiratory, or neoplastic diseases; reduced ambulation; and frequent exposure to broad-spectrum antibiotics. **Silent aspiration of oropharyngeal secretions,** the most common mechanism of pulmonary infection, is often related to alcoholism, use of sedatives or narcotics, cerebrovascular disease, esophageal disorders, and nasogastric intubation.

Inhalation pneumonia: Aerosolized organisms inhaled into the lower airways as microparticles include *Mycobacterium tuberculosis, Legionella* spp, and the influenza virus. *M. tuberculosis* and the influenza virus are transmitted via aerosolized secretions produced by coughing. Although most cases of pneumococcal pneumonia are acquired by aspiration, inhalation of the organism can also occur, especially in the occasional epidemic. *Legionella* organisms are not passed from person to person but are usually aerosolized from a waterborne source (eg, air conditioners or shower heads). Other waterborne organisms may be introduced into the lower airways by instrumentation or delivered by small-particle aerosols from reservoir nebulizers used with ventilation equipment. Bacteria that survive well in water include *P. aeruginosa*, other pseudomonas, *Serratia marcescens, Achromobacter, Flavobacterium*, and *Acinetobacter* spp.

Aspiration pneumonia: Pneumonia-causing pathogens in the elderly are often aspirated, but the organisms involved vary in different circumstances. In community-acquired aspiration pneumonia, the usual pathogens are the anaerobic bacteria that normally reside in the gingival crevices (eg, peptostreptococci, fusobacteria, and black-pigmented anaerobes formerly referred to as *B. melaninogenicus*). In institutionally acquired aspiration pneumonia, the usual pathogens are gram-negative bacilli, sometimes in association with anaerobes. Most cases of pneumococcal and gram-negative bacillary pneumonia presumably follow microaspiration, an occult event resulting in a fairly small inoculum of more virulent bacteria from the posterior pharynx. Large-volume aspiration results in a relatively large inoculum of oropharyngeal bacteria into the lower airways and is associated with conditions that compromise consciousness or cause dysphagia.

Changes with aging (see also Ch. 45): Many factors contribute to the increased incidence of pneumonia in elderly patients and to the resultant high morbidity and mortality. Changes in pulmonary function that occur with aging include decreased cough effectiveness, increased residual volume, decreased compliance, increased closing volume, decreased diffusing capacity, and reduced oxygen saturation. Although these changes do not constitute a substantial risk for pneumonia, they markedly increase susceptibility to complications. This is also true for both chronic obstructive pulmonary disease and chronic bronchitis, which are especially common in older persons. Other conditions that appear to be associated with increased risk for pneumonia as well as increased morbidity in the elderly patient include severe hypoxia, pulmonary edema, acidosis, alcohol intoxication, and azotemia.

Host defenses (see also Chs. 45 and 84): Invasion by microorganisms involves a complex interplay of the mucociliary elevator, alveolar macrophages, polymorphonuclear leukocytes, humoral defenses, and cell-mediated immunity. For most of these defense mechanisms, functional capacity remains intact or is only mildly reduced. The most clearly defined and pronounced deficiency correlated with aging concerns T-cell function (ie, **cell-mediated immunity**). This defect, readily demonstrated by an increased rate of anergy using common skin test antigens, may contribute to the increased incidence of tuberculosis (see TUBERCULOSIS, below). Other opportunistic pathogens reflecting defective cell-mediated immunity are relatively uncommon unless modifying factors are superimposed, such as administration of corticosteroids, cancer chemotherapy, or lymphoma. A possible exception is *Pneumocystis carinii* pneumonia, which has been described in a few otherwise healthy elderly patients.

Humoral defenses as measured by serum antibody response to tetanus or pneumococcal vaccine show a somewhat blunted response that is nevertheless generally sufficient to provide protective levels. The response to influenza vaccine is clearly suboptimal in terms of both antibody titers and clinical protection conferred. The loss of protection afforded by antigens confronted during childhood presumably accounts for the enhanced susceptibility of the elderly to parainfluenza viruses, respiratory syncytial virus, and possibly the influenza viruses.

Symptoms, Signs, and Diagnosis

The typical clinical features of pneumonia are cough, fever, and sputum production. They tend to be deceptively subtle in elderly patients, even in cases with an ominous prognosis. The fever pattern may be particularly misleading. Elderly patients have a lower basal temperature and a reduced ability to mount a significant fever in response to infection. To emphasize this point, Dr. Louis Weinstein often states, "The older, the colder." The cough associated with pneumonia is frequently mistaken for chronic lung disease or an upper respiratory infection with bronchitis. The expected findings on physical examination are rales and signs of consolidation over the involved area.

The symptoms and signs, combined with a pulmonary infiltrate on chest x-ray (see Laboratory Findings, below), are diagnostic of pneumonia. *The greatest diagnostic challenge is not establishing the presence of pneumonia but sorting out the causative agent.* Identifying the causative organism guides the selection of antimicrobial drugs. The major clinical clues to the cause of the infection are the **tempo of the disease process, changes on chest x-ray,** and **the epidemiologic setting.**

The onset of pneumococcal pneumonia in the elderly is rarely marked by the typical shaking chill, although it is an acute pulmonary infection. Few clinical features distinguish pneumococcal pneumonia from gram-negative bacillary pneumonia except that the latter is more often acquired in institutions and has a higher mortality rate. Legionnaires' disease also tends to be an acute infection, but the initial feature is often fever *without* prominent pulmonary symptoms.

When pulmonary infection occurs during an influenza epidemic in any setting, the influenza virus should be considered the cause, regardless of the host's immunization status. Distinguishing primary influenza pneumonia from influenza associated with a superimposed bacterial infection may be virtually impossible. However, primary influenza pneumonia typically has a relentless and hectic progression, and influenza with a superimposed bacterial infection is often an acute febrile illness followed by clinical improvement and subsequent deterioration with a new infiltrate on chest x-ray.

A different array of pathogens, primarily *M. tuberculosis*, fungi, and anaerobic bacteria, is more likely involved in **chronic pneumonia.** These infections are associated with fever and symptoms of chronic disease, such as weight loss and anemia.

Anaerobic pulmonary infections tend to involve lung segments that are dependent when the patient is recumbent, primarily the superior segments of the lower lobes or the posterior segments of the upper lobes. The long-term sequelae are suppurative complications such as lung abscess and empyema. The patient often has putrid sputum or breath, which is suggestive of anaerobic infection.

Another recognized form of what is probably anaerobic pneumonitis is a condition previously referred to as **hypostatic pneumonia** or **nursing home pneumonia.** It is characterized by subtle clinical findings and evidence of pulmonary infiltrates in the lower lobes on chest x-ray. This condition has not been sufficiently studied bacteriologically, but the suspected pathogens are anaerobic bacteria, *S. pneumoniae, H. influenzae,* and gram-negative bacilli.

Differential diagnosis: Other conditions with similar findings include atelectasis, heart failure, and pulmonary embolism, with or without infarction.

Laboratory Findings

The most useful tests in evaluating suspected pneumonia are the CBC count, the chest x-ray, and microbiologic studies of respiratory secretions.

Complete blood count: A leukocyte count is seldom useful unless it is very high (> 25,000/μL), suggesting overwhelming pneumonia, or very low (< 3,000/μL), suggesting a viral infection or overwhelming bacterial pneumonia. A low hemoglobin value suggests a chronic disease, which may be a component of the current condition, such as tuberculosis or anaerobic pulmonary infection, or another underlying condition. Blood cultures should be performed whether or not the patient is febrile.

Chest x-ray: The diagnosis of pneumonia requires that an infiltrate be evident on chest x-ray. Although the x-ray may be normal early in the disease course, an infiltrate is almost invariably present 24 h after the onset of symptoms. Cough, fever, and sputum production with a normal chest x-ray usually indicate bronchitis or a noninfectious problem. Thus the x-ray becomes pivotal in management decisions, since pneumonia is virtually always treatable with specific antimicrobial agents. Chest x-rays showing cavity formation raise the probability of specific causes, primarily tuberculosis or anaerobic bacterial infection. Patients with pleural effusions on chest x-ray should have a thoracentesis, which is often helpful in microbiologic diagnosis and is essential for detecting and managing empyema.

Respiratory secretions: Expectorated sputum is unreliable when cultured; even when a potential pathogen is recovered, it may not be responsible for the pulmonary infection. Exceptions to this are *M. tuberculosis*, pathogenic fungi (*Histoplasma, Blastomyces,* and *Coccidioides*), and *Legionella* spp; the special techniques required for detection virtually always identify them as causative agents. An expectorated sputum culture will usually detect gram-negative bacilli and *S. aureus*; however, expectorated sputum also has a high rate of false-negative results for *S. pneumoniae* and *H. influenzae* and of false-positive results for gram-negative bacilli and *S. aureus* (although negative results eliminate gram-negative bacilli and *S. aureus* as causes). Gram stain of expectorated specimens may actually provide more useful information than culture, especially for making therapeutic decisions.

Alternatively, more reliable procedures for recovering conventional bacteria and anaerobes include transtracheal aspiration (a cannula is passed to the lower airways after percutaneous puncture through the cricothyroid membrane), transthoracic aspiration, and fiberoptic bronchoscopy using the protected brush, but these procedures are rarely used for routine diagnostic evaluation.

Specific recommendations for microbiologic studies include the following techniques. (1) **Conventional bacteria:** One expectorated sputum sample should be obtained for Gram stain and culture before antibiotic treatment. (2) ***Legionella* spp:** Two expectorated sputum samples (or other respiratory secretions) should be obtained for direct fluorescent antibody stain and culture using special media, preferably before erythromycin therapy or after no more than 3 days of such therapy. Urine evaluation for *L. pneumophila* antigen appears to be the most sensitive test. (3) **Anaerobic bacteria:** An uncontaminated specimen should be obtained before antibiotic therapy by transtracheal aspiration, transthoracic needle aspiration, thoracentesis, or fiberoptic bronchoscopy using the protected brush. Gram stain of expectorated sputum is of limited value, and culture in anaerobic conditions is not recommended. (4) ***M. tuberculosis:*** Three expectorated sputum samples are needed for acid-fast bacillus stain and culture on special media. (5) **Influenza virus:** Viral culture specimens may be obtained from throat washings, and serologic tests can be done using paired serum specimens collected 3 wk apart. Influenza is usually a presumed diagnosis based on typical symptoms that occur during an epidemic.

Prophylaxis

Preventive measures include the use of vaccines, judicious use of antibiotics, and intervention during epidemics. **Influenza vaccine** provides protection against infection; even when the vaccine fails, the severity of disease and the frequency of complications are reduced. **Pneumococcal vaccine** is also advocated for persons > 65 yr old. Serologic studies indicate that elderly patients develop protective antibody titers following immunization with the commercially available 23-valent pneumococcal vaccine; clinical trials show a 60% rate of protection in immunocompetent adults (see Ch. 85).

Patients who are prone to aspiration may benefit from the head-down position, and those who repeatedly aspirate food may benefit from a feeding gastrostomy. Unconscious patients, who are susceptible to aspiration pneumonia, do *not* appear to benefit from prophylactic antibiotics. These agents seem to predispose such patients to infection with resistant strains and should be restricted to those with clinical evidence of pneumonia.

Epidemics of pneumonia in institutions such as hospitals or nursing homes are most often caused by the influenza virus. Unlike bacterial infections, influenza tends to affect all exposed persons rather than just debilitated persons. Acquisition is from an exogenous rather than an endogenous source, and concurrent outbreaks usually occur in the community. Preventive measures include restriction of visitors, afflicted health care workers, and elective admissions and use of respiratory precautions in patients with documented infection. Outbreaks may be reduced or prevented by immunizing patients and staff with influenza vaccine and using amantadine or rimantadine in exposed patients. When amantadine is given prophylactically, the usual dose for persons with normal renal function is 100 mg/day; however, the drug may cause delirium, especially in persons with reduced renal function in whom doses should be reduced (see also Ch. 47).

When *Legionella* spp are responsible for outbreaks of pneumonia, the waterborne source must be determined. A source is found in about half of *Legionella* epidemics; the principal sources are cooling towers of air-conditioning systems and the potable water leading to contaminated shower heads. Once identified, *Legionella* spp must be eradicated using either heat or high chlorine concentrations. In pneumonia epidemics involving waterborne gram-negative bacilli, the source is usually contaminated respiratory therapy equipment or instruments such as bronchoscopes.

Treatment

The principal therapeutic modalities are antimicrobial agents, respiratory and other forms of supportive care, and drainage of empyemas and large pleural collections. The selection of antimicrobial agents is difficult but important; it is far easier when the causative organism is identified. Recommendations by specific organism are given in TABLE 46–1.

When no likely causative organism is identified **(enigmatic pneumonia)**, the recommendation is a regimen that includes erythromycin. This antibiotic alone is usually satisfactory in patients who are not seriously ill with community-acquired pulmonary infections. In seriously ill patients, especially those with institutionally acquired pneumonia, the antimicrobial spectrum should be extended with a regimen such as erythromycin and a third-generation cephalosporin, with or without an aminoglycoside.

These recommendations are similar to those for younger patients with pneumonia, *although the elderly require closer therapeutic monitoring*. Potentially nephrotoxic drugs, primarily aminoglycosides, require particular caution, including serum monitoring and frequent measurements of renal function, and should probably be avoided unless an alternative nonnephrotoxic drug cannot be used. Because older persons have reduced cardiac reserve, IV fluids and electrolytes and other forms of osmotic loading must be given cautiously. Hypersensitivity reactions are no more frequent in elderly than in younger patients, al-

TABLE 46–1. ANTIMICROBIAL AGENTS RECOMMENDED FOR SPECIFIC PNEUMONIAS

Causative Organism	*Antimicrobial Agent*
Streptococcus pneumoniae	Penicillin, 1st-generation cephalosporins, or erythromycin
Hemophilus influenzae	Cefuroxime, 3rd-generation cephalosporins, or trimethoprim-sulfamethoxazole
Pseudomonas aeruginosa	An antipseudomonad penicillin or ceftazidime plus an aminoglycoside (tobramycin or amikacin). Sensitivity tests required
Legionella spp	Erythromycin with or without rifampin
Staphylococcus aureus	An antistaphylococcal penicillin (nafcillin or oxacillin), cephalothin, cefamandole, or vancomycin. Vancomycin preferred for methicillin-resistant strains
Gram-negative bacilli	3rd-generation cephalosporins, imipenem, or aztreonam; an aminoglycoside is often added. Sensitivity tests required
Anaerobic bacilli	Penicillin or clindamycin
Influenza A virus	Amantadine and an antibiotic if superimposed bacterial infection is suspected

though an age-related risk of antibiotic-associated diarrhea or colitis is common with ampicillin, cephalosporins, or clindamycin. Drug interactions may also occur between antibiotics and other therapeutic agents (eg, warfarin sodium) commonly used in the elderly.

TUBERCULOSIS

An infectious disease caused by Mycobacterium tuberculosis.

Remarkable progress has been made in the control of tuberculosis **(TB)** in the USA and other industrialized countries. The mortality rate for TB patients declined from about 200/100,000 population at the turn of the century to about 1.5/100,000 in the 1980s. However, since 1985 this steady downward trend has reversed, and the number of active cases of TB is now increasing in the USA. This increase is attributed largely but not exclusively to the AIDS epidemic. In addition, the number of cases involving multidrug-resistant strains is increasing alarmingly. Persons > 65 yr account for 25% to 30% of newly diagnosed TB cases. The reasons are threefold: (1) Many older persons became infected when the prevalence of TB was substantially higher. (2) The loss of cell-mediated immunity that accompanies aging favors reactivation of dormant foci. (3) Prolonged contact with a large number of susceptible hosts, as occurs in chronic-care facilities, favors person-to-person spread.

Pathogenesis

Tuberculosis infection is acquired by inhaling droplet nuclei containing microorganisms aerosolized from untreated persons. The risk of transmission is remarkably lower once treatment has begun, even when sputum cultures continue to yield the microbe. Also, the duration of contact is important. Under ordinary circumstances, sustained exposure for at least 2 mo is required to achieve the inoculum necessary for transmission.

The inhaled organisms are deposited in the alveoli, most commonly in the lower lobes, which are the best-ventilated portions of the lung. There the organisms replicate slowly, about once every 24 h. They gain access to lymphatic channels, involving the regional lymph nodes in the chest, and then pass through the thoracic duct to the bloodstream, where widespread hematogenous dissemination may occur.

With the initial infection, known as **primary TB,** the patient may have a bronchopneumonia, usually involving the lower lobes and often the regional lymph nodes, or a unilateral pleural effusion. More frequently, the patient remains asymptomatic and the infection is detected later by a positive skin test, sometimes associated with x-ray changes that usually consist of a solitary nodule or a nodule accompanied by hilar adenopathy **(Ghon complex).** The nodule is often calcified, which helps distinguish it from carcinoma.

Patients with positive skin tests generally harbor viable organisms within macrophages, and they can retain a balanced host-parasite relationship for decades. Most TB cases in elderly patients involve reactivation of dormant organisms and are referred to as **reactivation TB.** Reactivation TB tends to occur at sites with relatively high oxygen concentrations, presumably because the organism is an obligate aerobe. A typical site is the lung's upper lobe, where ventilation-perfusion ratios provide high oxygen concentrations. Even so, elderly people (especially those in nursing homes) often express TB as a pneumonitis in the lungs' lower and middle portions.

Reactivation usually occurs when immune defenses, primarily cell-mediated immunity, are compromised (see Ch. 84). Cell-mediated immunity appears to be the most important factor in a balanced host-parasite relationship, and immunity is often compromised as the thymus atrophies with aging. By the fifth decade, a person has minimal thymic tissue, although lymphocytes and monocytes capable of antigenic recall continue to circulate for two to three more decades. Standard skin tests for cell-mediated immunity reveal a relatively high rate of anergy in the elderly. Despite this loss, most elderly patients are not more susceptible to the pathogens associated with other conditions characterized by anergy, such as immunosuppression from corticosteroid therapy, cancer chemotherapy, lymphomas, or AIDS. Rather, TB appears to be the exception.

Symptoms and Signs

Because TB in the elderly is often subtle, many of the clinical complaints, including weight loss, cough, weakness, and dyspnea, may be attributed to other conditions or even to aging itself. Fever is generally low grade and may not be apparent to the patient unless the temperature is measured. Night sweats and hemoptysis, which specifically suggest TB, are often not present or not pursued.

Diagnosis

The major diagnostic studies are the skin test, chest x-ray, and sputum culture. Because chest x-ray findings may be atypical, some authorities recommend that any elderly person who requires hospitalization for pneumonitis have at least one sputum culture for TB. All new employees and new residents in chronic-care facilities should have routine skin tests and chest x-rays; skin tests should usually be repeated annually.

Skin test: The preferred skin test is performed by injecting 5 tuberculin units of 0.1 mL purified protein derivative **(PPD)** into the volar or dorsal skin of the forearm. Results should be measured on the second or third day. The size of the reaction correlates to some extent with the probability of TB; induration of $\geq$ 10 mm is significant. A smaller reaction (5 to 10 mm of induration) is suspect in high-risk populations. BCG vaccine given in childhood does not account for a positive PPD skin test decades later.

Since reactivity wanes with time, a test that produces a negative result in the elderly should be repeated (using the same dose) a week later to detect the **booster phenomenon.** Most patients with active TB have positive tests, although some are anergic to all skin test reagents. A small percentage with active disease are selectively anergic only to tuberculin. The second-strength (250 tuberculin units) PPD test *should not be used,* and patients with a history of a positive test should not be retested. A **positive test** indicates that the person harbors viable organisms, although the test does not distinguish dormant from active disease. This distinction is made by symptoms, chest x-ray, and cultures.

Chest x-ray: All patients with a newly detected positive PPD test and those with anergy should have a chest x-ray and clinical evaluation. When x-ray findings indicate TB, they should be compared with the patient's past x-rays. The disease is considered active if symptoms and progressive changes on chest x-rays are attributed to current infection or if a culture yields *M. tuberculosis*.

Sputum culture: All patients suspected of having TB should have three morning sputum samples stained and cultured for acid-fast bacillus (AFB). Sputum stains for AFB identify about half the patients who subsequently have positive cultures without cavitary disease. Most patients with cavitary disease have a large mycobacterial load and positive AFB sputum smears. Patients who cannot expectorate sputum should have sputum production induced; if this is unsuccessful, they should undergo bronchoscopy.

Prophylaxis

High-risk persons who do not have active disease should undergo preventive therapy with isoniazid, 300 mg/day orally for 6 to 12 mo. This therapy is recommended for household members and other close contacts of potentially infectious persons; for newly infected persons (those who have had a tuberculin skin test conversion within the previous 2 yr); for persons with positive skin tests and abnormal chest x-rays compatible with previous TB; and for persons with positive skin tests in certain clinical situations, such as silicosis, diabetes, immunosuppression (including that resulting from corticosteroid administration and cancer chemotherapy), HIV-positive serologic findings, hematologic and reticuloendothelial malignancies, end-stage renal disease, and associated conditions characterized by rapid weight loss or chronic malnutrition.

Treatment

Patients with active TB require four antituberculous drugs: isoniazid, rifampin, pyrazinamide, and ethambutol. Treatment is given for 2 mo, until sensitivity test results are available. All *M. tuberculosis* isolates should undergo sensitivity testing for resistance. Patients with strains of TB sensitive to isoniazid and rifampin should receive these drugs for an additional 4 mo. Since most elderly patients acquired their original strains many decades before, when resistance was nonexistent, this treatment regimen is usually appropriate. Pyridoxine 25 to 50 mg/day is given to prevent peripheral neuropathy from isoniazid.

These recommendations are modified if in vitro sensitivity tests indicate infection with **resistant strains.** The current recommendation for multidrug-resistant strains (resistant to isoniazid and rifampin) is to give two drugs that are active in vitro for at least 18 mo. Resistance is suspected in patients who have undergone previous courses of treatment (especially if compliance was poor), in those with recently acquired disease, in immigrants from areas endemic for resistant strains, and in persons who acquire the infection from contact with these sources.

All patients with TB should remain under observation until compliance with their treatment regimen is established. **Monitoring during treatment** includes baseline measurements of liver enzyme, bilirubin, and serum creatinine levels; a CBC count; and a platelet count or estimate. Serum uric acid concentration should be measured when pyrazinamide is used. *Patients should be monitored for adverse reactions, with specific attention to symptoms suggesting hepatitis (eg, jaundice, fever, anorexia, and dark urine).* Such monitoring is especially important in elderly patients receiving isoniazid, since the frequency of hepatitis as an adverse effect shows an age-related correlation. Patients should be seen or contacted at least monthly during treatment and specifically questioned about these symptoms.

Routine laboratory testing is not recommended if there are no symptoms, although some physicians assess liver function monthly, especially during the first 6 mo of treatment when hepatitis is most likely to occur. Transaminase levels at least three times higher than the upper limit of normal values contraindicate further isoniazid treatment. For patients with active disease, sputum should be examined at least monthly until cultures convert to negative. In about 90% of patients, cultures convert within 3 mo of initiating the recommended regimens.

47. INFLUENZA

Infection with influenza A or B virus, which causes an acute febrile illness of the respiratory tract.

Epidemiology and Pathogenesis

Infections with influenza viruses occur every year, either sporadically as local outbreaks or as a widespread epidemic. In the Northern Hemisphere epidemics occur almost exclusively during the winter months (December through April), and in the Southern Hemisphere they occur during the summer months (May through September). Attack rates during such outbreaks may be as high as 10% to 40% over 5 to 6 wk. The overall annual risk of dying of influenza is about 1/5,000 to 1/10,000, although death rates are higher among elderly persons and among those with chronic diseases. Older persons, especially those with chronic medical conditions, account for at least 50% of all hospitalizations and 75% to 80% of all deaths attributed to influenza.

A unique feature of influenza virus is the frequency with which changes in antigenicity occur (principally involving the two external viral glycoproteins, hemagglutinin and neuraminidase). Changes in antigenicity occur almost annually with influenza A but less often with influenza B virus. Because of these alterations, variants of the viruses develop to which the population at risk has little or no resistance, which helps explain why influenza epidemics continue. Antigenic variations are referred to as **antigenic drift;** major variations that herald pandemic influenza and create a virus to which the population has no immunity are called **antigenic shift.**

Influenza is spread by aerosol droplets expelled during coughing or sneezing. Low relative humidity and low environmental temperature foster the survival of airborne virus. After being deposited on respiratory tract epithelium, the virus attaches to its cellular receptor via hemagglutinin and penetrates columnar epithelial cells, unless it is prevented from doing so by secretory IgA, by its attachment to nonspecific nucleoproteins, or by the action of the mucociliary apparatus. The virion then initiates a replication cycle within the cell, releasing virus for several hours before the cell dies. Released virus can infect nearby cells. Therefore, within a short period, many cells within the respiratory tract are either being infected, releasing virus, or dying.

The severity of illness correlates temporally with the amount of virus shed, suggesting that a major mechanism of illness is cell death resulting from viral replication. Shedding of virus precedes by 1 to 2 days the appearance of interferon in both nasal secretions and serum. The appearance of interferon coincides with an improvement in symptoms and a decrease in viral titers, suggesting that interferon may be active in the recovery process between the third and sixth days (before serum or secretory antibody is detected).

Symptoms and Signs

The clinical manifestations of influenza A and B viruses are similar. Influenza A is generally more severe, and five times as many persons with it require hospitalization compared to those with influenza B.

Many patients present with the classic flu-like syndrome, characterized by the abrupt onset of fever, chills, rigors, headache, myalgias, malaise, and anorexia. Early in the course of illness, the patient appears to be in a toxic condition: The face is flushed, and the skin is hot and moist. Prostration may occur in severe cases.

Fever is a consistent feature of influenza infection. Among elderly persons, fever is common, although the temperature may not rise as high as it does in children and young adults. The temperature usually rises rapidly within 12 h on the first day of illness, concurrently with the onset of systemic symptoms. The most troublesome initial symptoms are often headache and myalgias, which are related to the severity of the fever. Myalgias may involve the extremities or the long muscles of the back. Arthralgias, but not frank arthritis, are also common. Lateral gaze may elicit pain in the eye muscles; photophobia and other ocular symptoms (including injected, watery, and burning eyes) occur in up to 20% of patients. Diarrhea is a feature in $< 5\%$ of patients. Respiratory symptoms (ie, dry cough and a clear nasal discharge) are usually present at the onset of illness but are overshadowed by nonrespiratory symptoms. Nasal obstruction, hoarseness, and a dry or sore throat may also occur. Hyperemia of the mucous membranes of the nose and throat develops, but exudate generally does not. Most persons with influenza develop bronchitis without other involvement of the lower respiratory tract. Small, tender cervical lymph nodes develop in about 25% of patients.

On the second and third days of illness, the fever begins to diminish, along with reduction of systemic symptoms. As systemic symptoms and signs decline, respiratory complaints and findings, especially cough, become more apparent. The cough, which is nonproductive, may be accompanied by substernal discomfort or burning. Scattered wheezes or localized crackles are observed in < 20% of patients. Nasal obstruction and discharge can occur with pharyngeal pain and injection. These symptoms and signs usually persist for 3 to 4 days after the fever subsides, although full recovery can take 2 wk or more.

Complications

Numerous complications, especially pneumonia and severe bronchitis, can occur in elderly patients with influenza. The rate of occurrence is low in patients < 50 yr old but increases progressively with age and is high in those > 70 yr old. This higher rate of severe pulmonary involvement may be attributed to the decline in cell-mediated immunity with aging.

Pneumonia may be a consequence of primary influenza viral infection or secondary bacterial infection (see PNEUMONIA in Ch. 46). **Primary influenza pneumonia** most often affects persons with cardiovascular disease, especially rheumatic heart disease with mitral stenosis, which is associated with increased pulmonary blood flow or pressure. Other chronic illnesses may increase risk as well. Healthy adults of any age may develop this deadly syndrome, although it occurs infrequently. The onset of influenza is usually typical, followed by rapid progression of fever, cough, dyspnea, and cyanosis; hemoptysis may occur. Auscultation reveals fine inspiratory crackles and inspiratory and expiratory wheezes. Chest x-rays usually show diffuse perihilar infiltrates. The mortality rate of primary influenza pneumonia is high.

Patients at risk for **secondary bacterial pneumonia** often have chronic pulmonary, cardiac, metabolic, or other diseases. A classic influenza illness is followed by a period of improvement (over 4 to 14 days) before the clinical course worsens and symptoms and signs of bacterial pneumonia appear. The syndrome consists of fever, productive cough, and an area of consolidation found on physical examination. Chest x-rays show lobar or lobular infiltrates. Bacterial causes of pneumonia include the pneumococcus, *Staphylococcus aureus, Hemophilus influenzae,* and other gram-positive and gram-negative organisms.

Many **nonpulmonary complications** have been described in patients with influenza, including myositis (sometimes with myoglobinuria and renal failure), myocarditis and pericarditis, a toxic shock syndrome (probably from colonization of the trachea with *S. aureus*), Goodpasture's syndrome, and CNS complications such as Guillain-Barré syndrome, transverse myelitis, and encephalitis. Anosmia and ageusia (loss of smell and taste) can develop and, although usually temporary, may last months.

Diagnosis

The local or state health department or the Centers for Disease Control and Prevention often will confirm that influenza virus is affecting a region or community. When this happens, most persons with fever, muscle aches, and cough are likely to have influenza. Although rarely indicated, specific diagnostic procedures can be used to detect virus or viral antigens in respiratory secretions. Early in the course of illness, virus can be isolated from nasal or throat swab specimens, nasal washes, or sputum; bronchoalveolar lavage and lung tissue specimens can also be used to isolate virus. Specimens are inoculated onto cell cultures and examined for cytopathic effect or hemadsorption. Positive results appear in about ⅔ of cases within 3 days of testing and in the remainder of cases by 5 to 7 days. Virus can also be cultured by the inoculation of embryonated hens' eggs. Serologic tests, although sensitive and specific, do not yield data within a clinically relevant time because sera must be obtained from convalescing patients at least 10 days after the onset of illness. Complement-fixing antibody tests are most commonly used for serologic diagnosis. A fourfold or greater change in titer is considered diagnostic of infection.

Prophylaxis

Prevention of influenza is best accomplished by using **inactivated virus vaccines** (see also INFLUENZA VACCINE in Ch. 85). Antigenic drift makes disease prevention with vaccine a challenge. Each year the Public Health Service Advisory Committee on Immunization Practices makes recommendations regarding the composition of the influenza vaccine. Generally the vaccines contain both A and B inactivated viruses, usually the ones isolated from the previous influenza season.

Persons at highest risk of infection—those with chronic diseases, all persons ≥ 65 yr of age, and the medical personnel who provide their care—should be immunized annually with influenza vaccine. In addition, immunization may be advisable for all persons who have extensive contact with elderly persons. Vaccination should be given in October, several weeks before the start of the influenza season. However, vaccination can be provided throughout the influenza season until the late winter. Efficacy rates vary from 67% to 92%; the vaccine is about 75% effective in reducing deaths from influenza in hospitalized, high-risk elderly persons. Diminished responses to the vaccine may be seen in very elderly persons and in those who have renal failure or who are immunocompromised.

The only contraindication to vaccination is hypersensitivity to hens' eggs; vaccination is generally safe in persons who can eat eggs or egg-containing products. About 25% to 50% of patients experience some discomfort at the vaccine site 8 to 24 h after vaccination. About 1% to 2% of patients have fever or other systemic reactions. No further association of Guillain-Barré syndrome with influenza vaccination has been reported (the syndrome occurred sporadically in 1976 with the swine influenza immunization program). The vaccine cannot cause influenza or other respiratory infection.

Amantadine and **rimantadine** are approved for use as prophylactic agents against influenza; their efficacy is about 75% to 90%, similar to that of the influenza vaccine. In clinical studies, rimantadine is as effective as amantadine in preventing clinical influenza, and rimantadine has a lower incidence of side effects. The drugs are currently recommended as short-term (5 to 7 wk) prophylaxis during a presumed outbreak of influenza A for persons who did not receive the vaccine or for vaccinated persons (especially in a nursing home) who are becoming ill at a high rate; they should be used for only 2 wk if vaccine is given simultaneously. The suggested dose for either amantadine or rimantadine is 100 mg once daily. Prophylaxis with amantadine or rimantadine may be particularly useful in nursing homes to protect unvaccinated residents when others in the institution have become infected. In addition, the drugs may be used to supplement protection in patients expected to have a poor antibody response to vaccination. Household contacts of a person infected with the virus may also be given prophylaxis, as may staff and patients in hospitals or institutions, to prevent an outbreak.

Treatment

The only drugs approved by the Food and Drug Administration for the treatment of influenza A infection are **amantadine** and **rimantadine.** These drugs can reduce the symptoms and signs of influenza A infection and shorten its course by 1 or 2 days if given within 48 h of the onset of illness. Neither inhibits influenza B virus. For healthy elderly persons with normal renal function, the usual dose of amantadine is 200 mg initially, then 100 mg/day. The usual dose of rimantadine is 100 mg/day. When the index of suspicion is high (ie, during the winter months and when influenza has been reported in or near the community), patients who have an influenza-like illness and temperature > 37.7° C (> 100° F) are given amantadine or rimantadine for 3 to 5 days.

Amantadine is associated with minor, reversible CNS side effects such as nervousness, insomnia, dizziness, and difficulty in concentration. These side effects of amantadine therapy are common in the elderly. Nonetheless, the prevention or relief of influenza symptoms is generally greater than the toxicity of side effects, so that patients receive an overall net benefit with treatment. In patients with a known seizure disorder, seizures occur more often even when anticonvulsant therapy is maintained. Side effects occur less often with rimantadine than with amantadine, and rimantadine may eventually replace amantadine for treatment of uncomplicated influenza.

No controlled trials have been conducted of amantadine or rimantadine in the treatment of influenza viral pneumonia; their use in this situation is based on anecdotal case reports and on data indicating that the drugs reduce peripheral airway resistance in uncomplicated influenza. Amantadine-resistant and rimantadine-resistant influenza A virus has been reported, although the long-term clinical significance of resistant virus has yet to be determined.

Adjunctive therapy for influenza includes measures to provide symptomatic relief. Patients should remain at bed rest and receive additional fluids. Aspirin or acetaminophen is effective in reducing fever. Patients with proven or suspected bacterial pneumonia should receive antibiotics (see PNEUMONIA in Ch. 46).

48. CHRONIC OBSTRUCTIVE PULMONARY DISEASE

A group of diseases, including chronic bronchitis, emphysema, small airway disease, asthma, and bronchiectasis, characterized by chronic airflow obstruction with reversible and/or irreversible components. Airflow obstruction is a reduction in the ratio of forced expiratory volume in the first second to forced vital capacity **(FEV_1/FVC)**. Although each type of chronic obstructive pulmonary disease **(COPD)** is a distinct clinical entity, patients commonly have two or more types. In clinical practice, COPD usually refers to some combination of chronic bronchitis, emphysema, and small airway disease, while asthma and bronchiectasis are usually considered separate entities.

Chronic bronchitis is characterized by a chronic, productive cough occurring most days of the month for at least 3 mo of the year for two consecutive years. Mucous-gland hyperplasia occurs in the airways. **Emphysema** is characterized by its morphologic abnormalities, including enlarged alveolar spaces and destructive changes in the alveolar walls, which reduce the surface area for gas exchange. **Small airway disease** is characterized by physiologic test abnormalities compatible with dysfunction of airways $\simeq$ 2 mm in diameter. **Asthma** is characterized by increased bronchial and bronchiolar responsiveness to various stimuli resulting in widespread airway narrowing. Changes in severity may occur spontaneously or as a result of therapy. **Bronchiectasis,** a permanent dilatation of one or more bronchi, is characterized clinically by production of copious sputum that separates into distinct layers.

Incidence and Etiology

In the USA, COPD ranks among the ten leading causes of death. Over the last 15 yr, the incidence of COPD has risen more rapidly than that of any of the other nine leading causes of death. As a cause of Social Security–compensated disability, COPD ranks second only to coronary artery disease.

About 3% of the US population has chronic bronchitis, which is 1.2 to 2.3 times more prevalent in older persons than in younger persons; about 1% of the US population has emphysema. However, only 5% of those with chronic bronchitis and about 40% of those with emphysema have clinically significant airway obstruction. Asthma beginning in old age is uncommon.

A combination of genetic predisposition and environmental exposure leads to COPD. Cigarette smoking, the most common environmental risk factor, is believed to contribute to COPD in > 80% of cases. Smoking contributes to airway obstruction by causing an inflammatory reaction with or without mucus production in the airways; by promoting the influx of polymorphonuclear leukocytes, which release inflammatory mediators and elastases that break down lung elastin, leading to emphysema; and by inhibiting the body's endogenous elastases. Pollution, occupational contacts, and other environmental exposures are less important contributors to airway obstruction. Other risk factors for COPD include being male, having a low socioeconomic status, and having had a childhood respiratory illness.

Pathophysiology

Cigarette smoke leads to inflammatory changes in the lungs, which present clinically as chronic bronchitis and emphysema. Patients with **chronic bronchitis, emphysema,** and **asthma** invariably have an increased ratio of mucous glands to bronchial wall thickness (the Reid index). This is primarily due to an increase in the number of glands (hyperplasia), rather than an increase in the size of existing glands (hypertrophy). No strong relationship exists between the degree of glandular hyperplasia and the degree of airway obstruction, suggesting that other factors, including smooth muscle hyperplasia and reduced structural support of the airway, are more important in the development of airway obstruction.

The most common forms of **emphysema** are centrilobular and panacinar. Centrilobular emphysema is proximal acinar emphysema involving the respiratory bronchioles; it most commonly occurs in the upper zones of the lung. Panacinar emphysema involves the entire acinus and is more evenly distributed throughout the lungs. Patients with severe emphysema may have large bullous lesions scattered throughout the lungs.

The pathologic transition from normal lung to emphysema is gradual but may begin with smoking-induced respiratory bronchiolitis. Other changes that may occur during the transition include increased peribronchial muscle, fibrosis, goblet cell metaplasia, and increased intraluminal mucus. At autopsy, mild emphysema is commonly found in older persons with no history of dyspnea or smoking. Although the severity of emphysema does not correlate with symptoms as highly as might be expected, it does appear to correlate with airway obstruction.

Symptoms and Signs

The most common symptoms of COPD are cough, increased sputum production, dyspnea, and wheezing. Disabling symptoms increase rapidly in patients over age 50 and are more frequent in men than in women. A **productive cough** usually begins several years after a person starts to smoke. The cough may be mild, or it may be disabling, causing posttussive syncope, vomiting, or stress incontinence. In frail elderly persons, especially osteoporotic women, coughing can cause painful rib fractures. Usually opalescent, the **sputum** varies from < 1 tsp to several tablespoons. Larger quantities or color variations (eg, green or yellow) suggest infection or, less commonly, bronchiectasis.

Dyspnea, the most disabling symptom, usually begins at about age 50 and progresses. Day-to-day variation in the degree of dyspnea usually indicates bronchospasm. Dyspnea is more severe and frequent in men than in women. **Wheezing,** not present in all COPD patients, is usually first noted when the patient is supine. Later, it may occur with the patient in any position and is usually associated with bronchospasm.

As airway obstruction progresses, hypoxemia may slowly develop, resulting in subtle signs of brain dysfunction, such as an inability to concentrate and reduced short-term memory. If the airway obstruction goes unrecognized, hypercapnia may develop and slowly lead to brain swelling and further dysfunction, resulting in confusion, lethargy, and increasing somnolence.

Although signs of severe obstruction do not occur in all patients with COPD, they are specific when they do appear. A characteristic sign, **pursed lips breathing** delays airway closure so that a larger tidal volume can be maintained and respiratory muscles can function more efficiently. Breathing in the sitting position with elbows resting on the thighs is another common sign of severe obstruction. This position may fixate the upper thorax and increase the curvature of the diaphragm, making breathing more efficient. Breathing with extrathoracic muscles suggests severe obstruction, which may result from either emphysema or asthma.

Exacerbations of bronchitis in COPD patients usually result from viruses and from *Hemophilus influenzae* and *Streptococcus pneumoniae*. Fever and leukocytosis may not appear in patients with acute infections. Acute hypoxemia accompanying a respiratory infection may lead to confusion and restlessness, which may be misinterpreted as senility in older patients. Uncorrected hypoxemia leads to pulmonary hypertension, cor pulmonale, reduced free water clearance in the kidney, arrhythmias, polycythemia, and altered cognitive function.

Physical Examination

Prolonged forced expiration may be the first measurable change in early or moderate COPD. Therefore, patients should be asked to inhale as deeply as possible, then exhale as rapidly and fully as possible. Auscultation allows the physician to time the expiration (which should be < 4 sec) and to hear wheezing. Obvious inspiratory noises, heard with the unaided ear or with the stethoscope over the trachea, are common in patients with bronchitis.

Two stereotypes of patients with severe COPD—the pink puffer and the blue bloater—help define the extremes of the COPD spectrum. Actually, most patients have features of both stereotypes.

The **pink puffer** is typically an asthenic, barrel-chested emphysematous patient who exhibits pursed lips breathing and has no cyanosis or edema. Usually, such a patient uses extrathoracic muscles to breathe, produces minimal sputum, and experiences little fluctuation in the day-to-day level of dyspnea. Diaphragmatic excursions are reduced, and breath and heart sounds are distant. Arterial blood gas studies show only mild to moderate hypoxemia and normal or slightly reduced $PaCO_2$. The barrel-shaped chest is nonspecific because older persons commonly have increased lung compliance and larger resting lung volumes.

The **blue bloater** is typically overweight, cyanotic, and edematous and exhibits a chronic productive cough (chronic bronchitis). Arterial blood gas levels show hypoxemia and hypercapnia. Nocturnal hypoxemia may be profound. Elderly blue bloaters are uncommon because blue bloaters often have cor pulmonale, which rapidly leads to death if not treated appropriately.

Laboratory Findings

Chest x-rays are not sensitive to early or moderate obstructive disease. Typical findings in severe emphysema are a flattened diaphragm, a narrow heart, enlarged lungs, decreased peripheral vascular markings, and an increased retrosternal air space. These findings may also appear during acute bronchospasm. Patients with bronchitis may have normal chest x-rays or increased interstitial markings and enlarged pulmonary arteries.

Spirometry documents the obstructive component of the disease. Pulmonary function is measured after an aerosolized bronchodilator is administered to help determine the reversibility of the airway narrowing. Obstruction is present when the FEV_1 is $< 80\%$ of the FVC. Patients are usually not dyspneic until the FEV_1 approaches 1.5 L. With emphysema, a determination of lung volume by the helium dilution technique or body plethysmography shows an increased functional residual capacity (FRC) and residual volume (RV); with bronchitis, FRC and RV may be nearly normal. Normal aging is also associated with slight increases in FRC and RV. The diffusing capacity is low in emphysema but near normal in chronic bronchitis. An increased dead space is often found in patients with emphysema.

Arterial blood gas levels are typically abnormal in moderate and severe COPD. Hypoxemia, when present, results from ventilation-perfusion mismatching because of bronchospasm, intrabronchial mucus, or premature airway collapse. True shunting of blood is uncommon in COPD. When hypoventilation is present, reflected by hypercapnia, hypoxemia may result from reduced alveolar oxygen pressure. Chronic hypercapnia in these instances is confirmed by a near-normal blood pH and an elevated serum HCO_3^-. Care must be taken in diagnosing hypoxemia in older persons because the normal PO_2 of a 75-yr-old is about 75 mm Hg.

Prognosis

Close monitoring and intensive rehabilitation programs, including drug therapy and reconditioning through exercise, can improve the quality of life and reduce the number of hospitalizations for COPD patients. However, longevity probably cannot be improved significantly except in patients with hypoxemia.

Smokers developing COPD lose FEV_1 at the rate of 50 to 100 mL/yr, while nonsmokers lose only 25 to 30 mL/yr. Survival rates correlate with FEV_1. An $FEV_1 > 1.5$ L is usually associated with a normal adjusted life span; an FEV_1 of ≤ 1 L is associated with an average survival of ≤ 5 yr. Other poor prognostic signs include resting tachycardia, ventricular arrhythmias, and hypercapnia.

Treatment

The therapeutic goal for geriatric patients with COPD is to maintain functional independence and avoid repeated hospitalizations. Respiratory compromise eventually leads to functional impairment and loss of independence, often accompanied by anxiety, lowered self-esteem, depression, role reversal, and sexual dysfunction.

The chances of successful rehabilitation are enhanced when the patient has a positive attitude as well as a caring family and physician. Education about exercise, nutrition, avoidance of infections, and appropriate use of drugs can help improve the patient's quality of life.

Sexual function often improves if the person is rested, schedules sexual activity for the "best-breathing" time of day, uses a bronchodilator 20 to 30 min beforehand, avoids consuming large amounts of food or alcohol, and assumes a position that does not put pressure on the chest or abdomen or require arm support.

Typically, a COPD patient is in poor physical condition. The physician should determine if this condition results from end-stage lung disease or other causes. If the patient has no respiratory reserve, exercise is unwarranted, and the work of daily living should be decreased to minimize oxygen requirements. The physician may suggest that the patient live on a single level of his home, not wear shoes that require tying, and so on.

If the patient appears to have a respiratory reserve, a graduated exercise program should be instituted. Simultaneous supplemental oxygen may be required to allow the patient to exercise long enough to benefit from the program; however, Medicare requires a resting PO_2 of < 55 mm Hg for reimbursement for home oxygen therapy. The most efficient and inexpensive device for supplying supplemental oxygen in the home is an oxygen concentrator. This device, which plugs into a standard electrical outlet, extracts oxygen from the air and concentrates it for delivery through a nasal catheter that can allow the patient to move throughout one floor of a home. Outside the home, a patient can use a small tank of liquid oxygen that can be concealed in a bag with a shoulder strap. Such a tank allows patient mobility for 3 to 8 h, depending on its size, the flow rate, and the method of delivery (oxygen may be delivered continuously or through a valve that opens only when the patient inhales). Exercise should be continued year-round. Activities may include walking outdoors in nice weather, in malls in bad weather, and up and down stairs in the house in winter, as well as using an exercise bicycle.

Drug therapy is directed primarily at reducing dyspnea. Other therapeutic goals include controlling cough and sputum production. Because treatment is not curative, it is considered successful when it produces a favorable balance between symptomatic relief and drug-related side effects. Clear, written directions are important for older patients because their age-adjusted cognitive skills are further impaired by hypoxemia, leading to poor short-term memory and an inability to concentrate.

Preventing infection: Preventive measures include receiving annual influenza vaccinations and a lifetime polyvalent pneumococcal vaccine immunization, washing hands after contact with persons who have viral syndromes, and avoiding crowds in poorly ventilated spaces during influenza epidemics. At the first sign of purulent sputum, an antibiotic such as tetracycline 500 mg qid for 10 days, ampicillin 500 mg qid for 10 days, erythromycin 500 mg orally qid for 10 days, or trimethoprim-sulfamethoxazole 160 mg-800 mg (one double-strength tablet) orally bid should be started, even though the efficacy of such therapy is controversial. Increased administration of bronchodilators and oral corticosteroids may also be necessary during acute infections.

Managing bronchospasm: A reversible component of bronchospasm is documented when spirometry shows about a 15% improvement in FEV_1 after the patient inhales a bronchodilator. However, a lack of improvement in FEV_1 on a single test does *not* mean that the bronchodilator offers no therapeutic benefit. On the contrary, most bronchodilators (whether oral **theophylline preparations** or oral or aerosolized **β_2-sympathomimetics**) improve mucociliary clearance, delay fatigue of the diaphragm, and improve myocardial contractility. Theophylline may also be a mild respiratory stimulant and a diuretic. In older patients, the half-life of theophylline preparations is prolonged, so the dosage must be reduced appropriately, often to half the amount younger patients can tolerate. Plasma levels should be checked periodically.

Aerosolized β_2-sympathomimetics may be preferable to oral ones because they are less likely to produce cardiovascular side effects. The disadvantage of hand-held, metered-dose, aerosolized bronchodilators is that some older persons may not be able to synchronize drug aerosolization with inspiration because of musculoskeletal problems, such as rheumatoid arthritis. Using either a spacer, which is attached to the metered-dose inhaler, or a compressor nebulizer, which does not require patient coordination, helps improve administration. A compressor nebulizer delivers a continuous fine mist of sterile saline mixed with a bronchodilator. This device allows more controlled administration of higher doses of medicine and provides patient reassurance because most hospitals use this method of delivery.

An atropine derivative, **ipratropium bromide,** reverses bronchospasm in COPD; however, adverse effects may occur in patients with glaucoma or prostatic hypertrophy. **Corticosteroids** are beneficial during acute exacerbations of bronchospasm in patients with severe COPD and may reduce the length of stay in the intensive care unit and in the hospital. Long-term corticosteroid therapy is also beneficial in selected patients with end-stage COPD in whom all other forms of therapy are ineffective. Prolonged use of high-dose corticosteroids should be avoided in most older patients because of the risk of osteopenia, cataracts, subcutaneous hemorrhage, hyperglycemia, cutaneous fragility, and cardiovascular disease.

Controlling cough and sputum: When these signs are not caused by infection, avoiding irritants is the most important and effective therapy. Because cough is a natural protective mechanism, it should not be completely suppressed pharmacologically; however, forceful or frequent coughing can cause rib fractures or syncope. Over-the-counter drugs containing dextromethorphan often provide moderate cough suppression. When necessary, stronger narcotic derivatives may be useful for short periods.

Liquefaction and expectoration of sputum may be aided by adequate hydration and, occasionally, by potassium iodine solutions. Older persons tend to become dehydrated because of altered renal function, so they must be told to drink adequate amounts of fluids daily. Mucolytic agents have not been proved effective when inhaled, nor have expectorants been proved effective in removing secretions. Postural drainage after bronchodilator inhalation is effective in patients with bronchiectasis.

Reducing dyspnea: This symptom is thought to result in part from respiratory muscle fatigue caused by an inappropriate amount of work for a given level of ventilation. Therefore, attempts are made to (1) reduce the amount of work, (2) reduce the propensity for muscle fatigue, and (3) reduce the oxygen requirements. The work of breathing is reduced by dilating the narrowed airways using bronchodilators, corticosteroids, and a regimen of pulmonary care.

Diaphragm-strengthening exercises done several times a day for 10 to 15 min appear to decrease respiratory fatigue. To perform these exercises, the patient lies supine and places one hand on the abdomen and the other on the chest. The patient then inhales deeply through the nose while concentrating on making the hand on the abdomen move upward, using the diaphragm. The patient breathes out through pursed lips. Placing a 5- to 8-lb book on the abdomen facilitates diaphragm movement during expiration and forces the diaphragm to work harder on inspiration. Adequate nutrition and theophylline preparations may also reduce the propensity for muscle fatigue.

Oxygen requirements for a given level of activity can be reduced by conditioning exercises (and theoretically by ingesting a low carbohydrate, high fat diet), thereby decreasing the work of breathing. Anxiety associated with dyspnea can often be diminished by showing the patient how to use pursed lips breathing.

Correcting hypoxemia: The physician should determine if and when hypoxemia ($PO_2 < 60$ mm Hg) occurs (ie, at rest, during exercise, or during sleep). If hypoxemia occurs at rest, oxygen should be administered continuously. If hypoxemia does not occur at rest, oximetry measurements during exercise and sleep may be clinically indicated. If hypoxemia is documented, the lowest oxygen concentration capable of raising the PO_2 to about 65 mm Hg should be given; usually oxygen can be given by nasal cannula (1 to 2 L/min). A 5 to 10 mm Hg rise in PCO_2 is acceptable, provided no significant mental status changes occur.

Managing hypercapnia: This condition, which reflects reduced ventilation, commonly accompanies severe airway obstruction, but it generally is not dangerous when the blood pH is near normal. A rapid rise in PCO_2 with a drop in pH suggests that the patient has fatigued respiratory muscles and needs more intensive therapy, perhaps including ventilatory support.

Treating heart failure: Right-sided heart failure and biventricular failure are the two most common forms of cardiac decompensation in older patients with COPD. Right-sided heart failure usually results from hypoxemia-induced pulmonary hypertension; treatment includes administering oxygen, giving diuretics judiciously, and correcting electrolyte imbalances (eg, hypokalemia). Unless evidence of left-sided systolic dysfunction is present, digitalis preparations should be avoided. Pulmonary vasodilators (eg, nifedipine and hydralazine) may be helpful in selected patients with severe pulmonary and systemic hypertension.

49. PULMONARY EMBOLISM

An obstruction of the pulmonary arteries caused by a blood clot (embolus) or other material carried to the pulmonary vasculature by the circulatory system. Although a blood clot is the most common cause of pulmonary embolism, air, fat, bone marrow, foreign bodies, amniotic fluid, and tumor cells also can obstruct the pulmonary vessels.

Common but difficult to diagnose, pulmonary embolism can be effectively treated. In the USA, the incidence is about 650,000 cases annually. Pulmonary embolism is estimated to be the primary cause of death in 100,000 persons and a contributory factor in perhaps another 100,000 deaths annually. Statistics for the elderly are not available. Because the symptoms and signs are nonspecific, pulmonary embolism may be overdiagnosed or underdiagnosed, especially in the elderly. Perhaps 30% of cases are misdiagnosed, with overdiagnosis particularly common in patients who have cardiac and other respiratory conditions, as elderly patients frequently do. Accurate diagnosis minimizes the risks of both untreated pulmonary embolism and unnecessary anticoagulant therapy.

Pathophysiology

About 90% of blood clots that cause pulmonary embolism originate in the legs. The risk that a clot will embolize and lodge in the lung is greater if it is in the popliteal or iliofemoral vein (about 50%) than if it is in the calf veins (< 5%). Other, less common sites of thrombosis that may give rise to pulmonary embolism are the right atrium; the right ventricle; and the pelvic, renal, hepatic, subclavian, and jugular veins. Risk factors for venous thrombosis are vessel wall injury, stasis, and conditions that increase the tendency of the blood to clot, including deficiencies of antithrombin III, protein C, and protein S, as well as disseminated intravascular coagulation, polycythemia vera, and presence of the lupus anticoagulant or anti-cardiolipin antibody. Common medical conditions (eg, trauma to leg vessels, obesity, heart failure, malignancy, hip fracture, and myeloproliferative disorders) also predispose a person to venous thrombosis, as do estrogen use, the presence of a femoral venous catheter, surgery, and immobility, which is common among the elderly.

Symptoms and Signs

The degree of pulmonary vascular obstruction caused by the embolus and the patient's prior cardiopulmonary function affect the symptoms and signs. Patients who have small thromboemboli may be asymptomatic, although asymptomatic pulmonary embolism is rare in the elderly. In the general population, the most common symptoms are shortness of breath (80%), chest pain that may be pleuritic (70%), anxiety (60%), leg pain or swelling (40%), hemoptysis (35%), and syncope (15%). The most common physical findings are tachypnea (90%), tachycardia (50%), fever (40%), leg edema or tenderness (33%), cyanosis (20%), and a pleural friction rub (18%). Percentages for the elderly are not available. Although most patients with pulmonary embolism have deep venous thrombosis, only 33% have clinical signs of thrombosis—eg, leg swelling, tenderness, increased warmth, or Homans' sign.

Patients with pulmonary embolism usually present with one of the following patterns: (1) diagnostically confusing syndromes (confusion, unexplained fever, wheezing, resistant heart failure, or unexplained arrhythmias); (2) transient shortness of breath and tachypnea only; (3) pulmonary infarction (pleuritic pain, cough, hemoptysis, pleural effusion, and pulmonary infiltrate); (4) right-sided heart failure with shortness of breath and tachypnea; or (5) cardiovascular collapse with hypotension and syncope. Less than 20% of patients have the **classic triad of dyspnea, chest pain, and hemoptysis.** However, most patients do have tachypnea (respiratory rate > 16/min), shortness of breath, and chest discomfort. In fact, *if tachypnea is absent, pulmonary embolism is unlikely*.

About 33% of patients with pulmonary embolism have **pleural effusions,** which are usually unilateral but may be bilateral. About 67% are bloody (RBCs > 100,000/μL). The differential diagnosis of bloody effusion is limited to three principal conditions: pulmonary embolism, cancer, and trauma. Patients with pulmonary embolism and a bloody pleural effusion generally have a **pulmonary infiltrate** on chest x-ray that suggests hemorrhagic consolidation of the lung parenchyma. Most of these patients have only pulmonary hemorrhage, and the infiltrate resolves over several days. About 10% of patients with pulmonary emboli, especially those with severe heart failure, develop pulmonary infarction. About 67% of nonbloody effusions due to pulmonary embolism are exudates with elevated WBC counts (up to 75,000/μL), which mimic infected pleural effusions.

Mechanical obstruction of part of the pulmonary circulation may lead to **increased pulmonary vascular resistance,** although vasoconstriction secondary to alveolar capillary hypoxemia and mediator release may contribute. This increased resistance causes right ventricular and pulmonary arterial pressures to increase in order to maintain cardiac output. In patients with no prior cardiopulmonary disease, the pulmonary arterial pressure correlates with the percentage of the pulmonary vascular bed occluded by the emboli. Thus, pulmonary hypertension (> 25 mm Hg) in a patient with previously normal heart and lungs indicates extensive obstruction (> 40% to 50%) of the pulmonary vascular bed. However, in patients with prior cardiopulmonary disease, the pulmonary arterial pressure does not correlate with the percentage of vascular bed obstruction. In these patients, a small clot may be enough to produce a marked hemodynamic effect because of the limited cardiac reserve.

Syncope, a systolic blood pressure < 100 mm Hg, or a marked decrease in the systolic blood pressure in a hypertensive patient suggests the possibility of a massive pulmonary embolism or a hemodynamically significant embolus in a patient with marginal cardiopulmonary function. When a sudden increase in pulmonary vascular resistance prevents the right ventricle from generating sufficient forward flow, right ventricular failure, decreased cardiac output, and hypotension result. The latter is ominous because the decrease in aortic diastolic pressure may significantly reduce coronary blood flow to the overworked right ventricle, establishing a vicious circle.

A patient who is hypotensive because of pulmonary embolism will have elevated right atrial and ventricular pressures (as measured by a Swan-Ganz catheter). Thus, a normal right atrial or ventricular pressure in a patient with hypotension excludes pulmonary embolism as the cause.

Laboratory Findings

After a history is obtained and a physical examination is performed on a patient with suspected pulmonary embolism, a chest x-ray, an ECG, and arterial blood gas values should be obtained. If pulmonary embolism is still considered likely, the next step is usually to obtain a ventilation-perfusion lung scan. If deep venous thrombosis is strongly suspected or if the lung scan is likely to be indeterminate (because of underlying lung disease), an alternative approach might be to order an impedance plethysmogram or a venogram. However, the gold standard for diagnosing pulmonary embolism is pulmonary angiography.

Chest x-rays: Chest x-rays may be normal or may show nonspecific abnormalities, eg, atelectasis, an elevated hemidiaphragm, pleural effusion, or an infiltrate. Findings such as an enlarged pulmonary artery on one side or hyperlucency of one lung because of reduced pulmonary vascular markings are infrequent. Such findings are more commonly produced by rotation of the patient than by pulmonary embolism. However, a pleural-based pyramidal infiltrate that points toward the hilus (Hampton hump) is an infrequent finding that suggests pulmonary embolism. Although the chest x-ray cannot establish or exclude a diagnosis of pulmonary embolism, it can help diagnose other conditions that may explain the patient's symptoms, eg, pneumothorax, rib fracture, or heart failure.

Electrocardiography: Generally ECG findings are nonspecific; as many as 33% of patients with pulmonary embolism have a normal ECG. The most common abnormal findings are sinus tachycardia and nonspecific ST-segment and T-wave changes. Infrequent changes that strongly suggest pulmonary embolism indicate strain on the right side of the heart; these changes include T-wave inversion in precordial leads V_1 to V_4, transient right bundle branch block, right or left deviation of the QRS axis, sudden onset of atrial fibrillation or other atrial arrhythmia, and ECG signs of right ventricular hypertrophy or right atrial enlargement. The $S_1Q_3T_3$ pattern (deep S wave in lead I and a new Q wave and inverted T wave in lead III) also suggests pulmonary embolism. This pattern of right-sided heart strain is usually accompanied by T-wave inversion in the precordial leads.

Arterial blood gas studies: Pulmonary embolism often results in arterial hypoxemia because a low ventilation-perfusion ratio develops secondary to airway closure and bronchoconstriction in lung segments adjacent to the emboli. Intrapulmonary shunting of blood and a reduced mixed venous oxygen tension also contribute to the arterial hypoxemia. Rarely, right-to-left shunting of blood may occur because of a patent foramen ovale due to right atrial hypertension from massive pulmonary embolism. Of course, in very old people without pulmonary embolism, a decreased PaO_2 may not indicate disease.

Although pulmonary embolism often causes marked hypoxemia, some elderly patients with pulmonary embolism may have a PaO_2 of > 70 mm Hg while breathing room air. Therefore, a normal PaO_2 does not exclude an embolus. Perhaps more significant is a sudden decrease in PaO_2 that cannot be easily explained by another diagnosis. Because pulmonary embolism generally causes tachypnea and respiratory alkalosis, arterial blood gas values typically show a decrease in $PaCO_2$.

Lung scan: A lung scan showing no perfusion defect excludes pulmonary embolism. One showing a perfusion defect as large as or larger than a lung segment without a matching ventilation defect indicates an 85% to 90% probability of pulmonary embolism. Such a scan with a matching ventilation defect indicates a 30% to 45% likelihood of pulmonary embolism.

A lung scan with a subsegmental perfusion defect, with or without a matching ventilation defect, is often labeled a low-probability scan, but the probability of pulmonary embolism is still 20% to 30%. The lung scan is termed indeterminate if matching ventilation and perfusion defects correspond with an infiltrate on the chest x-ray; this type of scan has a 25% to 40% association with pulmonary embolism.

Pulmonary angiography: As mentioned, pulmonary angiography is the gold standard for diagnosing pulmonary embolism. Two findings are pathognomonic: a constant intraluminal filling defect and a sharp cutoff of a vessel. Experimental studies designed to test the sensitivity of pulmonary angiography indicate that a single, small embolus may be missed but that many emboli rarely are missed. Because most patients with pulmonary embolism have many emboli, the incidence of false-negative pulmonary angiograms is believed to be low. Follow-up clinical and laboratory studies in patients with negative pulmonary angiograms also suggest that false-negative angiograms are rare.

Pulmonary angiography is safe for patients who do not have severe pulmonary hypertension or cardiopulmonary decompensation. These conditions, which increase the risk of the procedure, are relative contraindications. When performed by an experienced angiographer, the procedure is associated with minimal morbidity and a mortality rate of only about 0.2%. However, the dye can induce significant renal injury, so patients should be well hydrated, and the use of mannitol should be considered. Several authorities believe that in an elderly patient, the risks associated with anticoagulation exceed those associated with pulmonary angiography performed by an experienced examiner.

Venography and impedance plethysmography: Venography is the gold standard for diagnosing venous thrombosis, although it may be impossible to perform in patients who have significant edema. Side effects, including allergic reactions and thrombophlebitis, occur in 2% of patients.

Impedance plethysmography, combined with Doppler ultrasonography, is a helpful noninvasive diagnostic test for deep venous thrombosis. Studies correlating results of impedance plethysmography with venography indicate that impedance plethysmography has a sensitivity of 86%, a specificity of 97%, a positive predictive value of 97%, and a negative predictive value of 85%. Impedance plethysmography is an excellent procedure for detecting a clot in the popliteal or iliofemoral vein, but it can miss a clot in the calf veins. Fortunately, the risk of pulmonary embolism from a clot confined to the calf veins is small. However, a calf-vein clot can extend into the popliteal and femoral systems, where the risk of pulmonary embolism is much higher. Serial impedance plethysmograms may be needed to exclude extension of a calf-vein clot.

Because 33% of people with negative pulmonary angiography findings have deep venous thrombosis, venography or impedance plethysmography can provide useful therapeutic information. Although these tests can help diagnose peripheral clots, they cannot directly establish the diagnosis of pulmonary embolism.

Digital subtraction angiography, magnetic resonance imaging, and fiberoptic angioscopy: These tests are being evaluated as diagnostic tools. Digital subtraction angiography and magnetic resonance imaging are less invasive and use less dye than pulmonary angiography. Though invasive, fiberoptic angioscopy provides direct visualization of the pulmonary vessels and clot as well as a means of removing the clot.

Diagnosis

The commonly asked diagnostic question is: *Does this patient have pulmonary embolism*? But prospective studies indicate that about 33% of patients with negative pulmonary angiography findings have deep venous thrombosis documented by venography. Therefore, a better diagnostic question would be: *Does this patient have evidence of either a pulmonary embolus or venous thrombosis*?

The likelihood of pulmonary embolism should be estimated using both clinical assessment and laboratory studies, including the lung scan. If the lung scan shows no perfusion abnormality, pulmonary embolism can be excluded. If the lung scan shows a perfusion defect smaller than a subsegment of the lung and the clinical likelihood of pulmonary embolism is low, many clinicians would not pursue the diagnosis further. Conversely, if the lung scan reveals a perfusion defect that is segmental or larger without a matching ventilation defect, and the clinical likelihood of pulmonary embolism is high, most clinicians would treat the patient unless special circumstances required a definitive diagnosis by pulmonary angiography.

Prospective clinical studies indicate that about 10% of patients evaluated for pulmonary embolism have both a low-probability lung scan and an unlikely clinical assessment. At the other extreme, about 30% of patients have both a high-probability lung scan and a likely clinical assessment. Management of patients at either extreme is clear, but the appropriate management for the other 60% of patients is not. Several approaches are available: Obtain a pulmonary angiogram, empirically anticoagulate, obtain an impedance plethysmogram or venogram, or observe.

In patients with a low-probability lung scan, impedance plethysmography may help determine whether anticoagulant therapy is appropriate. Generally, patients with positive impedance plethysmography results should be treated with heparin for deep venous thrombosis. In patients with less than a high-probability lung scan, only a moderate clinical probability of pulmonary embolism, an adequate cardiopulmonary reserve, and negative impedance plethysmography results, observation and serial plethysmograms may be appropriate. In general, the greater the risk of not treating the patient for pulmonary embolism or the greater the risk of therapy, the greater the need for definitive angiographic diagnosis. The elderly, especially women and those who tend to fall or confuse medications, are particularly vulnerable to the side effects of anticoagulant medications.

Prognosis

The mortality rate for patients with pulmonary embolism who receive anticoagulant therapy is only 8%; the rate for those who do not receive treatment is 30%. In the elderly, the difference between these mortality rates may be even greater. Prognosis is poorest in patients with severe underlying cardiac or pulmonary disease. Between 75% and 90% of deaths from pulmonary embolism occur within the first few hours. After that, death usually results from a recurrent embolic event.

Pulmonary embolism is believed to recur in 5% to 10% of patients despite heparin therapy. The likelihood of recurrent emboli is greatest in those who have massive pulmonary embolization and those in whom anticoagulant therapy has been inadequate. If recurrence develops in the first few days of heparin or thrombolytic therapy, treatment is usually continued. If recurrent episodes or massive embolization occurs from a clot in the legs, interruption of the inferior vena cava should be considered.

The long-term prognosis for patients surviving pulmonary embolism is determined by underlying medical problems and cardiopulmonary status. Recurrent pulmonary embolism leading to chronic pulmonary hypertension and cor pulmonale is uncommon, occurring in perhaps $< 2\%$ of patients; the exact frequency in the elderly is not known.

Treatment

The general principles of therapy are to provide enough supplemental oxygen to achieve a PaO_2 of 60 to 70 mm Hg, to relieve pain with morphine or other analgesics, to provide adequate intravascular fluid for maintaining cardiac output, to monitor the patient for evidence of bleeding from anticoagulant therapy, and to avoid drugs that adversely affect platelet function (eg, aspirin or other cyclooxygenase blockers).

The **hypotensive patient with pulmonary embolism** should be treated with volume expanders, streptokinase to speed clot lysis, and an infusion of enough norepinephrine to increase aortic diastolic pressure and coronary blood flow. Studies in experimental animals indicate that norepinephrine is much more effective than volume loading or isoproterenol infusion in reversing shock in pulmonary embolism. Rarely, immediate surgery to remove a large clot from a major vessel may be attempted, but survival rates are poor.

Generally, the first medication used to treat deep venous thrombosis or pulmonary embolism, **heparin** prevents clot formation and extension but does not lyse clots. Because the risk of death from pulmonary embolism is greatest in the first few hours and because diagnostic test results often are not available for 8 to 12 h, it is generally advisable to begin heparin therapy in patients with a high clinical probability of pulmonary embolism or deep vein thrombosis before obtaining all diagnostic results.

For pulmonary embolism, heparin is usually infused IV for 7 to 10 days. A loading dose of 75 to 100 u./kg (usually 5000 u.) is given as a bolus, followed by a continuous infusion of 15 u./kg/h, with a range of 10 to 30 u./kg/h. In the elderly, the usual initial infusion rate is 800 to 1000 u./h. The partial thromboplastin time should be checked 4 to 6 h after beginning therapy, and the infusion rate should be adjusted to achieve a value of 1.5 times the control. For the first 24 to 48 h, elderly patients have a standard response to heparin therapy. Subsequently, their partial thromboplastin time may become abnormally elevated, requiring a decrease in the infusion rate, often by 25% or more. Heparin can also be infused intermittently, although the risk of bleeding is believed to be reduced by continuous administration. Adjusting the dose to maintain the partial thromboplastin time at 1.5 times the control value reduces the risk of bleeding.

The **major complications** of heparin therapy are reversible thrombocytopenia and bleeding. Risk factors for bleeding during therapy include uremia, liver disease, surgery in the previous 2 wk, GI bleeding in the previous 6 mo, diastolic blood pressure > 110 mm Hg, and age > 60 yr. The risk of bleeding during therapy appears particularly high in women > 60 yr. About 5% to 15% of patients who receive heparin therapy require blood transfusion because of bleeding.

If major bleeding occurs, the usual approach is to stop administering heparin and allow the anticoagulant effect to dissipate over a few hours. Blood transfusions do not correct the anticoagulant effect of heparin. Protamine can inactivate heparin but generally is not used because of the risk of acute hypotension, dyspnea, and bradycardia.

Heparin can also be administered subcutaneously. Low-dose heparin, 5000 u. s.c. bid, reduces the incidence of deep venous thrombosis, pulmonary embolism, and death from pulmonary embolism in patients undergoing abdominal surgery. Subcutaneous heparin is also used to prevent deep venous thrombosis in medical patients who are at risk of thrombosis—for example, bedridden patients and those who have severe heart failure, hemiparesis after a stroke, or a history of venous thrombosis.

Long-term anticoagulation is usually started in the hospital and continued after discharge using **warfarin.** With elderly patients, some physicians wait 24 to 48 h after starting heparin to begin warfarin. However, clinical studies indicate that warfarin therapy can safely begin at the same time as heparin therapy and that starting them at the same time substantially decreases the length and cost of hospital stay. Although warfarin administration for only 24 h may increase the prothrombin time, 3 to 7 days of therapy (5 to 10 mg daily) are generally needed to achieve a stable antithrombic state. For persons who cannot tolerate warfarin, heparin s.c., usually 10,000 u. q 12 h, may be given. Heparin should be continued for at least 3 days after the prothrombin time has become therapeutic.

How long anticoagulation should continue is unclear. In a patient with a temporary predisposing factor who has not had a previous clot, therapy is usually continued for 4 to 8 wk. In a patient who has had previous episodes of thrombosis, anticoagulant therapy is often given for 3 to 6 mo or continued indefinitely. The need for ongoing warfarin therapy should be reassessed periodically because such therapy poses at least a 10% risk of serious bleeding in the elderly.

Thrombolytic therapy should be considered for patients with deep venous thrombosis involving the iliofemoral system and for patients with massive pulmonary embolism who have significant pulmonary hypertension, obstruction of multiple segments of the pulmonary circulation, or systemic hypotension. Thrombolytic therapy is used in patients with severe proximal deep venous thrombosis because it can achieve greater revascularization of the deep veins in the leg than can heparin therapy.

Clot lysis may reduce the incidence of recurrent thrombi and postphlebitic syndrome. A controlled clinical trial indicated that thrombolytic therapy causes a faster return to normal pulmonary arterial pressure than heparin therapy does. Thrombolytic therapy also relieves strain on the right side of the heart more quickly than heparin does. However, thrombolytic therapy does not improve survival. The potential benefits of this therapy have to be weighed against the greater possibility of hemorrhage, including an approximately 1% to 2% risk of intracranial bleeding. Thrombolytic therapy for deep venous thrombosis or pulmonary emboli has not been compared with heparin therapy in the elderly.

Streptokinase is the most commonly used thrombolytic agent, although **urokinase** is also effective and may be used in patients who are allergic or resistant to streptokinase. **Tissue plasminogen activators** are also useful; however, they offer no advantage over the thrombolytics while costing more. Streptokinase is administered initially as a rapid infusion (bolus) IV of 250,000 u. over 30 min, followed by a continuous infusion of 100,000 u./h for 1 to 3 days. The bolus neutralizes antistreptococcal antibody from previous streptococcal infections. Thrombolytic therapy is generally monitored by measuring thrombin time before therapy, 4 h after therapy begins, and then every 12 h. The objective is to increase the thrombin time to two to four times the baseline value.

After 1 to 3 days of streptokinase therapy, heparin is typically infused at the standard dose for 5 to 7 days. The heparin therapy should be started without a loading dose 4 h after discontinuing the streptokinase.

If **major bleeding** occurs, whole blood or fresh frozen plasma reverses the effect of streptokinase or urokinase.

Contraindications to thrombolytic therapy include eye or central nervous system surgery within the preceding 2 wk, intracranial neoplasms or vascular abnormalities, stroke within the preceding 2 mo, active bleeding, severe hypertension, and allergy to thrombolytic agents. Age alone is not known to be a contraindication, but experience with thrombolytic therapy in the elderly is limited.

Interruption of the inferior vena cava may be required in a small number of patients who have a contraindication to anticoagulation, fail to respond to anticoagulant therapy as demonstrated by recurrent emboli, or have pulmonary emboli from septic thrombophlebitis. The most common technique is to place a filter in the inferior vena cava. The filter is introduced percutaneously into the jugular vein, then advanced to a position below the level of the renal veins. This procedure eliminates the immediate risk of further embolization from a clot in the legs. However, the immediate benefit must be balanced against possible complications, including chronic leg edema, thrombosis formation above the filter, recurrent embolization through collateral veins, perforation of the vena cava, and migration of the filter.

Endarterectomy may be helpful in patients who have chronic pulmonary hypertension because of a clot occluding the main or lobar pulmonary arteries.

50. LUNG CANCER

North Americans have the highest rates of lung cancer worldwide, with age-standardized rates of 74 per 100,000 for men and 29 per 100,000 for women. In the USA, lung cancer is the most common cause of cancer deaths among both men and women. Since the 1940s, the increase in lung cancer mortality by sex has followed historic patterns of cigarette smoking with a 20-yr time lag. With age, the incidence increases, reaching 482 per 100,000 men in the US population > 65 yr. About 65% of all lung cancer deaths occur in persons ≥ 65 yr.

About 90% of male lung cancer deaths and 80% of female lung cancer deaths are attributable to cigarette smoking. Smoking cessation reduces the risk of lung cancer mortality at any age, and the elderly can lower their lung cancer risk substantially by quitting. However, the earlier a smoker quits, the better. For example, the lung cancer risk for 75-yr-old former smokers who quit in their early 60s was 45% of that for lifelong smokers; for those who quit in their early 50s, about 20%; and for those who quit in their early 30s, < 10%. For those who never smoked, the lung cancer risk at age 75 is < 5%. The risk of lung cancer in the elderly may be explained by total years of exposure to carcinogens and promoting agents (both present in cigarette smoke) and the age-related decline in cellular DNA repair activity.

Natural History and Pathology

From exposure to clinical presentation, lung cancer probably has a 15- to 20-yr natural history. Much of this time is spent in carcinogenesis, when metabolic activation of inhaled carcinogen leads to binding with DNA, genomic instability and mutation, perhaps including mutation of a proto-oncogene. Later during carcinogenesis, altered oncogene proteins may lead to structural alterations, which can be detected as atypia by the light microscope. Daughter cells with inherited genomic instability may continue to mutate and proliferate as independent clones. Finally, the transformed, promoted, proliferating clones become malignant and invade local structures.

Under light microscopy, the four major cell types of lung cancer may be distinguished: squamous cell carcinoma, adenocarcinoma, large-cell carcinoma, and small-cell (oat cell) carcinoma. Often, lung cancer shows two or more histologic patterns simultaneously.

Squamous cell carcinoma: Once the most common type, squamous cell carcinoma now accounts for 25% to 30% of lung cancers overall, but it remains the most common (45%) among the elderly. Arising in proximal bronchi, this cell type often progresses from metaplasia to dysplasia and carcinoma in situ before invading. Atypical and neoplastic cells characterized by intracellular keratin formation may exfoliate and be detected at an early stage by cytologic examination of the sputum. These tumors are often among the most slow growing.

Adenocarcinoma: Once the predominant cell type only among women and nonsmokers, adenocarcinoma is now the most common (40%) of all lung cancers and the second most common among the elderly. Reasons for the increased incidence of this cell type remain unknown. Arising from the peripheral bronchiolar epithelium, mucosal glands, or scar, adenocarcinoma frequently forms glands and produces mucin. Except for stage I lesions, this tumor generally has a worse prognosis than squamous cell cancer (see TABLE 50–1).

Large-cell carcinoma: The least common type, large-cell carcinoma accounts for 15% of all lung cancers. Usually, it is distinguished by the absence of distinctive characteristics. Lacking the keratin or gland and mucin characteristics of the better differentiated non–small-cell lung tumors, many large-cell tumors now are reclassified by newer staining techniques as poorly differentiated squamous cell carcinoma or adenocarcinoma. The site of origin and prognosis for large-cell carcinoma are similar to those for adenocarcinoma.

Small-cell (oat cell) carcinoma: This type accounts for about 20% of lung cancers. Arising from basal neuroendocrine (Kulchitsky's) cells in midsized bronchi, small-cell cancers are often characterized by stainable neurosecretory granules and the expression of neuroendocrine peptides. Invading the submucosa early in their growth, these tumors present with regional or distant metastases and usually are considered a

TABLE 50–1. LUNG CANCER TNM STAGING SYSTEM

Stage	*Description*	*5-Yr Survival (%)**
0	Carcinoma in situ, no involvement of nodes, no distant metastases (Tis, N0, M0)	90.0
I	Tumor ≤ 3 cm, no involvement of nodes, no distant metastases (T1, N0, M0)	68.5
	Tumor > 3 cm or any size tumor either invading visceral pleura or causing obstructive pneumonitis and atelectasis to hilum and ≥ 2 cm from carina at bronchoscopy, no involvement of nodes, no distant metastases (T2, N0, M0)	59.0
II	Tumor ≤ 3 cm, node involvement limited to peribronchial or ipsilateral hilum, no distant metastases (T1, N1, M0)	54.1
	Tumor > 3 cm or any size tumor invading visceral pleura or causing obstructive pneumonitis and atelectasis to hilum and ≥ 2 cm from carina at bronchoscopy, node involvement limited to peribronchial or ipsilateral hilum, no distant metastases (T2, N1, M0)	40.0
IIIa	Tumor extending beyond visceral pleura, ie, into chest wall, diaphragm, pericardium, or < 2 cm from carina at bronchoscopy; no involvement of nodes; no distant metastases (T3, N0, M0)	44.2
	Tumor extending beyond visceral pleura, ie, into chest wall, diaphragm, pericardium, or < 2 cm from carina at bronchoscopy; node involvement limited to peribronchial or ipsilateral hilum; no distant metastases (T3, N1, M0)	17.6
	Tumor of any size with involvement of subcarinal or ipsilateral mediastinal nodes, no distant metastases (T1-3, N2, M0)	28.8
IIIb	Tumor invasion of mediastinal structures or malignant pleural effusion, involvement of any nodes (Any T4)	< 5
	Tumor of any size with involvement of contralateral intrathoracic or any scalene or supraclavicular nodes, no distant metastases (Any N3M0)	< 5
IV	Tumor of any size with distant metastases, eg, brain, bone, liver (Any M1)	< 5

T = tumor, N = node, M = metastases.
* 5-yr survivals refer only to non–small-cell lung cancer.
Modified from Mountain CF: "A new international staging system for lung cancer." *Chest* 89(Suppl):225S–233S, 1986; used with permission.

systemic (metastatic) disease at diagnosis. Small-cell cancer is the most rapidly growing and most chemoresponsive of all lung cancers. Management of small-cell cancer follows its own staging system. While prognosis is poor, current chemotherapy regimens have unequivocally prolonged survival; about 10% of those treated remain free of disease 2 yr after therapy.

Screening

Screening for markers of early lung cancer among asymptomatic smokers is a sound concept but not yet a practical one. In a large study sponsored by the National Cancer Institute, 30,000 middle-aged, male cigarette smokers were screened by chest x-ray, with or without sputum cytologic analysis. Only squamous cell cancer cases were detected in sputum at an early stage. Thus, cytologic evaluation may be particularly useful in detecting squamous cell cancer in elderly cigarette smokers. Overall, however, routine cytologic screening failed to detect lung cancer cells at a stage early enough to perform surgical resection or to reduce mortality.

Recent advances in tumor biology have led to the development of immunohistochemical probes and polymerase chain reaction techniques for detecting sputum cells undergoing carcinogenesis. Until these newer techniques are validated for mass screening, however, physician-directed case detection using radiographic and cytologic methods offer the only hope for timely curative treatment among elderly cigarette smokers.

Symptoms, Signs, and Diagnosis

The symptoms and signs that commonly accompany local and regional lung cancer growth are shown in TABLE 50–2. Pulmonary symptoms and radiographic changes in the elderly patient should trigger a high degree of suspicion. Patients ≥ 50 yr who are current or former smokers and who present with community-acquired pneumonia should raise particular concern. The routine practice of waiting up to 3 mo for clearance of a community-acquired pneumonia in elderly smokers may delay early detection and unnecessarily limit treatment options.

Treatment

Therapy for non–small-cell lung cancer follows the international TNM staging system presented in TABLE 50–1.

Pulmonary resection: Curative surgical treatment for non–small-cell lung cancer may be considered for patients with stage I or stage II disease and for those few with stage III disease that can be completely resected. Age alone is not a contraindication to potentially curative surgery; however, the elderly cigarette smokers most likely to develop lung cancer commonly have coronary artery disease and ventilatory obstruction as well. Yet even these high-risk patients have undergone thoracotomy successfully with limited and nonanatomic resections. Perioperative pulmonary complications in the elderly can be minimized

TABLE 50–2. SYMPTOMS AND SIGNS OF LOCAL AND REGIONAL LUNG CANCER GROWTH

Type of Growth	*Description*	*Symptoms and Signs*
Local tumor growth	Endobronchial growth	Cough Dyspnea (secondary to endobronchial obstruction) Chest pain Hemoptysis Wheeze or stridor Pneumonic symptoms (fever, productive cough)
	Peripheral growth	Pain (pleural or chest wall) Cough Dyspnea (secondary to restriction, effusion)
Regional tumor growth	Nerve entrapment	Hoarseness (recurrent laryngeal nerve) Hemidiaphragm elevation with dyspnea (phrenic nerve)
	Vascular obstruction	Superior vena cava syndrome
	Pericardial or cardiac extension	Tamponade Arrhythmia Cardiac failure
	Pleural involvement	Pleural effusion
	Mediastinal extension	Esophageal compression with dysphagia Bronchoesophageal fistula Lymphatic obstruction with pleural effusion

Modified from Cohen MH: "Signs and symptoms of bronchogenic carcinoma," in *Lung Cancer: Clinical Diagnosis and Treatment*, ed. 2, edited by MJ Straus. New York, Grune & Stratton, 1983, pp 97–111; used with permission.

by preoperative smoking cessation, intensive pulmonary physical therapy, antibiotic therapy (for existing bronchitis), bronchodilator therapy, and postoperative pulmonary rehabilitation.

The Lung Cancer Study Group reports a 1.3% postoperative mortality rate for patients < 60 yr, a 4.1% rate for patients 60 to 69 yr, and a 7.1% rate for patients ≥ 70 yr. Respiratory complications occur twice as often in patients ≥ 75 yr, current smokers, and those who experience dyspnea on mild exertion. Those who are unable to walk > 100 yd on a level surface without a rest, who are dyspneic on talking or dressing, or who are unable to leave the house because of dyspnea have twice the complication rate of patients without dyspnea. Perioperative complications correlate with preoperative physiologic measurements (ie, FEV_1, especially when supplemented by maximum minute ventilation and maximal oxygen consumption). General quality-of-life questionnaires add little prognostic information regarding surgical complications.

The key element of the preoperative assessment is a prediction of postoperative pulmonary function. Although no prospective studies have documented a safe lower limit of postoperative pulmonary function, a predicted postoperative FEV_1 of > 800 mL has been suggested as a minimum because hypercapnia often occurs below this level. Hypoxia (Pa_{O_2} < 50 mm Hg) and hypercapnia (Pa_{CO_2} > 45 mm Hg) are also risk factors for perioperative mortality. For patients with no or mild obstruction without atelectasis, hilar mass, or other suggestion of endobronchial disease, postoperative pulmonary function may be predicted, based on a loss of 5.26% for each lung segment resected. Thus, the mortality rate for pneumonectomy is much higher than that for a lobectomy, and the mortality rate for a lobectomy is higher than that for a segmental resection. For patients with more significant obstruction or endobronchial disease, perfusion lung scanning helps predict postoperative pulmonary function.

The success of lung cancer resection, the choice of adjuvant therapy, and the prognosis for resected non–small-cell lung cancer depend on the extent of metastasis. For the patient with adequate pulmonary reserve and no evidence of extrathoracic (bone, brain, or liver) metastases, the extent of mediastinal and thoracic lymph node involvement determines whether curative resection is possible. In 33% to 50% of lung cancer patients, the cancer has spread to the mediastinal lymph nodes before the initial evaluation. The history and physical examination may identify symptoms of hypercalcemia (nausea, mental decline) or other suggestions of local or regional tumor invasion (see TABLE 50–2). Improvements have made computed tomography **(CT)** scanning a valuable addition to chest radiography for determining mediastinal tumor extension. Yet staging by mediastinoscopy has shown that CT scanning may be falsely negative in 9% of cases in which it had indicated only local involvement. Magnetic resonance imaging **(MRI)** is superior to CT only for assessing vascular invasion. The use of the Wang transbronchial needle biopsy for mediastinal staging is promising but not yet validated in clinical trials. Routine hematoxylin-eosin (H&E) staining of mediastinal lymph node biopsy specimens has a substantial false-negative rate (63% in one study) for detection of metastases.

Chemotherapy: For most patients with advanced (stage IIIb, stage IV) non–small-cell lung cancer, nonsurgical therapies are often recommended. Although complete response rates are low for advanced lung cancer, more than one quarter of patients may be expected to receive some benefit (see TABLE 50–3). Recent reports of combined chemotherapy and radiotherapy suggest that even higher response rates may be possible. Cure is rarely possible.

TABLE 50–3. CHEMOTHERAPY TOXICITY AND RESPONSE RATES FOR ELDERLY PATIENTS WITH ADVANCED LUNG CANCER TREATED WITH DOXORUBICIN AND CYCLOPHOSPHAMIDE OR SEMUSTINE AND CYCLOPHOSPHAMIDE

	Age < 70 yr	*Age ≥ 70 yr*
Number of cases	966	104
Percentage with severe toxicity		
Hematologic effects Leukocytes < 2,000/μL, platelets < 50,000/μL, neutrophils < 1,000/μL, or need for transfusions	14%	13%
Vomiting Intractable	7%	7%
Infection Debilitating or life-threatening	1%	2%
Cardiac effects Mild heart failure, multifocal premature ventricular contractions, pericarditis, or worse reactions	1%	2%
Percentage with complete response	4%	5%
Percentage with complete or partial response	26%	21%

Modified from Begg CB, Carbone PP: "Clinical trials and drug toxicity in the elderly. The experience of the Eastern Cooperative Oncology Group." *Cancer* 52:1986–1992, 1983; used with permission.

The Eastern Cooperative Oncology Group (ECOG) reported that elderly patients and younger patients with advanced lung cancer who undergo chemotherapy have similar response rates. Rates of severe toxicity are also the same in these groups. The only exception is that methotrexate and semustine cause more hematologic reactions in elderly patients. The ECOG report concludes that elderly patients should be treated as aggressively as younger patients. Instead of using an arbitrary age limit to exclude patients from aggressive chemotherapy, ECOG investigators recommend using physiologic functional parameters such as renal, liver, and marrow function. Thoughtful decisions on the appropriateness of chemotherapy for older lung cancer patients are supported through frank discussions of possible benefits, toxicity, lifestyle, and personal preferences.

Small-cell lung cancer is usually metastatic; thus, treatment is based on whether cancer is limited or extensive, rather than on whether it is localized or metastatic. A small-cell tumor confined to a hemithorax (including the mediastinum or supraclavicular lymph nodes) that can be reached by a single radiation therapy port, is defined as limited disease. When negative CT scans of the brain and abdomen and negative bone marrow aspirate and biopsy findings confirm that small-cell cancer is limited, reported median survival is 10 to 16 mo with treatment. However, two thirds of patients with small-cell lung cancer have extensive disease; reported median survival is 6 to 12 mo with currently available therapy.

Radiotherapy: Radiotherapy can be used as primary therapy or for palliation and pain control in advanced disease. Local control of unresectable disease often can be achieved with radiation, although control of metastases and cure are uncommon. Patients with resectable non–small-cell lung cancer who have medical contraindications to surgery can be considered for curative radiotherapy; the expected cure rate at 5 yr is about 20%. Patients with locally (T3, T4) or regionally (N2, N3) advanced non–small-cell cancer often receive radiotherapy alone or radiotherapy and chemotherapy as primary treatment. Patients with distant metastases (M1) receive radiotherapy for symptom palliation.

When measured by caloric intake, adequacy of energy intake, total radiation dose tolerated, or concurrent illnesses, susceptibility to the effects of radiation therapy is no different for patients ≥ 65 yr than for those < 65 yr. Similarly, no significant differences occur in weight, body mass index, or multidimensional functional status. Just as with chemotherapy, with radiotherapy elderly patients did not experience therapy-related problems any differently than younger patients did, indicating that age alone is not a sufficient criterion for judging a patient's ability to undergo curative or palliative treatment.

§3. ORGAN SYSTEMS: GASTROINTESTINAL DISORDERS

51. EFFECTS OF AGING ON THE GASTROINTESTINAL SYSTEM

A major obstacle to the advancement of geriatric gastroenterology is our ignorance of the basic science of aging. This handicap is analogous to doing research in infectious disease without having the basic science of bacteriology. Nevertheless, some progress has been made in understanding the effects of aging on GI physiology and pathophysiology.

The primary functions of the GI system are digestion and absorption; the secondary functions that subserve these activities are secretion and motility. Throughout life, the gut is constantly and rapidly changing. Epithelial cell turnover occurs as often as every 24 to 48 h. Absorption and secretion are almost constant. Myoelectric and motor activity are continuous.

Aging is associated with physiologic and pathophysiologic changes in many organ systems (eg, endocrine, vascular, nervous) that affect GI structure and function and produce variations in the presentation of GI illness. Aging also allows for the superimposition of altered alimentary function by extraintestinal diseases. When such diseases are common, the observed changes may appear to result from the aging process. A prime example is the esophageal motility changes in octogenarians that for decades were assumed to result from age-determined esophageal muscle changes. Recently, these changes have been shown to result from extraintestinal disorders (eg, diabetes mellitus and neurologic and vascular changes that supervene with age). In fact, research has shown that most age-related changes in GI motility result from neurologic rather than muscular changes.

The intricate interaction among psychologic and social stress and physiologic function is especially pertinent in the elderly, who are subject not only to the usual stresses of adulthood but also stresses such as loss of spouse, family members, friends, and job at a time of increasing mental and physical limitations. The interplay of psychosocial stresses and anatomic, motor, and secretory changes often leads to GI symptoms, sometimes atypical ones. Some patients deny or downplay their GI symptoms; others exaggerate them.

Constipation, incontinence, and diverticular disease are the most commonly recognized GI problems in the elderly. Each has different underlying causes, and the specific pathogenesis dictates specific treatment.

Age may alter the presentation of malabsorption, and chronic diarrhea may affect an older patient differently and more severely than it affects a younger patient. For example, the increased incidence of nutritional deficiencies among the elderly makes them particularly vulnerable to the effects of malabsorption. Also, the concentration of the brush border enzyme, lactase, decreases gradually with age, increasing lactose intolerance and intestinal gas and diarrhea. When malabsorption is superimposed, the symptoms are augmented. This situation is particularly bothersome when the patient has associated disabilities, such as a mobility disorder that makes reaching the bathroom difficult. If incontinence is also present, the foul-smelling, pasty steatorrhea is much less tolerable than the odor of otherwise normal stool. Besides diarrhea from lactase deficiency, osmotic diarrhea caused by laxatives is common among the elderly and readily leads to dehydration, particularly because the thirst mechanism may be impaired.

Cancer of various intestinal organs is common in elderly persons, and special considerations are required for successful surgical management. For example, elderly patients may have arthritis, stroke, or other impairments of dexterity, which may interfere with proper management of colostomies and ileostomies. Benign lesions in the elderly also require a specialized approach. Elderly patients are more fragile, and they often have coexisting cerebrovascular, cardiovascular, renal, or hepatic disorders that increase their risk for any type of surgery. Nevertheless, treatment of brisk GI bleeding should not be delayed in the elderly, who do not tolerate prolonged bleeding as well as younger persons.

Diagnostic approaches are also influenced by aging. When undertaking diagnostic studies or therapeutic regimens, the physician must take into account the special needs of the elderly. A number of factors must be considered in deciding on the advisability of endoscopy and in determining the appropriate preparation and techniques. When determining the premedication requirement for endoscopy, the physician must consider the increased sensitivity to sedatives and analgesic medication and the susceptibility to respiratory depression and hypotension. Careful monitoring is essential. Also, the lateral rather than the supine position must be maintained to minimize the risk of aspiration.

52. DENTAL AND ORAL DISORDERS

Two major functions of the oral cavity are to initiate digestion and to allow the production of speech. All oral tissues have evolved to permit these activities: The teeth, supporting periodontal tissues, and temporomandibular joint aid in mechanical food processing; the tongue with its finely coordinated movements not only mixes and assists in translocating food but also is central to phonation.

Although the mouth is exposed to the outside environment, the oral mucosa provides a barrier against pathogens. Saliva protects oral tissues with its lubricatory, antimicrobial, and dental-remineralizing proteins. Saliva also helps to break down food and to transform it into a swallow-ready bolus. The mouth has an intricate sensory control system, including exquisitely developed receptors for pain, taste, texture, and temperature.

Dental and oral disorders affect all of the tissues and functions mentioned above. Most problems are not life threatening, but they may be serious and may impact greatly on the quality of life.

DENTAL CARIES

A disease characterized by decalcification of the tooth's inorganic portion and accompanied or followed by disintegration of the organic portion, resulting from the action of microorganisms.

In the past, elderly persons were likely to be edentulous. With advances in dental preservation, they are more often dentate and dental caries is seen more often.

Pathophysiology

Dental caries results from dissolution of the tooth surface by microbial by-products found in dental plaque. The type of caries most often affecting the elderly occurs on the root surface **(root caries).** Loss of alveolar (supporting) bone around teeth is seen in older persons, and root surfaces become exposed to the oral milieu (see FIG. 52–1). Cementum, the mineralized substance surrounding the root surface, is an extracellular matrix with about 50% less mineral content than the enamel matrix covering the crown. Thus, root surfaces in older persons may be increasingly susceptible to abrasion, attrition, and demineralization.

Root caries is about four times more prevalent in elderly than in younger persons. **Coronal caries** (*decay on the crown of the tooth*) is more common among children, adolescents, and young adults. However, older persons are still susceptible to coronal caries, which usually recurs around restorations. Generally, root caries is more difficult to repair than coronal caries. The rapid and extensive appearance of root caries in an elderly patient often signals marked salivary dysfunction (see SALIVARY GLAND DISORDERS, below).

Prophylaxis and Treatment

All forms of caries should be treated promptly. Untreated caries will progress and penetrate the dental pulp; may cause considerable pain, discomfort, and local infection; and ultimately will entail more extensive therapy—eg, an **exodontic procedure** (extraction) or **endodontic procedure** (root canal therapy). The elderly should have regular dental care, including prophylaxis (fluoride rinses, plaque and tartar removal) to limit caries. A dental examination once every 6 mo is usually adequate, but a history of rapidly developing carious lesions or conservatively managed periodontal disease may require more frequent check-

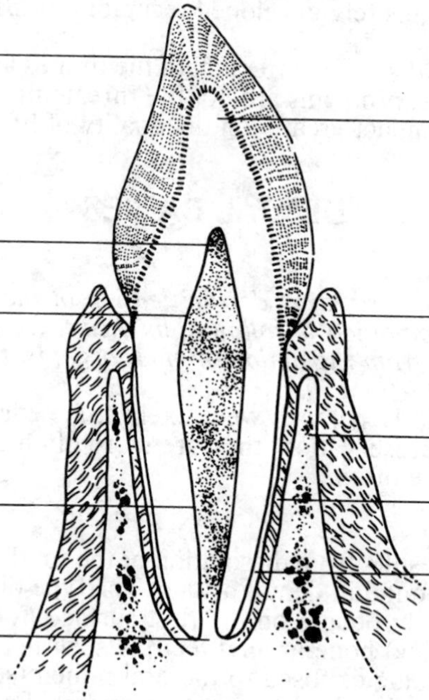

FIG. 52–1. Anatomic structures of a tooth shown from sagittal section through a mandibular cuspid and surrounding hard and soft tissues. Redrawn from Berkey DB, Shay K: "General dental care for the elderly." *Clinics in Geriatric Medicine* 8(3):579–597, 1992; used with permission.

ups. Older persons with diminished dexterity may need professional prophylaxis more often and individually tailored techniques for oral hygiene.

PERIODONTAL DISEASE

Disease of the tooth's supporting structure, including the gingiva, alveolar bone, and periodontal ligament.

Pathophysiology, Symptoms, and Signs

Most tooth loss in adults stems from periodontal disease, usually associated with gingival recession. Like dental caries, periodontal disease is caused by bacterial plaque that accumulates and adheres to the teeth. Bacterial antigens penetrate periodontal tissues; this penetration initiates an inflammatory response and results in local immunopathologic destruction of connective tissues.

Periodontal disease tends to progress slowly, in an episodic pattern. Initially, gingiva bleeds and becomes edematous—a hallmark sign **(gingivitis).** Later, destruction of alveolar bone and the periodontal ligament **(periodontitis)** results in loss of support for the tooth (see FIG. 52–1). A person's periodontal status represents the accumulation of lesions over a lifetime.

Many common clinical situations can aggravate periodontal disease; eg, diabetes may cause an exaggerated inflammatory reaction with poor tissue response and healing. Drugs also can affect periodontal status. Some (eg, cyclosporine, nifedipine, and phenytoin) may irritate the gums and cause **gingival hyperplasia.** Others (eg, antihypertensives, psychoactive drugs, and anticholinergics) can reduce saliva production and thereby diminish the key endogenous protective mechanism in the mouth (see SALIVARY GLAND DISORDERS, below).

Prophylaxis and Treatment

Principal prophylactic measures involve good oral hygiene. An antimicrobial (antiplaque) mouthwash containing chlorhexidine is effective and is particularly useful for persons who have difficulty with dental hygiene because of diminished dexterity. However, regular use may stain teeth and composite resin dental restorations. These tenacious stains can be removed from the teeth by professional prophylaxis. However, resin restorations may be permanently discolored.

Local or systemic antibiotics in conjunction with periodontal debridement have been suggested for aggressive periodontitis. Because both mixed anaerobic and facultative bacteria are associated with adult periodontitis, no single antibiotic is completely suitable. Nevertheless, after analysis of the microbial population, appropriate short-term systemic antibiotic therapy is useful for some older patients (eg, tetracycline 250 mg/day for 7 to 21 days; doxycycline 100 mg/day for 14 to 21 days; metronidazole 200 to 250 mg tid for 5 to 14 days; or amoxicillin and clavulanate potassium 250 mg tid for 10 to 14 days).

Surgery may not be necessary because *active* periodontal disease seems to be less common in older persons, and confounding systemic factors (eg, use of anticoagulant or immunosuppressive drugs) may contraindicate it. Nonsteroidal anti-inflammatory drugs, as an adjunct to traditional prophylaxis, appear to help slow periodontal tissue destruction.

ORAL MUCOSAL DISORDERS

Oral mucosa in older persons has been stereotypically characterized as pale, thin, atrophic, dry, and readily traumatized. However, little hard evidence is available to support this. Despite quantitative histologic evidence of epithelial atrophy with age, there is no indication that this is clinically significant. Many age-related local changes, such as varicosities and Fordyce's granules, also have no clinical significance. For example, varicosities in the floor of the mouth, the ventral surface of the tongue, and the hypopharynx rarely bleed. In general, the critical barrier function of the oral mucosa is well maintained in healthy adults, regardless of age.

Most complaints are probably manifestations of a systemic disease (Sjögren's syndrome) or conditions (side effects of drugs or head and neck irradiation) that diminish salivary gland performance (see below). Other conditions (eg, certain endocrinopathies and nutritional deficiencies) can also adversely affect the oral mucosa.

Older edentulous or partially edentulous persons frequently present with traumatic **lesions—erythematous, hyperplastic, hyperkeratotic, or ulcerative—secondary to ill-fitting dental prostheses.** Patients with such lesions should be referred to a dentist for a new prosthesis or repair of the old one.

If painful ulcerations occur, palliative topical agents may be helpful, eg, 0.5% dyclonine elixir combined with an equal amount of diphenhydramine elixir. This combination requires compounding by a pharmacist. It can be applied with a cotton-tipped applicator directly to intraoral ulcerations if there are only a few. However, as an oral rinse, 5 mL of the mixture as needed can relieve the pain of a generalized stomatitis. Nutritional counseling (to avoid spicy and irritating foods) may also be required until the mucositis is alleviated. If tissue is considerably hyperplastic, surgery may be necessary to allow normal chewing.

Burning sensations of the oral mucosa have been reported, particularly by postmenopausal women. These symptoms are rare, and their etiology is unclear. Patients with so-called burning mouth syndrome represent a spectrum of problems. Psychologic factors are considered important in the course of this syndrome, but many patients show signs of neurologic dysfunction, vitamin deficiency, poor oral hygiene, or salivary hypofunction. Some burning mouth complaints are associated with candidiasis (see below). Some patients with burning mouth syndrome can be difficult and frustrating to manage, but they may benefit from referral to an expert in treating chronic pain syndromes. Complete, apparently spontaneous, remission is not uncommon.

Oral candidiasis can occur in older persons with dental prostheses (under a denture or at the labial commissures), in those with salivary hypofunction, and in those taking antibiotic or immunosuppressive drugs long term. Candidal hyphae indicate that the oral mucosal barrier has been breached; therefore, the patient is at risk for systemic infection. Treatment with anticandidal agents is required, eg, an oral suspension of nystatin 100,000 to 400,000 u. 3 to 6 times/day for 14 days or clotrimazole troches 10 mg 5 times/day for 14 days.

ORAL CARCINOMA

Oral carcinoma, which represents 3% to 5% of all forms of cancer, is a serious concern in the elderly. Its prevalence is low until middle age but increases sharply thereafter. Oral cancers tend to occur twice as often in men as in women.

Close attention should be directed at persons with clearly defined **risk factors,** ie, those who smoke cigarettes and those who regularly drink alcoholic beverages. Less common risk factors are pipe and cigar smoking. Smokeless (chewing) tobacco appears to be related to verrucous carcinoma (a highly differentiated variant of squamous cell carcinoma).

The **diagnosis** of oral cancer is often problematic because of the many ill-defined or variable-appearing lesions that can occur in the mouth. Most are benign, though they may easily be confused clinically with a malignancy. Conversely, malignant changes can appear quite benign. Typically, the chief complaint is a sore in the mouth. White, red, or ulcerated lesions that persist > 3 wk should be evaluated by a dentist or oral surgeon. Induration, fixation, and lymphadenopathy indicate advanced lesions. The lesion's clinical history and other oral findings dictate whether biopsy is indicated. Carcinoma should be part of the differential diagnosis of many oral lesions.

About 90% of oral cancers are detected in the following high-risk sites: the floor of the mouth, the oral and basal portions of the tongue, the oropharynx, and the lips. Buccal and labial vestibular carcinoma should be considered in people who use smokeless tobacco. Patients with an oral cancer are at high risk (up to 33%) for developing a second primary neoplasm in the mouth, pharynx, larynx, esophagus, or lung. Therefore, patients identified as having an oral cancer should be screened in all these sites (eg, using indirect laryngoscopy, chest x-ray) and reexamined annually.

More than any other factor, the stage of these cancers determines the **prognosis.** While oral cancers < 1 cm in diameter are easily cured, most lesions are *not* diagnosed before they have metastasized to lymph nodes. Therefore, 5-yr survival rates remain at 30% to 40%. This unfortunate situation appears to result from inadequate knowledge of appropriate screening procedures.

NONDENTAL MINERALIZED TISSUE LOSS

Alveolar Bone

Alveolar bone, an important component of the periodontium, provides support for the teeth and is clearly different from the underlying jawbone (mandible and maxilla). Although a general loss of bone mass occurs with age, **resorption of alveolar bone** is a result of local factors rather than a part of the aging process. Once dentition (part or all) is lost, alveolar bone is not needed and atrophy quickly ensues. This problem will likely decline as dentition is better preserved.

Fabricating an effective dental prosthesis for patients with severely resorbed alveolar bony ridges is difficult. Upper dentures with a large surface area on the hard palate can usually be adjusted to fit satisfactorily. However, the mandibular arch may be particularly hard to fit. Endosseous metallic implants (typically titanium) or posts can be surgically placed (especially in edentulous lower jaws) to support dental prostheses and should be considered for patients who report increasing difficulty in retaining dentures.

The installation and proper fit of dentures is important. The loss of dentition and supporting bone affects facial height and results in a tendency toward prognathism, which may contribute to a diminished self-image. Loss of teeth or improperly fitted dentures may adversely affect the patient's dietary selection and nutrition.

Temporomandibular Joint

The temporomandibular joint **(TMJ)** is located between the maxillary glenoid fossa and the condylar process of the mandible and is structurally unique. It is essential to all articulated maxillary and mandibular functions and is involved in many craniofacial pain disorders. Temporomandibular disorders are *a constellation of symptoms involving the TMJ and muscles of mastication*. Most affected persons are in their third, fourth, and early fifth decades, and temporomandibular disorders decrease with advancing age. A commonly held view that patients with these disorders have a higher incidence of psychopathology is not well supported in controlled research.

The TMJ is subject to the symptoms and signs associated with most arthritides. Osteoarthritis is often detectable by the presence of crepitus and degenerative changes on tomographic imaging. Other common temporomandibular disorders include displacement of the TMJ disk and myofascial pain in the masseter and temporal muscles. Clinical signs include jaw clicking and a reduced range of mandibular motion (< 40 mm intraincisal distance). Pain is the most common complaint and can include otalgia and neck pain as well as pain referred to otherwise healthy teeth.

The clinician should examine the preauricular areas for joint noises (click, crepitus) and for tenderness in the TMJ and in the masseter, temporal, and pterygoid muscles. Gross evaluation of the occlusion is indicated, although the degree to which occlusion is causative in temporomandibular disorders is controversial. Magnetic resonance, tomographic, or panoramic imaging may rule out intra-articular or bone disease. A diagnosis of temporomandibular disorder should be deferred until more serious extra- and intracranial abnormalities have been excluded (eg, common geriatric conditions such as trigeminal neuralgia and temporal arteritis).

Treatment should be directed toward providing support to the affected structures and reducing and eliminating aggravating factors such as teeth clenching (bruxism). Specialists should include a dentist with expertise in temporomandibular disorders, a physical therapist, and when indicated, a psychiatrist or psychologist. Typical treatment consists of an interocclusal appliance, short-term physical therapy, behavior modification, and nonsteroidal anti-inflammatory drugs; therapy can include a soft diet, muscle relaxants, and moist heat. Complete or partial edentulism (anodontia) may complicate treatment.

ORAL MOTOR DYSFUNCTION

The oral motor apparatus is involved in finely coordinated functions, including speaking, chewing, swallowing, and facial posture. In general, aging is associated with morphologic and biochemical alterations in neuromuscular systems. Several studies of oral motor function in healthy adults demonstrate measurable changes in motor performance with age. **Reduced masticatory muscle performance** is common and appears to lead to an increased tendency to swallow larger food particles than usually attempted at a younger age. This practice could result in choking or aspiration. A **prolonged oral phase of swallowing** similarly may interfere with deglutition.

Motor changes are of greater concern in nonhealthy, elderly patients. Obviously, frank neuropathies may markedly affect the oral-maxillofacial musculature. However, most oral motor dysfunctions are iatrogenic and not necessarily directly related to the neuromuscular apparatus; thus, any treatment that diminishes salivary gland function may negatively affect the timing and pattern of the oral swallowing phase. Drugs (eg, antihypertensives, anticholinergics, antipsychotics, and antidepressants) can significantly affect salivary performance (see TABLE 52–1). Diminished saliva is also seen in patients after irradiation or surgery for head and neck neoplasms. Additionally, some drugs (eg, phenothiazines) are often associated with tardive dyskinesia in the oral and maxillofacial region.

Certain characteristic **changes in voice and speech production** occur with age. However, aging is not normally associated with impaired ability to produce speech and thus is not a general clinical concern.

Many **postural alterations** occur with age. The lower face and lips may droop because of decreased tone of the circumoral muscles and (in edentulous persons) reduced bone support. This change is both an aesthetic concern and a potential source of embarrassment, since it can lead to drooling or food spills. Healthy older persons may also have difficulty closing their lips competently while eating, sleeping, or even

TABLE 52–1. DRUGS THAT DECREASE SALIVARY FLOW

Drug Class	*Marked Decrease*	*Moderate Decrease*	*Minimal or No Decrease*
Antidepressant	Amitriptyline Nortriptyline Clomipramine Imipramine Desipramine Maprotiline Chlorpromazine Triflupromazine Doxepin	Dothiepin Zimelidine Nomifensine Lofepramine Haloperidol Thioridazine	Citalopram Lithium
Antianxiety	—	—	Lorazepam
Antihypertensive	Clonidine	—	Propranolol Metoprolol Verapamil Timolol maleate
Diuretic	—	—	Bendroflumethiazide Amiloride Hydrochlorothiazide
Anticholinergic/ antireflux	Atropine Scopolamine Propantheline	Hyoscyamine	Pirenzepine Cimetidine Ranitidine Bethanechol Metoclopramide
Antihistamine	Diphenhydramine	—	—

Modified from Kaplan MD, Baum BJ: "The functions of saliva." *Dysphagia* 8:225–229, 1993; used with permission.

resting. Loss of circumoral muscle tone is often first recognized when the person complains of excessive saliva.

Oral motor dysfunction is best managed by a multidisciplinary approach. Coordinated referrals to specialists in prosthetic dentistry, rehabilitative medicine, speech pathology, and gastroenterology may be needed.

GUSTATORY DYSFUNCTION

(See also TASTE AND SMELL DISORDERS in Ch. 104)

Adequate taste and smell not only ensure proper food selection but also protect against ingesting spoiled food. Anecdotally, gustatory function declines with age, although recent data suggest that changes in healthy older persons are modest and tend to affect a specific quality of taste (ie, too sweet, sour, salty, or bitter).

Food enjoyment also requires olfactory and textural sensory cues. Textural sensory function appears to undergo little or no change with aging. Conversely, olfactory function is markedly impaired. Thus, olfactory function must be assessed in any evaluation of gustatory or food enjoyment complaints.

Hypogeusia, *a decreased ability to taste,* or **dysgeusia,** *a persistent bad taste in the mouth,* may be associated with neuropathy, upper respiratory infection, drug use (eg, captopril, penicillamine, vinblastine), dental extractions, trauma, menopause, and a host of systemic diseases, but the linkages are weak. Most gustatory complaints are likely to be related to dental status and poor oral hygiene; eg, purulent material from a dental or periodontal abscess may distort gustatory signals. Also, many elderly persons have difficulty maintaining good oral hygiene. Poor hygiene, particularly around teeth with extensive restorations or dental prostheses, may result in chronic unpleasant taste sensations.

Diagnosis

Assessment of gustatory complaints begins with the history. Patients should be asked if they can taste salt when added to soup, the sweetness of sugar when added to tea, the sourness of lemon juice, and the bitter taste of coffee. Affirmative answers indicate a likely olfactory deficit rather than taste loss. Gross taste function can be assessed using these simple chemicals, which define the four basic taste qualities. When a patient complains of an unpleasant taste (and if it is usually associated with meals or can be rinsed away with water), suspicion should center on dental disease and dental hygiene. If no local cause seems likely, history of head trauma or upper respiratory disease should be checked. Cranial nerve evaluation should include the first (olfactory), seventh (facial), ninth (glossopharyngeal), and tenth (vagus) nerves.

Tests for taste: Detailed, meaningful tests of gustatory function are difficult to administer in a typical clinical setting. If the above screening procedures are inadequate, referral to a chemosensory center for intensive testing may be necessary.

Tests for olfaction: A reliable and easy-to-use odor recognition test is the University of Pennsylvania Smell Identification Test. It is a prepackaged, scratch-and-sniff test that requires minimal supervision during administration and is easy to score.

Treatment

There are no good therapies for gustatory dysfunction. Zinc preparations appear to have little more than a placebo effect. If olfactory disorders relate to airway obstruction, surgical correction may be possible. Meticulously documenting complaints and reassuring patients that measurable sensory deficits are noted often helps and is appreciated.

SALIVARY GLAND DISORDERS

Adequate salivary gland function is essential to all aspects of oral health. Saliva is necessary to form and translocate food boluses, to lubricate and maintain the integrity of the oral mucosa, and to prevent demineralization and promote remineralization of teeth. It contains at least six antimicrobial proteins that control bacterial colonization and limit fungal and viral growth. Saliva buffers acids produced by bacteria and mechanically cleanses the mouth.

Many studies have suggested that salivary gland morphologic appearance is altered in older people, with parallel reductions in saliva production. However, recent studies in carefully defined populations indicate that no general reduction in salivary performance occurs with age; resting and stimulated parotid gland function remains intact. Reductions in submandibular-sublingual saliva seen in the well elderly are probably not biologically significant. Most age-related changes in salivary function are attributed to systemic disorders or their treatment.

Etiology

Salivary gland disorders are usually iatrogenic or caused by Sjögren's syndrome. Less frequently observed conditions that affect salivary glands include bacterial infections, sialoliths, trauma, and neoplasms.

Iatrogenic: Salivary gland dysfunction is usually drug related. Xerostomia is a potential side effect of > 400 drugs (see TABLE 52–1), many of which are often used by the elderly. In addition, head and neck irradiation (in particular) and cytotoxic chemotherapy for neoplasms directly and dramatically affect salivary gland performance.

Sjögren's syndrome, *an autoimmune exocrinopathy afflicting primarily women,* is the most common disease affecting salivary glands in older persons. It may occur as a primary disorder (affecting only the salivary and lacrimal glands) or in a secondary form (with glandular dysfunction and connective tissue disease).

Symptoms and Signs

Xerostomia, *dryness of the mouth,* is the most common condition linked with salivary dysfunction. It may be associated with reduced salivary output or could result from altered lubricatory factors, defective sensory receptors, or impaired cognition. Patients with true salivary gland dysfunction typically have difficulty swallowing dry foods, a need to drink while attempting to swallow, dryness of the mouth and lips while eating, and difficulty in speaking at length. Important signs include an unexpected recent increase in dental caries and ulcerated, erythematous, or furrowed mucosa. However, mucosa may appear normal even when glands are dysfunctional.

Diagnosis

Salivary gland status should first be evaluated by oral examination. Attempts should be made to assess major gland duct patency and to express saliva from each orifice. Saliva production should be measured quantitatively under basal and stimulated conditions. For evaluation of total saliva flow, patients should be instructed to have nothing by mouth for 90 min. Ask the patient to swallow any saliva present, then to let saliva passively accumulate in the mouth for a set time (1 to 5 min), followed by expectoration into a calibrated vessel. The volume per minute is the whole saliva resting flow rate. Stimulated saliva is collected in a similar manner except that saliva production is stimulated with lemon juice or by chewing a rubber band. Typically, basal function is severely reduced in affected persons, although many show some stimulated saliva production, indicating the presence of functional gland parenchyma. Absence of stimulated secretions indicates the loss of fluid-secreting cells.

Retrograde sialography is a particularly useful diagnostic imaging method when inflammatory or obstructive disorders are suspected. **Sodium pertechnetate Tc 99m scintigraphy** is useful when acinar function needs to be assessed objectively. The radionuclide parallels water movement; both an uptake phase (which shows acinar parenchyma) and an efflux phase (which shows secretion into the mouth) are clearly visualized.

If Sjögren's syndrome is suspected, biopsy of minor labial salivary glands should be performed (usually by an oral surgeon) and lacrimal gland function should be evaluated. Additionally, serologic markers of autoimmune disease (particularly anti–SS-A, anti–SS-B, and rheumatoid factor) should be analyzed.

Clinical features of **sialadenitis** (salivary gland inflammation) can include fever and swelling, pain, and erythema over the affected gland. When the gland is palpated, a purulent discharge that can be gram-stained and cultured is expressed from the ducts; the most common organism is *Staphylococcus aureus.*

Treatment

Drug-induced gland dysfunction is almost always fully reversible. If action is warranted because of oral complications, either reducing drug levels or using alternative drugs may help. In patients with basal secretory deficits who have some stimulated responses, pharmacologic stimulation of salivary glands has been achieved with the cholinergic agent pilocarpine 5 mg orally tid. There is no satisfactory treatment for the autoimmune component of gland hypofunction.

Patients without functional gland parenchyma have no fluid-transporting cells and do not respond to any directed salivary or systemic therapy. They should have frequent, comprehensive, preventive dental care.

Salivary substitutes are helpful in limiting hard tissue problems but unsatisfactory for soft tissue complaints. For the latter, only palliative therapy is available. Mouthwashes, including topical analgesics and antimicrobials noted above, are helpful.

Treatment of sialadenitis consists of rehydration and antibiotic administration. Occasionally, an abscess requires surgical drainage.

53. FUNCTIONAL DISORDERS OF THE GASTROINTESTINAL TRACT

Disturbances of gut physiology arising as part of an array of adaptive reactions, often to stress, nongastrointestinal illness, or drugs. Patients with such disturbances account for about 60% of all consultations for GI symptoms and about 2.4% of all hospital admissions. Functional GI disorders are common in patients of all ages, but often the presentation is different in elderly patients. Instead of intermittent cramping and diarrhea, older patients more commonly develop constipation, bloating, eructation, swallowing disorders, fecal incontinence, and sensations of bad taste.

Several age-related changes in the GI tract predispose the elderly to such complaints. Although transit time does not change much with aging, illness, depression, and medication slow transit time more profoundly in the old than in the young. Also, the myenteric reflexes that help prevent constipation become less effective with age. The capacity of the rectum to store feces increases, making impaction more likely. Acid secretion in the stomach decreases, and gastrin levels increase. Substantial changes occur in esophageal motility, with intrinsic slow waves slowing and decreasing in amplitude, a condition sometimes called **presbyesophagus.** Also, some evidence indicates that sphincter pressure at the esophagogastric junction decreases, more readily allowing reflux.

Disease and medical interventions are more common with age, and many of them affect GI function. Diabetes may impair the autonomic nervous system and voluntary innervation of the anus. Heart failure can cause fluid shifts, producing edema of the GI tract. Many medications affect GI function. Anticholinergics substantially slow transit time and commonly cause constipation; diuretics may dehydrate the feces; and other drugs may cause GI upset.

The relationship between functional GI problems and psychologic imbalance is strong at all ages, and psychosocial stress commonly causes or exacerbates functional GI disturbances in the elderly. Loss of a spouse, emotional adjustment to retirement, admission to a hospital or nursing home, and frustration resulting from disease and the aging process all contribute to psychophysiologic stresses in elderly patients. Depression often goes undiagnosed and untreated. Also, poor dietary habits and lack of physical activity may cause or compound problems.

Approach to the Patient

An evaluation of GI disturbances requires a thorough review of traditional medical issues as well as a review of prescription and over-the-counter drugs, diet, physical activities, and psychologic issues. The history should be obtained in an open-ended interview, which encourages the patient to respond spontaneously and helps prevent physician bias. Leading questions or those that elicit yes or no answers should be avoided at first. At all times, the questions should communicate the physician's willingness to consider all aspects of the illness, whether biologic or psychogenic.

Rather than asking, "Are you under stress?" at the end of the history, the physician should make an open-ended request early in the interview, eg, "Tell me what happened and how you felt during your last attack." This type of request is less threatening and allows the patient to offer medical and psychologic data concurrently.

The history should explore the patient's eating habits, especially the timing of meals, the amount of fiber consumed, the amount of liquid consumed daily, the relationships of particular foods with symptoms, and stressful factors that might be related to eating.

Medication use must be fully explored. Questions should cover both prescription and over-the-counter drugs. Special attention should be paid to the correlation between symptoms and medications taken on an as needed basis.

Physicians should resist the tendency to order unneeded studies or treatments just to do something for an insistent patient. When the initial examination and studies are unrevealing and the patient is clinically stable, the wise course is to tolerate the diagnostic uncertainty and monitor the patient. However, a nonthreatening behavioral disorder causing GI symptoms does not preclude the presence or development of a medical disease that presents as a GI or other complaint. Complete objectivity must guide the approach to even the most vague, dramatic, or bizarre symptom complex.

In persons of all ages, GI symptoms may have adaptive value to the patient. In younger patients, secondary gain may include obtaining disability pay, avoiding family chores, and receiving attention. In the elderly, the gain is more likely to be receiving attention from family, friends, and the physician. Giving up the benefits of the illness may be a greater loss than the presumed benefits of symptom relief. Suspicion should be high when the patient overtly or covertly resists management. Management can be frustrating for the physician, and therapeutic interventions can cause more harm than good.

Frequently, older persons with GI complaints are given psychoactive drugs. Such therapy is often warranted, especially when depression or chronic anxiety is at the root of the problem. However, these medications are also overused. Medication cannot replace counseling or psychotherapy and can cause serious side effects. In fact, many psychoactive drugs, especially the tricyclic antidepressants and antipsychotics, are strongly anticholinergic and can worsen GI disturbances. Thus, they must be used judiciously and only after thorough evaluation.

NONCARDIAC CHEST PAIN

Typical angina-like pain is not always cardiac in origin, especially in the elderly. Noncardiac causes are most common in older women whose chest pain is unrelated to exertion. Long-term follow-up studies in > 2500 patients showed that myocardial infarctions (1.6%) and cardiac death (0.5%) were rare in this group. Nevertheless, these patients suffer real disability and often undergo repeated, unnecessary testing and treatments if their conditions are not properly diagnosed.

Etiology

The most common identifiable causes of noncardiac chest pain are **musculoskeletal** and **esophageal problems.** Other, less common causes include pulmonary embolism, pneumonia, peptic ulcer, biliary tract disease, thoracic conditions, and colon problems (usually irritable bowel syndrome). A large proportion of elderly patients with noncardiac chest pain have an esophageal problem, although new studies suggest that esophageal causes of noncardiac chest pain may not be as common as once thought. Among esophageal causes, gastroesophageal reflux is more common than esophageal motility disorders.

Most patients with gastroesophageal reflux complain of heartburn, but 5% to 20% present with only atypical chest pain. Although acid reflux may cause esophageal motility dysfunction, the pain probably results from stimulation of acid-sensitive chemoreceptors. Theoretically, esophageal motility disorders could stimulate chest pain by high-amplitude, nonperistaltic contractions producing esophageal myoischemia or retarding bolus movement. The most common esophageal motility disorder associated with chest pain is **nutcracker esophagus,** a syndrome characterized by high-amplitude peristaltic contractions confined to the distal esophagus.

Psychologic factors and stress may contribute to or cause chest pain. Studies suggest that persons with noncardiac chest pain have more physical complaints than age-matched controls and score higher on psychologic measures of neuroticism and depression. Two studies in patients with noncardiac chest pain and esophageal motility disorders also confirm a high frequency of psychiatric diagnoses, primarily depression, anxiety, and somatization. These psychologic profiles are similar to those reported in patients with irritable bowel syndrome.

Diagnosis

The differential diagnosis of noncardiac chest pain first demands that cardiac disease be excluded. In older patients, evaluation is not always easy. Baseline ECGs may not correlate with active symptomatic disease; stress testing or coronary angiography is required. Occasionally, pericarditis and mitral valve prolapse may cause recurrent chest pain. A normal erythrocyte sedimentation rate (ESR) helps exclude pericarditis, and the presence of a click and murmur or use of echocardiography may help diagnose mitral valve prolapse.

After cardiac disease is excluded, emphasis should be placed on the musculoskeletal and upper GI systems. Clinical history alone is usually not helpful in separating diseases of these systems from cardiac problems. A thorough musculoskeletal examination should be performed with particular attention to locating trigger points that replicate the patient's pain syndrome. Trigger points painful to palpation suggest the **fibromyositis syndrome.** An elevated ESR also supports an inflammatory cause for pain.

Structural lesions of the upper GI tract should be excluded by barium studies or endoscopy. Radiographic studies should include the esophagus to exclude webs, constrictions, or achalasia. Rarely, gallstones cause chest pain. When they are suspected, cholecystography or abdominal ultrasonography is useful; however, many gallstones are silent, and their discovery does not prove that they are the cause of chest pain. If esophagitis or an ulcer is found, further testing is not needed.

Occasionally, the failure to make a diagnosis requires further evaluation for an esophageal cause, which may be done with a provocative test, such as the esophageal acid perfusion test (Bernstein test) or the edrophonium test (Tensilon 80 mg/kg IV). Generally, these tests are performed in the office without esophageal manometry. However, the validity, safety, and reliability of these tests in the elderly have not been determined. If the tests reproduce the patient's typical chest pain, a diagnosis of an esophageal cause is likely. If the tests are negative, additional studies with manometry and prolonged ambulatory pH monitoring may be warranted.

Treatment

When a favorable patient-doctor relationship is established, most patients respond to confident reassurance based on thorough diagnostic studies. This supportive approach results in better patient acceptance of symptoms, fewer limitations on lifestyle, and frequently a decrease in or even a resolution of the chest pain.

More specific therapy should be directed at identifiable causes of noncardiac chest pain. Patients with musculoskeletal problems can be treated with nonsteroidal anti-inflammatory drugs (NSAIDs) and monitored closely for both GI and renal side effects. If gastroesophageal reflux is a possibility, it should be vigorously treated. Elevating the head of the bed at night and eating smaller, more frequent meals are often helpful. Antacids, histamine H_2-receptor blockers, or omeprazole can also be used with appropriate dose reductions for the elderly. Esophageal motility disorders may respond to sublingual nitroglycerin, anticholinergics (eg, dicyclomine 20 mg tid), or calcium channel blocking agents (nifedipine 10 to 20 mg tid or diltiazem 60 to 90 mg tid); however, the anticholinergics usually should be avoided because of their potent side effects in the elderly. Although not extensively studied, especially in the elderly, behavior-modification programs and biofeedback may also help in long-term management of noncardiac chest pain.

GLOBUS HYSTERICUS

The subjective sensation of a lump in the throat. No specific cause or physiologic mechanism has been identified for this condition, and little information about globus hystericus in the elderly exists. Some studies suggest that elevated pressure in the upper esophageal sphincter or abnormal hypopharyngeal motility is present when symptoms occur. Other reports suggest an increased incidence of gastroesophageal reflux. Aerophagia and drying of the throat associated with emotional states may also contribute to globus hystericus.

Medical disorders that can be confused with globus hystericus include esophageal webs, esophageal motility disorders (especially achalasia), gastroesophageal reflux, musculoskeletal disorders (eg, myasthenia gravis, myotonic dystrophy, and polymyositis), and mass lesions in the neck or mediastinum causing esophageal compression. Most often, history and physical examination can exclude these disorders. Globus hystericus occurs during certain emotional states and does not worsen during swallowing. Food does not stick in the throat, a determination that can be made by carefully observing the patient eat, and the symptom is occasionally relieved with eating. No pain or weight loss occurs. True dysphagia from a structural or motor disorder of the pharynx or esophagus must be ruled out. The best approach is to obtain cineesophagography.

Treatment primarily involves reassurance. No drug has proved beneficial, and commonly prescribed anticholinergics can aggravate the situation. Underlying depression or anxiety should be managed. Providing support and pointing out the association between the symptom and the patient's mood or life situation can be very beneficial. When the problem disrupts the patient's lifestyle or functional level, psychiatric referral is indicated.

NONULCER DYSPEPSIA

A symptom complex, often related to eating, including intermittent epigastric pain, bloating, fullness, gaseousness, nausea, and heartburn. In the elderly, such complaints may indicate peptic ulcer disease but are often misdiagnosed and left untreated until more serious complications develop. The terms nonulcer dyspepsia, functional dyspepsia, flatulent dyspepsia, Moynihan's symptom complex, and indigestion are all used to indicate a heterogenous group of symptoms.

Pathophysiology

Older studies show that 10% to 40% of patients with normal x-rays and dyspepsia later develop peptic ulcer disease, suggesting that the condition is really an early form of peptic disease. The relationship to *Helicobacter pylori* infection remains uncertain.

Abnormalities in GI motility may contribute to the symptoms of nonulcer dyspepsia. In some patients with **flatulent dyspepsia,** delayed gastric emptying has been demonstrated by scintigraphy. Nonetheless, most flatulence in the elderly is caused by diet. When flatulence is severe and accompanied by diarrhea, lactose intolerance should be considered. The best way to confirm this diagnosis is a trial lactose-free diet. Sometimes, a hydrogen breath test after a meal of lactose may support the diagnosis.

Eructation is often part of dyspepsia. Frequent belching may be caused by aerophagia that occurs while eating or when anxious, depressed, or under stress. Commonly, air is swallowed as patients sigh. Aerophagia can lead to bloating, early satiety, and abdominal pain. Air swallowing is not easy to detect, even when watching for it closely.

Intolerance to foods, especially fats and poorly digested carbohydrates in beans, vegetables, and dairy products, may produce gas. A patient should be instructed to avoid such foods for several weeks. If the symptoms disappear, the patient can start eating these foods one at a time until the offending one is identified.

The **sensation of bad taste** is another common complaint, particularly in older persons. With age, xerostomia becomes more prevalent, not because less saliva is produced but because it is not as well retained in the mouth. Dry mouth can alter the taste of food, producing a bitter, sour taste. Poorly fitting and poorly cleaned dentures can also produce bad tastes. Sometimes, drugs cause bad tastes. Diuretics and anticholinergics further dry the oral mucosa, and some antihypertensives and antibiotics cause a bitter taste. If a drug is suspected, it should be stopped and another substituted. Otherwise, the frequent use of lozenges is usually the best solution. A dental evaluation is usually warranted, and dentists can often recommend medicaments that further alleviate the problem.

Dyspepsia may be caused by reflux of alkaline duodenal contents into the stomach. Epigastric discomfort can be produced by distention of the transverse colon by food or gas. Fats and many drugs, including NSAIDs, aspirin, alcohol, and tobacco, may also cause dyspepsia without producing an ulcer or gastritis.

Although scientific data are limited, emotional factors generally play an important role in the genesis of dyspepsia. Several studies confirm a higher prevalence of anxiety, neuroticism, and depression in nonulcer dyspepsia patients than in the general population. Dyspeptic patients are reported to have more negative life stresses associated with the onset of symptoms and to view life as more stressful than do control subjects.

Diagnosis

Identified during the patient's history, dyspepsia has varied presentations, but the pain is usually epigastric and described as burning or gnawing and intermittent. Generally, the pain is not relieved by meals and does not awaken patients at night, although those with reflux may complain of pain shortly after lying down. If the pain is associated with heartburn, gastroesophageal reflux should be suspected. Pain associated with defecation or abnormal bowel movements suggests irritable bowel syndrome. The presence or absence of epigastric tenderness is not a reliable indicator of peptic ulcer disease. Routine hematologic and biochemical tests are usually normal in dyspeptic patients.

Upper GI endoscopy is the most sensitive and specific method of excluding organic lesions of the esophagus, stomach, and duodenum. Although barium studies may miss 10% to 20% of peptic ulcers and most mucosal lesions, they are still commonly used. Whether the frail elderly more easily tolerate an upper GI barium study or endoscopy is not known; choosing the appropriate test requires a consideration of sensitivity, specificity, and the condition of the patient. If symptoms persist or are associated with weight loss, endoscopy is usually best. Older persons with severe, persistent pain should also be evaluated by CT scan to rule out pancreatic cancer and by barium enema or colonoscopy to rule out a colonic lesion in the transverse colon.

Treatment

The most important component in treating dyspepsia is reassurance. Many patients have an inordinate fear of cancer or ulcers that reinforces and magnifies symptoms.

Four controlled studies have been done on the efficacy of antacids in chronic nonulcer dyspepsia; all report negative results. The studies on histamine H_2-receptor blockers are contradictory: about half show no benefit, but the studies with the largest numbers of patients show that cimetidine and ranitidine have a statistically significant benefit over the placebo. Data specific to the elderly are lacking, and because these drugs more often cause side effects in the elderly, they cannot be recommended without evidence of gastritis or ulcer. Other drugs, such as metoclopramide (10 mg tid before meals) and cisapride (10 mg tid before meals) may be useful in flatulent patients with delayed gastric emptying, but side effects (eg, parkinsonism and tardive dyskinesia with metoclopramide) are particularly common in the elderly and may be severe. In patients with flatulence caused by dietary intolerance, these drugs are not helpful. Thus, in general, they should not be used. The role of sucralfate in nonulcer dyspepsia remains to be tested.

IRRITABLE BOWEL SYNDROME

A motility disorder consisting of altered bowel habits, abdominal pain, and no detectable organic pathologic abnormalities.

Irritable bowel syndrome accounts for 20% to 50% of all GI complaints in private and institutional care facilities. Women outnumber men 2:1, and whites outnumber nonwhites. The preponderance of women with this diagnosis may reflect their greater tendency to seek health care rather than the actual incidence. In 50% of patients, symptoms begin before age 35, and 40% of patients are 35 to 50 yr of age. Neither the incidence nor prevalence in the elderly has been well defined. Geriatric patients with this condition usually have a long history of bowel dysfunction, often beginning in childhood.

Pathophysiology

Although irritable bowel syndrome is considered by many to be a disorder of intestinal motility, the motor dysfunctions recorded in the laboratory do not correlate well with the clinical pattern and frequently may be simple exaggerations of normal responses. Abdominal pain, which originates in stretch receptors in the distal colon, is caused by bowel distention from gas and stool or spastic contractions of the bowel. Under baseline conditions, the colonic motility of patients with irritable bowel syndrome and that of patients without are indistinguishable. However, patients with irritable bowel syndrome show greater colonic motility in response to emotional arousal, pain, balloon distention, eating, and stimulation by cholecystokinin or pentagastrin. These motility changes differ quantitatively rather than qualitatively from those in patients without the syndrome, suggesting that irritable bowel syndrome patients are hyperreactive to many stimuli.

Psychometric tests show that patients with irritable bowel syndrome are more psychologically disturbed than those without, but they do not show a pattern of psychologic traits specific to the syndrome. Psychiatric diagnoses are noted in 70% to 90% of irritable bowel syndrome patients, although the proportion has not been defined in the elderly. The most common diagnoses are depression, anxiety, and somatization (the conversion of depression or anxiety into bodily complaints). Evidence suggests that psychogenic factors do not result from the disorder but rather contribute to the onset and exacerbation of symptoms. In 85% of patients, psychologic factors either precede or coincide with the onset of symptoms. Moreover, 50% of patients also note an association between stress and an exacerbation of symptoms. Most of the stressors mentioned by patients are everyday concerns about family, work relations, or finances. In the elderly, cancer phobias may predominate and need to be addressed.

Symptoms and Signs

Characteristic symptoms of irritable bowel syndrome include abdominal pain, erratic bowel habits, and a variation in stool consistency with a passage of mucus. More nonspecific symptoms include bloating, gas dyspepsia, headache, fatigue, lassitude, and flatulence. Patients with irritable bowel syndrome are divided into two major groups. In the first, the spastic colon group, most patients have pain over one or more areas of the colon associated with periodic constipation or diarrhea; in some patients, constipation and diarrhea alternate. Most complain of colicky or dull lower abdominal pain or discomfort over the sigmoid colon, commonly triggered by meals, especially breakfast, and often relieved by a bowel movement. The second group of patients complain primarily of painless diarrhea. They usually have urgent diarrhea that occurs immediately upon arising or, more typically, during or immediately after a meal. Incontinence may occur, but nocturnal diarrhea is unusual.

On physical examination, patients with either type generally appear to be in good health. However, they are frequently tense and anxious, with autonomic lability evidenced by a rapid, labile pulse; elevated blood pressure; or sweaty palms. In the elderly, these findings may be masked. Palpation of the abdomen may reveal tenderness, particularly in the left lower quadrant over the sigmoid colon.

Diagnosis

De novo irritable bowel syndrome symptoms are distinctly uncommon in the geriatric patient. Therefore, organic diseases must be excluded before symptomatic therapy is begun. Older patients with irritable bowel syndrome usually have a long history of bowel problems, but they need to be reevaluated periodically to rule out any intercurrent pathologic process. A diagnosis of irritable bowel syndrome can usually be established within the first few visits.

Evaluation includes a CBC and erythrocyte sedimentation rate to rule out anemia and inflammation. Stools should be cultured and examined for occult blood, ova, and parasites. In a geriatric patient with new complaints, sigmoidoscopy and barium enema examination are essential to rule out more serious underlying disease. Sigmoidoscopy usually reveals normal mucosa except for mild hyperemia and increased mucus. Reproduction of symptoms with air insufflation is a further suggestive finding. Mucosal biopsies may help exclude early ulcerative colitis or collagenous colitis. A double-contrast barium enema may show exaggerated haustral contractions, particularly in the descending colon, or conversely, an absence of normal haustral markings, often with a narrowed lumen.

The patient may have coexisting diverticulosis, and in the elderly, irritable bowel syndrome may be the precursor of diverticular disease. If weight loss or obstructive symptoms are present, an abdominal CT scan and small-bowel series should be obtained to exclude malignancy, Crohn's disease, and adhesions. For patients who complain of distention, bloating, or diarrhea, a 3-wk trial lactose-free diet is recommended. Transient lactase deficiency, often precipitated by a viral gastroenteritis, may mimic irritable bowel syndrome in older persons.

Treatment

The patient should be reassured that the necessary tests have been performed to exclude organic disease, particularly cancer. The simple act of applying a name to the disorder may provide comfort. The physician should emphasize that the colonic spasm and resulting pain are real and that they are influenced by several factors that must be managed to control symptoms. The patient should be assured that irritable bowel syndrome does not lead to more serious illness or a shortened life span.

In general, a **high-fiber diet** should be followed. Psyllium preparations bind water, thus preventing excessive dehydration of stool as well as excessive liquidity. Fiber can also be obtained by eating bran cereals or fiber-rich snack bars. Some people respond better to one form than another, and some people find liquid preparations intolerable. Diabetic patients should avoid preparations high in sugar, and obese patients should be advised that bran cereals are often high in calories. Fiber is useful in irritable bowel syndrome patients who have diarrhea or constipation.

Antispasmodics such as dicyclomine, propantheline bromide, and tincture of belladonna should *not* be used in the elderly. These drugs have never been shown to provide substantial relief, and their potent anticholinergic properties may cause constipation, confusion, dry mouth, blurred vision, orthostatic hypotension, and urinary retention. When diarrhea is severe, frequent small doses of **bismuth subsalicylate** may be helpful. Patients should be warned that it turns stool black. Alternatively, **diphenoxylate** 2.5 to 5.0 mg q 4 to 6 h or **loperamide** 2 mg q 4 to 8 h can be prescribed. **Aromatic oils,** such as spirit of peppermint, may help relieve cramping.

PSYCHOGENIC ABDOMINAL PAIN

Very few patients with chronic abdominal pain who are referred to diagnostic centers are given a specific medical diagnosis. When such patients are studied psychologically, personality and behavioral abnormalities, which presumably explain their symptoms, are often reported. However, patients with psychogenic abdominal pain may commonly be treated by nonpsychiatric physicians.

The problem occurs four times more often in women than in men, and most patients are < 50 yr. Geriatric patients may constitute 10% to 20% of this group. However, the actual prevalence of psychogenic abdominal pain in the elderly is unknown, and differences between the elderly and younger adults have not been well studied.

Chronic, unrelenting pain, usually lasting > 6 mo and unrelieved by bowel movements, characterizes this syndrome. Patients often describe their symptoms with vague statements, but when they are questioned, the descriptions become more personalized and often bizarre, eg, "like blowing out my side" or "a hot poker sticking into my belly." Many patients also have nonspecific symptoms including nausea, bloating, dizziness, fatigue, and musculoskeletal complaints. Up to 30% may have associated symptoms compatible with irritable bowel syndrome.

Diagnosis

The diagnosis of psychogenic abdominal pain is difficult because physicians vary in their ability to obtain psychologic data, and many patients resist referrals to psychiatrists and psychologists. When sensitively and sympathetically questioned, most patients report antecedent events involving personal losses, eg, the death of a close family member. Symptoms frequently appear during times of personal stress (eg, the anniversary of a traumatic event, a meaningful birthday, or the Thanksgiving-Christmas holiday season). In other cases, sexual or physical abuse may be the inciting event. Depression, hypochondriasis, histrionic or pain-prone personality, or a combination of these disorders may be identified by psychologic testing.

Treatment

These patients are difficult to manage and often frustrate the physician. They see themselves as medical patients and are reluctant to obtain psychiatric evaluation and treatment. A psychiatric consultant can help the primary care physician confirm the diagnosis and provide treatment guidelines, but general management is best directed by the nonpsychiatric physician.

For such patients, a reasonably successful outcome is improved psychosocial function (eg, return to work, church, or social activities), rather than complete pain resolution. For some patients with a relatively short duration of symptoms and without evidence of a personality disorder, greater improvement and even pain resolution can be anticipated.

When symptoms are related to grieving, a physician's empathetic listening can provide considerable relief. If the grief reaction or recurrence manifested by the somatic complaint is severe and prolonged, antidepressant medication may be helpful.

FECAL INCONTINENCE

(See also FECAL INCONTINENCE in Ch. 55)

An inability to control defecation. Fecal incontinence is much less common than urinary incontinence, but when it occurs, it is a humiliating regression in bodily function, severely impairing activity and socialization. It may lead to institutionalization; 16% to 60% of institutionalized older persons have some fecal incontinence.

Etiology

The maintenance of continence is complex, and incontinence can have several causes. Sometimes, it results from dementia that causes an inability to react normally to the sensation of a full rectum. Incontinence may also be caused by impaired voluntary contraction of the external sphincter resulting from nerve damage that occurred in traumatic vaginal childbirth, rectal prolapse (procidentia), previous anal surgery (hemorrhoidectomy, anal dilation, sphincterotomy), or spinal cord injury. Diabetes and autonomic neuropathy may produce internal sphincter dysfunction.

Diarrhea from any cause may contribute to incontinence, particularly in the elderly, who frequently have decreased sphincteric pressures and continence for liquids compared with younger persons. Fecal impaction commonly causes diarrhea and incontinence, especially in institutionalized elders, because the stool proximal to the obstructing fecal mass becomes liquefied and oozes around it. Because many such patients have long-standing constipation and megacolon, they cannot sense the movement of stool into the rectal vault, and the fecal impaction tonically inhibits the internal anal sphincter, leading to fecal incontinence.

Diagnosis and Treatment

Evaluation should begin with a consideration of the underlying causes. Examination of the rectum may show decreased sphincter tone, although the correlation between digital examination of rectal tone and objective measurements is poor. The examination also helps exclude fecal impaction. Appropriate GI, neurologic, and endocrine studies should be done, and treatment should be individualized.

When constipation and fecal impaction are present, the mass must be removed either digitally or with tap water enemas. (A Fleet enema usually is not useful because the volume is insufficient.) Also, bowel habits should be normalized by administering bulking agents, stool softeners (eg, docusate sodium 50 to 200 mg/day), or mild laxatives (eg, milk of magnesia 1 to 2 tbsp/day or lactulose or sorbitol 1 tbsp bid) to produce one to two soft bowel movements daily. All these doses can be adjusted to control constipation.

If diarrhea is a contributing factor, underlying causes should be treated. Nonspecific diarrhea can be treated with bulking agents and antidiarrheal drugs (bismuth, loperamide, or diphenoxylate). If sphincter tone is markedly decreased, enemas may be used regularly to cleanse the bowel. Surgical treatment of incontinence has yielded inconsistent results.

Biofeedback therapy is the most exciting advance in the treatment of fecal incontinence. Successful treatment requires a well-motivated patient who can follow directions and who has an external anal sphincter capable of responding to rectal distention. Using a balloon pressure monitor placed in the rectum, patients watch a physiologic tracing and try to improve their anal contractions. The image of the rectal manometric recording provides the biofeedback. Because patients frequently improve after a single session, reinforcement sessions are often unnecessary.

Biofeedback has been successful in treating > 70% of patients with incontinence caused by sensory or motor impairment. In one study of 18 geriatric patients who received biofeedback training, 15 improved by at least 50%, and 6 became continent. However, some types of incontinence, such as incontinence from severe sensory loss (eg, diabetes, spinal cord injury) or incontinence from poor rectal compliance (eg, rectal trauma, radiation injury), do not respond to biofeedback. Also, many elderly patients with fecal incontinence suffer from dementia and are not suitable candidates for biofeedback training.

54. UPPER GASTROINTESTINAL TRACT DISORDERS

Most disorders of the upper GI tract seen in elderly patients also occur in younger patients. However, GI disorders more common to the elderly should be considered when geriatric patients present with appropriate symptoms.

DYSPHAGIA SYNDROMES

Dysphagia, or *difficulty in swallowing,* may occur at any age and may be caused by several conditions. In the elderly, vascular disease, malignancy, and other degenerative conditions are particularly important. Dysphagia can be divided into two distinct syndromes: **oropharyngeal dysphagia,** produced by abnormalities affecting the finely tuned neuromuscular mechanism of the pharynx and upper esophageal sphincter, and **esophageal dysphagia,** caused by various disorders affecting the esophagus itself.

OROPHARYNGEAL DYSPHAGIA

Etiology

In the elderly, five types of abnormalities may cause oropharyngeal dysphagia: cerebrovascular accidents, other neuromuscular disorders, oropharyngeal tumors, Zenker's diverticulum, and cervical hypertrophic osteoarthropathy (see TABLE 54–1).

Cerebrovascular accidents: Patients who have had a major stroke often have dysphagia, particularly if the lesion involves critical areas in the brain stem that affect the swallowing center. Dysphagia may occur in **Wallenberg's syndrome** (occlusion of the posterior inferior cerebellar artery, which supplies blood to the lateral area of the medulla that innervates the homolateral palatal muscles) or in **pseudobulbar palsy** (impairment of the muscles supplied by the medulla oblongata caused by bilateral multiple cerebral infarctions). Dysphagia may also occur in **bulbar palsy** (paralysis or weakness of the muscles supplied by the medulla oblongata not caused by cerebral infarctions). In patients with these syndromes, dysphagia may be the primary symptom, making the specific diagnosis difficult. Patients with poststroke dysphagia occasionally respond to retraining of the physical aspects of swallowing. Such rehabilitation is best performed in conjunction with a videotaped barium swallow to assess the effects of difficult foods (ie, semisolid, solid) on swallowing and to evaluate for aspiration.

Other neuromuscular disorders: Several neurologic and muscular disorders that affect movement of the tongue, pharynx, or upper esophageal sphincter may produce oropharyngeal dysphagia. In the elderly patient, likely candidates include **Parkinson's disease, myasthenia gravis, hypothyroidism** or **hyperthyroidism,** and **amyotrophic lateral sclerosis.** With these disorders, dysphagia may be the only symptom. Diagnosis may be difficult, particularly with hyperthyroidism, which may not have typical manifestations in the elderly.

Oropharyngeal tumors: Head and neck tumors may cause oropharyngeal dysphagia, particularly in the elderly. If such a tumor is suspected after a thorough history and examination, direct laryngoscopy complemented by CT should be performed.

Zenker's diverticulum: Transient pre-esophageal dysphagia may be the earliest symptom of this outpouching of one or more layers of the esophageal wall immediately above the upper esophageal sphincter. When the sac becomes large enough to retain food, patients develop the typical symptoms of persistent cough, fullness in the neck, gurgling in the throat, postprandial regurgitation, aspiration, and an offensive odor and taste. Some diverticula become so large that patients must perform various maneuvers, such as applying pressure to the neck and coughing

TABLE 54–1. COMMON CAUSES OF OROPHARYNGEAL DYSPHAGIA IN THE ELDERLY

Cerebrovascular accidents (particularly with brain stem involvement)
Bulbar palsy
Pseudobulbar palsy
Wallenberg's syndrome
Other neuromuscular disorders
Parkinson's disease
Myasthenia gravis
Hypothyroidism or hyperthyroidism
Amyotrophic lateral sclerosis
Oropharyngeal tumors
Zenker's diverticulum
Cervical hypertrophic osteoarthropathy

repeatedly, to empty them. These sacs can become large enough to produce a visible mass in the neck or to obstruct the esophagus by compression.

Much controversy surrounds the pathogenesis of these diverticula. Diminished opening of the upper esophageal sphincter because of decreased elasticity is currently thought to play a major role. If symptoms become disabling or repeated tracheal aspiration occurs, surgical diverticulectomy and cricopharyngeal myotomy is the treatment.

Cervical hypertrophic osteoarthropathy: Although asymptomatic cervical osteophytes (spurs) may occur in 20% to 30% of the population, only about 75 cases of osteophyte-induced dysphagia have been reported. Most are secondary to diffuse idiopathic skeletal hyperostosis, in which flowing calcification occurs within at least four contiguous vertebrae in conjunction with minimal degenerative disk disease and an absence of apophyseal joint ankylosis. In the elderly, cervical osteophytes may be related to dysphagia when they are extraordinarily large, when they occur in the cricoid cartilage region (C6) where the esophagus is relatively immobile, or when periesophagitis occurs secondary to rapid expansion of the osteophyte.

Diagnostic studies should include plain cervical spine films with lateral views, as well as barium videofluoroscopy with food bolus to determine the degree of compression during swallowing. Most patients can be managed with reassurance and support; if the dysphagia is unremitting, surgical removal of the osteophyte may be necessary.

Diagnosis

Identifying the cause of oropharyngeal dysphagia requires close attention to the history, physical examination, and appropriate diagnostic tests. **Barium x-ray studies** of the pharynx and upper esophageal sphincter are little help without **videofluoroscopy.** Because the sequence of muscular changes needed to transfer ingested material from mouth to upper esophagus occurs in about 1 sec, rapid-sequence pictures must be obtained. **Manometric studies** of the pharynx and upper esophageal sphincter are only occasionally helpful, but as manometric techniques continue to improve, these studies should provide better diagnostic information.

Treatment

Treatment depends on the underlying cause. Treatable disorders, including Parkinson's disease, myasthenia gravis, and thyroid abnormalities, should receive the appropriate therapy. Depending on the degree of dysphagia, medical treatment for parkinsonism and myasthenia gravis may not completely restore swallowing. Tumors should be resected, if possible, or should be treated with chemotherapy or radiation therapy. However, surgical resection or radiation therapy for a tumor can cause a subsequent stricture that may precipitate dysphagia.

For a patient with an otherwise untreatable neuromuscular disorder, such as a stroke, rehabilitation techniques are often effective (eg, altering the diet or eating with the head held in different positions). These approaches should be determined after consultation with a speech pathologist that includes radiographic assessment of the patient's ability to swallow various types of food (liquid, semisolid, solid) while maintaining different head positions.

ESOPHAGEAL DYSPHAGIA

Neuromuscular (motility) defects or mechanical obstructing lesions can cause esophageal dysphagia by interfering with the transport of ingested material down the esophagus. These two types of disorders can usually be differentiated by taking a detailed history. Motility disorders are more likely to cause dysphagia for solids and liquids; obstructing lesions usually produce dysphagia for solids only, but sometimes dysphagia for liquids develops late in the course of the disease if the esophageal lumen becomes subtotally occluded (see TABLE 54–2).

Obstructive dysphagia can also result when a foreign object lodges in the esophagus. Many elderly persons are susceptible to this problem because they have poor vision and wear dentures, which decrease their ability to feel objects in the mouth (especially bones in meat). Sometimes, the foreign object is the dentures.

Motility Disorders

Achalasia: Most patients with achalasia present between ages 20 and 40, but a second peak occurs in the elderly. Neurologic in origin,

TABLE 54–2. DIFFERENTIATING CAUSES OF ESOPHAGEAL DYSPHAGIA

Type of Dysphagia	*Common Associated Symptoms*	*Cause*
Intermittent dysphagia		
Solid foods only	Steakhouse syndrome (initial episode of dysphagia while eating steak and bread)	Rings or webs
Solids and liquids	Chest pain	Diffuse esophageal spasm
Progressive dysphagia		
Solid foods only	Malaise Weight loss	Carcinoma
	Chronic heartburn	Peptic stricture
Solids and liquids	Nocturnal aspiration	Achalasia
	Chronic heartburn	Scleroderma

achalasia results from defects of the ganglion cells in Auerbach's plexus of the esophageal wall. The disorder causes slowly progressive dysphagia for solids and liquids and insidious weight loss. Regurgitation of undigested foods may cause nocturnal coughing and aspiration. An elderly patient may have had symptoms for months or years before diagnosis.

Chest x-ray may show a dilated esophagus with an air-fluid level from retained food and saliva. About 50% of patients do not have the normal gastric air bubble. Barium swallow studies reveal a dilated, sometimes tortuous esophagus with a smooth, "bird-beak" narrowing at the gastroesophageal junction. Esophageal manometry usually provides the diagnostic findings of increased lower esophageal sphincter pressure with incomplete sphincteric relaxation during swallowing and an aperistaltic esophagus. These defects result in a major functional obstruction of food passing from the esophagus.

In the elderly, differentiating between **idiopathic achalasia** and **secondary achalasia** from cancer (which rarely produces identical radiographic and manometric findings) is particularly important. Gastric, pancreatic, or lung cancer or lymphoma may be associated with such findings. Therefore, endoscopy with biopsy of any suspicious area is mandatory in all patients with achalasia. The clinical triad that suggests secondary achalasia is age > 50 yr, dysphagia for < 1 yr, and weight loss > 15 lb.

Treatment for achalasia may be medical or surgical. Generally, good results can be obtained with either approach, and the choice should be based on the physician's skills, the patient's health, and the patient's preference after being informed about the techniques, risks, and expected outcomes. Medical management may be more suitable for older patients in poor health.

Initial medical treatment usually consists of pneumatic dilation of the lower esophageal sphincter. Although such dilation is not quite as effective as Heller myotomy (80% vs. 95% success rate), it is associated with less morbidity (particularly gastroesophageal reflux), does not require general anesthesia, and is a same-day procedure.

Surgery is indicated when several balloon dilations over a relatively short period are needed to maintain lower esophageal sphincter patency. Surgical intervention is also indicated when pneumatic dilation causes esophageal perforation. This complication occurs in about 5% of cases and requires surgical closure of the perforated area along with myotomy.

Occasionally, dysphagia can be sufficiently relieved by giving a smooth-muscle–relaxing drug just before meals. Either nitroglycerin tablets 0.4 mg sublingually 5 min before meals or nifedipine capsules 10 mg bitten and held sublingually 15 min before meals may be effective. The rapid action of these drugs enhances lower esophageal sphincter relaxation and may improve dysphagia during the meal. However, most achalasia patients require the more definitive procedures discussed above to open the esophagogastric junction. Because the elderly patient with other serious medical problems may not be a candidate for pneumatic dilation or surgery, treatment with smooth-muscle–relaxing drugs should be considered definitive therapy. These drugs may cause transient symptomatic hypotension; patients should be told that lightheadedness, weakness, and other manifestations of postural hypotension occasionally develop after taking them.

Scleroderma (progressive systemic sclerosis): Esophageal involvement occurs in > 80% of scleroderma cases and seems to correlate with Raynaud's phenomenon. Scleroderma produces a slowly progressive dysphagia for liquids and solids, as in achalasia; heartburn is also a prominent symptom. Up to 40% of these patients develop a peptic esophageal stricture. Manometric findings include decreased peristalsis in the lower esophagus (smooth muscle) and normal peristalsis in the upper esophagus (striated muscle). Also, lower esophageal sphincter pressure is very low.

Treatment consists of acid suppression with omeprazole 20 mg/day orally. In patients with severe reflux, 24-h pH monitoring can be used to ascertain the effectiveness of treatment, and the omeprazole dosage can be increased as needed to control reflux.

Diffuse esophageal spasm and related disorders: Diffuse esophageal spasm is an esophageal motility disorder manifested by dysphagia, chest pain, or in some cases, both. Dysphagia usually occurs intermittently for liquids and solids. Both symptoms may be induced by stress and may be exacerbated by hot or cold foods or drinks.

This disorder may be related to several nonspecific esophageal motility disorders that can progress to achalasia. One such disorder, **nutcracker esophagus,** is characterized by high-amplitude peristaltic contractions (> 180 mm Hg) and associated symptoms of dysphagia, chest pain, or both.

Treatment of diffuse esophageal spasm and related conditions includes administering nitrates (isosorbide dinitrate 10 to 30 mg orally tid) or calcium channel blockers (preferably nifedipine 10 to 30 mg orally tid or diltiazem 30 to 90 mg orally qid). Use of longer-acting nitrates or sustained-release calcium channel blockers may increase patient compliance because of decreased dosing frequency. Esophageal dilation may also be helpful, and in severe, refractory cases, esophageal myotomy may be considered. Many patients benefit from learning that their pain originates in the esophagus, not in the heart, and from learning how to cope better with stress.

Obstructing Lesions

Esophageal carcinoma (see also Ch. 60): Patients with esophageal carcinoma are generally > 50 yr and present with rapidly progressive dysphagia (solids first, then liquids) and weight loss. Typically, they have no history of heartburn, although it may occur. A history of heavy alcohol and tobacco use is common. Barium x-ray studies often suggest the diagnosis, but endoscopy (with biopsy and cytologic evaluation) is necessary for a more definitive diagnosis.

Treatment depends on the extent of the disease. When possible, surgical resection is the treatment of choice. CT scanning may help determine resectability. Radiation therapy, chemotherapy, or both may be palliative. The prognosis is grim, with a 5-yr survival rate of < 5%.

Peptic stricture: This condition is characterized by progressive dysphagia for solids and usually follows a long history of heartburn or other reflux symptoms. The diagnosis is made by barium radiography, but endoscopy is needed to rule out carcinoma. The strictures are smooth, tapered, and of varying lengths. If they are located above the distal esophagus, **Barrett's esophagus** (metaplastic columnar epithelium lining the distal esophagus) may be present. Patients with this condition, which is related to chronic gastroesophageal reflux, have an increased risk of cancer.

Treatment for patients with peptic stricture consists of long-term antireflux therapy. Intermittent esophageal dilation is often necessary as well, and occasionally surgery is required.

Rings and webs: These disorders, associated with intermittent dysphagia for solids, are best diagnosed by barium swallow. Endoscopic evaluation is indicated if the diagnosis is in doubt. Because the first episode frequently occurs while the patient is eating steak and bread, these disorders have been termed **steakhouse syndrome.** The bolus is usually forced down by drinking liquids but occasionally must be regurgitated, and then the meal can usually be finished without difficulty.

The most common structural lesion is **Schatzki's ring,** composed of invaginated mucosa. The ring, located at the gastroesophageal mucosal junction, is seen on barium swallow about 3 to 4 cm above the diaphragm. It most often produces symptoms when the lumen is narrowed to $\leq$ 12 mm.

Treatment consists of a single esophageal dilation with a large-caliber bougie. If the symptoms occur infrequently, more careful eating habits may suffice.

Vascular causes: Esophageal dysphagia may also be caused by vascular anomalies that compress the esophagus. The more common lesions are congenital aortic-arch abnormalities associated with dysphagia presenting in early childhood, such as dysphagia lusoria (dysphagia caused by a retroesophageal aberrant right subclavian artery and an anomalous left pulmonary artery). Occasionally, symptoms present in adulthood. **Dysphagia aortica** is a disorder of the elderly resulting from esophageal compression by either a large thoracic aortic aneurysm or an atherosclerotic, rigid aorta posteriorly and the heart or esophageal hiatus anteriorly.

DISORDERS OF THE STOMACH AND DUODENUM

Gastric and duodenal acid peptic disorders frequently occur in the elderly. With age, the incidence of duodenal ulcers appears to decrease; this may be related to diminishing gastric acid secretion. Secretory studies have repeatedly demonstrated decreased acid output and a relative increase in achlorhydria with aging. In association with decreased acid output, basal serum gastrin concentrations tend to increase with age. The incidence of gastric ulcers may actually increase in the elderly, particularly in those chronically taking nonsteroidal anti-inflammatory drugs (NSAIDs). Both duodenal and gastric ulcers tend to develop more complications in older patients, making surgery more likely.

Other disorders of the stomach and duodenum affecting the elderly include atrophic gastritis, gastric atrophy, hypertrophic gastropathy, bezoars, gastric volvulus, and gastric tumors. For a discussion of gastric tumors, see Ch. 60.

ATROPHIC GASTRITIS AND GASTRIC ATROPHY

Atrophic gastritis is characterized by an increased number of inflammatory cells in the stomach wall and varying degrees of atrophy of the gastric mucosa. This gastritis appears to be progressive and may eventually develop into **gastric atrophy**—a more diffuse disorder characterized by a decreased number of secretory cells (both chief and parietal) in the mucosa of the gastric body and fundus. Generally, these age-related gastric mucosal changes correlate with decreased gastric secretion.

Two types of atrophic gastritis exist. **Type A,** a more diffuse gastritis, is antral sparing and usually associated with decreased acid output, elevated serum gastrin levels, and circulating antibodies to parietal cells. This type of gastritis may evolve into characteristic pernicious anemia. **Type B** is a more focal, antral gastritis caused by *Helicobacter pylori* infection. This type is associated with a smaller reduction in acid secretion, normal serum gastrin levels, and an absence of antibodies to parietal cells.

Patients with these conditions are usually asymptomatic, although benign gastric ulcer may develop. *Both atrophic gastritis and gastric atrophy, which share the premalignant status of pernicious anemia, have the potential for malignancy.* Managing patients with these conditions, therefore, usually includes periodic endoscopic cytologic evaluation and biopsy for carcinoma. Although the optimal interval for these examinations has not been determined, they are generally performed every year or two.

Pernicious anemia is the end-stage condition in type A chronic gastritis. It usually presents as a hematologic abnormality in the elderly, and GI symptoms are unusual. The diagnosis, however, is strongly supported by the finding of characteristic **achlorhydria,** *an absence of gastric acid secretion in response to maximal stimulation.* Up to 10% of patients with pernicious anemia eventually are found to have carcinoma of the stomach, which occurs three to five times more often in these patients than in the general population of similar age.

HYPERTROPHIC GASTROPATHY

Enlarged gastric rugae involving part or all of the stomach characterize **Ménétrier's disease,** a relatively unusual condition that is not unique to the elderly. A number of conditions mimicking Ménétrier's disease are more likely to occur in older persons, including gastric lymphoma, infiltrative carcinoma, granulomatous disorders such as tuberculosis, and other infiltrative conditions such as amyloidosis. These conditions may be associated with vague epigastric pain and weight loss. More important, however, may be the frequent finding of hypoalbuminemia secondary to protein loss across the gastric mucosa.

On barium x-ray studies, all these conditions, including Ménétrier's disease, may show large gastric folds appearing as polypoid filling defects along the greater curvature of the stomach. Endoscopy with adequate biopsy helps the differential diagnosis. Treatment depends on the diagnosis. Sometimes, anticholinergics decrease the gastric protein loss in Ménétrier's disease. Occasionally, gastrectomy is required.

PEPTIC ULCER

An ulceration of the mucous membrane penetrating the muscularis mucosa and occurring in the areas bathed in acid and pepsin. In younger persons, duodenal ulcer is the predominant form of peptic ulceration, but in the elderly, the proportion of gastric ulcer increases. Peptic ulcer presentation later in life may be more acute, including severe hemorrhage, perforation, and obstruction. Aggressive therapy is often needed in older patients, and surgery should not be delayed or withheld solely because of age. All gastric ulcers should be evaluated endoscopically to differentiate benign ulcers from carcinoma. Furthermore, multiple biopsies of benign-appearing gastric ulcers are needed to rule out malignancy (4 to 6 biopsies at the ulcer margins and biopsy of the ulcer base); endoscopy should be repeated in 2 to 3 mo to ensure healing and to exclude gastric carcinoma.

Giant duodenal ulcers in some elderly men cause upper abdominal pain, often radiating to the back. These ulcers may exceed 2 cm in diameter and may involve most of the surface of the duodenal bulb as well as contiguous organs such as the pancreas, gallbladder, and liver. Frequently, GI bleeding occurs. A giant duodenal ulcer is diagnosed using barium x-ray studies or endoscopy. Surgery is usually preferable to medical treatment.

Treatment

Therapy for peptic ulcer in the elderly is similar to that in younger patients. However, certain principles require closer attention when treating older patients. For treatment of complications (hemorrhage, perforation, obstruction), see Ch. 62.

Antacids: Although these medications are used frequently for symptoms of peptic ulcer disease, *their high sodium content can cause sodium overload in the elderly.* Titralac Plus Liquid is the antacid with the lowest sodium content. Other possible side effects are diarrhea (predominantly with antacids containing magnesium), constipation (predominantly with antacids containing calcium), and altered absorption of other drugs, including digoxin, quinidine, isoniazid, and broad-spectrum antibiotics.

Histamine H_2-receptor blockers: The primary drugs currently used to treat peptic ulcer disease are the histamine H_2-receptor blockers. These drugs may produce mental confusion in the elderly patient, particularly when given parenterally. Also, cimetidine is associated with several important drug interactions and may increase blood levels of diazepam, warfarin, theophylline, and phenytoin.

Sucralfate: By enhancing the protective mechanisms of the gastric mucosa, sucralfate provides an effective alternative therapy for acute peptic ulcer. In the elderly, this drug offers the advantage of being potentially free of the systemic side effects produced by histamine H_2-receptor blockers. The recommended dosage of sucralfate for duodenal ulcer is 1 gm orally qid for 4 to 6 wk; for gastric ulcer, 1 gm orally qid for 12 wk.

Omeprazole: This proton-pump inhibitor is the treatment of choice for patients with ulcer refractory to high-dose histamine H_2-receptor blockers. Although the side effect profile has been favorable in humans, more long-term studies are needed before chronic acid suppressive therapy can be recommended.

Misoprostol: This prostaglandin E_1 analog has both antisecretory and mucosal protective properties that may prevent gastric ulcer formation caused by nonsteroidal anti-inflammatory drugs (NSAIDs). Adverse effects of misoprostol include diarrhea and abdominal pain, which may interfere with compliance in the elderly population.

ZOLLINGER-ELLISON SYNDROME

Zollinger-Ellison syndrome was initially described as a triad of recurring peptic ulcer disease, marked gastric hypersecretion of acid, and a pancreatic adenoma. Later, the adenoma was found to produce a high gastrin output, resulting in continuous stimulation of the parietal cells to produce excessive acid. Because about 33% of patients with this syndrome are over age 60, it should be considered in any patient with persistent or recurring peptic ulcer disease. If Zollinger-Ellison syndrome remains a possibility after a serum gastrin determination, gastric secretory studies should be performed. Traditionally, patients with this syndrome have a basal acid output > 15 mEq/L, and maximal stimulation does not double the output. Provocative testing with IV secretin is definitive. In normal subjects, IV secretin slightly increases, slightly decreases, or has no effect on serum gastrin levels. In patients with gastrinoma, within 10 min after the secretin injection, serum gastrin levels increase by at least 200 pg/mL and then gradually decrease to baseline levels. Once the diagnosis of Zollinger-Ellison syndrome is made, all candidates for surgery need evaluation with abdominal ultrasonography, computed tomography, and selective arteriography to localize tumors and to exclude metastases.

Treatment

Surgery is the treatment of choice, with cure rates approaching 40% in patients who have undergone successful resections. Contraindications to surgery include unresectable metastatic disease.

Omeprazole is the medical treatment of choice because of its potency, long duration of action, and favorable side effect profile. Initially, the dose is usually 60 mg/day orally; gastric acid secretion is monitored, and the dose is adjusted as necessary. Goals for gastric acid suppression are basal acid output < 10 mEq/h in patients who are not operative candidates, < 5 mEq/h in patients with gastric resection, and < 1 mEq/h in patients with severe reflux.

Octreotide, a synthetic analog of somatostatin, decreases serum gastrin levels and gastric acid production in patients with Zollinger-Ellison syndrome but can be given only parenterally. Furthermore, long-term studies have not shown any increased benefit of octreotide over omeprazole. Chemotherapy with streptozocin and 5-FU has been shown to decrease serum gastrin levels in patients with metastatic disease but is usually reserved for patients with liver metastases to provide symptomatic relief from mass effects of the tumor.

BEZOARS

Intragastric masses consisting of extrinsic substances such as hair, fruit and vegetable fibers, or a mixture of such substances. Bezoars are seen with increased frequency in the elderly, especially after vagotomy or subtotal gastrectomy, and may be related to reduced gastric motility. They occur often in elderly diabetic patients because of severely abnormal gastric emptying. An edentulous patient may be at risk because food fibers are insufficiently broken up. Pulpy fruits or vegetables—especially citrus fruits but also figs, coconuts, apples, green beans, sauerkraut, berries, potato peels, and brussels sprouts—most commonly lead to bezoars.

Diagnosis begins by ruling out mechanical obstruction. Barium x-ray studies may indicate a mass lesion in the stomach, which may mimic a cancer. Treatment with endoscopy, including attempts to break up the lesion with a biopsy forceps or a jet spray of water, is often successful.

GASTRIC VOLVULUS

This relatively rare condition is more common in the elderly because the ligaments supporting the stomach are relaxed. A complete twist of the organ can result in strangulation of the blood supply, which can lead to gangrene. Patients often present with severe epigastric pain of abrupt onset followed by retching with an inability to vomit or belch.

Two types of gastric volvulus occur. The more common **organoaxial volvulus** involves a rotation of the stomach on its longitudinal axis (from cardia to pylorus); an x-ray often shows an "upside-down stomach" and double air-fluid levels (fundus and antrum). The less common **mesenteroaxial volvulus** results from rotation around a vertical axis passing through the center of the lesser and greater curvatures. Patients usually present with a distended upper abdomen, which hampers passage of a nasogastric tube. The combination of an inability to vomit, upper abdominal pain and distention, and an impediment to nasogastric tube insertion is known as **Borchardt's triad.** Diagnostic clues are usually obtained on x-ray examination, either with a plain film of the abdomen or with contrast material added. *Acute gastric volvulus requires emergency surgery.*

VASCULAR LESIONS

Occult GI bleeding may occur secondary to **angiodysplasia** in the mucosa of the stomach or duodenum. These lesions occur more frequently with age and are more common in the colon (see Ch. 55); they often cause upper GI bleeding in patients with chronic renal failure. Occasionally, they can be identified on endoscopy, but often angiographic confirmation is needed. Choosing appropriate therapy can be difficult. If bleeding is severe enough to require transfusion, endoscopy with electrocoagulation is the treatment of choice. Refractory bleeding requires surgery. In patients at increased surgical risk, a trial of hormonal therapy with a combination of 0.05 mg ethinyl estradiol and 1 mg norethindrone daily may be warranted, but whether hormonal therapy is truly effective remains controversial.

---

55. LOWER GASTROINTESTINAL TRACT DISORDERS

The principal functions of the colon and rectum are to store fecal waste for prolonged periods and expel it appropriately. Storage is facilitated by adaptive compliance of the intestine and by contractions of colonic smooth muscle, which slow the movement of stool, thereby promoting water absorption and reducing stool volume. Stool moves by relatively infrequent peristaltic contractions. Defecation and continence are maintained by the ability to sense rectal filling and by the coordinated function of the internal and external anal sphincters and the pelvic floor muscles. Colonic motility and transit in healthy elderly persons are similar to those in younger persons; however, aging is associated with diminished anal sphincter tone and strength and decreased rectal compliance. The latter may increase susceptibility to fecal incontinence in the elderly.

The major symptoms of colonic and rectal disorders are constipation, diarrhea, pain, rectal bleeding, and fecal incontinence. Colonic and rectal disorders that occur more commonly in the elderly include diverticular disease, vascular ectasias, colonic ischemia, antibiotic-associated diarrhea and colitis, fecal incontinence, and constipation. Inflammatory bowel diseases occur in all age groups, but new onset is more likely in the elderly and in persons in their 20s. Constipation is discussed in Ch. 56.

DIVERTICULAR DISEASE

Colonic diverticula are *herniations of colonic mucosa through the smooth muscle layers.* **Diverticulosis** is *the presence of diverticula without inflammation.* **Painful diverticular disease** is *diverticulosis accompanied by painful spasm or other symptoms.* **Diverticulitis** is *an infection arising from colonic diverticula.*

Diverticula develop in areas where circular smooth muscle has been weakened by the penetration of blood vessels to the submucosa. Usually, diverticula are found in the sigmoid and descending colons and rarely in the rectum.

Diverticula are associated with aging, which may lead to structural weakening of colonic muscle. Diverticular disease occurs in about 40% of those > 65 yr and about 50% of those > 80 yr in Western countries. Diverticula have been found with increasing frequency in Western populations, probably because of increased longevity and insufficient dietary fiber. Low fiber diets may increase colonic motor activity and intraluminal pressures; therefore, fiber supplements are recommended for diverticulosis and painful diverticular disease.

The incidence of diverticulitis increases with the duration of diverticulosis. Diverticulitis develops in 15% to 25% of persons with diverticulosis who are followed up ≥ 10 yr. The organisms that cause diverticulitis include usual colonic flora (eg, aerobic and anaerobic gram-negative bacilli); the role of enterococci is unknown.

Symptoms and Signs

Colonic diverticulosis is asymptomatic. **Painful diverticular disease** is characterized by crampy discomfort in the left lower abdomen without infection or inflammation. Symptoms often are associated with constipation or diarrhea and tenderness over the affected areas; symptoms increase after eating and may be partially relieved by defecating or passing flatus. Excessive colonic motility is the underlying mechanism producing symptoms. Symptoms of painful diverticular disease are similar to those of irritable bowel syndrome and partial bowel obstruction caused by tumors or ischemia. In contrast to diverticulitis, painful diverticular disease is not characterized by fever, leukocytosis, or rebound tenderness.

In **diverticulitis,** inflammation begins at the apex of a diverticulum when the opening becomes obstructed with stool. Fever, leukocytosis, or rebound tenderness indicates inflammation, which often remains localized in the adjacent pericolic tissues but may progress to a peridiverticular abscess. Other complications include fibrosis and bowel obstruction; fistula formation to the bladder (most common), vagina, or adjacent small intestine; perforation with peritonitis; and sepsis. Frank rectal bleeding is *not* characteristic of diverticulitis.

The clinical distinction between painful diverticular disease and diverticulitis carries a sizable rate of error. In an elderly or debilitated patient, the absence of fever, leukocytosis, or rebound tenderness does not exclude diverticulitis.

Bleeding associated with diverticula is usually brisk and painless. The origin of most diverticular bleeding, when known, is the right colon. Bleeding usually stops spontaneously, although 10% to 20% of patients have persistent hemorrhage. Bleeding results from rupture of the penetrating arteriole in its course around the diverticular sac.

Diagnosis

Because diverticula are asymptomatic in most persons and are common in the elderly, other possible causes of nonspecific GI symptoms should be considered before attributing these symptoms to diverticula.

Other disorders that occur in the elderly may cause presenting symptoms similar to those of diverticular disease. For example, carcinoma of the colon, inflammatory bowel disease, and ischemia may mimic diverticulitis; a patient with vascular ectasias of the colon may present with brisk, painless bleeding.

If diverticulitis, abscess, or extraintestinal complications are suspected (eg, if a palpable mass is present), **barium enema** should usually be delayed about 1 wk to allow some resolution of the inflammatory process. A single contrast study should be done with precautions to minimize the risk of perforation and extravasation of contrast material. **Computed tomography** or **ultrasonic imaging** of the abdomen are safe studies that provide better definition of colonic wall thickness and extraluminal structures.

Colonoscopy is a less attractive option during an acute episode. It is best used to exclude tumors or other conditions when other diagnostic tests are inconclusive. When contrast studies fail to identify the source of bleeding, colonoscopy is indicated. Before colonoscopy, colon cleansing is necessary; once the patient is stabilized and bleeding has slowed or stopped, balanced electrolyte solutions containing polyethylene glycol are given orally or by nasogastric tube. If bleeding remains brisk or the patient is unstable, **selective mesenteric angiography** can be used to locate the site of bleeding and to infuse vasoactive substances to control bleeding. If bleeding is intermittent or too slow to be detected by angiography, serial abdominal scans preceded by injection of **technetium Tc 99m red blood cells** can be used.

Treatment

The rationale for treating **diverticulosis** is to prevent complications such as diverticulitis or bleeding. However, there is no evidence that treatment prevents complications.

TABLE 55–1. MEDICAL TREATMENT OF DIVERTICULAR DISEASE

Measures	*Painful Diverticular Disease*	*Diverticulitis*
Diet	Increase fiber	Reduce fiber (or NPO)
Bulk laxatives	Probably effective	Not indicated
Analgesics	Nonnarcotic analgesic (NSAIDs are preferred); if a narcotic is needed, choose meperidine or ketorolac over morphine	Nonnarcotic analgesic (NSAIDs are preferred); if a narcotic is needed, choose meperidine or ketorolac over morphine
Antispasmodics (Note: High risk of adverse effects in the elderly)	Propantheline bromide 15 mg tid Dicyclomine hydrochloride 20 mg tid Hyoscyamine sulfate 0.125–0.250 mg q 4 h Glucagon 2 mg IV	Not indicated
Antibiotics	Not indicated	Oral Amoxicillin and potassium clavulanate 750 mg tid Parenteral (choice) 1. Gentamicin sulfate or tobramycin 5 mg/kg/day plus clindamycin 1.2–2.4 gm/day or mezlocillin 4 gm qid 2. Cefoxitin 4–6 gm/day 3. Ampicillin sodium and sulbactam sodium 6–12 gm/day

From Wald A: "Colonic diverticulosis," in *Management of Gastrointestinal Diseases*, edited by SJ Winawer. Published by Wolfe Publishing, an imprint of Times Mirror International Publishers; 1992, chapter 34, pp 1–18.

The treatment of **painful diverticular disease** is designed to reduce symptoms related to smooth muscle spasm; the treatment of **diverticulitis** is designed to manage bacterial infection (see TABLE 55–1). If the clinical picture is mild, the diverticulitis patient may be treated as an outpatient with oral antibiotics and oral intake restrictions. If the patient is more acutely ill, the need for hospitalization will be apparent.

Surgery is recommended for patients with diverticulitis who fail to respond to medical therapy within 72 h, for many patients who have had two or more attacks of diverticulitis, for many immunocompromised patients, and for patients whose first attack occurs before age 40. The preferred procedure is a one-stage operation in which the diseased segment of bowel is resected and continuity restored by a primary anastomosis. If this procedure is not feasible, a two-stage one that requires a diverting colostomy should be used.

Before elective surgery, large abscesses often can be drained percutaneously by an interventional radiologist using computed tomography or ultrasonography. After successful drainage and 2 to 3 wk after antibiotic therapy, surgery may be performed.

Emergency surgery is required for generalized peritonitis, persistent high-grade bowel obstruction, or rapid, unremitting GI bleeding. *Elderly patients with generalized peritonitis require immediate excision of the perforation site; giving antibiotics and waiting for resolution is associated with an extremely high mortality.* Most patients with complicated diverticular disease require surgery even if clinical recovery occurs because of the high risk of recurrent attacks with complications and increased morbidity.

VASCULAR ECTASIAS
(Angiodysplasia)

Small clusters of dilated and tortuous veins in the mucosa of the colon and small intestine. Found in > 25% of those > 60 yr, vascular ectasias are an important cause of lower GI bleeding in the elderly. The main theory concerning their development is that repeated episodes of low-grade, partial obstruction of submucosal veins occur when colonic muscles contract or when intraluminal pressure increases, resulting in venous dilation and tortuosity. Mucosal veins drained by the submucosal vein may also be affected. In the final stage of development, the precapillary sphincter becomes incompetent, and a small arteriovenous communication with the ectatic tuft of vessels develops. Vascular ectasias usually develop in the right colon, probably because of the greater tension on the bowel wall, as expressed by Laplace's law relating tension to the diameter of the bowel lumen. A putative causal association between vascular ectasias and aortic stenosis has been questioned after a thorough review of the literature.

Symptoms and Signs

Mucosal vascular ectasias are asymptomatic in most persons. Patients usually present with painless, subacute, and recurrent bleeding, which stops spontaneously in the vast majority of cases. Bleeding may consist of bright red blood, maroon stools, or melena, or it may be occult. About 10% to 15% of patients have episodes of brisk blood loss.

Diagnosis

Diagnosis may be made by colonoscopy or angiography. **Colonoscopy** is preferred because it can exclude other causes of bleeding and also can be used as a therapeutic intervention. Because lesions are small, often multiple, and difficult to see, the colon must be thoroughly cleansed to allow adequate visualization of the mucosa. Cleansing is usually done after bleeding has stopped; it should be done within 48 h so that other sources of bleeding, such as diverticula or ischemia, can be identified. Meperidine should not be used to sedate patients undergoing colonoscopy because it makes identification of ectasias more difficult; if meperidine is required, naloxone can be administered during the procedure to enhance visualization.

Mesenteric angiography is preferable when acute bleeding is brisk. A finding of tortuous, densely opacified clusters of small veins that empty slowly indicates advanced ectasias. Early filling of the vein, indicating an arteriovenous communication, is found in most patients who are studied for bleeding. When bleeding is active (≥ 0.5 to 1.0 mL/min), the contrast medium is extravasated into the bowel lumen, but because bleeding is often intermittent, extravasation is seen in only a minority of patients. In such cases, scintigraphy with technetium Tc 99m red blood cells may locate a bleeding site. This technique detects active bleeding at rates of 0.05 to 0.1 mL/min, and the patient can be serially scanned for up to 36 h if bleeding is intermittent.

Treatment

Conservative treatment, consisting of blood or iron replacement as appropriate, should be used whenever possible. When bleeding is recurrent, transcolonoscopic electrocoagulation or laser coagulation may be attempted. Difficulties include identifying the ectatic lesions and excluding other causes of blood loss if bleeding has stopped. Also, perforation of the right colon is a recognized hazard of coagulation therapy.

Active, severe bleeding may be controlled quickly by intra-arterial or IV administration of vasopressin 0.2 to 0.6 u./min. This therapy often stabilizes the patient for more definitive treatment. If coagulation therapy is not technically possible or if acute bleeding cannot be controlled, surgery is required. If the right colon is the only identified source of bleeding, a right hemicolectomy is performed. However, after surgery, bleeding recurs in up to 20% of patients, who then require a more extensive colonic resection or exploratory laparotomy. **Small-bowel enteroscopy** may eventually reduce the need for diagnostic laparotomy in patients with recurrent bleeding from obscure sites.

INFLAMMATORY BOWEL DISEASE

Although ulcerative colitis and Crohn's disease are more common in early adulthood, they are not uncommon in the elderly, partly because more patients with inflammatory bowel disease are living into old age. Also, both diseases have a bimodal age of onset; the first occurs during the 20s, and the second occurs between ages 50 and 80. This pattern persists even when diseases that mimic inflammatory bowel disease (eg, ischemic and infectious colitis) have been excluded. The reasons for this bimodality are unknown.

ULCERATIVE COLITIS

A chronic inflammatory process of unknown cause that affects the superficial layers of the colonic wall in a continuous distribution.

Histologic examination reveals diffuse ulcerations, epithelial necrosis, depletion of goblet cells, and polymorphonuclear cell infiltration extending from the superficial layers of the colon to the muscularis mucosa. Crypt abscesses are characteristic but not pathognomonic. The inflammatory process invariably involves the rectum and extends proximally for variable distances but not beyond the colon.

Symptoms and Signs

Symptoms in the elderly are similar to those in younger persons. Ulcerative colitis may be classified as mild, moderate, or severe (see TABLE 55–2). Most patients have diarrhea with or without blood in the stool, although older patients occasionally present with constipation or hematochezia. Systemic manifestations occur during more severe attacks and indicate a poorer prognosis. Though the disease may be less extensive in older patients, they present with a severe initial attack more often and have higher mortality and morbidity rates than younger patients.

Extraintestinal manifestations of ulcerative colitis include arthralgias, erythema nodosum, pyoderma gangrenosum, uveitis, and migratory polyarthritis. These conditions are usually associated with increased disease activity and occur less often in ulcerative colitis than in Crohn's disease.

Complications

Toxic megacolon is a serious complication of ulcerative colitis that occurs more often in elderly patients. Abdominal x-rays show colonic dilation; patients may be confused and have high fever, abdominal distention, and overall deterioration.

TABLE 55–2. CRITERIA FOR ASSESSING SEVERITY OF ULCERATIVE COLITIS

Factor	*Severe Disease*	*Mild Disease**
Frequency of bowel movements	≥ 6/day	≤ 4/day
Blood in stool	+ +	±
Temperature	> 37.5° C (99.5° F) on 2 of 4 days	Normal
Pulse rate	> 90 beats/min	Normal
Hemoglobin (allow for transfusion)	≤ 75%	Normal or near normal
Erythrocyte sedimentation rate	> 30 mm/h	≤ 30 mm/h

* Values for moderate disease are between those for mild and severe disease.

Based on data from Truelove SC, Witts LJ: "Cortisone in ulcerative colitis: Final report on a therapeutic trial." *British Medical Journal* 2:1041–1048, 1955.

The risk of developing **colorectal cancer** is about nine times greater in elderly patients with ulcerative colitis than in elderly persons in the general population. The risk increases substantially in patients of all ages about 8 yr after the onset of the disease; carcinoma almost always develops after many years of even quiescent disease. The risk is greatest in those with universal colitis. Carcinoma occurs at an earlier age in patients with ulcerative colitis than in the general population. For these reasons, despite some shortcomings in the interpretation of biopsies and in the outcome of surveillance programs, all patients with longstanding ulcerative colitis should have an annual colonoscopy with biopsy to detect mucosal dysplasia, which is considered a premalignant lesion in ulcerative colitis. Biopsies should be taken randomly throughout the colon and in areas that appear suspicious. If high-grade dysplasia is found, proctocolectomy is indicated.

Diagnosis

The diagnosis is made by sigmoidoscopy and rectal mucosal biopsies because the disease always involves the rectum. The extent of the disease is determined by colonoscopy or barium x-ray; both procedures should be avoided in patients who are severely ill because of the risk of perforation and toxic megacolon. The characteristic findings are diffuse erythema, granularity, and friability of the mucosa without intervening areas of normal mucosa (skip areas). Inflammatory pseudopolyps indicate more severe erosion of the mucosa and must be distinguished from true polyps.

Diseases that may mimic ulcerative colitis must be excluded, particularly in the elderly. These include Crohn's disease, ischemic colitis, radiation coloproctitis, and diverticulitis. In acutely ill patients, stool cultures should be obtained to exclude infectious agents, including *Salmonella, Campylobacter, Shigella,* amebiasis, *Yersinia,* and *Escherichia coli* 0157:H7. *Clostridium difficile*–associated diarrhea and pseudomembranous colitis should be considered in elderly persons, particularly those who recently have been treated with antibiotics, reside in institutions, or have been recently hospitalized.

Treatment

The treatment of ulcerative colitis is based on the extent and severity of the disease (see TABLE 55–3). A number of effective drugs (eg, corticosteroids, 5-aminosalicylic acid, and immunosuppressive agents) can be administered IV, orally, or rectally.

Severe disease: Patients with severe or fulminant disease, including toxic megacolon, should be hospitalized and receive IV hydrocortisone or corticotropin infused in fluids containing enough potassium to avoid hypokalemia. One study suggests that corticotropin is more effective in patients who have not been treated previously with corticosteroids, whereas hydrocortisone may be more effective in those who have. If corticotropin does not produce significant improvement in 2 to 3 days, IV cyclosporine may be tried, but renal function should be closely monitored, especially in the elderly. When improvement is noted, IV therapy should be replaced with oral therapy.

Moderately severe disease: Oral corticosteroids are used to achieve a remission or to sustain one after IV therapy. Therapy consists of prednisone 40 to 60 mg/day initially given in two doses, then in a single morning dose. Corticosteroids should not be used for long-term maintenance therapy because of significant side effects related to both the dose and duration of therapy. These drugs may exacerbate diabetes mellitus, heart failure, osteoporosis, and hypertension, which are common in the elderly. When the disease is controlled, the prednisone dose should be tapered rapidly to 20 mg every morning. Then it can be tapered by 5 mg/day each week until the drug is discontinued, if the disease remains quiescent. The corticosteroid dose should be tapered while clinical activity and appropriate laboratory studies are monitored.

5-Aminosalicylates (5-ASA) should be given with oral corticosteroids. Sulfasalazine is effective and inexpensive, but its use is limited by side effects in up to 30% of patients. The side effects, which are often dose dependent, include nausea, anorexia, headache, and sometimes a generalized rash; in most cases, these effects result from the

TABLE 55–3. TREATMENT OF ULCERATIVE COLITIS

Indication	*Drug*	*Dosage*
Severe disease (patient has previously received corticosteroids)	Prednisone	60–80 mg/day IV
	Hydrocortisone	300 mg/day IV
Severe disease (patient has not previously received corticosteroids)	Corticotropin	120 u./day IV
Mild to moderate disease (proximal to sigmoid)	Sulfasalazine	2–4 gm/day orally
	Mesalamine*	2.4–4.8 gm/day orally
	Prednisone	40–60 mg/day orally
Active distal disease	Hydrocortisone cream	One application (1% in 30 gm) 1–2 times per day
	Hydrocortisone aerosol foam	One application (1% in 10 gm) 3–4 times per day
	Mesalamine enema	60 mL (4 gm mesalamine) rectally once a day
	Sulfasalazine	4–6 gm/day orally
Maintenance of remission		
Distal disease	Mesalamine enema	Every night to every 3rd night
Pancolonic disease	Sulfasalazine	1 gm bid orally
	Olsalazine*	500 mg bid orally

* If sulfasalazine is not tolerated

inactive sulfapyridine carrier rather than the 5-ASA. If side effects occur, sulfasalazine should be replaced with a more expensive 5-ASA drug, such as olsalazine or mesalamine. Diarrhea is a potential side effect of all 5-ASA drugs.

Mild disease: Patients with mild disease may be treated effectively with 5-ASA drugs that can be given by mouth, by enema in patients with left-sided disease, or by suppositories in patients with limited proctitis. Rectal corticosteroids are also effective in left-sided disease, but in general, they are not more effective than 5-ASA drugs. Because about 60% of a rectal corticosteroid may be absorbed, it is less suitable for maintenance therapy. Several poorly absorbed corticosteroid enemas and corticosteroids that do not affect the adrenal-pituitary-hypothalamic axis are under investigation.

Maintenance therapy: For patients in remission, long-term maintenance with a 5-ASA drug reduces the frequency of relapses. The usual maintenance dose of sulfasalazine (1 gm bid) produces few or no long-term adverse effects. For patients who cannot tolerate sulfasalazine, olsalazine 500 mg bid with meals is effective. For those with ulcerative proctitis or left-sided colitis, 5-ASA suppositories and enemas are effective when given every night to every third night. Nonsteroidal anti-inflammatory drugs have been reported to activate quiescent inflammatory bowel disease and should be avoided if possible.

Surgery: Surgery is indicated when medical therapy for acute fulminant disease fails, when patients cannot be weaned from long-term corticosteroid therapy, when surveillance studies reveal precancerous colonic lesions, and when medical therapy for chronic ulcerative colitis produces a suboptimal response.

In all age groups, the most common operation for acute fulminant colitis is subtotal colectomy and ileostomy. In elderly patients, proctocolectomy and ileostomy is the procedure of choice when long-term medical therapy fails or when premalignant changes develop. Procedures that avoid ileostomy, such as the ileoanal reservoir, are a good choice for many younger patients. However, the increased morbidity rate associated with this procedure limits its use in the elderly, who are already at greater risk for fecal incontinence because of age-associated changes in anal sphincter function.

CROHN'S DISEASE
(Regional Enteritis)

A chronic inflammatory process of unknown cause that most often affects the terminal ileum or colon and that is characterized by transmural inflammation, often with linear ulcerations and granulomas.

Histologic examination reveals transmural inflammation affecting all layers of the bowel and often associated with submucosal fibrosis. Other features that distinguish Crohn's disease from ulcerative colitis are linear ulcerations, fissures, fistulas, discrete mucosal ulcers, granulomas, and skip areas. Unlike ulcerative colitis, Crohn's disease frequently does not affect the rectum. The disease can involve any area of the GI tract from the mouth to the anus but most often involves the ileum and colon. Crohn's disease confined to the colon **(Crohn's colitis)** occurs more often in the elderly than in younger persons, and left-sided colitis appears to be prevalent in elderly women.

Symptoms and Signs

The clinical picture in the elderly is similar to that in younger persons; it includes rectal bleeding, diarrhea, fever, abdominal pain, and weight loss. In patients with colorectal involvement, perianal disease, a feature of Crohn's disease, may be an early manifestation. A person with perianal disease may present with rectal or anal strictures, fissures, fistulas, abscesses, prominent skin tags, or ulcers. The prevalence of extraintestinal manifestations such as migratory arthritis, pyoderma gangrenosum, iritis, and erythema nodosum is similar in older and younger patients. Common laboratory abnormalities such as leukocytosis, hypoalbuminemia, elevated erythrocyte sedimentation rate, and abnormalities indicating anemia vary with the severity of the illness. Rarely, the patient presents with peritonitis caused by bowel perforation, although it is more common with ileal involvement. An elderly patient with peritonitis may present atypically with mild abdominal pain, few abdominal findings, and mental confusion. Uncommonly, a patient with Crohn's colitis presents with massive lower GI bleeding or bowel obstruction.

Diagnosis

Prolonged delays in diagnosis probably occur more often in the elderly. A possible explanation is that Crohn's colitis, which is common in the elderly, tends to present more indolently than ileal or ileocolonic involvement.

Because the rectum is often unaffected and the distribution in the colon is often discontinuous, colonoscopy and barium x-ray are the diagnostic tests of choice. Both procedures can identify the characteristic ulcerations, skip lesions, and areas of colonic narrowing. Barium studies are better able to identify fistulas to adjacent visceral organs, whereas colonoscopy provides better visualization of the mucosa and allows mucosal biopsies to be taken. Biopsies should be taken from mucosa that appears grossly normal and from affected areas. Biopsies help to distinguish Crohn's colitis from diseases that mimic it. Such differentiation is particularly important because diverticula are common in the elderly and because ischemic colitis often occurs in a discontinuous distribution.

Computed tomography provides better definition of the colonic wall than colonoscopy and can identify extraintestinal abdominal abnormalities such as abscesses in patients with fever or palpable masses. Computed tomography and ultrasonography may also identify renal lithiasis and ureteral obstruction, which often occur silently.

Venereal disease, which is uncommon in the elderly, and carcinoma, which may complicate long-standing Crohn's proctitis, should be excluded. Infectious agents should be excluded by appropriate studies.

TABLE 55–4. MEDICAL TREATMENT OF CROHN'S DISEASE

Indication	*Drug*	*Dosage*
Ileocolonic and colonic involvement	Sulfasalazine	4–6 gm/day orally
	Mesalamine*	2.4–4.8 gm/day orally
	Metronidazole	125–250 mg tid orally
	Prednisone	20–30 mg bid orally
Perianal involvement	Metronidazole	1.5–2 gm/day orally
	Mercaptopurine or	50 mg/day up to 1.5 mg/kg/day orally
	Azathioprine	50 mg/day up to 2 mg/kg/day orally
	Ciprofloxacin	500 mg bid orally
Refractory disease	Mercaptopurine or	50 mg/day up to 2 mg/kg/day orally
	Azathioprine	50 mg/day up to 2 mg/kg/day orally
Maintenance of remission	Sulfasalazine	2 gm/day orally
	Mesalamine*	500 mg/day orally
	Mercaptopurine or	50 mg/day orally
	Azathioprine	50 mg/day orally
	Olsalazine*	500 mg bid orally

* If sulfasalazine is not tolerated

Treatment

Treatment of Crohn's disease is based on its extent, severity, distribution, and complications. Medical therapy includes all the drugs used for ulcerative colitis; in some patients, selected antibiotics are also useful (see TABLE 55–4).

Ileocolitis and colitis: Patients with mild to moderate disease often respond to sulfasalazine; those who cannot tolerate it may respond to one of the newer 5-ASA drugs. Dosages are similar to those used for ulcerative colitis. If the patient responds inadequately to 5-ASA drugs and the disease remains mild or moderate, metronidazole 125 to 250 mg tid may be tried before immunosuppressive agents.

If the disease worsens despite conservative therapy or if the patient has moderate to severe symptoms, prednisone 20 to 30 mg bid is given, followed by conversion to a single morning dose when disease activity significantly lessens. After remission is induced, the prednisone dose should be reduced by 5 to 10 mg/wk until it is 20 mg/day. Subsequently, the dose should be tapered about 5 mg/day every 3 wk while clinical activity and laboratory parameters are monitored until the patient is weaned.

About 60% of patients who cannot be weaned from oral corticosteroids respond to azathioprine (up to 2 mg/kg/day) or mercaptopurine (up to 1.5 mg/kg/day). A therapeutic response may not develop for 6 to 9 mo. These drugs may be continued indefinitely, but at least one attempt to discontinue them should be made after 1 yr of therapy to determine if remission can be maintained.

Perianal disease: Perianal fistulas and abscesses can be debilitating and frustrating to treat. Although perianal disease often improves with standard therapy for bowel inflammation and control of diarrhea, perianal symptoms persist in some patients. Short-term success has been reported with metronidazole 1.5 to 2.0 gm/day; however, side effects are common at these doses, and relapses occur when the drug is stopped or the dosage is tapered. Ciprofloxacin 500 mg bid, a more expensive alternative, also has a high relapse rate. If an abscess develops, it should be incised and drained.

If perianal disease does not respond to therapy, the colon may be diverted surgically, but surgery may also fail to heal the disease. Azathioprine or mercaptopurine may be useful in some patients with refractory disease.

Surgery: Unlike ulcerative colitis, Crohn's disease is not cured by surgery. Therefore, surgery should be reserved for patients who do not respond to medical therapy.

For patients with extensive Crohn's colitis, proctocolectomy with ileostomy is the best surgical option. For elderly patients who are debilitated or malnourished, an initial subtotal colectomy with ileostomy is less debilitating; it also gives the patient an opportunity to gain weight and to improve physically. If a subsequent proctectomy is required, the risk of complications is reduced; if rectal disease is mild or absent, a proctectomy may not be needed. More limited colonic resections may be appropriate if severe disease is localized or if obstructive symptoms are caused by relatively circumscribed bowel involvement.

Patients with small bowel disease may require laparotomy for intestinal obstruction, peritonitis, abscess formation, or occasionally for a suspicion of malignancy. Indications for surgery in older patients with Crohn's disease are the same as those for younger patients.

Surgery for ileal disease is generally well tolerated in the elderly, and the prognosis is comparable to that in younger patients. Elderly patients with extensive colitis or severe ileocolitis have higher morbidity and mortality, especially when emergency surgery is needed.

Recurrence rates after surgical resection for Crohn's disease vary; this variation is related in part to the initial site of disease. Proximal extension of distal colonic disease appears to be uncommon in older patients, and data suggest that recurrence rates are lower in older patients than in younger ones. Mortality rates associated with Crohn's disease do not appear to be significantly higher in the elderly.

COLONIC ISCHEMIA

Impairment of blood supply to the colon that results in inflammation and edema.

The colon is supplied with blood mainly by branches of the superior and inferior mesenteric arteries; collateral circulation, particularly by the marginal artery of Drummond and arc of Riolan, is extensive. Thus, if a major artery is occluded, collateral vessels open immediately to maintain an adequate blood supply to the bowel. Colonic ischemia may result from a generalized reduction in blood flow (nonocclusive ischemia), from inadequate distribution of blood flow (ie, vessel obstruction with poor collateral circulation), or a combination of the two. The splenic flexure is the most vulnerable point in the colon; about 80% of ischemic colitis occurs there. Colonic ischemia is the most common vascular disorder of the intestines in the elderly; it is often misdiagnosed unless it is strongly suspected and an aggressive diagnostic approach is used.

In most cases, the cause of colonic ischemia cannot be established with certainty and no vascular occlusions can be identified. In a significant minority of patients, a potential obstruction, such as a benign stricture, diverticulitis, or carcinoma, is found in the colon. Other contributing factors include hypotension, dehydration, heart failure, use of digitalis, polycythemia, volvulus, and cardiac arrhythmias.

Symptoms and Signs

The clinical manifestations of colonic ischemia are varied. The most common presentation is the sudden onset of mild to moderately severe cramping pain in the left lower abdomen. Often, this pain is accompanied by bloody diarrhea or hematochezia that may not appear until 24 h later. Frank hemorrhage is not characteristic of ischemia. Physical examination reveals tenderness over the involved bowel. In about ⅔ of patients, tenderness occurs over the splenic flexure or the distal transverse or descending colon. Peritoneal signs may last for several hours; if they last longer, a bowel infarction may have occurred. Fever, leukocytosis, absence of bowel sounds, and abdominal distention also suggest the possibility of bowel infarction.

Ischemia may be classified as reversible or irreversible. Reversible ischemia may present with submucosal or intramural hemorrhage or transient ischemic colitis, which completely resolves within weeks to months, depending on the severity. Irreversible ischemia may present with chronic ulcerations, strictures of varying lengths, colonic gangrene, or fulminant transmural colitis.

Recurrent episodes of colonic ischemia occur in < 10% of patients. Attempts should be made to correct or remove underlying conditions that predispose patients to colonic ischemia.

Diagnosis

If colonic ischemia is suspected clinically, a gentle barium enema or colonoscopy with minimal insufflation of air should be done within 48 h. Barium studies may show **thumbprinting** in the affected areas of the colon, which represents submucosal or mucosal hemorrhages during early ischemia. This thumbprinting corresponds to the purplish blebs seen on colonoscopy. X-ray findings from later stages of ischemia include segmental ischemia, which may or may not return to normal within weeks or months; this finding corresponds to segmental necrosis, inflammation, ulcerations, or mucosal sloughing on colonoscopy. Mesenteric angiography is not useful in patients with colonic ischemia in contrast to those with suspected mesenteric ischemia of the small intestine.

Treatment

Treatment includes bowel rest, IV fluids or plasma expanders, and in severe cases, systemic antibiotics such as gentamicin and clindamycin. Corticosteroids are *not* beneficial and should *not* be given. In mild disease, symptoms resolve within several days, and radiologic healing usually occurs within several weeks, although some patients may not heal for up to 6 mo.

If the patient continues to have diarrhea, bleeding, or significant obstructive symptoms for more than several weeks, surgical resection is usually indicated. *If colonic infarction is suspected, emergency laparotomy with resection of nonviable bowel is required.*

ANTIBIOTIC–ASSOCIATED DIARRHEA AND COLITIS

Diarrhea and colonic inflammation that occurs during or shortly after the administration of antibiotics or chemotherapy.

The vast majority of cases are mediated by a cytotoxin produced by *Clostridium difficile;* this cytotoxin triggers epithelial necrosis and a characteristic inflammatory process. *C. difficile,* the most common agent of nosocomial diarrhea, is acquired most often by elderly persons in hospitals or nursing homes. Nosocomial transmission involving environmental contamination with *C. difficile* and carriage of the organism on the hands of hospital personnel has been documented. Acquisition of *C. difficile* is often asymptomatic, but it may have clinical consequences if elderly patients receive certain antibiotics or chemotherapeutic agents. Other possible risk factors include surgery, intensive care, nasogastric intubation, and length of hospital stay. Some patients have antibiotic-associated diarrhea without evidence of *C. difficile* infection.

Although almost all antibiotics have been implicated, cephalosporins, extended-spectrum penicillins (eg, ampicillin), and clindamycin are implicated most often. Other penicillins and erythromycin are involved less often.

Symptoms and Signs

The disease spectrum ranges from mild diarrhea (with little or no inflammation) to severe colitis often associated with pseudomembranes, which adhere to necrotic colonic epithelium. The typical clinical picture of antibiotic-associated colitis includes watery nonbloody diarrhea, lower abdominal cramps, fever, and leukocytosis. Fever is usually low grade, although occasionally it can be high. In severe cases, dehydration, hypotension, hypoproteinemia, toxic megacolon, or colonic perforation may occur. When diarrhea occurs without colitis, constitutional symptoms are usually absent.

Diagnosis

Diagnostic studies are used to define anatomic and histopathologic changes and to identify the causative organism. Certain tests can identify *C. difficile* or its toxin. The tissue culture assay for a cytopathic toxin neutralized by specific antitoxins is the standard, but many hospitals lack the facilities for these assays and must submit stool specimens to reference laboratories. The preferred alternative is an enzyme immunoassay that yields results comparable to the tissue culture assay. Stool cultures for *C. difficile* require selective growth media, and inexperienced laboratories have reported difficulties in recovering the organism. Moreover, whether *C. difficile* can be implicated in antibiotic-associated diarrhea without identifying the cytotoxin is unknown.

In general, endoscopy should be performed in severely ill patients who present atypically and require a rapid diagnosis to expedite treatment. In severely ill patients, flexible sigmoidoscopy is usually satisfactory because the distal colon is involved in most cases. However, changes may be confined to the right colon in up to ⅓ of cases, making colonoscopy necessary when less extensive procedures do not confirm a diagnosis that is strongly suspected. The yellowish-gray pseudomembranes are dense and adhere to the underlying colonic mucosa, but the mucosa between the pseudomembranes appears normal. When pseudomembranes are not grossly visible, mucosal biopsies may exhibit characteristic findings. Barium x-rays and computed tomography are less useful. Barium enemas should be performed gently to reduce the risk of colonic perforation.

Treatment

In patients with *C. difficile*-associated diarrhea or colitis, the implicated drug should be stopped, if possible. If symptoms persist or the disease is clinically severe, patients should receive metronidazole 500 mg orally bid for 7 to 14 days or vancomycin 125 mg orally qid for 7 to 14 days. If oral administration is not possible, metronidazole 500 mg IV q 6 h should be given until oral administration is possible. Metronidazole and vancomycin appear to be therapeutically comparable, but metronidazole costs substantially less. However, if the patient is seriously ill, oral vancomycin is usually recommended. Fever usually resolves within 24 h, and diarrhea decreases over 4 to 5 days.

Relapse rates average 20% to 25% after successful treatment with either agent. Patients who have one relapse are more likely to have another. This phenomenon cannot be explained by antibiotic resistance but may involve sporulation, which leads to relapse within 4 wk after successful treatment. Relapses invariably respond to another course of antibiotic therapy. In the 5% to 10% of patients who have multiple relapses, metronidazole or vancomycin in conventional doses should be followed by a 3-wk course of cholestyramine 4 gm tid and/or lactobacillus 500 mg orally qid, or vancomycin 125 mg orally every other day. The efficacy of a nonpathogenic yeast, *Saccharomyces boulardii,* is being investigated, and preliminary results appear promising.

FECAL INCONTINENCE

(See also FECAL INCONTINENCE in Ch. 53)

Loss of voluntary control of defecation. Continence requires rectal and anal sensation to detect rectal filling and to discriminate among fluid, feces, and flatus; the reservoir capacity of the rectum and distal colon to store feces for variable periods of time; and the coordination of the internal and external anal sphincters to prevent unwanted defecation. The pelvic floor muscles, especially the puborectal muscle, preserve continence by retarding stool passage by mechanical means. The motivation to maintain continence is also important, especially among the elderly because cognitive dysfunction is more prevalent. The causes of fecal incontinence in elderly persons are listed in TABLE 55–5.

The effects of impaired contractile strength of the puborectal muscle or the external anal sphincter become more important as rectal viscoelasticity and resting pressures of the internal anal sphincter decrease with aging. Because a given volume of rectal distention elicits higher rectal pressures, rectal urgency is experienced at smaller distention volumes. Furthermore, smaller distention volumes are able to inhibit anal sphincter tone. All of these changes predispose the elderly to fecal incontinence and add stress to the striated muscles of the anorectum.

TABLE 55–5. CAUSES OF FECAL INCONTINENCE IN THE ELDERLY

Fecal impaction	**Decreased rectal sensation**
	Diabetes mellitus
Functional impairment	Megarectum
Mental (dementia, confusion)	Fecal impaction
Physical (weakness, immobility)	
	Impaired anal sphincter and puborectal muscle function
Decreased reservoir capacity	
Aging	Idiopathic (perineal descent)
Radiation	Trauma, surgery
Tumor	Spinal cord or pudendal lesions
Ischemia	
Surgical resection	

From Wald A: "Constipation and fecal incontinence in the elderly." *Gastroenterology Clinics of North America* 19:405–418, 1990; used with permission.

In **institutionalized, physically or mentally impaired elderly patients,** the most common cause of fecal incontinence is leakage of liquid stool around an impacted fecal mass. Fecal incontinence probably results from a failure to sense rectal volumes that are large enough to inhibit the internal anal sphincter. Thus, these patients do not consciously contract the striated muscles to prevent incontinence. Anal sphincter pressures are usually normal after disimpaction. In patients with global dementia, fecal incontinence may occur after meals or other activities that stimulate the gastrocolonic response because these patients simply do not suppress the urge to defecate.

In **ambulatory, noninstitutionalized elderly patients,** fecal incontinence is often associated with abnormal anorectal continence mechanisms, which may involve decreased contractile strength or impaired automaticity of the puborectal and external anal sphincter muscles. These changes may result from age-related muscle weakness; however, in elderly women, they often result from a partial denervation injury from pudendal neuropathy. In many women with a diagnosis of idiopathic fecal incontinence, the injury to the pudendal nerve appears to be even more severe; this injury is associated with prolonged nerve conduction and evidence of a denervation-reinnervation injury to the external anal sphincter or puborectal muscle.

The cause of pudendal neuropathy is unknown. Suggested causes include repetitive stretching of the pudendal nerves in middle-aged and elderly women because of chronic constipation and defecatory straining, weaker pelvic floor muscles caused by a hormonal effect, and spondylitic compression of nerve roots.

TABLE 55–6. EVALUATION OF FECAL INCONTINENCE

Studies	*Information Obtained*
Proctosigmoidoscopy	Inflammation, melanosis coli (laxative abuse), tumors, strictures
Proctography	Rectal capacity and diameter Anorectal angle (puborectal muscle function) Perineal descent (pelvic floor function)
Anorectal manometry	Anal sphincter pressures Rectal sensation Rectal compliance External sphincter responses (cough, distention, voluntary)

From Wald A: "Constipation and fecal incontinence in the elderly." *Gastroenterology Clinics of North America* 19:405–418, 1990; used with permission.

Diagnosis

Patients with fecal impaction and incontinence do not require extensive testing. However, incontinent persons without fecal impaction require a comprehensive evaluation of possible underlying causes. This evaluation usually includes diagnostic studies to assess anorectal continence mechanisms such as proctosigmoidoscopy, barium enema, proctography, and anorectal manometry (see TABLE 55–6).

Treatment

After removal of a **fecal impaction,** treatment continues with daily or twice-daily enemas. Because failure to empty the colon increases the risk of recurrent impaction, colonic irrigation with large volumes of a balanced electrolyte solution can be used after initial enemas. After the colon is cleansed, **immobilized or functionally impaired patients** should be placed on a restricted fiber diet and have enemas administered once or twice weekly to prevent recurrent soiling.

In **nonconstipated, intact elderly patients,** biofeedback techniques, drugs, and surgery may be used to treat incontinence.

Biofeedback is a simple and often effective treatment for incontinence associated with **rectosphincteric abnormalities.** An anorectal manometer attached to a visual display allows the patient to see when sphincteric responses are appropriate; the patient then tries to reproduce the appropriate response. In essence, biofeedback is a trial-and-error learning process. Many elderly patients have difficulties because of anxiety about the procedure and short-term memory loss.

However, the technique has been successful in up to 70% of patients who meet the criteria for biofeedback (motivation, ability to comprehend and remember directions, and some degree of rectal sensation), including patients with incontinence caused by prior sphincter surgery or anorectal diseases, idiopathic incontinence, and diabetes mellitus. Similar results have been reported when patients use an intra-anal plug containing two electrodes attached to an electrometer. With this device, electrical impulses generated by the contracting anal sphincter provide the patient with audible or visual feedback concerning sphincteric responses.

For fecal incontinence associated with **chronic diarrhea,** opiate derivatives are often helpful. Studies suggest that loperamide is superior to codeine and diphenoxylate in reducing incontinence. When incontinence is associated with impaired reservoir capacity or with neurogenic abnormalities affecting colorectal function, a program of planned regular defecation and fiber restriction to reduce stool volume often reduces incontinence. If incontinence persists, loperamide can be taken. The dosage (maximum 16 mg/day in divided doses) is titrated to decrease stool frequency or eliminate defecation altogether. To prevent fecal impaction when defecation is eliminated, enemas should be administered once or twice weekly.

When fecal incontinence is associated with **rectal prolapse,** surgery is the procedure of choice. Rectal prolapse is caused by an intussusception of the rectum through the pelvic floor; resuspension or proctopexy can prevent further intussusception and can be combined with rectosigmoidectomy to restore continence in up to ⅔ of patients. However, when prolapse is severe or prolonged, permanent neuropathic sphincter impairment may preclude a good surgical result.

For patients who have fecal incontinence without full-thickness rectal prolapse, surgery should be considered if conservative therapy is unsatisfactory. However, the decision to treat surgically and the choice of surgical procedure must be made carefully because none of the procedures is easy to perform or without complications. Also, few controlled studies have compared the long-term outcomes of the various procedures with those of conservative treatment. In one study, 65% of those who underwent surgery had a successful outcome compared with 40% of those who received nonsurgical treatment. However, biofeedback techniques were not used in this study. When surgery is selected, the procedure should be designed to correct abnormal continence mechanisms identified by preoperative studies.

56. CONSTIPATION

No precise definition of constipation exists, but patients often define it as a need to strain in order to defecate or as infrequent or incomplete bowel movements.

The frequency of constipation gradually increases with age; after age 65, the prevalence dramatically increases. At all ages, constipation occurs more frequently in women than in men, in nonwhites than in whites, and in persons with lower income and less education.

A recent study suggests that elderly patients with chronic constipation fall into two major groups: those with functional megarectum (with or without megacolon), who frequently present with fecal impaction, and those with a hypertonic distal bowel, who frequently complain of difficult passage of hard small stools.

Constipation in the elderly may be related to many medical and surgical conditions as well as many medications (see TABLE 56–1). Often, several contributing factors are involved. For example, inactivity and bed rest may slow colonic transit, while the use of a bedpan, an inability to respond to the urge to defecate, inadequate dietary fiber intake, depression, or confusion may cause or aggravate constipation. Neuromuscular disorders may cause constipation because of neurogenic bowel dysfunction, generalized muscle weakness, or incoordination. Dietary modifications prescribed for other conditions may also produce constipation.

TABLE 56–1. CAUSES OF CONSTIPATION IN ELDERLY PATIENTS

Dietary causes	Low fiber intake Poor caloric or fluid intake
Functional causes	Depression Confusion Inadequate toilet arrangements Weakness Immobility

Secondary causes (secondary to other diseases)	Neurogenic disorders
	  Spinal cord lesions
	  Parkinson's disease
	  Cerebrovascular accidents
	  Dementia
	Endocrine disorders
	  Hypothyroidism
	  Hyperparathyroidism
	Colonic obstruction
	  Ischemia
	  Diverticulitis
	  Tumors
	  Radiation

(continued)

TABLE 56–1. CAUSES OF CONSTIPATION IN ELDERLY PATIENTS *(Continued)*

Other cause	Misperception (patient views normal variation as constipation)

Pharmacologic causes	Opioids
	Anticholinergics
	  Antidepressants
	  Antihistamines
	  Antiparkinsonian drugs
	  Antipsychotics
	  GI antispasmodics
	  Muscle relaxants
	Cation-containing agents
	  Aluminum (antacids, sucralfate)
	  Calcium (antacids, supplements)
	  Iron supplements
	Neurally active agents
	  Anticonvulsants
	  Antihypertensives
	  Calcium channel blockers
	  Ganglionic blockers
	  Opiates
	  Vinca alkaloids
	Diuretics

Modified from Wald A: "Constipation and fecal incontinence in the elderly." *Gastroenterology Clinics of North America* 19:405–18, 1990; and Wald A: "Constipation in elderly patients: Pathogenesis and management." *Drugs and Aging* 3(3):220–231, 1993; used with permission.

Complications

In the elderly, straining may have serious adverse effects on the cerebral, coronary, and peripheral arterial circulations. In these persons, who often have cerebrovascular disease or impaired baroreceptor reflexes, excessive straining can lead to transient ischemic attacks and syncope. Any person, young or old, can develop hemorrhoids or other anal disorders from straining, but the elderly develop them more commonly.

A major complication of constipation in the elderly, **fecal impaction** can result in intestinal obstruction, stercoral ulceration (colonic ulceration caused by pressure and irritation from retained feces), urinary retention, and fecal incontinence with spurious diarrhea. Fecal impaction is often regarded as a consequence of the mental and physical decline of the elderly person. The elderly are predisposed to impaction by changes in anorectal physiology, including impaired rectal, anal, and perianal sensations so that larger rectal volumes are needed to produce the urge to defecate and to generate rectal contractions. For the same reason, recurrence of fecal impaction after disimpaction and bowel cleansing is common.

Fecal impaction can be treated satisfactorily by using a warm water enema or by *cautiously* using a sodium phosphate and biphosphate enema. Soap enemas should be avoided because they may damage the mucosa. Thoroughly emptying the distal colon is critically important and can be achieved by giving large amounts of polyethylene glycol–electrolyte solutions orally or by nasogastric tube.

Because impaired rectal sensation predisposes patients to recurrent impaction, regular enemas have been recommended to keep the rectum empty for 5 to 6 wk. However, no data suggest that rectal sensation returns to normal during this time. Thus, periodic monitoring and purgation may be required indefinitely after disimpaction.

Idiopathic megacolon occasionally occurs in geriatric patients with chronic constipation; this condition predisposes patients to volvulus of the sigmoid colon. In such persons, fiber supplements are not helpful. Rather, a fiber-restricted diet with cleansing enemas once or twice weekly minimizes fecal buildup and impaction and may reduce the risk of volvulus.

Diagnosis

Excluding an underlying cause of constipation such as malignancy, intestinal obstruction, or hypothyroidism is always important. Such conditions are typical in elderly patients who have had a recent change in bowel habits. However, colonoscopic or barium studies should not be performed repeatedly in patients with chronic symptoms because the studies are expensive, time consuming, potentially debilitating, occasionally associated with complications, and unlikely to yield important information after an initial negative finding. Besides reviewing underlying illnesses, medications, diet, activity, and other potential contributors to constipation, the physician should assess mental status and psychosocial parameters. A self-administered behavioral test designed for the nonpsychiatric practitioner, such as the Hopkins Symptom Checklist (SCL-90-R) or the Millon test for depression, may be used. These tests can detect marked depression, a frequently overlooked diagnosis.

In patients with intractable symptoms, objective studies of colonic and anorectal function may provide clues to the underlying mechanisms.

Abdominal x-rays are used to measure colonic transit. The patient swallows radiopaque markers on 3 successive days. Then x-rays are obtained 4 and 7 days after ingestion of the first set of markers, and the markers are counted in three abdominal regions corresponding to the right, left, and rectosigmoid colon. A study of 30 ambulatory, constipated elderly persons found normal colonic transit in 8 persons, slowing in only the left colon in 5 persons, and rectal stasis in 17 persons.

Similar findings have been reported by others using similar techniques, suggesting that constipation is most often associated with distal colonic or anorectal dysfunction in ambulatory elderly persons and that colonic transit is normal in a sizable percentage of patients.

Evacuation proctography (defecography) permits defecation to be studied by measuring the evacuation of thickened barium with cineradiography. This test determines rectal diameter and emptying. Also, abnormalities not apparent at rest may be seen with straining; these abnormalities include rectoceles, intussusceptions, poor relaxation of the puborectal muscle, and excessive perineal descent.

Similarly, **anorectal manometry** has documented impaired rectal sensation, megarectum, and abnormal expulsion dynamics in many patients with severe constipation. However, the relevance of radiologic or manometric abnormalities is not always certain because they may also occur in asymptomatic persons.

Treatment

Ideally, the treatment of chronic constipation should be based on the presumed pathophysiologic mechanisms in each patient. Practically speaking, effective treatment in elderly persons consists of dietary approaches such as fiber supplementation, laxatives and enemas, and surgery in selected and carefully defined circumstances.

Dietary approaches: Adding bran to the diet of nonconstipated persons increases stool weight, shortens colonic transit time, and increases the frequency of defecation. In several controlled studies, constipation improved in institutionalized elderly persons after fiber and fluids were added to their diets. In these studies, bran 6 to 20 gm/day was well tolerated. During the initial stages of bran supplementation, patients may complain of abdominal discomfort or excessive flatulence, but these symptoms usually diminish with time. If bran is not tolerated, synthetic bulk laxatives such as methylcellulose or calcium polycarbophil may be substituted.

Before fiber supplementation is initiated, any fecal impaction should be removed. Patients with obstructive lesions anywhere in the GI tract should *not* be given fiber supplements. Fiber also is not indicated for patients with megacolon or megarectum, especially if they are confined to bed, are demented, or have neurogenic constipation. On the contrary, such patients are better managed by *reducing* colonic contents and using periodic timed evacuation, ie, evacuating several days per week either spontaneously or with laxatives or enemas.

Compliance remains a major problem with fiber therapy. Patients should be advised that fiber helps prevent constipation.

Laxatives: The use of laxatives is deeply rooted in medical and social traditions, and vast amounts of laxatives are consumed, often inappropriately, by elderly persons. Nonbulk laxatives are classified in four groups on the basis of their presumed mode of action: hyperosmolar, saline, stimulant, and emollient laxatives (see TABLE 56–2).

TABLE 56–2. COMPARISON OF LAXATIVES

Laxatives	*Usual Daily Dose*	*Adverse Effects*
Hyperosmolar laxatives		
Polyethylene glycol	240–480 mL orally	Abdominal bloating
Lactulose	15–45 mL orally 1–2 times daily	Abdominal bloating
	Long-term therapy: 30–45 mL orally 1–2 times daily to produce 1–2 soft stools daily	
Sorbitol	30–150 mL of 70% solution orally	Abdominal bloating
Glycerine	1 adult (3 gm) suppository	Rectal irritation
	5–15 mL enema	Rectal irritation
Saline laxatives		
Magnesium sulfate	15 gm orally	Magnesium toxicity (with renal insufficiency)
Magnesium citrate	200 mL orally	Magnesium toxicity (with renal insufficiency)
Magnesium hydroxide	30–60 mL orally	Magnesium toxicity (with renal insufficiency)
Sodium phosphate	20–30 mL orally	Phosphate toxicity (with renal insufficiency and sodium-restricted diet)
Sodium phosphate, sodium biphosphate	118 mL enema	Phosphate toxicity (with renal insufficiency and sodium-restricted diet)
Stimulant laxatives		
Castor oil	15–60 mL orally	Nutrient malabsorption
Diphenylmethanes		
Phenolphthalein	60–100 mg orally	Skin rashes
Bisacodyl	10–15 (up to 30) mg orally	Gastric irritation
	10 mg rectally	Gastric irritation

(continued)

TABLE 56–2. COMPARISON OF LAXATIVES *(Continued)*

Laxatives	*Usual Daily Dose*	*Adverse Effects*
Stimulant laxatives *(continued)*		
Anthraquinones		
Cascara sagrada	1 tablet or 5 mL orally at bedtime	Melanosis coli, injury to submucosal and myenteric plexuses
Senna	1–2 tablets at bedtime (up to 8 tablets/day); 1 suppository at bedtime; 5–15 mL liquid orally at bedtime (up to 30 mL/day); 1/4–1 teaspoon granules (up to 4 teaspoons/day)	Melanosis coli, injury to submucosal and myenteric plexuses
Casanthrol	1–2 capsules at bedtime	Melanosis coli, injury to submucosal and myenteric plexuses
Emollient laxatives		
Docusate salts	50–500 mg orally	Skin rashes

Modified from Wald A: "Constipation in elderly patients: Pathogenesis and management." *Drugs and Aging* 3(3):220–231, 1993; used with permission.

Hyperosmolar laxatives include mixed electrolyte solutions containing polyethylene glycol and nonabsorbable sugars such as lactulose and sorbitol. The latter are degraded by colonic bacteria to low-molecular-weight acids, thereby increasing stool acidity and osmolarity.

This type of laxative can be used for prevention or treatment as long as GI motility is not substantially impaired; such impairment may result from a narcotic or an anticholinergic drug. Lactulose or sorbitol is recommended for long-term use if fiber supplements are ineffective or poorly tolerated. Doses should be adjusted to minimize side effects (eg, bloating, flatulence, diarrhea) and modulate defecation.

The high cost of lactulose has limited its use. A recent study of elderly men with chronic constipation found that sorbitol produced effects comparable to lactulose, making sorbitol a cost-effective alternative.

Saline laxatives contain relatively nonabsorbable cations and anions, which exert an osmotic effect to increase intraluminal water content. Some oral preparations contain magnesium, which may also stimulate the release of cholecystokinin to increase intestinal motility. Because an appreciable amount of magnesium may be absorbed, possibly leading to magnesium toxicity, these agents are contraindicated in patients with renal insufficiency. Saline laxatives can also be administered as sodium phosphate enemas or suppositories, but they should be given cautiously to elderly patients at risk for salt and water retention.

Stimulant laxatives include castor oil, anthraquinones (cascara sagrada, senna, and casanthranol) and diphenylmethanes (phenolphthalein and bisacodyl). They are particularly useful in treating constipation caused by narcotic or anticholinergic drug use. Castor oil is hydrolyzed by intestinal lipases to ricinoleic acid, which stimulates intestinal secretion, decreases glucose absorption, and increases intestinal motility.

Anthraquinone laxatives increase fluid and electrolyte accumulation in the distal ileum and colon by actions that are not completely understood. Long-term anthraquinone use produces pathologic changes in the colon, such as melanosis coli, a benign and reversible condition, and perhaps damage to the myenteric plexus.

An appreciable amount of phenolphthalein is absorbed from the small intestine and enters enterohepatic circulation, which explains its often prolonged duration of action. The drug both stimulates colonic motor activity and increases intraluminal fluid content. Occasional side effects include fixed drug eruptions, erythema multiforme, and photosensitive bullous skin lesions. Bisacodyl is structurally and pharmacologically similar to phenolphthalein.

In general, the long-term use of stimulant laxatives should be discouraged. These laxatives are the most commonly abused cathartics, and their long-term use may lead to abdominal cramps, fluid and electrolyte disturbances, malabsorption, and cathartic colon. However, these laxatives are readily available as over-the-counter medications, and many elderly persons are unwilling to change long-standing patterns of use. With such persons, a reasonable approach is to achieve a compromise by limiting use of these cathartics to once or twice weekly. This approach may help minimize adverse effects.

Emollient laxatives include mineral oil and docusate salts. Mineral oil, administered orally or by enema, penetrates and softens the stool. Because mineral oil may decrease the absorption of fat-soluble vitamins, it should be given between meals. It should not be given at bedtime. Aspiration with lipid pneumonia is a recognized hazard; mineral oil is *contraindicated* in patients with esophageal dysmotility or dysphagia and in elderly debilitated patients.

Docusate salts are anionic surfactants that lower the surface tension of stool to allow mixing of aqueous and fatty substances. This mixing softens the stool to permit easier defecation. However, controlled studies have not demonstrated changes in stool water content, stool weight, frequency of defecation, or colonic transit when docusate salts were given in recommended doses. Thus, the efficacy of stool softeners is controversial. They may be tried for short periods in patients with hard stools who report excessive straining during defecation, but they have marginal value in treating chronic constipation and are useless in treating drug-induced constipation.

Surgery: A proctologic examination or evacuation proctography in an elderly patient with constipation may identify a rectocele, intussusception, or rectal prolapse. However, these conditions are common in older nonconstipated persons, and the constipation should not be attributed to the condition without closer consideration.

Rectocele repairs often do not alleviate constipation. A rectocele repair consists of reducing or eliminating the pouch with posterior colporrhaphy. A helpful maneuver is to observe rectal evacuation for improvement when the patient exerts pressure on the posterior wall of the vagina during defecography.

Surgical approaches to rectal intussusceptions and prolapse consist of various resuspension procedures. But for most patients who undergo surgery, constipation does not improve, and surgical repair should be recommended with caution. Unless rectal prolapses are frequent, severe, or irreducible, medical treatment of constipation should be tried before undertaking surgery.

57. DIARRHEA

An increase in the frequency of defecation (more than three stools per day) associated with increased stool volume (> 300 mL), increased fluidity, and abnormal sensations such as urgency and pain.

Diarrhea can be classified on the basis of pathophysiologic processes and disorders. A simple classification uses six general processes: **(1) osmotic diarrhea** secondary to ingestion of osmotically active ingredients in foods and drugs; **(2) infectious diarrhea** including **toxigenic diarrhea** from infection caused by bacteria or viruses, which elaborate toxins that cause the intestinal epithelial cells to secrete water and electrolytes into the intestinal lumen, and **invasive diarrhea** caused by invasive pathogens affecting the distal ileum and colon; **(3) maldigestive diarrhea** secondary to pancreatic exocrine insufficiency (especially lipase deficiency) and bile acid insufficiency and bacterial overgrowth syndromes; **(4) malabsorptive diarrhea** encountered in celiac disease, tropical sprue, giardiasis, and Whipple's disease; **(5) diarrhea secondary to increased secretion of hormones, peptides, or biogenic amines from tumors,** including carcinoid tumors, medullary carcinoma of the thyroid, islet-cell tumor of the pancreas (vipoma), gastrinoma (Zollinger-Ellison syndrome), parathyroid adenoma, and small cell carcinoma of the lung; and **(6) colonic diarrhea** secondary to ulcerative colitis,

Crohn's disease, ischemic colitis, carcinoma of the colon, villous adenoma, radiation colitis, and resection of < 100 cm of the distal ileum (bile-acid–induced diarrhea).

Supportive Treatment

Elderly persons with acute, nonspecific diarrhea should reduce their activity. To prevent pressure sores, they should change position frequently and get out of bed for meals. For the first 24 h, clear liquids (such as ginger ale, decaffeinated cola, decaffeinated tea, broth, and Gatorade) and gelatin should be given. The patient should consume 2 to 3 L of fluid because most diarrhea-associated complications result from fluid and electrolyte loss. After 24 h, the patient should eat bland foods, such as cooked cereals, rice, soup, bread, crackers, baked potatoes, eggs, and applesauce. Fruits, vegetables, fried or spicy foods, bran, candy, and caffeinated and alcoholic beverages should be avoided. After 2 or 3 days, patients can progress to their regular diet.

Non-antimicrobial agents used to treat acute diarrhea include bismuth subsalicylate (effective for traveler's diarrhea), tincture of opium, diphenoxylate with atropine, and loperamide (highly effective at a daily dose of 8 mg). Both diphenoxylate with atropine and loperamide should be avoided in patients with fever or blood in the stool.

OSMOTIC DIARRHEA

In the elderly, osmotic diarrhea is caused by the ingestion of poorly absorbable solutes such as magnesium sulfate, sodium sulfate, laxatives containing citrate, antacids containing magnesium hydroxide and mannitol, and sorbitol (chewing gum and diet candy). Disaccharidase deficiencies, especially lactase deficiency, can cause osmotic diarrhea. About 80% of the world population has primary lactase deficiency. Although it begins in childhood, people do not outgrow it. The highest incidence of lactase deficiency occurs in black Americans and Jews. Osmotic diarrhea also occurs after a gastrectomy or vagotomy, in dumping syndrome, in short bowel syndrome, and with chronic small intestinal ischemia.

The diarrhea begins abruptly and is characterized by increased stool volume and an absence of blood and fat in the stool. Nausea, vomiting, and crampy abdominal pain do not occur in osmotic diarrhea. The diarrhea stops when the patient fasts or stops ingesting the poorly absorbable solute.

Diagnosis

The history of symptoms after ingestion of milk or milk products is essential. In patients with lactase deficiency, the stool pH is usually 4 to 6 (normal is > 6) with an associated increase in short-chain fatty acids. A lactose-hydrogen breath test reveals breath hydrogen > 20 ppm within 3 h after lactose ingestion. Measuring magnesium (normal is

< 12 mmol), sulfate (normal is < 5 mmol) and phosphate (normal is < 12 mmol) in stool water may be necessary, especially in cases of surreptitious laxative abuse, a problem more common in elderly women.

Treatment

Treatment consists of having the patient avoid the offending solute and explaining why this is necessary. Lactase deficiency is treated by having the patient avoid foods with lactose and drugs with lactose fillers. Low-lactose milk or milk with lactase added are recommended. Lactase caplets can be prescribed, but they are expensive.

INFECTIOUS DIARRHEA

The exact incidence of infectious diarrhea in the elderly is unknown, but it is higher than in younger adults and has a higher mortality. Age-related anatomic and physiologic changes, chronic illnesses, and increased drug use make the elderly more susceptible to gastrointestinal infections. Gastric acidity, which helps inactivate ingested bacteria, is generally decreased because of mucosal atrophy, frequent use of H_2-receptor blockers and antacids, and in some cases, gastric resection. Intestinal motility, another defense mechanism, is also decreased secondary to intrinsic neuronal degeneration, vascular ischemia, diabetes mellitus, and frequent use of anticholinergic drugs or narcotics. As a result, pathogenic organisms and their toxins can remain in the gut for an extended period and thus may overgrow. Intestinal mucosal immunity (ie, IgA secretion) is also believed to be decreased, although such a decrease has not been proved.

Viruses responsible for infectious diarrhea include the Norwalk virus-like agents and, less commonly, rotavirus. The exact pathogenetic mechanism is unclear. Diarrhea is caused by Norwalk virus throughout the year, whereas rotavirus infection occurs more often in the cooler months. Both agents have caused epidemic diarrhea in nursing homes and are easily spread by the fecal-oral route.

TOXIGENIC DIARRHEAS

Toxigenic diarrheas are caused by several microorganisms that usually produce an enterotoxin or enterotoxin-like substance. These microorganisms include *Staphylococcus aureus, Bacillus cereus, Clostridium perfringens, Escherichia coli, Vibrio cholerae, Clostridium botulinum, Clostridium difficile,* and *Vibrio parahaemolyticus*.

Staphylococcus Aureus Food Poisoning

Staphylococcus aureus food poisoning is caused by heat-stable enterotoxin B that is preformed by a toxigenic strain of *S. aureus* growing in contaminated food. The onset is explosive, generally within 2 to 6 h after ingesting a contaminated food, such as cream pastries, coleslaw, or potato salad. Severe vomiting precedes the passage of loose, foul-smelling stools. Moderate to diffuse abdominal cramps occur without tenesmus and fever. The self-limited clinical course usually resolves in 12 to 24 h.

Diagnosis is made on the characteristic clinical picture, a finding of $> 10^5$ colony-forming units (CFU)/gm of staphylococci in the food, and a test identifying enterotoxin B. **Treatment** is supportive. Antimicrobial therapy is not indicated.

Bacillus Cereus Food Poisoning

Bacillus cereus, a frequent cause of food poisoning, is usually associated with contaminated refried rice or vegetables. This type of poisoning is characterized by two clinical syndromes: **short-incubation emesis syndrome** and **long-incubation diarrheal syndrome.** The emesis syndrome mimics *Staphylococcus aureus* poisoning; vomiting associated with abdominal pain and diarrhea begins about 6 h after the ingestion of the contaminated food. The diarrheal syndrome mimics *Clostridium perfringens* poisoning, occurring 8 to 16 h after the ingestion of contaminated food; it is not associated with vomiting, but nausea occasionally occurs. This syndrome includes abdominal pain with some tenesmus and profuse, foul-smelling watery diarrhea. In one long-incubation *B. cereus* outbreak involving elderly patients in a chronic disease hospital, the mean duration of illness was 2.3 days; in one patient the illness lasted 10 days.

Diagnosis is made by finding 10^5 CFU/gm of the organism in the stool. **Treatment** is supportive; both forms of the illness subside in 12 to 24 h.

Clostridium Perfringens Food Poisoning

Clostridium perfringens is a gram-positive, spore-forming bacillus producing a potent thermolabile exotoxin. It exerts its effect on the proximal small intestine by activating adenylate cyclase, producing increased intestinal fluid secretion and decreased reabsorption. *C. perfringens* poisoning is associated with contaminated beef, beef products, and poultry and is characterized by the sudden onset of unusually foul-smelling diarrheal stools without blood or mucus, moderately severe colicky abdominal pain, and no vomiting. The self-limited disorder usually lasts less than 24 h.

Diagnosis is established by finding $> 10^5$ CFU/gm of the organism in food or stool. **Treatment** is supportive.

Escherichia Coli Diarrhea

At least five types of *Escherichia coli* can cause GI infections, including enterotoxigenic, enteropathogenic, enteroinvasive, enterohemorrhagic, and enteroadherent *E. coli*. Enterotoxigenic *E. coli* comes from contaminated water and causes a subacute illness with a 24- to 72-h incubation period. This illness is associated with diffuse, mild abdominal pain; foul-smelling, profuse watery diarrhea; and occasional vomiting. The duration of the illness is less than a week.

Diagnosis is based on the clinical picture. **Treatment** primarily consists of fluid replacement. In severe cases, oral tetracycline 250 mg qid for 2 days may be given. When enterotoxigenic *E. coli* is the causative pathogen in **traveler's diarrhea,** rehydration should be provided immediately. Bismuth subsalicyate 30 to 60 mL (or 2 tablets) qid significantly reduces diarrhea. In severe cases associated with nausea, vomiting, abdominal cramps, fever, or bloody stool, antibiotics can be used to reduce the duration of the illness. Trimethoprim-sulfamethoxazole **(TMP-SMX)** 960 mg (TMP 160 mg, SMX 800 mg) should be administered bid for 3 to 5 days. Ciprofloxacin 500 mg bid for 5 days and norfloxacin 400 mg bid for 5 days are also effective.

Elderly patients, especially those in nursing homes, are more susceptible to ***E. coli* 0157:H7 infection,** which has high morbidity and mortality rates. The incubation period is about 8 days. The clinical picture is hemorrhagic colitis, which begins with watery diarrhea; hours to days later, the stool becomes grossly bloody. The diarrhea is accompanied by abdominal cramps and vomiting; fever is not a prominent feature. Risk factors include reduced gastric acidity, antacid and H_2-receptor antagonist use, and antibiotic therapy. The development of fever and leukocytosis may herald complications including hemolytic-uremic syndrome, thrombotic thrombocytopenic purpura, and death. Fatality rates in two nursing home outbreaks were 16% and 35%. (By contrast, the rate among younger persons is typically 5% to 10%.)

Diagnosis is established by stool culture for *E. coli* 0157:H7 in the first 4 days of the illness; stool filtrates should be tested for verotoxin activity. **Treatment** is supportive with IV fluid replacement.

INVASIVE DIARRHEA

The principal pathogens include *Shigella, Salmonella, Campylobacter,* and *Yersinia*. The latter two are seen predominantly in children and young adults. These four invasive pathogens involve the distal ileum and colon, producing mucosal ulceration.

SHIGELLOSIS

Shigellae are a group of gram-negative enteric organisms. Four major subgroups exist: group A-serotypes of *Shigella dysenteriae,* group B-serotypes of *Shigella flexneri,* group C-serotypes of *Shigella boydii,* and group D-serotypes of *Shigella sonnei*. The most common serotype is *S. sonnei*, which is responsible for 60% to 80% of *Shigella* dysentery in the USA.

Symptoms and Signs

The illness is characterized by lower abdominal pain, rectal burning, tenesmus, and diarrhea. In about 33% of patients, dysentery stool contains blood and mucus; in about 40%, fever occurs. Severe disease causes toxicity, and patients are highly febrile. The duration of symptoms is variable, but in the elderly, the average is 7 days.

Diagnosis and Treatment

Microscopic examination of fecal samples reveals multiple polymorphonuclear leukocytes and RBCs. Stool should be cultured, and antibiotic sensitivity testing should be performed. Sigmoidoscopy and biopsy are generally not performed.

Therapy consists of rehydration with oral and IV fluids for high-volume diarrhea and excessive vomiting. Opiate and atropine derivatives should be avoided because an inhibition of peristalsis prevents the removal of the pathogen and can exacerbate the gastroenteritis. Moderate to severe cases require ampicillin 500 mg orally qid or 1 gm IV q 6 h. In communities where isolates are known to be resistant to ampicillin, TMP-SMX at a dosage of 10 mg/kg/day TMP and 50 mg/kg/day SMX for 5 days should be prescribed. Alternatively, TMP-SMX 960 mg (TMP 160 mg, SMX 800 mg) orally or IV q 12 h for 5 days may be given.

SALMONELLOSIS

Salmonellae are gram-negative, non–spore-forming bacilli that belong to the family of Enterobacteriaceae. Three species exist: *Salmonella typhi, Salmonella choleraesuis,* and *Salmonella enteritidis. S. enteritidis typhimurium* is the serotype most commonly causing infection in humans. It invades mucosal cells and multiplies within them, eliciting a polymorphonuclear leukocyte response. Fluid accumulation within the intestinal lumen is related to the elaboration of heat-labile and heat-stable enterotoxins.

Gastroenteritis caused by *Salmonella* is found more frequently in patients > 60 yr, partially because of reduced gastric acidity. *Salmonella* bacteremia also occurs more often in the elderly than in young adults with *Salmonella* gastroenteritis and is potentially more harmful because it tends to colonize the endothelial surfaces of atherosclerotic aortic aneurysms. An outbreak in a long-term care facility may cause a local epidemic.

Symptoms and Signs

The initial clinical manifestations of *S. enteritidis typhimurium* in the elderly include nausea, vomiting, and a chill followed by colicky abdominal pain, diarrhea, and vomiting. The diarrhea ranges from a few loose stools to as many as 30 bowel movements daily. Characteristically, the stools are watery, green, and malodorous, with varying amounts of mucus. Some patients present with high fever and bloody, mucoid diarrhea, suggesting significant colonic involvement. The illness may last only a week or as long as 3 mo. The average course is 3 wk. The main complications are bleeding, toxic megacolon, and overwhelming sepsis.

Diagnosis and Treatment

Microscopic examination of methylene blue–stained specimens reveals moderate numbers of polymorphonuclear leukocytes. Stool should be cultured on selective or differential media.

Usually, antimicrobial therapy is not used for *Salmonella* gastroenteritis. However, elderly patients—especially those with underlying malignancies, lymphoproliferative disorders, cardiovascular diseases, aneurysms, and vascular grafts—should be given ampicillin 50 to 100 mg/kg/day in divided doses orally or parenterally for 10 to 14 days. Based on the incidence of relapse, such therapy may be continued for up to 21 days. Alternatively, TMP-SMX is given at a dosage of 10 mg/kg/day TMP and 50 mg/kg/day SMX to a maximum of 4 tablets/day (320 mg and 1600 mg) for 2 wk. Other alternatives include ciprofloxacin and several other third-generation cephalosporins.

58. MALABSORPTION SYNDROMES

A spectrum of symptoms and signs usually resulting from excessive fat excretion (steatorrhea); varying degrees of panmalabsorption of fat-soluble vitamins, water-soluble vitamins, electrolytes, and water; and maldigestion of carbohydrates and proteins.

The nutritional status of elderly persons is influenced by the effects of age on nutrient digestion and absorption. Aging does not significantly affect the structure and function of the exocrine pancreas, nor does it impair digestive capacity. Maldigestion and malabsorption occur only when more than 90% of pancreatic function is lost. Similarly, the small intestine has a large reserve capacity, and aging has only subtle influences on the digestive and absorptive processes.

The well-nourished elderly person has a reduced mucosal surface area with a slight reduction in villus height but normal enterocyte height, intraepithelial lymphocyte counts, and lamina propria cellularity. Jejunal brush border lactase and alkaline phosphatase levels decrease with age; other disaccharidase values are relatively stable, until after the seventh decade, when they decline. Fat absorption is normal, but absorption of fat-soluble vitamins A and K increases, while absorption of vitamin D decreases.

Measurement of breath hydrogen to determine carbohydrate absorption shows excess hydrogen excretion in one third of those over age 65. This abnormality may have several causes and is due in part to achlorhydria, abnormal bacterial flora, delayed gastric emptying, and slow intestinal transit; the key element is bacterial overgrowth. Vitamin B_{12} and folate absorption remain normal, while nonheme iron absorption decreases. Thus, absorption and digestion disorders in the elderly are not related to physiologic processes but to disease states.

Malabsorption falls into three pathophysiologic categories: **intraluminal maldigestion** secondary to pancreatic insufficiency, intraluminal bacterial overgrowth, and biliary tract disease; **mucosal lesions** resulting from celiac disease, Crohn's disease, and ileal resection > 100 cm; and **lymphatic dysfunction** such as retroperitoneal fibrosis, intestinal lymphangiectasia, and retroperitoneal malignancy. In the elderly, malabsorption has three main causes: celiac disease, bacterial overgrowth syndrome, and pancreatic insufficiency.

CELIAC DISEASE

(Celiac Sprue; Gluten-Induced Enteropathy; Idiopathic Steatorrhea; Nontropical Sprue; Sprue Syndrome)

A genetic disease involving malabsorption of many nutrients, resulting from characteristic, if not specific, pathologic changes in the small intestinal mucosa induced by ingestion of the gliadin fraction of gluten. Gliadin is a mixture of high-molecular-weight cereal proteins found in wheat, rye, oats, and barley. In most patients, prompt clinical, biochemical, and histologic improvement follows the withdrawal of gliadin-containing cereal from the diet.

Celiac disease occurs throughout the world, but its prevalence is unknown. The incidence, which varies considerably in different parts of the world, is highest in western Ireland (1:300). Recent research indicates that the affected population is older than previously recorded; many cases are diagnosed during or after the seventh decade. This age-related skew—seen in the USA, Sweden, Scotland, and Ireland—probably reflects clinicians' increased willingness to consider the diagnosis in the elderly.

Etiology and Pathogenesis

Celiac disease is closely associated with the human leukocyte antigens HLA-DQw2, HLA-DR3, and (to a lesser degree) HLA-B8.

Various mechanisms of etiology and pathogenesis have been proposed. One theory holds that the small intestinal absorptive cell lacks one or more enzymes that normally break down gliadin peptides, and the residual polypeptides injure the epithelial absorbing cells. Another theory suggests that susceptible patients absorb gliadin, which causes a humoral and a T-lymphocyte–dependent immune reaction, resulting in lysis and death of absorptive cells with a compensatory increase in crypt cell proliferation and a flat mucosal lesion. A third theory holds that gluten behaves like a lectin and binds to pathologically altered carbohydrate structures of the luminal small intestinal cells.

Also, an amino acid sequence homology has been shown between a protein of the human adenovirus and a major α-gliadin component. This finding suggests that the immune response to antigenic determinants produced during a previous intestinal viral infection may be important in the pathogenesis of celiac disease. However, studies in animals and humans have failed to support this hypothesis and suggest that persistence of the adenovirus is not a major element in the pathogenesis of celiac disease. Thus, this disease probably has many causes, with genetic, immunologic, biochemical, and perhaps environmental factors all playing a role.

Symptoms and Signs

The clinical manifestations of celiac disease in the elderly are subtle and variable. Most patients have steatorrhea, diarrhea, weight loss, and malnutrition, which may be mild. Certain nutritional deficiencies such as iron deficiency, osteomalacia with bone pain, or hypoprothrombinemia; or fatigue with mild hematologic abnormalities such as unexplained macrocytosis, low folate reserve, a peripheral smear showing Howell-Jolly bodies (splenic atrophy), target cells, or thrombocytopenia may obscure the underlying disorder and prevent early diagnosis.

Physical findings vary among patients. Some appear chronically emaciated with pale mucous membranes and dry, scaly skin; in a small number, the dry, scaly skin is hyperpigmented. Blood pressure is normal or low, and peripheral edema often occurs. The hair may be thin, and the fingers may be clubbed. Usually, glossitis and cheilosis are present. The striking finding is abdominal distention with hyperactive bowel sounds. Other findings include positive Trousseau's and Chvostek's signs (associated with hypocalcemia), ecchymoses and hematomas resulting from decreased vitamin K absorption, skeletal deformities secondary to osteoporosis and osteomalacia, loss of height, evidence of peripheral neuropathy, and subacute combined degeneration.

Laboratory Findings

With **fat malabsorption,** microscopic examination of a stool specimen stained with Sudan III reveals increased fat droplets. A 24-h stool specimen usually weighs more than the normal 200 gm. Chemical fat determination of a 3- to 6-day stool specimen obtained while the patient ingests a 100-gm fat diet shows fat excretion of 10 to 40 gm/24 h (normal is < 6 gm/24 h). A ^{14}C-labeled triolein breath test showing an increase in labeled breath carbon dioxide suggests fat malabsorption.

A **5-h urinary xylose excretion** after ingesting 25 gm D-xylose is 0.5 to 2.5 gm (normal is > 4.5 gm), and the blood level of xylose at 1 h is < 30 mg/dL (normal is > 30 mg/dL). Because of decreased renal function in the elderly, both urinary excretion and blood levels of xylose should be obtained. **Hematologic findings** include iron deficiency anemia with hypochromia and microcytosis on blood smear. Some patients have a megaloblastic anemia secondary to folic acid or vitamin B_{12} deficiency or both. Serum folate levels range from 0.7 to 3.5 ng/mL (normal is > 3.5 ng/mL).

In patients with severe ileal damage, the **Schilling test** reveals an excretion of < 8% of ^{57}Co-cyanocobalamin. This finding cannot be corrected by administering intrinsic factor or broad-spectrum antibiotics, thus differentiating celiac disease from pernicious anemia and blind-loop variants, respectively.

A useful screening test, serum carotene measurement invariably reveals levels < 50 μg/dL. Low levels of serum albumin, cholesterol, and vitamin A and a low prothrombin time (which can be corrected with IV vitamin K) may be found. In patients with osteomalacia, serum calcium is low, serum phosphorus is normal or low, and bone alkaline phosphatase is elevated. A bone biopsy revealing increased osteoid foci and widened osteoid seams confirms the diagnosis of osteomalacia. A generalized deficiency of intestinal disaccharidase activity occurs secondary to brush border damage. Lactase is most affected. A lactose-hydrogen breath test after lactose ingestion shows an increase in breath hydrogen > 20 ppm within 3 h.

Diagnosis

Diagnosis is based on characteristic histologic changes in a blind or endoscopic peroral jejunal mucosal biopsy. These changes include a loss of villus architecture, markedly elongated intestinal crypts, cuboidal luminal epithelial cells with a loss of nuclear polarity, cytoplasmic basophilia, and vacuolization. The brush border is markedly attenuated. There is an apparent increase in intraepithelial cells. In the lamina propria, increased cellularity consists of immunoglobulin-producing plasma cells (IgM), lymphocytes, and some eosinophils and polymorphonuclear leukocytes.

Characteristically, the abnormal mucosa is confined to the proximal small intestine, but in severe cases, it extends to the entire small intestine. The lesions are not specific for celiac disease, but most patients who have them and who live in the temperate zone have this disease and respond clinically, biochemically, and histologically to a gluten-free diet. Clinical or biochemical relapse or worsening of jejunal biopsy findings with a gluten or gliadin challenge confirms the diagnosis.

Measurement of circulating endomysial, reticulin, and gliadin antibodies is an important advance in the serologic diagnosis of celiac disease. The IgA-class endomysial and reticulin antibodies are both sensitive and specific markers; the IgA-class gliadin antibodies are specific but less sensitive markers. All these markers may help in monitoring patient compliance with a gluten-free diet.

Treatment

The treatment of choice is a well-balanced diet containing normal amounts of fat, protein, and carbohydrate but *no* foods containing

TABLE 58–1. ORAL CALCIUM SUPPLEMENTATION PRODUCTS

Preparation	*Tablet Size (mg)*	*Elemental Calcium/ Tablet (mg)*
Calcium carbonate (40% elemental calcium)		
Generic	650	260
Cal-Sup	750	300
Caltrate	1500	600
Os-Cal 500	1250	500
Tums	500	200
Titralac	420	168
Generic calcium gluconate (9% elemental calcium)	650	58.5
Generic calcium lactate (13% elemental calcium)	650	84.5
Generic dibasic calcium phosphate (23% elemental calcium)	500	115

Modified from Bauwens SF: "Osteomalacia and osteoporosis," in *Pharmacotherapy: A Pathophysiologic Approach*, ed. 2, edited by JT DiPiro, RL Talbert, PE Hayes, et al. Norwalk, Conn., Appleton & Lange, 1993, p 1305; used with permission.

wheat, rye, barley, or oats. Lactose-free milk is recommended for patients with lactase deficiency. Symptoms and signs usually show improvement within days or weeks but may take months.

Most patients who do not respond either are not adhering to the diet or have another disease such as giardiasis, lymphoma, Whipple's disease, or collagenous sprue. (A rare disease, **collagenous sprue** is characterized by a severe lesion similar to the celiac disease lesion but with broad bands of fibrosis and collagen beneath the basement membrane. The prognosis is generally poor.)

A few patients respond initially to gluten withdrawal but then relapse despite strict adherence to the diet. Some of these refractory or unclassified celiac disease patients may respond to treatment with high doses of corticosteroids (such as prednisone 60 mg/day for about 1 mo) or other immunosuppressive drugs, such as azathioprine or cyclophosphamide. Others, despite such therapy, have a relentless course usually culminating in death.

Supplemental therapy: Patients with iron deficiency anemia should receive supplemental ferrous sulfate 325 mg tid, while those with folic acid deficiency should receive folic acid 5 mg/day for 1 mo, followed by a maintenance dosage of 1 mg/day. Patients with vitamin B_{12} deficiency should receive 100 μg vitamin B_{12} IM daily for 2 wk, then 100 μg monthly. About 1200 mg/day of elemental calcium corrects calcium deficiency (see TABLE 58–1); 1 to 4 gm/day of magnesium gluconate corrects magnesium deficiency.

Patients with radiologic evidence of osteopenic bone disease require 1 to 3 gm/day of elemental calcium plus 50,000 u./day of vitamin D. Vitamin K 10 mg IV should be given *slowly* (ie, 1 mg/min) to correct prolonged prothrombin time. Severe reactions, including fatalities, have occurred during or immediately after IV injection. Thus, IV vitamin K should be given only to quickly correct prothrombin time; then oral vitamin K (phytonadione 10 mg once a day) should be given. Therapeutic formula multivitamin preparations containing vitamin A, thiamine, riboflavin, niacin, pyridoxine, vitamin C, and vitamin E should be administered to patients with prolonged, severe malabsorption.

BACTERIAL OVERGROWTH SYNDROME

Intraluminal small intestinal bacterial overgrowth accompanied by nutrient malabsorption secondary to carbohydrate catabolism by gram-negative aerobes, bile acid deconjugation by anaerobes, cobalamin binding by anaerobes, and patchy damage to small intestinal epithelial cells.

Etiology

In healthy adults, the proximal lumen of the small intestine contains 0 to 10^4 microorganisms per milliliter, consisting of aerobes and facultative anaerobes, which are largely oral flora. This relative sterility is maintained by normal gastric acid secretion, normal peristalsis of the proximal small intestine, and luminal immunoglobulins. In persons age 70 and older, however, hypochlorhydria or achlorhydria commonly allow bacterial overgrowth.

Several conditions can lead to stagnation of the small intestine, including a large duodenal diverticulum, multiple jejunal diverticula, stricture, fistulas, radiation enteritis, afferent loop of Billroth II partial gastrectomy, surgical blind loop, and resection of the ileocecal valve. Motor abnormalities secondary to scleroderma, idiopathic intestinal pseudo-obstruction, and diabetic autonomic neuropathy also can lead to bacterial overgrowth in the small intestine.

About 20% of patients over age 65 who undergo an upper GI series have a duodenal diverticulum. A similar percentage is found in postmortem studies using plaster casts of the duodenum. By contrast, jejunal diverticulosis is uncommon, with an autopsy prevalence of 0.5%. Although patients with this disease are usually asymptomatic, they may have many large jejunal diverticula, leading to bacterial overgrowth and malabsorption of fat and vitamin B_{12}. Severe malabsorption has been described in patients with duodenal and jejunal diverticulosis who also have chronic pancreatic insufficiency; these patients did not respond to broad-spectrum antibiotics alone but did respond when pancreatic enzymes were added.

Symptoms and Signs

Patients may be asymptomatic or may present with watery diarrhea secondary to deconjugated bile acids, hydroxy fatty acids, and organic acids; clinically significant steatorrhea resulting in weight loss; bone pain and pathologic fractures; easy bruising from vitamin K deficiency; night blindness from vitamin A deficiency; hypocalcemic tetany; and weakness and easy fatigability from cobalamin deficiency. Some patients may present with a dimorphic anemia, both macrocytic and microcytic, the latter resulting from microulcerations of the stagnant loop that produce occult blood loss and guaiac-positive stools. Patients with strictures and small intestinal pseudo-obstruction have symptoms of abdominal distention (nausea and crampy periumbilical pain) before the onset of diarrhea, steatorrhea, and anemia.

Diagnosis

An increase in stool weight and evidence of excessive fat (on Sudan III stain, 72-h stool fat, or ^{14}C-labeled triolein breath test) should be documented. An upper GI series with small intestine follow-through identifies duodenal diverticulum, jejunal diverticula, stricture, gastrojejunocolic fistulas, afferent loop syndrome, intestinal pseudo-obstruction, scleroderma, and Crohn's disease. A small intestine biopsy excludes celiac disease, Whipple's disease, eosinophilic gastroenteritis, and giardiasis. Reduced excretion of labeled cobalamin that is not corrected by intrinsic factor but is corrected by broad-spectrum antibiotics confirms vitamin B_{12} deficiency secondary to bacterial overgrowth.

The 1-gm ^{14}C-labeled xylose breath test is the test of choice for detecting bacterial overgrowth; it reveals elevated $^{14}CO_2$ levels within the first 60 min. Although culture of the small intestine's contents has excellent specificity, it is cumbersome. The ^{14}C-labeled cholylglycine breath test is easy to perform but lacks specificity.

Treatment

The recommended treatment is a 10-day course of cephalexin 250 mg qid and metronidazole 250 mg tid orally. Many patients respond to treatment in 7 to 10 days, a few require repeat therapy, and rarely a patient needs continuous therapy for months. Chloramphenicol 50 mg/kg/day orally in four divided doses for 7 to 14 days is recommended for patients who do not respond to cephalexin and metronidazole. Cobalamin deficiency in malabsorption responds to monthly IM injections of 100 μg vitamin B_{12}. Deficiencies of calcium, vitamin D, and vitamin K should be corrected as in celiac disease (see above).

CHRONIC PANCREATITIS WITH PANCREATIC INSUFFICIENCY

Recurrent or chronic pancreatic inflammation resulting in recurrent or persistent abdominal pain secondary to anatomic damage (calcification, ductal changes, fibrosis) or functional damage (exocrine or endocrine insufficiency) to the pancreas. Pancreatic exocrine or endocrine insufficiency develops without pain in some patients, especially elderly patients, many of whom have associated pancreatic calcification.

Etiology

In the elderly, the most common forms of chronic pancreatitis with pancreatic insufficiency result from heavy alcohol intake for more than 15 yr, trauma, vascular disease, abdominal radiation therapy, and pancreatic carcinoma. Rarely, primary pancreatic atrophy and pancreatic lipomatosis cause steatorrhea and diabetes mellitus. However, a few of these patients are alcoholics without abdominal pain, thus raising the question whether this is a true entity.

Symptoms and Signs

In 90% of younger patients with chronic pancreatitis, the predominant symptom is recurrent, severe abdominal pain. In elderly patients, the pain is mild or absent—except in those with pancreatic carcinoma and secondary pancreatic insufficiency. Characteristically, the elderly have an abrupt onset of frequent bowel movements producing bulky, malodorous, greasy stools that are difficult to flush. Rectal seepage of oil and oil in the toilet bowl may be the presenting complaints. A weight loss of 6 to 20 kg occurs secondary to malabsorption and poor oral intake. Polyuria and polydipsia may precede the abnormal bowel movements. Less common clinical manifestations include arthritis, subcutaneous fat necrosis, and intramedullary fat necrosis with associated bone pain.

Diagnosis

Diffuse, stippled pancreatic calcification on a flat plate film of the abdomen is diagnostic. Ultrasonography and CT scan should be performed on patients with abdominal pain to rule out pancreatic pseudocyst and pancreatic carcinoma. Pancreatic insufficiency is documented by a **bentiromide urinary excretion test** in which the cumulative 6-h excretion of aminobenzoic acid (PABA) is < 50% of the ingested synthetic peptide bentiromide. The serum trypsin-like immunoreactivity test reveals a value < 20 ng/mL (normal is 20 to 80 ng/mL), which is characteristic of pancreatic insufficiency. However, this test is less sensitive than the bentiromide test.

Endoscopic retrograde cholangiopancreatography shows an irregularly strictured, dilated main pancreatic duct with a beaded appearance that is almost diagnostic of chronic pancreatitis. Steatorrhea can be documented by the Sudan III stain for qualitative fat or by a quantitative stool fat or ^{14}C-labeled triolein breath test.

Treatment

Alcohol ingestion should be eliminated. Patients with pain should be given nonaddictive analgesics—salicylates, acetaminophen, and nonsteroidal anti-inflammatory drugs. Large doses of potent pancreatic enzyme preparations high in lipase and proteolytic enzymes are required: 6 to 8 tablets (Ilozyme, Viokase), 6 to 8 capsules (Ku-Zyme HP, Cotazym), or 3 microencapsulated capsules (Pancrease) with each meal. Because gastric acid inactivates lipase, the non-microencapsulated forms of pancreatic enzymes (eg, Viokase, Cotazym) may be given with H_2-receptor antagonists. However, enteric-coated preparations (eg, Pancrease, Creon) are used more commonly because of fewer GI side effects, lower cost, and greater convenience. The prognosis is generally good except in patients with pancreatic carcinoma and in those incapable of discontinuing alcohol consumption.

59. THE AGING LIVER

In clinical medicine, attempting to separate the effects of aging from those of disease is a recurring challenge. The elderly who have no significant disease but whose biologic age appears greater than their chronologic age (as determined largely by functional assessment) are described as "frail." Understanding the role of such frailty in liver aging is just beginning. Most research on changes in the aging liver has been done in rodents and may not necessarily be extrapolated to humans.

There are no peculiar or characteristic diseases of the aged liver. Furthermore, the liver ages gracefully, without producing changes in the results of so-called liver function tests. In this context, the effects of aging on liver appearance, histologic characteristics, physiology, drug metabolism, and response to stress require more detailed comment.

Appearance

Autopsy studies and peritoneoscopy show that the liver becomes **brown** and **more fibrotic** with age. The increased capsular and parenchymal fibrosis should not be confused with cirrhosis. With age, hepatic weight declines; autopsy studies show a decrease of about 25% between ages 20 and 70 in men and women. In vivo ultrasound studies also show that liver volume is 17% to 28% lower in those over age 65 than in those under age 40.

Histologic Characteristics

Studies of age-related changes in hepatic fine structure have reported disparate results. Historically, it has been believed that human hepatocytes enlarge with age; however, some studies report no change in size. Several studies on rodents report that hepatocytes enlarge with age, whereas others report that they enlarge with maturation but diminish with senescence.

Some studies report polyploidy and increases in nuclear size and binuclear liver cells with aging, although other studies report no significant changes. The structural changes found in hepatocyte mitochondria have been as disparate as an increased number of swollen, vacuolated mitochondria and a decreased number of mitochondria per liver volume. Unlike other components of hepatocytes, lysosomes and dense bodies increase consistently with age.

The brown pigment buildup with aging represents a lifetime accumulation of unexcretable metabolic residue and generally has no physiologic significance. An increased number of lipofuscin granules in hepatocytes accounts for much of this pigment. Lipofuscin is a brown pigment resulting from the accumulation of end-stage metabolic products of lipids and proteins; thus, it is a wear and tear pigment.

Hepatic changes caused by malnutrition and those caused by aging are similar in some ways. Both are associated with a brown, atrophic-appearing liver. However, in malnutrition the number of hepatocytes is normal, but they are smaller; in aging there are fewer hepatocytes, but they are usually larger.

Physiology

Decreased hepatic weight is accompanied by **diminished hepatic blood flow** (resulting from decreased splanchnic blood flow). In dye elimination tests using indocyanine green, the apparent hepatic blood flow declined by 35% in persons over age 65 compared with those under age 40. The diminished liver mass and blood flow may account for some changes in drug elimination in aging patients.

Protein synthesis and degradation appear to decrease with age. Several methods have been used to study hepatic protein synthesis, including cell-free systems, in vivo studies, hepatocyte suspensions, and liver perfusion systems. Although the results of the studies do not completely agree, most evidence points to **decreased protein synthesis** with age. However, the degree of decrease appears to vary widely among various proteins. No sex-related differences are apparent in studies involving male and female rodents.

Degradation of several proteins, including some enzymes, has been studied by following radiolabeled amino acids, using several techniques. The results suggest a **decreased rate of degradation** with age. The accumulation of abnormal proteins with aging may reflect a decreased ability of cells to degrade these proteins. In the only study on abnormal liver proteins as a function of age, a significant increase in their half-life was observed in mice. The extent to which these abnormal proteins are functional or represent inadequately broken down, deteriorated "junk" proteins is unclear.

As the liver ages, regeneration is delayed but not greatly impaired. In older rats mitotic activity is decreased more than in younger rats after partial hepatectomy. Although mitotic activity decreases, the hepatocytes that do divide appear to undergo more cell cycles, and thus regeneration catches up.

Aging does not alter results of the so-called liver function tests, which measure hepatic damage, eg, hepatocellular injury (aminotransferases), selected protein synthesis (alkaline phosphatase), or transport of hepatocytes (bilirubin), rather than overall function. Thus, abnormal values for these tests in the elderly reflect disease, not the effects of aging.

Drug Distribution and Metabolism

Because the elderly take more prescription medications than any other age group, they are more likely to have adverse drug reactions. Therefore, much effort has been directed toward understanding the changes in drug metabolism that occur with aging. Many factors may influence drug disposition in the elderly, including changes in body composition (decreased lean body mass and increased fat), a general decrease in serum albumin concentration, decreased renal function, and environmental influences including dietary changes (see Ch. 21).

With the age-related increase in body fat, the distribution of lipid-soluble drugs increases. If plasma clearance remains unchanged, the half-life of the drug is prolonged, and the potential for toxic concentrations increases unless the dosing interval is modified appropriately.

With drugs that have a high rate of **hepatic extraction,** a significant change in bioavailability can occur with aging. Such drugs usually undergo significant metabolism before reaching the systemic circulation. Although absorption across the gut does not change significantly with aging, first-pass metabolism may decrease, most likely from reduced intrinsic clearance, and lead to increased bioavailability. Oral doses of nifedipine, propranolol, morphine, and labetalol, for example, achieve significantly higher plasma concentrations in the elderly.

The two major drug-binding proteins in serum are human serum albumin and α_1-acid glycoprotein. With increasing age, serum albumin tends to decrease, whereas α_1-acid glycoprotein tends to remain the same. Thus, in older patients there is less albumin-bound drug and more free drug. Because therapeutic effect is usually related to the amount of free drug, decreased serum albumin can result in increased levels of active drug. The clinical significance of this depends on the size of the increased free fraction, pharmacokinetics, and the drug's therapeutic index. Although large increases in the free fraction have been reported after acute administration of a few drugs (including naproxen, salicylate, and valproic acid) in the elderly, once steady state is achieved (chronic administration), increased total body clearance minimizes the clinical impact.

With aging, hepatic clearance changes for many drugs. Factors that may influence hepatic drug clearance in the elderly include decreased hepatic blood flow, altered oxidative microsomal enzyme activity, and decreased functional hepatic mass. Elimination of high-clearance drugs is influenced primarily by decreased hepatic blood flow. Elimination of low-clearance drugs is affected primarily by hepatic metabolism (intrinsic clearance), which in turn depends on hepatic enzymes and total liver mass.

Located in the smooth endoplasmic reticulum of hepatocytes, the **microsomal enzymes** are responsible for much of the biotransformation of drugs. Enzymatic actions are classified as phase 1 and phase 2 reactions. Phase 1 reactions involve oxidation, reduction, or hydrolysis; they convert the parent drug into more polar metabolites. Phase 2 reactions involve conjugation of the parent drug or metabolite with an additional substrate (for example, glucuronic acid, sulfate), achieving the same result. In humans, unlike in rodents, phase 1 reactions decrease very rarely with age, and phase 2 reactions remain essentially unchanged.

The precise cause of any altered microsomal oxidative enzyme activity is unknown. Most studies suggest that phase 1 enzyme activity per gram of liver is actually preserved and that decreased phase 1 activity results primarily from an age-related decline in liver mass. However, why phase 2 reactions are relatively preserved despite the decline in liver mass is unclear. Could it be because of compensatory extrahepatic conjugation? The body of knowledge on hepatic drug metabolism makes clear that age-related changes are quite variable, with significant differences among species, drugs, and individuals.

Response to Stress

The liver's ability to withstand stress may decrease with age. It has been suggested that the aged liver is less responsive to induction with some agents and therefore is less adaptable. Drugs and toxins such as benoxaprofen and allyl alcohol cause more severe injury in the older liver. However, if transplantation is considered a significant stress to the donor organ, the older liver may be more resilient than expected.

As more **liver transplants** have been performed, it has become apparent that livers > 50 yr are suitable donor organs. A review of all cadaveric donor transplants at centers participating in the United Network of Organ Sharing (UNOS) from October 1987 to December 1989 shows that 1-yr survival rates of recipients of donor organs 16 to 45 yr and recipients of donor organs > 45 yr differ by only 10.8%. Furthermore, a higher percentage of older donor livers were transplanted into sicker, higher-risk patients, helping to explain the difference in 1-yr survival. More recent data on donor livers > 55 yr show lower graft survival rates at 4 mo and 1 yr, but the differences are not statistically significant. The differences are even less marked for patient survival rates. Thus, transplantation provides further evidence that, unlike other vital organs, the liver is relatively resistant to senescent change.

60. GASTROINTESTINAL NEOPLASMS

Cancer is second only to heart disease as the leading cause of death in the elderly, and GI tract cancer accounts for > 25% of all cancer deaths. The causes of GI tract cancer remain elusive, and worldwide variations in incidence of cancer at specific sites are enormous. In the elderly, environmental factors (eg, dietary content of animal fat, fiber, minerals, and carcinogens) probably play a much greater role than hereditary factors.

The more common primary neoplasms of the GI tract among the elderly are discussed below.

NEOPLASMS OF THE ESOPHAGUS

Fewer than 10% of esophageal neoplasms are benign. Esophageal cancer accounts for only 4% of all GI cancers in the USA but is more common in China, Iran, Ceylon, and Russia.

BENIGN NEOPLASMS

Leiomyoma is the most common tumor. Rare lesions include inflammatory polyps, squamous papilloma, lymphangioma, granular cell tumor, fibromyxoma, fibrolipoma, and lipoma. Usually asymptomatic, these tumors are often found incidentally on examination for unrelated complaints or at autopsy. Symptomatic tumors may produce dysphagia or upper GI bleeding. Diagnosis often is established by barium swallow followed by esophagoscopy and biopsy. Endoscopic ultrasonography may help evaluate these tumors. If the tumor produces bleeding or obstruction, surgical resection usually is indicated.

MALIGNANT NEOPLASMS

A number of carcinogenic factors and disease states have been associated with esophageal cancer, including chronic thermal injury (eg, from drinking very hot tea); poor oral hygiene; esophageal stasis associated with achalasia; intake of exogenous toxins (eg, alcohol, tobacco, silica, nitrates, nitrosamines, and zinc); a history of ionizing radiation; lye stricture; severe reflux esophagitis and associated Barrett's epithelium; and the Plummer-Vinson syndrome associated with esophageal webs.

Esophageal cancer occurs predominantly in men between ages 50 and 70 and is more common in smokers and blacks. It usually involves the middle and lower thirds of the esophagus. The tumor may be infiltrative, ulcerative, or polypoid and may cause a stricture or mass.

While squamous cell carcinoma predominates in the upper and middle esophagus, adenocarcinoma is more common in the distal esophagus. In the past decade, adenocarcinoma at the cardioesophageal junction has been increasing in spite of a level incidence of proximal esophageal cancer and a continued decline of distal gastric adenocarcinoma. The reasons for this trend are not known.

Symptoms and Signs

The most common symptoms are progressive dysphagia and weight loss. Others include pain on swallowing, hoarseness, recurrent respiratory infections, and hematemesis. Signs appear late in the course of disease and include regional lymphadenopathy, vocal cord paralysis, and pulmonary findings (eg, wheezes or rales).

Diagnosis

Initially, the diagnosis is often made by barium swallow followed by endoscopy. The upper GI series often shows a stricture or an eccentric or asymmetric mucosal irregularity. Endoscopy provides direct visualization of the lesion and tissue for microscopic examination. The combination of biopsy and brush cytology yields the diagnosis in > 95% of cases. In high-risk areas, such as Northern China, mass screening using balloon cytologic techniques that reveal early lesions seems to improve the prognosis. In selected cases, endoscopic ultrasonography, CT, and laparoscopy are useful for tumor staging.

Treatment

Surgical resection is usually the primary treatment, although lesions in the upper third of the esophagus may be inoperable. In high-risk surgical patients, some mid-esophageal cancers can be treated with radiation. Combined radiotherapy and chemotherapy have yielded poor results. This approach is reserved for patients with metastatic disease and for high-risk surgical patients, especially those with squamous cell carcinoma. Combinations of surgery, radiotherapy, and chemotherapy are under continued investigation.

Palliative measures for recurrent luminal obstruction or inoperable cancer (eg, dilatation, laser fulguration of tumor and placement of an esophageal prosthesis) may be performed endoscopically. In advanced cases, nutritional support may be accomplished by percutaneous endoscopic gastrostomy or jejunostomy tube feedings.

The prognosis is dismal. The overall 5-yr survival rate is 5%, although selected series show nearly a 25% survival rate in those with cancer of the lower esophagus. About 50% of US patients who have curative surgery are ≥ 65 yr. Surgical treatment is discussed in Ch. 62.

NEOPLASMS OF THE STOMACH

Fewer than 5% of all gastric tumors are benign. The incidence of gastric cancer increases with age.

BENIGN NEOPLASMS

Although **leiomyoma** is the most common benign gastric tumor in the general population, hyperplastic and adenomatous polyps are also common among the elderly. Other benign neoplasms include carcinoids, fibromas, lipomas, and neural tumors.

Hyperplastic polyps are small (usually < 1 cm in diameter), flat lesions that account for about 95% of all gastric epithelial polyps. The remaining 5% are predominantly **adenomatous polyps,** which can attain a diameter > 4 cm. Hyperplastic polyps carry no malignant potential, whereas adenomatous polyps do, usually when they are > 2 cm in diameter.

Gastric polyps most often develop in association with chronic atrophic gastritis and intestinal metaplasia of the gastric mucosa, as in pernicious anemia. The **Cronkhite-Canada syndrome,** the only GI polyposis syndrome found in the elderly, includes ectodermal changes (eg, increased pigmentation, alopecia, and atrophic nails). The polyps consist of dilated, cystic glands and markedly edematous stroma. This nonhereditary syndrome occurs equally in men and women. The lesions are not premalignant, but progressive diarrhea commonly leads to cachexia and death in women, while men tend to have spontaneous remissions.

Symptoms, Signs, and Diagnosis

Most benign gastric tumors are asymptomatic and are found during barium studies or endoscopy performed for other conditions. The most common presenting finding is anemia from chronic occult bleeding. Less commonly, epigastric pain or acute GI bleeding from ulceration of the tumor occurs. If the cardia is involved, dysphagia may occur. If the prepyloric antrum is involved, gastric outlet obstruction may occur.

An upper GI series using the double-contrast technique can provide clear x-ray definition of small gastric mucosal lesions. Endoscopy provides direct visualization and tissue specimens for biopsy and cytology; with endoscopy, diagnosis can be made in 90% of patients.

Treatment

Treatment usually consists of endoscopic excision or fulguration. If the lesion is submucosal or if its size or location prohibits endoscopic resection, surgery may be warranted if significant blood loss or other symptoms have developed.

MALIGNANT NEOPLASMS

In the USA, about 24,000 new cases and 13,000 deaths from gastric cancer occur annually, and the incidence increases with age. The mean age at the time of diagnosis is 55 yr. Gastric cancer is more common in blacks and among poor socioeconomic groups; the male:female ratio is 2:1.

Adenocarcinoma accounts for 95% of all gastric malignancies. The worldwide incidence varies dramatically with low rates in the USA and high rates in Japan, Chile, and Costa Rica. Although an unexplained worldwide reduction has occurred over the past 50 yr (except in black men), the incidence around the gastroesophageal junction has increased. The cause of this increase is not clear, but the increase may result in part from an increase in Barrett's epithelium in the esophagus.

Lymphoma accounts for about 4% of gastric malignancies. The stomach is the most common site of primary extranodal lymphoma, accounting for up to 75% of all cases of primary GI tract lymphomas. Most are histiocytic. Gastric lymphoma occurs mainly in men in the sixth decade.

Other malignancies, including leiomyosarcoma, carcinoid tumor, and Kaposi's sarcoma, account for < 1% of all gastric malignancies.

Gastric abnormalities with malignant potential include adenoma, mucosal atrophy with intestinal metaplasia (with or without associated pernicious anemia), and hypertrophic gastropathy. *Helicobacter pylori* infection may also be a risk factor for gastric adenocarcinoma and lymphoma. Gastroduodenal peptic ulcer disease has no etiologic association with gastric cancer, although a gastric ulcer that appears benign on endoscopy can have a microscopic malignant focus.

Pathology

Gastric cancer is generally classified as early or advanced, according to its gross appearance. **Early gastric cancer** is confined to the mucosa or submucosa and is divided into three types: (1) protruded, either polypoid or fungating; (2) superficial, either elevated, flat, or depressed; and (3) excavated. **Advanced gastric cancer** is defined as disease penetrating the muscularis propria with lymph node involvement; the prognosis is poor. It is divided into three types: (1) a mass lesion, either polypoid or fungating; (2) diffuse or infiltrating; and (3) ulcerated. Advanced gastric cancer may have more than one of these characteristics. If the tumor infiltration is diffuse and associated with a fibrous reaction, **linitis plastica** (leather-bottle stomach) may occur.

Gastric cancer develops predominantly in the distal portion of the stomach and is rarely multicentric. Cancer spreads by direct extension or metastasis via the lymphatics or the bloodstream.

Symptoms and Signs

In the early stages, symptoms may be insidious and dismissed as indigestion. The most common presenting symptom is vague epigastric discomfort followed by anorexia, early satiety, weight loss, hematemesis, melena, and severe abdominal pain as the tumor progresses. If the cardia is involved, dysphagia may occur. If the prepyloric antrum is involved, symptoms of partial or complete gastric outlet obstruction (eg, epigastric fullness, nausea, and vomiting) may occur.

In the early stages, there are no specific signs of gastric cancer. In the later stages, weight loss, a palpable mass, and lymphadenopathy in the left supraclavicular region **(Virchow's node)** may be noted. Liver metastases can present as hepatomegaly. Dermatologic signs of gastric cancer include acanthosis nigricans and dermatomyositis.

Diagnosis

An **upper GI tract barium study** is usually the initial test, but lesions are frequently missed. The double-contrast technique can improve detection, so that a mass, an infiltrating ulcer, or only thickened rugae can be seen.

Upper GI endoscopy allows visualization of most lesions, provides a means of obtaining tissue for biopsy and cytologic examination, and yields the diagnosis in > 90% of cases. Endoscopic ultrasonography may provide information regarding the depth of invasion. When older patients can tolerate only one test, endoscopy is generally preferred to x-ray studies.

Other laboratory procedures provide little help. Elevated levels of carcinoembryonic antigen (CEA) and fetal sulfoglycoprotein and decreased levels of pepsinogen have been noted in about 15% of patients with gastric cancer, but because of poor sensitivity and specificity, these measures have no clinical role. An abdominal CT scan helps evaluate the extent of disease.

The differential diagnosis includes peptic ulcer and pancreaticobiliary tract disease. Patients who have undergone partial gastrectomy or gastroenterostomy for peptic ulcer disease more often have gastric polyps, epithelial dysplasia, and carcinoma in the remaining gastric pouch beginning 10 to 15 yr after surgery. The only real chance of curing gastric cancer is early diagnosis and surgical excision.

The patient with gastric lymphoma presents with symptoms similar to those of gastric carcinoma. The radiographic appearance may also be similar, although large gastric folds and evidence of infiltration into the duodenum are more typical of lymphoma than of carcinoma. Endoscopy may confirm the diagnosis if multiple directed biopsies combined with brush cytology yield positive results. Because the lesions are submucosal, this approach may be unsuccessful, and laparotomy may be needed.

Treatment

Surgery is widely accepted as the initial therapy for early gastric cancer. **Radiation therapy** alone is ineffective for adenocarcinoma. Radiation therapy after resection is commonly used with good results in patients with gastric lymphoma. **Chemotherapy** for metastatic adenocarcinoma has a poor response rate. Chemotherapy for gastric lymphoma is much more effective, although it must be used cautiously because free perforation can occur during tumor lysis.

Palliation of gastric carcinoma causing distal esophageal or gastric outlet obstruction has been achieved in selected cases using **endoscopic laser photoablation.**

The overall 5-yr survival rate for patients with adenocarcinoma is < 10%. With early gastric cancer, 5-yr survival rates of up to 95% have been reported. With primary gastric lymphoma, the 5-yr survival rate approaches 50%. However, the prognosis is adversely affected by age; the 5-yr survival rate for patients < 45 yr with gastric lymphoma is 57%; for those > 65 yr, it is 32%.

NEOPLASMS OF THE SMALL INTESTINE

Benign neoplasms of the small intestine are rare, accounting for < 5% of all GI tumors. Fewer than 3% of all GI tract cancers originate in the small intestine.

BENIGN NEOPLASMS

Usually these benign neoplasms occur in the fifth, sixth, and seventh decades of life. About 80% of them occur in the jejunum and ileum. Adenomatous polyps are the most common benign neoplasms, followed by leiomyoma, lipoma, and hemangioma. In the small intestine, as in the rest of the GI tract, adenomatous polyps are premalignant. Villous adenomas, which occur in the duodenum, usually in association with familial polyposis, may undergo malignant change.

Most often, benign lesions are asymptomatic and are found during investigation for unrelated symptoms or at autopsy. However, patients may present with recurrent abdominal pain, GI hemorrhage, abdominal mass, or intestinal obstruction—often because of intussusception. Diagnosis can be made by small-bowel x-ray. When the duodenum or terminal ileum is involved, small-bowel endoscopy may provide visualization and tissue for diagnosis. A new, longer enteroscope can be used to examine the entire small intestine. Arteriography provides visualization of vascular tumors.

Surgical resection is usually the treatment of choice.

MALIGNANT NEOPLASMS

Cancers originating in the small intestine usually occur in the sixth and seventh decades. The most common malignancy is carcinoid tumor followed by adenocarcinoma, lymphoma, and leiomyosarcoma.

The small intestine ranks second only to the appendix as the most common site of **carcinoid tumors.** Only 25% to 30% of these carcinoid tumors are symptomatic. **Adenocarcinoma** produces symptoms more often than other small-intestine tumors. Adenocarcinoma is generally found in the proximal small intestine, predominantly in the duodenum. Predisposing factors include gluten enteropathy, Crohn's disease, and the GI polyposis syndromes, such as Gardner's syndrome. Tumors are usually annular and constricting. **Lymphoma** occurs predominantly in the ileum and is usually of B-cell origin; lymphoma of T-cell origin is associated with adult celiac disease. **Leiomyosarcoma** is as common as lymphoma.

Symptoms, Signs, and Diagnosis

Although most small-intestine malignancies are asymptomatic, 60% to 75% of symptomatic small-intestine tumors are malignant. Patients with advanced disease present with abdominal pain resulting from intestinal obstruction, recurrent intussusception, mesenteric thrombosis, perforation, GI hemorrhage, or a palpable abdominal mass. The **carcinoid syndrome,** characterized by diarrhea and flushing, occurs usually when hepatic metastases develop. Lymphoma, especially Hodgkin's disease, may present as **malabsorption syndrome** with weight loss, diarrhea, malaise, weakness, and edema.

Preoperative diagnosis is generally made by small-intestine x-ray and CT scan. Endoscopy may provide visualization and tissue for diagnosis, and arteriography may show vascular malignancies. With advanced carcinoid tumors, urinary 5-hydroxyindoleacetic acid (5-HIAA) levels may be elevated.

Treatment

The usual treatment is surgical resection. Radiation therapy and chemotherapy are potentially effective only for lymphoma. The 5-yr survival rate for patients with adenocarcinoma is 30%; for those with lymphoma and leiomyosarcoma, it approaches 50%. The prognosis for patients with carcinoid tumors can be good with survival commonly exceeding 10 yr. Octreotide is often effective in treating severe flushing and diarrhea in patients with the carcinoid syndrome.

NEOPLASMS OF THE COLON

Benign colonic tumors have a high prevalence in the USA and Western Europe. Colorectal cancer is the second most common malignancy in the USA and Western Europe.

BENIGN NEOPLASMS

Incidence figures vary from 7% to 75% of the population > 50 yr, increasing with age and peaking in the seventh decade. Most benign tumors are polyps (a clinical term without pathologic significance that refers to any mass of tissue arising from a mucosal surface and protruding into the lumen). The relationship of colonic polyps to age, diet, geographic distribution, family history, and prior neoplasms is similar to that of adenocarcinoma of the colon, which is discussed below. Hamartomas, juvenile polyps, and congenital lesions usually do not occur in the elderly.

Adenomatous polyps, the most common colorectal neoplasms, are found in 50% to 60% of persons > 60 yr at autopsy. Although they may involve the entire colon, they are more concentrated in the distal region. Lesions may be sessile or pedunculated. Synchronous lesions (more than one at the same time) occur in about 50% of cases and are classified histologically as tubular, tubulovillous, or villous adenomas, depending on the proportion of villous elements. These polyps are true neoplasms with malignant potential, which varies with the size, proportion of villous elements, and degree of dysplasia. The overall risk for malignant change within an adenomatous polyp is about 1% to 2%.

Hyperplastic polyps are common benign tumors of the colon. They are small, dome-shaped, sessile lesions. Often a person has several of these lesions. These polyps have no inherent malignant potential.

Inflammatory polyps usually occur in persons with no associated disease; however, those with inflammatory bowel disorders, ischemic colitis, specific infections (eg, amebiasis and tuberculosis), toxic reactions to mineral oil and barium, and colitis cystica profunda are especially prone to such polyps.

Lipomas, the second most common benign tumors of the colon, usually occur at or near the ileocecal valve. Incidence peaks in the seventh to eighth decades. Colonic **hemangiomas** are predominantly found with advancing age. Frequently, many lesions appear. They may be classified as capillary, cavernous, or mixed and are a common cause of hemorrhage and a rare cause of intussusception. The incidence of **leiomyomas** seems to peak in the sixth decade and decline sharply thereafter.

Cronkhite-Canada syndrome is the only multiple polyposis syndrome affecting the elderly. The average age at diagnosis is 60, and the lesions resemble juvenile polyps. The syndrome occurs in both men and women, but it runs a relentless course in women with death occurring in 6 to 18 mo, whereas men tend to have spontaneous remissions.

Symptoms and Signs

Most polyps are asymptomatic and are found incidentally during evaluation for another disorder. The usual symptom is **rectal bleeding,** which most commonly is occult and rarely is massive; however, massive bleeding is more common with hemangiomas. Rarely, large villous adenomas cause a severe mucoid rectal discharge and diarrhea, which may result in hypokalemia and hyponatremia. Even more unusual are constipation caused by large, bulky tumors and rectal prolapse caused by distal lesions. In patients with Cronkhite-Canada syndrome, diarrhea is progressive, leading to inanition and cachexia, especially in women.

Patients with submucosal tumors (eg, lipomas, hemangiomas, and leiomyomas) may present with an abdominal mass or abdominal pain from intussusception.

Diagnosis and Treatment

Polyps are usually detected by fecal occult blood testing, sigmoidoscopy, barium enema, or colonoscopy. Although air-contrast barium enema is far superior to the single-contrast technique, it can miss up to 50% of polyps. With colonoscopy, polypectomy can be performed, and tissue can be obtained for diagnosis. Colonoscopy is usually performed when an adenomatous polyp is found on sigmoidoscopy because of the high frequency of additional polyps. Surgical excision may be necessary for submucosal tumors or polyps that cannot be removed endoscopically.

When well-differentiated carcinoma is detected in a polyp and no vascular, lymphatic, or stalk invasion exists and a clear resection margin does exist, the only treatment usually needed is endoscopic polypectomy. If these conditions are not met, surgery may be considered, depending on the location of the adenoma and other factors.

For patients with adenomatous polyps, repeated examinations every 3 to 5 yr after polypectomy are needed because additional lesions develop.

MALIGNANT NEOPLASMS

Colorectal cancer is second only to lung cancer as the most common malignancy among US and Western European men and women. In the USA, about 150,000 new cases of and 60,000 deaths from this disease occur annually.

The incidence of colorectal cancer begins rising at age 40 and doubles every 5 yr thereafter, peaking in the eighth decade. Adenocarcinoma constitutes 95% of all colorectal cancers. Rectal cancer is more common in men; colon cancer apparently occurs equally in men and women. Synchronous colon cancers appear in about 3.5% of patients followed for > 25 yr, and metachronous lesions appear in 5% of such patients. Colonoscopic polypectomy in these patients will undoubtedly reduce these percentages.

Colorectal carcinoma is more common in upper socioeconomic classes. High-risk populations consume a diet higher in animal fat and refined sugar and lower in fiber than that consumed by low-risk populations. Other predisposing factors include age > 40, a history of colonic adenomatous polyps or cancer of the colon without follow-up colonoscopy surveillance, cancer of the breast or female genital tract, first-degree relative with colon cancer, inflammatory bowel disease (eg, ulcerative colitis, Crohn's disease, or radiation proctocolitis), and certain chronic parasitic infections (eg, schistosomiasis). Hereditary disorders (eg, familial polyposis) also are associated with a high incidence of colorectal carcinoma, but they are rare in the elderly.

The extent of tumor spread is graded by a modified Dukes classification. Dukes A lesions involve the mucosa; B lesions extend through the wall but do not involve lymph nodes; C lesions involve lymph nodes; and D lesions have distant metastases. Many modifications of this staging system exist.

Other colorectal malignancies include lymphoma, leiomyosarcoma, and carcinoid tumors.

Symptoms and Signs

Because colon cancer is asymptomatic in its early stages, screening is performed using routine sigmoidoscopic examination every 3 to 5 yr and annual fecal occult blood testing.

The location of a tumor in the colon influences the symptoms. **Right-colon lesions** are usually large, fungating, bleeding masses that cause iron deficiency anemia, fatigue, and weakness, and the large-caliber, thin-walled right colon contains fluid-like feces. These tumors usually do not cause obstruction but may grow large enough to be palpable on abdominal examination. **Left-colon lesions** are usually "napkin-ring," obstructive tumors that cause rectal bleeding, crampy abdominal pain, or altered bowel habits because of the narrower caliber of the left colon and the semisolid consistency of the feces. Patients with **rectal lesions** generally present with stool streaked or mixed with blood. They may also complain of tenesmus or a sensation of incomplete evacuation. Palpable lymphadenopathy, hepatomegaly, or both occur only in the late stages and suggest a very poor prognosis.

Diagnosis

Diagnosis is made by x-ray or endoscopy. A **rigid sigmoidoscope** may not be able to detect colon cancer because the instrument may not even reach its 25-cm length. The **fiberoptic sigmoidoscope** can detect lesions in the rectum, the sigmoid colon, and the distal descending colon, the region where > 50% of cancers occur. The more proximal segments of the colon are examined by barium enema x-ray or colonoscopy. **Air-contrast barium enema** is usually superior to the single-contrast technique in detecting colon cancer. **Colonoscopy** provides visualization and tissue for diagnosis and also allows inspection of the entire colon for synchronous polyps or cancers.

Fecal occult blood testing helps detect colonic tumors. Screening of elderly patients with annual fecal occult blood testing using six guaiac-impregnated slides over 3 days and sigmoidoscopy every 3 to 5 yr aids detection of early stage colon cancer, which is potentially curable. With both screening tests, the positive predictive value is better in persons > 60 yr. Screening with fecal occult blood testing can reduce the mortality rate of colorectal cancer.

Carcinoembryonic antigen (CEA) levels may be elevated in patients with cancer of the colon, pancreas, breast, lung, prostate, stomach, or bladder as well as in those with benign conditions and thus are nonspecific. An elevated CEA level is especially insensitive for early stage cancers. However, if the CEA level is elevated before surgery and decreases after it, a subsequent rise may indicate a recurrence.

Treatment

Treatment of colorectal cancer consists primarily of anatomic surgical resection (see Ch. 62). Except with lymphoma, radiation therapy and chemotherapy do not cure. In Dukes C colon cancer and in Dukes B_2 and C rectal cancer, adjuvant chemotherapy with 5-fluorouracil and levamisole combined with radiation therapy improves survival.

In patients with adenocarcinoma, the 5-yr survival rate is about 90% for patients with Dukes A lesions, 50% to 80% for those with B lesions, 30% to 40% for those with C lesions, and < 5% for those with D lesions. Primary GI tract lymphoma has an overall 5-yr survival rate of > 50%.

NEOPLASMS OF THE ANORECTUM

Cancer may develop in the perianal skin, the anal canal, or the lower rectum. **Epidermoid carcinoma** accounts for 2% of colorectal cancers and 90% of anal cancers. The histologic types of anal carcinoma include squamous cell, basal cell, basaloid squamous, and cloacogenic carcinomas. Other malignant neoplasms include Bowen's disease (intraepithelial squamous cell carcinoma in situ), extramammary Paget's disease, carcinoid tumor, and malignant melanoma. Cloacogenic carcinoma is most prevalent in patients ages 60 to 70. Factors predisposing persons to anorectal cancer include infections from human papillomavirus types 16 and 18 or human immunodeficiency virus, leukoplakia, lymphogranuloma venereum, chronic fistula formation, irradiation of the anal skin, and organ transplantation.

Symptoms, Signs, and Diagnosis

Bleeding is the most common symptom. Other frequent complaints are anal discomfort, constipation, and diminished stool caliber. The presenting feature may be a mass on digital rectal examination, inguinal adenopathy, or perianal dermatitis. Cancer should be considered with all nonhealing ulcers or fistulas. Biopsy of all suspicious lesions is essential.

Treatment

The treatment of choice is local surgical excision preceded by a course of radiation therapy and chemotherapy to debulk a large tumor mass. Such radiation therapy and chemotherapy may obviate abdominoperineal resection in many patients. Fulguration with electrocautery and laser photocoagulation are palliative measures in selected cases.

NEOPLASMS OF THE APPENDIX

The most common tumor of the appendix is a **carcinoid tumor,** which is found in about 1 in 1000 resected appendixes. Rarely malignant, carcinoid tumors are treated by appendectomy. If they are > 2 cm in diameter or show evidence of lymphatic or lymph node involvement, a right colectomy should be performed.

Primary adenocarcinoma of the appendix is rare, even though the appendix is lined with colonic mucosa. This tumor may block the lumen, leading to acute appendicitis and perforation.

Mucoceles produce appendiceal distention and outlet obstruction because of the intraluminal accumulation of mucus. The symptoms suggest early appendicitis. A mucocele may be demonstrated by CT scan. Although mucoceles are usually benign and treatable by appendectomy, some are associated with low-grade adenocarcinoma; if these mucoceles perforate, a form of carcinomatosis known as **pseudomyxoma peritonei** results. Patients who have this indolent tumor present with increased abdominal girth and a doughy abdomen. They can survive for several years, but repeated accumulation of intraperitoneal mucus or intestinal obstruction occurs. Palliative surgery often prolongs life and makes the patient more comfortable.

NEOPLASMS OF THE PANCREAS

Neoplasms of the pancreas include both exocrine and endocrine tumors.

EXOCRINE NEOPLASMS

The only significant benign exocrine pancreatic neoplasm is **cystadenoma,** which usually occurs in the body and tail of the pancreas in middle-aged and elderly women. Surgical resection may be needed for diagnosis and relief of symptoms from a large mass.

Pancreatic cancer is the second most common GI cancer in the USA with about 28,000 new cases diagnosed annually. The incidence increases with age and is 10 times greater in men > 75 yr than in the general population. Risk factors include cigarette smoking, diabetes mellitus, and a diet high in animal fat and alcohol.

Ductal cell adenocarcinoma accounts for 75% to 96% of all cancers arising from the pancreas. Others include giant cell carcinoma, adenosquamous carcinoma, cystadenocarcinoma, and lymphoma. **Giant cell carcinoma,** also called carcinosarcoma, is a highly malignant lesion with distant metastases occurring early. **Adenosquamous carcinoma** occurs predominantly in men, more often in patients with a history of radiation therapy. **Cystadenocarcinoma,** a low-grade malignancy, has the best prognosis because only 20% have metastasized by the time of surgery. **Lymphoma** of the pancreas accounts for 2% of all non-Hodgkin's lymphoma and may be of B-cell or T-cell origin.

Symptoms and Signs

The clinical features of pancreatic cancer often depend on the location of the lesions; 80% occur in the head of the pancreas, and 20% in the body and tail. Patients with lesions of the pancreatic head often present with painless jaundice and acholic stools from common duct obstruction or with nausea and vomiting from gastric outlet obstruction. Itching may accompany jaundice. The onset of symptoms in those with lesions of the body and tail is more insidious, amounting to little more than weight loss and vague abdominal or back pain. Symptoms precede diagnosis by about 3 to 6 mo. In 90% of patients with ductal cell adenocarcinoma, metastases are present at diagnosis, so death often occurs within 6 mo.

Findings associated with pancreatic cancer include depression, thromboembolic phenomena associated with **Trousseau's syndrome,** GI bleeding from gastric varices secondary to splenic vein thrombosis, polyarthritis, diarrhea caused by exocrine pancreatic insufficiency, superior vena cava syndrome caused by mediastinal metastases, and Horner's syndrome caused by thoracic outlet metastasis. The onset of diabetes mellitus or a worsening of preexisting diabetes warrants an evaluation for pancreatic cancer.

Early in the disease the physical examination is negative. Later, an epigastric mass, supraclavicular lymphadenopathy, hepatomegaly from biliary stasis or metastasis, or a large, palpable gallbladder may be noted. Painless jaundice and a palpable gallbladder (Courvoisier's sign) combined with acholic stools are diagnostic. Silver-colored stools may be noted in cancer of the ampulla of Vater because of the combination of mild bleeding and acholic stools.

Diagnosis

Early diagnosis when the tumor is still resectable is rarely possible. It is possible only with cancer of the pancreatic head associated with jaundice and with cancer of the ampulla of Vater, which may cause early jaundice. Diagnosis may be suggested by upper abdominal sonography, although a CT scan of the abdomen can better visualize a pancreatic mass. In up to 90% of cases, endoscopic retrograde cholangiopancreatography can detect the tumor with the characteristic findings of ductal irregularity and cutoff. Although tissue for diagnosis can usually be obtained by needle biopsy, exploratory laparotomy is often necessary. Serologic tumor markers including CEA, CA19-9, and galactosyltransferase isoenzyme II (GI-II) may be elevated in some cases but are rarely useful clinically.

Treatment

Patients who have nonmetastatic, resectable lesions in the pancreatic head may be candidates for pancreatoduodenectomy (Whipple's operation). Only 10% of patients with ductal cell carcinoma have localized tumors. In most patients, the only procedure that can be performed is a palliative bypass (eg, cholecystojejunostomy for distal bile duct obstruction or gastrojejunostomy for gastric outlet obstruction); however, surgery is usually not warranted, and obstructive jaundice can be managed with an endoscopically placed stent. In older persons with nonresectable tumors, forgoing all attempts at cure is often best.

Chemotherapy produces little response and no long-term benefit in patients with adenocarcinoma. Radiation therapy offers minimal benefit, except for palliation of retroperitoneal pain. Palliative treatment with a biliary stent (placed endoscopically or radiologically using transhepatic cholangiography) may reduce jaundice and itching.

Generally, abdominal pain is treated with analgesics and oral narcotics. However, a celiac axis nerve block may be needed for severe, unrelenting pain. Pruritus from jaundice may be relieved with antihistamines or cholestyramine 4 gm orally 1 to 4 times daily. Pancreatic insufficiency can be managed with pancreatic enzymes (lipase, protease, and amylase).

The overall prognosis is dismal for adenocarcinoma; the 1-yr survival rate is $< 10\%$, and the 5-yr survival rate is only 2%. Cystadenocarcinoma, which has a low incidence of metastasis at diagnosis, has a 5-yr survival rate of 65% with aggressive surgery. Lymphoma also has a good prognosis.

ENDOCRINE NEOPLASMS

Endocrine tumors arise from the neuroendocrine cells of the pancreas predominantly in the islets of the pancreatic body and tail. However, enterochromaffin cells and other neuroendocrine cells can arise anywhere in the GI tract. Endocrine tumors are rare in older persons.

These tumors are indistinguishable microscopically without special immunochemical staining. Localization of tumors can be aided by CT scan, portal venous sampling, and intraoperative ultrasonography. They may be either nonfunctioning or functioning (ie, hormone secreting).

Nonfunctioning tumors may cause obstruction of the biliary tract or duodenum, bleeding into the GI tract, or an abdominal mass. Functioning tumors produce various syndromes.

Insulinomas, which may be single or multiple, produce insulin and are identified by episodes of hypoglycemia, which may progress to coma in severe cases. Insulinomas are rarely malignant. Removal of all tumor tissue results in complete cure.

Gastrinomas produce the Zollinger-Ellison syndrome, an extremely virulent ulcer diathesis with excessive gastric acid secretion and diarrhea. The tumors can occur near the ampulla of Vater or the antrum as well as in the pancreas and are malignant in about 90% of cases. If metastasis does not occur, complete excision of the tumor is curative. If metastasis does occur, various therapeutic modalities may be used, including administration of large doses of H_2-receptor blockers or omeprazole and, if medical therapy fails, gastric surgery to reduce acid secretion.

Glucagonomas secrete glucagon and have a high potential for malignancy. They lead to mild diabetes mellitus and a severe dermatitis involving portions of the lower half of the body. Although complete removal may not be possible, debulking the tumor may help relieve symptoms. Streptozocin can help treat the residual tumor.

Vipomas produce vasoactive intestinal polypeptide, pancreatic polypeptide, and perhaps other hormones. Because the primary characteristics are watery diarrhea, hypokalemia, and achlorhydria, the disease is also known as the **WDHA syndrome.** Half of the tumors are malignant. As much tumor as possible should be resected, and the residual tumor should be treated with streptozocin.

Somatostatinomas are rare tumors that secrete somatostatin. Clinical findings include diabetes, steatorrhea, and achlorhydria.

These clinical conditions can sometimes present as multiple endocrine neoplasia syndromes, in which tumors or hyperplasia occurs in two or more endocrine glands. Usually, these conditions are associated with tumors or hyperplasia of the parathyroid, pituitary, thyroid, or adrenal glands.

NEOPLASMS OF THE LIVER

Benign neoplasms of the liver are usually asymptomatic. By far, the most common form of hepatic tumor is metastatic carcinoma.

BENIGN NEOPLASMS

Hemangioma, the most common benign neoplasm of the liver, is found in about 5% of adult autopsies. Other benign tumors include **hepatocellular adenoma** and **focal nodular hyperplasia,** which are most often associated with oral contraceptives and are not usually seen in elderly persons. **Bile duct adenomas** and **cystadenomas** and rare **mesenchymal tumors** have also been reported.

Symptoms and Signs

Usually, these tumors are asymptomatic and are found incidentally at laparotomy or when a CT scan, ultrasonography, or angiography is performed for unrelated symptoms. Rarely, patients with hemangiomas present with massive hemorrhage from rupture or consumptive coagulopathy **(Kasabach-Merritt syndrome).**

Diagnosis and Treatment

Liver function test results are normal or slightly abnormal. The diagnosis can be established by routine liver biopsy in nonvascular lesions, although laparoscopy or laparotomy is often necessary. Therapy for nonvascular tumors usually consists of segmental resection.

MALIGNANT NEOPLASMS

The liver is the most common site of metastasis from other cancers. Liver metastases are found at autopsy in 30% to 50% of patients with cancer.

Primary malignancy of the liver is rare in the USA and Western Europe but common in Africa and Asia. About 90% of primary adult hepatic cancers originate in the hepatocyte and are called **hepatocellular carcinoma** or **hepatoma;** 5% to 10% originate in the bile ducts as **cholangiocarcinoma** or are a mixed type, **cholangiohepatoma.** Other primary liver cancers are exceedingly rare and include **cystadenocarcinoma, angiosarcoma,** and **hepatoblastoma.** Hepatic malignancies are more common in men than in women and occur between ages 50 and 70.

Hepatocellular carcinoma may be nodular, massive, or diffuse. The nodular type, which is the most common, consists of multiple discrete nodules. The massive type, which essentially accounts for the rest, develops as a large, often necrotic, hemorrhagic mass. The diffuse type is most often associated with cirrhosis and consists of minute lesions scattered throughout the liver. Predisposing factors include hepatitis B, hepatitis C, alcohol or tobacco use, cirrhosis, and aflatoxin exposure.

Symptoms and Signs

About 70% of patients present with right upper quadrant or epigastric pain and weight loss. With progressive liver dysfunction, mental status may deteriorate. Pulmonary symptoms and pathologic fractures may result from metastases. A rare tumor rupture with intra-abdominal hemorrhage and symptoms of an acute abdomen is life threatening.

Physical examination may reveal hepatomegaly, a right upper quadrant mass, or ascites. Splenomegaly is less common. Lymphadenopathy, especially in the right supraclavicular region, can occur. Gynecomastia is rare.

Paraneoplastic syndromes associated with hepatocellular carcinoma include erythrocytosis, hypercalcemia, hypoglycemia, hyperlipidemia, porphyria cutanea tarda, and dysfibrinoginemia.

Diagnosis

Liver function test results are usually abnormal. Elevated serum alkaline phosphatase levels are common, but elevated serum aminotransferases and bilirubin levels are less so. Hepatitis B surface antigen and hepatitis C virus markers may be positive. Elevated levels of α-fetoprotein are noted in 90% of patients with hepatocellular carcinoma.

Diagnosis is often made with a combination of abdominal ultrasonography and CT scan, angiography, and biopsy. Though CT scan is more sensitive and specific than ultrasonography, it may miss 10% of the tumors. Lipiodol intrahepatic injection followed in 2 wk by CT scan can identify tumors 0.2 to 0.3 cm in size.

Needle aspiration guided by CT scan or ultrasonography is a safe, reliable technique. Angiography usually shows a typical capillary blush. Laparoscopy allows inspection of the abdominal cavity for secondary tumor and for directed biopsy.

Treatment

Treatment of hepatocellular carcinoma is unsatisfactory, with a 5-yr survival rate near 0%. However, surgical resection of a localized tumor and hepatic transplantation are associated with longer survival. Radiation therapy and chemotherapy are unsatisfactory, though intrahepatic arterial infusion of chemotherapeutic agents and angiographic embolization of vascular tumors prolong survival in some patients.

NEOPLASMS OF THE GALLBLADDER

Benign gallbladder tumors are found at cholecystectomy in about 1% of patients; the incidence is not higher among the elderly. Gallbladder cancer has been reported at cholecystectomy in 0.2% to 5% of patients.

BENIGN NEOPLASMS

These tumors include adenomas, cystadenomas, fibroadenomas, adenomyomas, and hamartomas. Adenomas, which are frequently associated with gallstones and cholecystitis, may have malignant potential.

Symptoms and signs may be nonexistent, vague, or typical of acute or chronic cholecystitis. Diagnosis is made by demonstrating a filling defect in the gallbladder. For small lesions, follow-up consists of ultrasound examination every 3 to 6 mo. If the lesions do not grow, treatment is not necessary. If the lesions grow, cholecystectomy is recommended because of the uncertain premalignant nature of some lesions.

MALIGNANT NEOPLASMS

Gallbladder malignancy has been reported in 0.2% to 5% of patients undergoing cholecystectomy, mostly women between ages 60 and 70. Adenocarcinoma accounts for 80% of gallbladder malignancies; squamous cell carcinoma and adenoacanthoma account for the remaining

20%. Metastasis is found in 75% of cases at the time of diagnosis. Workers in rubber and automotive plants have a particularly high risk of gallbladder cancer.

Gallstones are associated with the development of gallbladder carcinoma, and preventing such carcinoma may justify early cholecystectomy in patients with cholelithiasis.

Symptoms, Signs, and Diagnosis

Symptoms include intermittent pain and dyspepsia similar to that of chronic cholecystitis. In the late stages, weight loss and jaundice develop. Often a firm, tender mass is palpable in the right upper quadrant. Abdominal ultrasonography and CT scan provide visualization of the tumor. Endoscopic retrograde cholangiopancreatography or percutaneous transhepatic cholangiography is useful for a complete evaluation of the biliary tree.

Treatment

Radical cholecystectomy is the treatment of choice for localized disease. Radiation therapy and chemotherapy are ineffective. The prognosis is dismal; the 5-yr survival rate is only 5%. Biliary stenting by endoscopic retrograde cholangiopancreatography or percutaneous transhepatic cholangiography may provide limited palliation of an obstruction.

NEOPLASMS OF EXTRAHEPATIC BILE DUCTS

Malignant neoplasms of the bile ducts are rare and often difficult to diagnose.

BENIGN NEOPLASMS

Papilloma and adenoma are the most common benign neoplasms of the bile ducts, although fibroadenoma, adenomyoma, leiomyoma, granular cell myoblastoma, neurinoma, and hamartoma also occur. Intermittent jaundice and right upper quadrant pain are the most common symptoms. The treatment of choice is local excision.

MALIGNANT NEOPLASMS

By far the most common malignant neoplasm is adenocarcinoma. Bile duct cancer is more common in men; the average age at diagnosis is 60 yr. Tumors of the upper portion of the ducts (50% of all lesions) are intimately related to the liver; those of the middle portion, to the portal vein and hepatic artery; and those of the lower portion, to the pancreas and duodenum. Such localization has both diagnostic and prognostic implications.

Predisposing factors include primary sclerosing cholangitis, *Clonorchis sinensis* infestation, and industrial exposure (in automobile and rubber manufacturing plant workers).

Symptoms, Signs, and Diagnosis

Because of their location, malignant tumors usually cause early symptoms. Jaundice occurs in almost all patients. Right upper quadrant pain occurs in > 50%. Other associated symptoms and signs include weight loss, nausea, vomiting, anorexia, fever, chills, diarrhea, constipation, clay-colored stools, and hepatomegaly. If obstruction occurs below the cystic duct, a distended gallbladder (Courvoisier's sign) may be palpated.

Diagnosis of large tumors is made by ultrasonography and CT scan. However, percutaneous transhepatic cholangiography or endoscopic retrograde cholangiopancreatography frequently is more important in making the diagnosis and localizing the tumor. Liver function test results are consistent with extrahepatic obstruction.

Treatment

The prognosis for bile duct cancer is poor with a 5-yr survival rate of only 5%. Tumors in the proximal portion of the bile duct system rarely are operable. When they are, complex liver and duct resections are required, and there are few long-term survivors. Palliation may be accomplished by dilation and stent insertion either endoscopically or via transhepatic cholangiography. Resectable tumors of the central portion of the bile ducts may be treated by local en bloc excision. Bile duct drainage is reestablished by hepaticojejunostomy.

For resectable tumors of the distal ducts, radical resection and pancreatoduodenectomy (Whipple's operation) provide some promising benefit with 5-yr survival rates of 20% to 30%. With nonresectable tumors, palliation may be accomplished by hepaticojejunostomy or by stent placement followed by internal radiation via endoscopic retrograde cholangiopancreatography or percutaneous catheter insertion into the ducts. Chemotherapy, radiation therapy, and liver transplantation are ineffective.

NEOPLASMS OF THE MESENTERY AND PERITONEUM

Benign neoplasms of the mesentery and peritoneum are twice as common as malignant neoplasms; however, they are still rare.

BENIGN NEOPLASMS

The most common benign neoplasms are fibromas and lipomas. Most often found incidentally during routine examination, these tumors frequently grow large before causing symptoms. The most common symptoms are vague abdominal pain and bloating caused by compression or traction of adjacent structures. Intestinal obstruction may occur.

Diagnosis is usually made by x-rays that reveal extrinsic compression of the large or small bowel. Surgical excision is curative.

MALIGNANT NEOPLASMS

Malignant neoplasms of the mesentery and peritoneum, which are rare, usually include mesothelioma, fibrosarcoma, or leiomyosarcoma. Symptoms and signs include vague abdominal pain and bloating caused by traction or compression of adjacent structures and intestinal obstruction. Weight loss, anorexia, and weakness can also occur. Mesothelioma is associated with asbestos exposure.

Diagnosis is made by x-rays, including an upper GI series, barium enema, and CT scan, that reveal extrinsic compression or signs of invasion of the small or large bowel and other local structures. Surgery is the only effective treatment for cure or palliation. However, chemotherapy and radiation therapy may improve results for mesothelioma.

61. GASTROINTESTINAL ENDOSCOPY

Endoscopy is a general term for *the visual inspection of body cavities by instrumentation*. Specific terms are derived from the area being examined; thus, esophagogastroduodenoscopy refers to upper GI endoscopy, and colonoscopy refers to lower GI endoscopy.

Although originally considered a procedure complementary to a barium x-ray, endoscopy is now often used as the primary tool for evaluation of the GI tract. Conventional x-rays cannot identify color changes (eg, gastritis), bleeding, or vascular malformations, and during endoscopic examination, both biopsy and therapeutic maneuvers can be performed.

Gastrointestinal endoscopy is particularly valuable in elderly patients because their symptoms may be atypical. Usually, the elderly tolerate GI endoscopy well. However, it should be performed only for appropriate indications because complications are more common in the elderly than in younger persons. Not only are older tissues more fragile and more easily traumatized, but older patients generally have other medical problems besides the GI complaint.

Early endoscopy for GI bleeding may help the physician select patients for whom early surgery is lifesaving. The diagnostic accuracy of endoscopic retrograde cholangiopancreatography **(ERCP)** in a patient with jaundice is unsurpassed, and the techniques for removing stones from the bile duct and placing a stent through a bile duct compressed by a malignant tumor may avoid the need for surgery altogether. The source of unexplained GI bleeding or iron deficiency anemia is frequently determined by colonoscopy because the blood loss often originates in the colon, an area in which x-rays may be inaccurate.

Proper training in the use of endoscopes for diagnosis and therapy is necessary to attain the experience and knowledge needed to diagnose pathologic conditions correctly and prevent complications. Short courses or weekend training sessions are not adequate for this purpose.

Most endoscopes vary in length from 30 to 185 cm; a special 300-cm enteroscope is used for the small intestine. These flexible instruments have operator-controlled tip deflection capability, which permits guidance through the intestinal lumen. A high-intensity external light source illuminates the field under examination, while the image is transmitted through fiberoptic bundles to the operator's eye or via digitized signals (videoendoscope) to a television screen. An internal channel permits the passage of biopsy or grasping forceps, wire snares (for polypectomy), injection needles, and electrocoagulation or laser probes. The channel also allows fluid instillation (for flushing debris from the intestinal wall) and suction aspiration.

Before GI endoscopy, the physician may prohibit food and drink to empty the stomach or order a purgative to cleanse the colon. Most endoscopic procedures are performed with the patient under sedation. Because transient bacteremia infrequently occurs during endoscopy, patients at high risk for infection—those with valvular heart disease (rheumatic heart disease and valvular prosthesis), neutropenia, or artificial joint implants—should receive antibiotics, usually ampicillin and gentamicin, before the examination.

Because older patients are more sensitive to sedative and analgesic drugs, doses must be adjusted to prevent adverse reactions. Benzodiazepines are commonly used to induce preendoscopic sedation, and doses may need to be reduced by 50% to 75% to guard against cardiorespiratory depression. During endoscopy in the sedated elderly patient, the physician should frequently check skin color, pulse, and respirations to monitor the depressant effects of premedication. Continuous mechanical monitoring of oxygen saturation levels with a pulse oximeter may benefit the elderly patient. Close monitoring is even more important during emergency endoscopy because events occur quickly, and the patient's homeostatic mechanisms may be only marginally functioning.

ESOPHAGOGASTRODUODENOSCOPY

The goal of esophagogastroduodenoscopy is to visualize the entire upper GI tract (to the second portion of the duodenum).

Indications

Both diagnostic and therapeutic maneuvers can be performed during the procedure. Fluid and tissue specimens can be obtained.

Diagnostic indications: Esophagogastroduodenoscopy may be used to explore upper GI symptoms or abnormalities seen on an upper GI x-ray series. An x-ray is not a prerequisite for upper GI endoscopy because the gastroscope can be passed safely under direct vision even in patients with dysphagia and a possible Zenker's diverticulum. Any pathologic process (ulcer, mass, irregularity) can be characterized by inspection and biopsy. Brush cytology may increase the diagnostic findings in malignant disease.

Esophagogastroduodenoscopy may be used to monitor the healing rate of gastric ulcer but is usually unnecessary with duodenal ulcer. Periodic endoscopy and biopsy in Barrett's syndrome, a premalignant process, can detect early evidence of cancer. The best way to identify the site of upper GI bleeding, esophagogastroduodenoscopy should be performed as soon as the patient is stable.

Therapeutic indications: These indications include dilating **esophageal strictures** using a dilator threaded over an endoscopically placed guide wire or using a balloon catheter passed through the endoscope. In a patient who is not a surgical candidate, an obstructive **esophageal or gastric neoplasm** may be vaporized with a laser wave guide passed through the gastroscope or with a bipolar tumor probe under endoscopic guidance. With a more extensive obstructive tumor, enteral nutrition can be reestablished by precisely locating the tumor endoscopically and placing an esophageal stent prosthesis with the aid of a guide wire.

Endoscopic therapy for bleeding has markedly enhanced the value of esophagogastroduodenoscopy. Almost all episodes of upper GI bleeding can be controlled by using injection therapy with epinephrine or absolute alcohol or by using a thermal coagulation device. **Sclerotherapy for esophageal varices** and injection therapy for bleeding vessels may be performed during the initial diagnostic examination by passing a long, flexible needle-tipped catheter through the endoscope. **Polyps** may be resected using a wire snare loop and an electrocoagulation current to prevent bleeding.

Usually, **submucosal lesions** cannot be resected endoscopically. **Removing foreign bodies** from the esophagus or stomach may require special maneuvers, including attaching a shield that folds over sharp objects to the tip of the endoscope to prevent esophageal injury during extraction. Foreign bodies smaller than a dime frequently pass spontaneously and may not require endoscopic removal. Food **bezoars** can sometimes be broken up with the snare, biopsy forceps, or a strong jet of water. Percutaneous endoscopic gastrostomy has largely replaced surgical creation of a **feeding gastrostomy** and can be accomplished at the bedside with little risk.

Contraindications and Risks

Absolute contraindications are a recent myocardial infarction and an acute perforated viscus. Patients with cardiorespiratory disease and dyspnea are at special risk. Even without sedation, these patients have a slightly lowered PO_2; with sedation, some are particularly vulnerable to respiratory depression. In these patients, using a small-caliber endoscope and administering additional oxygen during the procedure may be beneficial.

Procedure

For most patients, the only preparation is a restriction on eating and drinking for 6 h before the examination. Those with either achalasia or gastric outlet obstruction may have retained food for days and may require lavage to empty the esophagus or stomach. Light sedation with an IV narcotic or a benzodiazepine may be combined with a local anesthetic applied to the posterior pharynx. The procedure is usually performed with the patient in the left lateral position. The examiner passes the instrument under direct vision through the pharynx to examine the entire esophagus, stomach, and duodenum. The entire procedure can be performed in 15 to 30 min.

Complications

Perforation occurs in 0.03% of examinations, and death from complications occurs in about 0.006% of cases. Most complications are caused by medication and include arrhythmias, aspiration, and cardiac arrest.

COLONOSCOPY

The goal of colonoscopy is to visualize the entire colon, including the cecal caput. With training and experience, the examiner accomplishes this in > 90% of cases, but the inexperienced examiner may achieve total intubation in < 80%. Every colonoscopist should be capable of removing polyps during a diagnostic examination because repeating the preparation and examination causes the patient additional discomfort and places the patient at additional risk.

Indications

Diagnostic indications: Most colonoscopic examinations are performed to evaluate an abnormality detected on a barium enema x-ray. During colonoscopy, the mucosa and all lesions are inspected directly, biopsies may be performed on tumors, and polyps may be removed. The risk of colorectal cancer increases with age, but with colonoscopy, the physician can detect such cancer in its earliest phases and remove the polyps.

Not all patients need an initial x-ray. Occasionally, elderly patients are unable to retain barium for an x-ray but tolerate colonoscopy well. Also, primary colonoscopy should be considered in those with a positive fecal occult blood test or iron deficiency anemia and in those at high risk for colorectal cancer (patients with a previous colonic polyp, previous colon cancer, strong family history of colon cancer, or ulcerative colitis for > 8 yr). Colonoscopy of the large bowel is the most straightforward approach to a positive fecal occult blood test or anemia because the colon is the most common site of occult bleeding. Colonoscopy may be difficult during acute, massive lower GI bleeding, but its use in such cases has been advocated by some investigators. If colonoscopy findings are negative, the patient should undergo upper GI endoscopy. This schema provides answers rapidly and efficiently, thereby decreasing the time needed for a diagnosis and minimizing the inconvenience to the patient.

Therapeutic indications: Colonic polyps can be removed without surgery in most patients. Bleeding sites (eg, arteriovenous malformations) may be treated with electrocoagulation, and volvulus may be decompressed, as may the dilated colon in **Ogilvie's syndrome** (acute colonic pseudo-obstruction). Laser vaporization of obstructive rectosigmoid neoplasms may provide symptomatic relief. Strictures may be dilated with balloons or bougies.

Contraindications

Absolute contraindications are fulminant colitis, acute diverticulitis, perforated viscus, and a recent myocardial infarction. Poor colon preparation is a relative contraindication. Colonoscopy has a low diagnostic yield when used to identify the cause of chronic abdominal pain.

Procedure

The colon must be clean. One or two days of a liquid diet and a potent cathartic (castor oil or citrate of magnesia) with enemas on the day of colonoscopy usually suffice. Enemas are unnecessary if two oral doses of sodium phosphate or a 4-L electrolyte solution containing polyethylene glycol is administered. Electrolyte and fluid shift must be carefully considered in the elderly patient with cardiovascular and renal instability. Usually, an IV narcotic or a benzodiazepine is given for sedation. General anesthesia is unnecessary and undesirable.

The colonoscope is passed to the cecum under direct vision with a combination of dial-control manipulation, advancement and withdrawal of the instrument, and air instillation. Fluoroscopy, once considered vital for successful colonoscopy, is now rarely necessary. Every centimeter of the colon's surface may be inspected, but the examiner must ensure that potentially blind areas just behind acute bends or colonic flexures are not missed. Once the cecum is reached, the small bowel frequently can be entered, and a biopsy performed.

Therapy is performed as in esophagogastroduodenoscopy. A polyp is resected by lassoing its base with a wire snare loop and then tightening the snare. Electrocautery current passed through the wire loop during polyp removal prevents bleeding.

Complications

Medication complications are similar to those with esophagogastroduodenoscopy. During routine colonoscopy, the risk of perforation is about 0.1%, and the risk of bleeding is nil. Following polypectomy, perforation occurs in 0.3% of patients and bleeding in 1.5%.

ENDOSCOPIC RETROGRADE CHOLANGIOPANCREATOGRAPHY

In endoscopic retrograde cholangiopancreatography (ERCP), a lateral-view endoscope is passed orally to the duodenum for visualization of the ampulla of Vater. Then under direct vision, a cannula is placed into the ampulla of Vater. Under fluoroscopic monitoring, a dye is injected so that it flows retrograde (or counter) to the normal flow of secretions and makes the common bile duct and its tributaries or the pancreatic duct and its tributaries opaque. Because of the position of the biliary tree, a cholangiogram is more difficult to obtain than a pancreatogram, but an experienced endoscopist can visualize the desired duct in > 90% of cases. An ultrathin fiberscope, the size of a cannula, which can be passed through the ERCP instrument directly into the ducts for direct intraductal visualization, is under investigation.

Indications

Diagnostic indications: With ERCP, the examiner can determine the cause of jaundice and identify the site of an obstruction with a high degree of accuracy. The procedure also is useful in demonstrating ductal abnormalities in a nonjaundiced patient when the clinical presentation suggests biliary disease, pancreatic malignancy, or pancreatitis, and it helps evaluate chronic pancreatitis or pancreatic pseudocyst preoperatively. If symptoms, signs, or laboratory tests suggest common bile duct stones, ERCP is indicated before laparoscopy to diagnose and remove the stones because exploring the common bile duct during laparoscopic cholecystectomy is difficult. Pressure measurements, performed in highly specialized medical centers, help diagnose dysfunction in Oddi's sphincter.

Therapeutic indications: In endoscopic sphincterotomy, the muscular fibers at the distal bile duct sphincter are cut to allow the passage of stones that cannot pass spontaneously because of the narrow orifice or large stone size. Emergency sphincterotomy is the procedure of choice for acute gallstone pancreatitis. Large stones may be crushed by a lithotriptor or may be dissolved over several days by chemical instillation via an indwelling nasobiliary tube placed through the sphincterotomy. A benign stricture may be dilated with a balloon, and a malignant obstruction may be treated symptomatically by placing a stent. Therapeutic ERCP is often used for biliary complications of laparoscopic cholecystectomy, such as duct obstruction from clips, bile leakage from the cystic duct stump, or removal of retained stones. Currently, stones in the gallbladder cannot be treated endoscopically.

Contraindications

Absolute contraindications include a recent myocardial infarction and perforated viscus. Also, ERCP is not indicated for evaluating abdominal pain in the absence of symptoms, signs, or laboratory findings that suggest biliary tract or pancreatic disease, nor is it indicated for evaluating suspected gallbladder disease without evidence of bile duct disease. The procedure has little value when pancreatic malignancy has already been demonstrated by ultrasonography or CT scan.

Procedure

The patient should not eat or drink for 6 h to empty the stomach and duodenum. If the patient has recently ingested barium, an x-ray should be obtained to ensure that the barium is not superimposed on the areas of interest. An IV narcotic and/or a benzodiazepine is given for sedation.

The lateral-view endoscope provides only partial vision through the esophagus, although the stomach can be adequately visualized. With the endoscope tip at the papilla of Vater, a plastic cannula is inserted into the ductal orifice—a challenging feat since neither of the ductal lumens may be discernible. A lever on the instrument's control head helps direct the cannula tip. Fluoroscopic monitoring during retrograde injection of the water-soluble contrast material is essential to ensure cannulation of the desired duct and to prevent overfilling. X-rays should be taken for a permanent record of the examination.

A fine wire may be passed into the biliary tree; when heated with an electrocautery current, the wire incises Oddi's sphincter (sphincterotomy), opening the lower end of the bile duct. Stones may be removed by passing a basket or balloon into the bile duct after an incision into the papilla of Vater (papillotomy). A lithotriptor, laser, or electrohydraulic shock waves may be used to crush large stones trapped in the basket. Indwelling cannulas or drainage stents may be left in the papilla of Vater to instill drugs or drain an obstructed duct.

Complications

Besides perforation (which is rare) and drug reactions, the major complications of ERCP are pancreatitis and infection. Pancreatitis occurs in $< 1\%$ of patients and is usually mild. Infection is less common, occurring in patients with duct obstruction. Sphincterotomy has a 1.5% mortality rate and an overall complication rate (including bleeding) of < 10%, which is lower than that of similar surgical procedures.

SIGMOIDOSCOPY AND ANOSCOPY

These procedures permit examination of the distal large bowel without extensive preparation or sedation. Disease within the anal canal is best seen with an anoscope—a short, tubular instrument with a sharply angulated bevel that allows direct visualization of the canal and the distal rectum. The rigid sigmoidoscope, when passed to its full length of 25 cm, permits inspection of the rectum and distal sigmoid colon. The 30-cm flexible sigmoidoscope allows inspection of most of the sigmoid colon; the 60-cm flexible sigmoidoscope allows inspection of most of the descending colon.

Facility in using the flexible sigmoidoscope requires training and experience. Performing a digital rectal examination along with sigmoidoscopy and anoscopy allows the physician to discover and treat precancerous polyps. It is important to discover lesions within 6 cm of the anus (the area in which cancer usually requires removal of the rectum and anus) and thus avoid the need for colostomy.

Indications

The flexible sigmoidoscope may be used to screen the left side of the colon, where ⅔ of neoplasms appear. Rigid or flexible sigmoidoscopy can evaluate the distal colon for suspected disease; either procedure may complement a barium enema. Anoscopy is best suited for visualizing perianal problems, eg, fissures, fistulas, or hemorrhoids.

Because of the age-related increase in colorectal polyps and cancer and the predominantly left-sided distribution, these procedures are valuable for early detection. For an asymptomatic person, the American Cancer Society recommends sigmoidoscopy every 3 yr to diagnose adenomas at a stage when their removal will prevent the development of colorectal cancer.

Contraindications

A recent myocardial infarction contraindicates this procedure. When indications for colonoscopy (anemia, positive results in a fecal occult blood test, polypectomy) are present, flexible sigmoidoscopy should not be substituted. In general, polyps should not be removed during flexible sigmoidoscopy because more extensive colon preparation is required for safety and because total colon evaluation is recommended whenever a polyp is identified.

Procedure

Sedation is not required. One or two phosphate enemas cleanse the bowel adequately. The patient usually lies on the left side for flexible sigmoidoscopy but assumes the knee-chest position for rigid sigmoidoscopy or anoscopy.

Complications

Complications are extremely rare but may include perforation and infection. Air insufflation or instrument looping in the colon may cause cramps and discomfort.

---

62. SURGERY OF THE GASTROINTESTINAL TRACT

In many ways, surgical problems of the abdomen are different in geriatric patients from those in younger patients. Diagnosis, particularly in emergencies, is more difficult because sensations are not as acute as in the young, and pathophysiologic reactions (eg, pain, tenderness, and response to inflammation) are not as quick or effective. Thus, minimal symptoms may accompany a potentially fatal intestinal perforation, and the first sign may be free subphrenic gas on the plain abdominal x-ray.

Acute abdomen should be suspected in patients who complain of only minimal abdominal pain. Peritonitis caused by perforation of the sigmoid, stomach, or duodenum may be present even if the patient has only slight abdominal tenderness. Vascular lesions (eg, mesenteric artery thrombosis) also are common. With appendicitis, acute cholecystitis, and strangulated hernias, the interval between onset and gangrene may be only a few hours.

The physical examination is extremely important. Old incisional scars suggest the possibility of intestinal obstruction. Thorough examination of potential hernia sites is essential. Absence of bowel sounds indicates aperistalsis, a serious finding that requires other diagnostic tests to be performed expeditiously.

Massive GI hemorrhage is tolerated poorly by older patients. A quick diagnosis must be made, and treatment must be started sooner than with younger patients, who can better tolerate repeated episodes of bleeding.

A high percentage of abdominal operations result from emergencies. In recent years at Massachusetts General Hospital, 60% of operations for peptic ulcers in patients ≥ 70 yr were emergency procedures for massive hemorrhage or acute perforation, 19% were urgent operations, and 11% were elective operations.

The major indications for **emergency surgery** are perforation of a viscus, appendicitis, intestinal obstruction, and massive hemorrhage. Acute cholecystitis usually requires an urgent operation. Most **elective**

surgery is for malignant disease. Excluding hernia repairs, more than 90% of abdominal procedures involve the colon, the gallbladder, and the stomach, with procedures divided almost equally among the three organs.

Optimal treatment of hernias can be controversial. Obviously, all patients with strangulated inguinal hernias need immediate surgery. Femoral hernias also are prone to strangulation and should be repaired electively, if possible. Many small, direct inguinal hernias and painless, indirect inguinal hernias with relatively large openings do not represent immediate threats. However, the *only* hernias that are safe to simply observe are small, direct, nonpainful hernias that reduce spontaneously when the patient is recumbent. Otherwise, hernias should be repaired, unless surgery is contraindicated. Frequently, the operation can be done using local anesthesia.

Generally, the elderly tolerate a single operation well, provided the offending lesion is removed. However, complications from second or third operations performed soon after the first carry a high mortality rate. Staged procedures should be spaced apart to allow complete recovery. These considerations are particularly important in surgical diseases of the gastrointestinal tract.

GASTROINTESTINAL BLEEDING

(See also GASTROINTESTINAL BLEEDING in Ch. 4)

Bleeding of the GI tract may be manifested clinically by **hematemesis** (*vomiting of blood*), **melena** (*passage of black, tarry stools*), or **hematochezia** (*passage of red bloody stools*). Bleeding may be either occult (detectable only by chemical means) or overt. Some persons do not recognize overt bleeding; eg, they may not be aware that coffee-ground vomit contains blood altered by gastric juice. Color blindness may also prevent a person from identifying red blood. Other ocular diseases common in the elderly (eg, cataracts and presbyopia) also limit the ability to recognize bleeding.

The GI tract has many potential sites of bleeding. The most common sites, in descending order, are the anorectum, stomach, colon, small intestine, and esophagus. Blood that originates in the mouth, the nasopharynx, or the lung can be swallowed and mimic gastric bleeding. The liver, pancreas, and aorta are unusual bleeding sites.

In the elderly, hemorrhoids and colorectal cancer are the most common causes of minor bleeding; peptic ulcer, diverticular disease, and angiodysplasia are the most common causes of major hemorrhages.

Diagnosis

Diagnosis consists of documentation of bleeding and identification of the bleeding site. The history, physical examination, blood tests, endoscopy, selective arteriography, radionuclide studies, barium contrast studies, and exploratory laparotomy aid in making the diagnosis. Often, identifying the bleeding site is difficult, but therapy must nonetheless proceed.

The **history** provides important clinical information. Alcoholism and a previous massive upper GI hemorrhage suggest bleeding caused by esophageal varices in young adults, but in older patients, the more likely cause is peptic ulcer. If a patient has an aortic aneurysm or an abdominal aortic graft, erosion into the duodenum should be suspected. Massive colonic bleeding is most likely caused by diverticular disease or angiodysplasia. Streaks of red blood on the toilet paper usually indicate hemorrhoids, but polyps and cancer must be ruled out.

The cause of the bleeding may not be in the GI tract. For example, a history of aspirin ingestion may explain GI bleeding. One aspirin tablet can prolong bleeding times for at least 6 days, while a larger dose can cause aspirin-induced gastritis. Nevertheless, the physician should not be influenced too strongly by such a history because many patients who take aspirin bleed from other causes. Alcohol, anticoagulants, and anti-inflammatory agents such as ibuprofen as well as coagulopathies such as those associated with metastatic disease or chemotherapy may cause gastritis or bleeding, and the origin of such bleeding cannot be determined by either endoscopy or operation.

Physical examination can help estimate the amount of bleeding. As a rough guide, orthostatic hypotension suggests a 25% loss of blood; shock while recumbent represents at least a 50% loss. Pulse and blood pressure must be monitored closely whenever continued or recurrent bleeding is suspected. Hepatomegaly suggests portal hypertension or metastatic disease. Palpable masses along the course of the colon or in the left hypogastrium suggest colonic or gastric cancer, respectively. Rectal and vaginal examinations are essential.

Blood tests include serial hematocrit or hemoglobin levels, red blood cell and platelet counts, and smears for red blood cell, white blood cell, and platelet morphologic studies. Microcytosis can indicate chronic bleeding, even if acute bleeding is superimposed. Determinations of prothrombin time and partial thromboplastin time should be performed routinely; they are essential if the patient has been taking anticoagulants or has jaundice.

Endoscopy includes esophagogastroduodenoscopy, anoscopy, rigid sigmoidoscopy, flexible sigmoidoscopy, and colonoscopy. Both upper and lower GI endoscopy can be used with exploratory laparotomy. Endoscopy is most valuable when the patient is bleeding slowly enough to allow adequate observation.

Selective arteriography is an important aid in identifying the bleeding site, provided blood loss is ≥ 1 mL/min. This procedure helps localize lesions in the stomach, small bowel, and colon and may be combined with exploratory laparotomy.

Two types of **radionuclide studies** are generally used in adults. The most common requires withdrawing about 10 mL of blood, labeling it with a technetium radionuclide, and reinjecting it into the patient. The procedure, which takes about an hour, demonstrates the bleeding site if the loss is ≥ 1 mL/min, even if bleeding is intermittent. The second study involves injecting the patient with a prepared sulfur colloid radionuclide. If the patient is bleeding, the bleeding site can be identified in a few minutes. Both methods are less useful with upper GI bleeding because of the amount of background scatter. Technetium scans occasionally demonstrate Meckel's diverticulum because of selective uptake by gastric mucosa, which may be present in the lesion; however, this is a rare cause of bleeding in geriatric patients.

Barium contrast studies can be sensitive and specific diagnostic evaluations that can be used when endoscopy, selective arteriography, and radionuclide studies are not available. The barium upper GI series, often with small bowel visualization together with air contrast barium enema studies, can identify potential bleeding sources. Commonly identified lesions include peptic ulcer, gastritis, gastroesophageal varices, polyps, diverticula, or GI tumors. These barium studies do not provide histologic diagnosis by biopsy, nor do they specifically identify that bleeding originates with the lesion. Despite these limitations, definitive treatments can be designed, based on these studies when other diagnostic studies are not available. When endoscopy, selective arteriography, or other more specific studies are available, they should be used, and barium studies should be delayed. The presence of barium in the GI tract can obscure the findings of these more sensitive and specific studies.

Exploratory laparotomy is the definitive diagnostic method, although it was used more frequently before arteriography became available. Examination of the abdominal viscera, especially the small bowel, can identify many lesions (eg, angiomas, leiomyomas, and diverticula). If a long peroral endoscope is introduced during the laparotomy, the whole small-bowel lumen can be examined. Likewise, selective arteriography during exploratory laparotomy can help identify bleeding lesions in the small bowel, allowing resection of the involved segment.

Treatment

The physician first needs to decide whether hospital admission is necessary. Treating someone with more than minor rectal bleeding, tarry stools, or hematemesis as an outpatient is dangerous. Bleeding assumed to be from hemorrhoids or other limited rectal bleeding requiring only diagnostic colonoscopy or barium enema may be treated in an outpatient setting, provided time is not lost making the diagnosis.

Often, determining whether bleeding originates in the upper or lower GI tract is difficult. Thus, ongoing diagnostic evaluation is essential while bleeding continues. A nasogastric tube should be passed and the gastric contents aspirated. If the aspirate is grossly bloody or guaiac-positive, iced saline solution is used to irrigate the stomach until bleeding slows significantly. Then esophagogastroduodenoscopy is performed. However, if the gastric aspirate remains bright red, a choice must be made between selective arteriography and immediate exploratory laparotomy; patients with massive GI bleeding can experience cardiovascular collapse in the angiographic suite.

Essentially the same therapeutic choices are applicable, whether the bleeding site is in the stomach, duodenum, or colon. The specific choice depends on the patient's age and cardiovascular status, the rate and quantity of blood loss, and the treatment modalities available. Options include expectant treatment by medical measures (eg, intubation, ice water instillation), endoscopy using electrocoagulation or laser, selective arteriography with local or peripheral vasopressin infusion or embolization, and surgery.

When the bleeding site has been identified using selective arteriography, the catheter may be used to inject vasopressin directly. This injection immediately controls bleeding in > 80% of cases. Peripheral vasopressin 0.4 u./min is also an option, although cardiac arrhythmias occur more frequently, and caution is necessary. If the vasopressin infusion fails, embolization with Gelfoam or coils may be attempted. However, the danger of postembolic necrosis arising in either the wall of a viscus or the liver from a dislodged embolus must be recognized.

At times, bleeding is so massive that emergency surgery is the only reasonable treatment. If a patient is apparently bleeding from the stomach or the colon but the bleeding site cannot be determined and severe blood loss continues, the only option is to perform a blind gastrectomy or colectomy. Fortunately, these situations are not as common today as they were in the past.

In one prospective study of gastroduodenal bleeding, the mortality rate was extremely low for patients < 60 yr who were treated either medically or surgically. For patients > 60 yr, the mortality rate was about 0% if they underwent immediate surgery and 15% if they were first treated medically and then surgically for persistent or recurrent hemorrhage.

SPECIFIC BLEEDING SITES

Gastrointestinal bleeding may originate in the esophagus, stomach, small intestine, colon, liver, or pancreas or at an abdominal aortic graft site.

Esophagus

Varices secondary to portal hypertension are not common in the elderly. When they occur, the primary treatment is sclerotherapy. Recurrent bleeding in a patient who is a reasonable surgical risk is treated by portosystemic shunt.

Esophagitis often is associated with benign ulcers of the distal esophagus and with a sliding hiatus hernia. Slow but persistent bleeding may occur. Treatment with H_2-receptor blockers or omeprazole usually is very helpful because the ulceration results from acid reflux. However, cancer must be excluded by endoscopy and biopsy. Severe bleeding requiring surgery rarely occurs in the elderly.

Stomach

Mallory-Weiss tears occur radially at or just below the esophagogastric junction and usually result from repeated vomiting. They involve the gastric mucosa and can be identified and often cauterized through the endoscope. When necessary, surgery involves suturing the lacerations.

In the elderly, bleeding is more common from **gastric ulcers** than from **duodenal ulcers,** and controlling bleeding by conservative measures is less certain in gastric than in duodenal ulcers. The usual operation for intractable gastric ulcer hemorrhage is partial gastrectomy with or without vagotomy; for duodenal ulcer bleeding, the usual procedure is ligation of the bleeding vessel and either gastric resection or pyloroplasty and vagotomy.

Anastomotic ulcers may occur just distal to the suture line of previous peptic surgery even after medical measures stop the bleeding. This is particularly common when a vagotomy and posterior gastroenterostomy have been performed. Gastric resection and vagotomy are usually indicated. In the case of vagotomy with either a posterior gastroenterostomy or pyloroplasty, a resection of the gastric antrum is usually sufficient; in the case of vagotomy with antrectomy, further gastric resection is usually necessary and sufficient.

Gastritis is troublesome when it involves the mucous membrane of the entire stomach; if bleeding is not controlled medically, only a radical subtotal gastrectomy with vagotomy or total gastrectomy achieves hemostasis. **Stress ulcers** are similar to gastritis but occur after trauma, surgery, burns, or infections. Nasogastric suction, sucralfate, IV H_2-receptor blockers, omeprazole, or oral antacids to control gastric pH, and IV alimentation are the main medical treatments for bleeding from stress ulcers, gastritis, or peptic ulcer disease. Endoscopic electrocoagulation often is successful. Laser coagulation is dangerous because of the risk of perforation. Nasogastric intubation is necessary to keep the stomach empty, to monitor bleeding, and to administer antacids.

Vascular lesions (cirsoid or racemose aneurysm, or Dieulafoy's disease) are localized arteriovenous malformations and communications in the gastric mucosa. More common in the fundus, they may be impossible to see during endoscopy or surgery unless they are bleeding. If they are bleeding, endoscopic therapy is possible, but high or total gastrectomy is necessary to achieve hemostasis in some patients.

Tumors may cause any type of bleeding. Slow, persistent bleeding is more typical of malignant tumors than benign tumors. Benign leiomyomas often lead to massive hemorrhage that requires emergency laparotomy.

Small Intestine

Tumors, though uncommon in the small intestine, may produce bleeding. Massive bleeding usually results from large leiomyomas. Slow, persistent bleeding is more typical of angiomas.

Diverticular disease of the jejunum may be extensive and can lead to massive bleeding as well as malnutrition.

Varices secondary to portal hypertension at times may involve the small intestine and lead to bleeding. **Multiple arteriovenous malformations** usually are discovered in children but also may develop later in life.

Colon

Anemia may be the first indication of **carcinoma of the cecum.** Many neoplasms are diagnosed on the basis of a positive stool occult blood test. With cancer or a polyp, the amount of visible blood in the stool is usually small.

Angiodysplasia and diverticular disease cause massive bleeding with equal frequency. **Angiodysplasia** refers to small (1 to 5 mm in diameter) single or multiple lesions found chiefly in the cecum or ascending colon and resembling submucous arteriovenous malformations on microscopy (see Ch. 55). **Bleeding diverticula** occur proximal to the splenic flexure in nearly 66% of cases, whereas nonbleeding diverticula occur distal to it in > 90% of cases. The average age at diagnosis for angiodysplasia and bleeding diverticula is 70 yr. The diagnosis of angiodysplasia can be made by colonoscopy in some cases, and the lesions can be destroyed by electrocoagulation. However, if bleeding is profuse, selective arteriography is the best diagnostic modality. The characteristic angiographic finding in angiodysplasia is an early-filling vein in the region of the ileocecal valve. Angiodysplasia can coexist with other colonic lesions such as cancer.

The exact cause of massive bleeding from the colon cannot be determined in about 10% of cases. In these cases, the surgeon performs a subtotal colectomy; the ileorectal anastomosis is placed within reach of the rigid sigmoidoscope, or < 25 cm from the anal verge.

Liver and Pancreas

In nearly all cases, bleeding from the liver and pancreas results from **trauma.** Usually, the diagnosis is made by selective arteriography; during the procedure, embolization may be able to stop the bleeding. If bleeding continues, the vessels must be ligated.

Aortic Graft Site

In older patients, a relatively sudden onset of massive GI bleeding can occur months or years after an abdominal aortic aneurysm has been excised and replaced with a vascular graft. In such cases, a **fistula** between the graft and the small intestine is the most likely cause. Although aortoduodenal fistulas predominate, erosion into any section of the small intestine may occur.

Endoscopy extending to the distal duodenum usually is diagnostic. A membrane between the graft and the intestine can be visualized on CT; if this membrane is absent, graft erosion into the intestinal wall is certain. Arteriography also may be helpful. Treatment is difficult because infection, which accompanies an established fistula, is a strong deterrent to graft replacement. The usual procedure is to remove the graft and establish an extra-anatomic bypass graft, usually between an axillary artery and the distal aorta; the proximal aorta is ligated with suture.

INTESTINAL OBSTRUCTION

A blockage of the alimentary tract between the ligament of Treitz and the anus, preventing the passage of intestinal contents. The obstruction may be acute or chronic, mechanical or adynamic, simple or strangulated; it may occur in the small intestine or the large intestine. Certain features are common to all types, but the choice of therapy depends on a specific diagnosis.

An acute intestinal obstruction has several possible mechanical causes. In the elderly, adhesions and hernias are the most common lesions of the small intestine; cancer predominates in the colon. Adynamic ileus occurs when the absence of reflex nerve stimulation precludes peristalsis in an otherwise normal bowel. In a simple obstruction, the blood supply to the intestine is not compromised; in a strangulated obstruction, the vessels to a segment are occluded, usually by adhesions or bands.

Symptoms and Signs

Symptoms and signs are highly variable and depend chiefly on the site and cause of the obstruction, as well as on the amount of time since onset.

A patient with an acute obstruction characteristically presents with a rapid onset of abdominal cramps, vomiting, distention, and obstipation. Cramps tend to recur about every 3 min and are associated with high-pitched bowel sounds caused by peristalsis (borborygmi). Although wide individual variation may exist, crampy pain usually occurs in the epigastrium with small-bowel obstruction and in the lower abdomen with colonic obstruction; cramps may not occur with high jejunal obstruction. Abdominal distention usually occurs and increases with time. In a simple obstruction, the abdomen is not tender; when abdominal tenderness is elicited and intermittent cramps change to continuous pain, strangulation almost certainly has occurred. Because a simple obstruction can lead to strangulation in as little as 6 h, every patient with a suspected intestinal obstruction should be hospitalized immediately.

With a small-bowel obstruction, vomiting usually occurs early; it may progress to fecal emesis, which can be distinguished from coffee-ground vomit (caused by upper GI hemorrhage) with a guaiac test. With a large-bowel obstruction, vomiting occurs much later or not at all and is usually preceded by distention and cramps. Initially, scanty diarrhea may occur; *complete* obstruction is followed by obstipation.

Diagnosis

The physician performs a complete **physical examination,** placing particular emphasis on the cardiorespiratory system, state of consciousness, vital signs, and urine output. The most important area, of course, is the abdomen. Besides inspecting it for scars from previous abdominal operations and for groin or incisional hernias, the physician auscultates the abdomen for several minutes to detect bowel sounds, palpates it for tenderness or masses, and performs a rectal examination and, in women, a vaginal examination.

A complete blood cell count, blood chemistry tests, and urinalysis should be performed; urine output, degree of hydration, and respiratory status should be determined to establish baselines and to detect impending shock. An indwelling bladder catheter and central venous pressure line are usually advisable.

The **x-ray examination** is extremely important but should be performed after a nasogastric tube has been inserted. Plain abdominal films should be taken in both the supine and upright positions. Lateral decubitus films sometimes are helpful, particularly in cases of external hernias.

With a typical small-bowel obstruction, a ladderlike pattern of distended intestinal loops appears. With strangulation, however, a mass rather than distended loops may be visible. Distended loops may also be absent in a high jejunal obstruction, particularly if the patient has had a gastric resection.

Obstruction of the ascending colon may resemble a small-bowel obstruction when reflux occurs through an incompetent ileocecal valve. Obstruction of the descending colon leads to distention of the entire proximal large bowel because of gas. A single large gas-filled loop of colon in the midabdomen or left upper quadrant usually results from a cecal volvulus, and a single loop of distended sigmoid usually results from a sigmoid volvulus. If gas appears in the intrahepatic bile ducts, a gallstone obstruction is likely.

Colonoscopy or a **barium enema** is used when the site of a colonic obstruction is unclear or when determining whether an obstruction is in the small or large intestine is difficult. Oral barium may be administered to confirm the diagnosis and to localize the site of small-bowel obstruction but should not be used with a colonic obstruction. Barium that remains in the ascending colon above the obstruction becomes inspissated and forms an almost irremovable concrete-like mass.

Differential diagnosis: Many abdominal diseases simulate intestinal obstruction (eg, acute appendicitis, acute cholecystitis, diverticulitis, and pancreatitis). Also, thoracic disease (eg, pneumonia) may cause adynamic ileus.

Treatment

Acute mechanical obstruction calls for surgery, which ideally corrects the underlying cause as well as relieves the obstruction. However, with obstructing carcinoma of the descending colon, often priority must be given to relieving the obstruction. Thus, unless the surgeon is extremely skilled and either can perform a subtotal colectomy and ileocolic or ileorectal anastomosis beyond the cancer site in nondilated bowel or can empty the colon and perform a more limited resection, a proximal colostomy is performed first; resection of the tumor is deferred for 1 or 2 wk. Nasogastric intubation and preoperative antibiotics are needed.

Certain types of intestinal obstruction can be treated by GI intubation and IV alimentation. These types include adynamic ileus, early postoperative obstruction, and recurrent obstruction caused by adhesions from previous intra-abdominal surgery. Some surgeons believe that simple obstruction can be treated by intubation, but others believe that surgery is the treatment of choice for all intestinal obstructions except those mentioned above.

In cases of small-bowel obstruction without evidence of strangulation (ie, audible peristalsis and no abdominal tenderness) but with marked dehydration, several hours may be needed to rehydrate the patient and establish adequate urinary output. However, severely dehydrated patients who have advanced strangulation and are in shock may require immediate surgery.

TYPES OF OBSTRUCTION

An intestinal obstruction may result from adynamic ileus or mechanical blockage.

Adynamic Ileus

This disorder should be suspected in patients with symptoms of obstruction and a history of recent surgery, back injury, severe trauma, or thoracic or renal disease. Peristalsis is absent or infrequent, and abdominal films show gas in scattered areas of the small intestine and colon. Treatment consists of nasogastric suction and IV alimentation. Administration of metoclopramide or vasopressin usually is not beneficial.

In **colonic ileus,** the colon may become enormously distended with gas, but the competent ileocecal valve prevents reflux into the small bowel, which remains collapsed. In **Ogilvie's syndrome,** the distention extends from the cecum to the splenic flexure; because no mechanical obstruction exists at this site, this syndrome also has been called **pseudo-obstruction of the colon.** In these cases, the patient apparently has acute colonic obstruction. A supine x-ray film of the abdomen shows a dilated proximal colon with a cutoff at the splenic flexure and a nondilated distal colon. However, colonoscopy, a barium enema, or surgery reveals no obstructing lesion. The cause of Ogilvie's syndrome is unknown but is thought to be kinking of the colon from proximal distention at the splenic flexure. Usually, advanced colonic ileus can be treated effectively by colonoscopy, which may need to be repeated.

Mechanical Obstruction

A few symptom complexes can lead to early diagnosis. For example, a history of gallstone colic before intestinal obstruction develops or tenderness over the gallbladder and intestinal obstruction probably results from an impacted **gallstone** in the terminal ileum; the stone may not appear on x-ray or may appear considerably smaller than it actually is. However, *gas in the intrahepatic biliary tree is diagnostic*.

A patient with false teeth and a partial gastrectomy is likely to swallow masses of indigestible fiber, such as orange pulp, that form an **obstructing bezoar** in the small intestine. Bezoars also can cause obstruction in patients treated in the intensive care unit with large doses of antacid to prevent bleeding stress ulcers. Compounds containing laxatives, such as magnesium, minimize this risk.

Richter's hernia is a nonpalpable, small inguinal hernia involving strangulation of only part of the intestinal wall in a small hernial sac.

In the elderly, apparent intestinal obstruction accompanied by shock, marked leukocytosis, and variable abdominal tenderness is probably caused by **mesenteric artery occlusion** from thrombosis or embolism. This condition is not a true mechanical obstruction but an ileus caused by aperistalsis. During surgery, carrying out any reparative procedure is usually impossible, although in a few cases, thrombectomy may result in survival.

In elderly patients with signs of intestinal obstruction, a low-grade fever, and slight abdominal tenderness, **acute appendicitis, diverticulitis,** or **cholecystitis** should be suspected. Patients with a single dilated loop of jejunum or transverse colon (the so-called **sentinel loop**) in the epigastrium may have **pancreatitis.**

Fecal impaction is common and rarely produces complete obstruction. More commonly, repeated attempts to evacuate produce small, diarrheal stools. If the condition is detected early by rectal examination, the impaction can be removed digitally or with warm mineral oil retention enemas. If the condition is advanced, the patient may require sedation to facilitate complete removal. Fecal impaction high in the rectum or in the sigmoid can lead to obstruction, perforation, and fecal peritonitis.

VASCULAR DISORDERS OF THE GASTROINTESTINAL TRACT

Common in elderly patients, vascular disorders of the GI tract often require surgery, and the mortality rate is high. The disorders may be classified as ischemic syndromes or aneurysmal disease.

Ischemic Syndromes

These syndromes occur more often in the colon than in the stomach or small intestine because collateral circulation is not as well developed in the colon.

Colonic ischemia may result in gangrene of the colon—a fulminating, undiagnosable abdominal catastrophe—or a milder version called ischemic colitis—a nongangrenous, spontaneously resolving process that results in a fibrous colonic stricture. In the stomach and small intestine, acute mesenteric ischemia from arterial occlusion results from either a thrombosis or an embolus in the celiac axis or superior mesenteric artery and causes midgut necrosis that is almost uniformly lethal. In a series of 136 patients with acute intestinal ischemia treated at Massachusetts General Hospital, only 11 patients (8%) survived. Less commonly, chronic arterial occlusive disease and acute venous thrombosis can lead to ischemic syndromes.

Colonic ischemia: The gangrenous form more likely involves the entire colon with the splenic flexure being most severely affected; in contrast, the milder ischemic colitis more likely involves only a segment of the colon. These syndromes often result from ligation of a major colic artery, aortic reconstructive surgery, thrombi, or emboli; occasionally, they occur without any vascular occlusion. Particularly common in those in their 60s and 70s, these syndromes are frequently associated with cardiovascular disorders (including heart failure, myocardial infarction, and pulmonary embolism) and with severe hemorrhage and the postoperative state. Gangrene of the colon commonly occurs in elderly patients in intensive care units who are experiencing low flow states associated with conditions such as heart failure and sepsis.

Symptoms of a gangrenous colon are generalized abdominal pain (particularly in the left iliac fossa and left hypochondrium), nausea, vomiting, diarrhea, and occasionally frank rectal bleeding. The physical findings suggest an abdominal catastrophe with generalized peritonitis in a patient who is extremely ill. These findings include generalized abdominal tenderness, aperistalsis, and hypotension with cardiovascular collapse. The diagnosis is often confused with perforation of a hollow viscus, fulminant pancreatitis, or mesenteric ischemia. At operation, the colon is edematous and discolored with the worst changes at the splenic flexure. Usually, pulses are easily seen and felt within the small intestine vessels. A subtotal colectomy is required.

Ischemic (nongangrenous) colitis produces milder symptoms and signs, and an exploratory laparotomy usually is not performed. The acute pain is usually in the left iliac fossa; fever and a moderate amount of dark rectal bleeding frequently occur. On examination, localized left-sided peritonitis suggestive of diverticulitis is found. However, these two conditions can be distinguished, based on the degree and quality of the rectal bleeding. The rectal bleeding associated with ischemic colitis usually is bright red, whereas the rectal bleeding associated with diverticulitis is usually occult. Massive rectal bleeding usually occurs in patients with diverticulosis without clinical evidence of diverticulitis. If colonoscopy is performed on a patient with ischemic colitis, the mucosa appears bluish and edematous with mucosal ulcerations and contact bleeding. A barium enema may show thumbprinting, a series of blunt semiopaque projections into the lumen.

Acute mesenteric ischemia: This ischemic syndrome is characterized by a *sudden onset of severe abdominal colic followed by rectal passage of mucus and blood and circulatory collapse within a few hours.* One hallmark of this syndrome is that the severe pain at onset is well out of proportion to the physical findings. However, peritonitis follows promptly with dramatic physical findings and leads to circulatory shock. With the onset of peritonitis, the initial colic is replaced by a generalized abdominal pain, ileus, and distention. Without treatment, this abdominal catastrophe commonly leads to death within 48 h. The key to a successful outcome is very early operative intervention before peritonitis and irreversible shock become established. Unfortunately, in most cases, the presentation is not characteristic, and the diagnosis is made very late.

None of the simple diagnostic tools specifically identify acute mesenteric ischemia. The plain x-ray film of the abdomen shows a pattern of ileus with gas-filled loops of edematous small intestine. By the time the diagnostic finding of air in the mesenteric veins appears, irreversible changes have already taken place. Laboratory findings, except for a nonspecific leukocytosis, are not helpful in making an early diagnosis. *Laparotomy is necessary to make a diagnosis; laparoscopy is not recommended.*

The only definitive treatment is early surgery that reestablishes blood flow by removing the embolus or bypassing the thrombosis in the visceral vessel and that resects the nonviable intestine. Generally, the ends of the remaining intestine should be exteriorized, and primary intestinal anastomoses should not be attempted. A "second look" laparotomy should be performed in 24 h to reevaluate the viability of the remaining intestine. After extensive small intestine resections, parenteral nutrition is necessary, especially in the elderly. Perioperative management is especially difficult and requires close attention to fluid balance, antibiotic therapy, anticoagulation, and frequently, control of metabolic acidosis.

Chronic arterial obstruction in the celiac axis or superior mesenteric artery: Such obstruction can result in profound weight loss and pain suggesting abdominal angina. The pain, which is midabdominal or epigastric, often is exacerbated postprandially. These features make this condition indistinguishable from many other more common abdominal conditions, such as peptic ulcer disease. However, this diagnosis should be considered, and an arteriogram should be performed in elderly patients who have profound weight loss, severe abdominal pain of obscure origin, and no evidence for carcinomatosis.

Acute mesenteric venous thrombosis: In this condition, the patient has generalized superior mesenteric vein thrombosis. Because of the well-developed collateral venous circulation, thromboses affecting less of the superior mesenteric vein seldom have much effect. This syndrome is usually lethal. Occasionally, a near total resection of the small intestine allows survival in children with short-bowel syndrome, but it is particularly devastating in the elderly.

Abdominal Aortic Aneurysms

These aneurysms are common among the elderly, and their frequency and size increase with age. The likelihood that an aneurysm will lead to death is directly related to its size. In an autopsy study from Massachusetts General Hospital, when the aneurysm was < 7 cm in diameter, it caused death in 25% of cases; when the aneurysm was ≥ 10 cm, it caused death in 61% of cases. Since the operative risk for elective aneurysm repair is dramatically lower than the operative risk for rupture, age should not be a determining consideration for elective repair of a large abdominal aortic aneurysm in a healthy elderly patient. Because the operative risk is so high after a rupture, detecting these aneurysms in asymptomatic patients is imperative. Therefore, *no examination of an elderly patient is complete without abdominal palpation for an aneurysm.*

The pain pattern of abdominal aortic aneurysm can be misleading. Usually, the pain is referred to the back and is indistinguishable from general backache. Because the elderly frequently have other causes of backache, a symptomatic abdominal aortic aneurysm can be easily overlooked. *No examination for backache in the elderly is complete without palpation of the abdomen for an aneurysm.*

About 98% of abdominal aortic aneurysms are infrarenal in origin; the remaining ones are thoracoabdominal or involve the celiac axis, the superior mesenteric artery, or the renal arteries. The diagnosis of an infrarenal aneurysm is best made by *gentle* abdominal palpation. (NOTE: A plain abdominal x-ray often shows the thin calcification within the aneurysm wall, but this calcification can be better seen on a lateral abdominal film.) Abdominal ultrasonography is usually helpful; in most cases, diagnosis can be based on ultrasound and physical examination findings. Usually, abdominal CT scans are helpful only to distinguish an infrarenal aneurysm from the more complicated ones.

DISORDERS OF THE LOWER ESOPHAGUS

(See also Ch. 54)

The normal esophagus is lined with squamous epithelium, but islands of gastric mucosa (columnar epithelium) also can appear above the gastroesophageal junction **(Barrett's esophagus).** The lower esophageal sphincter, lying just above this junction, normally exerts about 13 cm of water pressure, preventing gastric reflux. Squamous epithelium is less resistant to the caustic effects of hydrochloric acid than gastric mucosa, so reflux leads to inflammation, erosion, ulceration, and bleeding and later to scarring and stenosis.

Other disorders affecting the esophagus include obstruction (which may result from cancer), webs (Schatzki's ring being the major example), and motility disturbances. Emetic injuries and iatrogenic trauma (chiefly from endoscopy) may lead to perforation. Portal hypertension causes esophageal varices. Large epiphrenic diverticula can form just above the esophageal hiatus.

The distal 5 cm of the esophagus and the cardia share similar disease patterns and symptoms because of their proximity.

Symptoms and Signs

Dysphagia is the most common symptom of esophageal disease. If the patient has had it intermittently for many years, a benign cause is probable; if the patient has had it for a short time and must swallow increasingly smaller food boluses, cancer is the most likely diagnosis. Regurgitation of gastric contents, heartburn, and aerophagia frequently accompany reflux. Pain deep behind the lower end of the sternum suggests esophagitis.

Diagnosis

Endoscopy and biopsy are the most effective methods of diagnosis. Barium studies help identify the site and degree of obstruction or the presence of a hiatus hernia or Schatzki's ring. Reflux usually can be documented by the radiologist. Hiatus hernias are demonstrated best by x-ray and may or may not be associated with reflux. If a perforation is suspected, a diatrizoate meglumine swallow usually shows the site.

Differential diagnosis: Coronary artery disease and esophageal reflux can produce similar symptoms. Esophageal motility studies and 24-h esophageal pH monitoring can help diagnose esophagitis; stress testing and other assessments of cardiac status can rule out coronary artery disease. Prompt relief of pain by nitroglycerin suggests angina pectoris.

Treatment

Depending on the diagnosis, treatment may consist of dietary modification, dilations with bougies, fracture of webs by endoscopy, laser sclerotherapy, or surgery. Surgery, which may be either curative or palliative, is emphasized in the following discussion of the various disorders.

SPECIFIC DISORDERS

Lower esophageal disorders that may require surgery include cancer, esophagitis, perforation, motility disturbances, Schatzki's ring, epiphrenic diverticula, and esophageal varices.

Cancer

(See also NEOPLASMS OF THE ESOPHAGUS in Ch. 60)

Many carcinomas that arise in the cardia or in hiatus hernias invade the lower esophagus; these adenocarcinomas appear to have a slightly better prognosis than squamous cell lesions, which account for 65% of esophageal malignancies. An estimated 10% of patients with Barrett's esophagus eventually develop cancer.

Carcinomas metastasize to lymph nodes (including the left gastric, thoracic, and cervical nodes) and to liver, lung, and bone marrow. If scans and x-rays show no metastases, the lesion is approached through a left thoracotomy. At least 5 cm and preferably 10 cm of apparently normal esophagus above the lesion and 5 cm of stomach below it are resected. Continuity is restored by anastomosing the esophagus to the distal stomach or, occasionally, by using a segment of colon to bridge the gap.

Although the overall cure rate for esophageal cancer is only about 5%, selected series show nearly a 25% survival rate in patients with cancer of the distal portion. Because the cure rate is so low, experimental protocols have been designed that combine radiation therapy and chemotherapy, using cisplatin and other drugs; in some cases remarkable tumor regression has occurred.

Esophageal cancer causes an especially miserable death, chiefly because patients cannot swallow their saliva. Therefore, palliative procedures are frequently offered, even when cure is unlikely. Resection and esophagogastrectomy, when possible, are preferred. If the tumor cannot be resected, the favored procedure is colonic bypass, in which the esophagus is left in place. Rigid tubes (Celestin's or Souttar's) may be inserted through the tumor, but they tend to become displaced and cause perforation, so they are not often used. Laser therapy or radiation therapy and chemotherapy can debulk obstructing tumors. Gastrostomy allows feeding but does not alleviate dysphagia.

Esophagitis

Although acid reflux is by far the most common cause of esophagitis, bile reflux frequently occurs after total gastrectomy unless bile diversion has been accomplished by a Roux-en-Y anastomosis or enteroenterostomy. In patients who have not had antireflux surgery, symptoms depend on the amount of reflux. Pain is most common when the patient lies flat but also may occur when he bends over. Conservative therapy, effective in most cases, includes losing weight, elevating the head at night using at least two pillows, restricting food intake after 6 PM, and taking H_2-receptor blockers, omeprazole, or antacids before bedtime. Acid reflux can be more effectively controlled with full doses of H_2-receptor blockers, such as cimetidine 300 mg qid or ranitidine 150 mg bid, or with omeprazole 20 mg daily. Intractable esophagitis requires surgery.

Perforation

Iatrogenic injury: Perforation by an endoscope may occur either in the proximal or the distal esophagus. The perforation is almost always above the diaphragm rather than below it. Perforation is rare with flexible scopes but not with rigid scopes, which still must be used in many circumstances. Overinflation of Sengstaken-Blakemore tubes, balloon dilation for achalasia, and surgery on the upper stomach or esophagus (eg, vagotomy or hiatus hernia repair) may also cause perforation.

Perforation is an emergency. Pain and fever are the important clinical findings in a patient with a previously undetected perforation; if they develop after the procedures mentioned, esophageal perforation is the probable cause. An x-ray of the chest probably shows mediastinal emphysema, and later extensive subcutaneous emphysema involving chest, neck, abdomen, and scrotum may occur. A diatrizoate meglumine swallow should be performed immediately; it will nearly always show an existing perforation. The perforation must be closed immediately, and the closure reinforced by the stomach, a flap of parietal pleura, or a muscle flap from the chest wall. Drainage is provided by a chest tube.

Emetic injury: Vomiting when the stomach is full can significantly increase the pressure in the lower esophagus, particularly if there is a concurrent hiatus hernia and reflux. Such pressure can rupture the distal esophagus, leading to rapid contamination of the left pleural cavity **(Boerhaave's syndrome)** or peritonitis. Complaints of severe pain in the left upper quadrant, chest, or shoulder after vomiting or subcutaneous emphysema mandates the same emergency diagnostic and therapeutic measures as required for iatrogenic perforation.

Motility Disturbances

These common disturbances produce dysphagia and severe substernal pain secondary to esophageal spasm. **Achalasia,** a condition in which ganglion cells are absent near the esophagogastric junction, prevents smooth muscle from relaxing. The treatment of early, uncomplicated achalasia is pneumatic dilation, which can be repeated as required. If it fails, or if achalasia is untreated, enormous esophageal distention or an epiphrenic diverticulum may develop. Aspiration of food from the lower esophagus or diverticulum may occur. Rarely, attempted balloon dilation of the sphincter has led to rupture. Surgical resection of a diverticulum and myomotomy of the distal esophagus are the usual procedures. Often, an antireflux procedure is also performed to prevent later esophagitis.

Disorders of peristalsis can be diagnosed by special techniques using multiple balloons. Some motility disorders respond to calcium channel blockers; others, such as scleroderma, are progressive. In some cases, an antireflux procedure is necessary.

Schatzki's Ring

A ring of mucosa and submucosa that causes narrowing at the esophagogastric junction. Because it denotes the proximal end of the stomach, it proves the presence or absence of a hiatus hernia but not of reflux. The ring tends to become smaller with advancing age. When the lumen becomes as small as 15 mm, intermittent dysphagia may occur; a luminal diameter of 11 mm is considered dangerous. When Schatzki's ring is symptomatic, dilation with bougies is usually successful. If surgery is necessary, the ring can be broken with a finger inserted into the esophagus, and any associated hernia can be repaired.

Epiphrenic Diverticula

These diverticula develop just above the diaphragm and are associated with hyperactivity of the lower esophageal sphincter and often with a sliding hiatus hernia. Some may become ≥ 5 cm in diameter. Not only are they subject to food retention and infection, but also cancer may develop in the mucosa. If pain or regurgitation occurs, excision is necessary; if the diverticula are asymptomatic, they probably should be followed up endoscopically. Accompanying distal esophageal spasm is treated with pneumatic dilation.

Esophageal Varices

Very few patients with portal hypertension and esophageal varices reach old age. The initial symptom is usually massive upper GI hemorrhage. Treatment is immediate endoscopic sclerotherapy. If this treatment is not available, a Sengstaken-Blakemore tube is inserted; the balloon is inflated for 24 to 48 h and then deflated. Sclerotherapy is then performed. If sclerotherapy fails, a portosystemic shunt may be performed in patients who are good surgical risks.

DISORDERS OF THE STOMACH AND DUODENUM

Disorders of the stomach and duodenum that may require surgery include diaphragmatic hernias, peptic ulcer disease and its complications, stress ulcers, gastritis, stomach cancer, duodenal tumors, and diverticula of the stomach and duodenum. Stomach cancer and duodenal cancer are discussed in Ch. 60.

Diaphragmatic Hernia

The stomach is involved in nearly every type of diaphragmatic hernia except congenital hernias. In the most common type, the sliding hiatus hernia, the portion of the stomach just below the esophagogastric junction and the abdominal esophagus rise into the chest. In paraesophageal hernia, the esophagogastric junction remains in place, but the stomach rises alongside the esophagus. Combinations of sliding and paraesophageal hernias also occur.

Sliding hiatus hernia: A small hiatus hernia can be detected in most older people. Such hernias are almost always asymptomatic, unless the patient has reflux esophagitis. However, mild flatulence or substernal discomfort may occur, and if a Schatzki's ring tightens to a diameter < 11 mm, esophageal obstruction can develop.

The diagnosis of a sliding hiatus hernia is based on barium contrast studies and endoscopy. The differential diagnosis includes coronary artery disease, esophageal spasm, gallbladder disease, gastritis, peptic ulcer, and functional complaints for which no organic cause can be found. Symptoms that appear suddenly always suggest malignant disease, not only of the esophagus but of an abdominal organ. Consequently, an abdominal rather than a thoracic approach is used for repair because an unexpected tumor may be found.

Asymptomatic hernias should not be repaired. Mild complaints are treated by conservative measures, including a bland diet, weight reduction, antacids, and nighttime elevation of the head and chest on several pillows.

Controversy continues concerning the best surgical procedure for hiatus hernia associated with esophagitis. Each procedure restores a proper length of abdominal esophagus and strengthens the lower esophageal sphincter. In the Nissen repair, the fundus of the stomach is wrapped around the lower esophagus. In the Belsey repair, a valve is created by suturing the stomach to the anterior surface of the esophagus. In the Hill repair, the part of the stomach at the gastroesophageal junction is anchored to the median arcuate ligament, which lies just anterior to the aorta; a valve is created by anterior sutures through the junction, drawing it back toward the ligament. The abdominal approach is used more frequently, but some surgeons prefer the thoracic approach. The more recent Angelchik procedure uses a plastic collar around the lower esophagus to prevent reflux; migration of the prosthesis and late stenosis have limited the usefulness of this method.

Regardless of the procedure, postoperative recurrences after several years are not uncommon because of the negative intrathoracic pressure that occurs with every inspiration. Nevertheless, surgery offers great relief for long periods in selected patients. In a few cases, esophagitis is so marked that resection and replacement with a section of jejunum or colon is necessary. In some older patients, recurrent strictures at the gastroesophageal junction can be treated by periodic dilation with bougies.

Paraesophageal hernia: These hernias can be huge, with the entire stomach in the chest. Both the esophagogastric junction and the pylorus may be level with the diaphragm as the gastric fundus rotates upward into the left or right side of the chest. On chest x-ray, a large gas bubble can be seen and the diagnosis is confirmed by barium contrast studies.

Paraesophageal hernias can cause complete pyloric obstruction and gastric incarceration, strangulation, and perforation. Unless the patient is a poor surgical risk, these hernias should be repaired.

Traumatic rupture of the diaphragm: After an injury to the left side of the chest or the left upper abdominal quadrant, a chest x-ray may show a gas bubble above the diaphragm on the left side. The possibility of a diaphragmatic rupture should be suspected, and barium contrast studies should be performed. The stomach is the usual organ found to be injured, but the colon, spleen, and even other viscera can be identified in some cases. Immediate repair is necessary.

Peptic Ulcer Disease

(See also Ch. 54)

The introduction of H_2-receptor blockers has shifted the treatment of uncomplicated ulcers strongly toward pharmacologic control. Today, peptic ulcer surgery is performed essentially for unhealed gastric ulcers, anastomotic ulcers, and complications of ulcers. In a recent study, 23% of those requiring surgery for peptic ulcer were ≥ 70 yr.

Gastric and anastomotic ulcers: Gastric ulcers present special problems because a small percentage of malignant ulcers appear benign. Endoscopic biopsies cannot always differentiate; any persistent ulcer must be regarded with suspicion and treated surgically. Because benign ulcers heal more slowly in the elderly, if the patient has no complications, at least 6 wk of medical treatment should be allowed before resection.

Anastomotic ulcers frequently cause hemorrhage. The best method of diagnosis is endoscopy; often barium studies do not reveal these ulcers. Anastomotic ulcers respond poorly to conservative therapy. The most effective surgery is gastric resection with vagotomy.

Complications of ulcers: Elderly patients are at particular risk for the major complications: hemorrhage, perforation, and obstruction. Though unusual in the elderly, intractable pain may also develop.

The most common complication of peptic ulcers in the elderly is **hemorrhage.** In a recent study, 38% of all surgery for massive hemorrhage from ulcers was performed in patients ≥ 70 yr. Methods of diagnosis are discussed under GASTROINTESTINAL BLEEDING, above.

The choice of treatment is controversial, but some authorities believe that geriatric patients who have lost ≥ 5 u. of blood have a better chance of survival with early surgery—ie, gastric resection for gastric ulcer and either gastric resection or vagotomy-pyloroplasty with ligation of the bleeding vessel for duodenal ulcer. Alternative treatments include angiographic control with vasopressin or embolization, which may be hazardous in ulcer disease, and endoscopic thermal coagulation or laser coagulation of the bleeding vessel. The laser can be hazardous because of the danger of perforation.

The second most common complication of peptic ulcer disease is **perforation.** Often the typical clinical finding of abdominal rigidity is absent, and the patient may have only minimal tenderness on examination. This paucity of clinical findings may inordinately delay diagnosis. Acute ulcer perforation usually produces acute upper abdominal pain followed in a few hours by a rapid progression of shock to cardiovascular collapse. An x-ray taken with the patient erect usually reveals free gas beneath the diaphragm. In doubtful cases, a diatrizoate meglumine swallow demonstrates extravasation from the stomach or duodenum.

The prognosis is poor in older patients. About 30% of perforations occur in those ≥ 70 yr, and the overall mortality rate is 20%.

Immediate surgery is necessary except in the few patients who are so ill from other causes that they probably would not survive laparotomy. For example, a patient who sustains a perforated ulcer a day or two after an acute myocardial infarction can be treated by nasogastric intubation and suction as well as antibiotics if the perforation is small or apparently walled off. Treatment involves primarily closure of the perforation. However, because the incidence of ulcer recurrence is high, if optimal operating conditions prevail, either gastric resection or pyloroplasty combined with vagotomy should also be performed.

Pyloric **obstruction** occurs from cicatricial stenosis of a chronic duodenal ulcer or from gastric ulcers located near the pylorus. Symptoms include recurring vomiting, weight loss, and metabolic alkalosis. Attempts must be made to rule out a malignant obstructive lesion. A gastric resection with a vagotomy is preferred; however, in the elderly, vagotomy may produce gastric paresis.

Intractable pain is unusual in older patients with peptic ulcer disease. Conservative therapy is not likely to be successful; gastric resection is the treatment of choice. Older patients who have been receiving long-term H_2-receptor blocker therapy often develop prolonged postoperative gastric stasis if vagotomy is also performed.

Stress Ulcers

Stress ulcers are peptic ulcers, usually gastric, resulting from stress. Typically, they are small (1 to 3 mm) and superficial (limited to the mucosa). Frequently, a patient has many stress ulcers, and they are associated with gastritis. Predisposing causes include recent serious operations, trauma, shock, infections, and burns. Although the exact cause is not clear, certain factors besides the predisposing causes enhance the development of these dangerous ulcers: gastric dilation, ventilatory insufficiency, and a reduction in the mucosa's ability to withstand the effects of hydrochloric acid. The important symptom is hemorrhage, which can be massive and life threatening. Most of these lesions are encountered in intensive care units.

Because treatment is difficult and often unsatisfactory, prophylaxis is extremely important. The stomach should be kept as empty as possible with a nasogastric sump tube placed on suction. Pulmonary function, if not adequate as determined by blood gas values, must be aided by intratracheal intubation and assisted ventilation, possibly including positive end-expiratory pressure (PEEP).

One of several methods may be used to reduce the level of gastric acid and maintain the intragastric pH at ≥ 4.0. An effective method is to give oral doses of an antacid–anti-gas combination drug. Before each administration, a nurse withdraws acid from the stomach and measures the pH to keep it between 5 and 7. This method requires intensive nursing care; therefore, another method—administering cimetidine 300 mg IV q 6 h or by constant drip—is usually used, although it may be slightly less effective. Since cimetidine may cause confusion in the elderly, parenteral ranitidine 50 mg q 6 to 8 h may be substituted. Studies have shown that sucralfate effectively prevents bleeding by creating a physical barrier to acid and pepsinogens. Sucralfate has a theoretical advantage because it does not raise the pH of the stomach. Therefore, the bactericidal effect of natural gastric acidity could keep the stomach relatively free of bacteria.

If prophylaxis has not been used or if gastric bleeding occurs despite treatment, the possibility of a typical peptic ulcer must be considered. Endoscopy is indicated to determine the exact source. Small bleeding points may be treated by electrocoagulation. If a typical peptic ulcer is found, treatment should be administered as discussed in Ch. 54. When stress bleeding is encountered, the source of persistent sepsis should be sought and then drained without delay.

If multiple bleeding points are found and bleeding continues after cauterization, selective arteriography should be used; if possible, the catheter should be placed in the left gastric artery rather than the celiac axis. This procedure confirms the diagnosis if bleeding continues. Selective vasopressin infusion stops the bleeding in about 80% of cases. If bleeding is not stopped, surgery is required, as a last resort; either total gastrectomy or high subtotal gastrectomy with vagotomy may be selected.

Gastritis

(See also Ch. 54)

Frequently, gastritis leads to massive upper GI hemorrhage. In most uncomplicated cases, gastritis can be handled medically. All gastric irritants should be eliminated; the common ones include aspirin, alcohol, ibuprofen, and excessive caffeine intake. Smoking is contraindicated (see also GASTROINTESTINAL BLEEDING, above).

Treatment frequently includes an antacid and an H_2-receptor blocker or omeprazole. Sucralfate may be given 1 gm qid on an empty stomach; if it is given with an H_2-receptor blocker, the activity of the H_2-receptor blocker is reduced. Massive bleeding can usually be treated with selective arteriography and an injection of vasopressin into the left gastric artery. Endoscopy is not likely to be satisfactory because many bleeding points usually exist. Every attempt should be made to avoid surgery. If it is required, distal gastrectomy and vagotomy can be performed if just the distal stomach is involved. If gastritis extends throughout the stomach, total gastrectomy may be necessary.

Diverticula of the Stomach and Duodenum

In the stomach, these lesions are rare and tend to occur on the lesser curvature just below the diaphragm. In the duodenum, they are common and often occur near Oddi's sphincter; in some cases, the common duct empties into a diverticulum. Unless symptoms clearly arise from diverticula, they are best left untreated. Surgical extirpation is difficult and may be dangerous. If food becomes impacted in a large duodenal diverticulum, gastric resection with a Roux-en-Y anastomosis is probably safer than excision of the diverticulum.

DISORDERS OF THE JEJUNUM AND ILEUM

Disorders of the jejunum and ileum may exist alone or may coexist with disorders of other viscera (such as gastroenteritis or Crohn's disease). Many of these disorders are treated medically, but some are also treated surgically and must be considered in the differential diagnosis of surgical abdomen.

Disorders of the small intestine may be caused by congenital, acquired, or iatrogenic factors; inflammatory or toxic agents; malabsorption; motility defects; or tumors. Tumors of the small intestine are discussed in Ch. 60.

Congenital Lesions

Meckel's diverticulum, the only congenital lesion common in geriatric patients, is nearly always an incidental finding, and symptoms are rare in the elderly.

Acquired Lesions

The most common acquired lesion is **diverticulosis,** in which saclike projections of the mucosa protrude through the muscularis of the bowel. These projections are most common in the jejunum of older patients. Diverticulosis may be asymptomatic or may be associated with massive bleeding, malabsorption, or inflammation (diverticulitis). In cases of massive bleeding, locating the involved bowel segment is desirable. Selective arteriography, which may be combined with exploratory laparotomy, is the best diagnostic tool. It allows resection of the shortest possible segment of bowel. Perforation is uncommon, but if it occurs, resection and reanastomosis are the procedures of choice (see also Ch. 55).

Iatrogenic Lesions

The most common iatrogenic lesion problems are excessive enterectomy, radiation enterocolitis, and blind loop syndrome. For a discussion of excessive enterectomy, see Malabsorption, below.

Radiation enterocolitis: Radiation therapy is used frequently for cancer of the bladder, prostate, rectum, colon, and female genitalia. The small intestine is damaged by 50 Gy; the colon is slightly more resistant.

The symptoms of radiation enteritis are indistinguishable from those of chronic intestinal obstruction. Radiation colitis produces bleeding and diarrhea. Conservative therapy usually is indicated at the outset because some acute symptoms may subside with IV alimentation and restriction of oral intake.

Minor colonic ulceration may be treated with a bland diet and psyllium hydrophilic mucilloid. Surgery to treat radiation colitis is often unsuccessful because radiation diminishes the intestinal blood supply and anastomoses heal poorly unless made in normal intestine. Furthermore, because dense pelvic adhesions are likely to be encountered, dissection is arduous; leakage and fistula formation are occasional sequelae. Thus, resection may be difficult or impossible, and palliative enteroenterostomy may be required. However, in severe cases, resection of the involved segment with reanastomosis may be possible; in other cases, a permanent colostomy may have to be combined with resection of the involved rectum or colon.

Blind loop syndrome: This syndrome develops when a surgeon creates a bowel loop in which intestinal contents collect and stagnate. Poor drainage leads to secondary infection and occasionally to deficiency syndromes. The typical example is a side-to-side anastomosis that sidetracks a long segment of small intestine. Similar problems may occur after a gastrectomy in which the terminal ileum rather than the jejunum is erroneously anastomosed to the stomach. Long afferent loops after a gastric resection and gastrojejunostomy may lead to major dilation of the afferent loop **(afferent loop syndrome).** In some cases, side-to-side small-intestine anastomosis is followed by marked dilation of the blind ends of the two segments.

Typical symptoms include indigestion, gas, cramps, and diarrhea. Antibiotic therapy (eg, tetracycline) has not been satisfactory.

Inflammatory Lesions

Diseases that mimic surgical emergencies are common. Acute gastroenteritis with its typical acute onset, nausea, vomiting, and diarrhea can mimic a surgical abdomen. Persistent symptoms, localized tenderness, and silent abdomen in elderly patients with abdominal scars or evidence of hernias are signals to reconsider the diagnosis of gastroenteritis.

Unusual infections can also mimic a surgical abdomen. Giardiasis is endemic to some areas of the USA. *Yersinia* infections can cause acute ileitis that is not diagnosed until a laparotomy is performed. Acute amebiasis is a threat to travelers and is endemic to many areas of the USA. Probably the most common and dangerous of all infections is salmonellosis. Patients treated with antibiotics and those receiving immunosuppressive drugs are at particular risk of developing salmonellosis.

Toxic Lesions of the Intestine

Organisms that produce toxins (eg, staphylococci, *Vibrio cholerae, Campylobacter* spp, and *Clostridium perfringens*) can cause severe enteritis or colitis. From the surgeon's viewpoint, the most common disease is pseudomembranous enterocolitis from *Clostridium difficile*.

Malabsorption

Malabsorption may result from gastrointestinal surgery or from an underlying disease. Nutritional deficiencies after a **gastrectomy** result from diminished absorption of iron, calcium, fat, and protein and are related to the extent of gastrectomy and the type of anastomosis. Total gastrectomy does not necessarily lead to inanition, but specific nutritional deficiencies (eg, loss of intrinsic factor) must be treated. After an **enterectomy,** absorption of all nutrients is diminished, depending on the extent of resection. As a general rule, 1/3 of the jejunum and ileum may be excised without seriously impairing nutrient absorption. More radical resection is tolerated poorly, and adults who have lost 2/3 of the small intestine usually develop severe metabolic problems. Total parenteral nutrition has improved survival. After **resection of the distal ileum,** absorption of vitamin B_{12} and cholesterol is reduced. A loss of 30 cm usually is well tolerated, but regular supplementation with parenteral vitamin B_{12} (cyanocobalamin) may be needed after more extensive resection. **Right colectomy** temporarily diminishes the absorption of water and some electrolytes. **Total proctocolectomy** produces only temporary malabsorption.

Gastrinomas produce the **Zollinger-Ellison syndrome,** which causes diarrhea and malabsorption. Unexplained diarrhea should suggest other **neuroendocrine tumors of the pancreas or the gut,** such as somatostatinomas or vipomas. Malabsorption of fat may be an early sign of **pancreatic cancer. Crohn's disease** can lead to malabsorption from an inflamed mucosa or a surgically shortened bowel. Fistulas from the stomach or gastrocolic and proximal enterocolic fistulas, most commonly caused by peptic ulcer disease and colonic cancer, respectively, can produce malabsorption.

Symptoms common to most of these syndromes are diarrhea and inanition. Gas, abdominal distention, nausea, and cramps generally develop as well.

Celiac disease (nontropical sprue) is a gluten-induced enteropathy characterized by atrophy of intestinal villi. Cramps, diarrhea, and abdominal distention may mimic intestinal obstruction (see Ch. 58). In chronic cases, **lymphoma** or **carcinoma** of the small intestine may develop and must be considered in elderly patients.

Lactase deficiency produces abdominal distention, gas, bloating, nausea, and diarrhea after ingestion of lactose-containing dairy products. Varying degrees of lactase deficiency occur in nearly all geriatric patients.

Motility Disorders

Intestinal motility is affected by many agents, including laxatives, antidiarrheal drugs, poisons, and food additives (eg, monosodium glutamate and sodium sulfite). Ingesting mushrooms and shellfish can lead to severe diarrhea.

Scleroderma is a well-recognized cause of diminished intestinal motility. In the small intestine, it usually involves the duodenum, leading to megaduodenum. A surgical bypass of the duodenum may provide relief, but other segments of the intestine may become involved. Scleroderma of the colon produces severe constipation with episodes of fecal blockage that usually can be relieved by laxatives. Diagnosis is aided by barium enema, which often shows short, broad-based diverticula scattered throughout the colon.

Chagas' disease, common in Brazil and other tropical areas of South America, is caused by infection with *Trypanosoma cruzi*. The disease leads to megaesophagus, megacolon, and megaduodenum. For extreme distention of the colon and unremitting constipation, colectomy may be needed.

Uncommon motility disorders include amyloidosis, mesenteric lipomatosis, desmoid tumors of the mesentery, and Whipple's disease. **Amyloidosis of the mesentery** produces symptoms of intestinal obstruction, but laparotomy usually shows such wide infiltration that surgical cure is impossible. **Mesenteric lipomatosis** also produces symptoms of intestinal obstruction; if the disease is not too extensive, a bypass of the mesenteric mass may be possible, but excision usually is not. **Desmoid tumors of the mesentery** usually cannot be resected. Improvement after vitamin C use has been reported. **Whipple's disease** (intestinal lipodystrophy) occurs in men and usually is associated with arthritis, diarrhea, and fat malabsorption. It is caused by a bacillary infection, and diagnosis should be confirmed by peroral intestinal biopsy before surgery.

Neuroendocrine tumors of the gut are a diagnostic challenge because they can produce a wide variety of symptoms. The primary tumor may be located near the intestine or in the pancreas, liver, or elsewhere. About ⅔ are functioning tumors producing several peptides and amines, some of which may cause colic and diarrhea. Malignant carcinoid, insulinoma, gastrinoma, vipoma, glucagonoma, somatostatinoma, adrenal cortical adenomas, and multiple endocrine adenopathy are among the lesions that have been identified. Though these tumors are rare in older people, they must be considered when no other cause of persistent diarrhea can be found.

Functional disturbances of the jejunum and ileum may account for motility disorders. Many patients complain of some degree of nonspecific constipation or diarrhea combined with abdominal distention and flatulence. In nearly all cases, intestinal transit is normal. Patients with permanent ileostomies do not report these symptoms; thus, most of these functional complaints apparently arise from the colon, not the small intestine.

DISORDERS OF THE APPENDIX

Disorders of the appendix that may require surgery include appendicitis and tumors. Tumors of the appendix are discussed in Ch. 60.

Appendicitis

Characteristically, the initial symptom of appendicitis is epigastric pain, followed by nausea and then by localization of pain and tenderness in the right lower quadrant. Low-grade fever and leukocytosis also typically occur. However, in older patients, pain more often *begins* in the right lower quadrant and may not be severe until perforation occurs. Because the blood supply to the appendix is generally less adequate in older patients, the course of the disease can be fulminant. In some instances, symptoms and signs may be minimal, and chronic infection occurs marked by low-grade fever and poorly defined localization of abdominal signs.

The treatment is appendectomy. Antibiotics should be given before surgery and continued for at least 48 h afterwards. If perforation has already occurred and peritonitis is spreading, the value of drainage is controversial. Simple drainage is recommended for a localized abscess, and appendectomy should follow in a few weeks. In nearly all other cases, however, the appendix is removed during the initial operation.

In the elderly, appendicitis occasionally occurs in association with colon cancer. Low-grade obstruction can lead to appendiceal distention that mimics true appendicitis. If the patient who has had a simple appendectomy fails to recover promptly, the colon should be examined by endoscopy or barium enema.

DISORDERS OF THE COLORECTUM

The most common colorectal disorders requiring surgery in the elderly are cancer, volvulus, diverticular disease, and angiodysplasia. (Diverticular disease and angiodysplasia are discussed in Ch. 55.) Ulcerative colitis is an uncommon but serious problem.

Colorectal Cancer

(See also Ch. 60)

Cancers of the colon and upper rectum preferably are treated by segmental resection and reanastomosis in a single operation. Multiple tumors may require subtotal colectomy. However, because low ileorectal anastomoses may lead to severe diarrhea in older patients, an adequate amount of large bowel should be left when possible. Preferably, wide excision of the mesentery and regional lymph nodes is performed concurrently. The distal line of resection preferably should be at least 2 cm beyond the tumor.

Cancers of the middle and lower rectum are more problematic in the elderly because the operation most likely to cure—abdominoperineal resection with permanent colostomy—requires lifestyle changes that may be unsatisfactory to some patients. Fortunately, use of a stapling device permits anastomosis lower than is possible with hand-suturing techniques. However, the anal sphincter can be preserved in only about 5% of lower rectal cancers.

Favorable cancers of the lower rectum can be treated with procedures other than proctectomy (eg, local excision, intracavitary radiation therapy, and electrocoagulation). In cases of carcinoma of the anal canal, remarkable local tumor control with chemoradiation therapy has been demonstrated.

Local excision is satisfactory for polypoid rectal tumors that are not fixed, not > 2 cm in diameter, and of low or moderate differentiation. Specimens must include the entire tumor and underlying rectal wall; the margins of the specimen must be free of cancer. In one series, recurrence was noted in only 8% of cases. However, if the tumor is larger or attached to the underlying muscularis, the recurrence rate rises (about 23% in this study).

Papillon's method of **intracavitary radiation,** in which about 150 Gy are delivered to the tumor through a special scope, was successful in his hands with small, polypoid, freely movable neoplasms. Others have found that attempts to extend Papillon's method to the more common larger, fixed tumors is less effective and usually results in recurrence.

Electrocoagulation also may be effective for small lesions. However, according to one study, when it was used for cancers > 4 cm in diameter, the results were poor.

A combination of radiation therapy and surgical resection is helpful in many patients. Preoperative radiation allows many fixed and otherwise inoperable rectal cancers to be resected. For the usual rectal cancer, postoperative radiation reduces the local recurrence rate in B_2 and C lesions; some studies have shown increased survival. Intraoperative radiation, although still investigational, appears to have a favorable influence, particularly in reducing local recurrence.

Chemotherapy has proved valuable in reducing local recurrence of rectal cancer. Fluorouracil combined with radiation therapy is recommended. Adenocarcinoma of the colorectum responds much less favorably than squamous cell cancer of the perianal area.

Immunotherapy has not played any significant role in the treatment of colorectal cancer.

Follow-up: Patient follow-up after resection of colorectal cancer is not standardized. Nevertheless, the removal of all cancer and polyps from the bowel should be ascertained. Patients should be examined every 6 mo using rigid sigmoidoscopy, guaiac stool tests, and carcinoembryonic antigen (CEA) determinations. Anastomotic recurrences are most common after low rectal anastomoses and can be detected by rigid sigmoidoscopy. The best marker for recurrent colorectal cancer, CEA determinations are especially valuable postoperatively, when a rise above baseline usually indicates recurrence. Other recurrent cancers, particularly those of the rectum, may not produce an elevated CEA level. Some patients can be cured by a second operation for a recurrence diagnosed by a rising CEA level. For at least 5 yr, an annual colonoscopy should be performed. If it is not, an annual barium enema is indicated.

Palliative procedures: In many cases, only palliative procedures are possible, either initially or when cancer recurs. A colostomy may help relieve unremitting tenesmus. Radiation therapy can ease the pain of recurrent rectal cancer. Laser therapy has been used to reduce inoperable rectal tumors and prevent obstruction.

Prognosis: The crude 5-yr survival rate for colorectal cancer is about 50% to 55% in most major medical centers. When deaths from other causes are excluded, the adjusted 5-yr survival rate is 90% for class A disease, about 60% to 70% for class B, 40% for class C, and < 20% for class D. Local recurrence of rectal cancer has been reduced significantly by preoperative and postoperative radiation and chemotherapy; in several recent studies, life expectancy has increased beyond that for patients treated by surgery alone.

Volvulus

Volvulus arises from *a twist of the colon on its mesentery sufficient to produce intestinal obstruction.* An unusually long, mobile mesentery in the affected segment or a lack of fixation is needed for the twist to occur. Unless the obstruction is relieved, it progresses proximally and distally because of gas formation within the occluded segment. As a result, the mesenteric vasculature supplying the involved segment is also occluded, and gangrene and perforation can follow.

Common in the elderly, volvulus is most prevalent in inactive women who have restricted mental capabilities and live in nursing homes. The combination of an unusually large, long colon and inadequate bowel hygiene is a contributing factor.

Sigmoid volvulus: Volvulus occurs most commonly in the sigmoid. Obstipation, cramps, and marked abdominal distention are the usual complaints. Abdominal x-ray shows a large, distended colon. Distention may be limited to the sigmoid loop but occasionally extends above the liver. A barium enema shows the typical bird-beak deformity at the level of the twist.

Usually, a long rectal tube can be passed through a sigmoidoscope (or colonoscope) beyond the obstruction; this can produce explosive deflation. If deflation is incomplete or indications of gangrene are noted, immediate laparotomy is necessary. The colonoscope is useful in determining if gangrene is present.

If deflation occurs, resection of the involved colonic segment is done electively during the same hospitalization, unless overriding reasons to defer surgery exist. If surgery is not performed, the probability of recurrence is very high.

Cecal volvulus: The cecum is another likely site for volvulus. Diagnosis is made on the basis of abdominal cramps, nausea, vomiting, distention, and obstipation. Abdominal x-ray shows a large gas bubble in the midabdomen or the left upper quadrant. Barium enema shows the typical bird-beak deformity in the ascending colon and no reflux into the ileum. *Gangrene supervenes rapidly, so immediate surgery is essential.* If no evidence of gangrene exists, the cecum can be anchored by a cecostomy tube after the twist has been reduced. The alternative for low-risk patients is immediate resection and reanastomosis. When gangrene occurs in a high-risk patient, resection and the formation of ileal and colonic fistulas is necessary. Intestinal continuity is reestablished later.

Ulcerative Colitis
(See also Ch. 55)

This disease is treated primarily by gastroenterologists. The major complications requiring surgery include failure to respond to medical therapy, hemorrhage, toxic megacolon, perforation, and late-developing cancer. Ulcerative colitis often pursues a more virulent course in patients > 60 yr; with late onset, the mortality in severe cases is > 20%.

In severe cases, medical therapy almost always includes corticosteroids. However, these drugs increase the risk of spontaneous perforation, which may be painless and diagnosed only when an upright abdominal x-ray shows subdiaphragmatic gas.

Surgery is usually a subtotal colectomy or a total proctocolectomy, both of which require a permanent ileostomy. The most common cause of mortality is a long delay before surgery.

DISORDERS OF THE ANORECTUM

These disorders occur in the distal 3 cm of rectum, the anal canal, and the area (5 cm in diameter) around the anal verge. Some 50 dermatologic disorders can affect the perianal area, the most common being pruritus ani. Crypts and papillae, which mark the proximal end of the canal, and deep rectal glands may show pathologic changes, such as inflammation. Fecal incontinence is discussed in Chs. 53 and 55, and cancer is discussed in Ch. 60.

Pruritus Ani

Intense chronic itching in the anal region. Pruritus ani is a common symptom with many causes. Many people, in their zeal for cleanliness, excoriate the delicate perianal skin. Using harsh soaps or sensitizing perfumes or deodorizers, wiping excessively with toilet paper, and wearing nylon underwear and tight, warm clothing that promote sweating are the most common exogenous causes. Fungal diseases (eg, epidermophytosis) and parasitism (eg, with pinworms) are examples of infections and infestations that cause pruritus ani. Pruritus may accompany local manifestations of more widespread diseases (eg, psoriasis). Psychologic problems may also contribute to perianal itching.

Some topical drugs used to treat anal diseases (eg, anesthetic compounds such as lidocaine and benzocaine) may produce contact dermatitis. Some oral antibiotics can cause an overgrowth of intestinal *Candida* by suppressing the normal bowel flora, resulting in pruritus from perianal candidiasis.

On physical examination, the perianal area may appear normal, but usually excoriations from involuntary scratching during sleep can be seen. In advanced cases, secondary bacterial infection may be present.

Treatment: The underlying cause of pruritus should be determined and treated. Systemic diseases should be identified, and fungal infections should be treated with over-the-counter topical antifungal powders. Nylon underwear and deodorizers should be avoided. After defecation, the perianal area should be cleaned gently with moist cotton and little wiping. In mild cases caused by simple irritation, such cleansing followed by petroleum jelly application can be very effective. Oral antibiotics should be discontinued, if possible.

The most effective local therapy is hydrocortisone cream; several preparations containing 0.5% or 1% hydrocortisone are available. Usually, the cream is applied only at night, when itching occurs. Severe cases may require application several times a day. The cream is discontinued as soon as itching is controlled. Although recurrence is common, re-treatment in the same manner is successful.

Surgery is rarely indicated. Injection of 95% alcohol is effective but may lead to local necrosis. Excision of skin tags and biopsy of refractory lesions to rule out malignant disease are indicated in refractory cases. Hemorrhoidectomy is not helpful.

Hemorrhoids

Abnormally large or symptomatic conglomerates of blood vessels, supporting tissues, and overlying mucous membrane or anorectal skin. Internal hemorrhoids occur above the anorectal (dentate) line. Prolapsed internal hemorrhoids extend down into the anal canal or through the anus. External hemorrhoids occur below the anorectal line and form so-called piles. A thrombosed external hemorrhoid is a localized clot that either forms in the vein of a hemorrhoid or arises from a ruptured hemorrhoidal blood vessel. Skin tags representing irregular remnants of external hemorrhoids interfere with proper hygiene. Combined hemorrhoids include both internal and external hemorrhoids.

Internal hemorrhoids occur because the vena cava and iliac veins have no valves; thus, erect posture, heavy lifting, and straining all distend the veins. These hemorrhoids develop in three veins, which can be observed anoscopically in the right anterior, right posterior, and left posterior positions.

Internal hemorrhoids may be asymptomatic in the early stages, but later they tend to bleed. The bleeding may vary, but usually it is minimal and appears as bright red blood on the stool or toilet paper. Rarely, significant bleeding occurs; if the blood is retained above the sphincter, a large amount can be expelled at one time. Continued blood loss even in small increments can lead to anemia.

Internal hemorrhoids may lead to external or combined hemorrhoids, which exhibit the same symptoms. Pain occurs only with prolapsed internal hemorrhoids and thrombosed external hemorrhoids. With the latter, perianal pain is sudden and severe.

Diagnosis of internal hemorrhoids requires proctoscopy; hemorrhoids are soft and cannot be reliably detected digitally. Hemorrhoids may be a symptom of a lesion higher in the colorectum. In geriatric patients, rectal bleeding requires a complete examination, including either proctosigmoidoscopy and barium enema or total colonoscopy. External hemorrhoids can be noted on inspection and nearly always indicate the presence of combined hemorrhoids. They are asymptomatic unless a thrombosis or hematoma forms. On inspection, a thrombosed external hemorrhoid appears as a tense, blue subcutaneous mass.

Treatment: Mild hemorrhoids are treated with a soft diet and a bulk producer, such as psyllium hydrophilic mucilloid. Straining at stool and heavy lifting should be avoided.

Hemorrhoidectomy is the most effective treatment for combined hemorrhoids or internal hemorrhoids with major prolapse. Hemorrhoidectomy can relieve symptoms immediately and provides excellent long-term results. Patients' main objection to surgery—fear of postoperative pain—indicates the need for long-lasting local anesthetics at the time of surgery.

Rubber bands can be used in the office to treat internal hemorrhoids that have bled or are mildly prolapsed. The bands are placed under tension around the base of each major hemorrhoid in one or more sessions. The bands should be positioned above the anal canal or great pain results. Several instruments have been devised that make placement relatively simple. Properly performed, the procedure involves no postoperative pain, and long-term results are good.

Sclerotherapy produces good early results, although later secondary hemorrhoids tend to develop. Hemorrhoidectomy of such secondary hemorrhoids is more difficult. Quinine urea hydrochloride 5% is a widely used sclerosing solution.

Cryosurgery and **laser therapy** also have been used, but the small amount of tissue removed and delayed healing have made these modalities less popular.

Subcutaneous injection of a local anesthetic and **evacuation** of a thrombosed external hemorrhoid provide immediate relief. A small section of skin also should be excised to allow adequate drainage in case of further bleeding. If the patient is not seen within 48 h of onset, the clot may be difficult to remove. Some small clots resolve without much discomfort, but large ones, if not evacuated, are slow to improve and are painful for many days. Warm sitz baths and analgesics are beneficial.

Fissures

Longitudinal breaks in the squamous epithelium of the anal canal. The breaks may be superficial or deep; with deep fissures, the internal sphincter is exposed. An external skin tag, called a sentinel pile, often forms at the lower end of a chronic fissure. **Causes** are assumed to be large or hard bowel movements, rough fecal debris, straining at stool, diarrhea, and trauma to the anal canal from rough wiping or foreign bodies (eg, thermometers and enema nozzles).

The major **symptom** is severe pain, which is aggravated by defecation and persists for several minutes afterward. Relative relief occurs until the next bowel movement. In adults, bleeding is rare.

Diagnosis usually can be made by separating the buttocks and having the patient strain so the fissure can be seen. Characteristically, it is in the posterior midline, but occasionally it is in the anterior midline. If the fissure is not visible, it can be seen on anoscopy (if the patient can tolerate the procedure). In some cases, the examination is so painful and associated with so much spasm of the sphincter that local or general anesthesia is needed.

Treatment depends on chronicity. Superficial lesions respond to stool softeners (eg, psyllium hydrophilic mucilloid) and warm sitz baths. Topical agents (not suppositories) may be helpful. Creams or ointments containing local anesthetics or simple protectants may provide relief when applied after bowel movements.

Chronic fissures require one of two surgical procedures. The first consists of anal dilation and excision of the fibrotic margins of the ulcer, the sentinel pile, and the accompanying papilla at the upper end of the fissure. The hazard in older patients is that excessive dilation may tear the sphincter muscle, causing permanent incontinence.

The second, more commonly used, method is internal sphincterotomy, a relatively simple procedure that can be accomplished under local anesthesia. A tight band, which is readily palpable at the lower end of the internal sphincter, is divided, relieving pain and allowing healing. The division must be done on the lateral anus; if it is done posteriorly, permanent incontinence can result. Incontinence after lateral sphincterotomy is uncommon. There are two variants: In one, an incision is made over the internal sphincter through the mucous membrane, and the muscle band is cut under direct vision; in the other, a scalpel is inserted from below and the band is cut beneath the intact mucosa.

Perianal and Ischiorectal Abscesses

Localized collections of pus in cavities resulting from infections, followed by tissue disintegration. Perianal abscesses are located close to the anus and are relatively superficial; ischiorectal abscesses are deep and located at a higher level.

Perianal abscesses, the more common type, usually develop from inflammation of glands located between the sphincters at the dentate line or from inflammation in the crypts at the same level. Pus tends to track into the lower rectum just above the anal canal and externally, forming a tender swelling that usually is posterior to the midline of the anus but may be anywhere within several centimeters of the anal verge. **Ischiorectal abscesses** are more difficult to diagnose, are usually larger, and are accompanied by marked systemic symptoms (such as severe pain and fever). They usually develop from a break between the extraperitoneal rectum and the fatty tissue in the fossa; however, the source of infection may lie within the peritoneal cavity. In older patients, diverticulitis is the most likely cause.

The cardinal symptom is pain, which warrants drainage. If surgery is delayed, signs of sepsis (eg, chills and fever), local swelling, induration, and tenderness follow. Spontaneous rupture may occur if the abscess is superficial, but it should not be expected or awaited. Antibiotics are given but cannot substitute for drainage. Both aerobic and anaerobic organisms similar to those found in feces can be obtained from the pus for culture. Delayed drainage may lead to life-threatening clostridial infections.

Since nearly all abscesses originate from a break in the rectal mucous membrane, a persistent fistula is common after simple incision and drainage. Consequently, a fistula should be sought during the original operation. However, if a fistula is not readily found, awaiting further developments is preferable to risking damage to the anorectal mucosa and sphincter.

Anal Fistula

(Fistula in Ano)

A sinus tract between the rectum and the skin. Fistulas form for several reasons. The most common follow inflammation in rectal crypts or glands, progressing to perirectal abscesses that track internally into the rectum and externally to the skin. Other diseases (eg, Crohn's disease, tuberculosis, and lymphogranuloma) may involve the rectum and cause fistulas. Intraperitoneal lesions (eg, diverticulitis or Crohn's disease of the small intestine or colon) may cause fistulas that track into the perineum. Trauma, including iatrogenic injuries, childbirth, and cancer, can produce fistulas that track into the vagina. Because of these many possibilities, microscopic examination of excised tissue is imperative.

Usually, an anal fistula opens near the anus. If the external opening is adjacent to the posterior half of the anus, the tract almost always runs into the rectum exactly in the posterior midline. However, if the external opening is adjacent to the anterior half of the anus, the tract runs radially into the rectum. During initial examination, probing the entire tract may be possible, but usually determining the site of the internal opening is difficult until surgery.

Most fistulas connect with the rectum just above the anal canal, so that exposing the tract sacrifices very little of the sphincter; this simple procedure is curative. However, if the internal opening is high, the use of a seton is advised to avoid damaging the sphincter and causing incontinence. The seton (either a silk suture or a rubber band) is passed through the tract into the rectum and tied. It gradually cuts through the tissues and leads to fibrosis and fixation, thus avoiding incontinence.

Prolapse and Procidentia

Protrusion of part of the rectum through the anus. **Mucosal prolapse** involves only the mucosa; all other layers of the rectum remain in place.

Complete prolapse involves all layers. In the most severe form, called **procidentia,** several inches of rectum may pass through the anus, and the pouch of Douglas descends to the level of the anal canal, which remains in place.

Prolapse is common in elderly persons, more so in women than in men. The underlying defect is a long, lax sigmoidorectal mesentery; therefore, the rectum is not fixed in the pelvis in its normal position.

Symptoms include protrusion of either mucous membrane or several inches of rectum. Initially, manual reduction is possible, but later, protrusion occurs whenever the patient stands, causing pain and discharge of mucus and blood from the inflamed mucosa. Physical examination includes inspection and palpation of the protrusion when the patient is standing or squatting or immediately after a bowel movement to determine the degree of prolapse.

Unless surgical repair is performed early, continued dilation of the anal sphincters leads to incontinence; the weakened muscular ring often remains incompetent despite later attempts at repair. Mucosal prolapse is treated by excision of the redundant tissue, similar to standard hemorrhoidectomy. When prolapse is complete, conservative therapy—avoidance of straining at stool, lifting, and excessive standing and, when necessary, manual reduction—gives temporary relief. Attempts can be made to maintain normal anatomy by strapping the buttocks. However, surgery is necessary and should not be delayed.

Many operations have been devised, but surgeons do not agree on which is best. For a low-risk patient, the best procedure is a transabdominal resection of the redundant colon and rectum together with the corresponding mesentery. After a low anastomosis, the rectum is anchored in the pelvis in its normal position. Resection of excess bowel and a coloanal anastomosis are also possible through a perineal approach, which is less taxing on the patient. Another technique is to anchor the rectum by means of a plastic sling, using an abdominal approach; however, this method makes subsequent sigmoidoscopy or colonoscopy difficult or impossible. The Thiersch procedure, in which a wire loop is passed about the upper end of the anal canal and tightened appropriately, is the simplest operation but has been abandoned. The problems include intestinal obstruction if the wire is tied too tightly and recurrence if the wire breaks.

Postoperative fecal incontinence is common, particularly if it existed preoperatively. Procedures in which the sphincters are tightened have been helpful in some cases.

DISORDERS OF THE GALLBLADDER AND BILIARY TREE

Disorders of the gallbladder and biliary tree account for about 1/3 of abdominal operations performed in patients > 70 yr. Gallstones, cholecystitis, and carcinoma of the gallbladder are the most important disorders. Carcinoma of the gallbladder and biliary tree are discussed in Ch. 60.

Gallstones

Calculi in the gallbladder **(cholelithiasis)** is an extremely common disorder. According to estimates, 25% of persons > 50 yr will develop gallstones, the indication for nearly all 475,000 cholecystectomies done annually in the USA (1 in every 500 people). The incidence rises with age; calculi are found at autopsy in about 1/3 of persons > 70 yr.

Diagnosis: The primary symptom of gallstones is biliary colic. Colic, or steady pain, usually is felt in the right subcostal area but often radiates to the right scapula or the right shoulder and, in some instances, is similar to angina. At times, the pain may be felt anywhere in the abdomen. Vomiting may occur but is not repetitive. Usually, slight tenderness occurs in the right upper quadrant. Epigastric distention, gas, and vague dyspepsia occur in so many people that these findings cannot be considered specific for gallbladder disease.

Acute cholecystitis, a complication of gallstones, is characterized by increased local tenderness, fever, and leukocytosis. The gallbladder frequently is palpable. Migration of a stone into the common duct can lead to jaundice, chills and fever, and gallstone pancreatitis. **Pancreatitis** is accompanied by more diffuse epigastric tenderness and elevated serum amylase levels.

Ultrasonography shows gallstones in > 95% of cases and shows distended intrahepatic ducts when a patient has a common duct obstruction. However, ultrasonography does not visualize the distal common duct adequately, and CT scan is better for diagnosing pancreatic lesions. Transhepatic cholangiography and endoscopic retrograde cholangiopancreatography are valuable when common duct involvement is suspected.

Treatment: The patient may decide to live with the stones. If not, the first surgical choice is cholecystectomy. Laparoscopic cholecystectomy is widely used, although damage to the common duct is much more common with this procedure than with open cholecystectomy. Other methods, such as stone dissolution by chenodeoxycholic acid, are successful in some cases but require continued medication. The recurrence rate for lithotripsy is so high that the procedure has been abandoned. Cholecystectomy combined with common duct exploration is the preferred operation for common duct stones. Endoscopic papillotomy and basket removal of an obstructing stone from the common duct may be advisable if the patient is very ill or the gallbladder already has been removed.

Treatment may need to be modified because of complications. If the gallbladder is acutely inflamed, antibiotics are given for a longer period; surgery should be performed within 2 or 3 days of the onset of acute cholecystitis. With diabetic patients, glucose levels should be controlled, and surgery should be performed as soon as possible because the danger of perforation is high. In some instances, the pathologic changes at the base of the gallbladder are so great that the surgeon should perform a cholecystostomy, leaving the elective cholecystectomy for later. The common duct should be explored if the patient has had chills and fever suggestive of cholangitis, the gallbladder contains small stones, the patient is jaundiced, or there is evidence of pancreatitis.

Many people have asymptomatic gallstones, and the indication for prophylactic surgery is controversial. Surgeons tend to advise patients to undergo cholecystectomy for several reasons: The mortality rate associated with elective operations is about $1/10$ that associated with emergency procedures, severe complications (common duct stones and pancreatitis) are avoided, and cancer of the gallbladder is prevented. If a patient travels extensively, elective cholecystectomy precludes the need for an emergency operation far from home.

One study has shown that asymptomatic gallstones lead to biliary colic in $1/3$ of patients within 2 yr. The mortality rate from elective cholecystectomy in patients < 70 yr is < 1%. Cancer of the gallbladder is associated with gallstones in 75% of cases and is an incidental finding in about 1 of every 100 cholecystectomies. These are strong arguments for cholecystectomy in patients < 70 yr who are otherwise healthy. However, in patients > 70 yr, the mortality rate for elective cholecystectomy has been estimated at 5%, and many other considerations are important. Thus, surgery for asymptomatic gallstones in patients > 70 yr rarely is advised.

If an initial attack of biliary colic occurs, a second attack is probable within 2 yr in $2/3$ of patients. The argument for cholecystectomy therefore becomes more compelling. However, the diagnosis should be confirmed and symptoms of other diseases (eg, coronary insufficiency) ruled out, especially in elderly patients. In equivocal cases, waiting for at least one more attack before recommending surgery is advisable. Usually, patients have several attacks before surgery is advised.

Specific Syndromes

Acute cholangitis: This syndrome usually results from a stone impacted in the ampulla of Vater, but it may be secondary to pancreatic cancer. Other causes, such as ascending infection after sphincterotomy of Oddi's sphincter or infection secondary to stricture from a previous choledochoduodenostomy or choledochojejunostomy, are rare. In the Far East, Oriental cholangitis results from either ascending infection from the intestinal tract or parasites.

Treatment varies, depending on the patient's condition. Patients in septic shock on admission must be treated vigorously with antibiotics before surgery. Gentamicin 1 to 1.5 mg/kg IV q 8 h, ampicillin 1 to 2 gm IV q 6 h, and clindamycin 600 mg IV q 6 h are recommended, although in the future third-generation cephalosporins may become the preferred antibiotics. Fluid balance must be restored. Emergency operations that precede stabilization are associated with a high mortality.

Alternatively, **endoscopic sphincterotomy** has been valuable in treating Oriental cholangitis and is used widely in the USA and Europe for stones impacted in the distal common duct. Skill in endoscopy is essential because of the hazards of perforation, bleeding, and infection.

Gallstone pancreatitis: Patients present with symptoms and signs similar to those of acute cholecystitis, except that the pain is more likely to be epigastric and is associated with elevated serum amylase levels and often with increased bilirubin and alkaline phosphatase levels. Initial treatment is conservative with the patient taking nothing by mouth and receiving IV alimentation. Typically, pain subsides rapidly, and cholecystectomy is performed 5 to 7 days after admission.

Acalculous cholecystitis: This condition tends to occur in patients in intensive care units and in those whose oral intake is poor (eg, because of total IV alimentation). Symptoms are minimal. Unexplained fever and vague abdominal distress warrant ultrasound examination of the gallbladder, which may show edema of the gallbladder wall and increasing distention on successive examinations. Either cholecystectomy or cholecystostomy is the usual procedure. Percutaneous catheter drainage of the gallbladder has been used, but the frequent occurrence of coexisting gangrene makes this procedure somewhat questionable.

Retained stones in the common duct: These stones are common, particularly if multiple hepatic duct stones were found during the initial exploration. The surgeon prepares for this possibility in questionable cases by placing a large T-tube (No. 14 French) to drain the common duct. The radiologist can extract the stones later. As mentioned above, endoscopic removal also is feasible.

Fistulas: Fistulas form between the gallbladder and the intestine, allowing gallstones to migrate and causing intestinal obstruction. Patients usually present with signs of distal small-bowel obstruction, often with tenderness over the gallbladder. Abdominal x-ray may show the stone and usually shows gas in the biliary tree. The proper surgical procedure is removal of the stones (if one is faceted, others are present) and cholecystectomy. Cholecystectomy may be deferred if the patient is very ill.

Iatrogenic stricture of the common duct: A major complication of cholecystectomy is damage to the common bile duct. Usually, the problem is manifested very early by protracted biliary drainage; diagnosis is made by fistulogram. Surgical repair is a Roux-en-Y anastomosis of the upper duct to the jejunum. A stricture may form at the anastomosis and cause symptoms many years later. Intermittent attacks of pain, fever, and jaundice suggest the diagnosis, which can be confirmed by transhepatic cholangiography. Surgical repair is necessary. Balloon dilation through a transhepatic catheter has been attempted by radiologists, but the stricture is usually too tight to yield a good result.

Polyps of the gallbladder: Usually small and filiform, these polyps have no malignant potential. Many defects shown on ultrasonography simulate polyps but actually are small stones.

Jaundice: The differential diagnosis of jaundice is extensive, and many diagnostic methods are available. The first task is to determine whether jaundice is obstructive. Often, the history is helpful, and the physical examination can give important information. A symmetrically enlarged liver in an alcoholic usually results from cirrhosis; in a temperate or abstaining elderly person, from metastatic cancer involving the liver. A palpable gallbladder in a jaundiced patient usually signifies pancreatic cancer. Obstructive jaundice is manifested by bile in the urine and acholic stools. In jaundice caused by hepatitis, the stools are brown, and the urine contains little or no bile. Serum bilirubin and alkaline phosphatase values document the degree of jaundice; elevations of enzymes such as AST (SGOT) and LDH confirm intrinsic liver disease.

When more sophisticated tests are needed, noninvasive procedures should be done first. Ultrasonography determines the presence of gallstones and the size of the intrahepatic and common bile ducts. If necessary, endoscopy follows, providing direct visualization of the lumen of the stomach and duodenum. Endoscopic retrograde cholangiopancreatography usually can be done safely, and if required, transhepatic cholangiography can follow. Fine-needle percutaneous biopsy is positive in nearly 80% of pancreatic cancer cases.

Both endoscopic retrograde cholangiopancreatography and transhepatic cholangiography carry the hazards of perforation, infection, and hemorrhage. Furthermore, in many cases, establishing a differential diagnosis is impossible without exploratory laparotomy. The value of radioisotope scans using dyes (eg, HIDA) that are excreted with the bile is controversial. If the patient has low-grade jaundice and the dye passes through the common duct into the duodenum, obstructive jaundice is unlikely. Some authorities believe that such scans do not reliably detect acute cholecystitis, although others believe that an inability to visualize the gallbladder after giving the dye is a presumptive sign of a blocked cystic duct and, when associated with local tenderness, a presumptive sign of acute cholecystitis. (See also NEOPLASMS OF EXTRAHEPATIC BILE DUCTS in Ch. 60.)

DISORDERS OF THE LIVER

In the elderly, the most common hepatic lesion requiring surgery is metastatic cancer. (Cirrhosis and its complications are more common in younger persons.) Because hepatic surgery is not well tolerated in the elderly, heroic measures that might enable long-term survival but that carry a high mortality rate are not attempted frequently. Hepatic neoplasms are discussed in Ch. 60.

Cysts

Cysts may be congenital or acquired. Often, multiple **congenital cysts** are associated with polycystic disease of the kidney and pancreas. Usually, they are not significant, and if found during surgery, they can merely be unroofed and left in place. Very rarely, a cyst enlarges during periodic follow-up because it is a cystadenocarcinoma; excision is necessary.

Hydatid cysts, the single important acquired type, are common in many parts of the world. Because they develop slowly, symptoms (such as epigastric pain, liver enlargement, jaundice, and anaphylactic reactions) may not be noted for many years. These cysts may be huge and are diagnosed by CT scan or ultrasonography. Aspiration must be *avoided*. Treatment is excision of the entire cyst; care must be taken to avoid spilling daughter cysts or scoleces into the abdomen.

Abscesses

Pyogenic abscesses and **amebic abscesses** must be differentiated because the treatment differs. Pyogenic abscesses occur in the biliary tree in about 40% of cases; because of the widespread use of antibiotics, pylephlebitis and secondary abscesses from appendicitis are rare. Diverticulitis and sepsis following hemorrhoidal banding are other known causes. Aerobic and anaerobic gram-negative bacteria predominate. Symptoms include upper abdominal pain, chills and fever, and in many cases, right upper quadrant tenderness and mild jaundice.

Diagnosis of hepatic abscess is usually made by CT scan, although both ultrasonography and radionuclide scan may also be helpful. In nearly half the cases, multiple abscesses occur. Aspiration helps establish the cause.

Treatment of pyogenic abscess consists of vigorous antibiotic therapy and drainage (at times, using a percutaneous catheter). The cause should be identified and, if possible, treated. For example, cholangitis, a common finding, requires transperitoneal exploration of the biliary tree, cholecystectomy, and T-tube drainage of the common duct.

Amebic abscesses nearly always respond to metronidazole 500 to 750 mg orally tid; metronidazole may also be given IV. Percutaneous aspiration may be required to diagnose amebic abscesses. Rupture of the abscess into the peritoneal cavity requires surgery. A few surgeons recommend more frequent use of drainage than is customary in the USA today.

DISORDERS OF THE PANCREAS

In older patients, the major disorders of the pancreas are injuries from blunt trauma, gallstone pancreatitis, and cancer. Exocrine and endocrine neoplasms of the pancreas are discussed in Ch. 60.

Traumatic Injury

Diagnosing and treating penetrating wounds present no problems. However, diagnosing an injury from blunt trauma is often difficult, and the treatment is controversial.

The most common cause of blunt trauma is a steering-wheel injury. At first, the patient may be asymptomatic, but within a few hours epigastric pain and tenderness supervene. Hyperamylasemia is noted in > 90% of cases. Most transections of the gland are identified on CT scan. Because retroperitoneal rupture of the duodenum often accompanies pancreatic injuries, a diatrizoate meglumine swallow is desirable before surgery. Also, endoscopic retrograde cholangiopancreatography is advisable to identify or rule out injury of the pancreatic duct. Other tests, such as ultrasonography and peritoneal lavage, have not proved helpful.

Operation is indicated for all suspected pancreatic injuries; the procedure depends on the pathologic changes. Contusions without evidence of ductal or duodenal injury or with minor ductal disruptions are drained. If the gland has been completely divided or the duct is disrupted, the portion of the gland distal to the injury is resected. Serious injuries involving the head of the pancreas *and* the duodenum may require pancreatoduodenectomy or temporary defunctioning of the duodenum as a passage for gastric secretions by closing the pylorus with a temporary suture and emptying the stomach by a gastroenterostomy.

Postoperative complications include abscess, pancreatic or duodenal fistulas, persistent pancreatitis, hemorrhage, and pseudocyst formation.

Pancreatitis

Acute pancreatitis: The major causes are alcohol, gallstones, and postoperative inflammation. The incidence varies with the circumstances and the patient's age. In metropolitan areas, patients tend to be younger, and alcoholism is the most common cause. In rural areas and in geriatric patients, gallstones predominate. The mortality rate for acute pancreatitis rises with age.

Diagnosis is based on the sudden onset of severe epigastric pain that may radiate to the back or later involve the whole abdomen. Vomiting and epigastric tenderness follow. In severe cases, shock, mild jaundice, and respiratory distress may then develop. Serum amylase levels are elevated early on in 95% of cases but may fall thereafter. Serum calcium levels also may fall. Leukocytosis is noted and if bleeding occurs, hematocrit is lowered. Hyperglycemia and hypocalcemia are common in severe cases.

Abdominal x-ray often shows a sentinel loop of gas-filled jejunum in the left upper quadrant. Ultrasonography is particularly valuable in detecting gallstones but not in evaluating the pancreas. For this purpose, CT scan is the best method by far; if the patient fails to improve rapidly, serial examinations should be performed.

Other diseases must be excluded. **Perforated peptic ulcer** may be excluded by an upper GI series using a diatrizoate meglumine swallow rather than barium, but **strangulating intestinal obstruction** or **ischemic bowel disease** may be more difficult to diagnose. At times, laparotomy is necessary. **Gallstone pancreatitis** must also be excluded because it requires surgery; if the disease follows the usual course, in which the severe pain subsides rapidly, surgery is performed a few days after the initial episode. No chemical tests can reliably determine the cause of pancreatitis, but CT scan shows a comparatively normal gland in gallstone pancreatitis compared with severe alcoholic pancreatitis. **Vascular disease** (mesenteric thrombosis or embolism) can lead rapidly to gangrene of the intestine; it mimics acute pancreatitis with pain and leaking toxins.

Treatment is supportive, unless the patient has gallstone pancreatitis. Nasogastric suction, IV alimentation, and fluid replacement are essential. Antibiotics are not used in the early stages. In Europe, total pancreatectomy is often performed immediately, but this procedure is not used in the USA. For patients with gallstone pancreatitis, early surgery is recommended. Endoscopic retrograde cholangiopancreatography and endoscopic papillotomy are not used by most surgeons because of the risk of exacerbating the pancreatitis.

Following therapy, the course varies greatly. Many patients, including nearly all those with gallstone pancreatitis, improve rapidly. Those whose condition worsens require ongoing reevaluations with CT scan and surgical treatment of the serious complications that can follow.

Chronic pancreatitis: Cases of acute pancreatitis that continue or ones that subside and recur are considered chronic pancreatitis. The most severe form is pancreatolithiasis, in which patients have such severe persistent pain that many become addicted to narcotic analgesics. Weight loss, diarrhea caused by loss of enzymes, and diabetes caused by fibrosis of the islets of Langerhans are late complications. A few patients have hyperparathyroidism too. Appropriate studies include measurements of AST (SGOT), LDH, alkaline phosphatase, serum bilirubin, amylase, glucose, calcium, and phosphate levels.

Several tests have been used to establish the pain as pancreatic. The Nardi test involves subcutaneous injection of morphine and neostigmine; the development of typical pain together with elevated serum amylase and lipase levels suggests obstruction at Oddi's sphincter. After subcutaneous injection of secretin, dilation of the duct of Wirsung seen on ultrasonography also suggests a sphincter abnormality. No consensus has been reached on the value of these tests. When endoscopic retrograde cholangiopancreatography shows a large, uniformly dilated duct, obstruction of the ampulla is probable, and anastomosis of a Roux-en-Y loop of jejunum to the pancreas (pancreaticojejunostomy) usually has good results.

Various extirpative procedures may also be required. These include distal pancreatectomy when the disease is in the tail of the gland, Whipple's procedure when only the head is involved, and total pancreatectomy in extreme cases of pancreatolithiasis. Splanchnic nerve section for pain relief has had only sporadic success. In all cases, the patient must abstain from alcohol.

Pancreatic Cysts

Several types of cysts occur in the pancreas. **Congenital cysts** are rare but can be found in some cases of polycystic disease. The gland may contain many small cysts from which cystadenocarcinoma can develop. Excision or resection of a portion of the pancreas may be necessary.

Pseudocysts are formed by extravasation of pancreatic secretions into the lesser peritoneal sac. Characteristically, they follow trauma. The patient complains of left upper quadrant pain and tenderness, and a mass may be palpable. Diagnosis may be made by CT scan or, if the cyst is large, by an upper GI series showing displacement of the stomach or other viscera. In the early stages, only a weak wall surrounds the collection of fluid; generally, surgery is deferred. If it is necessary, drainage is all that can be done. Later, as the surrounding wall thickens, or matures, the pseudocyst can be drained internally by anastomosis to the stomach or intestine.

Cysts frequently form in the pancreas, or pseudocysts develop in adjacent tissue of patients with alcoholic pancreatitis. Many of these cysts resolve spontaneously, as shown by serial CT scans. If they do not resolve after 6 wk, surgery is indicated. Depending on its location, the cyst is anastomosed to the stomach, the jejunum, or the duodenum.

DISORDERS OF THE SPLEEN

Surgery is limited in the treatment of splenic disorders. Operative measures include splenectomy, repair of injuries by methods other than splenectomy, and drainage of abscesses.

The main indications for **splenectomy** are trauma (either blunt, penetrating, or iatrogenic), disease of adjacent organs (such as the stomach, pancreas, or colon), idiopathic thrombocytopenic purpura, and advanced splenomegaly. Rarely in the elderly, splenectomy is performed for hypersplenism and splenic artery aneurysms, as a staging procedure for Hodgkin's disease, or as a requirement of splenorenal shunt for portal hypertension.

Trauma

Iatrogenic damage to the spleen commonly results from vagotomy and operations involving the stomach, tail of the pancreas, or the colon. Such trauma as well as blunt and penetrating trauma frequently requires splenectomy.

The surgeon decides whether the injury is severe enough to warrant splenectomy or whether simple suturing or hemostasis is possible. Although the matter is controversial, several facts are clear. Older patients tolerate splenectomy better than younger patients and have a much lower incidence of subsequent fatal sepsis. However, older patients do not tolerate continued bleeding as well as younger patients do. Therefore, in an elderly patient, unless hemostasis is absolute, splenectomy should be performed.

Idiopathic Thrombocytopenic Purpura

Idiopathic thrombocytopenic purpura usually is treated with corticosteroids; however, older patients do not respond to such therapy or to splenectomy as well as younger patients do. In a series of > 200 splenectomies for this disease, 12% of patients were > 70 yr. Splenectomy alone cured only about half the older patients; the others required continued corticosteroid therapy.

Massive Splenomegaly

A huge spleen is subject to repeated episodes of minor thromboses, which add to the pain and discomfort of the mass and the pressure on adjacent organs. Such episodes can occur, for example, with splenomegaly resulting from lymphocytic or myelogenous leukemia. In these diseases, splenectomy usually is contraindicated because of high postoperative mortality; patients rarely live for more than a few months after such an operation. However, in some medical centers, splenectomy now is recommended for pain relief.

Gaucher's disease results from the accumulation of glucocerebrosides in the spleen. As the spleen enlarges, hypersplenism may follow (see below). Therapy is now available in which the deficient enzyme (glucosylceramidase) is replaced with periodic IV infusions of recombinant human placental glucocerebrosidase. Limited patient studies have shown clinical improvement in the hematologic and splenic findings. Some of the largest spleens excised have been removed for Gaucher's disease. After splenectomy, the typical lipid-laden macrophages continue to accumulate in the liver and bone marrow.

Disease of Adjacent Organs

Surgical treatment of gastric cancer often includes splenectomy because of the frequency of splenic lymph node metastases. Other reasons for splenectomy include cancer of the splenic flexure of the colon, which also may invade the spleen; large cysts of the distal pancreas; and splenic artery aneurysms.

Hypersplenism

Enlargement of the spleen is associated with any combination of anemia, leukopenia, or thrombocytopenia. Many diseases, such as bacterial infections, malaria, kala-azar, and Gaucher's disease, may be associated with hypersplenism. In the USA, portal hypertension and the various lymphomas are the most important.

Abscesses

Abscesses may form in the spleen secondary to sepsis. Formerly, diagnosis was difficult and could be established only by splenectomy. Currently, CT scan is helpful in making the diagnosis. Many abscesses can be drained by using percutaneous catheters guided by CT scan.

§3. ORGAN SYSTEMS: GENITOURINARY AND GYNECOLOGIC DISORDERS

HEMATOLOGIC DISORDERS

§3. ORGAN SYSTEMS: GENITOURINARY AND GYNECOLOGIC DISORDERS

63. RENAL CHANGES AND DISORDERS

A substantial reduction in renal function accompanies normal aging, although the senescent kidney ordinarily functions sufficiently to remove wastes and adequately regulate the volume and composition of extracellular fluid. Nevertheless, changes in renal function reduce the older person's capacity to respond to a variety of physiologic and pathologic stresses, with important clinical implications.

Renal Anatomy

Without hypertension or marked vascular disease, the senescent kidney maintains its relatively smooth contour. However, renal mass is progressively lost, and kidney weight decreases from 250 to 270 gm in young adulthood to 180 to 200 gm in the eighth decade. The loss of renal mass is primarily cortical, with relative sparing of the medulla. The number of identifiable glomeruli decreases, roughly in accordance with the decline in kidney weight. In addition, the proportion of sclerotic glomeruli increases from 1% to 2% in middle age to > 12% after age 70. The glomerular tuft becomes less lobulated, the number of mesangial cells increases, and the number of epithelial cells decreases, thus reducing the surface area available for filtration. On the other hand, glomerular permeability does not change with age, as shown by dextran clearance studies.

Several minor microscopic changes occur in the renal tubule with age. Of particular interest is the appearance of diverticula in the distal nephron, reaching a high of about three per tubule by age 90 yr. These diverticula may evolve as the simple retention cysts that are common in the elderly.

The walls of the larger renal vessels undergo various sclerotic changes with age. The sclerosis does not encroach on the lumen and is augmented by hypertension. Smaller vessels appear to be spared; only 15% of older normotensive persons have sclerotic changes in the renal arterioles. X-ray studies show that normotensive persons > 70 yr of age have an increasing prevalence of abnormalities similar to those seen in younger hypertensive persons, such as abnormal tapering of interlobar arteries, abnormal arcuate arteries, and increased tortuosity of intralobular arteries.

Two distinctive age-related patterns of change occur in arteriolar-glomerular units. The first pattern, seen primarily in the cortical area, consists of hyalinization and collapse of the glomerular tuft. The lumen of the preglomerular arteriole becomes obliterated, with a resultant loss in blood flow. The second pattern, seen primarily in the juxtamedullary area, is characterized by glomerular sclerosis and the development of anatomic continuity between the afferent and efferent arterioles. The end point is shunting of blood flow from afferent to efferent arterioles and loss of glomeruli. Blood flow is maintained to the arteriolae rectae vera, the medulla's primary vascular supply; these arterioles do not decrease in number with age.

Renal Physiology

Renal blood flow: Blood flow through the kidneys progressively decreases from 1200 mL/min in young adulthood to 600 mL/min by age 80 yr. The primary underlying factor is the decreased renovascular bed. However, the reduction in flow does not simply reflect decreased renal mass, since flow per gram of tissue falls progressively after the fourth decade. The age-related decline in renal blood flow is due to fixed anatomic changes rather than to reversible vasospasm, as shown by studies with vasoactive agents. Of significance, cortical blood flow decreases and medullary flow is preserved, a finding consistent with histologic studies that show selective loss of cortical vasculature with age. These vascular changes probably account for the patchy cortical defects commonly seen on renal scans in healthy elderly adults.

Glomerular filtration rate: The major clinically relevant functional defect arising from the age-related anatomic and histologic changes described above is a progressive decline in the glomerular filtration rate as measured by **creatinine clearance** (see formula under Drug Doses, below). Creatinine clearance is stable until the middle of the fourth decade, when it declines linearly at about 8 mL/min/1.73 m^2/decade.

Longitudinal studies indicate that aging's effect on creatinine clearance varies substantially, with as many as ⅓ of older persons showing *no* decline in glomerular filtration rate. This variability suggests that factors other than aging may be responsible for the apparent loss of renal function. For example, increases in blood pressure still within the normotensive range are associated with an accelerated, age-related loss of renal function.

Tubular function: The argument that entire nephrons disappear with advancing age is supported by the striking parallel decline in glomerular filtration rate and several proximal tubular functions, including maximal excretion of *p*-aminohippurate and iodopyracet and maximal absorption of glucose. The renal threshold for glycosuria, which relates inversely to the degree of splay in reabsorptive capacity of individual nephrons, increases with age. Thus, glucose generally spills into the urine at a lower blood glucose level in a young diabetic patient than in an elderly one.

Drug Doses

Although muscle mass, from which creatinine is derived, decreases with age, serum creatinine level does not usually decline with normal aging because the reduction in renal function (ie, the decline in glomerular filtration rate and creatinine clearance) balances the decreased production of creatinine. For example, the average healthy 80-yr-old man has a creatinine clearance 32 mL/min less than that of his 30-yr-old counterpart but the same serum creatinine value. Depression of glomerular filtration sufficient to raise the serum creatinine level above 1.5 mg/dL is rarely due to normal aging and therefore indicates renal disease.

In clinical practice, the doses of many drugs excreted primarily by the kidneys (eg, digoxin preparations and aminoglycoside antibiotics) require adjustment to compensate for changes in renal function (see also Ch. 21). However, adjustments are too often based on serum creatinine values, with the resultant predictable drug overdose in elderly patients. Ideally, dose adjustments should be based on creatinine clearance, which does not require absolute 24-h urine collection but can be estimated using a sample collected after 8 h (eg, overnight).

When only the serum creatinine level is available, creatinine clearance can be estimated by using the following formula:

$$\text{Creatinine clearance (mL/min)} = \frac{(140 - \text{age [yr]}) \times \text{body wt (kg)}}{72 \times \text{serum creatinine (mg/dL)}}$$

In women, the calculated value is multiplied by 0.85.

Renin–Angiotensin–Aldosterone System

Whether estimated by plasma renin concentration or renin activity, basal renin is diminished by 30% to 50% in the elderly despite normal levels of renin substrate. Certain therapies and maneuvers (eg, salt restriction, diuretic administration, and upright posture) augment renin secretion, further lowering the renin level.

Lower renin levels are associated with 30% to 50% reductions in plasma concentrations of aldosterone; the secretion and clearance rates of aldosterone are also significantly reduced. Plasma aldosterone and cortisol responses after corticotropin (ACTH) stimulation are not impaired with age. Therefore, aldosterone deficiency in the elderly is usually a function of the coexisting renin deficiency and not secondary to intrinsic adrenal changes.

The impact of normal aging on plasma renin must be considered when categorizing hypertensive patients according to renin level. A hypertensive geriatric patient, or occasionally a patient with modestly elevated systolic blood pressure, may be categorized as having low-renin hypertension, when actually the renin level is normal for the patient's age.

Age-related decreases in renin and aldosterone contribute to the elderly's increased risk for **hyperkalemia** in a variety of clinical settings (see HYPERKALEMIA in Ch. 3). Through its action on the distal renal tubule, aldosterone increases sodium reabsorption and facilitates potassium excretion. Aldosterone is one of the major protective mechanisms in preventing hyperkalemia during periods of potassium challenge. Since glomerular filtration rate (another major determinant of potassium excretion) is also impaired in older patients, plasma potassium levels are likely to become seriously elevated, especially in the presence of GI bleeding (a major source of potassium) or when potassium salts are given IV.

The tendency toward hyperkalemia is enhanced by any clinical setting associated with acidosis, since the senescent kidney is sluggish in its response to acid loading, resulting in prolonged depression of serum pH and concomitant potassium elevation. Potent antagonists of renal potassium excretion (eg, spironolactone or triamterene), as well as most nonsteroidal anti-inflammatory drugs, β-adrenergic blockers, and angiotensin converting enzyme inhibitors, which also inhibit potassium elimination, should be administered *with caution* in the elderly. The concomitant administration of these agents and potassium should be *avoided*.

RENAL DISEASES

The most common renal diseases in the elderly are the nephrotic syndrome, acute glomerulonephritis, renal embolism, renal artery thrombosis, and both acute and chronic renal failure.

NEPHROTIC SYNDROME

A condition characterized by generalized edema, heavy proteinuria, hypoalbuminemia, and susceptibility to infections.

Traditionally, age was thought to play an important role in the pathogenesis of nephrotic syndromes (eg, the likelihood of minimal-change disease decreases and that of amyloidosis increases with age). However, clinical and biopsy data from a large number of elderly nephrotic patients now indicate that, in general, age has *no* impact on the frequency of any pathologic glomerular change.

The most common nephrotic lesion in old age is **membranous glomerulonephritis;** the second most common is **minimal-change disease.** Membranous glomerulonephritis is often associated with carcinoma of the lung, colon, or stomach. Nonsteroidal anti-inflammatory drugs are emerging as an important preventable cause of nephrotic syndrome in the elderly.

Elderly patients with minimal-change disease generally have an excellent response to corticosteroids and immunosuppressants. In addition, some elderly patients with membranous glomerulonephritis respond to corticosteroid or cyclophosphamide therapy. In many cases, cyclophosphamide may be the treatment of choice to avoid having corticosteroids exacerbate other conditions (eg, glucose intolerance, hypertension, osteoporosis, and cataracts). Focal sclerosis often has a more aggressive clinical course in the elderly than in younger adults.

ACUTE GLOMERULONEPHRITIS

A disease characterized by diffuse inflammation in the glomeruli.

Acute glomerulonephritis has a clear age-related presentation and prognosis. **In children and young adults,** acute glomerulonephritis is often associated with recent streptococcal infection, producing hematuria, heavy proteinuria, edema, hypertension, and in many cases, the development of pulmonary congestion. The prognosis is generally good in poststreptococcal disease but variable in nonpoststreptococcal cases.

In elderly patients, the nonspecific clinical features (such as nausea, malaise, arthralgias, and a striking predilection for pulmonary infiltrates initially) are thought to represent worsening of a preexisting illness, especially heart failure. Proteinuria is generally moderate. Hypertension or edema, although unusual, indicates a streptococcal cause, more often a pyodermal streptococcal infection rather than pharyngitis; the prognosis is favorable. Otherwise, the prognosis is poor, with crescentic glomerulonephritis associated with focal, segmental, necrotizing, or fibrosing glomerulitis the most common histologic finding.

The value of treatment with corticosteroids, immunosuppressive agents, anticoagulants, and plasmapheresis remains controversial. In view of the poor prognosis of rapidly progressive glomerulonephritis in the elderly, the potential benefits of high-dose pulse corticosteroid therapy are likely to outweigh the risks.

RENAL EMBOLISM

An occlusive arterial disease that is an important cause of both acute and chronic renal failure in the elderly.

Renal arterial emboli can occur in any clinical setting that is associated with peripheral embolization (eg, acute myocardial infarction, chronic atrial fibrillation, subacute bacterial endocarditis, and aortic surgery or aortography). The manifestations of renal embolism may vary from essentially no symptoms and signs to a full-blown syndrome of severe flank pain and tenderness, hematuria, hypertension, spiking fevers, markedly reduced renal function, and elevated serum lactic dehydrogenase levels.

Small emboli are difficult to detect, since renal scans show focal perfusion defects in many apparently healthy elderly patients. Major emboli may be suggested by differential contrast excretion on urography and confirmed by renal scanning and aortography.

Surgery is generally not indicated, and anticoagulant therapy is unlikely to offer major benefit. In many cases in which renal function is discernibly impaired, improvement may occur over a period of several days to weeks.

Renal cholesterol embolization is a specific geriatric syndrome that may occur spontaneously or after aortic surgery or angiography in patients with diffuse atherosclerosis. Definitive diagnosis may be difficult, requiring visualization of cholesterol crystals on renal biopsy; a presumptive diagnosis is often masked by other possible causes of reduced renal function (eg, hypotension or administration of angiographic contrast material). The clinical course varies, with most patients developing progressive renal failure. However, some have only moderate impairment and may regain renal function over time. No specific treatment is available.

RENAL ARTERY THROMBOSIS

Thrombotic occlusive renal artery disease often complicates severe aortic and renal arterial atherosclerosis, especially when renal blood flow is reduced because of heart failure or volume depletion. Symptoms of renal artery occlusion may be notably absent. If renal function previously was good, the only manifestation of unilateral thrombosis may be an increase in BUN and serum creatinine levels and perhaps a modest increase in blood pressure. In patients with preexisting renal impairment and azotemia, renal artery occlusion may precipitate heart failure, marked hypertension, and the uremic syndrome.

Renal scanning is usually more informative than IV urography in evaluating a patient with possible renal artery thrombosis. It is also safer. However, definitive diagnosis requires angiography. A coexisting abdominal aortic aneurysm should be sought, because it may lead to renal artery occlusion by extension of atheroma or dissection. In angiography, the least possible amount of contrast material should be used to minimize the likelihood of a nephrotoxic reaction; such a reaction, while generally limited to several days of oliguria and mild azotemia, may take the form of acute oliguric renal failure.

When technically feasible, surgical revascularization should be considered. Prompt revascularization can lead to a substantial return of renal function, and some patients recover even if surgery is delayed several months.

ACUTE RENAL FAILURE

The clinical conditions associated with rapid, steadily increasing azotemia, with or without oliguria (< 500 mL/day).

The conditions that often precipitate acute renal failure include hypotension associated with marked volume depletion, heart failure, major surgery, sepsis, angiographic procedures (because the radiocontrast agents are nephrotoxic), and the injudicious use of nephrotoxic antibiotics. These conditions are more common in the elderly, especially those who have many impairments, who are often at increased risk because of preexisting moderate renal insufficiency.

Although **acute tubular necrosis** (2 to 10 days of oliguria followed by a diuretic phase before function is recovered) is typical in the elderly, **nonoliguric acute renal failure** is being diagnosed more often. In either case, renal function, as reflected by BUN and serum creatinine levels, is impaired for several days after a brief hypotensive episode. After this brief period of azotemia, renal function gradually returns to its previous level.

Despite the transient loss of renal function, oliguria is not a prominent part of the clinical picture. Since the clinical hallmark of renal failure is generally thought to be a dramatic reduction in urine output, nonoliguric acute renal failure may go unrecognized. Therefore, drugs excreted predominantly via renal mechanisms may inadvertently accumulate during the period of impaired renal function.

The same general principles used in younger patients guide the management of elderly patients with full-blown acute renal failure complicated by oliguria. *Most important is the rapid exclusion of urinary obstruction as a cause of the renal failure,* particularly in men with prostatic hypertrophy or carcinoma and in women with gynecologic malignancy.

Treatment

The management of acute renal failure is complex and demanding. The aging kidney retains the capacity to recover from acute ischemic or toxic insults over the course of several weeks.

Dialysis: Dialysis often simplifies management considerably. **Hemodialysis, peritoneal dialysis,** and the recently introduced forms of **hemofiltration** are effective, and the complication rate seems to result more from concurrent cardiovascular disease than from age. It is usually more prudent to initiate dialysis early in a patient with acute renal failure than to wait for an emergency. The indications for emergency dialysis or ultrafiltration therapy include pulmonary edema unresponsive to diuretics, hyperkalemia, uremic pericarditis, seizures, and uncontrolled bleeding due to uremia.

Femoral vein catheterization for dialysis is a major advance. These catheters are easily placed, may be left in situ for several days to a week with a very low incidence of infection or thrombosis, and circumvent the need for implantation of arteriovenous shunts.

Water and electrolyte balance: **Water and sodium balance** is also important (see also VOLUME DEPLETION AND DEHYDRATION in Ch. 3). A patient with acute renal failure typically loses about 1 lb of body mass daily because of catabolism. Attempts to keep body weight constant result in gradual expansion of extracellular fluid volume and a consequent increase in blood pressure, with the risk of precipitating heart failure. Similarly, overzealous fluid restriction impairs the patient's general condition and CNS function and may delay the recovery of renal function. In general, the administration of about 600 mL fluid daily, in addition to insensible losses, provides adequate water and sodium balance.

Potassium balance is critical. *Hyperkalemia must be avoided if possible* and treated promptly if present (see HYPERKALEMIA in Ch. 3). Gastrointestinal bleeding, which is often aggravated by azotemia, is a common cause of hyperkalemia because potassium is absorbed from lysed red cells in the gut. **Acidosis** progresses with the duration and degree of renal failure, and sodium bicarbonate should be administered to maintain circulating HCO_3^- levels in the range of 15 to 20 mEq/L. Because sodium bicarbonate may expand extracellular fluid volume, patients should be observed for evidence of heart failure.

Other treatment measures: Additional routine measures include the administration of oral phosphate-binding agents to minimize the elevation of serum phosphate and the provision of a low-protein diet to blunt the rise in BUN. Particular attention should be paid to changing the dose interval of drugs excreted renally and recognizing the enhanced sensitivity of elderly uremic patients to psychoactive drugs (eg, hypnotics and major tranquilizers).

Complications

Volume overload precipitating acute pulmonary edema, hypertensive crisis, hyperkalemia, and infection are the major causes of death during acute renal failure. Urinary infection secondary to bladder catheterization is a particularly common infection. Little is gained from placing a urinary catheter in an oliguric patient; volume status and BUN, creatinine, and potassium levels are better guides to treatment than the urinary output. Infection from IV lines is also common; IV lines should be monitored scrupulously and discontinued as soon as possible. As always, the best treatment is prevention; awareness of these risks and careful management as indicated are critical.

CHRONIC RENAL FAILURE

The clinical condition resulting from many pathologic processes that lead to derangement and insufficiency of renal excretory and regulatory function.

Many forms of chronic renal failure are more common late in life, because renal disease is often secondary to other age-dependent illnesses. For example, prostatic hypertrophy or cancer may lead to hydronephrosis; renovascular hypertension or renal failure may be secondary to atherosclerosis, multiple myeloma, or amyloidosis; drug use may cause renal insufficiency; and perhaps most common, heart failure or volume depletion may lead to prerenal azotemia.

Diagnosis

One factor that often delays recognition of chronic renal failure in the elderly is its presentation as decompensation of a previously impaired organ system before specific symptoms of uremia emerge. Examples include worsening of heart failure because sodium and water cannot be excreted, GI bleeding in a patient with a GI malignancy or ulcer, and mental confusion in a borderline demented patient who becomes increasingly azotemic.

Once chronic renal failure is established, the cause should be identified. Generally, renal failure in the elderly is due to chronic glomerulonephritis, hypertensive and atherosclerotic vascular disease, diabetes, or in some cases, late-presenting polycystic kidney disease. The most important diagnostic consideration is strict exclusion of potentially reversible causes, such as urinary tract obstruction, particularly in men with symptoms of prostatism; renal artery occlusion that may be reparable; hypercalcemia; and the administration of nephrotoxic agents. If a reversible cause is not identified, the patient should be monitored every several months or perhaps more frequently, depending on how quickly creatinine rises, until the rate of renal function loss can be accurately assessed.

Treatment

While general principles of management are similar in young and old adults, the geriatric patient with chronic renal insufficiency requires several special considerations. Appropriate adjustments should be made in the doses and dosing schedules of all drugs, especially digoxin and aminoglycoside antibiotics, and hypertension should be controlled.

Dietary management: The diet of an elderly patient with chronic renal failure is often *overmanaged,* compounding the nutritional impact of renal failure. Protein and salt restriction to suppress the volume expansion and BUN elevation is often unnecessary because many elderly patients normally ingest only 60 to 70 gm of protein and 4 to 5 gm of salt daily. Similarly, although dietary potassium intake should be controlled to avoid hyperkalemia, the reductions required in the elderly are often moderate. The best approach is altering the diet to meet the patient's individual needs.

As serum phosphate concentration rises, phosphate-binding antacids should be given with meals to suppress the parathyroid hormone. As serum phosphate falls in response to treatment, serum calcium generally rises toward the normal range. Hypocalcemia that persists after phosphate levels return to normal should be treated with preparations of vitamin D or its congeners (vitamin D_2 tablets 50,000 u. bid or tid; dihydrotachysterol 0.2 to 0.4 mg bid; 1,25-dihydroxycholecalciferol [1,25-dihydroxyvitamin D_3] 0.25 to 0.5 μg bid) to increase intestinal calcium absorption.

Dialysis: Chronic maintenance dialysis (generally, hemodialysis but occasionally chronic ambulatory peritoneal dialysis) remains the mainstay of treatment for uremic patients. Many elderly persons do very well on dialysis, with the frequency of complications seemingly related more to the adequacy of the dialysis treatment and the coexisting extrarenal diseases than to age itself. Psychologically, elderly patients often are better able to adapt to chronic dialysis than are younger persons. Once it is clear that a patient needs hemodialysis, an arteriovenous fistula should be created, since such fistulas often mature slowly in older persons. **Renal transplantation** is increasingly used in persons > 60 yr of age, with the criteria for selection increasingly emphasizing the patient's overall health status and degree of extrarenal disease (comorbidity) rather than age per se.

Complications

Anemia associated with chronic renal failure often requires more aggressive treatment in elderly patients because of coexisting cardiac disease. Red blood cell indexes are not a reliable estimate of iron deficiency in uremia. Iron deficiency should be excluded by evaluation of serum iron and ferritin levels, and oral or parenteral iron supplements should be administered, if indicated. Non-iron deficiency anemia associated with chronic renal failure can be treated with monthly injections of androgens (eg, nandrolone decanoate 200 mg IM). Erythropoietins developed through genetic engineering are now available and are very effective in controlling the anemia of renal failure, thus often markedly enhancing patients' functional status. Epoetin alfa (erythropoietin, EPO) is generally started at a dose of 50 to 100 u./kg three times per week, intravenously in dialysis patients and subcutaneously in others. Maintenance therapy is adjusted by hematocrit; the average dose is 25 u./kg three times per week.

Pruritus is a major problem in elderly uremic patients, especially if xerosis coexists. In addition to skin moisturizers, ultraviolet treatments are effective and safe. Antipruritic agents (eg, antihistamines and ataractics) are rarely helpful, since they act primarily by causing sedation and may have adverse central nervous system effects.

64. DISORDERS OF THE LOWER GENITOURINARY TRACT: BLADDER, PROSTATE, AND TESTICLES

Symptoms of GU tract dysfunction, such as nocturia and urinary frequency, are common in the elderly. Large urine volumes result from insufficient urinary concentrating ability, and many age-related changes occur in neuromuscular coordination of the bladder (described in Ch. 15). However, since aging alone is an insufficient explanation for GU tract dysfunction, the conditions listed in TABLE 64–1 must be considered as possible causes.

DRUG-RELATED URINARY PROBLEMS

Nocturia is reported in ⅔ of women and men > 65 yr of age who are not taking drugs; for those who take drugs or have more than three chronic diseases, the incidence is > 80%. Nocturia contributes to sleep disturbance, a problem for > 20% of elderly persons (see Ch. 11).

Many older patients suffer from loss of bladder distensibility and urinary concentrating ability. Therefore, if chronic diuretic therapy is required for hypertension or heart failure, two options should be considered: (1) For hypertension control, the smallest effective dose (eg, 12.5 or 25 mg hydrochlorothiazide) should be used once daily in the morning. (2) For treatment of heart failure, 1 h of recumbency in the morning after the dose of loop diuretic often obviates the need for twice-daily dosing. Excessive fluid intake or the use of "natural" diuretics (alcohol and caffeine) before bedtime should be avoided whenever nocturia is a significant problem.

The internal urinary sphincter is innervated in part by α-adrenergic fibers. Thus, it is important in men with bladder outlet obstruction that this sphincter not be tightened by excess α-adrenergic stimulation. Excessive sympathetic (α-adrenergic) nervous system activity from sympathomimetics (eg, decongestants) can tighten the sphincter and lead to imbalance of the micturition reflex. On the other hand, α-blocking agents, such as prazosin (prescribed for hypertension), may sometimes lead to incontinence because it reduces the tone of the sphincter.

The cholinergic system contracts the detrusor muscle. Thus, anticholinergic drugs, such as psychoactives, antidepressants, antihistamines, and certain antiarrhythmics, should be avoided to prevent weakening the contraction, which can lead to inadequate emptying.

TABLE 64–1. SYMPTOMS AND CAUSES OF GENITOURINARY TRACT DYSFUNCTION IN MEN

Symptom Group	*Common Causes*	*Less Common Causes*
Lower GU tract irritative symptoms		
Dysuria: Painful urination Frequency: Urinating more than 6 times/day Urgency: Inability to delay urination once the sensation to void is felt Nocturia: Interrupting sleep to urinate	**If dysuria present:** Cystitis, prostatitis **If dysuria absent:** Diuretic therapy; heart failure; outlet obstruction from prostatic hypertrophy or urethral stricture; detrusor instability; alcohol, coffee, or excessive fluids before bedtime	**If dysuria present:** Cancer of bladder or prostate, prostatism **If dysuria absent:** Cancer of bladder or prostate, neurogenic bladder, uncontrolled diabetes, renal insufficiency, hypercalcemia, extrinsic bladder compression
Lower GU tract obstructive symptoms		
Hesitancy, intermittency, postvoiding dribbling, inability to void, and decrease in force and caliber of the urinary stream	Diuretic therapy; prostatic hypertrophy; urethral stricture; therapy with α-agonists, narcotics, anticholinergic drugs	Bladder stone, prostate cancer
Scrotal mass	Epididymitis, varicocele, hydrocele, bowel from hernia	Cancer (lymphoma, spermatocytic seminoma, and seminoma)
Hematuria: Blood, gross or microscopic (> 5 RBCs/high-power field)	Cystitis, bladder cancer, prostatic hypertrophy, or unknown	Prostatitis, renal disease (cancer or glomerulonephritis), bladder stone, prostate cancer

The drugs listed in TABLE 64–2 have two characteristics in common: (1) They may weaken the detrusor muscle, inhibit internal sphincter relaxation, or both. (2) They are often prescribed at unnecessarily high doses (particularly antidepressants and psychoactives), or they may be unnecessary (particularly antihistamines and other strongly anticholinergic drugs).

TABLE 64–2. DRUGS THAT AFFECT BLADDER FUNCTION*

Classification	*Most Problematic*	*Preferred Alternatives*
Antidepressants†	Amitriptyline Imipramine	Desipramine Fluoxetine Trazodone
Antipsychotics	Phenothiazines and haloperidol in high doses	When prescribed for agitation, consider benzodiazepines with short half-lives
Antihistamines	All OTC types, particularly when combined with a sympathomimetic drug‡	Astemizole Terfenadine

* In addition to the drugs listed in the table, all drugs with anticholinergic effects cause potential problems and should be discontinued whenever possible.

† Desipramine is not very sedative; trazodone is somewhat sedative. The more sedative the antidepressant, the more pronounced the anticholinergic effect. Lower dosages may be therapeutic in older persons, eg, desipramine 75 mg daily and trazodone 100 to 150 mg daily.

‡ Discontinue whenever possible.

URINARY TRACT INFECTION/ PROSTATITIS

The diagnosis and treatment of urinary tract infection are described in Ch. 65. Chronic asymptomatic bacteriuria in the elderly usually does not require any therapy. When exacerbation of urinary symptoms coincides with prostatic pyuria and bacteriuria, a trial of antibiotics is indicated. Chronic infection suggests significant urinary retention, calculi, or chronic bacterial prostatitis in men. Reducing the amount of urine retained and removing stones increase the effectiveness of antibiotic therapy.

URETHRAL STRICTURE

Persistent hesitancy and decreased force of stream suggest urethral stricture, which is often a result of urethral trauma following catheterization, endoscopy, or prostatic surgery. Rarely, a history of gonococcal urethritis is noted.

Direct visualization confirms the diagnosis, excludes urethral cancer, and avoids creating false channels by blind passage of a urethral sound. Repeated dilatation or direct vision urethrotomy is usually effective.

BENIGN PROSTATIC HYPERPLASIA

As men age, the normal golf ball–sized prostate increases in size due to hyperplasia of the prostatic epithelium. A subsequent increase in the fibromuscular stroma causes the prostate gland to encroach on the urethra. Why the prostate usually enlarges with age is unknown, though the action of androgens at a cellular level seems to have a major influence. The bladder compensates for the increased resistance by thickening its wall with hypertrophic muscle bundles that, when visualized cytoscopically, appear as trabeculation. Irritation may accompany obstructive symptoms because the thickened bladder wall is noncompliant and spontaneous bladder contractions occur with distention.

TABLE 64–3 lists the American Urological Association's scoring system for benign prostatic hyperplasia. A man with a score of ≥ 8 is considered to have moderate symptoms; a score ≥ 20 indicates severe symptoms. However, neither symptoms, flow rate, nor excessive postvoiding bladder volumes per se indicate the need for medical or surgical treatment. These symptoms and signs of benign prostatic hyperplasia are highly variable. The degree to which the problem bothers the patient is usually the best indication of his need for treatment.

Evaluation

A man with moderate symptoms (eight or more) should have at least a serum creatinine measurement and a urinalysis. Postvoiding residual is best measured by catheterization. More than 5 RBCs per high-power field in uninfected urine requires cystoscopy to rule out bladder cancer. Abnormal renal function should prompt ultrasound evaluation of the ureters and of the bladder after voiding for signs of obstruction. Hydronephrosis or a large postvoiding residual (> 350 mL) usually requires surgical intervention. Recurrent, severe urinary tract infection with a large postvoiding residual, or large bladder calculi in a patient with trabeculation and visible prostatic obstruction, also call for prostate surgery.

Treatment

The treatment of benign prostatic hyperplasia can be divided into three categories: surgery, medical therapy, and watchful waiting. For most men with advanced symptoms, surgery is the best and most effective option.

Surgery: The choice of surgical procedures includes open prostatectomy, transurethral incisions, and transurethral resection of the prostate **(TURP).** Surgery is recommended when creatinine levels are increasing, when hematuria or outflow obstruction recurs because of an enlarged prostate, or when other therapies fail. Surgery is also the most effective treatment for men with moderate to severe symptoms and significant distress from benign prostatic hyperplasia. Open prostatectomy is most appropriate for removal of exceedingly large prostate glands. Its advantage is that subsequent surgery is needed less often for recurrence of symptoms. However, it is associated with more short-term complications. TURP is usually performed under spinal anesthesia in an inpatient setting. Transurethral incision is most useful in men who have significant symptoms but a small prostate gland. Transurethral incision can be done under spinal or local anesthesia. Regardless of which procedure is used, frail older men may need longer inpatient stays. Since the length of surgery adds significantly to the risk, very ill older patients may do best with incisions or removal of small amounts of tissue by TURP.

A recent Veterans Administration Cooperative Trial compared TURP to close monitoring without surgical intervention in men with moderate symptoms of benign prostatic hyperplasia. It showed no mortality from TURP, although other studies suggest a mortality rate of about 1%. The most common postoperative complications were retention requiring recatheterization (4%) and hemorrhage requiring a transfusion (1%). Although uncontrolled studies have suggested that TURP causes incontinence in as many as 22% of patients and impotence in 2% to 12% of patients, these problems were not statistically associated with surgery in this controlled trial. About 10% of TURP patients developed bladder neck contracture or needed urethral dilatation or another TURP procedure within 3 yr.

Other invasive treatments are available for benign prostatic hyperplasia. Urethral stents may be placed in a frail man with severe obstruction and a limited life expectancy to avoid any need for general anesthesia. Laser prostatectomy may be as effective as TURP, but it is much more expensive, requires a long period of catheterization after treatment, and will probably have a similar profile of complications.

Medical therapy: Although TURP was superior to watchful waiting in preventing symptoms, most men did not suffer adverse events if they chose to delay surgery. Nevertheless, during the 3 yr of follow-up in the Veterans Administration trial, more than 20% of those in the watchful waiting group required surgical intervention, usually because of intolerable symptoms, the development of large postvoiding residuals, or acute urinary retention.

Nonsurgical treatment of benign prostatic hyperplasia in the elderly includes above all having the patient relax during urination; minimize fluid intake at bedtime; and avoid caffeine, unnecessary diuretics, and anticholinergic agents (see also Outlet Obstruction under TREATMENT

TABLE 64–3. AMERICAN UROLOGICAL ASSOCIATION SYMPTOM INDEX FOR BENIGN PROSTATIC HYPERPLASIA

	Not at all	*Less than 1 time in 5*	*Less than half the time*	*About half the time*	*More than half the time*	*Almost always*
1. Over the past month or so, how often have you had a sensation of not emptying your bladder completely after you finished urinating?	0	1	2	3	4	5
2. Over the past month or so, how often have you had to urinate again less than two hours after you finished urinating?	0	1	2	3	4	5
3. Over the past month or so, how often have you found you stopped and started again several times when you urinated?	0	1	2	3	4	5
4. Over the past month or so, how often have you found it difficult to postpone urination?	0	1	2	3	4	5
5. Over the past month or so, how often have you had a weak urinary stream?	0	1	2	3	4	5

6. Over the past month or so, how often have you had to push or strain to begin urination?	0	1	2	3	4	5
7. Over the last month, how many times did you most typically get up to urinate from the time you went to bed at night until the time you got up in the morning?	0 (none)	1 (1 time)	2 (2 times)	3 (3 times)	4 (4 times)	5 (≥ 5 times)

Score = sum of answers to questions 1 through 7.

From Barry M, Fowler F Jr, O'Leary M, et al: "The American Urological Association symptom index for benign prostatic hyperplasia." *Journal of Urology* 148:1549–1557, 1992; used with permission.

CONSIDERATIONS in Ch. 15). About 60% of men will claim that these approaches are helpful. Symptoms *may* be helped by α-adrenergic blocking (sphincter-relaxing) agents; prazosin 2 mg bid and terazosin 1 to 5 mg/day up to 20 mg/day are commonly prescribed for this purpose. Finasteride 5 mg/day, a drug that indirectly blocks testosterone's growth-enhancing effects on the prostate, reduces prostate size and may improve symptoms as well; however, response is likely to take several months.

PROSTATE CANCER

Although > 50% of men > 70 yr of age have histologic evidence of prostate cancer, most cancers never cause symptoms and < 3% of men with histologic evidence die of the disease. Nevertheless, prostate cancer is the second most common cause of cancer death in men. Cancer of the prostate can be anatomically staged as clinically localized or clinically advanced disease. Unfortunately, up to 50% of cancers may be clinically advanced at the time of discovery. The cancer is also usually graded histologically as either well, moderately, or poorly differentiated. Small, well-differentiated cancers are least likely to spread. Most clinically localized cancers are of moderate grade. Generally, poorly differentiated cancers are likely to have spread even when they seem to be clinically localized. The 10-yr cancer-specific death rates for the three grades of prostate cancer are as follows: < 10% for well differentiated, 10% to 20% for moderately differentiated, and 30% to 60% for poorly differentiated cancers.

Symptoms, Signs, and Diagnosis

Most patients are asymptomatic or have symptoms compatible with benign prostatic hyperplasia. Few present with acute retention, hematuria, or symptoms related to distant metastases (pain, weight loss, or lymphedema). Prostate cancer typically metastasizes to bone, leading to bone pain and anemia. An annual digital rectal examination can be performed to screen for this disease. The prostate-specific antigen **(PSA)** test is growing in popularity as a screening tool, and the American Urological Association and American Cancer Society recommend that it be performed annually. The National Cancer Institute and the U.S. Preventive Services Task Force have not endorsed its use. With the PSA test, more cancers are discovered at an earlier clinical stage; however, the benefits of early detection are unproved. Furthermore, the PSA test misses about ⅓ of clinically important cancers and is falsely positive in about 60% of cases, leading to unnecessary and costly diagnostic evaluations. A firm nodule or induration of the gland or an elevated PSA usually prompts referral to a urologist for prostate core biopsy or prostate aspiration if the patient believes that treatment is a reasonable option for him.

TABLE 64–4. PERSISTENT ADVERSE OUTCOMES AFTER TREATMENT OF LOCALIZED PROSTATE CANCER

Outcome	*Radical Surgery*	*Radiation Therapy*
Treatment mortality	0.3–2%	0–0.6%
Severe incontinence	6–7%	1–5%
Severe bowel injury	1%	1–3%
Recurrent strictures	9–12%	3–10%
Impotence	30*–100%	12–40%

* Lowest rates expected when nerve-sparing surgery can be performed.

Modified from Wasson JH, Cushman CC, Bruskewitz RC, et al: "A structured literature review of treatment for localized prostate cancer." *Archives of Family Medicine* 2(5):487–493, 1993. Copyright 1993, American Medical Association.

Treatment

A large percentage of men with prostate cancer will not die of it, in part because it often progresses slowly. Therefore, when a man is beyond his 60s, the potential advantages of invasive treatment are greatly diminished, as death from causes other than the prostate cancer become more likely.

Treatments for **clinically localized prostate cancer** include radical surgery, radiation, and watchful waiting. The unproven theory is that surgical and radiation treatments reduce the chance for spread of the disease. For men with well and moderately differentiated cancer whose PSA level is < 10, most tumors are confined to the prostate. For men with poorly differentiated cancers or a PSA level > 20, the likelihood that disease is confined to the prostate is much less. Complications of radical surgery and radiation are listed in TABLE 64–4. The patient must weigh potential harm of complications against potential benefits of treatment. The nerve-sparing radical prostatectomy may be attempted in a sexually potent man to reduce the risk of impotence. This technique is least likely to be successful for poorly differentiated or locally advanced disease.

For **locally invasive disease,** radiation and close monitoring are the customary options. Options for radiation therapy include both external beam radiation and radioactive implants. External beam is most commonly used, but the relative advantages of external beam vs. implants have not been well studied. Treatment for **symptomatic, advanced disease** with diethylstilbestrol 1 to 3 mg/day, gonadotropin-releasing hormone analogs, antiandrogens, and chemotherapeutic agents usually affords the patient temporary relief. Orchiectomy mitigates the risks of antiandrogen therapy but may not be acceptable to the patient. Although 3/4 of men with prostate cancer have some response to hormonal therapy, in up to 1/3 of men with advanced, symptomatic disease the cancer becomes refractory to hormonal manipulation within a year.

BLADDER CANCER

The annual incidence of bladder cancer is 20 cases per 100,000 persons $\geq$ 40 yr of age; the incidence in men is twice that in women. Exposure to dyes and cigarettes are particularly important risk factors. Bladder cancer represents a spectrum of pathologic processes with different tendencies for invasion, spread, and multicentric evolution.

The **diagnosis** of bladder cancer must be considered in any older patient complaining of gross hematuria not caused by urinary tract infection. A urinalysis revealing > 5 RBCs per high-power field or a positive test for hemoglobin should prompt cystoscopic evaluation. About 10% of older patients with hematuria have bladder cancer. Other common identifiable causes include urethral inflammation, benign prostatic hyperplasia, and bladder stone. Since renal cell or ureteral cancers occasionally cause hematuria that is missed by cystoscopy alone, renal ultrasonography, CT scanning, or IV urography is reasonable in the older patient whose hematuria is inadequately explained by cystoscopic findings. However, IV urogram and retrograde pyelogram are the best tests for finding transitional cell carcinoma; the retrograde study helps avoid the complications of IV dye loads. The insensitivity and nonspecificity of urine cytologic examination make it inadequate as the sole test for bladder, ureteral, or renal cancer.

In general, the depth of tumor penetration and histologic grade correspond best with metastatic potential. More than 70% of bladder cancers are discovered as superficial tumors. However, unpredictability of spread and recurrence makes **treatment** of even superficial tumors difficult. Usually, solitary superficial papillary tumors have the lowest recurrence rate; multiple superficial tumors, the highest. Although removal of the bladder would seem to be the simplest way to eliminate the risk for metastatic spread, cystectomy is fraught with significant morbid risks for local disease, infection, dehydration, and acidosis. Endoscopic excision, partial cystectomy, intravesical chemotherapy or BCG therapy, and repeated cystoscopic surveillance remain the most common therapies for disease limited to the bladder. Treatment for disease outside the bladder is experimental.

SCROTAL MASSES

Scrotal hernias, especially large, neglected ones, are difficult to correct surgically. However, for the physiologically healthy elderly man who has neither advanced chronic obstructive pulmonary disease nor prostatism, either primary surgical repair or secondary repair using autogenous fascia or a plastic mesh may be successful.

Hydroceles, which transilluminate, and **varicoceles,** which feel like "a bag of worms," occasionally present de novo in the elderly; testicular and renal cancer, respectively, should be ruled out. When the size of the hydrocele prompts the patient to request treatment, aspiration or surgical excision may be offered. However, aspiration is seldom permanently effective. Varicoceles are treated by ligation or embolectomy of the spermatic vein.

Epididymo-orchitis usually is a temporary sequela of a urinary tract infection, prostatectomy, cystoscopy, or indwelling catheterization. Treatment of this painful condition consists of bed rest, scrotal support, and an antibiotic effective against both gram-negative bacteria and *Chlamydia,* such as tetracycline. These infections occasionally form abscesses that require surgical drainage.

Although **testicular cancer** is rare in the elderly, painless testicular masses should always be considered neoplastic. At a minimum, ultrasound evaluation is indicated. **Lymphoma** is the most common testicular malignancy in the elderly. Unfortunately, even patients whose disease seems to be limited to the testicle may have systemic disease. Therefore, after orchiectomy establishes the local diagnosis, further evaluation (CT scan, bone marrow biopsy, chest x-ray) is usually necessary for staging and decisions regarding radiation therapy or chemotherapy. Of the germ cell tumors, **spermatocytic seminomas** occur most frequently in the elderly and carry a favorable prognosis. Orchiectomy is the only treatment required. Other germ cell tumors, including other seminomas, are usually aggressive and metastasize early.

---

65. URINARY TRACT INFECTION

Bacterial urinary tract infections **(UTIs)** are classified according to the following clinical criteria:

1. Localization, as **cystitis** in the bladder wall and **pyelonephritis** in the kidney.

2. Tendency to recur, as **recurrent** and **sporadic infections** (a term preferred to "acute" because recurrent infections often produce acute symptoms). There is no universally accepted definition of recurrent infection; one proposal is to call an infection recurrent *if the patient has more than one episode in a 6-mo period or more than two episodes in a* *year.* Recurrent infections are subclassified as **relapses** and **reinfections.** A relapse is caused by the same bacterial strain as the previous infection; ie, therapy failed to eradicate the bacteria or the patient developed a new infection with the same strain. A reinfection is caused by a bacterial strain different from the one that caused the previous infection.

3. Symptomatology, as **symptomatic** and **asymptomatic infections.** Asymptomatic bacteriuria is characterized by ≥ 10^5 colony-forming units (CFU)/mL without dysuria, urinary frequency, incontinence of recent onset, flank pain, fever, or other signs of infection during the week preceding the time the urine sample was obtained. Small numbers of WBCs are common.

4. Complicating factors, as **complicated** and **uncomplicated infections.** All UTIs occurring in men are considered complicated.

Epidemiology

The annual incidence of symptomatic bacterial UTIs in elderly persons is estimated to be as high as 10%. Since many of these infections are recurrent, the actual number of infected patients is lower. In younger populations, UTIs are much more prevalent in women; in the elderly, the sex difference narrows, in part because older men often suffer from bladder outlet obstruction from benign prostatic hyperplasia. Additionally, the reduced incidence of UTI in elderly women may be due to a decrease in sexual activity, which can introduce bacteria into the bladder. Severe UTIs, particularly septicemia originating from the urinary tract, become more common with advancing age (see UROSEPSIS, below), in part because of more frequent bladder catheterization and instrumentation and possibly from changes in the immune system. Recurrent and complicated infections are also more common because of the higher frequency of predisposing anatomic and pathophysiologic factors, such as prolapse, urolithiasis, and malignancies in the genitourinary tract and uterus.

Etiology

UTIs are almost always caused by **aerobic bacteria.** Anaerobes are isolated only from patients with rectovesical fistulas or other abnormal communications between the urinary tract and bowel, allowing the anaerobic fecal flora direct access to the urine. Bacteriologic findings vary according to previous antibiotic therapy, type of infection (complicated or uncomplicated, sporadic or recurrent), and whether the bacteriuria is community- or hospital-acquired.

Escherichia coli is the pathogen most commonly isolated. It accounts for up to 90% of bacteriuria in elderly female outpatients with uncomplicated sporadic cystitis and for about 40% in patients with indwelling bladder catheters, complicated infections, or hospital-acquired infections.

Klebsiella spp, especially *K. pneumoniae,* are the second most commonly isolated gram-negative, aerobic pathogens. *Proteus mirabilis, P. vulgaris, P. inconstans,* and *Morganella morganii* are more common in men than in women because these species tend to dominate the normal aerobic preputial flora. They are also commonly isolated from the urine of patients with calculi, since they grow best in an alkaline milieu, and from patients with urogenital tumors. *Proteus* spp, *M. morganii,* and *Providencia* spp are commonly isolated from patients who are chronically catheterized. *Serratia, Enterobacter, Citrobacter, Acinetobacter,* and *Pseudomonas* spp are seen mainly in patients with hospital-acquired UTIs.

In patients with **recurrent infections,** gram-negative bacteria other than *E. coli* and gram-positive bacteria tend to predominate. Of the latter, enterococci are commonly isolated, since many antibiotics used to treat bacteriuria (eg, cephalosporins and sulfonamides) are inactive against these organisms, resulting in enterococcal **superinfection.**

Pathogenesis

Host factors: **In aging women,** atrophic vaginal mucosa may predispose to bacteriuria, since the vault is often heavily colonized with gram-negative aerobes. Women have short urethras, which allow bacteria to be transported easily to the bladder. Atrophic urethritis adds further to the risk of UTI because the epithelium is thinner in the external portion of the urethra. **In aging men,** benign prostatic hyperplasia, carcinoma of the prostate, and urethral strictures predispose to UTIs.

Bacteria proliferate in stagnant bladder urine, and clinically important bacteriuria becomes established. A large amount of postvoiding residual urine is most common with a neurologic disorder, bladder outlet obstruction, or urethral stricture. A residual urine of 5 to 20 mL is not uncommon in otherwise healthy elderly persons. **Foreign bodies,** most commonly indwelling bladder catheters, also promote bacterial growth. In catheterized patients, important bacteriuria is established within 14 days unless a closed and aseptically handled system is used, in which case bacterial growth may be delayed for an additional, variable period of time. With time, indwelling catheters always lead to bacteriuria. Bladder calculi can also result in sustained bacteriuria that is difficult to treat even with antibiotics. Development of bacteriuria is facilitated by poorly controlled **diabetes mellitus;** increased urine glucose provides the substrate for bacterial growth.

Bacterial virulence factors: Bacterial species differ in their tendency to colonize urine. The most important bacterial virulence factor is the ability to adhere to epithelial cells in the urethra and the ureters. The bacterial antigen responsible for adherence is located in the pili (fimbriae) of *E. coli* and probably of other gram-negative species. The receptor is a glycosphingolipid on uroepithelial cells and erythrocytes. Persons who lack the blood group P (a rare situation) do not have this glycosphingolipid and are less prone to develop bacteriuria. Attachment of bacteria to epithelial cells in the urethra and the ureters facilitates transport to the bladder and kidneys, respectively. Bacterial attachment also causes the epithelial cells to release cytokines, mainly interleukin-1 and interleukin-6, with subsequent systemic reactions such as fever and increased levels of C-reactive protein. While adherence is an important virulence factor in patients with normal anatomy, it seems to be less important in those with abnormal anatomy.

Diagnosis

Bacteriologic diagnosis is usually based on the concept of **clinically important bacteriuria.** The usual definition of important bacteriuria, *$> 10^5$ colony-forming units (CFU)/mL of a midstream urine sample following > 4 h of bladder incubation,* still applies to complicated and recurrent UTIs and to asymptomatic bacteriuria. In women with uncomplicated cystitis, however, the highest diagnostic sensitivity and specificity are achieved when clinically important bacteriuria is defined as *$> 10^2$ CFU/mL with pyuria* (increased number of leukocytes in the urine) in a symptomatic patient. If the clinical importance of bacteriuria is doubtful (eg, when repeated samples yield more than one bacterial strain), urine may be obtained by **bladder puncture** (which is better than bladder catheterization because the risk of contamination is minimized). *Any number* of bacteria is then important.

For culture, urine samples should be obtained at least a few hours after the last voiding. Waiting is not necessary in patients with residual urine or in those with indwelling bladder catheters.

Rapid tests can provide a semiquantitative determination of bacteriuria. The best is the **nitrite test,** in which the conversion of nitrate to nitrite by bacteria in the urine is demonstrated by color change on a dipstick. This test has a high degree of sensitivity and specificity but does not demonstrate bacteriuria caused by *Pseudomonas* spp, staphylococci, or enterococci, which are incapable of metabolizing nitrate.

Quantitative urine cultures can be performed by bacteriology laboratories; the urine must be refrigerated if culture and incubation are delayed. The test identifies the species involved and determines antibiotic susceptibility. In outpatient clinics, a **dip-slide culture** may be used, in which an agar-covered slide is dipped in urine and incubated or even left at room temperature overnight. The number of bacteria in the sample is reliably quantified, and gram-negative and gram-positive organisms are differentiated. A positive dip-slide can later be sent to a bacteriology laboratory for identification of species and determination of antibiotic susceptibility.

ASYMPTOMATIC BACTERIURIA

Bacteriuria in a patient who had no symptoms of UTI during the week preceding the time the urine sample was obtained.

Diagnosis

The diagnosis is based on demonstration of *bacteriuria with limited or no pyuria in two or more consecutive samples.* Only about 70% of asymptomatic patients with high colony counts in a single urine sample have true bacteriuria as confirmed on the second sample. Asymptomatic bacteriuria is a common finding in the elderly, especially in women.

Treatment

The treatment of asymptomatic bacteriuria is generally not warranted, although neither the benefit of treating it nor the risk of withholding treatment has been demonstrated.

In women, asymptomatic bacteriuria should not be treated unless coexisting conditions may increase the risk of symptomatic invasive disease. In untreated asymptomatic bacteriuria, the organisms (especially *E. coli*) lose their virulence and become extremely susceptible to the bactericidal effect of normal human plasma. Large amounts of bacteria in the urine may therefore protect against symptomatic bacteriuria caused by more virulent strains. Additionally, *the bacteria in a patient with asymptomatic bacteriuria become more susceptible to antibiotics* and can be eradicated by antibiotics used for treating other infections, leaving the patient at higher risk for acquiring a symptomatic infection.

In men, asymptomatic bacteriuria should be investigated to exclude complicating factors such as residual urine, calculi, or tumors. While the diagnosis is being determined and causative factors are eliminated, treatment should be considered with the antibiotics indicated by sensitivity testing of identified bacteria.

Asymptomatic bacteriuria in elderly persons with chronic bladder catheterization may be associated with increased mortality, probably due to other diseases or general frailty. Urosepsis is more common in patients catheterized for prolonged periods. Yet, treating asymptomatic bacteriuria in persons with indwelling catheters is generally not advised; recolonization rapidly develops after treatment ends. Thus, to prevent increased mortality, catheter use must be minimized. *Catheters should be used only when medically indicated* and not as a remedy for urinary incontinence. Whenever possible, the conditions leading to a need for catheterization should be corrected.

CYSTITIS

Infection localized to the bladder wall.

Bacteriuria is the most common clinical manifestation of cystitis. The urethra is also often infected **(cystourethritis).** Symptoms are caused by inflammation of the urethral and bladder mucosa.

Symptoms and Signs

The onset of cystitis is usually acute, with urgency, dysuria (burning sensation during micturition), and frequency (pollakiuria). The patient often feels the urge to void three to four times per hour although little urine is excreted; the urine may be foul-smelling. In the elderly, cystitis sometimes presents more cryptically, with vague complaints, fever, or incontinence. Gross hematuria is more common in young women than in the elderly, especially with infections caused by *Staphylococcus saprophyticus*. Physical examination yields few positive findings; there may be suprapubic tenderness on palpation.

Diagnosis

The diagnosis is based on the history and the results of urinalysis, rapid tests such as the nitrite test for demonstration of bacteriuria, and urine culture. Urine microscopy shows a large number of polymorphonuclear leukocytes. Erythrocytes may be seen, but casts should not. Bacteria may be seen (a finding that is not diagnostic), and microscopy may allow differentiation between rods and cocci. Bacteriuria cannot be quantified by light microscopy. Proteinuria is common and is the result of the large cellular content (not renal disease).

The **differential diagnosis** is often difficult. Urethritis without bacteriuria may cause the same symptoms as cystitis. In patients with pyuria but whose routine bacterial culture shows no growth, tuberculosis of the urinary tract should be considered; centrifuged urine should be stained for acid-fast bacilli (Ziehl-Neelsen method) and cultured for mycobacteria. The most important differential diagnosis is between cystitis and pyelonephritis. WBC casts seen in the urine on microscopy strongly support a diagnosis of pyelonephritis, but the diagnosis is usually made from clinical signs of flank tenderness, fever, elevated WBC count, and sometimes positive blood culture (see PYELONEPHRITIS, below).

Prognosis

Uncomplicated cystitis recurs in $\geq$ 10% of cases, based on follow-up urine cultures obtained 3 to 5 wk after completion of treatment. Most recurrences are reinfections, and relapses are seen in $<$ 3% of properly treated patients. In patients with complicated cystitis (eg, those with residual urine), the frequency of recurrence is much higher (ie, $>$ 25%). Such patients are also at greater risk for ascending infections and development of pyelonephritis.

Treatment

Cystitis should be treated with renally excreted antibacterial agents active against the most frequently isolated pathogens, especially *E. coli* and enterococci. Coverage in the antibacterial spectrum of *S. saprophyticus* is not necessary in elderly patients. Since most cases of cystitis are uncomplicated, an antimicrobial should be chosen that causes a minimum of adverse reactions and, if possible, is inexpensive.

Patients with **community-acquired infections** can be treated with trimethoprim, a short course of trimethoprim-sulfamethoxazole (TMP-SMX), or an oral cephalosporin (eg, cephalexin, cefadroxil, loracarbef, cefuroxime). When organisms are resistant or when the risk of pyelonephritis is high, a fluorinated quinolone derivative (eg, norfloxacin, ofloxacin, ciprofloxacin, lomefloxacin) can be used, but these agents are expensive. Newer fluorinated quinolones are preferred over older nonfluorinated ones (eg, nalidixic acid and cinoxacin) because of their wider spectrum and lower incidence of emerging resistance. Ampicillin and amoxicillin are generally not preferred since at least 13% of *E. coli* strains are resistant to them.

In patients with **recurrent or complicated infections or hospital-acquired infections,** a fluoroquinolone or trimethoprim is recommended before the cephalosporins and amdinocillin pivoxil, since the first drugs are also active against enterococci. When renal function is markedly reduced, dosage should be decreased accordingly, either by lowering the dose at each administration or by prolonging the dose interval.

The **duration of treatment of uncomplicated cystitis** varies. Single-dose therapy, using two or three times the normal single dose, has been extensively evaluated. In all studies, single-dose treatment has been considerably less effective than treatment for 3 days or longer. Although 3 days of treatment with TMP-SMX has been shown to be as effective as and much safer than treatment for 5 days or more, expert opinion varies, with suggested duration ranging from 3 to 7 days. With cephalosporins and penicillins, treatment for 5 to 7 days is required. Trimethoprim and fluoroquinolones should be given for 3 to 7 days.

In persons with frequently recurring cystitis or in whom instrumentation of the lower genitourinary tract is planned, **prophylactic treatment** may be considered. Drugs recommended for prophylactic use are nitrofurantoin one 50- to 100-mg dose at night (lower doses should be given to patients with markedly reduced renal function), trimethoprim one 50- to 100-mg dose at night, or TMP-SMX 80 mg-400 mg (half or full tablet nightly or one tablet 3 times/wk). With nitrofurantoin, the risk of pulmonary hypersensitivity reactions should be kept in mind. Prophylactic therapy should *not* be used in patients with indwelling bladder catheters.

PYELONEPHRITIS

(Infectious Tubulointerstitial Nephritis)

Infection involving the renal parenchyma and renal pelvis.

Isolated pyelitis or infectious nephritis is extremely uncommon. **Chronic pyelonephritis** with renal scarring may develop in patients who had childhood pyelonephritis or who have renal tubular necrosis caused by overconsumption of phenacetin derivatives. Chronic phenacetin-associated pyelonephritis is usually found only in elderly patients with past exposure to phenacetin derivatives because these agents are no longer used in most countries.

In elderly patients with pyelonephritis, bacteria invade the renal parenchyma, usually from the renal pelvis. Reflux of urine from the bladder during micturition, ureteral or pelvic calculi, congenital or acquired pelvic deformity, or renal parenchymal disease all increase the risk of pyelonephritis. Infection of the renal parenchyma directly from a hematogenous source, although infrequent, may occur in debilitated, septic patients.

Symptoms and Signs

About 8% to 10% of all patients with symptomatic UTIs have pyelonephritis; the percentage in the elderly is unknown. These patients may present with an initial history of cystitis. Typical symptoms are fever, chills, and back pain, which may be unilateral or bilateral; bacteremia occurs in up to 25% to 30%. Sudden clinical deterioration may indicate septicemia.

Diagnosis

Bacteriuria is diagnosed as for cystitis (see above). Urine microscopy shows pyuria and often WBC casts. Most patients have leukocytosis with an absolute increase in polymorphonuclear leukocytes. Serum creatinine and BUN levels are sometimes elevated. Bacteriologic tests should always include identification of species and determination of antibiotic susceptibility. In most cases, the clinical features and microscopic findings in urine provide the diagnosis.

Blood cultures should be obtained in patients with fever, hypotension, or acute confusion. **Ultrasonography** or **radioisotope scanning** should be performed *only* if renal pelvic or ureteral obstruction due to a calculus is suspected. Intravenous dye studies pose great risk in frail elderly persons, and retrograde studies are generally preferable.

The **differential diagnosis** is often difficult. Renal pelvic or ureteral stones may produce a pattern of pain similar to that of pyelonephritis but do not normally cause fever. Acute appendicitis may simulate right-sided pyelonephritis. Cholangitis and cholecystitis should also be considered in patients with right-sided symptoms. Patients with lower lobe pneumonia may have back pain, fever, and leukocytosis similar to that of pyelonephritis.

Prognosis

The prognosis is good for an appropriately treated patient with pyelonephritis, and renal function returns to normal about 3 wk after treatment. However, a permanent reduction in renal function may remain in patients with previous renal damage, especially those who had recurrent episodes of pyelonephritis with renal scarring during childhood. Previous episodes of pyelonephritis that occurred only during adulthood do not normally worsen the prognosis. Patients who develop septicemia have a poor prognosis (see UROSEPSIS, below).

To prevent asymptomatic recurrences, all patients should be reevaluated with renal function tests and urine cultures at 1 wk and at 3 to 6 wk after treatment. A retrograde dye study may be indicated to detect renal scars if one was not performed during the previous 3 yr.

Treatment

Antibiotic treatment should be started as soon as urine and blood cultures are obtained, especially if there are signs of sepsis (eg, high fever, tachycardia, low blood pressure). Hospitalization is usually necessary unless the patient is otherwise healthy and can be monitored closely. Antibiotics should cover all important gram-negative uropathogens, pending identification. Therapy should be continued for at least 10 and preferably 14 days. Patients receiving initial treatment with parenteral antibiotics can be switched to oral drugs within a day after fever and pain resolve. Prolonged fever (5 days) is not uncommon in uncomplicated, properly treated pyelonephritis.

Suitable antibiotics for initial **oral treatment** include fluoroquinolones (eg, norfloxacin, ciprofloxacin, ofloxacin, lomefloxacin), oral cephalosporins (eg, cefadroxil, loracarbef), combinations of trimethoprim and sulfonamides, and amdinocillin pivoxil plus pivampicillin (not approved in the USA) or amoxicillin. Antibiotic sensitivity tests will guide follow-up treatment for those who began treatment with parenteral agents.

Patients requiring a **parenteral antibiotic** can be given a cephalosporin, pending results of culture and sensitivity tests. Aminoglycosides can also be used, but they pose more risk. In patients with community-acquired infections who have not received previous antibiotic treatment, a second-generation cephalosporin (eg, cefuroxime) will cover most pathogens; in patients with hospital-acquired infections, a third-generation cephalosporin (eg, cefotaxime, ceftazidime, ceftriaxone), aztreonam, or an aminoglycoside is preferred. Intravenous trimethoprim-sulfamethoxazole is an alternative. Amoxicillin or ampicillin alone is not recommended, since $\geq$ 13% of all urinary isolates of *E. coli* and even higher percentages of other gram-negative urinary pathogens are resistant to these antibiotics.

Reduced doses are often necessary in elderly patients because renal function is reduced by both aging and pyelonephritis. If aminoglycosides are used, serum concentrations must be monitored at regular intervals (ie, at least twice weekly) to avoid nephrotoxic or ototoxic reactions and to guarantee that therapeutic concentrations are achieved.

UROSEPSIS

Septicemia originating from the urinary tract.

Urosepsis is very common in the elderly, especially after initial insertion or change of a bladder catheter or after cystoscopy, during which bacteria in the urine enter the blood through traumatized urethral mucosa.

Symptoms and Signs

The patient may have a recent history of catheterization or cystoscopy; symptoms generally begin within 24 to 72 h. Onset is acute with fever, chills, and often signs of septic shock, although patients who develop septic shock may be afebrile on admission. Renal function is often seriously impaired, and anuria is common.

Diagnosis

The diagnosis is based on the history and physical findings. Bacteriologic confirmation is obtained from blood and urine cultures. Granulocytosis and elevations in ESR and C-reactive protein values are usually found. Electrolyte imbalance and elevated serum creatinine and BUN levels are common. Important differential diagnoses are hypovolemic shock and cardiogenic shock.

Prognosis and Treatment

The prognosis for geriatric patients with urosepsis is poor; 23% to 30% of those with positive blood cultures die. Early defervescence is a good prognostic sign.

Antibiotics should always be administered IV during the initial phase of treatment. The duration of IV treatment and oral follow-up is the same as for pyelonephritis (see above). First-line antibiotics are second- and third-generation cephalosporins, aztreonam, and aminoglycosides. Although the initial dose should always be maximal, subsequent doses usually need to be reduced substantially because of markedly decreased renal function. Maintenance of fluid and electrolyte balance as well as adequate blood pressure is critical.

---

66. FEMALE GENITOURINARY DISORDERS

(Genital atrophy as a result of estrogen deficiency is discussed in Ch. 83.)

Disorders of the gynecologic and lower urinary tract system, both benign and malignant, are very common in postmenopausal women. Symptoms typically include vaginal itching and burning, pain with intercourse, genital bleeding, pelvic pressure or protrusion, urinary frequency and urgency, and pelvic pain. Many older women are embarrassed to mention these symptoms to their primary care physicians, or they believe that the primary care provider may not know what to do about gynecologic problems. Thus, a basic gynecologic history and physical examination are important.

The **gynecologic examination** sometimes poses special problems for older women. If a patient has not had a pelvic examination for many years, she may find it embarrassing or uncomfortable. Women with arthritis or stiff joints may have difficulty assuming the lithotomy position and may find the left lateral position more comfortable. Additionally, the deep palpation needed to assess a small uterus and ovaries sometimes causes pain. Extra time, explanation, reassurance, and sensitivity are required.

The entire vulva and groin area should be palpated and visually inspected for specific lesions, nodal enlargement, vulvitis, or vulvar dystrophy. A speculum examination allows the vagina and cervix to be inspected for signs of atrophy or atrophic vaginitis, other types of vaginal inflammation, and vaginal or cervical lesions. The vaginal walls and cervix should be palpated for paravaginal masses and cervical abnormalities, and a bimanual examination should be performed to assess uterine size and shape, to evaluate pelvic and adnexal structures and the lower rectum, and to detect any adnexal lesions. A stool guaiac test should also be performed. If uterine or ovarian disease is suspected, then pelvic ultrasound evaluation may prove helpful.

Hematuria (blood in the urine) without evidence of infection is an indication for a full **urologic evaluation.** Although sometimes idiopathic, hematuria may signal a more serious condition such as transitional cell carcinoma, renal stones, or other renal neoplasias. Evaluation should include IV urography, renal ultrasonography, urine cytology, and cystourethroscopy. Intravenous urography must be performed with care in the elderly; hydration helps reduce the risk of renal impairment, but fluid overload and heart failure can follow.

POSTMENOPAUSAL BLEEDING

Postmenopausal bleeding may be associated with benign, premalignant, or malignant disease (see TABLE 66–1) and usually warrants thorough investigation. About 20% to 30% of patients with postmenopausal bleeding have endometrial carcinoma or atypical adenomatous hyperplasia. The history should include all medical conditions, drug use (especially exogenous estrogens), and previous gynecologic problems. A vulvovaginal examination, including a Papanicolaou (Pap) test and bimanual examination, should be performed to rule out trauma or bleeding from atrophic sites, as well as vulvar, vaginal, or cervical neoplasms.

For most patients, referral to a gynecologist is necessary, in part so that a sample of endometrium can be obtained by biopsy or full fractional dilatation and curettage (D & C). Which procedure is used depends on the physician's suspicion for pathologic findings and the patient's status. If the results of an office biopsy procedure are inconclusive, generally D & C with or without hysteroscopy is indicated.

TABLE 66–1. CAUSES OF POSTMENOPAUSAL BLEEDING

Atrophic vaginitis or cervicitis
Carcinoma of vulva, vagina, urethra, cervix, tube, or ovary
Endometrial atrophic bleeding
Endometrial stimulation by endogenous or exogenous estrogen
Endometrial polyps
Endometrial hyperplasia
Endometrial carcinoma, including sarcoma
Metastatic carcinoma to uterus, vagina, bladder, or urethra
Vaginal or vulvar trauma

PELVIC SUPPORT DISORDERS

Because women today are living longer, pelvic support disorders are becoming more prevalent. What causes pelvic support problems, or **pelvic relaxation,** is not known, although certain factors are known to exacerbate these problems (eg, trauma with childbirth; increased abdominal pressure because of obesity, chronic coughing, or straining at stool; and estrogen deficiency).

The most common symptom of pelvic relaxation is heaviness or pressure in the vaginal area. A mass may protrude at the introitus. These symptoms almost always occur when the patient is upright and are of little bother when she is supine.

Some of the more common pelvic support disorders include rectoceles, enteroceles, cystoceles, or a combination of these defects. **Rectoceles** occur when weakness in the muscular wall of the rectum and the perirectal fascia causes the rectum to protrude into the vaginal lumen (see FIG. 66–1). A patient with a rectocele may have difficulty passing stools, and manual manipulation may be needed for complete defecation. An **enterocele** is a herniation of the peritoneum and small bowel. Most enteroceles occur between the uterosacral ligaments downward into the rectovaginal space and may be visibly indistinguishable from rectoceles. Diagnosis is usually made by rectovaginal examination with the patient performing a Valsalva maneuver while standing; when the patient does so, the prolapsing small bowel can usually be felt to bulge downward (see FIG. 66–2). **Cystoceles** are hernial protrusions of the urinary bladder through the anterior vaginal wall; they usually occur when the pubocervical fascia weakens or detaches from its lat-

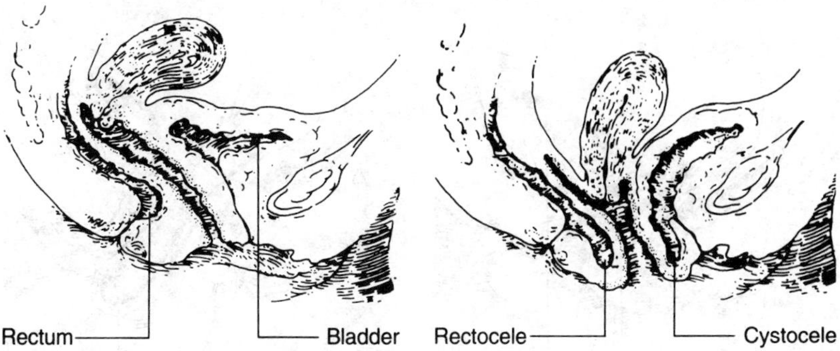

FIG. 66–1. ***Left,*** **sagittal section showing normal anatomy;** ***right,*** **cystocele and rectocele.**

eral or superior connecting points. Cystoceles may lead to stress or overflow urinary incontinence (see Ch. 15), incomplete bladder emptying, or urinary tract infection.

Other pelvic support disorders include uterine prolapse and procidentia. **Uterine prolapse** is generally the result of poor cardinal or uterosacral ligament support. Patients with uterine prolapse may have lower back or sacral pain while standing, although many patients are asymptomatic. Typically, uterine prolapse is classified as first degree when the cervix descends below the level of the ischial spine, second degree when the cervix descends to but not through the introitus, and third degree when the cervix descends through the introitus. **Procidentia,** which involves prolapse of the uterus and vagina, and **total vaginal vault prolapse,** which can occur after hysterectomy, represent eversion of the entire vagina (see FIG. 66–3). Because the vagina protrudes through the introitus, a patient with total vaginal vault prolapse may experience pain, especially when sitting. Both vault prolapse and third-degree uterine prolapse may lead to ulceration of the vaginal mucosa. Patients with total vaginal or uterine prolapse may have bladder or rectal dysfunction. For example, many patients have difficulty voiding and have chronic residual urine, problems that are often worse after prolonged standing and are presumably due to urethral kinking. Although $< 1/3$ of these patients develop urinary incontinence, at least $2/3$ demonstrate stress incontinence when the prolapse is reduced. In some patients, kinking of the urethra may be protective, as it stops urine from leaking when the anterior vagina and bladder protrude. Ureteral obstruction and subsequent renal damage are uncommon but should be sought if the patient has an enlarged uterus or a pelvic mass.

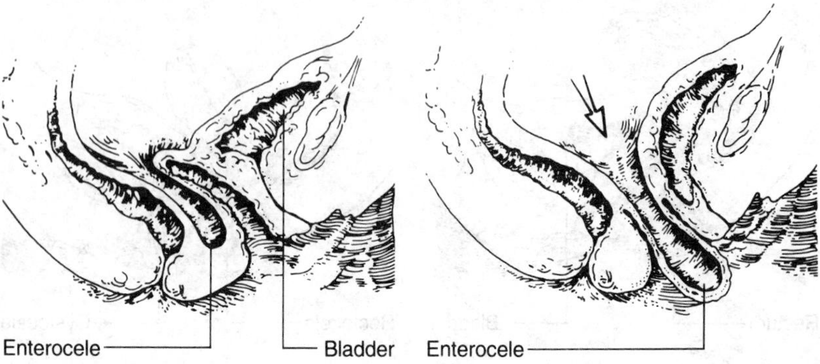

FIG. 66–2. ***Left,*** **posterior enterocele without eversion;** ***right,*** **enterocele with eversion.**

Anal sphincter tone and the bulbocavernosus reflex should be assessed in a patient whose uterus or vaginal vault prolapses through the introitus. Additional tests include residual urine measurement, urinalysis, urine culture and sensitivity, and bladder fill-testing and stress-testing with the prolapse reduced. Most patients with severe urinary leakage or symptoms and signs of complex bladder dysfunction should undergo full urodynamic assessment (see Ch. 15).

Treatment

The treatment of pelvic floor disorders may be medical or surgical. Medical management involves the use of a pessary. Several types of pessaries are available (see FIG. 66–4); some are placed and changed periodically by the physician, and others are placed each morning and removed each night by the patient. Although many patients find pessaries to be quite acceptable, some elderly women find them difficult to use. They are particularly useful for those in whom surgery is contraindicated. Surgical treatment involves a transvaginal or transabdominal approach and has numerous variations as discussed below.

Rectoceles are best repaired transvaginally with dissection of the rectovaginal space to fully expose the defect in the rectal wall or pararectal fascia. The defect is then closed with interrupted or running delayed absorbable sutures. Further plication of the pararectal fascia, paralevator fascia, and the fascia of the perineal body may be performed to maintain anterior positioning of the distal vagina.

Enteroceles may be repaired vaginally or abdominally. Repairs involve dissection and excision of the enterocele sac, then closure usually

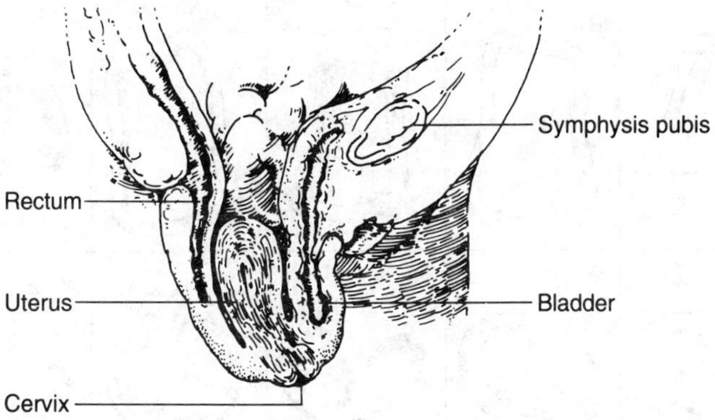

FIG. 66–3. Procidentia of uterus and vagina.

with pursestring sutures or occasionally with a series of vertically placed sutures (Halban procedure).

Cystoceles may be repaired either transabdominally or transvaginally. The vaginal approach involves dissection of the vesicovaginal space and plication of the pubocervical fascia, thereby correcting its attenuation. The abdominal approach is particularly useful for patients who have lateral detachment of the pubocervical fascia, in which case the fascia may be reapproximated to the arcus tendineus within the obturator fascia on the pelvic sidewall. For all cystocele repairs, the pubocervical fascia should be anchored firmly to the vaginal cuff or to the paravaginal fascia on the posterior side of the vaginal cuff to prevent future cuff defects.

For patients with **uterine prolapse, procidentia,** or **total vaginal vault prolapse,** the upper vagina should be attached to a stable structure within the pelvis. With vaginal procedures, the sacrospinous or sacrotuberous ligament on the posterior pelvic sidewall provides a good attachment point (sacrospinous or sacrotuberous vaginal suspension). With abdominal procedures, a synthetic or fascial graft secures the upper vagina to the anterior sacral ligament below the sacral prominence (sacrocolpo suspension).

Large defects, such as vaginal vault prolapse and procidentia, are best managed by surgeons experienced in repairing these problems. If the patient is to undergo surgery, then all pelvic support defects should be corrected. Minimal defects that are not repaired will likely become worse with time. Any lower urinary tract problems (notably stress incontinence) should also be corrected (see Ch. 15).

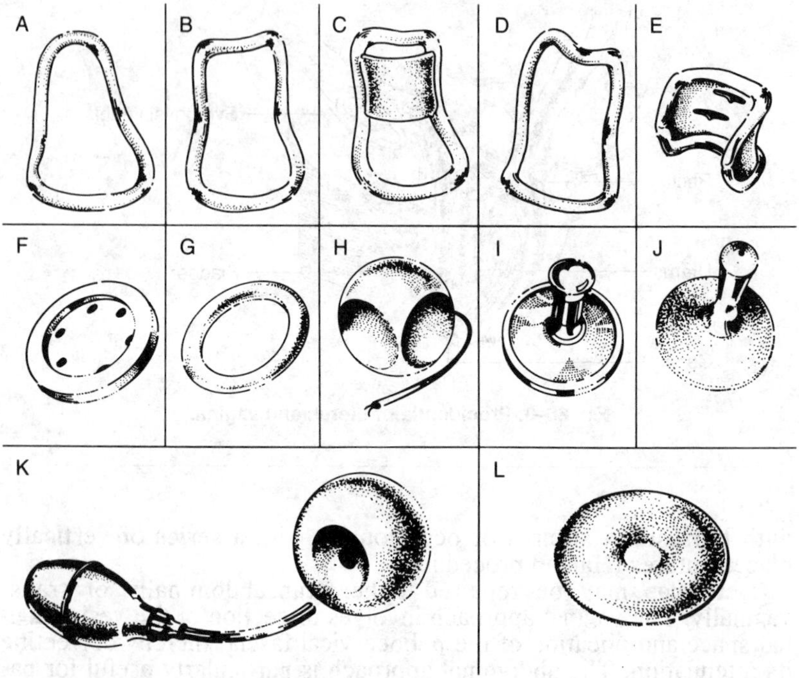

FIG. 66–4. Types of vaginal pessaries. (A) Smith's; (B) Hodge's; (C) Hodge's with web support; (D) Risser; (E) Gehrung; (F) ring with web support; (G) ring; (H) cube; (I) Gelhorn, rigid; (J) Gellhorn, flexible; (K) Inflatoball; (L) doughnut. Choice of pessary is a matter of physician and patient preference.

CARUNCLE

A caruncle, sometimes referred to as a prolapsed urethra, is characterized by erythematous urethral mucosa protruding through the external urethral orifice. Compared with a neoplasm, which is generally firm and nontender, a caruncle is soft and may be tender. The patient may have dysuria and bleeding. Asymptomatic caruncles generally require no treatment; symptomatic caruncles can be removed under local anesthesia.

FISTULAS

Genitourinary and enterourinary fistulas occur in elderly women under fairly well-defined circumstances.

Vesicovaginal and Ureterovaginal Fistulas

Vesicovaginal or ureterovaginal fistulas may follow hysterectomy for benign conditions or (rarely) other pelvic surgical procedures. Patients leak urine continuously or intermittently and have some vulvar excoriation and erythema. Vesicovaginal fistulas occasionally occur in elderly women many years after radiation therapy for pelvic malignancy; these patients typically present with total urinary incontinence. In this case, recurrent cancer is a strong possibility and must be excluded.

The diagnosis of a vesicovaginal fistula can be established by cystography (a cystogram with fluid containing a colored dye), cystoscopy, vaginal examination, or vaginography. However, none of these diagnostic tests is sufficiently sensitive to rule out a fistula if the result is negative. Intravenous or retrograde urography is the best test for diagnosing ureterovaginal fistula.

Fistulas that are caused by surgical or obstetric trauma are best managed by surgical correction. Fistulas that are caused by cancer or radiation-induced injury usually require a diversionary procedure.

Urethrovaginal Fistulas

Urethrovaginal fistulas are very rare but may occur in a patient who has had surgery for stress incontinence or urethral diverticula. If the bladder outlet is closed by a well-functioning sphincter and the fistula lies below the sphincter, urine pools in the vagina during voiding and results in postvoiding incontinence. Fistulas distal to the external sphincter are generally asymptomatic, although they may also result in postvoiding incontinence.

Diagnosis is made by endoscopy, urethrography, or both, sometimes using a double-balloon catheter to occlude both the internal and external urethral orifices. Many fistulas are missed on the first diagnostic attempt. Treatment is surgical, involving closure of the fistula, and often requires interposition of some vascularized tissue, such as a labial subcutaneous flap.

Colovesical Fistulas

Colovesical (enterovesical) fistulas in the elderly may be associated with diverticulitis or, less commonly, with a colonic malignancy. Symptoms include lower abdominal pain, cystitis, pneumaturia, and hematuria. Colovesical fistulas should be sought promptly if the patient has repeated urinary tract infections or infections that fail to respond to continuous suppressive antimicrobial therapy, especially when multiple bowel flora are cultured from the urine. Diagnosis is often difficult because the fistulas may intermittently seal, making them difficult to find on the first attempt. Diagnostic methods include barium enema, sigmoidoscopy, cystography, and oral ingestion of charcoal with subsequent examination of the urine for charcoal particles.

The treatment of colovesical fistulas associated with diverticulitis depends on the extent and nature of the inflammatory process. In some cases, the involved segment of sigmoid colon can be resected, with immediate reanastomosis and closure of the opening in the bladder. In other cases, a proximal diverting colostomy is safer, as it allows the inflammatory process to subside before the involved segment of colon is definitively repaired and resected. Fistulas associated with malignancy usually require excision, with proximal diversion and concurrent treatment of the tumor.

GYNECOLOGIC MALIGNANCIES

Cancers of the female reproductive organs include those of the endometrium, cervix, ovaries, vulva, and vagina.

ENDOMETRIAL CARCINOMA

Endometrial carcinoma is the most common gynecologic malignancy in the USA, affecting mostly postmenopausal women. Peak incidence occurs in women between the ages of 50 and 60. Risk factors include obesity, nulliparity, and using unopposed exogenous estrogens either continuously or cycled (ie, without periodic progesterone).

Postmenopausal bleeding is usually the first symptom in elderly women (see POSTMENOPAUSAL BLEEDING, above). **Diagnosis** is made by fractional biopsy (endometrial biopsy or endocervical curettage), which has a high rate for detecting carcinoma and does not require general anesthesia. Although dilatation and curettage (D & C) of the uterus requires anesthesia, the procedure might be performed because it helps determine whether the carcinoma has spread to the cervix, which may be important in planning therapy.

Treatment is primarily surgical, requiring hysterectomy and retroperitoneal lymph node sampling in the pelvic and para-aortic areas for staging. Upper vaginal or pelvic radiation therapy, chemotherapy, or both may be required for tumors at an advanced stage. Although the incidence of endometrial carcinoma appears to be increasing, early diagnosis and treatment have made the **prognosis** generally better than that for other gynecologic malignancies. Five-year survival rates range from 70% to 75% for those with stage I disease to 10% for those with stage IV disease. The combined 5-yr survival rate for all stages is about 65%.

CERVICAL CARCINOMA

The peak incidence of invasive cervical cancer, the second most common gynecologic tumor, occurs in the 5th and 6th decades. However, this cancer can affect women of all ages, including the elderly. Several human papillomavirus types have been implicated in the development of this disease.

Histologic changes in the cervical epithelium are classified as **minimal cervical dysplasia,** in which abnormal cells proliferate in the lower (basal) 1/3 of the epithelium; **severe dysplasia,** in which abnormal cells proliferate in 2/3 of the epithelium; **carcinoma in situ,** in which a full thickness of epithelium contains abnormal cells; or **invasive carcinoma,** in which cancer cells penetrate the basement membrane and invade the stroma. About 85% to 90% of cervical carcinomas are squamous cell tumors. Adenocarcinomas account for 10% to 15% of cervical tumors, but their incidence may be increasing.

Symptoms depend on the stage of the tumor. Some women with endometrial carcinoma have postcoital or postmenopausal bleeding, although many patients with premalignant or small lesions are asymptomatic. Routine **Papanicolaou (Pap) testing** is the best method of screening for cervical cancer, as it can detect about 90% of early cervical neoplasias. The American Cancer Society and the American College of Obstetricians and Gynecologists support annual Pap tests and pelvic examinations for all women, with no universal upper age limit. Some have proposed that patients who have had three or more consecutive normal results receive Pap tests every 2 to 3 yr until the age of 65. Any woman who has not had regular Pap tests should have at least two tests, a year apart, before the screening interval is lengthened. Women who have had a hysterectomy should receive Pap tests if they have any remaining cervical tissue; otherwise, Pap tests need to be obtained only every 2 to 3 yr to detect upper vaginal neoplasia. The pelvic examination also allows palpation of ovaries and performance of a rectal examination to screen for other cancers.

Colposcopic-directed biopsies and endocervical curettage are useful diagnostic tools when the Pap test result is positive. However, cervical conization may be required for diagnosis because the cervical transformation zone, where most early cancers originate, may not be visible on colposcopy in elderly women. Conization can often be accomplished using diathermy loops in an office setting under local anesthesia.

For early stages of cervical carcinoma, **treatment** involves surgery or radiation therapy, and cure rates using either modality approach 85%. More advanced disease is treated by radiation therapy alone. The combined cure rate for all cervical cancers is 50% to 60%. Chemotherapy is sometimes used as an adjuvant to surgery or radiation but data do not support any substantial added benefit; chemotherapy is not curative as the sole therapy.

OVARIAN CARCINOMA

Ovarian carcinomas most often occur in women in their 50s. Although ovarian cancer is less common than either endometrial or cervical cancer, it is much more deadly. Most malignant tumors of the ovary are either serous or mucinous in character, although many other types exist.

Symptoms develop late and are usually nonspecific, often nothing more than vague abdominal or GI discomfort. Patients may present with large abdominal or pelvic masses, ascites, or both. Ovaries in postmenopausal women are small and normally not palpable. Thus, any palpable ovary on pelvic examination in a postmenopausal patient suggests ovarian carcinoma, and prompt referral to a gynecologist is warranted. If carcinoma is confirmed by ultrasonography, laparoscopy with or without subsequent laparotomy is indicated for definitive diagnosis.

Treatment is first surgical, with the intent to remove all visible disease. Combination IV chemotherapy is given after the surgery, often for several months, except to patients with very early, small, or histologic borderline tumors. Treatment rarely includes radiotherapy.

Operability rates are high, even in women with advanced tumors, and chemotherapy can usually be tolerated. However, a woman who has advanced disease and is debilitated may not be able to withstand major surgery and rigorous chemotherapy. Clinical judgment is needed, and personal choices must also be discussed.

The CA-125 marker is useful for monitoring treatment and disease status in many women, especially those with serous tumors. Survival depends on tumor stage; but since most ovarian tumors are discovered at an advanced stage, the 5-yr survival rate is only about 30%. The survival rate is higher (50% to 80%) in women with germ cell tumors who receive combination therapy.

VULVAR CARCINOMA

Carcinoma of the vulva is the fourth most common gynecologic malignancy, with a peak incidence between the ages of 70 and 80 yr. **Premalignant vulvar lesions** (vulvar dystrophy) must be distinguished from malignant lesions, especially in the elderly. Premalignant lesions may be white patches, brown pigmented areas, or granular red lesions. Although pruritus vulvae is the most common presenting symptom, many patients are asymptomatic. **Malignant vulvar lesions** may be erythematous and flat, condylomatous, or ulcerated; many cause itching, discharge, or local discomfort.

Premalignant vulvar lesions are classified into three types: atrophic, hypertrophic, and mixed. Some physicians still use the term **lichen sclerosus et atrophicus** for atrophic dystrophy. Presumed dystrophic or inflammatory lesions that do not respond within a few weeks to topical therapy with estrogen or corticosteroids should undergo biopsy. Although the potential for malignancy is small, most vulvar lesions should be evaluated by a gynecologist or dermatologist. Some clinicians recommend staining flat or slightly raised ulcerative lesions with toluidine blue, which helps identify areas of nuclear crowding, or applying 3% acetic acid, which coagulates protein-rich neoplastic surface cells and whitens the suspicious area. If these tests are positive, a biopsy is performed. Raised or ulcerated lesions should undergo biopsy without such testing.

Treatment of vulvar lesions is primarily surgical. Topical therapy with cytotoxic agents (such as 5% 5-fluorouracil cream) may be useful for some in situ lesions. However, while treatment with 5-fluorouracil cream results in complete response in 50% of cases, it often causes vulvar irritation and painful superficial ulceration. Most women, no matter how debilitated, can have skin lesions removed under local anesthesia.

In situ lesions, as well as small, superficially microinvasive (1 or 2 mm) vulvar carcinomas, may be removed by wide local excision. Because microinvasive vulvar lesions seem to metastasize to regional lymph nodes more frequently than do comparably sized cervical lesions, consultation with a gynecologic oncologist is suggested, even for superficially invasive lesions. Radical vulvectomy, often combined with unilateral or bilateral inguinal lymphadenectomy, is required for larger or deeply invasive tumors. Radiation therapy occasionally has an adjunctive role; some investigators believe that preoperative radiotherapy can make extensive tumors resectable.

Prognosis is generally good if invasive lesions are treated in an early stage. Five-year survival rates of 80% to 90% are achieved if lymph nodes are negative; survival rates of 16% to 30% are achieved if lymph nodes are positive.

VAGINAL CARCINOMA

Vaginal carcinoma is a relatively rare malignancy that is almost always squamous cell in type, although adenocarcinoma may occur. Early **symptoms** include vaginal bleeding or discharge. Women with these cancers usually have nodular or ulcerated areas on the vaginal mucosa, and all such lesions should undergo biopsy.

Treatment usually consists of a combination of surgery, radiation, and topical chemotherapy, although radiotherapy is probably best for palpable or large lesions. **Prognosis** depends on the size and location of the lesions within the vagina; lesions in the upper third near the cervix may be resectable. Five-year survival rates vary from 25% to 48%.

67. BREAST CANCER

Breast cancer is a major cause of morbidity and mortality in older women. Pathologically, breast cancer may be classified as in situ or as invasive carcinoma. **Ductal carcinoma in situ,** the most common in situ carcinoma in older patients, is generally multicentric and has a high tendency to recur locally after partial mastectomy. Axillary lymph nodes are rarely involved (< 2%). **Lobular carcinoma in situ,** a multicentric lesion that often involves both breasts, is rare after menopause.

Of the invasive carcinomas, **intraductal carcinoma** is the most common in women of all ages. The incidence of **medullary carcinoma,** which is often bilateral, decreases with age, while the incidence of mucinous carcinoma increases. The prognostic significance of different histologic subtypes of breast cancer is unclear. **Inflammatory carcinoma** of the breast is a very aggressive tumor, occurring with equal frequency in pre- and postmenopausal women. Patients with inflammatory carcinoma present with diffuse and poorly defined erythema of the breast; histologically, the carcinoma may produce vascular dilatation, lymphoplasmacytic infiltration, and intralymphatic tumor emboli.

Paget's disease of the nipple, which may be considered a ductal carcinoma in situ, is associated with invasive carcinoma in more than 50% of cases. The incidence of this rare condition increases with age.

Incidence

Each year about 50% of the 175,000 new cases of breast cancer occur in women ≥ 65 yr. The incidence of breast cancer is almost comparable in black and white women > 65 yr. However, since 1970, in all age groups breast cancer incidence has risen more rapidly among black women. The incidence of breast cancer increases up to age 80, then plateaus until age 85, and may decline thereafter. The measured decline in women > 85 yr is difficult to interpret and may reflect the inadequacy of epidemiologic data. Breast cancer in men, which also increases in incidence with age, accounts for 1% of all new cases.

In the USA, a woman's cumulative risk of developing breast cancer is 10.2%, but that of dying from the disease is only about 3.6%. Much of this risk occurs after age 75 (see TABLE 67–1). For example, the oft-cited 10% lifetime risk of developing breast cancer is based on an actuarial analysis and calculated from birth to age 110. The cumulative risk for the disease in any 20-yr period is considerably lower; cumulative risks > 40% are rare for even the highest risk groups.

Risk Factors

The major risk factors for breast cancer are listed in TABLE 67–2. Of these, reproductive history, history of estrogen replacement therapy, and abdominal obesity suggest that estrogens have a role in the pathogenesis of breast cancer.

TABLE 67–1. BREAST CANCER RISKS IN WHITE WOMEN

Age	*Risk of Developing Breast Cancer (%)*	*Risk of Developing Invasive Breast Cancer (%)*	*Risk of Dying from Breast Cancer (%)*
Birth–110	10.2	9.8	3.6
20–30	0.04	0.04	0.00
20–40	0.49	0.42	0.09
20–110	10.34	9.94	3.05
35–45	0.88	0.83	0.14
35–55	2.53	2.37	0.56
35–110	10.27	9.82	3.56
50–60	1.95	1.86	0.33
50–70	4.67	4.48	1.04
50–110	8.96	8.66	2.75
65–75	3.17	3.08	0.43
65–85	5.48	5.29	1.01
65–110	6.53	6.29	1.53

Adapted from information appearing in Seidman H, Mushinski MH, Gelb SK, Silverberg E: "Probabilities of eventually developing or dying of cancer—United States, 1985." *CA—A Cancer Journal for Clinicians* 35(1):36–56, 1985; used with permission.

Family history of breast cancer is a risk factor for all women, not just premenopausal women as previously believed. A history of colon and endometrial cancer in first-degree relatives (in two consecutive generations of the same family) is also a risk factor (Lynch syndrome II).

Although the role of dietary fat in the pathogenesis of breast cancer is controversial, a diet in which fat represents ≤ 30% of the total calories is recommended in view of other health benefits. Breast cancer risk increases with android (abdominal) obesity (defined as a ratio ≥ 0.71 between the waist and hip circumferences), probably because of the associated lower concentration of circulating sex hormone–binding globulin. An increased prevalence of android obesity among older women may partly explain the higher risk of breast cancer with age.

TABLE 67–2. RISK FACTORS FOR BREAST CANCER

Age
Personal or family history of breast cancer
Reproductive history
Early menarche
Late menopause
No pregnancies or late first pregnancy (at age $\geq$ 31)
Diet
Regular consumption of alcohol
High fat diet*
Body size
Abdominal obesity
Postmenopausal estrogen use
Exposure to ionizing radiation

* Inconclusive evidence.

Postmenopausal estrogen replacement therapy at daily doses > 1.25 mg of conjugated estrogens (Premarin) modestly increases breast cancer risk. The risk is negligible for daily doses $\leq$ 0.625 mg, which are usually adequate for preventing coronary artery disease and osteoporosis but which may be inadequate for controlling hot flushes and treating atrophic vaginitis and cystitis. Ionizing radiation causes breast cancer, but the amount of radiation involved in screening mammography is negligible and very unlikely to induce breast cancer. The benefits of mammography definitely outweigh the minimal potential risks.

Prevention

Prevention is mainly the task of primary care physicians. The goal of primary prevention is to prevent or halt the carcinogenic process and that of secondary prevention is to detect breast cancer at an early and curable stage by screening asymptomatic women.

Primary prevention: Currently, primary prevention of breast cancer is investigational. Chemoprevention (the use of drugs to prevent cancer) is the most realistic form of primary prevention, and the drugs tamoxifen and 4-hydroxy-phenylretinamide are particularly promising.

Tamoxifen, a partial estrogen antagonist, prevents breast cancer in animal models and reduces by 1/3 the incidence of cancer in the contralateral breast of women who had a previous breast malignancy. Tamoxifen is usually well tolerated and may even help prevent osteoporosis and coronary artery disease, but bothersome hot flushes force about 15% of postmenopausal women to stop taking the drug. **4-Hydroxyphenylretinamide** is a retinoid that also prevents breast cancer in animal models, but its use in humans is still under study. The drug is synergistic with tamoxifen, has a more favorable toxicity profile than other retinoids, and is more suitable for long-term clinical use.

Chemoprevention of cancer may be more effective in older than in younger women because the concentration of cells undergoing carcinogenic changes susceptible to tamoxifen and 4-hydroxy-phenylretinamide may increase with age. At this time, however, chemoprevention is recommended only for women in clinical trials.

Secondary prevention: Most older women do not regularly perform **breast self-examination.** Additionally, older women tend not to have regular gynecologic examinations, and routine medical examination too often fails to include thorough breast examination. Elderly women may also be embarrassed by abnormalities that they find, thereby delaying assessment and treatment. For these reasons, primary care physicians and nurses must routinely evaluate elderly women for breast lesions. Although studies have not proved that breast self-examination is effective in older women, older women should probably be taught how to examine their breasts and encouraged to perform breast self-examination every month.

Screening asymptomatic women for breast cancer involves periodic **mammography** and **clinical breast examination.** Appropriate screening can reduce breast cancer–related mortality among women aged 50 to 75 by 20% to 25%. Regular screening may also be beneficial for women > 75, but which method is best (ie, whether they should receive mammography or clinical breast examinations or both) has not been established.

The ongoing debate over the most effective screening program is reflected in different guidelines promulgated by several organizations (see TABLE 67–3). The choice of screening program for older women should take the following into consideration: The results of biennial and yearly mammography are comparable; biennial examinations are cheaper and more convenient; the sensitivity of clinical breast examination may improve as the breast becomes more atrophic with age; a thorough examination may be performed in a short time in any ambulatory setting and may be the most effective way to screen older women; the value of breast self-examination has not been conclusively demonstrated; breast self-examination requires some skills and may be impossible for those with declining cognitive function.

Despite widespread public education about the benefits of screening mammography, most older women do not take advantage of screening

TABLE 67–3. BREAST CANCER SCREENING GUIDELINES FOR OLDER WOMEN

	American Cancer Society	*American Geriatric Society*	*United States Preventive Study Task Force*
Mammography	Yearly	Biennially*	Biennially*
Clinical breast examination	Yearly	Yearly	Yearly
Breast self-examination	Monthly	—	—
Upper age limit	None	85	75

* Every other year.

programs. Less than 50% of women ≥ 65 yr have ever undergone mammography, and an even smaller proportion is screened regularly. According to recent surveys, whether older women participate in screening programs is determined mostly by the support of primary physicians, who are in the best position to identify and to help patients overcome socioeconomic, cultural, and educational barriers. Not surprisingly, breast cancer is generally more advanced at diagnosis among older women.

Symptoms, Signs, and Diagnosis

Breast cancers have the same clinical characteristics in older as in younger women. Cancer is usually suspected when changes are noted on mammography or when a breast lesion is seen or felt. Lesions usually can be felt as firm nodules within the breast. Ulcerations may occur, and lesions within or near the nipple may produce discharge. Sometimes, breast cancer is discovered only after metastatic lesions cause bone fractures, neurologic changes, hypercalcemia, liver failure, or ascites.

When a tumor is detected by physical examination, bilateral mammograms should be obtained to rule out occult lesions. Certain radiographic images—such as speckled calcifications or tissue infiltration—suggest cancer, while a cystic appearance suggests a benign process. Even an apparently benign finding on mammogram requires further evaluation. Generally, the diagnosis is established by fine needle aspiration, a simple and safe procedure with 94% sensitivity. Fine needle aspiration allows collection and cytologic examination of cystic fluid and is extremely helpful in planning definitive treatment of breast cancer. Although a positive result on fine needle aspiration is diagnostic, a negative result usually should be followed by an open biopsy.

Chest x-ray, CBC count, and liver enzyme studies are performed on all patients. More complex and costly tests should be reserved for specific indications, such as hepatomegaly or abnormal liver enzymes, bone pain and tenderness, nocturnal headache, sixth-nerve paralysis, focal neurologic signs, and cranial hypertension.

The characteristics of metastatic breast cancer are the same in younger and older women. Metastases have a high affinity for bone; these metastases may cause pathologic fractures, especially in osteoporotic women, which require both radiation therapy and orthopedic pinning. Prophylactic orthopedic pinning is indicated for osteolytic metastases of weight-bearing long bones. Pathologic fractures can cause severe pain, especially when they lead to spinal compression. Bone metastases may also cause profound hypercalcemia, which can be the presenting symptom (most typically in women who have been on bed rest). Breast cancer also frequently metastasizes to brain and liver.

Clinical Course and Prognosis

Breast cancer may have a more indolent clinical course in women > 65 yr than in younger women. Several tumor and tumor-host observations support this hypothesis. Less aggressive hormone receptor–rich, well-differentiated tumors are more prevalent in older women, while life-threatening hepatic, cerebral, and lymphangitic metastases are less prevalent. In addition, the likelihood that a tumor is hormone receptor–rich increases with patient age. Overall, about 60% of tumors in postmenopausal women and > 80% of tumors in women ≥ 80 yr old are hormone receptor–rich. Also, slow-growing tumors, found mostly in the elderly, take longer to become detectable. Several age-related physiologic changes may slow neoplastic growth, including immune senescence and declining production of estrogens, growth hormone, and paracrine growth factors. As an example of how immune senescence affects tumor growth, one report showed that in older women the monocellular reaction to tumor is less intense and the secretion of a monocyte-derived tumor-stimulating cytokine is reduced.

However, the suggestion that tumors are less aggressive in older women should not prompt complacency. Breast cancer is a common cause of morbidity and death, which may be avoided by intensive preventive programs and timely treatment.

The **prognosis** of breast cancer is determined by the stage of the disease (see TABLE 67–4) and by different factors within each stage. In **stages I and II,** the number of axillary lymph nodes microscopically involved by the tumor is the most important prognostic factor. Ten years after diagnosis, 60% to 70% of women with involvement of three or fewer lymph nodes are alive and free of disease, compared with only 15% to 20% of those with involvement of eight or more lymph nodes. When the axillary lymph nodes are not involved, the best predictors of recurrence include size of the primary tumor (recurrence rate increases

TABLE 67–4. STAGING SYSTEM FOR BREAST CANCER

Stages

0	= Tis, N0, M0	IIIA	= T0, N2, M0
I	= T1, N0, M0		T1, N2, M0
II	= T0, N1, M0		T2, N2, M0
	T1, N1, M0		T3, N1, M0
	T2, N0, M0		T3, N2, M0
	T2, N1, M0	IIIB	= T4, any N, M0
	T3, N0, M0		Any T, N3, M0
		IV	= Any T, any N, M1

Staging Criteria

Primary tumor

Tx = Primary tumor cannot be assessed
T0 = No evidence of primary tumor
Tis = Carcinoma in situ or Paget's disease of the breast without tumor
T1 = Tumor ≤ 2 cm in largest dimension
T2 = Tumor 2–5 cm in largest dimension
T3 = Tumor > 5 cm in largest dimension
T4 = Fixation to the chest wall or skin (chest wall includes ribs, intercostal muscles, and the serratus anterior muscle, but not the pectoral muscle)

Regional lymph nodes

Nx = Lymph node not assessable clinically
N0 = No palpable axillary lymph nodes
N1 = Metastasis to movable ipsilateral axillary lymph node(s)
N2 = Metastasis to ipsilateral axillary lymph node(s) fixed to one another or to other structures
N3 = Metastasis to ipsilateral internal mammary lymph node(s)

Distant metastases

Mx = Presence of distant metastases cannot be assessed
M0 = No distant metastases
M1 = Distant metastases, including metastases to ipsilateral supraclavicular nodes

Modified from the American Joint Committee on Cancer, *Manual for Staging of Cancer*, ed. 4, edited by OH Beahrs, DE Henson, RVP Hutter, BJ Kennedy. Philadelphia, JB Lippincott Company, 1992, pp 151–152; used with permission.

with tumor size, when the largest diameter is > 1 cm), low concentration of hormone receptors, high histologic grade (ie, poor histologic differentiation), high cell proliferation rate, abnormalities of the P53 protein (which is encoded by the P53 antioncogene and controls cell growth), and expression of HER/2 oncogene (which encodes for epidermal growth factor receptor). In **stage III disease,** factors indicating a poor prognosis include palpable supraclavicular or infraclavicular lymph nodes, edema, ulceration, fixation to the chest wall, and inflammatory breast cancer. In **stage IV disease,** the prognosis varies markedly with the metastatic sites: the average survival is 3 to 6 mo if the patient has liver or lymphangitic lung metastases, 24 mo if the patient has nodular lung metastases or pleural effusions, and > 5 yr if the metastases are limited to the bones.

Treatment

Treatment is guided by the stage of the disease, the patient's general condition, and the patient's preferences. Local treatment modalities include partial (lumpectomy), total, or radical mastectomy; axillary lymph node dissection; and external beam irradiation. Systemic treatment includes hormonal therapy and cytotoxic chemotherapy (see TABLE 67–5).

Stages I and II breast cancer: The management of localized breast cancer includes local and systemic (adjuvant) treatment. Local treatment involves total or partial mastectomy (lumpectomy) and axillary lymph node dissection. Total or partial mastectomy may be performed under local anesthesia, with negligible risk even for women ≥ 90 yr. Partial mastectomy is not a good choice for patients who have large tumors or collagen-vascular diseases that hinder normal wound healing. To prevent local recurrence of cancer, partial mastectomy is usually followed by postoperative radiation therapy.

The choice of surgical procedure is the patient's prerogative. Partial mastectomy may be preferable in terms of body image and sexual attractiveness, but postoperative radiation therapy is a major inconvenience; its cost, both for treatment itself and transportation to and from treatment, may be substantial. Yet, partial mastectomy does not always have to be followed by breast irradiation. Postoperative radiation therapy helps prevent recurrences but does not affect survival. The risk of local recurrence over 5 yr without radiation therapy is about 30%. Additionally, tamoxifen may reduce the risk of local cancer recurrences and obviate the need for radiation therapy. Also, older women are less likely to have local recurrences. Provided with this information, 2/3 of women aged 65 to 79 yr opt for partial mastectomy, although most of those > 79 yr opt for total mastectomy. Whether axillary lymph node dissection helps eliminate residual tumor is uncertain; thus if nodes are not palpable, this procedure may be unnecessary in older women. However, tamoxifen is likely to be beneficial regardless of regional lymph node involvement.

TABLE 67–5. SYSTEMIC TREATMENT OF BREAST CANCER

Agents	*Doses*	*Complications*	*Precautions*
Endocrine treatment			
Estrogen antagonists			
Tamoxifen	10 mg bid	Deep vein thrombosis Hot flushes Retinal degeneration	Avoid if history of deep vein thrombosis Periodic ophthalmologic examinations
Progestins			
Megestrol acetate	40 mg qid	Increased appetite Weight gain Fluid retention	Avoid in obesity
Aromatase inhibitors			
Aminoglutethimide	250 mg bid	Hypoadrenocorticism Somnolence Skin rash	Hydrocortisone 100 mg/day for 2 wk; 40 mg/day thereafter because aminoglutethimide inhibits steroid synthesis

Cytotoxic chemotherapy			
CMF	Every 4 wk:	Alopecia Myelosuppression Mucositis Nausea and vomiting	Avoid for GFR ≤ 40 mL/min Adjust doses of methotrexate and cyclophosphamide to CrCl HGF for history of neutropenic fever Hospitalization for diarrhea and severe mucositis
Cyclophosphamide	100 mg/m² orally days 1 through 14		
Methotrexate	40 mg/m² IV days 1 and 8		
Fluorouracil	500 mg/m² IV days 1 and 8		
CAF	Every 3 wk:	Alopecia Myelosuppression Mucositis Heart failure Nausea and vomiting	Avoid in patients with heart failure Monitor ejection fraction by radionucleotide scan or echocardiogram HGF for history of neutropenic fever Hospitalization for diarrhea and severe mucositis
Cyclophosphamide	500 mg/m² IV days 1 through 14		
Doxorubicin (Adriamycin)*	50 mg/m² IV day 1		
Fluorouracil	500 mg/m² IV day 1		
Mitomycin C	12 mg/m² IV every 3 to 4 wk	Alopecia Myelosuppression Pneumonitis Cardiomyopathy Hemolytic-uremic syndrome	HGF for prophylaxis of neutropenia
Vinblastine	4 mg/m² IV weekly	Myelosuppression Mucositis	HGF for history of neutropenic fever Hospitalization for diarrhea and severe mucositis

CrCl = creatinine clearance; GFR = glomerular filtration rate; HGF = hematopoietic growth factor.
* Mitoxantrone (Novantrone) may be substituted (CNF) in a dose of 6 mg/m², with reduced risk of alopecia, nausea, and vomiting.

Adjuvant treatment with tamoxifen prolongs both *the disease-free survival* and *the overall survival* of postmenopausal patients, even in women ≥ 70 yr, women with hormone receptor–poor cancer, and women whose regional lymph nodes are cancer-free. Tamoxifen should be given for at least 2 yr; longer treatment may be beneficial. Administering progestin, estrogen, or clonidine may alleviate the disabling hot flushes some women experience with tamoxifen therapy. These treatments are, however, still experimental.

Primary treatment of localized breast cancer with tamoxifen in women ≥ 70 yr *without* surgery has been investigated. About 40% of those treated this way achieve breast cancer stabilization for 5 yr. Thus, this approach should be recommended only for those women who cannot or should not undergo surgery.

After treatment, patients with stage I or II breast cancer should be followed up yearly. These women are at risk for new breast cancer, as well as for recurrence of the original tumor. In addition to a general physical examination, patients should have annual clinical breast examinations and mammography. The value of serial chest radiographs, CBC count, and tests of liver enzymes and the tumor marker Ca 15-3 is controversial. With the possible exception of Ca 15-3, none of these tests allows early detection of recurrence.

Stage III breast cancer: Locally advanced breast cancer is best managed with a combination of systemic and local therapies. Systemic treatment with chemotherapy regimens that contain doxorubicin or mitoxantrone is the first step. When tumor size is adequately reduced, total mastectomy, radiation therapy, or both may be used. With this approach, about 50% of patients are alive and disease-free 5 yr after treatment. The combination of cyclophosphamide, methotrexate, and fluorouracil may be used in patients with cardiac dysfunction.

The role of hormonal treatment in locally advanced breast cancer is not established. A 6-wk course of tamoxifen or other hormonal agents in women ≥ 65 yr is reasonable. In the case of inflammatory breast cancer, hormonal therapy by itself is seldom effective, and combined chemotherapy and hormonal therapy is advisable.

Stage IV breast cancer: Along with surgical removal of the primary tumor, hormonal manipulation is the best treatment of metastatic breast cancer in women ≥ 65 yr, even in those with hormone receptor–poor tumors. Estrogen antagonists, progestins, and aromatase inhibitors have comparable activity. Aminoglutethimide may be the most active agent for bone metastases, but the high incidence of side effects limits its use. Progestins are well tolerated, but the associated weight gain may stimulate enhanced tumor growth. Thus, most practitioners prefer tamoxifen as initial endocrine treatment and use other agents if the disease progresses or if complications with tamoxifen occur. In about 15% of patients with bone metastases, tamoxifen causes tumor flare-up resulting in hypercalcemia. This transient complication can be managed with IV fluids and furosemide and does not warrant stopping the drug.

Chemotherapy is indicated when two forms of hormonal treatment have failed. Of course, some elderly women may not wish to undergo chemotherapy, and those with extensive comorbidity may not be appropriate candidates. When appropriate, if the patient has life-threatening metastases (liver and lymphangitic lung metastases), chemotherapy and hormonal therapy should be combined as the initial treatment. Chemotherapy choices include CAF (cyclophosphamide, doxorubicin [Adriamycin], fluorouracil), CMF (cyclophosphamide, methotrexate, fluorouracil), mitomycin C, and vinblastine (see TABLE 67–5). Particularly promising new drugs for breast cancer are the taxanes (paclitaxel [Taxol] and taxotere [not available in the USA]) and the topoisomerase I inhibitor topotecan. Cytotoxic chemotherapy is usually well tolerated by patients > 70 yr when the doses of renally excretable drugs are adjusted to creatinine clearance level and when cardiotoxic drugs are avoided in patients with cardiac dysfunction.

Supportive care is very important for patients with metastatic breast cancer. Pathologic fractures of long bones may be prevented by prophylactic fixation of lytic lesions. Bone pain may be managed with local radiation therapy, strontium 89, and pamidronate. Brain metastases are managed with corticosteroids and radiation therapy.

---

68. SEXUALITY

A comprehensive national survey of sexuality has never been done for any age group. Therefore, the nature and frequency of sexual activity among the elderly, including its association with marital or health status or any other variable, is unknown. Available data consist of the important but now historic and limited Kinsey studies (1948 to 1949), the physiologic investigations of Masters and Johnson, and the findings of both the Duke Longitudinal Studies and the Baltimore Longitudinal Study on Aging. Questionnaire surveys of self-reported sexual activity have been conducted by mail (eg, by Consumers Union). The most important conclusion is that contrary to prevailing beliefs, sexual desire and satisfaction are important to many elderly persons. A number of factors (eg, low intrinsic drive dating back to youth, physical disability, poor marital relationship, or the death of a spouse or companion) may be responsible for an older person's being disinterested in sex or having an inhibited sexual drive.

A sexual history, with emphasis on current sexual function, should be part of the general medical evaluation of an older person. Physicians should handle sexual issues with dignity and skill. The discomfort physicians may feel in discussing the subject is often the result of negative stereotypes, personal anxieties, objections to the expression of sexuality by the elderly, or simply ignorance.

SOCIAL, EMOTIONAL, AND PSYCHOLOGIC ISSUES

Sexuality is associated more with intimacy than just with the act of sexual intercourse. Sexuality in old age is often described in terms that include the opportunity to express passion, affection, admiration, and loyalty; the affirmation that one's body is functioning well; the maintenance of a strong sense of identity; a means of self-assertion; a protection from anxiety; a renewal of a sense of romance; a general affirmation of life, especially the expression of joy; and a continuing opportunity to search for new growth and experience.

However, not all older persons have such positive attitudes. Even physically and mentally healthy persons may internalize the negative image of the typical older person as a desexualized invalid. Another social prejudice is one that falsely characterizes an elderly person who seeks sexual satisfaction as either a "dirty old man" or a "lecherous old woman." The inability to come to terms with aging may lead some people to envy the young and to feel hostility and bitterness toward them, to show prejudice against other older people and refuse to associate with them, to reject an aging partner, and to make frantic attempts to appear young.

Feelings of guilt and shame may surface. Brought up during an era of Victorian-like prudery, some older persons are probably misinformed about issues of sexuality and feel guilty about their desires. They may refuse to discuss the issue of sexuality or to accept help when problems are obvious. Reassurance and information from a physician may help these persons achieve a more positive self-image.

Boredom, fear, fatigue, grief, and problems with a mate affect the sexual behavior of all persons. However, the elderly are also more likely to experience depression and illness or incapacitation of a partner. While some people look forward to the freedom of retirement, others react to it with feelings of low self-esteem and self-worth.

With advancing age, women outnumber men, and women living alone are more likely to be poor and to have complex physical and psychosocial problems. Over 50% of older women are widows, 7% have never married, and 2% are divorced. Thus, about 60% of older women are without a spouse, in contrast to about 20% of older men. Partners are in short supply, especially for women. When opportunities do arise, older persons often feel unfamiliar with the practices of dating and courtship. They may not have undertaken such activities for decades.

Physicians should be aware of their older patients' needs and should be especially sensitive about the reluctance of those who have lost their companions to reenter the world of dating.

Negative societal attitudes about masturbation and homosexuality also can interfere with sexual expression. Some men require sexually arousing photographs and videos to assist fantasy as well as physical manipulation by their partners to achieve an erection. Both men and women without partners, heterosexual or homosexual, may seek out pornography or prostitutes. An estimated 10% of the population including the elderly is homosexual, and while long-term relationships are common, many elderly homosexual persons have not publicly revealed their sexual preference. Their relationships and physical problems are not much different from those of heterosexuals and require the same thoughtful approach and treatment.

NORMAL CHANGES IN SEXUAL FUNCTION

Sexual change in old age is a process of gradual slowing; more time is needed to become sexually aroused and to reach sexual climax. This should not be considered an impairment, since it may permit a better response synchronization between the sexes, compared to that in earlier years when men responded more quickly than women. Men and women often converge in other ways as they grow older: women typically become more assertive and men become more nurturant.

Special Concerns of Men

In addition to gradual slowing, older men may notice less preejaculatory fluid and less forcefulness at ejaculation. In general, testosterone levels decline only gradually, and some very old men still have levels identical to those in younger men. However, chronic illness or alcoholism reduces testosterone levels markedly. Men do not undergo a physiologic climacteric, and they remain fertile until the end of life.

A common concern of men of all ages including older men is their ability to maintain sexual potency and performance. Impotence is distressing and is usually (although inaccurately) attributed to aging (see IMPOTENCE in Ch. 69). However, impotence may occur from time to time at any age for a variety of reasons (eg, stress, fatigue, tension, guilt, depression, illness, excessive drinking, and anxiety over performance). A comprehensive evaluation is needed to separate psychologic from organic causes. Recent studies suggest that organic causes are a major factor in ≥ 80% of persistent male sexual dysfunction, and psychologic factors alone probably account for only 10% of cases of erectile dysfunction. However, psychologic and organic factors are often intermixed; anxiety over an organic cause of impotence often aggravates the problem.

The diagnostic process begins with a history and physical examination. Depression, anxiety, and stress must also be evaluated. Sleep studies that measure nocturnal penile tumescence help distinguish psychogenic from organic impotence. Such studies can be conducted at home with a portable monitoring unit or in sleep clinics.

Impotence can be treated successfully in most cases, often without surgery. In the case of psychogenic impotence, sexual capacity may return spontaneously; reassurance reduces anxiety and speeds recovery, but psychotherapy or professional sex therapy may be required. Involving the partner in the diagnosis and treatment program is important. Much of the expense of professional sex therapy (including that for couples) may be covered by Medicare or private health insurance, but the cost may be a problem for many older people. Medicare now pays 50% of the allowable charges for psychotherapy whether performed by a physician, psychologist, or social worker. Increasingly, insurance companies are paying for diagnosis and treatment of sexual dysfunction.

Special Concerns of Women

Older women usually can continue their earlier patterns of sexual functioning until the end of life or until serious illness intervenes. Women tend to be less concerned about sexual performance than men but are more worried about loss of youthful appearance. Some women enjoy sex more without the possibility of pregnancy. The frequency of intercourse for heterosexual women is often related more to the age, health, and sexual function of their partners (or the availability of a partner) than to their own sexual capacity or interest.

For women, most sexual changes are associated with **menopause,** when estrogen production slows. The effects of menopause on sexuality may include vaginal dryness leading to irritation or pain, a change in vaginal shape (shortening and narrowing), less acidic vaginal secretions with greater possibility of vaginal infections, cystitis due to thinning of vaginal walls with less protection for bladder and urethra, reduction in clitoral size, stress incontinence, and increase in facial hair.

Estrogen replacement therapy has long been used for menopausal symptoms and is effective in treating all of these changes as well as in controlling hot flushes; the specific therapy is discussed in Ch. 83. However, given the risks associated with estrogen replacement therapy, many women are skeptical about its benefits and often experience "estrogen anxiety," a fairly new psychologic issue of midlife sexuality. Other measures, such as using water-based vaginal lubricants (eg, K-Y Jelly), can help prevent or control vaginal dryness and irritation during intercourse.

EFFECTS OF MEDICAL PROBLEMS ON SEXUALITY

A number of common medical problems can affect sexual functioning. Because sexual activity is often important to a person's well-being, physicians should include a thoughtful discussion of sexuality when treating the medical problem.

Heart Disease

People with angina or heart failure and those who have undergone coronary artery bypass surgery or have had a myocardial infarction may avoid sex because of an assumed risk to life, but studies indicate that cardiac death during or after sexual activity is rare. Under most circumstances, patients with heart disease have few reasons to abstain from sex and many reasons to continue (eg, an opportunity for mild exercise and release of physical and emotional tension).

After **myocardial infarction,** an 8- to 14-wk waiting period is generally recommended before resuming sexual intercourse. The period of abstinence depends more on the patient's interest, general fitness, and conditioning. Depression and anxiety are common up to 1 yr after myocardial infarction, and avoiding sexual activity may exacerbate depression. Antidepressant drugs may further reduce sexual libido and capacity. A physician's support and encouragement can greatly help patients overcome their fears.

When **heart failure** is managed effectively, the physical exercise and emotional release associated with sexual activity may contribute to a patient's improvement. After an episode of pulmonary edema, a 2- to 3-wk recovery period is usually advised before resuming sex.

Physical symptoms, side effects of medical treatment, or fear of sudden death from physical exertion causes many patients to become sexually dysfunctional even before they become candidates for **coronary artery bypass surgery.** Patients who have had surgery should be reassured about the safety of sexual activity within reasonable limits to prevent straining the surgical repair. The sternum usually requires 3 mo to heal completely. Self-stimulation or mutual masturbation may be a less strenuous alternative to intercourse and usually can be started earlier in the recovery period.

Prolonged sexual problems can occur after surgery if the patient is not closely monitored. Exercise programs to improve cardiac function (eg, increasingly strenuous walking) can reassure patients who are afraid to resume sexual activity. Even though surgery may eliminate the need for medication, some patients become psychologically dependent on nitroglycerin before sexual activity because of previous chest pain upon exertion. Patients with **arrhythmias** may need the reassurance of successfully performing a treadmill test to overcome anxiety about engaging in sexual activity.

Hypertension

Men and women with mild to moderate hypertension need not restrict sexual activity. In men with untreated hypertension, the incidence of impotence is about 15%; the effects of hypertension on female sexuality are not as well studied. Selection of antihypertensive drugs should focus on those that do not impair sexual response (see EFFECTS OF DRUGS ON SEXUALITY, below).

Stroke

Sexual activity has not been shown to cause stroke or to increase neurologic deficit after stroke. Unless a stroke causes severe brain damage, sexual desire is usually unimpaired. However, sexual performance is more likely to be affected. Some men experience impotence; others do not. The unaffected side of the body should be emphasized in lovemaking. The partner of a woman who has suffered a stroke may become impotent if he fears injuring her, in which case reassurance may be needed. The use of headboards and bedboards can greatly assist positioning necessary for sexual activity.

Diabetes Mellitus

Sexual problems are common in men with diabetes. Impotence occurs two to five times more often in diabetic men than in the general population, even though sexual desire is unaffected. Good control of the diabetes may reestablish potency; however, if the diabetes is already well controlled, the impotence is likely to be irreversible. Concurrent endocrine problems (eg, a thyroid condition) may reduce potency.

Arthritis

The physical disabilities associated with osteoarthritis and rheumatoid arthritis may interfere with sexual desire or performance, but drugs commonly used to treat arthritis do not. A program of exercise, rest, and warm baths is especially useful in reducing arthritic discomfort and in facilitating sexual performance. Experimenting with new sexual positions that do not aggravate joint pain is often helpful; the side-by-side position may be preferred by both partners, especially when the patient has many tender areas and pain trigger points. Since osteoarthritis tends to be less severe in the morning and rheumatoid arthritis less severe in the afternoon and evening, sexual activity can be planned for times of the day when pain and stiffness are diminished. Some patients find that regular sexual activity relieves the pain of rheumatoid arthritis for 4 to 8 h; such relief may be due to hormone production, release of endorphins, or the physical activity involved.

Chronic Prostatitis

Chronic prostatitis is associated with unusually frequent sexual intercourse as well as with abstinence, excessive preliminary sexual arousal, or an incomplete orgasm. The pain of chronic or recurrent prostatitis may diminish sexual desire. Mild prostatitis may cause some perineal pain after ejaculation.

Therapy for chronic or recurrent prostatitis includes antibiotics, warm sitz baths, and periodic gentle prostatic massage. Kegel's exercises, which involve contracting the pelvic floor muscles, may also help.

Cystitis and Urethritis

Some women experience recurrent episodes of cystitis and urethritis after intercourse. Although these problems are usually due to the introduction of bacteria into the urethra during thrusting, the cause may be unclear. A urologic or gynecologic evaluation is indicated to determine the cause, as is a discussion of therapeutic and preventive options.

Peyronie's Disease

Intercourse is painful for about 50% of men with Peyronie's disease. When the penis is angled too sharply, penetration may become impossible. However, tumescence is preserved in about 90% of cases, even though there may be some pain. Psychotherapy can help the patient adjust to the structural and functional changes in the penis. Medical or surgical intervention is not usually effective, but symptoms sometimes disappear spontaneously after several years.

Chronic Renal Disease

Men with chronic renal failure may have reduced levels of serum testosterone, although the reason is unknown, and they are often impotent. Such patients may be treatable when the problem is intensified by concomitant emotional reactions such as anxiety or depression; treatment of the associated, underlying anxiety or depression and couples counseling can be helpful. Kidney transplantation often restores sexual capacity in impotent dialysis patients.

Parkinson's Disease

Parkinsonism is commonly associated with depression, which may lead to impotence in men and lack of sexual desire in both men and women. Advanced organic involvement may also result in impotence. Sex drive and performance improve in some men treated with levodopa, probably because of greater mobility and an increased sense of well-being. There is little evidence that levodopa acts as an aphrodisiac, and it should not be prescribed as such.

Chronic Emphysema and Bronchitis

Shortness of breath brought on by chronic emphysema and bronchitis hinders physical activity, including sex. Solutions include resting at intervals, finding the least taxing ways to have sexual contact, and using oxygen during sexual activity.

EFFECTS OF SURGERY ON SEXUALITY

Rate of recovery and return to sexual activity after surgery varies. Thorough explanation of surgical procedures, together with practical advice and emotional support before and after surgery, can enhance recovery and the return to previous levels of sexual activity (see also Heart Disease under EFFECTS OF MEDICAL PROBLEMS ON SEXUALITY, above).

Hysterectomy

Refraining from sexual activity for 6 to 8 wk after hysterectomy is usually advised to allow the surgical wounds to heal. Feelings of depression after hysterectomy are common and usually last from 2 to 10 days, although some women report them for 6 mo or longer. Hysterectomy without oophorectomy does not usually impair sexual function. However, women who are highly sensitive to cervical and uterine sensations during orgasm are aware of the loss. Although oophorectomy decreases testosterone and other androgen levels (as well as estrogen and progesterone levels), the effects on sexuality have not been well studied.

Mastectomy

The loss of one or both breasts can make a woman feel sexually mutilated, and the psychologic effects may be severe. Sexual desire may be lost because of embarrassment, inability to accept the loss of the breast, or fear of being less attractive to a partner. Periodic depression is common and should be expected during the first year or two after mastectomy.

Rehabilitation programs, such as the American Cancer Society's Reach to Recovery program, help women and their spouses deal with the physical, psychologic, and cosmetic concerns of breast surgery. Couples should share feelings openly and support each other emotionally.

Prostatectomy

Potency is rarely affected by the most common form of prostatectomy, transurethral resection of the prostate, although retrograde ejaculation is common. Healing usually takes up to 6 wk, after which sexual activity can be resumed. Men often assume incorrectly that sexual impairment is inevitable because of the physical proximity of the prostate to the penis. Factual information from physicians can alleviate fears. About 10% of men lose some ability to achieve an erection, although most men return to their presurgery level of sexual functioning. Most impotence after transurethral resection of the prostate is psychologic; about 3% to 5% of men develop nonpsychologic impotence. Suprapubic or retropubic prostate surgery may result in impotence.

Orchiectomy

The psychologic impact of this procedure can be devastating. Emotional preparation before and counseling after surgery are essential. Physiologic impotence does occur, but some men are able to have normal erections. When testosterone can be given soon after orchiectomy, potency may be retained. However, replacement testosterone therapy is usually contraindicated because in the elderly, orchiectomy is usually performed to treat prostate cancer.

Colostomy and Ileostomy

Patients who are sexually active before surgery usually can continue to be so afterward, although the adjustment can be complex. Couples should be given medical guidance and offered psychologic counseling. Some 250 ostomy support groups throughout the USA provide information and help.

Rectal Cancer Surgery

In men, removal of the rectum and anus with a permanent colostomy may result in total impotence. The proximity of male genital organs to the lower rectum leaves essential nerve fibers vulnerable to damage. In women who undergo this procedure, capacity for sexual arousal and orgasm is usually retained, since essential nerves are further from the surgical site.

EFFECTS OF DRUGS ON SEXUALITY

Many drugs adversely affect sexuality (see TABLES 68–1 and 68–2). Some interfere with the autonomic nervous system, which is involved in the sexual response. Others affect mood and alertness or change the production or action of sex hormones. Assessing the effects of drugs on sexuality is more difficult in women than in men, since potency problems in men are more obvious. However, drugs that affect men may also affect women, and further studies in women are warranted.

A patient who suspects that medications are the cause of sexual problems may be tempted to discontinue the drugs or decrease the doses without informing the physician. The possibility of adverse drug effects on sexual function should be discussed openly with patients, who should be encouraged to report any side effects.

Although the effects of specific drugs on sexuality are outlined in TABLES 68–1 and 68–2, some drugs deserve special mention. **Antipsychotics,** such as thioridazine and other phenothiazines, may inhibit erection or ejaculation, even though the capacity for erection remains. **Tranquilizers** can depress the sexual responses of women and men, and some **antidepressants** can inhibit sexual desire.

TABLE 68–1. POSSIBLE DRUG EFFECTS ON FEMALE SEXUALITY

Increased libido	Androgens; benzodiazepines (antianxiety effect); mazindol
Decreased libido	See TABLE 68–2. Some of the drugs that decrease libido in men *may* reduce libido in women. The literature on this subject is sparse.
Impaired arousal and orgasm	Anticholinergics; clonidine; methyldopa; monoamine oxidase inhibitors; tricyclic antidepressants
Breast enlargement	Penicillamine; tricyclic antidepressants; estrogens
Galactorrhea (spontaneous flow of milk)	Amphetamines; chlorpromazine; cimetidine; haloperidol; heroin; methyldopa; metoclopramide; phenothiazines; reserpine; sulpiride; tricyclic antidepressants
Virilization (acne, hirsutism, lowering of voice, enlargement of clitoris)	Androgens; haloperidol

Adapted from Long JW: "Many common medications can affect sexual expression." *Generations* 6:32–34, 1981. Reprinted with permission from *Generations,* Journal of the American Society on Aging, 833 Market Street, Suite 512, San Francisco, California 94103. Copyright 1981, ASA.

Antihypertensive drugs are the most common pharmacologic cause of impaired erection. **Cardiac drugs** that are often implicated in erectile dysfunction include those with peripheral or central actions of sympatholytic or β-adrenergic blocking activity. Those that have less of an effect on sexual function include calcium channel blockers, angiotensin converting enzyme inhibitors, and peripheral vasodilators. Methyldopa reduces blood flow to the pelvic area, thereby inhibiting erection. When certain antiarrhythmic drugs and β-blockers cannot be avoided and sexual dysfunction results, patients may benefit from encouragement to explore other forms of intimacy and physical pleasure.

The excessive use of **alcohol** is a common yet seldom considered factor in sexual problems; although it may stimulate desire, alcohol inhibits performance. Up to 80% of men who drink heavily experience such effects as impotence, sterility, and loss of sexual desire. Alcohol with its depressant action can also affect a woman's sexual desire. Many of the effects of moderate to heavy drinking are reversible if the drinking is stopped in time. Since alcohol tolerance decreases with age, smaller

TABLE 68–2. POSSIBLE DRUG EFFECTS ON MALE SEXUALITY

Increased libido	Androgens (replacement therapy in deficiency states); baclofen (antianxiety effect); diazepam; chlordiazepoxide (antianxiety effect); haloperidol; levodopa (may be an indirect effect due to improved sense of well-being)
Decreased libido	Antihistamines; barbiturates; chlordiazepoxide (sedative effect); chlorpromazine (10–20% of users); cimetidine; clofibrate; clonidine (10–20% of users); diazepam (sedative effect); disulfiram; estrogens (therapy for prostate cancer); fenfluramine; heroin; licorice; medroxyprogesterone; methyldopa (10–15% of users); perhexiline; prazosin (15% of users); propranolol (rarely); reserpine; spironolactone; tricyclic antidepressants
Impotence	(see TABLE 69–2)
Impaired ejaculation	Anticholinergics; barbiturates (when abused); chlorpromazine; clonidine; estrogens (therapy for prostate cancer); guanethidine; heroin, mesoridazine; methyldopa; monoamine oxidase inhibitors; phenoxybenzamine; phentolamine; reserpine; thiazide diuretics; thioridazine; tricyclic antidepressants
Decreased plasma testosterone	Corticotropin; barbiturates; digoxin; haloperidol (increased testosterone with low dosage, decreased testosterone with high dosage); lithium, marijuana; medroxyprogesterone; monoamine oxidase inhibitors; spironolactone
Impaired spermatogenesis (reduced fertility)	Adrenocorticosteroids (eg, prednisone); androgens (moderate to high dosage, extended use); antimalarials; aspirin (abusive, chronic use); chlorambucil; cimetidine; colchicine; co-trimoxazole; cyclophosphamide; estrogens (therapy for prostate cancer); marijuana; medroxyprogesterone; methotrexate; monoamine oxidase inhibitors; niridazole; nitrofurantoin; spironolactone; sulfasalazine; testosterone (moderate to high dosage, extended use); vitamin C (in doses $\geq$ 1 gm)
Testicular disorders	*Swelling:* tricyclic antidepressants. *Inflammation:* oxyphenbutazone. *Atrophy:* androgens (moderate to high dosage, extended use); chlorpromazine; spironolactone
Penile disorders	*Priapism:* cocaine; heparin; phenothiazines. *Peyronie's disease:* metoprolol

(continued)

TABLE 68–2. POSSIBLE DRUG EFFECTS ON MALE SEXUALITY *(Continued)*

Gynecomastia (excessive development of the male breast)	Androgens (partial conversion to estrogen); carmustine; busulfan; chlormadinone; chlorpromazine, chlortetracycline; cimetidine; clonidine (infrequently); diethylstilbestrol; digitalis and its glycosides; estrogens (therapy for prostate cancer); ethionamide; griseofulvin; haloperidol; heroin; isoniazid; marijuana; methyldopa; phenelzine; reserpine; spironolactone; thioridazine; tricyclic antidepressants; vincristine

Adapted from Long JW: "Many common medications can affect sexual expression." *Generations* 6:32–34, 1981. Reprinted with permission from *Generations,* Journal of the American Society on Aging, 833 Market Street, Suite 512, San Francisco, California 94103. Copyright 1981, ASA.

and smaller amounts may produce negative effects. People who choose to drink regularly should avoid drinking for several hours before sexual activity and should limit themselves to 1.5 oz of hard liquor, 6 oz of wine, or 16 oz of beer in any 24-h period.

69. MALE HYPOGONADISM AND IMPOTENCE

Spermatogenesis is remarkably sustained throughout life if testicular androgen synthesis is adequate; however, androgen production does decline with age. The impact of this reduced androgen synthesis on health, well-being, and sexual function has not been determined.

As testosterone secretion diminishes, its diurnal variation is also blunted, resulting in a lower 6 to 8 AM peak. Mean gonadotropin levels rise slowly, but large pulses of luteinizing hormone are less frequent, which impairs pulsatile testicular response. Binding of testosterone to sex hormone–binding globulin increases with age, resulting in substantially less unbound, bioavailable testosterone. Also, metabolism of testosterone is slowed. Evidence suggests that androgens play an important role in libido (sexual appetite) and influence the frequency of nocturnal erections; however, erections produced by erotic stimuli can occur despite low levels of androgens.

Penile erection is accomplished through engorgement of the corpora cavernosa, two paired vascular bundles. Because each corpus cavernosum is surrounded by a tough, fibrous sheath (the tunica albuginea), engorgement leads to rigidity. Erection occurs when arterial blood flow into the corpora cavernosa exceeds venous outflow. The pudendal artery supplies blood to the corpora, and blood flow is controlled by relaxation and contraction of arterial smooth muscle. Venous drainage occurs through venules just below the tunica albuginea. These venules are easily compressed as the corpora fill. The penis is innervated by the T11-L2 sympathetic nerves and the S2-4 somatic and parasympathetic nerves.

MALE HYPOGONADISM

Inadequate testicular androgen synthesis.

Male hypogonadism is not common in the elderly, with surveys suggesting a prevalence of less than 4%. Most cases in elderly men have no ready explanation and are associated with a combination of pituitary and testicular hyporesponsiveness. However, as shown in TABLE 69–1, hypogonadism is also caused by exposure to many drugs and toxins and by a number of illnesses.

Symptoms and Signs

Mild hypogonadism has few or very vague and nonspecific symptoms and no physical findings. Severe and prolonged hypogonadism leads to reduced skeletal muscle mass and the loss of body hair and masculine habitus. Small, soft testes and a loss of scrotal pigmentation and rugae are important clues.

Laboratory Findings

Leydig cell function may be estimated by a morning measurement of bioavailable (free) testosterone; a value < 67 ng/dL signifies hypogonadism. A total testosterone value of < 300 ng/dL is also diagnostic of hypogonadism, but the free fraction is more sensitive because of the increased binding of testosterone to sex hormone–binding globulin in the elderly. The level of luteinizing hormone is normal or low in almost all hypogonadal men. Dynamic testing with gonadotropin-releasing hormone adds little information, because the response is usually proportional to the basal luteinizing hormone level. A normal prolactin level helps exclude a pituitary tumor as the cause of hypogonadism.

Treatment

Hypogonadism is treated with androgen therapy. Long-acting esters of testosterone and 19-nortestosterone (the enanthate and the cyclopentylpropionate) are administered IM in a dose of 100 to 200 mg every 1 to 3 wk (usually as 100 mg each week, 200 mg every 2 wk, or 300 mg every 3 wk). Alternatively, oral forms of testosterone derivatives, which have an alkyl group in the 17 position, are usually prescribed as 5 to 50 mg/day of methyltestosterone (10 to 50 mg orally or 5 to 25 mg bucally). The IM formulations are generally preferred because the oral agents

TABLE 69–1. CAUSES OF HYPOGONADISM

Acute stress (eg, with surgery, myocardial infarction, stroke, or severe burns—usually the hypogonadism is temporary)	Exposure to heavy metals, organic solvents, radiation, or chemotherapy
Androgen resistance	Hepatic cirrhosis
Chronic renal failure	Kallmann's syndrome
Cushing's syndrome	Klinefelter's syndrome
Diabetes	Mumps orchitis
Drugs (especially spironolactone, ketoconazole, medroxyprogesterone acetate, cimetidine, ranitidine, omeprazole, ethanol, heroin, and methadone)	Myotonic dystrophy
	Panhypopituitarism
	Testicular trauma

may cause hepatotoxicity with reversible elevation of hepatic enzymes, occasional episodes of cholestatic jaundice, and hepatic tumors. Sublingual forms of androgens may be safer than oral forms.

Testosterone therapy restores muscle strength, bone density, hair pattern, libido, sense of well-being, and mood in severely hypogonadal men. Its effectiveness in the elderly is not usually as clear-cut as in younger men, and a 3-mo trial is recommended to identify benefits before either proposing long-term therapy or terminating treatment because it seems ineffective.

Therapy stimulates erythropoietin secretion, increasing the hematocrit. By enhancing activity of hepatic triglyceride lipase, it also reduces HDL cholesterol levels and increases sensitivity to the anticoagulant action of warfarin derivatives. Some degree of prostate growth and an increase in prostate-specific antigen (PSA) level may occur, but development or exacerbation of obstructive symptoms is rare. Patients with elevated or borderline values of PSA probably should not be treated with androgens because of persistent, but unproved, concern that androgens promote the development of prostatic carcinoma. However, for many the benefit may outweigh the risk, so that therapy may still be appropriate after careful consideration.

IMPOTENCE
(Erectile Dysfunction)

The inability to develop and sustain an erection sufficient for satisfactory sexual intercourse.

Etiology and Pathogenesis

Impotence increases progressively in frequency with age. About 25% of 65-yr-old men and 50% of 80-yr-old men are impotent. Impotence can be caused by vascular, neurologic, and endocrine disorders and by structural abnormalities of the penis. Drugs also cause impotence in the elderly.

Vascular disorders that can affect sexual function include atherosclerosis and venous leakage. Any occlusion of the arterial supply to the corpora cavernosa—such as from atherosclerosis, a clot (as in Leriche's syndrome), or vascular surgery (eg, aortoiliac bypass surgery)—that results in inadequate arterial pressure to the penis can lead to impotence. Venous leakage, in which inadequate compression of the venous drainage of the corpora cavernosa results in excessive venous outflow, occurs in 75% of impotent men with normal neurologic and hormonal function.

Neurologic causes of impotence include trauma, diabetes, multiple sclerosis, and toxins. Trauma to the nerves of the penis can occur from lumbar disk disease and from surgical procedures such as rectal surgery and prostatectomy. Diabetic neuropathy is a particularly common cause of impotence in the elderly. Alcoholism can produce a similar peripheral neuropathy.

Endocrine causes of impotence are relatively rare in the elderly. However, testicular failure as a result of childhood exposure to mumps, Klinefelter's syndrome, radiation and chemotherapy, pituitary and adrenal tumors, and other conditions (see TABLE 69–1) can cause extremely low testosterone levels and impotence.

Structural abnormalities of the penis are not common causes of impotence in the elderly. Peyronie's disease, which is more common in younger men, is characterized by fibrous accumulation in the tunica albuginea, which leads to a deformed erection. Although not technically impotence, the deformed erection may not allow penetration.

Drugs cause an estimated 25% of cases of erectile dysfunction (see TABLE 69–2). Among the most common offenders are some antihypertensives (most notably reserpine, β-blockers, guanethidine, and methyldopa), alcohol, cimetidine, antipsychotics, antidepressants, lithium, sedative-hypnotics, and hormones.

Psychologic causes are less common than organic causes and account for a smaller proportion of impotence cases in the elderly than in younger men. The misperception that prostate surgery will result in impotence may actually cause psychogenic impotence, which may be prevented by thorough explanations both before and after the surgery. Depression can lead to impotence in the elderly, as in younger men, and older men can also experience performance anxiety, especially when having sexual intercourse with a new partner.

Diagnosis

Elderly men today are more likely than past generations to seek help for impotence, and physicians should make them feel comfortable discussing the problem. A comfortable environment can be established by

TABLE 69–2. DRUGS THAT MAY CAUSE ERECTILE DYSFUNCTION

Anticonvulsants	Levodopa
Anti-infective drugs	Lithium
Cardiovascular drugs	Narcotic analgesics
Antiarrhythmics	Gastrointestinal drugs
Antihypertensives	Anticholinergics and antispasmodics
β-Adrenergic blocking agents	H_2-receptor antagonists
Calcium channel blockers	Metoclopramide
Centrally acting antiadrenergics	Miscellaneous drugs
Direct vasodilators	Acetazolamide
Diuretics	Baclofen
Peripherally acting antiadrenergics	Clofibrate
Drugs affecting the CNS	Danazol
Alcohol	Disulfiram
Antianxiety agents and hypnotics	Estrogens
Antidepressants	Interferon
Antipsychotics	Naproxen
CNS stimulants	Progesterone

Adapted from Stanisic TH, Francisco GE: "Impotence," in *Geriatric Pharmacology,* edited by R Bressler and MD Katz. New York, McGraw-Hill, 1993, p 272; used with permission of McGraw-Hill.

explaining that impotence is a common problem and by reassuring the patient that treatment is often effective. In private, the patient should be asked if he would like to discuss the matter alone or have his sexual partner present.

History: Before beginning the physical examination, the physician should be relatively certain whether the problem is erectile dysfunction or some other sexual dysfunction. History begins by establishing whether libido is intact and if nocturnal or morning erections occur. A history of changes in secondary sex characteristics or of vascular, pelvic, rectal, or prostate surgery may give clues to the cause. Depression, anxiety, and stress must also be sought, and the physician should learn about changes in sexual partners or problems with relationships. A review of all medication use, including alcohol and over-the-counter and illicit drugs, is essential.

Physical examination: The physical examination is usually less revealing than the history, but it helps detect signs of severe hypogonadism, such as small, soft testes, loss of pubic hair, and gynecomastia.

The bulbocavernous reflex helps establish the normalcy of the peripheral nerves innervating the pelvis. Measuring penile arterial pressure is not generally useful, although measuring pressures in the legs may help establish whether the patient has peripheral arterial disease.

Laboratory evaluation: Laboratory tests generally include obtaining a free (or total) testosterone level. Other tests for the common diseases that can lead to impotence should be ordered, such as CBC count, fasting blood sugar, and thyroid-stimulating hormone (TSH) level. A **nocturnal penile tumescence** measurement is useful if the occurrence of spontaneous erections cannot be ascertained. The simplest and least expensive test uses a ring of postage stamps placed around the penis at night: if the perforations are broken in the morning, an erection has occurred. More sensitive and reliable measurements can be made at home using a portable computerized unit.

While several tests are available to assess the penile vascular system, **duplex ultrasonography with intracorporeal injections of vasoactive agents** is generally the best. A papaverine-phentolamine combination is injected into the corpus cavernosum. Because the drugs are arterial vasodilators, an erection should occur; if erection occurs, such injections could possibly be used therapeutically (see below). Failure to produce an erection indicates venous leakage.

Treatment

Erectile dysfunction can usually be treated successfully, often without surgery. Determining the cause of impotence helps in choosing the initial treatment.

Men whose impotence is the result of psychosocial problems may benefit from **psychologic counseling.** Even those with primary erectile dysfunction may need psychologic counseling, and it often helps to have the patient's partner involved. Referral to experts in treating sexual disorders may be helpful when explanations and reassurance are inadequate.

Several drugs may ameliorate impotence, although none is remarkably effective. **Yohimbine,** an α_2-adrenergic blocker taken orally at 5.4 mg tid, appears to help a small proportion of men, especially those with vascular causes. **Testosterone replacement therapy** benefits only those whose impotence is due to hypogonadism (see above).

Binding and vacuum tumescence devices are often useful for obtaining and maintaining erections, but *men who are taking anticoagulants or who have low platelet levels or bleeding disorders should not use these devices.* Binding devices, which slow venous outflow at the base of the penis, used alone often help those with mild impotence. The devices are made of metal, rubber, or leather with snaps and can be purchased from medical supply houses or pharmacies (see FIG. 69–1).

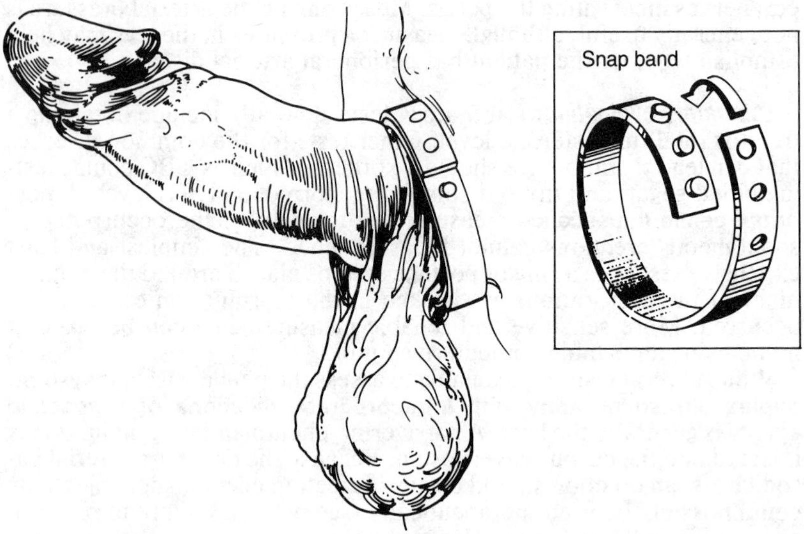

FIG. 69–1. Binding device used for maintaining an erection.

However, they can also be purchased less expensively at stores selling sexual paraphernalia, where they are known as "cock rings." The vacuum devices improve on the binder device by increasing arterial engorgement through vacuum assistance (see FIG. 69–2). A plastic cylinder vacuum device is fitted over the unerect penis, and a gentle vacuum is produced by sucking out air with a syringe, pump, or one's mouth (via tubing). Once an erection occurs, a wide rubber binding band is applied at the base of the penis and the vacuum device is removed. The band retards venous return and helps sustain the erection for up to 30 min. Binding devices can produce local discomfort and occasional difficulty with ejaculation, especially if too tight, and vacuum devices can produce petechiae if used excessively. Long-term safety and effectiveness are being evaluated.

Self-injection of vasoactive compounds **(intracavernous pharmacotherapy)** directly into the corpus cavernosum before sexual activity can help produce an erection (see FIG. 69–3). Self-injection therapy is usually effective when vascular disease is mild to moderate but not when it is severe. Furthermore, self-injection is not acceptable to all patients. A

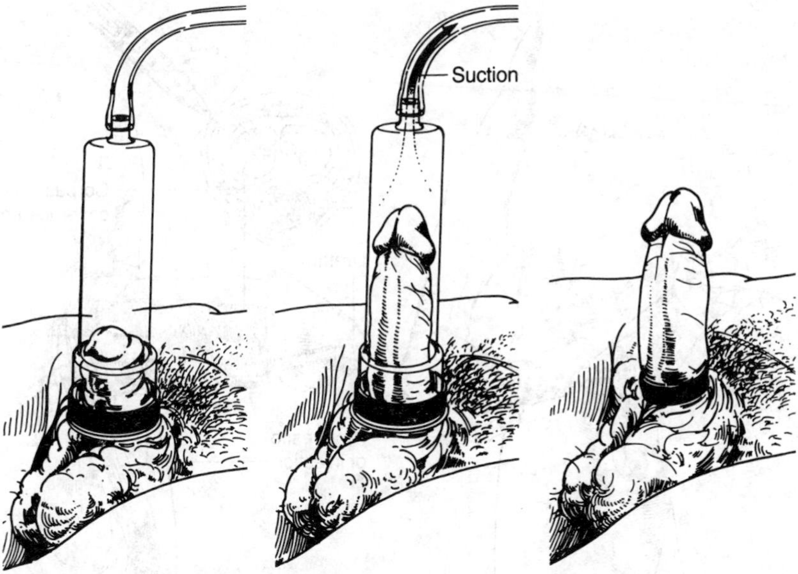

Fig. 69–2. Vacuum tumescence device. *Left,* A vacuum chamber is placed over the penis. *Middle,* Negative pressure draws blood into the penis to produce an erection. *Right,* A tension band is guided from the device to the base of the penis to entrap blood and maintain tumescence.

papaverine–phentolamine combination is often used, although the drugs do not have FDA approval. Alprostadil (prostaglandin E_1) is another drug that is used for intracavernous pharmacotherapy. The three agents may be given together, but no advantage of combined therapy over monotherapy has been established. The optimum combination of drugs to maximize effect while minimizing side effects is still being studied.

After injection, the patient should immediately initiate foreplay. He can expect to experience an erection after 5 to 10 min, and under ideal conditions, the erection will last up to 60 min. Problems include priapism, hematomas due to subcutaneous instead of intracavernosal injection, and pain. An injection of dilute epinephrine (20 μg/20 mL saline) or phenylephrine (500 μg/mL saline) usually reverses the priapism.

Permanent penile prostheses or implants may benefit patients with impotence that does not respond to other treatments, especially chronic organic impotence caused by diabetes. A prosthesis produces

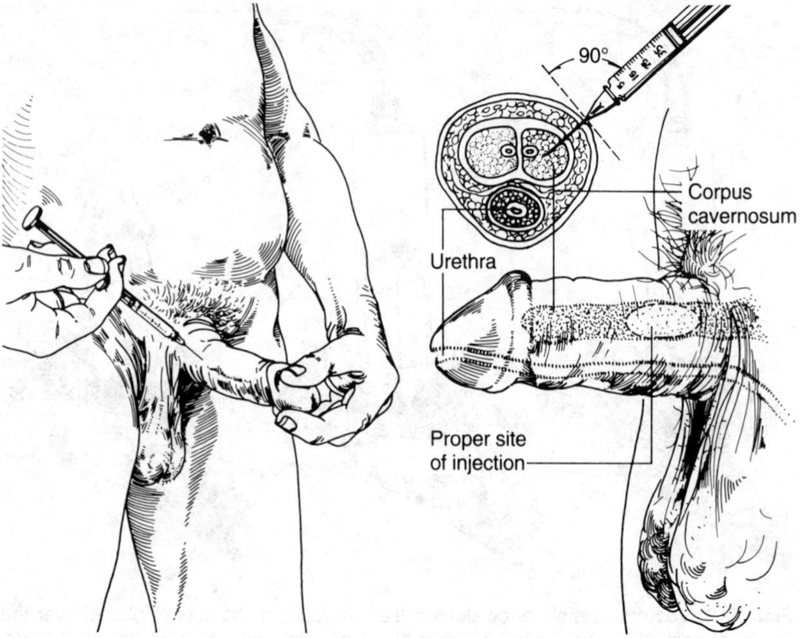

FIG. 69–3. Self-injection of vasoactive compounds (intracavernous pharmacotherapy).

an erection but cannot correct neurologic deficits that preclude normal sensation. Devices that produce a permanent erection include the Small Carrion semirigid rod prosthesis with a silicone sponge interior and the Flexi-rod II, a hinged modification of the Small Carrion device that allows the penis to be bent downward more easily when not being used for sexual activity. An inflatable (AMS 700 CX) prosthesis is also available. Contraindications to surgical implants include untreated depression, psychosis, severe personality disorder, and other severe psychiatric problems.

Penile revascularization surgery is still largely experimental. Surgery should be reserved for those with localized, identifiable lesions and performed only by highly skilled surgeons. Ligation of venous drainage is sometimes beneficial for those with impotence caused by venous leakage.

§3. ORGAN SYSTEMS: HEMATOLOGIC DISORDERS

70. AGE-RELATED HEMATOLOGIC CHANGES

The percentage of marrow space occupied by hematopoietic tissue varies throughout life, declining progressively from birth until about age 30, when it levels off. After about age 70, it again declines progressively. Whether this second decline results from a real reduction in blood-forming elements or a relative reduction caused by an increase in bone marrow fat is not known.

The following age-related changes occur in marrow function: (1) Marrow from older people can be maintained by serial transplantation in tissue culture just as long as marrow from younger people, but the number of stem cells in marrow decreases significantly with age. (2) Incorporation of iron in marrow culture from older people is comparable to that from younger people, but it increases less with erythropoietin stimulation. (3) Healthy older animals are unable to respond to bleeding or hypoxia as efficiently as younger animals because of ineffective erythropoiesis, but whether the defect lies with the hematopoietic elements, a decrease in growth factors, or age-related architectural changes in the marrow is unclear. (4) Although iron uptake from the intestines is normal in the elderly, slowed erythropoiesis reduces incorporation of iron into RBCs.

These changes in marrow function are not secondary to nutritional deficiencies since both total body and bone marrow iron increase with age, and both folate and vitamin B_{12} levels in healthy elderly people remain in the normal range.

Age-related changes in the peripheral blood include the following: (1) Average values of hemoglobin and hematocrit decrease slightly with age but remain within the normal adult range. (2) Mean corpuscular volume increases slightly with age, but RBC morphologic characteristics do not change significantly. (3) RBC content of 2,3-diphosphoglycerate decreases with age. (4) RBC osmotic fragility increases with age.

Factors that do not change with age include RBC life span, total blood volume, RBC volume, and platelet morphologic characteristics. Whether certain other factors change with age is uncertain: Lymphocyte and granulocyte counts have been reported as either normal or slightly decreased; platelet counts have been reported as either normal or slightly increased; and platelet function in healthy older people has been reported as normal, decreased, or increased.

71. ANEMIAS

Decreases in RBC or hemoglobin content resulting from blood loss, impaired production, or RBC destruction.

Anemia is common among elderly people, occurring in > 33% of outpatients. Because anemia is a symptom, not a diagnosis, an evaluation should be performed to identify the underlying cause. When older patients with significant anemia (ie, Hb < 12 gm/dL, Hct < 36%) are evaluated, an underlying disease is often discovered.

Symptoms and Signs

Generally symptoms and signs are similar to those in younger people; however, certain symptoms and signs may be more common in the elderly because of underlying, possibly unrelated, diseases. Fatigue, shortness of breath, worsening angina, and peripheral edema are more common when the patient has preexisting atherosclerotic heart disease or heart failure. Mental status changes, including confusion, depression, agitation, and apathy, may occur even in previously unimpaired persons. Dizziness is also common. Pallor may be less noticeable but often appears on the oral mucosa and the conjunctiva.

CLASSIFICATION

The most diagnostically useful way to classify anemias is probably by mean corpuscular volume **(MCV).** This method groups anemias into three categories: microcytic, normocytic, and macrocytic (see TABLE 71–1). However, some anemias may fall into more than one category; anemias of mixed etiologies have atypical presentations.

MICROCYTIC ANEMIAS

Anemia in which the MCV is < 80 fL. In the elderly, microcytic anemias include iron deficiency anemia, thalassemia minor, anemia of chronic disease, and myelodysplastic syndromes.

IRON DEFICIENCY ANEMIA

Characterized by small, pale RBCs and depleted iron stores, this chronic anemia accounts for almost 60% of all anemias in people > 65 yr. Iron deficiency is never normal in elderly persons. Because the body cannot eliminate excessive iron, total body and bone marrow iron stores increase with age.

TABLE 71–1. ANEMIAS CLASSIFIED BY USUAL MEAN CORPUSCULAR VOLUME

Microcytic anemia (MCV < 80 fL)	Iron deficiency anemia (can be normocytic) Myelodysplastic syndromes (can be normocytic) Anemia of chronic disease (usually normocytic) Thalassemia minor
Normocytic anemia (MCV 80–100 fL)	Iron deficiency anemia (usually microcytic) Anemia of chronic disease (can be microcytic) Myelodysplastic syndromes (can be microcytic) Hemolytic anemia (can be macrocytic) Unexplained anemia Aplastic anemia Bone marrow replacement by metastases Multiple myeloma Myeloid metaplasia Leukemia Endocrine disorders Chronic liver disease (usually macrocytic)
Macrocytic anemia (MCV > 100 fL)	Chronic liver disease (can be normocytic) Hemolytic anemia (can be normocytic) Vitamin B_{12} deficiency Folate deficiency

fL = femtoliter

Dietary iron deficiency in adults is virtually unknown in the USA, and iron malabsorption occurs only after total gastrectomy or with severe, generalized malabsorption. If these conditions do not exist, iron deficiency implies blood loss, most commonly from the GI or genitourinary tract, and evaluation is necessary. Possible causes include carcinoma, ulcer, atrophic gastritis, gastritis from drug ingestion, postmenopausal vaginal bleeding, bleeding hemorrhoids, and recurrent hemoptysis.

Pathophysiology

Iron deficiency affects many tissues, most notably those of the GI tract. Atrophy of the tongue and buccal mucosa as well as angular stomatitis may occur. Abnormalities of the gastric mucosa frequently develop; superficial gastritis accompanied by reduced hydrochloride secretion progresses to atrophic gastritis and achlorhydria. In those > 30 yr, iron therapy does not reverse achlorhydria. An inability to secrete intrinsic factor may also develop, resulting in vitamin B_{12} deficiency (see below).

Iron deficiency may lead to CNS dysfunction. Fatigue, irritability, and decreased cognitive function have been reported in younger people, but whether they occur in the elderly is unknown.

Diagnosis

In iron deficiency anemia, the peripheral blood smear is populated with microcytic hypochromic cells, and the MCV, the mean corpuscular hemoglobin (MCH), and the mean corpuscular hemoglobin concentration (MCHC) are usually reduced. In early iron deficiency, however, these values may still be normal. The RBC distribution width (RDW) may be elevated, but this elevation is not a reliable sign in the elderly. Many elderly people with iron deficiency anemia and chronic disease have normal RBC indices and distribution width. Chronic bleeding frequently results in an elevated platelet count, but the reticulocyte count does not increase. A transferrin saturation ratio (serum iron to total iron-binding capacity **[TIBC]**) < 16% may indicate iron deficiency. However, this ratio frequently is not useful because serum iron and TIBC decrease with age. Also, both serum iron and TIBC decrease in chronic disease, and the ratio decreases in the evening even in young adults without anemia.

Serum ferritin levels accurately reflect bone marrow iron stores. However, infection, inflammation, liver disease, and states of increased RBC turnover (eg, ineffective erythropoiesis and hemolysis) can falsely elevate serum ferritin levels. Serum ferritin levels < 10 μg/L are diagnostic of iron deficiency. A value of 10 to 30 μg/L is considered presumptive but not diagnostic. If an inflammatory disease is present, a level of < 100 μg/L raises suspicions of iron deficiency. In ambiguous cases, a combination of a decreased serum ferritin and an increased TIBC may help confirm the diagnosis of iron deficiency.

If a conclusive diagnosis still cannot be made, a bone marrow aspirate stained for iron may be performed. In iron deficiency, iron is either present in trace amounts or is absent. Another option is to give a 1-mo trial of oral iron in the form of ferrous salts (see Treatment, below). If the anemia results from iron deficiency, both hemoglobin and hematocrit will increase. If no increase occurs, either the patient is not iron deficient, blood loss is exceeding new blood formation, or an inflammatory or malignant process is contributing to the anemia.

Treatment

Treatment involves finding and eliminating the source of bleeding and correcting the iron deficiency. Because 150 to 200 mg of iron is needed per day, dietary replacement is impossible. But oral iron therapy is inexpensive, safe, and convenient. Only **ferrous iron salts** should be used; enteric-coated or sustained-release preparations should be avoided because they are not well absorbed. The simplest oral preparation is ferrous sulfate 300 mg, which contains 60 mg of elemental iron per tablet. One tablet tid taken 1 h before meals supplies 180 mg iron. To prevent constipation and gastric irritation, the patient may begin with 1 tablet/day and gradually increase the dose over 1 to 2 wk. Liquid preparations are available for patients unable to swallow tablets. Therapeutic response is monitored by serial levels of hemoglobin, hematocrit, and ferritin. Usually ≥ 6 mo of therapy is needed after bleeding has stopped to replenish iron stores.

In rare patients who have severe malabsorption, who cannot tolerate oral iron, whose iron stores need rapid replenishing, or whose bleeding continues, parenteral iron may be used. **Parenteral iron** is available as iron dextran and may be given IV or by deep IM injection. The maximum recommended dosage is 2 mL/day, which delivers 100 mg. An IV infusion should be given at a rate of ≤ 1 mL/min. *This therapy has been associated with anaphylactic shock, and a test dose of 0.5 mL IV should be given before treatment begins.* Other side effects include pain at the injection site, fever, and arthralgias. The most expensive and potentially hazardous way to replace iron, of course, is by **transfusion.** Each milliliter of transfused RBCs delivers 1 mg iron.

OTHER MICROCYTIC ANEMIAS

Except for **thalassemia minor,** anemias caused by abnormal hemoglobins are usually diagnosed in younger persons. Thalassemia minor occurs in those who are heterozygous for genes that produce few or no α- or β-globin chains. These conditions produce either microcytosis without anemia or a mild, microcytic anemia with hypochromia, target cells, anisocytosis, poikilocytosis, polychromatophilia, and basophilic stippling of RBCs on the peripheral smear. Reticulocytosis does not occur, and serum iron, TIBC, and serum ferritin are normal. Hemoglobin electrophoresis may reveal an increase in the minor hemoglobins, particularly fetal hemoglobin or hemoglobin A_2 in β-thalassemia; hemoglobin electrophoresis may be normal in α-thalassemia. No treatment is required for these conditions, and iron therapy is *contraindicated* because it may produce iron overload.

Anemia of chronic disease may be microcytic but is more commonly normocytic. **Myelodysplastic syndromes** may also be microcytic or normocytic and are discussed under MYELODYSPLASTIC SYNDROMES in Ch. 72.

NORMOCYTIC ANEMIAS

Anemia in which the MCV is 80 to 100 fL. The normocytic anemias include anemia of chronic disease, unexplained anemia, hemolytic anemia, aplastic anemia, and anemia caused by a malignancy.

Anemia of Chronic Disease

The most common normocytic anemia in the elderly, anemia of chronic disease accounts for up to 10% of the anemias in this population. The most common and most important causes include chronic infection or inflammation, renal insufficiency, chronic liver disease, and endocrine disorders.

Chronic Infection or Inflammation

Infection or inflammation commonly produces anemia, usually after 4 to 8 wk of illness. The anemia is usually mild, normochromic, and normocytic but may be slightly microcytic. It probably results from slightly decreased erythropoietin production, decreased RBC survival, and impairment in the delivery of iron from the reticuloendothelial system to the bone marrow. The reticulocyte count is low, serum iron and TIBC are normal or reduced, and serum ferritin is normal or increased. Treatment focuses on the underlying disorder.

Renal Insufficiency

This condition produces a normochromic, normocytic anemia resulting from decreased erythropoiesis and decreased RBC survival caused by decreased erythropoietin production. Serum iron stores are normal. In hemodialysis patients, injections of erythropoietin correct the anemia. In patients not being dialyzed, erythropoietin may not completely reverse the anemia because erythropoietic inhibitors can accumulate in uremia. Before erythropoietin is administered, nutritional deficiencies common in renal disease (eg, iron or folic acid deficiency) must be corrected. Erythropoietin is given IV to dialysis patients and subcutaneously or IV to nondialysis patients with renal failure. The starting dosage is 50 to 100 u./kg 3 times/wk. The target Hct is 30% to 33%. If the target hematocrit is reached or if the hematocrit increases 4 points in 2 wk, the dosage is reduced by 25 u./kg 3 times/wk. If the hematocrit does not increase by 5 to 6 points after 8 wk of therapy and the hematocrit is below the target, the dosage is increased by 25 u./kg 3 times/wk. Further increases of 25 u./kg 3 times/wk may be made at 4- to 6-wk intervals until the desired response is attained. The maximum recommended dosage is 300 u./kg 3 times/wk.

Chronic Liver Disease

This disorder produces a normochromic, normocytic anemia or a normochromic, macrocytic anemia resulting from decreased RBC production and survival. Large quantities of alcohol are toxic directly to the bone marrow as well as to the liver. Unless liver disease is complicated by bleeding, TIBC is decreased and serum iron is increased, resulting in an increased transferrin saturation. Serum ferritin is also increased and often reflects total body iron overload.

Endocrine Disorders

The endocrine disorders that commonly produce anemia are pituitary insufficiency, adrenal insufficiency, and hypothyroidism. In all three disorders, anemia is normocytic and normochromic. Hypothyroidism, however, is sometimes complicated by iron deficiency, producing microcytosis and hypochromia, or by associated megaloblastic anemia, producing macrocytosis and normochromia (see VITAMIN B_{12} DEFICIENCY and FOLATE DEFICIENCY, below). Unless a specific deficiency of iron, vitamin B_{12}, or folate is identified, treatment focuses on the underlying disorder.

UNEXPLAINED ANEMIA

A mild normochromic, normocytic anemia, with Hb usually between 11 and 12 gm/dL, has been reported in people > 70 yr and cannot be accounted for by any underlying disease or deficiency. The bone marrow does not contain ringed sideroblasts. This unexplained anemia accounts for up to 30% of the anemias in this age group. It may be associated with low neutrophil, lymphocyte, and platelet counts and with increased RBC 2,3-diphosphoglycerate levels, implying that this condition is not merely a normal, age-related variant. Its significance is unknown, but it is probably a myelodysplastic syndrome (see Ch. 72).

HEMOLYTIC ANEMIAS

Acquired hemolytic anemia (ie, *hemolysis not resulting from a congenital abnormality of the RBCs)* is a normochromic, normocytic anemia that may occur at any age, but its incidence increases with age. Increased peripheral destruction of RBCs results in increased production of immature RBCs by the bone marrow, producing an elevated reticulocyte count and polychromatophilia on the peripheral blood smear. If the reticulocytosis is marked, the RBC indices may become macrocytic because reticulocytes are larger than mature RBCs. Destruction of RBCs results in increased serum levels of unconjugated bilirubin, AST (SGOT), and LDH; decreased serum haptoglobin; and increased urine urobilinogen. If hemolysis is intravascular, urine hemosiderin increases as well. The direct antiglobulin (Coombs') test is used to detect antibody or complement on the RBC and can also identify the antigen to which the antibody is reacting.

Etiology

Idiopathic autoimmune hemolysis may result from warm-reactive antibodies of the IgG class; cold agglutinins that are usually of the IgM class but may be of the IgG class; or a nonagglutinating, cold-activated hemolysin of the IgG class. Idiopathic cold-agglutinin disease occurs primarily in old age.

TABLE 71–2. SELECTED DRUGS CAUSING HEMOLYTIC ANEMIA

Autoimmune Response	*Hapten-type Response*	*Immune Complex Response*
L-Dopa	Cephalosporins	*p*-Aminosalicylic acid
Methyldopa	Penicillins	Cephalosporins
Procainamide	Tetracyclines	Chlorpromazine
		Doxepin
		Insecticides
		Isoniazid
		Phenacetin
		Quinidine
		Quinine
		Rifampin
		Streptomycin
		Sulfonamides
		Sulfonylureas
		Tetracyclines
		Thiazides

Secondary immune hemolysis occurs in a wide variety of illnesses. About 30% of secondary immune hemolytic anemias are caused by lymphoproliferative diseases, including chronic lymphocytic leukemia, non-Hodgkin's lymphoma, Hodgkin's disease, and multiple myeloma (see Ch. 72). Agnogenic myeloid metaplasia, systemic lupus erythematosus, viral infections, *Mycoplasma pneumoniae* infection, syphilis, and various nonhematologic malignancies are also associated with immune hemolytic anemia.

Drug-induced hemolysis is another major cause of hemolytic anemia. The elderly are prone to this problem because they generally take more drugs than younger persons. Three types of drug-induced hemolysis have been described (see TABLE 71–2). Methyldopa causes autoantibody formation, with antibodies directed against normal RBC antigens, in 10% to 40% of people taking it. These antibodies attach to the RBC, resulting in a positive direct Coombs' test result against IgG; however, < 1% actually develop hemolysis. Discontinuing the drug usually corrects the anemia, but autoantibodies may persist for months to years. Other drugs that commonly produce autoantibodies but rarely produce autoimmune hemolysis include L-dopa and procainamide.

A second type of drug-induced, immune hemolytic anemia results when the drug binds to the surface of the RBC, acting as a hapten. Antibodies, usually IgG, are produced against the drug–RBC complex. The direct Coombs' test result is positive, and if the drug is added to test

RBCs, the indirect Coombs' test result is also positive. The drugs most commonly associated with this problem are the cephalosporins and penicillin. The anemia clears when the drug is discontinued.

A third type of drug-induced, immune hemolytic anemia occurs when a drug, either alone or bound to plasma protein, stimulates the production of antibodies to the drug. Drug-antibody immune complexes form in circulation and bind briefly to the RBC. Hemolysis occurs because the complex activates complement on the RBC surface. The Coombs' test result is positive for complement but not for IgG. The sulfonamides, quinidine, quinine, and many other drugs can produce this phenomenon. Hemolysis ceases when the drug is withdrawn.

Treatment

Idiopathic autoimmune hemolysis secondary to warm-reactive antibodies of the IgG class: In about 75% of cases, this condition responds to corticosteroid therapy. Prednisone 60 mg/day in divided doses is given initially, although occasionally 100 mg/day is needed. A rise in hemoglobin and hematocrit and a drop in the reticulocyte count usually occur within 3 to 14 days, but the response may be delayed up to 8 wk. Following remission, the dosage may be tapered by 5 mg/wk. A relapse requires increasing the dosage by 15 to 20 mg/day, followed by a more gradual tapering. Some patients continue to need a small daily dose or alternate-day therapy for long periods of time.

If after 4 to 8 wk, 60 mg/day of prednisone produces no response, higher doses may be tried or 200 mg bid to qid of the weak androgen **danazol** may be added. If this fails, the next step is usually **splenectomy,** which achieves long-term remission in 50% to 75% of cases. In patients who either do not respond to these measures or who are poor surgical candidates, the **immunosuppressive agent** cyclophosphamide (150 mg/day) or azathioprine (200 mg/day) may be useful.

Most patients with warm-antibody autoimmune hemolysis do not require **transfusion,** but for those who experience severe symptoms of anemia, transfusion can be considered. Blood compatibility testing is problematic, and the autoantibodies reduce the survival of the transfused RBCs. **Plasmapheresis** is usually not successful because IgG has a large volume of distribution in the body.

Idiopathic cold-agglutinin disease caused by IgM: This condition is treated by avoiding exposure to cold. **Corticosteroids** and **splenectomy** usually are *not* helpful, although they have been successful in a small number of patients with disease due either to low-titer IgM or to IgG. **Plasmapheresis** may lead to temporary improvement because IgM is confined to the intravascular space. **Transfusion** should be performed with warmed, washed RBCs.

Idiopathic disease caused by cold-activated IgG hemolysin: This condition is also treated by avoiding exposure to cold. **Transfusion** should be performed with warmed, washed RBCs.

TABLE 71–3. AGENTS CAUSING APLASTIC ANEMIA

Agents That Regularly Cause Aplasia If Enough Is Given	*Agents Occasionally Associated With Aplasia (20 or more cases)**
Benzene	Antimicrobials (chloramphenicol, organic arsenicals, quinacrine)
Ionizing radiation	Anticonvulsants (mephenytoin, trimethadione)
Sulfur or nitrogen mustard and congeners (busulfan, melphalan, cyclophosphamide)	Analgesics (phenylbutazone)
Antimetabolites (mercaptopurine, thioguanine, cytarabine)	Gold compounds
Antimitotics (colchicine, vincristine, vinblastine)	
Antibiotics (daunorubicin, doxorubicin hydrochloride)	
Inorganic arsenic	

* Many other agents have been implicated, but less than 20 cases have been reported.

Immune hemolytic anemia secondary to other diseases: This type of hemolytic anemia usually improves only with treatment of the underlying illness. If this approach is not possible, treatment may be tried as described above, but success is less likely than in idiopathic disease.

Drug-induced hemolytic anemia: Treatment usually consists of simply discontinuing the responsible drug. In rare instances, methyldopa-induced autoimmune hemolysis continues long enough to require corticosteroid therapy, as described above.

APLASTIC ANEMIA

Normochromic, normocytic anemia resulting from decreased bone marrow production of RBCs alone (pure RBC aplasia) or of all cell lines. In this disorder, the reticulocyte count is low; serum levels of iron, vitamin B_{12}, and folate are normal; and the bone marrow is hypoplastic. If thrombocytopenia occurs, bleeding may become a problem. Aplastic anemia is not very common; its overall mortality is > 50%.

Idiopathic aplastic anemia is usually a disease of adolescents and young adults. **Secondary aplastic anemia** can be caused by chemicals, radiation, or drugs, especially antibiotics, gold, and anticonvulsants (see TABLE 71–3). Because elderly persons frequently take several drugs, they are especially susceptible to this disorder. Thymoma and chronic lymphocytic leukemia are sometimes associated with pure RBC aplasia.

Treatment

All potentially offending drugs must be discontinued. An oral androgen (eg, oxymetholone 1 to 2 mg/kg/day) may be given, but such drugs are rarely successful. Bone marrow transplantation, the only effective therapy in younger adults, is not an option in older patients, who cannot tolerate transplant-related complications. Ongoing supportive treatment with transfusions is therefore required. Pure RBC aplasia may respond to prednisone or cyclophosphamide; if it is associated with thymoma, resection of the tumor may be helpful. The use of corticosteroids is controversial. Studies are being conducted using recombinant human granulocyte-macrophage colony stimulating factor (GM-CSF).

MALIGNANCY

Replacement of normal marrow by a neoplasm is a cause of normochromic, normocytic anemia. Serum iron, vitamin B_{12}, and folate values are normal or elevated, and the erythrocyte sedimentation rate is usually elevated. The neoplasm may be a primary disease of hematopoietic tissue or may metastasize from other sites.

MACROCYTIC ANEMIAS

Anemia in which the MCV is > 100 fL. With age, MCV increases slightly, but rarely does it increase enough to produce significant macrocytosis. Only a few disorders routinely produce macrocytic anemia. Anemia secondary to chronic liver disease and hemolytic anemia may be macrocytic. Megaloblastic anemias from vitamin B_{12} deficiency or folate deficiency also produce macrocytosis.

VITAMIN B_{12} DEFICIENCY

Vitamin B_{12} deficiency accounts for up to 9% of all anemias in elderly people. Potentially more important, 3% to 12% of all elderly people have low serum vitamin B_{12} levels. Because neurologic damage and dementia may occur before anemia or any hematologic changes are found, early detection of vitamin B_{12} deficiency is important.

Etiology

In elderly people, the most common cause of low serum vitamin B_{12} is an inability to split vitamin B_{12} from the so-called R proteins in food. This inability probably results from a deficiency of hydrochloric acid or pancreatic enzymes. Such a deficiency has also been reported in patients with AIDS.

Vitamin B_{12} deficiency anemia also results when a lack of intrinsic factor prevents vitamin B_{12} absorption and is known as **pernicious anemia.** In this autoimmune disease, antibodies are produced against parietal cells in which intrinsic factor is synthesized or against intrinsic factor itself. Pernicious anemia occurs in about 1% of people > 60 yr and is often associated with other autoimmune disorders. Other causes of vitamin B_{12} deficiency anemia include gastrectomy, intestinal disease, and intestinal bacterial overgrowth.

Symptoms, Signs, and Stages

Vitamin B_{12} deficiency takes years to develop, and its symptoms are subtle. Typically, patients develop glossitis with a smooth, red tongue; mild jaundice (lemon-yellow skin color); and neurologic changes. The latter includes paresthesias, abnormal position and vibration sensation, and gait ataxia from degeneration of the posterolateral columns of the spinal cord. Various psychiatric syndromes (including dementia, depression, and mania) may occur. The neuropsychiatric disorders may occur without anemia and often do not improve when the deficiency is treated. However, the hematologic problems are reversible.

Vitamin B_{12} deficiency has four stages: negative vitamin B_{12} balance, vitamin B_{12} depletion, vitamin B_{12} deficient erythropoiesis, and vitamin B_{12} deficiency anemia. The **first two stages** are characterized by a serum vitamin B_{12} level of < 300 pg/mL and a reduced holotranscobalamin II and transcobalamin II saturation. (The latter two tests are not commercially available.) Results of blood cell and deoxyuridine suppression tests are normal, as are levels of serum methylmalonic acid and homocysteine.

In the **third stage,** vitamin B_{12} deficient erythropoiesis, hypersegmented neutrophils appear, and the deoxyuridine suppression test becomes abnormal. The holotranscobalamin II and the transcobalamin II saturation fall further. The serum methylmalonic acid and homocysteine levels increase slightly. The patient is still not anemic, and the MCV is often normal. In the **fourth stage,** vitamin B_{12} deficiency anemia, all standard laboratory test results are abnormal, and the patient is anemic.

The stage at which myelin and brain damage occur is not known. Irreversible neurologic damage and dementia seem to occur before hypersegmentation develops and methylmalonic acid or homocysteine levels rise, so screening elderly persons for low serum vitamin B_{12} levels seems prudent. Because it is not known what proportion of cases will progress from the first to the fourth stage if untreated, treatment is currently recommended (see TABLE 71–4).

Diagnosis

The **serum vitamin B_{12} determination** is the most sensitive, practical way to discover early vitamin B_{12} depletion. Gallium, thyroid, and bone scans; RBC mass determinations; and ^{32}P (radioactive phosphorus) treatment produce falsely low levels. Also, pregnancy, folate deficiency, multiple myeloma, and ingestion of high doses of ascorbic acid have been reported to lower vitamin B_{12} levels. If serum vitamin B_{12} levels are low, serum methylmalonic acid and homocysteine levels may be used to evaluate the stage of deficiency.

TABLE 71–4. GUIDELINES FOR MANAGEMENT OF VITAMIN B12 DEFICIENCY

Until further research clarifies some controversial points, the following recommendations are offered:

1. Elderly patients should either undergo routine screening of serum vitamin B_{12} levels or take oral vitamin B_{12} on an empty stomach. A vitamin B_{12} level of < 200 pg/mL indicates vitamin B_{12} deficiency. A serum vitamin B_{12} level of 200 to 300 pg/mL suggests vitamin B_{12} depletion, and the test should be repeated in 1 to 3 mo.

2. When serum vitamin B_{12} levels are < 200 pg/mL, the peripheral blood smear should be examined for hypersegmented neutrophils, and if the patient is able to provide a 24-h urine specimen, a Schilling test should be performed. When available, a food Schilling test is useful. If a Schilling test is not possible, serum anti-intrinsic factor antibodies and antiparietal cells may be measured. Diagnosing true parietal cell-based intrinsic factor deficiency is important because patients with this disorder have a fourfold risk of gastric carcinoma. If methylmalonic acid and homocysteine levels are high, transcobalamin II binding of vitamin B_{12} is reduced or holotranscobalamin levels are low, or if the deoxyuridine suppression test result is abnormal, the patient should be treated for vitamin B_{12} deficiency. (These tests are not available in many clinical settings.)

3. Even if the patient has no hematologic abnormalities or the routine fasting Schilling test result is normal, a serum vitamin B_{12} level of < 200 pg/mL requires treatment.

4. Vitamin B_{12} 1000 μg/day should be given on an empty stomach until serum vitamin B_{12} levels increase to > 300 pg/mL.

5. A patient with an abnormal Schilling test result or one whose serum level of vitamin B_{12} does not increase to > 300 pg/mL with oral vitamin B_{12} should be treated with parenteral vitamin B_{12} (as if the patient has pernicious anemia).

The cause of vitamin B_{12} deficiency anemia can be determined by the **Schilling test.** This test measures the absorption of radiolabeled vitamin B_{12} before and after intrinsic factor is administered. If the patient has pernicious anemia, vitamin B_{12} absorption is abnormal before administering intrinsic factor and normal after administering it. If absorption remains abnormal after intrinsic factor is administered, the patient should be given a broad-spectrum antibiotic for 8 to 12 wk, then tested again. If absorption is normal, the problem was bacterial overgrowth. If the patient has pernicious anemia and chronic vitamin B_{12} deficiency, vitamin B_{12} malabsorption may result from a malfunction of the small intestine caused by the vitamin deficiency. If an intestinal malfunction is suspected, the Schilling test should be repeated after a few months of vitamin B_{12} supplementation.

If the standard Schilling test shows no abnormalities and the antibiotic therapy does not improve vitamin B_{12} absorption, the **food Schilling test** may be performed. In this test, radioactive vitamin B_{12} is mixed with a scrambled egg. Failure to absorb the vitamin B_{12} confirms an inability to split vitamin B_{12} from food proteins. NOTE: *A major* *problem with the Schilling tests is ensuring proper collection of a 24-h urine specimen, especially with elderly patients who have urinary incontinence or cognitive problems.*

Besides anemia, **laboratory abnormalities** associated with vitamin B_{12} deficiency anemia may include leukopenia and thrombocytopenia. The anemia is macrocytic, and hypersegmented polymorphonuclear leukocytes appear on peripheral smear. The platelets are large. The MCV and RBC distribution width (RDW) are typically elevated. Serum levels of bilirubin, ferritin, and LDH may be elevated because of ineffective erythropoiesis. When an anemia is present, bone marrow examination will show megaloblastic changes.

Treatment

Therapy for vitamin B_{12} deficiency from pernicious anemia consists of lifelong vitamin B_{12} administration. An initial regimen of 100 μg/day IM is sufficient for the first 5 days; however, a more convenient regimen is 1000 μg/day for the first week, then 1000 μg/wk for 4 wk or until the hematocrit is normal, and then 1000 μg/mo for life. The response to treatment is usually brisk reticulocytosis within 1 wk. While the anemia should be corrected within 1 mo, abnormalities in the peripheral smear may persist for 1 yr. Because hypokalemia and hypophosphatemia may occur early in therapy, serum phosphate and potassium levels should be monitored and supplements given, if necessary. Transfusion may produce volume overload; if it is necessary, it should be done slowly, and the patient should be monitored.

If the vitamin B_{12} deficiency results from an inability to split vitamin B_{12} from food proteins, 1000 μg/day of oral vitamin B_{12} may be given when the stomach is empty. Recent data have shown that even in patients with pernicious anemia, this is enough vitamin B_{12} to correct the deficiency by mass action absorption in the absence of intrinsic factor.

If the vitamin B_{12} deficiency is misdiagnosed as folate deficiency, treatment with folate alone may improve the hematologic disorder, but it will not affect the neurologic changes associated with vitamin B_{12} deficiency.

Folate Deficiency

Deficiency of folic acid produces changes in the peripheral blood smear and bone marrow that are indistinguishable from those caused by vitamin B_{12} deficiency. The incidence of folate deficiency in the elderly is controversial, partly because of varying definitions of the lower limits of the normal range and differences in radioimmunoassay and microbiologic methods used to measure both serum and RBC folate levels. Serum folate levels fluctuate rapidly and do not necessarily reflect body stores; RBC folate levels are more stable and, therefore, clinically reliable.

Normal body stores of folate can be depleted in < 6 mo. Rapid folate deficiency can be caused by malabsorption, poor nutrition, alcoholism, and states of increased folate utilization such as hemolytic anemia and neoplasia. Drugs (eg, anticonvulsants, trimethoprim, triamterene, and nitrofurantoin) also cause folate deficiency. Nevertheless, anemia resulting solely from folate deficiency does not seem to be common in the elderly.

Although traditional belief has been that folate deficiency alone does not produce neurologic abnormalities, evidence exists that pure folate deficiency may result in neurologic changes that are virtually indistinguishable from those caused by vitamin B_{12} deficiency. However, this problem does not seem to be common. A diagnosis of anemia caused by folate deficiency depends on macrocytic RBCs and hypersegmented neutrophils in the peripheral smear, a normal serum vitamin B_{12} level, and a low serum folate level (< 2 ng/mL) or a low RBC folate level (< 100 ng/mL). Bone marrow is histologically indistinguishable from that seen in vitamin B_{12} deficiency.

Treatment

Therapy consists of folic acid 1 mg/day orally. A parenteral form is available for patients with severe malabsorption. In a patient with megaloblastic anemia secondary to vitamin B_{12} deficiency, treatment with folate alone may correct the anemia but will not reverse neurologic damage.

---

72. MALIGNANCIES AND MYELOPROLIFERATIVE DISORDERS

ACUTE LEUKEMIAS

Accumulation of neoplastic, immature lymphoid or myeloid cells in the bone marrow and peripheral blood, tissue invasion by these cells, and associated bone marrow failure.

Classification

Acute leukemias are categorized as **acute lymphocytic leukemia** or **acute nonlymphocytic leukemia,** according to the morphologic characteristics of cells in peripheral blood and bone marrow smears, histochemical staining, and immunologic markers. The French-American-British (FAB) Cooperative Group classification, the system most widely used to facilitate clinical studies, allows some degree of prognostication (see TABLE 72–1).

TABLE 72–1. FRENCH–AMERICAN–BRITISH COOPERATIVE GROUP CLASSIFICATION OF ACUTE LEUKEMIAS

Acute Nonlymphocytic Leukemia	*Acute Lymphocytic Leukemia*
M1: Undifferentiated myelocytic	L1: Common childhood type (null or non-B, non-T; pre-B; T cell)
M2: Myelocytic	
M3: Promyelocytic	L2: Heterogeneous type (null or non-B, non-T; pre-B; T cell)
M4: Myelomonocytic	
M5: Monoblastic	L3: Burkitt's type (B cell)
M5 a: Monoblastic	
M5 b: Monocytic	
M6: Erythroleukemic	
Other: Megakaryoblastic, basophilic, eosinophilic	

Etiology

In most cases of acute leukemia, the etiology is unknown. Radiation exposure has been implicated as the cause in some cases. Data on atomic bomb survivors from Hiroshima and Nagasaki show a 10% to 20% increase in the incidence of acute nonlymphocytic leukemia. Likewise, studies show that the risk of developing acute nonlymphocytic leukemia is 2.5 times greater in diagnostic radiologists and 14 times greater in patients who received radiation therapy for ankylosing spondylitis earlier this century. High-level benzene exposure in the workplace has been strongly implicated as a risk factor for acute nonlymphocytic leukemia. Also, long-term, low-dose therapy with virtually any chemotherapeutic alkylating agent can cause acute leukemia, usually the nonlymphocytic type.

The combination of chemotherapeutic drugs and radiation therapy increases the risk of developing leukemia. Chronic bone marrow disorders (eg, the myelodysplastic syndromes, polycythemia vera, and aplastic anemia) are sometimes followed by a rapidly progressive leukemic phase. Viruses have long been suspected as the cause of some acute leukemias. Molecular genetic studies show that oncogenes, the cellular homologues of retroviral transforming genes, appear to have a role in inducing and maintaining the malignant state. Cytogenetic and molecular biologic techniques show that specific oncogenes are involved in nonrandom chromosome translocations or are found on deleted or reduplicated chromosomes.

Incidence

Acute leukemia is primarily a disease of the elderly. Although treatment and patient survival have significantly improved, the most dramatic results have been among the young. Leukemia has an incidence of about 15 per 100,000 across all age groups. But the incidence begins rising at age 40 and by age 80 is about 160 per 100,000. About 80% percent of adults with acute leukemia have the nonlymphocytic type, whereas 80% of children with acute leukemia have the lymphocytic type. Nevertheless, the incidence of acute lymphocytic leukemia is four times higher in the elderly than in children.

Pathophysiology

Primitive leukocytes (eg, lymphoblasts, myeloblasts) accumulate rapidly in the bone marrow and invade many tissues, including the liver, spleen, lymph nodes, and CNS. Normal bone marrow and normal leukocytes are replaced by these blasts, resulting in severe anemia, thrombocytopenia with marked bleeding, and great susceptibility to infection.

Symptoms and Signs

Acute leukemia frequently presents as an apparent infection with an acute onset and high fever. The associated thrombocytopenia usually is manifested by petechiae, ecchymoses, and bleeding from the nose, mouth, and GI and GU tracts. Often, the liver, spleen, and lymph nodes are enlarged. In the elderly, the disease can present insidiously with progressive weakness, pallor, an altered sense of well-being, and delirium.

Laboratory Findings and Diagnosis

The total peripheral WBC count may be low, normal, or elevated. Blasts are usually seen in the peripheral blood smear, but a bone marrow aspiration should be performed to confirm the diagnosis. The bone marrow shows excessive blast cells and an absence or decreased number of normal erythrocytic, granulocytic, and megakaryocytic cells. Histochemical stains and surface antigen markers help identify the type of acute leukemia.

Prognosis

An untreated patient dies, on average, within 4 to 6 mo of clinical onset. Some persons die within days. Infection, bleeding, advanced age, high blast counts, and chromosomal abnormalities have been proposed as indicators of a poor prognosis; Auer rods (in acute myelocytic leukemia) have been reported as an indicator of a good prognosis. Efforts have been made to define morphologic and in vitro growth characteristics as prognosticators; however, *data regarding all prognostic signs are contradictory.*

Advanced age (usually defined as > 60 yr) has typically been considered a bad sign. Much of the problem in treating the elderly seems to be their inability to tolerate the prolonged pancytopenia that accompanies aggressive induction chemotherapy regimens. The elderly also have more complex karyotypic abnormalities than younger patients, and they have more underlying primary marrow disorders (eg, polycythemia vera, myelodysplasia). A prior hematologic marrow disorder or leukemia secondary to prior therapy with an alkylating agent seems to indicate a poor prognosis.

Treatment

Acute lymphocytic leukemia: Older patients have a poor long-term survival rate compared with children, who have an excellent prognosis. The older patient is usually considered at high risk and often has one or more of the following: a WBC count > 20,000/μL, mediastinal mass, L2–L3 morphologic changes, T-cell or B-cell leukemia, and meningitis. Therapy usually consists of a combination of drugs, including vincristine, prednisone, an anthracycline, and asparaginase (which is tolerated poorly by older persons). Most older people relapse within the first year of treatment. Currently, there is no accepted standard therapy.

Bone marrow transplantation is rarely used in patients > 35 yr and not at all in elderly patients.

Acute nonlymphocytic leukemia: First, a complete remission—*the reduction of leukemic blasts to an undetectable level (in practice, < 5% marrow blasts)*—must be obtained. The induction phase is the most critical time because the patient is often infected and bleeding and has a large tumor burden with little normal hematopoiesis. Many induction regimens are being studied; the standard combination is cytarabine 100 to 200 mg/m²/day in a continuous IV infusion for 5 to 7 days and daunorubicin 45 mg/m²/day IV for the first 3 days. Attempts have been made to improve response rates in older people by giving low-dose cytarabine as attenuated doses of standard therapies. Although death rates are lower during induction, complete remission rates have not improved. Clearly, the regimen must be individualized for each patient. With the use of fresh, frozen platelets, packed RBCs, and antibiotics, the current complete remission rate in patients > 60 yr ranges from 40% to 76%. Median survival is 1 to 2 yr. The value of maintenance and consolidation chemotherapeutic regimens is under study. Recently, use of all-*trans*-retinoic acid in patients with acute promyelocytic leukemia has produced promising remission induction rates. Still experimental, this regimen has not been studied specifically in the elderly.

Bone marrow transplantation is rarely used in patients > 35 yr and not at all in elderly patients.

Complications of treatment: Infections are the major cause of morbidity and mortality in the acute leukemias. They result from the severe leukopenia and destruction of normal cutaneous and mucosal barriers. Polymorphonuclear leukocytes, about 500 to 1000/μL, are needed to protect against infection. In many patients, endogenous bowel flora is the source of infection, but the pharynx, lungs, perirectal area, and skin are also common sources. The GU tract and meninges are rare sites. Because the source of infection is internal, isolation has limited value. Viruses, protozoa, and anaerobic bacteria are uncommon pathogens early in therapy.

Fungal infections usually occur after 7 to 14 days of antibiotic therapy in neutropenic patients. The initial choice of antibiotics depends on the predominant organisms causing infection in a given hospital. An aminoglycoside plus a semisynthetic penicillin or a cephalosporin is usually the combination of choice because the most common organisms in most hospitals are *Pseudomonas* and *Escherichia coli*. Trimethoprim-sulfamethoxazole has been suggested as prophylaxis, particularly in patients who have had frequent admissions with fever and neutropenia.

Metabolic problems are common during induction therapy. Hyperuricemia should be treated prophylactically with allopurinol 300 mg/day. Often natriuresis and hyponatremia develop from increased osmolar clearance due to electrolytes, water, and urea released from dead blasts. Hypokalemia can occur from natriuresis, SIADH, physiologic hypervasopressinemia, or proximal renal tubular dysfunction. A renal tubular acidosis-like syndrome, with hypokalemia, aminoaciduria, and hyperphosphaturia, occurs but is probably not related to lysozyme. Metabolic alkalosis, metabolic acidosis, hypocalcemia, and hyperphosphatemia are also common complications. Oliguric renal failure will develop from uric acid nephropathy unless the patient is vigorously hydrated, treated with allopurinol, and has the urine alkalinized.

Aggregates of blasts and thrombi may occlude small blood vessels throughout the body, particularly in the brain and lungs. Therapy consists of hydration and rapid reduction of the blast count by promptly initiating chemotherapy. Leukapheresis and cranial irradiation may be temporizing measures.

The **CNS** is the most common site of extramedullary relapse in acute leukemia. The need for prophylactic meningeal therapy with cranial irradiation and intrathecal methotrexate or cytarabine has not been formally addressed in the elderly. Therefore, these methods currently must be used with extreme caution, if at all. Spinal cord compression, when it occurs, usually responds to local radiation. The acute T-cell lymphocytic leukemias are most likely to cause either CNS or gonadal invasion. However, the role of prophylactic testicular irradiation in the elderly is currently unclear.

Disseminated intravascular coagulation (DIC) is an uncommon complication seen mainly in promyelocytic (M3) leukemia. This bleeding disorder results from an underlying illness in which the clotting factors and platelets are consumed because of intravascular coagulation. The patient presents either with massive sudden bleeding (acute DIC) or, more usually, with slow bleeding (chronic DIC). Generally, DIC is self-limited and is most problematic during the rapid cell lysis of induction chemotherapy. The use of prophylactic heparin continues to be controversial.

CHRONIC LEUKEMIAS

Accumulation of neoplastic, mature lymphoid or myeloid cells in the blood that usually progresses more slowly than that in an acute leukemic process.

Classification

If the neoplastic cells are of the lymphoid type, the disease is called **chronic lymphocytic leukemia;** if they are of the myeloid type, it is called **chronic myeloid (myelocytic, myelogenous) leukemia.** Because chronic lymphocytic leukemia is primarily a disease of the elderly and chronic myeloid leukemia usually occurs in people in their 30s and 40s, this discussion concentrates on the former. In > 95% of cases, chronic lymphocytic leukemia involves the neoplastic proliferation of B cells.

Etiology

Ionizing radiation plays no part in the etiology of chronic lymphocytic leukemia. Rather, a genetic component seems to be involved because the illness is more common in certain families. Some of these families have immunologic abnormalities. Chronic viral infections (eg, Epstein-Barr virus) have been suggested as possible causes.

Incidence

Chronic lymphocytic leukemia is the most common leukemia in Western society, accounting for 25% to 40% of all leukemias. About 90% of all patients are > 50 yr, with the majority > 60 yr. Men are affected twice as often as women.

Pathophysiology

Monoclonal lymphocytes accumulate in the peripheral blood, bone marrow, lymphoid tissues, and sometimes other organs. Cells appear morphologically mature but have receptors for mouse erythrocytes, HLA-DR antigens, and small amounts of surface immunoglobulin, suggesting some degree of immaturity. Trisomy 12 has been identified in about 25% of cases. Infiltration of the bone marrow may eventually result in pancytopenia. Deficiency of normal B-cells often leads to bacterial infection. Transformation to a diffuse, large-cell lymphoma (Richter's syndrome) or to acute prolymphocytic leukemia may occur as a terminal event.

Symptoms and Signs

The presentation is highly variable. Over 25% of patients have asymptomatic disease discovered on routine physical examination or blood count. The most common initial symptoms are fatigue, malaise, and decreased exercise tolerance. In many elderly people, an exacerbation of coronary artery or cerebrovascular disease may be the initial manifestation.

Some patients complain of enlarged lymph nodes, abdominal pain, or early satiety, which is caused by splenomegaly. Lymphadenopathy is commonly found in the cervical, axillary, and supraclavicular areas, while inguinal adenopathy is rare. Splenomegaly is found in 50% of patients at presentation. Hepatomegaly may develop as the disease progresses. Lymphocytic infiltration can occur in any organ. Jaundice usually suggests hemolysis, although biliary obstruction can result from periportal lymph node enlargement. In the late stages, ecchymoses and petechiae may result from thrombocytopenia.

Fever is usually secondary to infection, but in the late stages, the development of acute prolymphocytic leukemia or aggressive lymphoma should be considered. Clinically significant hyperviscosity is rare, occurring only when the WBC count is ≥ 800,000/μL.

The most common **complications** of chronic lymphocytic leukemia are bacterial infections, especially of the lungs and urinary tract. Gram-positive coccal, gram-negative rod, fungal, *Listeria,* and *Pneumocystis carinii* infections may occur. In addition, patients have at least a fourfold risk of developing a carcinoma.

Laboratory Findings and Diagnosis

The diagnosis of chronic lymphocytic leukemia requires demonstration of sustained lymphocytosis and bone marrow lymphocyte infiltration in the absence of other causes. The absolute lymphocyte count is generally > 15,000/μL. The cells appear mature and tend to smudge when the blood smear is prepared.

In **B-cell chronic lymphocytic leukemia,** the number of T cells and B cells increases, but the B cells increase preferentially, accounting for 40% to 90% of all lymphocytes. They are of monoclonal origin and express the surface immunoglobulins of one light-chain class. The usual surface immunoglobulin is IgM, but less commonly it is IgD. In B-cell chronic lymphocytic leukemia, the ratio of helper (T4) to suppressor (T8) T cells is reversed because of an increased number of suppressor cells. This may account for the development of pure RBC aplasia that occurs in a few patients.

About 1% of patients have lymphocytes that form rosettes with sheep RBCs, and their disease is classified as **T-cell chronic lymphocytic leukemia.** In T-cell chronic lymphocytic leukemia, both T4 and T8 cells are seen. The lymphocytes often inhibit cytoplasmic azurophilic granules. Massive splenomegaly, marked neutropenia, skin infiltration, modest bone marrow infiltration, and a rapid clinical course leading to death occur in < 50% of these patients. There is a high concurrence with rheumatoid arthritis; however, most cases have an indolent course.

The RBC morphologic characteristics are usually normal. Anemia occurs in 10% to 20% of patients and is usually normochromic and normocytic. The anemia may result from marrow replacement, hypersplenism, or suppressor mechanisms. The Coombs' test reveals IgG coating of RBCs in about 20% of cases; however, an autoimmune hemolytic anemia is seen only 8% of the time. Thrombocytopenia, which is found in 10% to 20% of cases, may result from marrow replacement, hypersplenism, or antiplatelet antibodies. Bone marrow morphologic examination shows interstitial or nodular infiltration in the early stages of disease and diffuse infiltration in the advanced stages.

In about 5% of cases, the immunoglobulin found on the cell surface is also found in the serum as a monoclonal protein. Hypogammaglobulinemia or agammaglobulinemia is found in 50% to 75% of patients.

Prognosis

Clinical staging is based on the examination and CBC. Patients in stage A have fewer than three involved sites and usually survive > 7 yr. Those in stage B have three or more involved sites, which may include the cervical, axillary, supraclavicular, and inguinal lymph nodes, as well as the liver and spleen; these patients normally survive < 5 yr. Patients in stage C have anemia (Hb < 10 gm/dL) or thrombocytopenia (platelets < 100,000/μL) and usually survive < 2 yr. Generally, the disease progresses in a stepwise pattern from less severe to more severe.

Other poor prognostic signs include diffuse replacement of bone marrow, trisomy 12 plus other abnormal chromosomes, and surface IgM rather than IgD. Although many patients with chronic lymphocytic leukemia live 10 yr or more, the 5-yr survival rate is only about 50%.

Treatment

Stage A patients and **stage B patients** usually do not require treatment because the complications of chemotherapy (eg, infection, development of acute nonlymphocytic leukemia) may be more deleterious than the chronic lymphocytic leukemia. However, stage B patients are treated if they are troubled by progressive, disabling constitutional symptoms that are clearly attributable to the leukemia.

For **stage C patients,** chlorambucil is the most commonly used agent. It induces responses in 50% to 80% of patients and complete remission in 10% to 20%. **Chlorambucil** may be given at a daily dosage of 0.08 to 0.2 mg/kg orally or for 1 day every 4 wk at 0.4 to 0.8 mg/kg orally in 3 divided doses. The chlorambucil dosage is gradually reduced as the WBC count falls; the drug is discontinued when the lymphocyte count falls below 20,000/μL. **Prednisone** 0.8 mg/kg/day is often used concomitantly and may improve the response rate. Corticosteroids alone are used only in patients with autoimmune hemolytic anemia or thrombocytopenia. Some patients may benefit from fludarabine or pentostatin. Certain combination chemotherapy regimens such as cyclophosphamide, doxorubicin, vincristine, and prednisone may be useful in far advanced cases.

Radiation therapy is used to reduce local bulky disease, vital organ compromise, or painful bone lesions. Patients with refractory chronic lymphocytic leukemia may benefit from repeated **leukapheresis,** which lowers the WBC count, reduces organomegaly, and improves the cytopenia.

When transformation to either an acute prolymphocytic leukemia or an aggressive lymphoma occurs, response to chemotherapy or radiation is generally poor.

MULTIPLE MYELOMA

A neoplastic disorder resulting from the proliferation and accumulation of immature plasma cells in the bone marrow. Its major manifestations, which ultimately lead to death, result from the direct effect of these cells, the characteristic proteins they produce, and their secondary effects on other organ systems.

Classification

Neoplastic plasma cells almost always synthesize abnormal amounts of monoclonal immunoglobulin (IgG, IgA, IgD, or IgE) or κ or λ light chains. Therefore, they are usually classified according to their immunoglobulin class. Rarely, cases occur with no detectable production of immunoglobulin.

Incidence

The annual incidence is about 3 per 100,000 persons. The disease is more common in blacks than in whites. It occurs equally in men and women. Multiple myeloma usually occurs in people > 50 yr, and the incidence increases with age.

Etiology

An increased occurrence of myeloma in first-degree relatives and in blacks and the higher frequency of the 4C complex of HLA antigens in myeloma patients suggest that genetic factors play a role. The risk of developing myeloma seems to increase after high radiation exposure, as shown in Hiroshima and Nagasaki atomic bomb survivors. Other possibilities include chronic antigenic stimulation from factors such as cholecystitis, osteomyelitis, repeated allergen injections, rheumatoid arthritis, hereditary spherocytosis, or Gaucher's disease. Asbestos exposure and viral illnesses have also been suggested as possible etiologic factors.

Since myeloma is so age related, one potential influence may be the decrease in the T-lymphoid arm of the immune system. As T cells decrease, B-cell clones may proliferate excessively. Then because of such monoclonal expansion, spontaneous or externally induced genetic alteration of the clone may occur, allowing it to proliferate and produce its immunoglobulin. Since it would remain under some control of the immune system, it would be a **benign monoclonal gammopathy.** A second external oncogenic event could then result in uncontrolled proliferation of these cells (ie, multiple myeloma).

Pathophysiology

The consequences of abnormal plasma cell growth are plasma cell tumors, osteolysis, hematopoietic suppression, hypogammaglobulinemia, paraproteinemia, paraproteinuria, and renal disease.

Plasma cell tumors usually develop in areas of hematopoietically active bone marrow. They commonly occur in virtually any bone but rarely in extraskeletal sites. Even plasmacytomas that seem solitary usually become widespread eventually.

Osteolytic lesions, which are very common, are thought to result from the release of osteoclast-activating factor by the neoplastic plasma cell. This stimulates osteoclasts to resorb bone.

Marrow function is impaired in direct proportion to the number of plasma cells in the bone marrow. Anemia is most common, but neutropenia and thrombocytopenia also occur.

In multiple myeloma, the single clone of abnormal plasma cells produces an excess of a single type of immunoglobulin or a portion of the immunoglobulin molecule, and the other normal classes of immunoglobulins are suppressed, resulting in an actual or functional **hypogammaglobulinemia.** In > 50% of patients with monoclonal gammopathies, the monoclonal protein is an IgG; in 20%, an IgA; in 12%, an IgM (Waldenström's macroglobulinemia); and in 2%, an IgD. An IgE monoclonal protein is rare. About 10% of patients produce only light chains, and < 1% produce only heavy chains. Rarely, patients produce two or more monoclonal proteins, and about 1% of patients have no monoclonal protein in serum or urine.

Renal disease occurs in about 50% of patients with multiple myeloma. Glomerular amyloid deposits, urinary tract infections, calcium or uric acid calculi, and plasma cell infiltration of the kidney may occur. However, the major cause of renal failure is the tubular damage associated with the excretion of light chains. All light-chain proteins are not nephrotoxic, and some patients may excrete large amounts of light chains for years without developing renal failure. Patients who excrete λ light chains are at greater risk than those who excrete κ light chains.

Symptoms and Signs

Multiple myeloma is usually progressive. The abnormal plasma cells are estimated to double in 3 to 10 mo. In rare cases, however, the preclinical stage may last for years.

Bone pain is the most common symptom of multiple myeloma, occurring in about 70% of patients. Pain often occurs in the lower back or ribs and gradually increases in intensity. A sudden onset may mean that a vertebra has collapsed or that a spontaneous pathologic fracture has occurred (eg, in the shaft of a long bone, the pelvis, a rib, or a clavicle).

Systemic symptoms and signs include pallor, weakness, fatigue, dyspnea on exertion, and palpitations—all resulting from the anemia that occurs in about 70% of patients at the time of diagnosis. **Signs of thrombocytopenia** (eg, ecchymoses, purpura, epistaxis, and excessive bleeding from trauma) are common. **Infection** also occurs frequently because of neutropenia and immunoglobulin deficiency, and the patient may present with pneumonia, pyoderma, or pyelonephritis. **Cold sensitivity** and **urticaria** may result from cryoglobulinemia. Patients rarely present with **nephrotic syndrome.**

Hypercalcemia, common in patients with destructive bone lesions, may result in anorexia, nausea, vomiting, polyuria, polydipsia, constipation, and dehydration. Particularly in the elderly, hypercalcemia may produce drowsiness, confusion, and coma.

Renal disease may be acute or chronic. The acute disease is usually associated with azotemia, hypercalcemia, hypotension, dehydration, and infections treated with nephrotoxic antibiotics. Dehydration is frequently produced by fluid deprivation or IV use of hypertonic contrast media during a diagnostic procedure. In patients with multiple myeloma, procedures such as IV or retrograde pyelograms or open bone biopsies should *not* be performed unless urine flow is ample and hypercalcemia and hyperuricemia have been corrected.

Hyperviscosity syndrome occurs in about 50% of cases in which the monoclonal immunoglobulin is IgM (Waldenström's macroglobulinemia). The syndrome is uncommon in multiple myeloma with other immunoglobulin classes. Purpura, ecchymoses, epistaxis, GI bleeding, blurred vision associated with venous congestion, intraocular hemorrhages and exudates, and ischemic neurologic symptoms are common.

Neurologic symptoms and signs include mental confusion from hypercalcemia, spinal cord and nerve root compression, myelomatous meningitis, carpal tunnel syndrome from amyloid deposits, and sensorimotor polyneuropathy not due to amyloid or plasma cell infiltration. Rarer CNS symptoms include intracerebral plasmacytomas, herpes zoster, and multifocal leukoencephalopathy.

Laboratory Findings and Diagnosis

The order in which diagnostic tests are performed depends on the presentation of symptoms and signs. If a monoclonal protein is found on serum electrophoresis, the skeleton should be x-rayed, and a bone marrow aspiration should be performed. If neither lytic bone lesions nor plasma cell infiltration is found, a diagnosis of **benign monoclonal gammopathy** is likely. Confirming findings for this diagnosis include no significant amounts (< 60 mg/24 h) of a single type of light chain (ie, Bence Jones protein) in the urine and serum levels of monoclonal protein < 2 gm/dL.

Osteolytic bone lesions, monoclonal proteins in serum, and > 10% mature and immature plasma cells in the bone marrow are diagnostic of **multiple myeloma.** Excretion of light chain > 60 mg/24 h and serum levels of monoclonal protein > 2 gm/dL highly suggest multiple myeloma. If bone marrow plasmacytosis is not demonstrated along with these findings, repeated bone marrow aspirations and a search for an extraskeletal plasma cell tumor should be undertaken. Idiopathic monoclonal components occur with other cancers.

Prognosis

Only time will determine if a diagnosis of **benign monoclonal gammopathy** is really early multiple myeloma. Over 20 yr, about 33% of patients initially diagnosed with benign monoclonal gammopathy develop overt multiple myeloma. No evidence indicates that not treating these patients is harmful.

Once a diagnosis of **multiple myeloma** is made, the patient may be classified as a good or a poor risk for treatment. **Good-risk** patients have laboratory values of Hb ≥ 9.0 gm/dL, serum creatinine < 2 mg/dL, and Ca ≤ 12 mg/dL after hydration. **Poor-risk** patients fail to meet these criteria. With therapy, the good-risk group has a median survival of 42 mo; the poor-risk group, only 21 mo. The groups respond equally well to initial therapy.

In some good-risk elderly people, the disease progresses slowly. If the patient is asymptomatic or only mildly symptomatic, the disease can be followed over time to determine its pace. Occasionally, elderly patients with advanced-stage myeloma do well.

Treatment

If an elderly patient is feeling well, the physician should determine the pace of the disease before beginning treatment. Because multiple myeloma is a disseminated neoplastic disorder, the mainstay of treatment is chemotherapy. Radiation is useful for localized tumor burden and is widely used to relieve back pain from osteolytic lesions. However, if back pain results from extensive demineralization of bone, radiation usually will not relieve it, and chemotherapy should be begun promptly.

All patients should be encouraged to stay active to prevent further bone demineralization. Lumbar corsets and braces may help relieve pain and prevent further damage. Large osteolytic lesions should be irradiated before fractures occur. A fracture through a lytic lesion requires placement of an intramedullary pin and radiation therapy.

Patients must drink sufficient fluid (2 to 3 L/day) to increase urine output and excrete light chains, calcium, uric acid, and other metabolites. Hydration with saline or saline plus furosemide IV may also be used on a temporary basis. All infections must be treated promptly. Hyperuricemia should be treated with allopurinol 300 mg/day. Hypercalcemia is usually treated with calcitonin 4 to 8 IU/kg s.c. q 12 h, prednisone 40 to 100 mg/day, or both, until the serum calcium level returns to normal (usually in 1 to 5 days). If this approach is unsuccessful, plicamycin 25 μg/kg IV over 1 to 2 h may be used. Sodium or potassium phosphate 2 gm/day orally may also be useful in some patients with moderate hypercalcemia.

Many chemotherapeutic regimens are used for multiple myeloma. In elderly persons with decreased bone marrow reserve, the two most common regimens are high-dose, intermittent melphalan with prednisone and low-dose, continuous melphalan. In the high-dose, intermittent regimen, the dosage of melphalan is 0.25 mg/kg/day orally for 4 days, and the dosage of prednisone is 2 mg/kg/day for 4 days. This dosing is repeated every 4 to 6 wk, depending on the degree of bone marrow suppression. In the continuous regimen, the patient is generally first given melphalan 8 to 10 mg/day for about 1 wk (loading dose). The dosage is then reduced to 2 mg/day but must be adjusted frequently, depending on bone marrow sensitivity. In the very old, the loading dose is usually reduced to 4 mg/day for 1 wk.

For hyperviscosity, treatment with plasmapheresis may be effective in the short term.

LYMPHOMAS

Primary malignancies of the lymph nodes, including Hodgkin's disease and non-Hodgkin's lymphoma. These two lymphomas are distinct entities characterized by patterns of spread, clinical behavior, and cells of origin. Hodgkin's disease usually has a predictable pattern of spread to contiguous lymph node areas; non-Hodgkin's lymphoma is usually widespread at diagnosis and more likely to involve extranodal areas. Both can be subdivided into types based on the histologic appearance of the lymph nodes.

Classification

Fundamental to the diagnosis of **Hodgkin's disease** is the histologic finding in the lymph node of the giant **Reed-Sternberg cell,** usually with twin nuclei and nucleoli that give it the appearance of owl's eyes. The Reed-Sternberg cell is probably the malignant cell, and the surrounding cells probably represent tissue reaction.

Histologically, Hodgkin's disease is subdivided into four major types: **lymphocyte predominant** (mainly lymphocytes with few Reed-Sternberg cells); **mixed cellularity** (a cellular response of mature lymphoid cells, plasma cells, eosinophils, and Reed-Sternberg cells); **lymphocyte depleted** (few lymphoid cells with a majority of histiocytes, fibrotic reaction, and Reed-Sternberg cells); and **nodular sclerosis** (effacement of lymphoid structure by nodular aggregates of mature lymphoid cells and lacunar variants of Reed-Sternberg cells separated by bands of birefringent collagen).

The non-Hodgkin's lymphomas are a heterogeneous group of lymphoid malignancies that have some common but many different features. The classification of non-Hodgkin's lymphomas is controversial and has undergone many revisions. Currently, there are two complementary approaches: one based on descriptions of lymph node architecture and histologic features and the other based on the use of immunologic markers. TABLE 72–2 shows the histologic classification of Rappaport and the International Panel Working Formulation based on the type of lymphocyte seen.

TABLE 72–2. HISTOLOGIC CLASSIFICATION OF NON–HODGKIN'S LYMPHOMAS

Classification	*Working Formulation*	*Rappaport Classification*
Low grade	Small lymphocytic	Well-differentiated lymphocytic lymphoma
	Follicular small cleaved lymphocytic	Nodular poorly differentiated lymphocytic lymphoma
	Mixed follicular small cleaved cell and large cell	Nodular mixed lymphoma
Intermediate	Follicular, predominantly large cell	Nodular histiocytic lymphoma
	Diffuse small cleaved cell	Diffuse poorly differentiated lymphocytic lymphoma
	Diffuse large cells (cleaved or uncleaved)	Diffuse histiocytic lymphoma
High grade	Diffuse large cell immunoblasts (B cell, T cell, polymorphous, epithelial cell component)	Diffuse histiocytic lymphoma
	Lymphoblastic, convoluted or nonconvoluted	Lymphoblastic lymphoma
	Small noncleaved, Burkitt's or non-Burkitt's	Diffuse undifferentiated lymphoma

Etiology

The cause of Hodgkin's disease remains unknown. However, seroepidemiologic studies suggest that the Epstein-Barr virus may be involved. Patients with immunodeficiencies and autoimmune disease are at increased risk, suggesting that the immune system plays a role.

The cause of most non-Hodgkin's lymphomas is also unknown. However, immunosuppressed patients (eg, renal transplant recipients) and those with excessive immune function (eg, patients with Sjögren's syndrome) are at greater risk. A virus is involved in at least some cases. African Burkitt's lymphoma is associated with Epstein-Barr virus infection, and an aggressive T-cell leukemia–lymphoma is associated with human T-cell lymphotropic virus type I **(HTLV-I)** infection in Japan and the Caribbean. Similarly, patients with human immunodeficiency virus **(HIV)** infection often develop aggressive non-Hodgkin's lymphoma.

Incidence

The incidence of Hodgkin's disease is 2 per 100,000 persons annually in the USA. There is a bimodal age distribution with an initial peak between ages 15 and 35 and a second peak between ages 50 and 80. At age 25, the incidence is about 5 per 100,000 persons annually, and at age 75, it is 7 per 100,000 annually. The incidence is slightly greater in men. Hodgkin's disease appears to be associated with higher socioeconomic levels of the population. Geographic, occupational (woodworkers), and family clusters of Hodgkin's disease have been noted.

The age-adjusted incidence of non-Hodgkin's lymphoma ranges from 2.6 to 5.8 per 100,000 persons annually. The progressive age-related increase in incidence is similar to that of acute leukemia. At age 80, the incidence is about 40 per 100,000 persons annually. Some cases seem to be associated with viral infections.

The incidence of Hodgkin's disease and non-Hodgkin's lymphoma is increased in persons who have immune deficiencies or autoimmune disease and in those taking hydantoin drugs, such as phenytoin.

Pathophysiology

Normal lymphoid tissue is replaced by the malignant lymphoma, resulting in immunodeficiency and infections. The bone marrow may be replaced, resulting in pancytopenia and subsequent bleeding and infection. Tumor bulk may obstruct or invade vital organs, ultimately causing death.

Symptoms and Signs

Patients with **Hodgkin's disease** usually present with enlarged lymph nodes in the neck. Although any nodal group can be involved, the central or axial lymph nodes are most commonly affected. The patient may be asymptomatic or may exhibit the systemic symptoms of fever, night sweats, loss ≥ 10% of normal body weight, and pruritus, which are often associated with extensive disease. Patients with advanced disease may also present with diffuse adenopathy and involvement of the spleen, liver, bone marrow, or lung.

The **non-Hodgkin's lymphomas** appear to be multicentric in origin and widespread early in the disease process. A leukemic phase, detectable by peripheral blood testing, may occur. Most patients initially seek medical care because of cervical or inguinal lymph node enlargement. However, the skin, GI tract, bone, liver, and CNS make up 10% to 20% of the primary sites of lymphoma at presentation. Occasionally, splenomegaly, bone marrow failure, autoimmune hemolytic anemia, and autoimmune thrombocytopenia are presenting features. Systemic symptoms are not as common as in Hodgkin's disease. Waldeyer's tonsillar ring involvement has a high association with GI lesions. Hypercalcemia is prominent in HTLV-I–related non-Hodgkin's lymphoma but is rare in other types. Hypogammaglobulinemia may occur, but occasionally patients have a monoclonal serum M-component.

TABLE 72–3. CLINICAL STAGING OF HODGKIN'S DISEASE*

Stage	*Definition*
I	Disease limited to one anatomic region
II	Disease in ≥ 2 anatomic regions on the same side of the diaphragm
III	Disease on both sides of the diaphragm but limited to lymph nodes, spleen, and Waldeyer's tonsillar ring
III_1	Involvement limited to spleen, splenic nodes, and celiac and portal nodes, plus disease above the diaphragm
III_2	Involvement of paraaortic, pelvic, and disk nodes
IV	Extranodal disease not contiguous to a nodal area, ie, bone marrow, lung, pleura, liver, plus disease above the diaphragm

* All stages are subclassified as A if the patient is asymptomatic or B if the patient has unexplained fever, night sweats, loss of ≥ 10% of body weight.

Laboratory Findings and Diagnosis

The diagnosis is made by biopsy and the histologic picture of malignant lymphoma.

Clinical staging in **Hodgkin's disease** is extremely important in determining treatment. The currently accepted stages are listed in TABLE 72–3. Clinical staging is based on (1) a complete physical examination with special attention to all lymph node areas; (2) a routine blood chemistry profile and CBC; (3) CT scans of the abdomen, pelvis, and in some cases, the chest; (4) lymphangiograms via the pedal lymphatics to outline the femoral, inguinal, pelvic, and paraaortic nodes; and (5) in cases in which the clinical stage may change the treatment modality, laparotomy including splenectomy, liver biopsies, and biopsies of grossly suspicious lymph nodes, as needed. A bone marrow biopsy is also required if the findings will affect treatment. Clinical and pathologic stages change in up to 30% of patients after laparotomy. In the elderly, Hodgkin's disease is more likely to present as advanced disease (stage III or IV). Some authorities believe that patients > 40 yr, particularly those with mixed cellularity or lymphocyte depletion histologic findings, may not benefit from laparotomy.

In **non-Hodgkin's lymphoma,** clinical staging is similar to that of Hodgkin's disease, but staging laparotomy is rarely required. After a complete physical examination, CBC, blood chemistry profile, bone marrow aspirate, lymph node biopsy, chest x-ray, and abdominal CT scan, about 90% of patients are found to have stage III or IV disease. Other studies (eg, serum protein electrophoresis, skeletal x-rays, and IV urography) are sometimes useful.

Prognosis

With treatment, almost 70% of patients who have Hodgkin's disease are long-term survivors, regardless of histologic findings. Before the introduction of potentially curative treatment however, the lymphocyte predominant and nodular sclerosis types carried better prognoses than the other types. Success depends upon staging, identifying the spread pattern and the next potential site of involvement, and expertly using radiation and chemotherapy. Elderly persons in advanced stages do not do as well as younger persons because they are unable to tolerate maximum doses of radiation and chemotherapy; 30% to 40% of such elderly patients are long-term survivors.

In **non-Hodgkin's lymphoma,** indicators of a good prognosis are nodular histologic pattern, limited stage, and youth. Marrow involvement is a poor prognostic sign in the unfavorable histologic category but not in the favorable or intermediate histologic categories. Other poor prognostic signs are bulky abdominal disease, Hb < 12 gm/dL, and serum LDH > 250 u./L.

Treatment

In **Hodgkin's disease,** the primary intervention is treating the known disease and the next potential site of involvement. In general, limited area radiation therapy is recommended for stages I and II, and chemotherapy with or without radiation therapy is recommended for stages III and IV. The current recommendations are shown in TABLE 72–4. However, the regeneration of bone marrow after radiation therapy or chemotherapy is markedly diminished in patients > 40 yr, and the GI side effects are much more severe. Thus, consideration should be given to limiting the usual field of radiation in elderly patients with early-stage disease. Similarly, administering the optimum dose of chemotherapy may be impossible in older patients, even though the benefit of aggressive therapy outweighs the risk.

The survival rate of patients given palliative rather than aggressive therapy is dramatically lower. Many elderly patients can tolerate only 30% to 50% of the optimum doses of chemotherapy. The most frequently used regimens in the elderly are MOPP and British MOPP, each of which consists of four drugs (shown in TABLE 72–5). The duration of chemotherapy is 6 to 12 mo or for at least 2 mo after complete remission. The incidence of a second malignancy (usually acute leukemia or non-Hodgkin's lymphoma) increases in patients who have Hodgkin's disease and are receiving or have received chemotherapy, especially when combined with total nodal irradiation.

In **non-Hodgkin's lymphoma,** chemotherapeutic cures occur paradoxically only in patients in the intermediate and unfavorable prognosis histologic categories. In contrast, aggressive therapy does not seem to prolong survival in the favorable prognosis category lymphomas, even

TABLE 72–4. TREATMENT RECOMMENDATIONS FOR PATIENTS WITH HODGKIN'S DISEASE

Stage	*Therapy*	*Disease-Free Survival (%)*
IA, IIA, and II_1A	Mantle and paraaortic irradiation*	90
IIIA	Total nodal irradiation	50
	Chemotherapy and extended field irradiation*	85
IB and IIB	Similar to IA and IIA therapy	80–90
IIIA and IIIB	Chemotherapy and involved field irradiation**	80–85
IVA and IVB	Chemotherapy with or without irradiation of bulk disease	25–40

* If the mediastinal mass is > 1/3 the diameter of the chest, combined modality therapy consisting of chemotherapy and mantle irradiation is preferable to radiation alone.

** Some authorities reserve chemotherapy for stage IV disease and use only radiation therapy for stages I to III. The overall disease-free intervals are similar.

though they are extremely sensitive to chemotherapy. Therefore, therapy should be minimal in favorable prognosis disease and aggressive in unfavorable prognosis disease.

Favorable prognosis histologic category of non-Hodgkin's lymphoma: If any therapy is used in patients who appear to be in stage I or II disease, it should be regional radiation. However, most patients relapse because the disease is not truly in an early stage. In others, the disease is so indolent that it does not recur for 5 to 10 yr. Chemotherapy is rarely indicated in stage I or II; often, no therapy is needed. Particularly in the elderly, a practical approach is to withhold treatment and follow-up until problems develop.

In stages III and IV, the disease is still very indolent. Most patients respond to chemotherapy, but the relapse rate is 10% to 20% annually. Even though 80% to 90% of patients with favorable prognosis histologic findings achieve a complete remission, only 10% to 20% are without disease at the 10-yr mark. Thus, wisdom seems to favor avoiding both the serious systemic toxicity inherent in aggressive combination chemotherapy and the potential risk of acute nonlymphocytic leukemia associated with chronic low-dose alkylating agents. Most oncologists use a single alkylating agent (eg, chlorambucil 0.4 to 0.8 mg/kg in 3 divided

TABLE 72–5. CHEMOTHERAPY FOR HODGKIN'S DISEASE

*Regimen**	*Dosage*
MOPP	
Mechlorethamine (nitrogen mustard)	6 mg/m² IV on days 1 and 8
Oncovin (vincristine)	1.5 mg/m² IV on days 1 and 8
Prednisone	40 mg/m²/day orally on days 1 to 14 (cycles 1 and 4 only)
Procarbazine	100 mg/m²/day orally on days 1 to 14
British MOPP (ChlVPP)	
Chlorambucil	6 mg/m²/day orally on days 1 to 14
Vinblastine	6 mg/m² IV on days 1 and 8
Prednisone	40 mg/m²/day orally on days 1 to 14
Procarbazine	100 mg/m²/day orally on days 1 to 14

* Each regimen is given every 28 days.

doses for 1 day every 28 days). So-called pulse therapy has less myelotoxicity and, perhaps, less leukemogenic potential. Some physicians use relatively mild combination chemotherapy regimens (see TABLE 72–6).

Intermediate and unfavorable prognosis histologic categories of non-Hodgkin's lymphoma: These aggressive non-Hodgkin's lymphomas are rapidly growing tumors with a short natural history. Thus, the patients are usually treated with combination chemotherapy. Doxorubicin is not well tolerated in the elderly, nor is methotrexate, because of its renal complications. The chemotherapeutic regimens shown in TABLE 72–6 produce relatively low toxicity in the elderly.

Growth factors: There are now 15 characterized hemolymphopoietic growth factors. Currently, three of them—erythropoietin, granulocyte colony stimulating factor, and granulocyte-macrophage colony stimulating factor—are commercially available. The human granulocyte colony stimulating factor is used to decrease the incidence of infection in patients with nonmyeloid malignancies who are receiving myelosuppressive anticancer drugs associated with severe neutropenia. The recommended starting dose is 5 μg/kg/day s.c. or IV. The use of granulocyte colony stimulating factor varies with different chemotherapeutic

TABLE 72–6. CHEMOTHERAPY FOR NON–HODGKIN'S LYMPHOMA

*Regimen**	*Dosage*
CVP (COP)	
Cyclophosphamide	750 mg/m² IV on day 1
Vincristine	1.4 mg/m² IV on day 1**
Prednisone	60 mg/m²/day orally on days 1 to 5
C-MOPP	
Cyclophosphamide	650 mg/m² IV on days 1 and 8
Vincristine	1.4 mg/m² IV on days 1 and 8**
Prednisone	40 mg/m²/day orally on days 1 to 14
Procarbazine	100 mg/m²/day orally on days 1 to 14

* Cycles are repeated every 21 to 28 days.
** Maximum dose 2 mg.

regimens. Human granulocyte-macrophage colony stimulating factor has been used mainly after bone marrow transplantation and, therefore, no data exist on the elderly.

The use of other growth factors (including all the interleukins) is still experimental. However, this is one of the most promising areas of research in the treatment of malignancy.

MYELODYSPLASTIC SYNDROMES

A heterogeneous group of disorders in which the hematopoietic precursors are abundant but morphologically abnormal. Hematopoiesis is ineffective, and mature peripheral blood cells are not produced in normal numbers. The syndromes are vague, with refractory anemia often progressing to a refractory dysmyelopoietic anemia involving the red cell, white cell, and megakaryocytic lines.

Classification

The syndromes are classified by morphologic criteria (see TABLE 72–7). Involvement of the RBC line only with no ringed sideroblasts is **refractory anemia.** If there are > 15% ringed sideroblasts, the diagnosis

TABLE 72–7. FRENCH–AMERICAN–BRITISH COOPERATIVE GROUP CLASSIFICATION OF MYELODYSPLASTIC SYNDROMES

Refractory anemia	Chronic myelomonocytic leukemia (monocytosis, < 5% circulating blasts)
Refractory anemia with ringed sideroblasts (> 15% ringed forms in the marrow)	Refractory anemia with excess blasts in transformation (20% to 30% blasts in the marrow, ≥ 5% circulating blasts)
Refractory anemia with excess blasts (5% to 20% blasts in the marrow, < 5% circulating blasts)	

is **refractory anemia with ringed sideroblasts.** Excessive blasts in the marrow but not in the peripheral blood constitutes **refractory anemia with excess blasts.** Refractory anemia with excess blasts accompanied by peripheral blood monocytosis (monocytes > 1000/μL) is called **chronic myelomonocytic leukemia.** When ≥ 5% of peripheral blood cells are blasts, the diagnosis is **refractory anemia with excess blasts in transformation.** These terms have generally replaced the term preleukemia because only about 10% to 30% of patients with a myelodysplastic syndrome develop an acute leukemia. In refractory anemia and refractory anemia with ringed sideroblasts, platelets and white cells are usually normal. In refractory anemia with excess blasts, chronic myelomonocytic leukemia, and refractory anemia with excess blasts in transformation, these cell lines are often abnormal.

Etiology

In most patients, the cause is unknown, but treatment with alkylating agents is associated with an increased risk of myelodysplastic syndrome; the longer a patient is treated with an alkylating agent, the greater the likelihood of developing myelodysplastic syndrome. Long-term courses of melphalan for multiple myeloma or ovarian carcinoma or of chlorambucil or mechlorethamine plus radiation therapy for Hodgkin's disease lead to a 2% to 7% incidence of acute nonlymphocytic leukemia. Anemia or pancytopenia associated with changes in the bone marrow and peripheral blood identical to myelodysplastic syndrome develops 2 to 10 yr after therapy. The acute nonlymphocytic leukemia that may develop is invariably fatal. This long-term complication of successful chemotherapy may become more prevalent as more patients survive. Chemotherapeutic drugs that are not alkylating agents (eg, methotrexate or hydroxyurea) do not seem to produce this complication.

Other possible causes include RNA viruses, somatic mutations, radiation, and environmental toxins. Yet, the ability of any of these factors to induce cancer may be enhanced by aging. Accumulated genetic mutations from various causes, including aging, are more likely to result in malignant change than are single genetic insults, a concept sometimes called the "multihit theory."

Incidence

The actual incidence of these syndromes is not known, but they are fairly common in elderly people. Ineffective erythropoiesis increases with age, and in some studies, up to 20% of people > 65 yr have unexplained refractory anemia. The syndromes are twice as common in men and are rare in persons < 40 yr. A history of exposure to radiation or chemical leukemogens is common.

Pathophysiology

These syndromes are thought to arise from an undefined cytopathologic alteration of the pluripotential hematopoietic stem cell pool, evolving from the clonal expansion of a single stem cell (or a very small number of stem cells). The major pathophysiologic consequence is ineffective hematopoiesis because of defective maturation of marrow precursor cells. Proliferation of progenitor and early precursor cells is usually normal or enhanced (creating a hypercellular marrow), but circulating mature cells are deficient. The cells also have a slightly shorter life span, which contributes to the cytopenias.

Familial instances of such myelodysplastic syndromes are rare. A protracted myelodysplastic syndrome lasting up to 20 yr occurs before 5% to 10% of all cases of acute nonlymphocytic leukemia.

Symptoms and Signs

The patient generally seeks medical care for symptoms of anemia, thrombocytopenia, or leukopenia—eg, fatigue, decreased exercise tolerance, purpura, fever, or infections. Hepatomegaly occurs in about 5% of patients, splenomegaly in about 10%, and pallor in about 50%. Often the patient complains of arthralgias.

Because the cytopenias develop slowly, many patients are asymptomatic, and the diagnosis is made incidentally or the anemia is falsely attributed to aging. Most patients have increased iron stores, and many have clinical hemochromatosis with diabetes, cirrhosis, infiltrative heart disease, and pituitary dysfunction.

Laboratory Findings and Diagnosis

The hallmark of the syndromes is anemia with reticulocytopenia. The RBC morphologic appearance is usually abnormal. The RBCs are usually dimorphic; some cells are microcytic and hypochromic, and others are normochromic and normocytic or macrocytic. Basophilic stippling, target cells, schistocytes, siderocytes, and nucleated RBCs often appear.

Leukopenia is moderate, WBCs ranging from 1000 to 4000/μL, with neutropenia more pronounced than lymphopenia. Frequently, the neutrophils are sparsely granulated; the neutrophil alkaline phosphatase activity may be low; and the acquired Pelger-Huët nuclear anomaly (hypolobulation of the nuclei of mature neutrophils) may be present. The granulocytes often function abnormally, which further impairs resistance to infection. Since monocytosis occurs in 30% of patients, serum and urinary lysozyme levels may be elevated. Immature myeloid cells may be seen in the peripheral smear. Thrombocytopenia is common, although occasionally, patients have thrombocytosis. The platelets may have functional defects.

The **bone marrow is diagnostic** for the myelodysplastic syndromes. Erythroblasts may have double or fragmented nuclei or intranuclear bridging; budding, ringed sideroblasts may be prominent. These are usually found in patients with abnormalities in the RBC precursors. With primarily erythroid dysplasia, the ratio of myeloid to erythroid precursors (M:E ratio) is between 1:1 and 1:10 (normal is 3:1). Reticuloendothelial iron is increased, as are the serum iron and ferritin levels. Dyserythropoiesis results in moderately elevated levels of serum LDH and indirect bilirubin. Iron turnover studies reveal the ineffective erythropoiesis; the iron turnover rate is increased, but incorporation of iron into circulating erythrocytes is decreased. Iron stores are increased in most patients.

Marrow myeloid cells may show immature to mature neutrophils, may have the acquired Pelger-Huët nuclear anomaly, and are often sparsely granulated. Eosinophils and basophils may also be dysplastic. In patients with primarily myeloid dysplasia, the M:E ratio is between 3:1 and 20:1. Megakaryocytes may be immature and dysplastic as well.

Prognosis

Prognosis is *highly variable,* with survival ranging from a few months to 15 yr. The median survival is about 3 yr. Although about 10% to 30% of patients die as a result of acute blastic transformation (acute nonlymphocytic leukemia), individual prognosis cannot be predicted. Patients with primarily erythroid dysplasia are at lower risk than those with involvement of the other cell lines.

Treatment

Transfusion of blood products is the mainstay of treatment but should be limited. Transfusing packed RBCs causes the risk of iron overload; alloimmunization to RBC, WBC, and platelet antigens; and transmission of various infections. Washed RBCs may slow the development of alloimmunization. Platelets should be transfused only if the patient is bleeding or surgery is needed. Granulocyte transfusions should be given only to neutropenic patients with documented gram-negative infections that are unresponsive to antibiotics alone.

Occasionally, patients with ringed sideroblasts respond to oral **pyridoxine** 100 to 300 mg/day. However, the response is only partial, and an abnormal RBC morphologic appearance usually persists. **Androgens** and **corticosteroids** have benefited a small number of patients. Recombinant hematopoietic growth factors have been tried in the myelodysplastic syndromes, but no consistent improvement has yet been demonstrated. Continuous overnight (12 h) IV or subcutaneous administration of **deferoxamine** by portable pump should be considered when the patient is receiving blood transfusions monthly or more often. A convenient regimen is to give 2 gm of deferoxamine subcutaneously over 12 h by portable infusion pump for 5 days/wk.

Chemotherapy as early treatment of myelodysplasia with excessive blasts has not increased survival. Administering low-dose cytarabine to induce differentiation of blasts is controversial. In patients whose condition converts to acute nonlymphocytic leukemia, the remission rate is even lower than in patients with nonlymphocytic leukemia who did not previously have myelodysplasia. Patients with this secondary form of nonlymphocytic leukemia have prolonged marrow aplasia after chemotherapy. One approach in the elderly consists of giving supportive care with blood products and attempting to keep the WBC count $< 50{,}000/\mu L$ with oral hydroxyurea 10 to 100 mg/kg/day; the maximum daily dose is 4 gm.

MYELOPROLIFERATIVE DISORDERS

A group of disorders arising from a monoclonal proliferation of the hematopoietic pluripotential precursor cell. In this respect, the disorders may be considered malignancies. However, in most of the disorders, the pluripotential precursors retain the ability to differentiate and mature into functional cells, and the disorders are usually clinically benign and chronic.

Classification

The myeloproliferative disorders may be classified by degree of cell maturation, ranging from hyperplastic to dysplastic to malignant (see TABLE 72–8). This classification allows for overlap in the syndromes and the transition from more benign to more malignant phases. Variable amounts of fibrosis also occur in these disorders. Fibroblastic proliferation in myeloproliferative disorders has a polyclonal origin and is a reactive phenomenon.

The most **benign proliferative states** are characterized by panmyelosis of the central skeletal marrow and intact maturation of RBCs, WBCs, and platelets **(polycythemia vera** and **essential thrombocythemia).** The **dysplastic syndromes** are characterized by a reversion to a fetal distribution of the hematopoietic organ involving centrifugal expansion from the axial skeleton to the long bones and the reactivation of the extramedullary hematopoiesis in the spleen and liver **(myeloid metaplasia).** This occurs in **agnogenic myeloid metaplasia, polycythemia**

TABLE 72–8. MYELOPROLIFERATIVE DISORDERS CLASSIFIED BY DEGREE OF CELL MATURATION

Characteristics	*Hyperplastic Phase*	*Dysplastic Phase*	*Malignant Phase*
Typical syndrome	Polycythemia vera, essential thrombocythemia	Myeloid metaplasia (agnogenic, postpolycythemic)	Acute leukemia, paroxysmal nocturnal hemoglobinuria, aplastic anemia, acute myelosclerosis
Axial marrow			
Cellularity	Panhyperplasia	Panhyperplasia or hypocellularity	Primitive cell infiltration
Maturation	Intact	Mild to moderate impairment	Abnormal or absent
Architecture	Normal or slight increase in reticulin	Patchy or extensive fibrosis	Primitive cell infiltration
Peripheral marrow	Uninvolved or slight expansion	Moderate to marked expansion	Primitive cell infiltration
Extramedullary hematopoiesis	Slight or moderate splenomegaly	Marked splenomegaly, moderate hepatomegaly	Primitive cell infiltration
Circulating mature hemocytic cells	Increased	Variably increased or decreased	Absent or decreased
Complications	Thrombosis, hemorrhage	Thrombosis, hemorrhage, splenic infarction, hypersplenism, hydremia	Hemorrhage, infection, anemia

vera with myeloid metaplasia, and **postpolycythemia myeloid metaplasia.** Further **malignant deterioration** in myeloproliferative disease is characterized by ineffective erythropoiesis and decreased peripheral blood counts. Normal maturation is overtaken by abnormal cell production. During this phase, the hematopoietic picture may deteriorate into **aplastic anemia,** a **myelodysplastic syndrome,** or **paroxysmal nocturnal hemoglobinuria.** Final malignant deterioration is seen as **acute nonlymphocytic leukemia** or **lymphocytic leukemia.**

Etiology

The cause of these diseases is unknown. Rare cases with a familial history or a history of exposure to mutagens or bone marrow toxins (eg, benzene, radiation) suggest that a chromosomal abnormality may be involved.

Incidence

Accurate information on the incidence of myeloproliferative disorders is not available. These disorders occur in middle and late life. They are rare in the young. Men are affected slightly more frequently than women. An increased incidence among Ashkenazic Jews has been suggested but is questionable.

Pathophysiology

Uncontrolled production of mature RBCs is the predominant feature of **polycythemia vera.** The increased blood volume and circulating RBC mass lead to thrombosis and bleeding. Thrombosis may be arterial (coronary, cerebral, or peripheral) or venous (hepatic, portal, or peripheral). Small-vessel insufficiency produces cyanosis, erythromelalgia, or even frank gangrene of the fingers and toes. Mild hemorrhagic tendencies (eg, epistaxis, bruising, gingival bleeding) are common, but severe GI, GU, or pulmonary bleeding occurs in only about 10% of patients. The major causes of death in untreated patients are thrombosis and hemorrhage.

In **essential thrombocythemia,** hemorrhage and microvascular occlusions also occur. However, hemorrhage correlates poorly with the increased platelet count and in vitro platelet function abnormalities. The combination of erythrocytosis and thrombocytosis seems to predispose patients to large-vessel thrombosis. Thrombocythemia without an elevated RBC mass does not lead to large-vessel thrombosis. However, microvascular occlusion and bleeding occur frequently.

In **myeloid metaplasia,** the degree of splenic involvement by extramedullary hematopoiesis is independent of the degree of marrow fibrosis. This dissociation invalidates the concept that myeloid metaplasia compensates for diminished bone marrow function. Increased granulocytic stem cells showing fetal characteristics in peripheral blood suggests that myeloid metaplasia results from a return of these cells to a favorable environment in the spleen and liver. When myeloid metaplasia occurs de novo, it is referred to as **agnogenic myeloid metaplasia.**

About 10 yr after being diagnosed with polycythemia vera, 12% of patients develop myeloid metaplasia. This may occur more frequently after radioactive sodium phosphate P32 treatment. Myeloid metaplasia may also occur early in the course of polycythemia vera. It occurs far less commonly with essential thrombocythemia.

Patients with polycythemia and agnogenic myeloid metaplasia are at greater risk for developing **acute leukemia.** The leukemia may be acute lymphocytic, acute nonlymphocytic, or biphenotypic and is characteristically resistant to chemotherapy. Transformation to acute leukemia occurs in both treated and untreated patients, although it is more common in those who have received alkylating agents and radiation therapy.

Symptoms and Signs

The clinical effects of abnormal hyperplasia and dysplasia are shown in TABLE 72–9. **Polycythemia** is often discovered in asymptomatic persons with an elevated hematocrit. About 33% to 50% of patients exhibit plethora, headache, dizziness, visual disturbances, an inability to concentrate, and paresthesias. Many patients have hypertension or increased cardiac output and vascular stasis. Signs of large- or small-vessel thrombosis occur in about 33% to 50% of untreated patients. Major hemorrhage occurs in about 10% of patients. About 75% of patients have splenomegaly when diagnosed. Other symptoms include pruritus, peptic ulcer, and bowel hypermotility from the increase in WBCs. Hyperuricemia and hypermetabolic symptoms also occur.

Essential thrombocythemia is also frequently discovered in asymptomatic persons. Symptomatic patients have either hemorrhage or microvascular occlusions. Thus, they may be easily bruised and have epistaxis, GI or GU bleeding, or postoperative hemorrhage. Microvascular occlusion produces digital cyanosis, erythema, burning, headache, paresthesias, transient ischemic attacks, and visual disturbances.

About 30% of patients with **myeloid metaplasia** are asymptomatic when diagnosed. Usually, it is diagnosed by noting splenomegaly on physical examination. Hepatomegaly may follow splenomegaly. About 60% of symptomatic patients have anemia-related complaints (weakness, fatigue, angina, heart failure), 25% have splenomegaly-related complaints (abdominal pressure or pain, postprandial discomfort, and early satiety), and 20% have hemorrhage-related complaints (easy bruising, epistaxis, bleeding gums, GI bleeding, CNS hemorrhage from a single vessel, or DIC). Symptomatic splenomegaly may lead to weight loss and malnutrition. Splenic infarction is common and may be asymptomatic or may produce acute abdominal symptoms.

Malignant myelosclerosis, which causes death in 1 to 2 mo, is an acute illness with pancytopenia due to a fibrotic bone marrow with circulating myeloblasts; splenomegaly is usually absent. The patient is febrile but does not necessarily have an infection. Bone pain, arthritis, and generalized wasting are prominent. The symptoms and signs of acute leukemia are described above; the symptoms and signs of aplastic anemia are described in Ch. 71.

Laboratory Findings and Diagnosis

Polycythemia vera must be differentiated from other diseases causing erythrocytosis and from blood volume abnormalities. First, the RBC mass and blood volume must be measured. An increased RBC mass along with a normal arterial oxygen saturation and an enlarged spleen confirms the diagnosis of polycythemia. If splenomegaly is absent (as it is in 25% of patients at presentation), the presence of two other features

TABLE 72–9. EFFECTS OF ABNORMAL PROLIFERATION ON THE PATHOPHYSIOLOGY OF MYELOPROLIFERATIVE DISORDERS

	Hyperplastic Phase		*Dysplastic Phase*	
Cell Type	*Clinical Entity*	*Manifestations*	*Clinical Entity*	*Manifestations*
Erythrocyte	Polycythemia vera	Hyperviscosity, hypervolemia Circulatory overload, thrombosis, hemorrhage	Anemia	Cardiovascular compromise Transfusion requirement Iron overload, hepatitis
Megakaryocyte	Thrombocythemia	Thrombosis	Thrombocytopenia	Hemorrhage
	Thrombocytopathy	Thrombosis, hemorrhage	Thrombocytopathy	Hemorrhage
	Release of platelet-derived growth factor	? Fibrosis	Release of platelet-derived growth factor	? Fibrosis
Leukocyte	Basophilia	Histamine release Pruritus, ulcer, hyperacidity, bowel hypermotility, ? fibrosis	Neutrophil function defects Leukemic transformation	Infection
Pluripotential stem cell and progeny	Increased nucleoprotein turnover	Hyperuricemia, gout, tophi, uric acid stones, nephropathy	Myeloid metaplasia	Hypersplenism Anemia, cytopenia Splenic infarction Hydremia Anemia
	Hypocholesterolemia	? Effect on atherosclerosis, ? effect on cell membranes		
	Hypermetabolism	Fatigue, asthenia, weight loss, fever, diaphoresis		

of pluripotential cell involvement confirms the diagnosis; these features include an elevated neutrophil count (found in 50% to 80% of patients), thrombocytosis (in 35% to 50%), increased neutrophil alkaline phosphatase activity (in 80%), and increased vitamin B_{12} binding proteins (in 67%).

The bone marrow shows panmyelosis with erythroid hyperplasia and increased megakaryocytes. Increased reticulin occurs in 20% of patients, but fibrosis is rare. Cultured bone marrow produces erythroid colonies without added erythropoietin and a marked increase in erythroid colonies with added erythropoietin. Other laboratory findings include hyperuricemia, hypocholesterolemia, and an elevated blood histamine level.

The diagnosis of **essential thrombocythemia** is made by exclusion. The diagnosis may be made if the platelet count is > 1 million/μL and no cause of secondary thrombocytosis is found; the RBC mass is normal; the bone marrow contains iron but no bleeding occurs; no collagen fibrosis is found in the bone marrow biopsy; and no Philadelphia chromosome is found. Qualitative platelet defects are often found.

In **myeloid metaplasia,** anemia is the most consistent abnormality. The peripheral smear characteristically shows teardrop and elliptical RBCs and a leukoerythroblastic picture. The WBC count ranges from leukopenia to leukocytosis. Peripheral WBCs are immature with prominent metamyelocytes and myelocytes and < 5% promyelocytes or blasts. Circulating normoblasts are usually found. The platelet count ranges from thrombocytopenia to thrombocytosis. The platelets are large, and megakaryocyte fragments are seen. The combination of a leukoerythroblastic peripheral blood picture and splenomegaly strongly suggests myeloid metaplasia.

The bone marrow aspirate is often hypocellular, resulting in a dry tap. Bone marrow biopsy has a variable presentation, including hypercellularity, panmyelosis without fibrosis, patchy areas of hypercellularity and fibrosis, and panmyelosis with dense fibrosis with or without osteosclerosis. Megakaryocytes remain in the bone marrow even after the other hematopoietic elements disappear. No consistent association is found between the degree of marrow fibrosis and myeloid metaplasia.

Prognosis

The median survival for **polycythemia vera** and **primary thrombocythemia** patients who are treated is about 10 to 15 yr. The median survival for untreated patients with these diseases is only about 5 yr. **Myeloid metaplasia** patients have a 60% decrease in 5-yr survival compared with controls matched for age and sex. The **acute leukemias** and **myelosclerosis** are usually fatal within months.

Treatment

In **polycythemia vera,** restoring normal blood volume and hematocrit markedly reduces the incidence of complications. At diagnosis, the patient should undergo a series of phlebotomies of 250 to 500 mL every second or third day. For patients with cardiovascular disease and those > 75 yr, the volume usually should be only 250 to 350 mL each time. If hydration is maintained, the patient's plasma does not have to be administered. Once the Hct < 42%, phlebotomy should be repeated as required to maintain the desired level. Phlebotomy inevitably results in iron deficiency, which limits erythropoiesis and, therefore, the phlebotomy requirement to < 8 u./yr. Iron should *not* be given to correct the iron deficiency because it will stimulate erythropoiesis. A hematocrit measurement derived from an electronic cell counter may be underestimated by up to 7% when microcytosis is present.

Occasionally, a patient will not tolerate phlebotomies, or erythropoiesis is so active that phlebotomy frequency is unacceptable. In such patients, myelosuppression, either with chemotherapy or radiation therapy, must be achieved. However, treating patients with radioactive sodium phosphate P32 or chlorambucil introduces the risk of leukemia or a second malignancy. The peak incidence of leukemia approaches 30% in these patients 8 yr later (compared with < 1% in patients treated with phlebotomy alone). When myelosuppression is necessary, hydroxyurea 0.5 to 3.0 gm/day orally is used because mutagenicity has not yet been demonstrated with this agent.

In **essential thrombocythemia,** myelosuppression is indicated for patients > 60 yr who have marked thrombocythemia (platelet counts consistently > 1 million/μL) or who have a lower thrombocythemia with a history of thrombosis or hemorrhage or a coexisting condition that increases the risk of these complications. Myelosuppression is usually achieved with hydroxyurea 0.5 to 3.0 gm/day orally. The platelet count is usually reduced to between 500,000 and 800,000/μL. If surgery is needed, the platelet count should be reduced to < 500,000/μL. Postoperative bleeding should be managed with transfusion of normal platelets, regardless of the platelet count. If the patient with thrombocythemia is bleeding or has active thrombosis, the platelet count should be reduced rapidly with plateletpheresis and hydroxyurea.

In **asymptomatic myeloid metaplasia,** no therapy is needed unless the patient has thrombocythemia and is being prepared for surgery. Splenomegaly usually produces the major complications of myeloid metaplasia and responds to myelosuppression. Hydroxyurea 1 gm/day orally usually reduces spleen size without decreasing marrow function. Anemia is not a contraindication to myelosuppression because transfusion may be performed.

Myelosuppressive therapy cannot, however, be used in a patient with significant neutropenia and thrombocytopenia due to bone marrow hypoplasia or fibrosis. *Splenic irradiation must be used rarely and with extreme caution* because even localized therapy is myelosuppressive. The therapy of choice is splenectomy, but it is associated with significant mortality and morbidity in elderly patients with myeloid metaplasia. Indications for splenectomy include painful splenomegaly, repeated splenic infarction, a short-lived response to hydroxyurea or splenic irradiation, significant thrombocytopenia or neutropenia with bone marrow failure, refractory hemolytic anemia, and portal hypertension. When significant pancytopenia occurs, early splenectomy, performed before cardiovascular complications occur, has been advocated in the elderly. However, splenectomy is *contraindicated* if laboratory testing reveals DIC; 12% of patients with DIC have no clinical bleeding. Thrombocythemia should be treated with hydroxyurea before splenectomy.

Surgery is palliative therapy and usually should not be performed if the patient has a high serum alkaline phosphatase level, anemia and a spleen estimated to be > 3 kg, or anemia and a spleen estimated to be < 1 kg. Measurements of RBC production, survival, and splenic sequestration cannot predict the effect of splenectomy on the anemia. The anemia should be evaluated to determine whether deficiencies (eg, iron, folate, vitamin B_{12}) are present. Hemolysis may respond to corticosteroids and should be evaluated by radioactive chromium (^{51}Cr) RBC survival time. If erythropoiesis is ineffective (shown by ferrokinetics), pyridoxine and androgens may be tried.

The **malignant phases** of myeloproliferative disorders are notoriously resistant to therapy. However, treatment is similar to that described for other malignancies.

In all the myeloproliferative disorders, hyperuricemia is treated with allopurinol 300 mg/day orally. Hydration should be maintained, and hypertonic solutions for diagnostic purposes should be avoided as much as possible. Symptoms of histamine release (pruritus after baths) may be relieved by the potent antihistamine-antiserotonin agent cyproheptadine 4 mg orally. Other antihistaminics are usually not effective. Symptoms of GI hyperacidity may be controlled with H_2-receptor blockers or antacids.

§3. ORGAN SYSTEMS: MUSCULOSKELETAL DISORDERS

METABOLIC AND ENDOCRINE DISORDERS

§3. ORGAN SYSTEMS: MUSCULOSKELETAL DISORDERS

73. METABOLIC BONE DISEASE

(See also Chs. 8 and 82)

The skeleton is not simply an inanimate scaffold that supports the body, but a living, metabolically active organ. Thus, the structural integrity of the skeleton depends on the metabolic processes of its bony tissue.

The adult skeleton consists of two types of bone: cortical and trabecular. **Cortical bone** (compact or lamellar bone) forms the outer shell of long bones and the major portion of the cortex of other bones. It accounts for 75% of the total bone mass. The femoral neck is about 75% cortical bone; the midforearm, about 95%. **Trabecular bone** (spongy or cancellous bone) is formed by a network of intersecting plates (trabeculae), which in turn form the supporting infrastructure of bone. With its greater surface area, trabecular bone is more metabolically active and thus more sensitive to changes in the biochemical milieu. The vertebrae are more than 66% trabecular bone, with the center of the vertebral body being about 95% trabecular bone. The distal forearm is only 25% to 30% trabecular bone, and the femoral intertrochanteric region is about 50% trabecular bone and 50% cortical bone.

At the cellular level, specialized osteocytes effect the constant modeling and remodeling of bone. Osteoclasts resorb existing bone, and osteoblasts form new bone. These two closely linked processes are responsive to metabolic influences and to external agents and stresses.

Between the end of puberty and age 25 or 30, a person experiences a 10% to 15% turnover of the skeleton annually that results in a net **increase in bone density.** Although bone resorption and formation continue after age 30, the rate of resorption subsequently exceeds that of formation, resulting in a gradual net **loss of bone density** with age. In women between ages 50 and 60, an accelerated bone loss corresponds to the hormonal changes of menopause. In women, cortical bone density is lost at a rate of about 3% to 5% a decade; this rate increases to 10% to 20% a decade during the immediate postmenopausal period. In men, cortical bone loss occurs at a rate of about 3% to 5% a decade. Trabecular bone loss in the axial skeleton may start earlier and progress faster. After age 30, women may lose 50% of trabecular bone and 30% of cortical bone; men may lose 30% of trabecular bone and 20% of cortical bone. The higher risk of fracture in women may result from their smaller skeletons and greater bone loss.

Factors Affecting Bone Homeostasis

Bone metabolism is influenced by age, activity, dietary minerals, vitamin D, parathyroid hormone, sex hormones, thyroid metabolism, glucocorticoids, growth hormone, and other factors (see also Ch. 82). But the complex interactions of these factors are poorly understood. Recent information indicates that calcium intake, exercise, and sex hormones play important roles in normal skeletal aging.

Calcium intake: A person's intake of calcium is thought to influence age-related bone loss. Whether such intake helps more in achieving peak bone mass or in moderating subsequent bone loss is unclear.

Calcium intake tends to decrease in the elderly, especially in those with lactose intolerance. Also, aging decreases GI absorption of calcium as does inadequate dietary intake and impaired GI absorption of vitamin D and decreased exposure to sunlight. Age-related declines in vitamin D synthesis by the skin and 1,25-dihydroxycholecalciferol (calcitriol) production may also contribute to the inability to increase calcium absorption enough to compensate for reduced intake. Thus, an older person on a calcium-poor diet is more likely to have a calcium deficiency than a younger person on a similar diet.

Exercise: Bone density is greater in the parts of the skeleton that are directly stressed by activities. Thus, exercise helps achieve and maintain maximum bone density. In particular, weight-bearing exercise appears to decrease age-related bone loss. However, in premenopausal women, strenuous exercise leading to excessive weight loss and secondary amenorrhea (eg, long-distance running and ballet) is associated with reduced bone density and an increased risk of fracture. This suggests that estrogen sufficiency is more important than exercise in maintaining optimum bone density.

Estrogen deficiency: Although the exact mechanism is not completely understood, an estrogen deficiency from any cause is associated with accelerated bone loss. The reduced estrogen levels that occur at menopause cause increased bone turnover with greater bone resorption than bone formation. Most estrogen-related bone loss occurs in the first few years after menopause, but bone loss may continue for life. The therapeutic use of estrogen significantly retards bone resorption and decreases the risk of fracture. (Other benefits and risks of postmenopausal estrogen use are discussed in Ch. 83.)

Androgenic hormones: These hormones appear to slow age-associated osteopenia, although evidence for this association is not as strong as it is for the association between estrogen deficiency and bone loss. Osteoporosis occurs in men with hypogonadism (eg, Klinefelter's syndrome), and a slow decline in gonadal function may be partly responsible for the linear decreases in bone density in normal aging men.

OSTEOPOROSIS

A metabolic bone disorder characterized by a gradual decline in absolute bone mass with a preservation of the skeletal mineralization process. Decreasing bone density leads to an increased susceptibility to fractures, which may result from seemingly insignificant accidents and movements. The most common fractures occur in the vertebral bodies, the distal radius, and the proximal femur. These and other fractures are discussed in Ch. 8.

A major public health problem, osteoporosis affects more than 20 million Americans. The direct and indirect costs of osteoporosis are more than $10 billion annually in the USA.

Etiology

The elderly experience two types of **primary osteoporosis,** the most common metabolic bone disease (see TABLE 73–1). **Type 1 osteoporosis,** or **postmenopausal osteoporosis,** occurs between ages 51 and 75, affects six times as many women as men, and is largely responsible for the increased risk of osteoporotic fractures. Because it affects mainly trabecular bone, type 1 osteoporosis is largely responsible for vertebral crush fractures and Colles' fractures.

Type 2 osteoporosis is a gradual age-related bone loss. Also known as **involutional** or **senile osteoporosis,** it occurs mainly in persons > 70 yr and affects twice as many women as men. Because density decreases in both trabecular and cortical bone, type 2 osteoporosis results in femoral and vertebral fractures.

Postmenopausal endocrinologic changes probably cause type 1 osteoporosis; age-related changes in vitamin D synthesis are thought to lead to type 2 osteoporosis. In women, type 1 and type 2 may appear simultaneously, resulting in a biphasic pattern of bone loss.

Secondary osteoporosis may result from many causes including glucocorticoid excess, male hypogonadism, hyperparathyroidism, hyperthyroidism, malignancy, immobilization, hepatic insufficiency, gastrectomy, rheumatoid arthritis, acromegaly, chronic obstructive pulmonary disease, chronic renal failure, and heparin therapy. These secondary causes account for < 5% of all cases of osteoporosis in postmenopausal women (see TABLE 73–2). However, in young women and men of all ages with metabolic bone disease, the percentage is much higher. Furthermore, in the elderly, multiple causes must be considered.

Endogenous or exogenous glucocorticoid excess is a leading cause of premature osteoporosis. Corticosteroids inhibit osteoblastic function, stimulate bone resorption, increase parathyroid hormone secretion, inhibit intestinal calcium absorption, and cause decreased end-organ response to vitamin D.

TABLE 73–1. CHARACTERISTICS OF PRIMARY OSTEOPOROSIS

Characteristics	*Type 1*	*Type 2*
Age (yr)	51–75	> 70
Woman:man ratio	6:1	2:1
Type of bone loss	Primarily trabecular	Trabecular and cortical
Rate of bone loss	Accelerated; short duration	Not accelerated; long duration
Fracture sites	Vertebrae (crush) and distal radius	Vertebrae (multiple wedge) and hip
Laboratory values		
Serum calcium	Normal	Normal
Serum phosphate	Normal	Normal
Alkaline phosphatase	Normal (increased with fracture)	Normal (increased with fracture)
Urine calcium	Increased	Normal
Parathyroid hormone function	Decreased	Increased
Metabolism of $25(OH)D_3$* to $1,25(OH)_2D_3$†	Secondary decrease	Primary decrease
Calcium absorption	Decreased	Decreased

* $25(OH)D_3$ = 25-hydroxycholecalciferol
† $1,25(OH)_2D_3$ = 1,25-dihydroxycholecalciferol
Adapted from information appearing in Riggs BL, Melton LJ III: "Involutional osteoporosis." *The New England Journal of Medicine* 314(26):1676–1686, 1986; used with permission.

Risk Factors

The major risk factors for osteoporosis are age, female sex, white or Oriental race, family history of osteoporosis, thin habitus, early menopause (before age 45), oophorectomy, secondary amenorrhea, lifelong low calcium intake (including lactose intolerance), sedentary lifestyle, and immobilization. Other risk factors include nulliparity, protein-calorie malnutrition, gastrectomy, alcohol abuse, cigarette smoking, and a history of drug use or illness that predisposes a person to increased bone loss (eg, corticosteroid use, thyrotoxicosis).

TABLE 73–2. CAUSES OF SECONDARY OSTEOPOROSIS

Drugs	*Endocrinopathies*	*Other Conditions*
Alcohol	Hypercortisolism	Chronic obstructive pulmonary disease
Aluminum-containing antacids	Hyperparathyroidism	Chronic renal failure
Barbiturates	Hyperprolactinemia	Diabetes mellitus
Corticosteroids	Hyperthyroidism	Hepatic disease
Heparin	Hypogonadism	Immobility
Isoniazid		Malabsorption syndrome
Methotrexate		Osteogenesis imperfecta
Phenytoin		Osteomalacia
L-Thyroxine		Rheumatoid arthritis
Tobacco		Sarcoidosis
		Scurvy
		Systemic mastocytosis

Age: The chief single predictor for osteoporosis is age. However, the combination of age and other risk factors is insufficient for an accurate prediction of bone density or fracture risk.

Sex: Women have a lower peak bone mass at skeletal maturity and a greatly accelerated phase of bone loss for several years after menopause. By the sixth decade, their absolute bone density is significantly lower than that in men.

Race: Osteoporosis is more prevalent in whites and Orientals than in blacks, probably because blacks have a greater peak bone mass at skeletal maturity and possibly because of differences in nutrition, exercise, and body weight.

Family history: A family history of osteoporotic fractures is thought to be a major risk factor. Studies of twins suggest a significant genetic component to peak bone mass attainment and subsequent bone loss.

Body weight: Low body weight increases the risk of osteoporosis through unidentified mechanisms, which are thought to include decreased availability of biologically active estrogen in thin postmenopausal women and lower peak bone mass in thin young women. Obesity may provide protection because higher estrogen levels in obese men and women and increased skeletal weight bearing may stimulate bone formation.

Symptoms and Signs

Persons with osteoporosis are asymptomatic until a fracture occurs. The precipitating event may be as seemingly innocuous as turning over in bed, although falling and lifting are more common. Some patients cannot recall any precipitating event. In contrast, osteomalacia often causes diffuse bony tenderness and pain, even in the absence of radiographically evident fractures.

Diagnosis

Because no characteristic symptoms, signs, or laboratory abnormalities are associated with primary osteoporosis, diagnosis requires excluding other causes of metabolic bone disease, ie, osteomalacia, malignancy, and secondary osteoporosis. Usually, a history, physical examination, and a few laboratory studies will rule out other causes.

History and physical examination: The patient with a fracture or radiographic evidence of osteopenia should be questioned about the hallmarks of metabolic bone disease (eg, fractures, loss of height, bone pain, and muscle weakness) and specifically about drugs and disorders associated with vitamin D deficiency and osteomalacia (see below). The physician should also look for symptoms and signs of alcohol abuse, malabsorption, hypercortisolism, endocrinopathy, malignancy, and other diseases known to lead to secondary osteoporosis, particularly in men and women with premature osteoporosis.

Laboratory evaluation: If the history suggests metabolic bone disease, appropriate laboratory tests must be performed. If the history reveals no causes of secondary osteoporosis, the following tests usually exclude underlying disorders: a CBC count with differential, routine serum chemistry studies, thyroid function tests, serum protein electrophoresis, serum 25-hydroxycholecalciferol measurement, and 24-h urine calcium measurement. If osteomalacia cannot be excluded, an iliac crest bone biopsy with a double tetracycline-labeled histomorphometric analysis of undemineralized bone may be required. In an osteopenic patient, any blood count or protein electrophoresis abnormality raises the possibility of a malignancy involving bone marrow.

In primary osteoporosis, electrolyte, blood urea nitrogen, and creatinine levels are normal, unless the patient has coexisting renal disease. Serum and urine calcium levels are usually normal, although immobility from a recent fracture may increase urinary calcium excretion. An increased urine or serum calcium level may result from malignancy or hyperparathyroidism and should be promptly and thoroughly investigated. A low serum or urine calcium or phosphate level suggests malabsorption or osteomalacia.

In primary osteoporosis, serum phosphate and alkaline phosphatase values are also normal, although the latter may be elevated if the patient has a recent fracture, osteomalacia, Paget's disease, or skeletal metastases. Serum levels of vitamin D, 25-hydroxycholecalciferol, and 1,25-dihydroxycholecalciferol are normal in primary osteoporosis but may be low because of age-related changes in vitamin D metabolism. However, in elderly shut-ins, malnourished patients, and others at risk for vitamin D deficiency, osteomalacia and osteoporosis may coexist. The use of metabolic markers, such as serum osteocalcin, urinary excretion of pyridinium and deoxypyridinium, and urinary hydroxyproline, to assess bone turnover is under investigation.

Radiologic findings are insufficient for making a differential diagnosis of metabolic bone disease. Radiolucence is the hallmark of osteopenia on conventional x-rays, but it cannot be detected reliably until at least 30% of the bone is lost. However, incidental skeletal osteopenia on a chest x-ray is the most common clue to osteoporosis in asymptomatic postmenopausal women. Generally, the vertical trabeculae of vertebrae and vertebral end-plates appear more prominent because of the loss of horizontal trabeculae. In more advanced disease, the end-plates become concave as the intervertebral disks balloon ("codfishing"). Schmorl's nodes form when the nucleus pulposus breaks through the weakened end-plate and herniates into the osteopenic vertebral body. Although biconcavity of vertebral end-plates and fractures are common in all metabolic bone diseases, Schmorl's nodes are more common in primary osteoporosis and rarely appear in osteomalacia. A predominantly anterior compression of the vertebrae results in a wedge fracture; a collapse of the entire vertebral body results in a crush fracture. These compression fractures usually occur in the lower thoracic and upper lumbar vertebrae, although all vertebrae may be affected in severe disease. In long bones, cortical thinning and medullary space expansion may occur. Occasionally, x-ray findings may suggest other causes of metabolic bone disease, eg, the lytic lesions of multiple myeloma, the arthropathy of rheumatoid arthritis, and the pseudofractures of osteomalacia.

Prophylaxis

Given the success of estrogen replacement therapy in retarding bone loss and reducing the incidence of osteoporotic fractures, the perimenopausal patient should be evaluated for risk factors. No single risk factor or combination of risk factors accurately predicts the development of osteoporosis; however, bone density measurements predict fracture risk and help determine the need for preventive therapy.

Bone-density measurement: A bone-density determination at any site predicts the risk of fracture at all sites, although hip fractures more strongly correlate with proximal femoral bone mass and vertebral fractures more strongly correlate with vertebral bone mass. Generally, a bone density measurement of 1 SD below the mean for age is associated with an increased fracture risk and indicates the need for treatment. This is an arbitrary cutoff point, however, and longitudinal studies are needed to more accurately determine the density at which treatment should begin.

Cost-effective screening guidelines for asymptomatic perimenopausal women have not yet been established. Therefore, widespread screening for osteoporosis in asymptomatic women cannot be recommended. Bone-density measurements should be done in asymptomatic women only if the results will influence estrogen replacement therapy or other treatment. In patients with radiographic osteopenia or vertebral abnormalities, measurements can be used to diagnose osteoporosis if they will influence the diagnostic work-up or treatment. Bone densitometry may also be indicated for patients on long-term corticosteroid therapy if a measurement of spinal bone density will help in deciding whether to reduce the dose or add drugs to prevent bone loss. Other possible indications include a coexisting disease such as rheumatoid arthritis or primary hyperparathyroidism, which may reduce bone density, and the use of other medications that may affect bone density.

Serial bone density measurements to assess the rate of bone loss or the therapeutic response are controversial and cannot be routinely recommended. A recommendation has been made that women with a bone density between the mean and 1 SD below the mean should obtain a second measurement in 2 to 5 yr. However, this assumes that the second measurement is obtained by a similar technique at the same site under similar conditions so actual bone loss can be measured without machine variation and reproducibility problems. Also, serial measurements increase radiation exposure and cost. In the future, biochemical markers combined with bone density measurements may provide an estimation of the rate of bone loss.

Currently, four methods of measuring bone density are available: single-photon absorptiometry, dual-photon absorptiometry, quantitative computed tomography, and dual-energy x-ray absorptiometry (see TABLE 73–3).

Single-photon absorptiometry (SPA) of the radius, ulna, or heel is a widely available technique for measuring bone density. The procedure is inexpensive, exposes the patient to little radiation, and is reasonably accurate. However, it does not directly measure bone density in vertebrae or femurs, the most common and disabling sites of osteoporotic fractures.

Dual-photon absorptiometry (DPA) does directly measure vertebral and femoral bone density. But this technique is more expensive, is less widely available, and has a longer scanning time. This technique is most accurate in young and middle-aged persons. Falsely elevated values may occur with degenerative joint disease, compression fractures, or closely situated calcified vessels.

Quantitative computed tomography (CT) is used mainly to measure bone density at the lumbar spine but can be used at other sites as well. However, the accuracy, scanning time, and degree of radiation exposure may vary depending on the equipment and techniques. Because of the extremely high radiation exposure with quantitative CT, it should not be used in women of childbearing age or for serial measurements. The cost may be higher than that of other techniques. Reproducibility for serial measurements is poor.

TABLE 73–3. NONINVASIVE TECHNIQUES FOR MEASURING BONE DENSITY

Technique	*Site*	*Accuracy**	*Precision†*	*Absorbed Radiation (mrem)*	*Examination Time (min)*
SPA	Radius Ulna Heel	4–5%	1–3%	2–20	10–20
DPA	Spine‡ Hip Total body	4–10%	2–4%	5	20–60
QCT	Spine§	5–20%	2–5%	100–1000	10–20
DEXA	Radius Ulna Spine‡ Hip Total body	3–5%	0.5–2%	1–3	3–10

SPA = single-photon absorptiometry; DPA = dual-photon absorptiometry; QCT = quantitative computed tomography; DEXA = dual-energy x-ray absorptiometry; mrem = millirem.

* Accuracy is the tendency of test results to center around the true value.

† Precision is the tendency of test results to remain the same on repeated measurements.

‡ DPA and DEXA measure entire vertebral body.

§ QCT measures center of vertebral body.

Adapted from information in Johnston CC, Slemenda CW, Melton LJ III: "Clinical use of bone densitometry." *The New England Journal of Medicine* 324:1105–1109, 1991, used with permission; and from information in Fleming LA: "Osteoporosis: Clinical features, prevention, and treatment." *Journal of General Internal Medicine* 7:554–562, 1992.

Dual-energy x-ray absorptiometry (DEXA), the newest densitometry technique, is precise, exposes the patient to little radiation, and requires little scanning time. Together with its low cost, these characteristics make DEXA the technique of choice. It can measure bone density at the radius, ulna, spine, and femur and for the total body. Because it is more precise than other methods, DEXA is better suited to serial measurements. Although the ability of DEXA to predict fractures has not been as well studied as that of the other techniques, densitometric measurements with DEXA are almost identical to those with DPA; thus, they are assumed to have similar predictive values.

Treatment

Therapy for primary osteoporosis includes exercise and drugs such as calcium, vitamin D, estrogen, calcitonin, bisphosphonates, and fluoride. The drugs used to treat osteoporosis are classified as antiresorptive or formation-stimulating. Antiresorptive drugs—including calcium, estrogen, calcitonin, and bisphosphonates—are used mainly for prevention in perimenopausal women or for treatment of established osteoporosis. Fluoride is the only formation-stimulating agent. In the USA, only estrogen, calcitonin, and calcium (as adjunct therapy) are currently approved for osteoporosis therapy.

Other drugs, such as parathyroid hormone, calcitriol analogs, growth factors, thiazides, oral phosphate, and androgens, have not yet been proved to reduce the rate of osteoporotic fractures in randomized clinical trials.

Exercise: A regimen of moderate weight-bearing exercise—eg, walking for 45 to 60 min 3 to 5 times/wk—is safe and reasonable. Other forms of exercise must be evaluated for the particular patient.

Calcium: Among American women, the average dietary intake of calcium is about 400 mg/day, which is < 50% of the recommended daily allowance. Adequate calcium intake from childhood through the third decade is particularly important, and calcium supplements may be required for those who avoid milk products. In children, premenopausal women, and early postmenopausal women, calcium inhibits bone loss and may diminish the risk of fractures. Thus, 1000 mg/day of elemental calcium is recommended for premenopausal women, and 1500 mg/day is recommended for postmenopausal women, except for those with a history of renal calculi or hypercalciuria. Three glasses of milk provide about 900 mg of elemental calcium, but tablets may be easier to take and may be preferred in elderly persons who suffer some degree of lactose intolerance. Some orange juices and cereals are now fortified with calcium.

Calcium carbonate, the most widely available calcium supplement, is 40% elemental calcium by weight. However, it may cause constipation, rebound hyperacidity, abdominal bloating, and other GI side effects. **Calcium citrate,** which is 22% elemental calcium by weight, is better absorbed, particularly in elderly persons with achlorhydria, and has fewer GI side effects. Serum and urine calcium levels should be monitored before and after starting calcium supplementation in patients with renal impairment or a personal or family history of renal calculi.

Vitamin D: Vitamin D therapy has not been proved effective in treating osteoporosis, and pharmacologic doses pose the risk of hypervitaminosis D, which is associated with hypercalcemia, hypercalciuria, acute renal failure, and increased resorption of bone. However, a daily dose of 400 to 800 IU vitamin D, the amount found in many multivitamin tablets, is safe for most patients and prevents vitamin D deficiency. If vitamin D deficiency and osteomalacia are suspected (because of low sunlight exposure, avoidance of fortified dairy products, gastrectomy, small-bowel resection, malabsorption syndrome, hepatic disease, renal failure, or antiseizure medications), serum levels of 25-hydroxycholecalciferol and, in some patients with renal disease, 1,25-dihydroxycholecalciferol should be measured. Diagnostic bone histomorphometry and supplementation with appropriate vitamin D formulations should be considered (see OSTEOMALACIA, below).

In a recent study, women with established osteoporosis who took calcitriol (1,25-dihydroxycholecalciferol) 0.25 μg bid showed a significant reduction in new fractures. However, calcitriol therapy may lead to hypercalcemia, hypercalciuria, nephrocalcinosis, and renal insufficiency. Also, results of other studies with calcitriol are inconsistent, and the use of this drug for osteoporosis is not approved.

Estrogen: Currently, the only therapy that prevents the accelerated bone loss associated with menopause and other causes of ovarian failure is estrogen replacement. This therapy should be started within 4 to 6 yr of menopause to achieve its maximum effect. After that, significant, irreversible bone loss will have occurred. Nevertheless, some studies suggest that estrogen slows bone loss and decreases the fracture rate even when given well after the immediate postmenopausal period. Upon discontinuance of estrogen, bone loss begins anew. Therefore, in theory estrogen therapy alone or estrogen therapy followed by therapy with another antiresorptive agent should be continued indefinitely. See Ch. 83 for details of postmenopausal hormone replacement.

Calcitonin: Salmon calcitonin can be used to treat postmenopausal osteoporosis. Although studies demonstrate that it can increase total body calcium, transiently increase vertebral bone mass in postmenopausal women, and retard postmenopausal cortical bone loss, its long-term effect on bone density and fracture rate is still under investigation. Salmon calcitonin may have an analgesic effect on acute osteoporotic vertebral fractures and has few side effects, but it must be given parenterally and is expensive. Usual doses of salmon calcitonin are 50 to 100 IU subcutaneously every day or every other day after an initial low-dose skin test for sensitivity. Intranasally administered calcitonin is used in Europe but has not been approved in the USA.

Bisphosphonates: Etidronate is a bone resorption inhibitor; however, when used in doses that inhibit bone resorption, it also inhibits bone mineralization. Thus, long-term administration is discouraged. Studies using cyclic administration of etidronate for 2 wk followed by 11 to 13 wk of calcium supplementation show modest increases in vertebral bone density and a possible short-term decrease in vertebral fractures. The usual dosage of etidronate is 400 mg/day for 2 wk followed by 12 wk without medication. Because of its poor absorption, the drug should be taken on an empty stomach with no food consumed for 2 h before or after administration. Calcium 500 to 1000 mg/day should be taken to avoid mineralization defects. Calcium and etidronate administration should be separated by as much time as possible, ideally 12 h.

Newer generations of bisphosphonates are under investigation for the treatment of osteoporosis. Only one of these drugs, pamidronate, is available in the USA, where it has been approved for the treatment of malignant hypercalcemia. Because pamidronate is more potent than etidronate, the dose is less likely to produce the mineralization defects seen with etidronate. However, pamidronate may cause a transient hyperpyrexia in a small number of patients. Currently, pamidronate is available only in parenteral form.

Fluoride: Fluoride stimulates osteoblastic activity and increases new bone formation. When given without supplemental calcium, fluoride causes osteomalacia and secondary hyperparathyroidism. About 40% of patients receiving fluoride therapy experience adverse effects, including synovitis with ankle and knee pain, a painful plantar fascial syndrome (both probably secondary to microfractures of the leg because of rapid bone turnover), dyspepsia, recurrent vomiting, peptic ulcer, and iron deficiency anemia resulting from GI blood loss. Although fluoride increases bone density in the proximal femur and lumbar spine, radial bone density decreases. Because of the high frequency of side effects and the increase in nonvertebral fractures noted in at least one study, fluoride is not routinely recommended to treat osteoporosis. However, in a recent study, a lower dose, slow-release fluoride given in conjunction with calcium citrate inhibited new vertebral fractures. Further studies are needed on enteric-coated or slow-release fluoride.

Treatment of male osteoporosis: The treatment for osteoporosis in men depends on whether a secondary cause is identified. For example, in men with hypogonadism, androgenic hormones should be replaced, although whether this will reverse bone loss is unknown. Reversible risk factors such as alcohol and tobacco use should be addressed. Attempts should be made to taper corticosteroid therapy. Otherwise, calcium supplementation, exercise, a multivitamin preparation, and possibly calcitonin or bisphosphonate therapy, as described above, may be recommended. Further studies on the natural history and treatment of male osteoporosis are needed.

Treatment of drug-induced osteoporosis: Long-term corticosteroid therapy leads to osteoporosis. In patients receiving such therapy, the underlying illness should be treated, and the corticosteroid regimen should be reduced or discontinued as soon as possible. Exercise, calcium supplementation, vitamin D, calcitonin, bisphosphonates, and estrogen replacement may be considered.

Although anticonvulsants (eg, phenytoin and phenobarbital) contribute to the loss of bone density by decreasing serum levels of vitamin D metabolites, routine vitamin D supplementation is not recommended. After several years of anticonvulsant therapy, serum levels of 25-hydroxycholecalciferol should be measured and replacement therapy prescribed as necessary to prevent osteomalacia.

PAGET'S DISEASE OF BONE

(Osteitis Deformans)

A chronic, localized, metabolic bone disorder characterized by an early osteolytic process initiated by proliferating osteoclasts and a later osteoblastic phase resulting in abnormal histologic qualities and gross deformity of skeletal structures.

Etiology and Incidence

The cause of Paget's disease is unknown. With electron microscopy, abnormal inclusions resembling the nucleocapsids of viruses in the Paramyxoviridae family have been observed in osteoclasts, suggesting a slow viral process, but many hypotheses are being explored.

A common disease, it occurs equally in men and women, is more prevalent in English-speaking countries, and generally is rare in China, Japan, India, and the Scandinavian countries. In prevalent areas, radiologic evidence of Paget's disease is reported in 3% of the population > 40 yr and in 10% of those > 80 yr.

Pathophysiology

Characterized by multiple localized sites, the disease leaves most of the skeleton unaffected. In the early phase, an osteolytic process is initiated by the proliferation of multinucleated and often very large osteoclasts. Then enlarged osteoblasts line the bony trabeculae resorbed during the osteoclastic phase, initiating exuberant, though disordered, bone formation. The marrow may be filled with connective tissue, blood vessels, and fibroblasts that have displaced hematopoietic tissue. Thus, the resulting disordered bone may be extraordinarily vascular. A single bone may show evidence of osteolytic, osteoblastic, or "burnt-out" Paget's disease. The osteoblastic phase may occur simultaneously with the osteolytic phase in adjacent bone.

Symptoms and Signs

Asymptomatic in > 75% of patients, Paget's disease is often detected by an abnormal x-ray or an incidentally elevated serum alkaline phosphatase level. In symptomatic patients, the disease is characterized by deformities in the skull, long bones, and clavicles; pathologic fractures; bone pain; and hypervascularity. Gross enlargement of cranial structures can result in headaches, hearing loss, vertigo, and tinnitus. With bony impingement of the structures at the base of the skull, slurred speech, incontinence, diplopia, and deranged swallowing can occur.

Long-bone deformities, eg, tibial or femoral bowing, and acetabular deformation may also develop. When lumbar and thoracic vertebrae are involved, spinal nerve entrapment may occur.

Pain is usually described as vague, not severe, and may be difficult to distinguish from that of coexisting degenerative joint disease of the hips, knees, and lower back. However, pathologic fractures are characteristic of Paget's disease. Vertebral wedge and crush fractures may be heralded by back pain. Tibial and femoral fractures may occur after significant bowing but generally heal without delay.

The hypervascularity of pagetic bone may be detected as warmth of the overlying skin. When > 30% of the skeleton is involved or when skull involvement is extensive, high-output heart failure can result. With coexisting heart disease, less extensive bony involvement may compromise cardiac function enough to cause heart failure.

Angioid streaks, or defects in Bruch's membrane of the retina, may occur in 10% to 15% of patients but rarely impair vision. Neoplasms occasionally develop from pagetic bone. Osteosarcoma develops in < 1% of cases and may be heralded by a rapid enlargement of bone, increased bone mass, or an elevation in the serum alkaline phosphatase level. Giant cell tumors also may develop in some patients.

Diagnosis

In a patient with suggestive symptoms and signs, the diagnosis is confirmed by characteristic x-ray and bone scan findings and by elevated serum alkaline phosphatase and urine hydroxyproline levels. Serum alkaline phosphatase levels may reflect the extent of disease as established by x-rays and may be used to follow disease activity. Urine hydroxyproline levels may be especially helpful if serum alkaline phosphatase levels are confounded by the presence of other conditions. The serum calcium level is usually normal but may be elevated if the patient is immobilized or has a malignancy. If the patient is not immobilized, an elevated serum calcium level should be thoroughly investigated. Hypercalciuria, on the other hand, is a common finding and probably results from bone resorption. Immobilization exaggerates hypercalciuria. Hyperuricemia and gout are observed more frequently in patients with Paget's disease.

In the early, or osteolytic, phase of Paget's disease, a localized osteolytic lesion, particularly in the skull or on either end of long bones, may be seen on x-ray. When this lesion develops in the skull, it is called **osteoporosis circumscripta cranii.** In the extremities, lesions usually progress at the rate of about 1 cm/yr in a sharply delineated V shape. In the vertebrae, sclerotic margins may form a picture-frame appearance.

The radiologic findings of osteoblastic activity may not appear until years after the onset of the osteolytic phase but may be the first clue to the diagnosis of Paget's disease. In the skull, a honeycomb pattern may appear with patchy new bone filling in the underlying areas of osteoporosis circumscripta cranii. With increased bone formation and a thickened calvarium, a cotton-wool appearance may develop. In the extremities, x-rays reveal long bones with thickened irregular trabeculation. Thickening of the iliopectineal line in the pelvis is known as the brim sign. Though very sensitive, a **bone scan** is not specific for Paget's disease.

Treatment

For asymptomatic patients with minimal bony involvement, no treatment is needed. As bony involvement becomes more extensive, however, treatment may be initiated to prevent fractures and other complications. Treatment is indicated for patients with skeletal pain or deformity, neurologic or cardiac symptoms, or hypercalcemia and for orthopedic surgery candidates. For these patients, treatment usually begins about 3 to 4 mo before surgery.

Bisphosphonates: Bisphosphonates inhibit osteoclast activity, decreasing bone turnover, but they do not heal osteolytic lesions. These drugs improve skeletal, cardiac, and neurologic symptoms and reduce serum alkaline phosphatase and urine hydroxyproline levels. They reduce pain and increase mobility in most patients, although a small percentage experience a paradoxic increase in pain.

When etidronate is given in doses of 5 to 20 mg/kg/day, a biochemical plateau may be reached in 3 to 6 mo. At this point, remission may be sustained despite discontinuance of the drug. Generally, treatment for 6 mo at a time with drug-free intervals of 3 to 6 mo is effective. With larger doses, decreased osteoblastic activity predominates, reducing bone formation and leading to a mineralization defect and osteomalacia. Therefore, bisphosphonates are *not* the preferred treatment for orthopedic surgery candidates or those with osteolytic lesions. Adverse effects—including hyperphosphatemia, loose stools, and nausea—are uncommon.

Pamidronate, which is available in the USA, is under investigation for the treatment of Paget's disease. In studies, pamidronate 500 mg/day orally for 4 to 12 mo or 20 mg/day IV for 10 days has produced clinical remission in most patients. In many patients, remission may also be achieved by a single larger IV dose. Currently, pamidronate is available only in parenteral form.

Calcitonin: About 80% of patients respond to **salmon calcitonin**, making it as effective as etidronate. Unlike etidronate though, salmon calcitonin heals osteolytic lesions, so it is the preferred drug for patients anticipating orthopedic surgery. Its greatest drawback is that serum antidrug antibodies may form, inducing resistance to the drug. The usual dosage is 50 to 100 IU subcutaneously every day or every other day; some patients require more. Side effects, which include nausea, flushing, metallic taste, chills, perioral paresthesias, and polyuria, rarely require that the drug be discontinued.

In patients resistant to salmon calcitonin, **human calcitonin** appears to be effective, although resistance to it may develop after prolonged use. The recommended starting dose is 0.5 mg/day subcutaneously.

The dosage may be titrated to 0.25 mg/day or 0.5 mg 2 or 3 times/wk, but in patients with extensive osteolytic lesions, doses of up to 0.5 mg bid may be needed.

Both forms of calcitonin are expensive, with human calcitonin costing about twice as much as salmon calcitonin. Usually, the serum alkaline phosphatase level falls to about ½ of the pretreatment level within several weeks of therapy and subsequently maintains a plateau. Therapy may be discontinued in 6 to 12 mo and restarted when a relapse occurs.

Plicamycin: Not yet approved by the Food and Drug Administration for Paget's disease, plicamycin is a potent inhibitor of osteoclastic function. Usually given IV, the drug may cause renal, bone marrow, and hepatic toxicity. Occasionally, it may be used after other regimens fail.

Surgery: In some cases, surgery of pagetic bone may be necessary. Occipital craniectomy may relieve basilar and nerve compression. Osteotomy may be needed for extensive involvement of the tibia, and total hip replacement may be needed for severe degenerative joint disease.

OSTEOMALACIA

An osteopenic bone disorder caused by a failure of bone matrix to mineralize, resulting in a decreased mineralized bone:unmineralized matrix ratio. Total bone mass may be normal or increased. Osteomalacia differs from osteoporosis, which is characterized by a normal ratio of mineralized bone:unmineralized matrix and an absolute decrease in total bone mass.

Pathophysiology

The most common causes of osteomalacia are vitamin D deficiency, abnormal metabolism of vitamin D, and hypophosphatemia. The resulting hypocalcemia or hypophosphatemia probably impairs osteoid maturation, although the exact mechanism is unclear.

Vitamin D is obtained from the diet (vitamin D_2 [ergocalciferol]) and from the conversion of 7-dihydrocholesterol in skin to vitamin D_3 (cholecalciferol) after exposure to sunlight. Its metabolite 1,25-dihydroxycholecalciferol enhances GI absorption of calcium and phosphate, and 1,25-dihydroxycholecalciferol and 24,25-dihydroxycholecalciferol may have direct effects on the bone mineralization process, although this remains controversial. Vitamin D deficiency requires deficiency in both sources and may result from a restriction of foods (eg, dairy products, fish, and fortified flour), malabsorption of vitamin D, and insufficient exposure to ultraviolet radiation (eg, as occurs with shut-ins, residents in northern climates, and those who use sunblock or wear clothing that allows minimal skin exposure).

Dietary vitamin D (ie, vitamin D_2) is absorbed in the upper small bowel via fat-dependent absorption. Derangements in upper intestinal function or fat malabsorption can result in vitamin D deficiency. Such derangements include the sequelae of surgeries such as gastrectomy and intestinal resection, sprue, pancreatic insufficiency, biliary obstruction, and bile salt depletion that accompanies ileal disease or the chronic use of bile-salt–binding resins.

Once absorbed, vitamin D_2 or D_3 is hydroxylated in the liver to 25-hydroxycholecalciferol (calcifediol) and subsequently in the kidneys to 1,25-dihydroxycholecalciferol (calcitriol), the active metabolite. Interference with the metabolism of vitamin D may contribute to the development of osteomalacia. Liver disease, particularly cirrhosis of any cause, may interfere with hepatic 25-hydroxylation of vitamin D. In renal failure, the deficiency of renal 1α-hydroxylase activity may result in osteomalacia by producing a deficiency of 1,25-dihydroxycholecalciferol.

Increased vitamin D excretion or catabolism may also lead to osteomalacia. Drugs that increase the hepatic degradation of 25-hydroxycholecalciferol, particularly phenytoin and phenobarbital, are known to predispose patients to osteomalacia. In the nephrotic syndrome, an increase in vitamin D clearance and excretion may result in vitamin D deficiency.

Phosphorus is essential for the mineralization process. A dietary deficiency of phosphate is rare, but hypophosphatemia may result from a GI or renal loss of phosphate that is independent of parathyroid or vitamin D metabolism. Malabsorption and subsequent GI wasting of phosphates may be compounded by hyperparathyroidism and vitamin D deficiency and may also be exacerbated by phosphate-binding antacids. Renal wasting of phosphorus is a prominent feature of proximal renal tubular disorders that are associated with normal glomerular filtration rates. These disorders range from defects limited to increased phosphate clearance with a minimum of concomitant abnormalities to more widespread defects involving phosphorus, glucose, amino acids, uric acid, and potassium. The latter defects are typical of Fanconi's syndrome. In renal tubular acidosis, the acidotic state itself may also contribute to the development of osteomalacia. Osteomalacia and hypophosphatemia with high renal phosphate clearance also occur with many benign and malignant mesenchymal tumors, such as giant cell tumors, hemangiomas, and fibromas, as well as with prostatic carcinoma.

Symptoms and Signs

Bone pain, the hallmark of osteomalacia, may be generalized or localized to the vertebrae, ribs, hips, pelvis, or legs. The pain may be aggravated by movement, and bony tenderness is common. Although deformity is unusual in adults, leg bowing, gibbus deformity, and arthrokatadysis occasionally develop in severely affected persons. Pathologic fractures may occur, and when osteomalacia presents as vertebral wedge or crush fractures, distinguishing it from osteoporosis may be difficult. The two disorders may, in fact, exist simultaneously. Usually, muscle weakness and easy fatigability occur in osteomalacia but not in osteoporosis.

Diagnosis

In osteomalacia, serum alkaline phosphatase levels are usually elevated. Urine or serum calcium levels are usually low in patients with vitamin D deficiency, although serum calcium levels may be normal early in the disease. Because vitamin D deficiency can result in secondary hyperparathyroidism, urine levels of cAMP and hydroxyproline may increase. If vitamin D deficiency is suspected, 25-hydroxycholecalciferol levels should be measured directly. Serum levels of 25-hydroxycholecalciferol are usually low, and serum levels of 1,25-dihydroxycholecalciferol are usually normal, unless renal failure is a contributing cause of the osteomalacia. In hypophosphatemic osteomalacia, serum phosphate levels are low, but serum and urine calcium levels are usually normal.

Radiologic findings of osteomalacia are difficult to distinguish from those of osteoporosis. Vertebral biconcavity, ballooning of intervertebral disks, and vertebral compression fractures occur in both disorders. Occasionally, thin longitudinal bands of radiolucency may appear in the pubic rami, ribs, long bones, and scapulae; nonhealing results from impaired bone mineralization. These bands are known as pseudofractures, Looser's transformation zones, or Milkman's syndrome fractures and may show increased uptake on bone scan.

If the diagnosis is in doubt, a bone biopsy must be performed. Because the histopathologic findings are similar to those of hyperparathyroidism, hyperthyroidism, and Paget's disease of bone, histomorphometric techniques using double-tetracycline labeling are needed to identify the mineralization defect characteristic of osteomalacia. Although increased amounts of osteoid are seen in all metabolic bone disorders, the distance between the tetracycline bands is reduced or absent in osteomalacia, whereas it is normal or increased in other conditions.

Treatment

Treatment must be directed at the underlying cause and the resulting derangement in bone mineralization (see TABLE 73–4). The goal is to correct hypocalcemia without causing hypercalcemia. When the 24-h urine calcium level reaches > 200 mg/day, therapy should be kept at the same dose.

With any vitamin D regimen, improved calcium absorption may lead to vitamin D intoxication, hypercalcemia, and hypercalciuria. Therefore, close monitoring of urine and serum levels of calcium and vitamin D is recommended.

TABLE 73–4. TREATMENT OF OSTEOMALACIA

Cause	*Regimen*
Dietary deficiency of vitamin D	Vitamin D 2000–4000 IU/day for 3–4 mo, then 200–400 IU/day Elemental calcium 1–3 gm/day
Malabsorption syndrome	Treat underlying cause Vitamin D 50,000–100,000 IU/day to twice weekly Elemental calcium 1–3 gm/day
Hepatic disease	Calcifediol 50–100 μg/day or Vitamin D 5,000–10,000 IU/day and Elemental calcium 1–3 gm/day
Renal failure	Calcitriol 0.5–1.0 μg/day or Dihydrotachysterol 0.25–0.5 mg/day and Elemental calcium 1–3 gm/day Phosphate binders and low-phosphate diet
Renal tubular acidosis	Treat underlying disorder (alkalinization) and Vitamin D 50,000–100,000 IU/wk or Calcitriol 0.25 μg bid Vitamin D may be discontinued when alkalinization is achieved
Hypophosphatemia	Phosphate 1000–3000 mg/day in divided doses Calcitriol 0.25–1.0 μg/day (if deficient 1,25-dihydroxycholecalciferol)
Anticonvulsants	Routine therapy not recommended; serum vitamin D metabolites should be measured after the patient has been receiving anticonvulsant therapy for several years and should be replaced if deficient

Urine and serum calcium levels should be monitored closely in all cases to prevent the complications of hypervitaminosis D, which include hypercalcemia, hypercalciuria, and renal failure.

Dietary deficiency of vitamin D: A regimen of vitamin D 2000 to 4000 IU/day over 3 to 4 mo may be needed to restore a positive calcium balance and normal bone mineralization. After that, 400 IU/day, the amount in most multivitamin preparations, is usually enough to prevent subsequent vitamin D deficiency. All patients should also receive elemental calcium 1 to 3 gm/day during treatment.

Malabsorption syndrome: When osteomalacia results from malabsorption, the underlying GI disorder must be treated. In some patients, a relatively selective malabsorption of vitamin D may occur without overt steatorrhea or other symptoms (eg, celiac sprue). To overcome the malabsorption defect, the patient needs large doses of either vitamin D_2 or D_3, usually 50,000 IU twice a week in combination with calcium supplementation. Because the goal is to normalize serum 25-hydroxycholecalciferol (calcifediol) levels, up to 100,000 IU/day of vitamin D_2 or D_3 may be needed. Rarely, parenteral therapy is required. Because calcifediol is more polar than its parent compound, it may be more rapidly absorbed, facilitating a more reliable clinical response. Elemental calcium 1 to 3 gm/day is also required.

Treatment of osteomalacia from **increased catabolism or excretion of vitamin D** is similar to that of osteomalacia from malabsorption.

Hepatic disease: A regimen of vitamin D 5,000 to 10,000 IU/day may normalize serum 25-hydroxycholecalciferol levels. In patients with severe hepatic disease, the indicated treatment is calcifediol, which effectively bypasses the defective biochemical pathway. Calcifediol 50 to 100 μg/day or every other day may be used. Elemental calcium 1 to 3 gm/day may be used with either regimen.

Renal osteodystrophy: Osteodystrophy of chronic renal failure results from abnormalities of acid-base balance, vitamin D metabolism, and parathyroid function. Osteomalacia, a major component of renal osteodystrophy, results primarily from a deficiency in 1,25-dihydroxycholecalciferol. However, secondary hyperparathyroidism, acidosis, and aluminum toxicity may also contribute to the bone disease. This disorder is generally treated with calcitriol (1,25-dihydroxycholecalciferol) 0.5 to 1.0 μg/day or dihydrotachysterol (DHT) 0.25 to 0.5 mg/day. Elemental calcium 1 to 3 gm/day is also given. Finally, phosphate binders and a phosphate-restricted diet are needed to prevent the hyperphosphatemia of chronic renal failure.

Hypophosphatemia: Osteomalacia such as that seen in X-linked hypophosphatemia or with renal or GI phosphate loss must be treated with neutral phosphate salts. Diarrhea is a prominent adverse effect of this therapy, so the dose of a buffered phosphate solution should probably be increased gradually to 1 to 3 gm/day on a 4 to 6 times/day dosage schedule. Caution must be exercised because rapid phosphate repletion may result in hypocalcemia secondary to accelerated bone remineralization, particularly in patients with a coexisting deficiency of 1,25-

dihydroxycholecalciferol. Therefore, calcitriol 0.25 to 1.0 μg/day is added to this regimen. The metabolic bone disease seen in Fanconi's syndrome is related to the hypophosphatemia that is secondary to the underlying metabolic acidosis. When the acidosis is corrected, the metabolic bone disease will be ameliorated.

Anticonvulsant therapy: Patients receiving phenobarbital or phenytoin do not require routine administration of vitamin D. However, after a patient has been receiving anticonvulsant therapy for several years, serum vitamin D levels should be obtained and vitamin D supplements prescribed, as necessary.

---

74. GIANT CELL (TEMPORAL) ARTERITIS AND POLYMYALGIA RHEUMATICA

Giant cell arteritis, also called **temporal arteritis,** is a *chronic inflammatory process involving the extracranial arteries*. Temporal arteritis is a less satisfactory term because it de-emphasizes involvement of the more vital cranial blood vessels and ignores involvement of blood vessels other than those of the aortic arch and its tributaries. **Polymyalgia rheumatica** *is a syndrome characterized by pain and stiffness in muscles of the limb girdles and by responsiveness to corticosteroid therapy.* Since it has few pathologic features, its pathophysiology remains undefined. Rarer forms have little arterial or muscle involvement, and patients may present with cachexia, fever, or anemia; these are, respectively, the malignant, febrile, or anemic forms of the disorder.

Epidemiology and Etiology

Although giant cell arteritis and polymyalgia rheumatica may occur separately, 50% of patients with giant cell arteritis have clinical features of polymyalgia rheumatica, and 25% of patients with polymyalgia rheumatica have clinical or pathologic features of giant cell arteritis. In view of this overlap, most epidemiologic surveys group the two conditions together as one disorder.

The giant cell arteritis–polymyalgia rheumatica complex is twice as common in women as in men and its incidence increases strikingly with age: it is at least 10 times as common in patients > 80 yr of age as in those aged 50 to 59 yr (see FIG. 74–1). Hospital surveys report a wide variation in incidence: the number of cases per 100,000 people annually in Tennessee was 1.6; in Scotland, 4.2; in Minnesota, 11.7; and in Sweden, 18.3. The low incidence in Tennessee is partly attributable to the large black population in that state (the disorder is 6 times less common in blacks than in whites). The higher figures for Minnesota may be related to the large population of Scandinavian descent. However, these

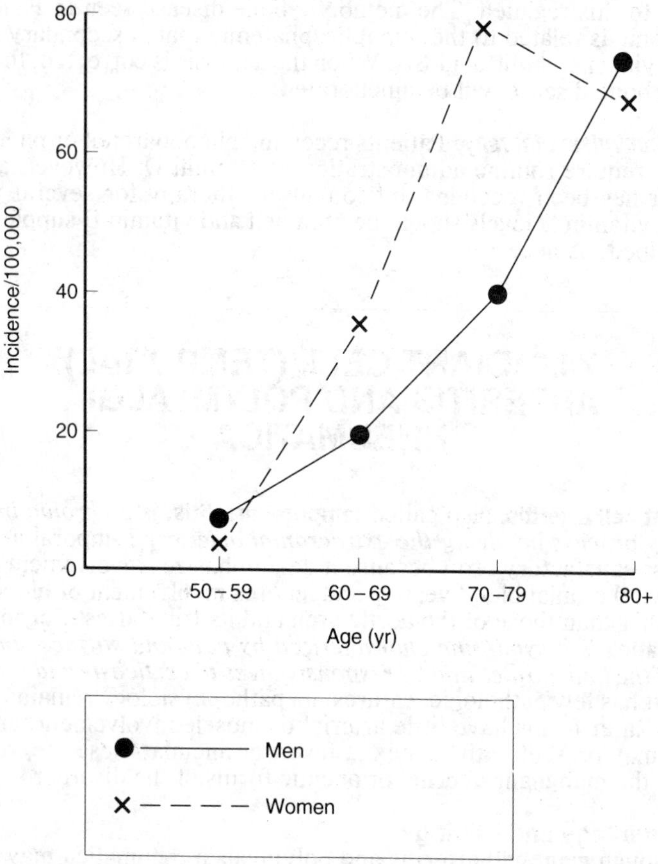

FIG. 74–1. Incidence of giant cell arteritis and polymyalgia rheumatica per 100,000 inhabitants > 50 yr of age in Sweden. (Based on data from Bengtsson BA, Malmvall BE: "The epidemiology of giant cell arteritis including temporal arteritis and polymyalgia rheumatica." *Arthritis and Rheumatism* 24:899–904, 1981.)

surveys may seriously underestimate the rate of occurrence; a recent survey of a British general practice in Cambridge revealed an annual incidence of 4/1000 in patients > 60 yr of age, a figure 20 times higher than that recorded in Swedish hospitals. Environmental factors have not been linked with the complex.

Reports suggesting that the disorder is rare in blacks could represent underdiagnosis in a group that often comes from a poor socioeconomic background; however, the difference in incidence between whites and blacks is so striking that other factors must be involved. Genetic factors appear to be important; several family clusters have been identified. Some centers have reported an increased prevalence in persons with the HLA-DR4 genotype, which is consistent with the low incidence in blacks, in whom the DR4 genotype is much less common. Associations with HLA-B8, B5, B14, and Bw38 genotypes have not been confirmed.

Pathology

Giant cell arteritis is characterized by round cell infiltration of the arterial intima and inner part of the media. Histiocytes, lymphocytes, and monocytes are the most numerous, but the presence of multinucleated Langhans' giant cells is more useful diagnostically. Many of the lymphocytes are helper/inducer T cells. This characteristic, combined with the rarity of immunoglobulin deposits around elastin fibers, suggests that the arterial lesion results from cell-mediated rather than humoral immunity.

The inflammatory process involves short segments of the artery, where it is usually circumferential. Smooth, often dilated, segments of normal artery taper to affected segments that are smooth and symmetrically stenosed or occluded. Although the accessibility of the superficial temporal artery for biopsy means that this vessel is most frequently associated with the disease, autopsy studies show that the vertebral, ophthalmic, and posterior ciliary arteries are often concurrently involved. Internal and external carotid and central retinal artery damage is less common, while the intracerebral vessels are rarely affected.

Various smaller arteries may also be involved. In the lungs, arteritis produces patchy granulomatous infiltration and necrosis, usually centered around a diseased blood vessel. Similar granulomatous lesions are common in the liver and have been reported in the pancreas, spleen, uterus, and breast. The kidneys may be affected with patchy vasculitis, and a membranous glomerulopathy has occasionally been identified.

Polymyalgia rheumatica is not associated with histologic abnormalities in skeletal muscle. Synovitis characterized by round cell infiltration and synovial proliferation is common, although the changes are much less severe than those found in rheumatoid arthritis. Usually the hips and shoulders are involved, but the knees and sternoclavicular joints may also be affected.

Symptoms and Signs

In giant cell arteritis, the typical presenting feature is a continuous, throbbing temporal headache. If branches of the external carotid artery are involved, necrosis and ulceration of the scalp may occur. Ischemia of the masseter muscles, tongue, and pharynx results in pain stimulated by chewing, talking, or swallowing and relieved by rest. Stenosis of the ophthalmic artery and its branches leads to ocular or orbital pain, transient loss of vision (amaurosis fugax), visual field defects, blurring, and hallucinations and may produce sudden blindness. Orbital muscle ischemia may cause diplopia.

In ⅔ of patients, **physical examination** may reveal characteristic tender, red, swollen, and nodular temporal arteries with diminished pulses. Reduced or absent pulses over other head and neck arteries are less common; focal necrosis of the scalp, tongue, or face occurs in severe cases. Ophthalmic artery involvement generally causes a central scotoma or total blindness; patchy peripheral visual field defects are less common. Ophthalmic artery blockage initially results in a pale, swollen optic disk surrounded by pericapillary hemorrhage, which progresses to a pale, atrophic disk. Patchy areas of retinal infarction are less common. Patients with orbital muscle damage present with varying degrees of ophthalmoplegia or ptosis.

In polymyalgia rheumatica, the most common symptoms are bilateral pain and stiffness of the shoulders and thighs, often severe and leading to immobility and other functional losses (eg, the ability to wash or dress). Symptoms lasting < 2 wk and morning stiffness lasting > 1 h usually suggest polymyalgia rheumatica. **Physical examination** elicits tenderness over the affected muscles and painful limitation of hip and shoulder movements.

Both giant cell arteritis and polymyalgia rheumatica are often associated with depression, weight loss, and fever. Weight loss or fever sometimes is the only finding, leading to a fruitless search for malignancy or infection. Thus, the concept of **malignant** or **febrile** forms of giant cell arteritis has evolved. Usually the symptoms and signs are not specific enough to make the diagnosis of giant cell arteritis or polymyalgia rheumatica, and laboratory tests are required (see below).

Complications

Eyes: *Any delay in starting treatment with corticosteroids may result in permanent unilateral or bilateral blindness.* Thus, every case is treated as a matter of urgency. In one survey, 12% of patients with giant cell arteritis suffered eye complications before treatment: 5% had transient visual impairment or diplopia, and another 7% had permanent visual impairment. Before routine use of corticosteroids, between 30% and 60% of patients developed visual complications. In extreme cases, edema from damaged blood vessels produces unilateral exophthalmos, suggesting an orbital tumor.

Aorta and related vessels: The aortic arch or one or more of its major branches is involved in about one of eight patients with giant cell arteritis. Subclavian or vertebral artery involvement may lead to brain stem ischemia. Coma with decerebrate rigidity may occur if arteritis is diffuse and progresses rapidly. Neurologic damage may be patchy, with abnormalities such as ataxia, nystagmus, or paralysis of upward gaze. Common or internal carotid artery damage may cause either a transient ischemic attack or a full-blown hemiparesis; involvement of both carotid arteries may produce bilateral neurologic signs, sometimes associated with a rapidly progressive form of multi-infarct dementia. Extremely rare are extrapyramidal signs such as tremor, rigidity, and akinesia. Cerebrovascular damage is a relatively uncommon complication of giant cell arteritis and polymyalgia rheumatica, especially if other clinical features are lacking. Thus, temporal artery biopsy should not be routinely performed in stroke patients.

Unilateral stenosis of the subclavian, axillary, or brachial artery may cause upper limb claudication associated with no pulse and zero blood pressure on the affected side. The diagnosis should be suspected when these features are associated with an elevated erythrocyte sedimentation rate.

Aortic arch involvement may lead to dilatation and incompetence of the aortic valve. Sometimes this complication appears years after the acute condition had resolved with corticosteroid therapy. Aortic arch aneurysms also may develop, and aortic dissection has been reported.

Angina pectoris may result from coincidental coronary atheroma or occasionally from obstruction of the coronary ostia by aortitis. Only rarely does arteritis directly involve the coronary arteries.

Proof that the aortic arch or its main tributaries are affected by giant cell arteritis requires contrast angiography. Findings are as follows: (1) long segments of smooth luminal stenosis alternating with segments of normal or dilated lumen, (2) smooth tapering of the lumen between normal and affected segments, and (3) no ulceration or irregular plaques within the lumen.

Joints: About 15% of patients with either giant cell arteritis or polymyalgia rheumatica have clinical evidence of arthritis affecting the knees or sternoclavicular joints. The usual features are pain, tenderness, swelling, redness, and limited mobility; evidence of effusion may be found in the knees. The rheumatoid factor test is invariably negative, and radiologic evidence of joint erosion is uncommon. Hip and shoulder joint involvement is usually clinically indistinguishable from the tenderness and limited movement associated with myalgia. On ultrasonography, up to 2/3 of patients have hip or glenohumeral joint effusions.

Respiratory tract: One in 10 patients with giant cell arteritis has cough, sore throat, or hoarseness. However, these are rarely the presenting features. These symptoms may result from arteritis in the pharyngeal and laryngeal muscles. The situation is particularly confusing in the very old, in whom many disorders including chronic obstructive pulmonary disease are common.

The disease may also produce radiologic changes, ranging from vague patches suggestive of infection to large solid lesions easily mistaken for "cannonball" metastases. Pleural effusion occasionally follows pleural involvement by arteritis.

Kidney: About 1 in 10 patients with giant cell arteritis has asymptomatic, microscopic hematuria; a few cases of chronic renal failure and nephrotic syndrome have also been reported.

Liver: One third of patients with polymyalgia rheumatica in one series had an increased antimitochondrial antibody titer and an increased serum alkaline phosphatase concentration. Although the pathophysiology has not been defined, the abnormalities may result from hepatic arteritis. Fortunately, clinical manifestations of liver involvement are rare.

Thyroid: Some reports show an increased prevalence of thyroid antibodies and hypothyroidism in patients with polymyalgia rheumatica and giant cell arteritis.

Other complications: Giant cell arteritis can affect almost any organ (eg, it can mimic breast carcinoma by producing a hard mass attached to surrounding tissue, with axillary lymphadenopathy). Uterine involvement, producing blood and pus in a vaginal smear, has also been reported. Arteritis of mesenteric vessels may cause infarction of small bowel segments; intestinal perforation has also been reported. Polyneuropathies, mononeuropathies, and even sensorineural hearing losses have been encountered. However, these clinical curiosities are rarely seen in everyday clinical practice.

Laboratory Findings

The most useful laboratory test is the erythrocyte sedimentation rate **(ESR).** In both giant cell arteritis and polymyalgia rheumatica, it is usually > 40 mm/h and often > 100 mm/h. Although the ESR is very sensitive, it occasionally falls within normal values, particularly for polymyalgia rheumatica. A common diagnostic pitfall is that the ESR is sometimes measured in patients already taking low doses of corticosteroids. C-reactive protein **(CRP)** levels are also usually elevated in the two disorders; however, there is little evidence that the CRP level has a greater specificity or sensitivity than the ESR.

Antibody titers (eg, rheumatoid and antinuclear factors) are normal; if they are elevated, the initial diagnosis should be reevaluated. Other biochemical tests are of no value in establishing the primary diagnosis.

Patients often have a normochromic, normocytic **anemia,** which is of diagnostic value when associated with other clinical features of giant cell arteritis and polymyalgia rheumatica. Anemia occurring as an isolated finding confuses the diagnosis; the disease is identified as the anemic form of giant cell arteritis only by a process of exclusion.

Temporal artery biopsy is the most specific test for giant cell arteritis. About 3 to 5 cm of artery should be excised; a shorter section may miss the involved segment. Round cell and Langhans' giant cell infiltration of the media confirms the diagnosis; if the biopsy is negative, there is a 5% to 10% chance that the diagnosis has been missed. Therefore, in exceptional circumstances, a biopsy of the contralateral artery may be justified. Biopsy rarely causes scalp necrosis, but the risk increases considerably if both arteries are removed.

While temporal artery biopsy should be performed in all patients with clinical features of giant cell arteritis, its role in those with symptoms of only polymyalgia rheumatica is controversial. A reasonable approach is to reserve biopsy for patients who fail to respond to corticosteroid therapy, although the corticosteroid therapy may have modified the histologic picture, making pathologic diagnosis more difficult.

Differential Diagnosis

The clinical features of giant cell arteritis and polymyalgia rheumatica are well defined, and even when they overlap, the diagnosis should be straightforward based on the symptoms, signs, ESR, and biopsy described above. Diagnostic problems arise in the few patients who lack evidence of temporal artery involvement.

Most elderly patients with a hemiparesis and an elevated ESR have **cerebral atherosclerosis** and an associated or coincidental disorder causing the high ESR. When most of these disorders have been excluded, a temporal artery biopsy should be considered.

Concurrent angina is usually the result of **coronary atherosclerosis,** even if a patient has convincing evidence of giant cell arteritis or polymyalgia rheumatica. However, the cause of the angina does not affect the decision to treat with corticosteroids. Coronary angiography is not routinely indicated.

Because giant cell arteritis is much less common than **Buerger's disease,** it may be overlooked as a cause of upper limb ischemia. Ischemia of the lower limbs is less common, and the diagnosis is likely to be missed unless other clinical manifestations of arteritis occur. As in other situations, the most useful screening test is the ESR.

In the rare situation in which clinical evidence of temporal arteritis is minimal and radiologic evidence shows extensive pulmonary involvement, **Wegener's granulomatosis** must be ruled out. Severe upper respiratory involvement (eg, rhinorrhea or epistaxis) and deteriorating renal function suggest the latter diagnosis. Although round cell and giant cell infiltration of arteries is found in Wegener's granulomatosis, the temporal arteries are rarely affected. A positive test for cytoplasmic antineutrophil antibodies further increases the likely diagnosis of granulomatosis.

Systemic lupus erythematosus is relatively uncommon in extreme old age, and most patients have high titers of antinuclear antibodies. If doubt remains, a temporal artery biopsy is usually conclusive.

Although **periarteritis nodosa** can involve almost any system, it usually causes fever, abdominal pain, hypertension, edema, and a polyneuropathy. Albuminuria and hematuria are also prominent. Renal biopsy should clarify the diagnosis.

Takayasu's disease, a rare form of arteritis, causes stenosis and occlusion of the major aortic branches, thus mimicking an atypical presentation of giant cell arteritis. However, because this disease affects primarily young women, it presents few diagnostic problems in the elderly.

Although about 15% of patients with giant cell arteritis have synovitis, only the large and sternoclavicular joints are involved, making the

TABLE 74–1. OTHER CAUSES OF POLYMYALGIA

Connective Tissue Disorders	*Neoplastic Disorders*	*Others*
Dermatomyositis Periarteritis nodosa	Carcinoma Multiple myeloma Waldenström's macroglobulinemia	Sarcoidosis Subacute bacterial endocarditis Osteomalacia Drug therapy (eg, HMG-CoA reductase inhibitors)

distribution totally different from that found in **rheumatoid arthritis.** Titers of rheumatoid factor are not increased. If a patient with rheumatoid arthritis develops polymyalgia rheumatica, this situation simply represents two concurrent diseases that are relatively common in old age. However, rheumatoid arthritis may mask concurrent polymyalgia rheumatica, causing a potentially reversible condition to go untreated.

Other causes of polymyalgia: TABLE 74–1 lists other causes of polymyalgia in the elderly. Most of these conditions rarely occur with polymyalgia. An exception is that pelvic girdle pain and tenderness is often the first manifestation of osteomalacia. Also, patients with carcinomatosis in advanced age can present with symptoms of polymyalgia.

Prognosis

Both giant cell arteritis and polymyalgia rheumatica are usually self-limited disorders, resolving within 5 yr of onset. In the interim, without treatment they may cause considerable discomfort and permanent incapacity. Recent longitudinal surveys suggest a standardized mortality rate of between 1 and 3 times normal, indicating a reduced life expectancy, even when the patient is treated with corticosteroids. More common causes of excess mortality are cerebrovascular disease, myocardial infarction, heart failure, rupture of an aortic aneurysm, and pulmonary embolism.

Treatment

Treatment with corticosteroids produces a dramatic response. The headache of temporal arteritis resolves, and even more serious problems (eg, blindness, angina, or upper-limb claudication) may remit within a few days if therapy is started soon enough. Symptoms of polymyalgia rheumatica also remit, and a person who was severely crippled may regain mobility and full independence within the first week of treatment.

The starting dose should be the equivalent of 60 to 80 mg prednisone daily for giant cell arteritis, and 30 to 40 mg daily for polymyalgia rheumatica for at least 2 mo. Efficacy should be monitored by serial determination of ESR. The dose can be gradually reduced to between 4 and 20 mg daily depending upon the ESR and clinical signs and symptoms. A larger initial dose of prednisone (eg, 120 mg daily) may be appropriate in a patient with such complications as scalp ulceration or hematuria.

If vision has recently deteriorated or disappeared, a larger dosage of corticosteroids may be effective (eg, 240 mg prednisone orally for 3 days). If this is ineffective, a massive IV infusion of 1000 mg prednisolone bid for 5 days may be indicated. The possible benefit of such treatment has to be balanced against the risk of serious complications (eg, GI hemorrhage, psychosis, or heart failure).

Maintenance therapy for both giant cell arteritis and polymyalgia rheumatica should be continued for 2 yr, then gradual withdrawal should be attempted. During this period, the patient should be closely monitored for an elevated ESR or a recurrence of symptoms. These effects occur in more than 50% of patients, and as many as 40% may still be taking corticosteroids 4 yr after starting treatment. After corticosteroids are discontinued, a patient should be monitored for at least 6 mo.

One way to reduce the cumulative dose of corticosteroids is to give depot methylprednisolone acetate. The starting dosage is 120 mg IM q 3 wk for 12 wk, which is reduced in response to changes in clinical features and the ESR. Another way to avoid serious side effects of long-term corticosteroid therapy is to treat patients concurrently with an immunosuppressant (eg, azathioprine or methotrexate). The added agent reduces the required dose of corticosteroid, and the drugs appear to be well tolerated. However, this approach should be further investigated before it can be generally advocated.

75. BONE, JOINT, AND RHEUMATIC DISORDERS

Musculoskeletal diseases are the leading cause of functional impairment in older patients. Incurable but rarely fatal, these disabling problems are chronic. However, musculoskeletal disease is not an inevitable consequence of aging and thus should be regarded as a specific disease process.

History and Physical Examination

The primary complaint of the patient with musculoskeletal disease is pain, the characteristics of which help narrow the differential diagnosis. The most important characteristics are the location (regional or diffuse), pattern (articular or nonarticular), timing (when it occurs), and

TABLE 75–1. DIFFERENTIAL DIAGNOSIS OF MUSCULOSKELETAL DISEASE BASED ON LOCATION AND QUALITY OF PAIN

Location	*Quality*	*Disease*
Generalized pain		
Articular	Noninflammatory	Osteoarthritis (distal and proximal interphalangeal joints, first carpometacarpal joints, knees, hips, toes)
	Inflammatory	Rheumatoid arthritis (proximal interphalangeal and metacarpophalangeal joints, wrists, shoulders, elbows, knees, ankles, feet) Systemic lupus erythematosus Polyarticular gout Calcium pyrophosphate dihydrate crystal disease Arthritis of malignancy
Nonarticular	Noninflammatory	Fibromyalgia Metastatic carcinoma Multiple myeloma
	Inflammatory	Polymyalgia rheumatica
Localized pain		
Articular	Noninflammatory	Fracture Osteoarthritis Aseptic necrosis Internal derangement
	Inflammatory	Septic arthritis Microcrystalline disease (gout, calcium pyrophosphate dihydrate crystal disease) Bursitis and tendonitis Knee (anserine, prepatellar) Shoulder (subdeltoid, bicipital) Elbow (olecranon)
Nonarticular	Noninflammatory	Carpal tunnel syndrome Nerve root compression Fracture Reflex sympathetic dystrophy Neuroarthropathy
	Inflammatory	Soft tissue infection

Adapted from Ettinger WH Jr: "Approach to the diagnosis and management of musculoskeletal disease." *Clinics in Geriatric Medicine* 4(2):269–277, 1988; used with permission.

association with other symptoms of the inflammatory process (ie, swelling, warmth, and stiffness). Considerations for differential diagnosis are listed in TABLE 75–1.

The clinician focuses on the symptomatic area, while examining the entire musculoskeletal system, noting tenderness, deformity, swelling, and loss of motion. An evaluation of asymptomatic joints is especially important because painless swelling or loss of motion in several joints may indicate a systemic or generalized inflammatory process not elicited by the history.

A **performance-oriented examination** should include evaluation of the back and all extremities. The clinician should test grip strength, the ability to hold objects (eg, eating utensils or writing instruments), and the ability to raise the arms over the head. The examination of the back includes assessing the ability to bend at the waist, to touch the feet, and to pick up objects from the floor. The examination of the legs focuses on mobility and includes testing the patient's ability to rise from a chair, to maintain balance, to initiate and maintain gait, to turn, and to return to the sitting position. The evaluation of endurance includes assessing the ability to climb stairs and to walk for 5 min.

Laboratory Tests

Laboratory testing has three potential pitfalls: (1) no definitive diagnostic tests exist for most musculoskeletal diseases; (2) many diagnostic tests have high sensitivity for disease but lack specificity; and (3) the normal values for certain laboratory tests may change with age, and certain test results (eg, those for autoantibodies) may be positive in older persons but may not indicate disease (see Ch. 113). Thus, *a clinician should not use laboratory tests to screen for rheumatic disease but rather should order specific tests to diagnose a disease when the pretest probability of the disease is high.*

Treatment

In treating the elderly patient, the clinician should separate the direct consequences of musculoskeletal disease from its effects on function. A helpful tool is a conceptual framework, such as the World Health Organization's International Classification of Impairments, Disabilities, and Handicaps. **Impairment** is defined as any psychologic, physiologic, or anatomic loss or abnormality, either temporary or permanent. Examples relevant to musculoskeletal disease include loss of a limb, loss of range of motion, or pain on motion. **Disability** is defined as the inability to perform an activity in the manner or within the range considered normal for a particular person. Thus, a disability almost always entails lost performance of compound or integrated tasks (eg, walking or combing one's hair). **Handicap** is defined as limited fulfillment of an individual's role based on age, sex, and social and cultural factors. A handicap, therefore, is a social disadvantage resulting from an impairment or disability (eg, loss of social interaction). Using this classification, a clinician can determine which disabilities or handicaps are most important to the person, rather than focus on impairments that do not affect function.

Three principles govern treatment of musculoskeletal disease in the elderly: (1) Therapy should be aimed at restoring function and improving the quality of life. (2) The patient should be involved in decision making, and his preferences should guide the goals of therapy. (3) A multifaceted approach to therapy should include pain treatment, physical therapy (including therapeutic exercise) or occupational therapy, psychologic support, and environmental manipulation.

The goals of therapy should be well defined and realistic. For example, a patient may be physically able to undergo rehabilitation after total joint replacement, but if appropriate social supports are lacking, the treatment goals may not be achieved.

OSTEOARTHRITIS

Primarily a disorder of hyaline cartilage and subchondral bone, though all tissues in and around involved joints are hypertrophic. Osteoarthritis is the most common joint disease. Although many persons with radiographic evidence of osteoarthritis have no symptoms, osteoarthritis is a leading cause of physical disability in persons > 65 yr.

Osteoarthritis is probably not one disease but several having similar clinical and pathologic features. Thus, the typical changes, which include both cartilage deterioration and bony remodeling, occur in a number of diarthrodial joints but may have different causes in each. Several factors are implicated. Aging alone does not cause osteoarthritis, although cellular or matrix alterations in cartilage that occur with aging probably predispose older persons to osteoarthritis. Other presumed factors include obesity (particularly for lower extremity osteoarthritis), trauma, congenital abnormalities (eg, hip dysplasia), and primary disorders of the joint (eg, inflammatory arthritis).

When no predisposing cause is known, the disorder is called primary osteoarthritis. When a clearly defined underlying condition (eg, trauma, metabolic disease, or inflammatory arthritis) is a contributing cause, the disorder is called secondary osteoarthritis.

Symptoms and Signs

Primary osteoarthritis is characterized by a slow progression of intermittent or constant joint pain that may be accompanied by limited movement and joint deformity. Pain is relieved by rest and exacerbated by movement and weight bearing; it is not associated with inflammatory symptoms. Primary osteoarthritis affects the distal and proximal interphalangeal joints, first carpometacarpal joint, cervical and lumbar spine, hips, knees, and toes. The metacarpophalangeal joints, wrists, elbows, shoulders, and ankles usually are spared in primary osteoarthritis.

Diagnosis

The diagnosis is based on clinical findings and the presence of osteoarthritic changes on x-ray. Characteristic x-ray features include osteophytes, subchondral sclerosis and cysts, and asymmetric loss of joint space (implying degeneration of cartilage). Conventional x-rays are not sensitive in detecting early osteoarthritis because they do not show pathologic changes in cartilage. Other imaging techniques such as magnetic resonance imaging and ultrasonography are more sensitive than conventional x-ray in detecting osteoarthritis but should not be used routinely. Other laboratory data are not helpful. The erythrocyte sedimentation rate and WBC count are normal, and no autoantibodies are found. Examination of synovial fluid from affected joints shows only a mild leukocytosis (a WBC count of $< 2000/\mu L$) and no other diagnostic features.

Treatment

When deciding on a therapeutic regimen, the physician must recognize that several factors may increase morbidity in the older patient. These factors include the physiologic changes of aging; other chronic diseases; and psychologic, environmental, social, and iatrogenic problems (see TABLE 75–2). Thus, the physician must decide if treating osteoarthritis alone will improve functioning or if other problems must also be treated. Also, other diseases (eg, renal disease, peptic ulcer, and hypertension) may make pharmacologic treatment of osteoarthritis more hazardous and difficult.

Comprehensive management involves a balance of psychotherapeutic, physical, pharmaceutical, and surgical measures. Specific goals of therapy must take into account the functional deficits and the patient's preferences for treatment. The patient should be taught the nature of the disease and realistic treatment expectations. Unrealistic expectations can lead to frustration, depression, and misunderstanding between the patient and the physician.

Pain relief is the cornerstone of therapy. Nonpharmacologic strategies include resting when pain is severe, altering activities to avoid repetitive movements that aggravate symptoms, and losing weight. A regimen of range-of-motion, strengthening, and endurance exercises is an important component in pain relief and functional restoration.

Pharmacologic therapy: The most commonly used drugs are acetaminophen and nonsteroidal anti-inflammatory drugs (NSAIDs; see TABLE 75–3). Acetaminophen is the first choice for pain relief because it is safer than the NSAIDs and often is effective. However, when patients do not respond to acetaminophen, an NSAID should be used. No evidence indicates that one NSAID is more efficacious than another in treating osteoarthritis. However, individual response to these drugs varies greatly, and several may be tried before relief is obtained. These drugs can be used on an as-needed basis; the lowest possible dose should be used.

TABLE 75–2. FACTORS THAT INCREASE MORBIDITY IN OSTEOARTHRITIS

Physiologic changes frequently associated with aging	Neurologic Motor system: Loss of muscle mass and strength; diminished balance reflexes Sensory system: Diminished proprioceptive and vibratory input; slowed reaction time Cardiovascular Blunted baroreflexes Decreased aerobic capacity
Chronic diseases	Musculoskeletal Fractures Primary muscle disease Painful foot conditions Neurologic Stroke Parkinson's disease Degenerative dementias Peripheral neuropathy Cardiovascular Heart failure Peripheral vascular disease Pulmonary Chronic obstructive pulmonary disease Other Blindness Severe systemic illness
Psychologic factors	Depression Cognitive impairment Poor motivation Poor coping skills
Environmental, social, and iatrogenic factors	Forced immobility Physical obstructions Lack of social support Drug side effects

Adapted from Ettinger WH Jr, Davis MA: "Osteoarthritis," in *Principles of Geriatric Medicine and Gerontology*, ed. 2, edited by WR Hazzard, R Andres, EL Bierman, JP Blass. New York, McGraw-Hill, 1990, pp 880–888; used with permission.

The dosage schedule for NSAIDs varies from one to four times per day; the major side effects of the different agents are similar. Each drug differs, however, in its propensity for side effects in individual patients. Consequently, the choice of drug should depend partially on the pa-

TABLE 75–3. NONSTEROIDAL ANTI-INFLAMMATORY DRUGS

Drug	*Usual Dosage Range*
Aspirin	625–1250 mg tid or qid
Diclofenac	50–75 mg bid
Diflunisal	250–500 mg bid
Etodolac	600–1200 mg/day in 2–4 doses
Fenoprofen	300–600 mg tid or qid
Flurbiprofen	200–300 mg/day in 2–4 doses
Ibuprofen	200–800 mg tid or qid
Indomethacin	25–50 mg tid or qid
Ketoprofen	25–75 mg tid or qid
Meclofenamate sodium	50–100 mg tid or qid
Nabumetone	500–2000 mg/day
Naproxen	250–500 mg bid
Naproxen sodium	275–550 mg bid
Nonacetylated salicylates	3–4 gm/day
Oxaprozin	600–1800 mg/day
Piroxicam	10–20 mg once a day
Sulindac	150–200 mg bid
Tolmetin sodium	200–600 mg tid

tient's tolerance or potential for developing a toxic reaction. The most common side effect is GI upset, which often occurs without evidence of ulceration or bleeding and may require discontinuance of the drug.

Ulcers and GI bleeding occur with all NSAIDs and are related to dose and frequency of use. Unfortunately, ulceration and bleeding do not correlate with subjective symptoms; thus, bleeding can occur without warning. Taking these medications with food may help minimize GI symptoms, and the concomitant use of cytoprotective agents, such as the prostaglandin misoprostol, may decrease the incidence of ulceration in high-risk patients.

The NSAIDs rank second to aminoglycosides as a cause of drug-induced acute renal failure. Therefore, they should be used cautiously in the elderly, particularly in those who have underlying renal disease, heart failure, volume depletion, or liver disease. Important, rare toxic effects in the elderly include cognitive dysfunction and personality changes. Patients and family should be questioned about CNS symptoms.

Other analgesics may be used occasionally. In general, systemic corticosteroids and narcotic analgesics should be *avoided*. However, intra-articular corticosteroids are indicated for a large, painful joint effusion unresponsive to other modalities. The most efficacious corticosteroid preparations are the least soluble ones, and a formulation of triamcinolone is recommended.

Surgery: **Total joint arthroplasty** is highly effective in managing osteoarthritis, and age alone should not be a contraindication. However, the decision to operate is complex; the goals to be achieved and the needs and capabilities of the patient must first be clearly defined.

Arthroscopy with lavage of the knee joint has been advocated as a therapy for osteoarthritis, but currently there are no adequately controlled trials to support its use. Arthroscopy may be used as a diagnostic and therapeutic technique for internal derangements, such as a torn meniscus.

RHEUMATOID ARTHRITIS

A chronic syndrome characterized by nonspecific, usually symmetric inflammation of the peripheral joints, possibly resulting in progressive destruction of articular and periarticular structures. The incidence of rheumatoid arthritis declines after age 65. However, because rheumatoid arthritis is a chronic illness, its prevalence is increased in older populations. The cause is unknown, but rheumatoid arthritis is characterized by intense inflammation of the synovium of the diarthrodial joints. Synovial tissue becomes hyperplastic and infiltrated with lymphocytes and plasma cells. A variety of inflammatory mediators, including cytokines, prostaglandins, and immunoglobulins, are found in the synovial fluid.

Symptoms and Signs

In most older patients with rheumatoid arthritis, the disease process began in middle age. Some patients have secondary joint deformities and degenerative changes even though the inflammation is inactive.

When rheumatoid arthritis develops de novo in an older person, the onset may be insidious or acute. In most patients, the arthritis is accompanied by mild or moderate constitutional symptoms. Usually, rheumatoid arthritis occurs primarily in the small joints of the hands (proximal interphalangeal, metacarpophalangeal), feet (metatarsophalangeal, interphalangeal), and the wrist; later, the disease involves the larger joints (eg, elbows, shoulders, knees). When an acute onset occurs, patients often experience constitutional symptoms, such as malaise, anorexia, and weight loss. Fever and night sweats occasionally are reported. Eventually, rheumatoid arthritis becomes a symmetric, additive disease of the joints, as in younger patients.

Laboratory Findings

Several abnormal test results occur in patients with rheumatoid arthritis; however, most are common to other inflammatory diseases. Abnormal findings include a normochromic, normocytic anemia; mild leukocytosis; and thrombocytosis. The erythrocyte sedimentation rate is elevated in about 80% of cases, and positive rheumatoid factor is present in about 50%. Rheumatoid factor in high titer (≥ 1:320) is highly specific for the disease; in contrast, low titers are seen with other diseases and in up to 25% of older patients without evidence of any disease. Initially, x-rays of involved joints usually show only soft tissue swelling. Characteristic late features include periarticular osteoporosis, joint-space narrowing, and marginal erosions.

Diagnosis

The diagnosis is based on clinical judgment and requires that the patient exhibit symmetric inflammatory arthritis involving the appropriate joints and prolonged morning stiffness lasting ≥ 1 h. Other diseases (eg, polymyalgia rheumatica, systemic lupus erythematosus, and the arthritis of malignancy) must be excluded.

Treatment

In general, the long-term prognosis for patients with rheumatoid arthritis is poor. Most become progressively disabled despite appropriate treatment, and higher rates of serious infections and perhaps cardiovascular disease increase mortality. Nevertheless, many patients do respond to treatment. Therapy should begin with **aspirin** or **another NSAID.** Also, physical and occupational therapy are essential along with exercise, the use of assistive devices, and possibly, physical modalities for pain relief (eg, locally applied heat or cold). Although rest should be encouraged when symptoms are severe, *prolonged bed rest may lead to irreversible immobility in an older patient*. Other chronic diseases and the loss of aerobic capacity and muscle strength associated with aging lower the threshold at which functional ability is so severely compromised that it cannot be restored.

An alternative to an NSAID is low-dose **prednisone** (eg, a 1-mo regimen starting at 25 mg/day and tapering to 5 to 10 mg/day). Because discontinuing corticosteroid therapy is difficult, the long-term effects (osteoporosis, cataracts, poor wound healing, hyperglycemia, hypertension, reactivation of tuberculosis, and increased risk of infection) must be balanced against the therapeutic benefits. **Intra-articular steroids** may be helpful in treating a single acutely inflamed rheumatoid joint.

Slow-acting antirheumatic drugs can be used when the response to an NSAID or low-dose prednisone is inadequate. These drugs appear to be effective in older people, but are associated with a high rate of side effects. Among the slow-acting agents, **methotrexate** is the first choice. It can be given at 7.5 mg/wk in 3 doses of 2.5 mg; the dosage may be increased to 15 mg/wk. The drug can also be given once weekly, beginning with a 5-mg dose and increasing it gradually. Patients receiving methotrexate need close monitoring because of the risks of hepatic toxicity, interstitial pneumonitis, bone marrow suppression, and GI ulceration and bleeding. The drug should not be given to patients with renal insufficiency. Aspirin may increase the toxicity of methotrexate by slowing its excretion rate.

The antimalarial **hydroxychloroquine** can be used in dosages of 6.5 mg/kg/day or 400 mg/day to treat rheumatoid arthritis that is not responding adequately to NSAIDs. Hydroxychloroquine can cause severe and sometimes irreversible adverse effects, particularly loss of vision. However, vision can be spared by having an ophthalmologist monitor vision at 6-mo intervals and discontinuing the drug at the first signs of retinal toxicity.

Gold therapy can be effective for mild to moderate rheumatoid arthritis. Gold sodium thiomalate and aurothioglucose are injectable; auranofin, the oral preparation, appears to be less toxic but may be less effective than the injectable forms. Injectable gold is administered in a test dose of 10 mg, followed by a therapeutic dose of 25 to 50 mg/wk for up to 20 wk. If the patient responds, treatment intervals are increased to 2 wk, then 3 wk, then 1 mo. Monthly therapy should be continued indefinitely to prevent a recurrence. The usual dosage of auranofin is 3 mg bid or 6 mg/day. The dosage may be increased to 3 mg tid after 6 mo if no therapeutic response occurs.

The most common side effects of gold therapy are skin rash, oral lesions, proteinuria, and falling peripheral blood counts. *Proteinuria, leukopenia, or thrombocytopenia requires permanent discontinuance of the drug.* Pruritus often precedes stomatitis and a diffuse rash, which may cause exfoliation. *When pruritus or a minor rash develops, gold therapy should be discontinued.* If the rash resolves, the drug may be restarted at a lower dose. Oral gold therapy causes less mucocutaneous and renal toxicity but more diarrhea and GI reactions.

The starting dosage of **penicillamine** is 125 to 250 mg/day, which is increased at 2- to 3-mo intervals by 125- to 250-mg increments to a total of 750 mg/day. Penicillamine should be taken between meals because food decreases absorption. Adverse effects include rash, proteinuria, dysgeusia, and thrombocytopenia; patients taking this medication must be monitored closely. More severe side effects (eg, pemphigus, myasthenia gravis, a lupus-like syndrome, and severe bone marrow suppression) have also been reported.

The cytotoxic drugs **azathioprine** and **cyclophosphamide** also have been used to treat patients with refractory rheumatoid arthritis.

SYSTEMIC LUPUS ERYTHEMATOSUS

An inflammatory connective tissue disorder that occurs mainly in women of childbearing age but also in older persons. The cause of systemic lupus erythematosus (SLE) is unknown, but its pathogenesis involves the formation of autoantibodies and immune complexes, resulting in damage to several organs. The incidence of SLE declines in old age, but in large series, patients > 50 yr account for about 12% of cases. Furthermore, the female:male ratio declines to about 3:1 in older populations. In contrast to idiopathic SLE, **drug-induced SLE** increases in prevalence with age, probably because of the greater use of predisposing drugs (eg, procainamide, hydralazine, and anticonvulsants).

Diagnosis

Diagnostic symptoms and signs are similar in elderly and younger persons. Typical clinical features include rash, asymmetric migratory arthritis, photosensitivity, pleurisy, pericarditis, pneumonitis, and Sjögren's syndrome. Some authorities contend that CNS manifestations, hematologic manifestations, and renal disease are unusual in older patients.

Clinical features of drug-induced SLE are similar to those of idiopathic SLE, although CNS and renal manifestations are uncommon.

Laboratory Tests

The antinuclear antibodies (ANA) test results are positive in 95% of patients with idiopathic SLE and in 100% with drug-induced SLE. About 50% of patients taking procainamide have a positive ANA test, and about 5% to 10% develop an SLE-like syndrome. Although patients with SLE have many other autoantibodies, these autoantibodies are not usually helpful in diagnosis. Serum complement levels may be depressed, particularly in patients with renal disease. The urinalysis may show proteinuria or cells and casts on microscopic examination, and the CBC count may show thrombocytopenia, leukopenia, and anemia.

Treatment

Treatment depends on the specific manifestations of SLE. Patients with mild disease, who have primarily arthritis or skin rash, may respond to treatment with an NSAID. Corticosteroids in high doses are indicated when the patient has CNS, renal, or severe hematologic manifestations. Usually, these drugs are also indicated when the patient has fever, weight loss, or severe pleurisy or pericarditis. Hydroxychloroquine may be useful in treating SLE, particularly in patients with marked skin involvement.

For drug-induced SLE, discontinuing the causative agent and administering an anti-inflammatory drug may be sufficient. However, some patients, particularly those with severe pericarditis, may need as much as 40 mg/day of prednisone for several weeks.

SJÖGREN'S SYNDROME

A cell-mediated autoimmune disease that results in inflammation, dysfunction, and destruction of the exocrine glands. This syndrome is characterized by decreased lacrimal and salivary gland activity **(sicca syndrome)** and a connective tissue disorder. Up to 25% of older people report xerophthalmia (dry eyes) and xerostomia (dry mouth), but most of these people have atrophic mucus-producing cells rather than an autoimmune disease.

Symptoms, Signs, and Diagnosis

The most common signs of Sjögren's syndrome are xerophthalmia and xerostomia. Patients complain of a foreign body sensation or grittiness in the eyes. Patients also have a need to drink copious amounts of fluids, a loss of taste, and excessive dental caries. Occasionally, Sjögren's syndrome is accompanied by systemic manifestations including Raynaud's phenomenon, polyarthritis, interstitial pneumonitis, vasculitis, neurologic and psychiatric manifestations, and loss of other exocrine functions.

The diagnosis is made from the clinical symptoms. The Schirmer's test (in which eye moisture is measured with a small strip of filter paper) has been advocated as a screening test for Sjögren's syndrome; however, this test is not standardized. Persons with Sjögren's syndrome exhibit focal or diffuse lymphocytic infiltration of the glands. Sjögren's syndrome may be accompanied by autoantibodies, including anti-Ro and anti-La, in the blood. The diagnosis can be confirmed by biopsy of the minor salivary gland of the lip, although it is rarely needed.

Treatment

Treatment of this syndrome is symptomatic. Artificial tears and lemon and glycerin mouth rinse are the standard therapies. For the systemic forms of Sjögren's syndrome, corticosteroids and other immunosuppressants have been tried with varied success.

SCLERODERMA
(Systemic Sclerosis)

An autoimmune disease characterized by fibrosis of the subcutaneous tissue and characteristic thickening of the skin over the fingers, arms, chest, and face. The cause of scleroderma is unknown. It is rare in older people.

Symptoms, Signs, and Diagnosis

Besides the characteristic skin thickening, symptoms include telangiectasis, Raynaud's phenomenon, esophageal dysmotility, pulmonary fibrosis, and occasionally vascular involvement of the heart and kidneys. Scleroderma sometimes occurs as part of an overlap syndrome, called mixed connective tissue disease. Autoantibodies are often found, especially anticentromere and anti-SCL-70.

Treatment

In early stages of scleroderma, treatment is largely symptomatic and includes the use of gloves and calcium channel blockers to prevent Raynaud's phenomenon. Penicillamine 250 to 500 mg/day has been advocated. However, no randomized clinical trials have shown this drug to be effective. It has significant side effects, and its toxicity may preclude use in older patients. Occasionally, patients present with acute renal failure and hypertensive crisis. This condition can be treated safely and effectively with angiotensin converting enzyme inhibitors.

GOUT

A recurrent acute arthritis of peripheral joints that results when crystals of monosodium urate from supersaturated hyperuricemic body fluids are deposited in and about the joints and tendons. **Primary gout** is most often a midlife disease of men; gout in women most often occurs after menopause. Gout correlates with hyperuricemia (usually serum urate levels > 7 mg/dL). Hyperuricemia represents an imbalance between endogenous uric acid production and renal urate excretion. Most cases of primary and most types of secondary hyperuricemia are characterized by a defect in renal handling of uric acid. Hyperuricemia may be exacerbated by drugs commonly taken by elderly patients (eg, thiazide diuretics and salicylates, even in small doses).

Symptoms, Signs, and Diagnosis

The onset of gout is marked by an acute inflammatory arthritis (acute gouty arthritis) that may follow trauma, illness, or surgery. The metatarsophalangeal joint of the great toe is the typical site of an acute attack **(podagra).** Other joints may be involved either as a monarthritis or in a polyarticular pattern including the ankle, knee, wrist, elbow, small joints of the hands or feet, and bursae (especially the bursa of olecranon).

Fever (temperature up to 39° C [102.2° F]) often develops. Tenderness is usually so exquisite that the patient cannot move the affected joint or tolerate the weight of bedclothes. The inflammatory process often extends beyond the joint, suggesting cellulitis in some cases. Untreated, the acute attack resolves in a few days to weeks. A history of recurrent acute episodes of arthritis, especially involving the great toe, should suggest the possibility of gout.

Chronic gouty arthritis may cause morning stiffness and achy joints, mimicking rheumatoid arthritis and other chronic polyarticular arthritides. It occurs primarily in patients who have tophaceous gout. Such patients often have x-ray evidence of urate deposits in soft tissue or bone adjacent to the joints. Sodium urate deposits in soft tissue increase with the severity of hyperuricemia. These deposits, called tophi, are commonly found in bursae, the articular cartilage, and bone. Tophi may be confused with rheumatoid nodules when they appear in the bursa of olecranon or over the extensor surface of the forearm.

Laboratory Findings

Acute gouty arthritis may be accompanied by leukocytosis and an elevated erythrocyte sedimentation rate. Elevated serum urate levels support the diagnosis but are not specific. The definitive finding is urate crystals in the synovial fluid of an affected joint. Synovial fluid should be analyzed, particularly when differentiating gout from infection is difficult. In acute gouty arthritis, the synovial fluid shows typical inflammatory changes with a WBC count in the 5000 to 50,000/μL range. In 90% of cases, urate crystals can be seen free in the fluid or engulfed by phagocytes. When viewed with a polarizing microscope, they are negatively birefringent.

Treatment

A simple, effective way to manage acute gouty arthritis is by giving an NSAID at the usual dosage (see TABLE 75–3). Relief occurs in 24 h, and symptoms usually resolve in 3 days, when the NSAID can be discontinued. Alternatively, colchicine can be given either IV or orally. Colchicine 1 to 2 mg diluted in 0.9% sodium chloride and injected IV over 20 min is highly effective in relieving acute symptoms. Oral colchicine at 0.5 mg bid to qid for 2 to 3 days may be necessary to provide complete relief. Oral colchicine 0.5 mg q 2 h also may be given until a favorable response is obtained or GI toxicity supervenes. However, because almost all patients must take colchicine until GI toxicity occurs, this treatment is not usually recommended.

An effective measure for treating acute gout of the large joints is withdrawing synovial fluid and injecting a long-lasting steroid (triamcinolone) at a dose of 20 to 40 mg. This treatment is especially effective in patients who are unable to take oral medications or who cannot tolerate NSAIDs or colchicine.

Uricosuric drugs and allopurinol should be *avoided* during the acute attack. The incidence of recurrent acute gouty arthritis may be lowered by long-term administration of colchicine 0.5 mg bid.

Measures to lower serum uric acid may be indicated for the presence of tophi, recurrent gouty arthritis uncontrolled by long-term colchicine administration, and the presence of renal urate stones.

Allopurinol blocks the metabolic pathway of uric acid production, specifically inhibiting xanthine oxidase. Because allopurinol does not produce its effect through the kidney and actually reduces the renal urate load, it is indicated in patients with renal calculi. The initial dosage of 100 mg bid may be increased gradually to 600 mg/day to achieve the desired effect.

Alternatives to allopurinol are the uricosuric agents, eg, probenecid, which should be administered initially at 500 mg q 12 h. This dosage may be increased to 3 gm/day to reduce the serum uric acid level to 6 mg/dL. An alternative to probenecid is sulfinpyrazone. This relatively short-acting drug must be given q 6 h in divided doses ranging from 300 to 1000 mg/day.

CALCIUM PYROPHOSPHATE DIHYDRATE CRYSTAL DISEASE

(Pseudogout)

A microcrystalline arthritis associated with calcification of hyaline and fibrous cartilage (chondrocalcinosis). Rare before the fifth decade, this disease is more common with advancing age. The mechanism of cartilage calcification is poorly understood; however, the association of chondrocalcinosis and arthritis with an array of diseases suggests that many factors play a role. Certain conditions predispose persons to calcium pyrophosphate dihydrate crystal disease, including hyperparathyroidism, acromegaly, and hypothyroidism.

Symptoms and Signs

The disease was originally called **pseudogout** to emphasize the acute, episodic, goutlike attacks of synovial inflammation. However, unlike gout, acute calcium pyrophosphate dihydrate crystal disease usually occurs in large joints, especially the knee. The shoulder, hip, wrist, and elbow may also be involved. This disease may cause a chronic, asymmetric, inflammatory polyarthritis, which in some cases mimics rheumatoid arthritis.

Laboratory Findings

Hematologic findings are nonspecific. Serum calcium levels are normal unless hyperparathyroidism is present. Hyperuricemia may be present and may play a role in pathogenesis. Chondrocalcinosis of the fibrocartilaginous menisci of the knees, the radial and ulnar joints, the symphysis pubis, and the articular disk of the sternoclavicular joint frequently appears on x-ray. In the acute form of this disease, the synovial fluid has a WBC count of 2,000 to 50,000/μL, which is typical of an inflammatory process. On examination, intracellular and extracellular calcium pyrophosphate dihydrate crystals can be identified in 90% of effusions. These crystals are generally rhomboid and, unlike urate crystals, are positively birefringent under polarized light.

Diagnosis

The diagnosis is based on a clinical history of recurrent, episodic acute attacks and the demonstration of calcium pyrophosphate dihydrate crystals in synovial fluid. A search for crystals using polarized light microscopy may be necessary, particularly when the patient has polyarticular chronic disease. The diagnosis is supported by x-ray demonstration of chondrocalcinosis of cartilage.

Treatment

As with gout, NSAID therapy is effective for an acute attack. Intra-articular corticosteroids may be useful when a large joint is involved, and colchicine therapy, as described above for gout, is also effective.

BURSITIS

Acute or chronic inflammation of a bursa. The causes of bursitis are varied and include acute and chronic trauma, crystal deposition disease, and infection. Occasionally, bursae are involved in systemic inflammatory diseases such as rheumatoid arthritis.

Symptoms, Signs, and Diagnosis

Subdeltoid (subacromial) bursitis: The subdeltoid bursa is located between the deltoid muscle and the joint capsule, extending under the acromion and coracoacromial ligament. Shoulder pain is a common problem in older adults, and bursitis is an important, common cause of nonarticular shoulder pain. Bursitis is often accompanied by inflammation of the supraspinatus tendon, and the two problems may be indistinguishable. Inflammation of the subdeltoid bursa results in painful shoulder movement, particularly abduction and extension. Pain mainly over the anterior shoulder aggravated by forearm supination against resistance is more likely to reflect bicipital tendinitis. Patients with subdeltoid bursitis tend to awaken at night when they turn on the affected shoulder. The pain often radiates down the arm in the C-5 dermatome.

Physical examination reveals tenderness over the lateral shoulder and the subacromial space. Pain can be elicited if the arm is abducted and then actively moved toward the body against resistance. Patients report pain on moving the arm downward through the arc of abduction at about 90°.

Trochanteric bursitis: The trochanteric bursa lies between the gluteus maximus and the tendon of the gluteus medius. The usual symptom of inflammation is a dull, aching pain or a burning, tingling sensation over the lateral hip. The pain may also be referred to the L-2 dermatome. Pain is worse with activity and after sitting with the affected leg crossed over the other. Sleep disturbances and an inability to lie on the affected side are common.

Physical examination reveals localized tenderness over the bony prominence of the greater trochanter. External rotation with abduction of the hip is often painful, although the range of motion is normal.

Anserine bursitis: The anserine bursa is located about 4 cm below the medial aspect of the knee joint. It lies under the pes anserinus (the combined insertion of the tendinous expansions of the sartorius, gracilis, and semitendinous muscles). The patient with anserine bursitis complains of knee pain that is worse at night. In bed, the patient needs a pillow between the knees. Physical examination may elicit point tenderness over the bursa and, occasionally, mild to moderate swelling.

Olecranon bursitis: The bursa of olecranon lies between the skin and the olecranon process. The usual presentation of this bursitis is swelling and tenderness over the most proximal part of the ulna. On physical examination, the elbow joint exhibits painless full range of motion.

Treatment

Before treating anserine and olecranon bursitis, determining the cause is important. If the history and physical examination do not yield an obvious degenerative or traumatic cause, aspiration and examination of the bursal fluid are indicated to determine if crystal deposits or infection is present. Aspiration and examination of subdeltoid or trochanteric bursae are rarely necessary before treatment unless signs of infection exist. A bursal fluid WBC count of $\geq$ 2000/μL suggests an inflammatory process. The fluid should be examined microscopically for crystals, and a Gram stain should be performed to exclude infection.

If infection is present, the most common organisms are those that colonize the skin: *Staphylococcus aureus* and group A streptococci. Antibiotic therapy should be used against these gram-positive organisms. If the patient is not having systemic symptoms such as high fever, antibiotics may be given orally. An infected bursa should not be drained openly but repeatedly aspirated.

If microcrystalline disease and infection have been excluded, the most successful treatment is fluid aspiration and injection of the bursal sac with a corticosteroid. Aspirin or another NSAID is also effective.

The patient should be encouraged to move the affected area, particularly the shoulder, but should avoid stressful exercise that may irritate it. Severe, long-term limitation of motion and frozen shoulder can occur if range-of-motion exercises are neglected.

SEPTIC ARTHRITIS

Arthritis resulting from infection of the synovial tissues with pyogenic bacteria or other infectious agents. Septic arthritis is most prevalent in patients > 65 yr. Bacterial infection occurs from direct inoculation or as a result of bacteremia from a known or unknown source. Infections occur more often in joints with preexisting disease, usually osteoarthritis or rheumatoid arthritis. Patients who are immunocompromised as a result of corticosteroid therapy, malignancy, or diabetes are also more likely to develop septic arthritis.

Symptoms, Signs, and Diagnosis

The disease usually presents as an acute febrile illness associated with monarticular or polyarticular arthritis. Primarily large joints are affected, most commonly the shoulder, elbow, wrist, hip, and knee. Notably, many patients may not look toxemic, particularly elderly persons, who may have a low-grade fever or no fever and whose peripheral WBC count may be < 14,000/μL. Diagnosis may be particularly difficult in debilitated or demented patients who cannot describe local symptoms. In febrile patients who cannot give a good history, all of the diarthrodial joints must be examined for a source of infection.

Infection is diagnosed by **aspiration of the joint** and **analysis of synovial fluid.** A WBC count > 50,000/μL indicates infection unless crystals are also seen. Infected fluid can have a WBC count of < 50,000/μL, although polymorphonuclear leukocytes predominate in most instances. The glucose level of synovial fluid is also low in most cases, and a difference of 40 mg/dL between serum and synovial fluid glucose is highly suggestive of infection. **Gram stain and culture** identify the organism in up to 50% of cases. **Blood cultures** should be obtained because the organism often grows in blood but not in synovial fluid. A specific organism is identified in > 80% of septic arthritis cases when all appropriate sites are cultured.

Other biochemical tests of synovial fluid include lactate level measurement, bacterial antigen detection, and nitroblue tetrazolium test. The most common organism is *Staphylococcus aureus,* as in younger patients; however, gram-negative bacteria are implicated in a significant number of cases in older patients.

Treatment

Treatment is urgently required to avoid destruction of cartilage and permanent joint damage. Joint fluid should be aspirated repeatedly and as completely as possible. If fever and the signs of arthritis are not substantially reduced in 48 to 72 h, surgical drainage of the joint may be necessary. Septic arthritis responds to appropriate systemic antibiotic therapy if the organism is sensitive and the dosage is adequate. Intra-articular antibiotics are not needed.

OSTEOMYELITIS

An infection of bone, usually caused by bacteria (occasionally mycobacteria), but sometimes by fungi. Symptoms and signs may include localized pain, nonhealing ulceration of overlying skin, persistent fever, and persistently elevated WBC count.

Hematogenous osteomyelitis is bimodal, often causing bone infection in children and in persons > 50 yr. Antecedent bacteremia may result from a concurrent urinary tract infection but often is untraceable. Although the vertebrae are most often involved, the long bones (eg, femur, tibia, humerus) may also become infected. About 60% of vertebral osteomyelitis cases occur in persons > 50 yr. Generally, only one organism is isolated. *Staphylococcus aureus* is the most common; however, gram-negative aerobic bacilli are frequently found. In vertebral osteomyelitis, *Escherichia coli* is the second most common isolate and most likely arises from genitourinary tract infection or instrumentation.

A contiguous focus of infection is more commonly associated with osteomyelitis in patients > 50 yr. Contiguous septic foci usually result from postoperative infections, decubitus ulcers, radiotherapy, or foreign bodies. In about 40% of cases, infection involves the head of the femur (often it is secondary to prosthetic hip infection). In 30% of cases, infection involves the tibia; in 16%, the mandible; and in 14%, the skull. The bacteria found in these infections are often mixed and frequently include *S. aureus, S. epidermidis,* gram-negative aerobic bacilli, and anaerobic species.

Vascular insufficiency is a common contributing factor to osteomyelitis of the foot in elderly patients because of the prevalence of associated conditions (eg, diabetes, atherosclerotic cardiovascular disease, vasculitis) in this population. The small bones of the feet and toes are most often involved. The infections are commonly mixed and may involve *S. aureus, S. epidemidis,* streptococci, gram-negative aerobic bacilli, and anaerobic organisms.

Diagnosis

The hallmark symptom of osteomyelitis, especially vertebral osteomyelitis, is pain. However, diabetic patients with osteomyelitis of the foot and debilitated patients with osteomyelitis from an overlying pressure sore may not have pain. Fever may not be present. The erythrocyte sedimentation rate is almost always elevated, but leukocytosis is variable.

Advanced osteomyelitis can be diagnosed by x-ray. During earlier stages, diagnosis requires a technetium bone or WBC scan with gallium or indium.

Treatment

Antibiotic therapy is the mainstay of treatment and may be required for weeks to months. Frequently, debridement is also needed for successful therapy. The choice of antibiotic should be based on organisms grown from blood cultures or a deep bone biopsy. Frequently, cultures of superficial bone or overlying wounds are inaccurate.

CARPAL TUNNEL SYNDROME

A syndrome of pain and motor and sensory symptoms that mainly affects the hand. The syndrome is caused by compression of the median nerve in the volar aspect of the wrist between the longitudinal tendons of forearm muscles that flex the hand and the transverse superficial carpal ligament. Carpal tunnel syndrome is relatively common, may be unilateral or bilateral, and occurs more often in women. In the elderly, it is more common in those whose activities require frequent flexion of the wrist and in those with diabetes or hypothyroidism.

Symptoms, Signs, and Diagnosis

Paresthesias occur in the radial palmar aspect of the hand. Pain, which may be more severe at night, may develop in the wrist, the palm, or the area proximal to the compression site in the forearm and shoulder. A sensory deficit in the palmar aspect of the first three digits and weakness and atrophy in the muscles responsible for thumb abduction and apposition may follow. In sedentary persons, symptoms may be minimal, although the use of crutches or a walker may aggravate them. The syndrome should be differentiated from C-6 root compression caused by cervical radiculopathy.

Treatment

Tasks requiring forceful wrist flexion should be avoided, if possible. Cock-up splints help relieve pain, especially at night, and can temporarily ease nerve pressure. Local corticosteroid injections may provide temporary relief. Progressive or unrelieved symptoms may require surgical decompression of the median nerve at the wrist, which can usually be carried out under local anesthesia.

CERVICAL SPONDYLOSIS

A condition in which the cervical canal or neural foramina are narrowed by degenerative changes in the intervertebral disk and the annulus and by the formation of bony osteophytes. Narrowing leads to cord compression, which typically causes a progressive myelopathy, characterized by a spastic gait. Patients with a congenitally narrow cervical canal are at increased risk.

Symptoms, Signs, and Diagnosis

If a painful cervical root syndrome predominates, radicular signs often indicate the most involved dermatome, usually one between C-5 and C-6 or between C-6 and C-7. Neural foraminal root compression causes arm weakness and atrophy with segmental reflex loss; spinal cord compression causes hyperreflexia, increased tone, vibratory impairment, and plantar extensor responses in the legs.

Spinal films, including oblique views of the neural foramina, reveal degenerative changes with osteophytes and disk-space narrowing. If the sagittal diameter of the cervical canal is < 10 mm, cord compression is likely. Computed tomography (CT) defines the diameter of the canal, and myelography shows the level and extent of the epidural compression, but magnetic resonance imaging (MRI) is rapidly becoming the diagnostic test of choice.

Treatment

Occasionally, signs improve spontaneously. Conservative therapy includes a soft collar, cervical traction, anti-inflammatory drugs, and symptomatic treatment with mild analgesics. Decompressive laminectomy is used sparingly to halt progressive signs or to stabilize the myelopathy.

76. MUSCULAR DISORDERS

Slowly progressive muscle wasting and decline in strength **(sarcopenia)** normally occurs between ages 30 and 75. In healthy young persons, 10% of body weight is bone, 30% is muscle, and 20% is adipose tissue. Muscle accounts for 50% of lean body mass and about 50% of the total amount of body nitrogen. By age 75, about 8% of body weight is bone, 15% is muscle, and 40% is adipose tissue. Half the muscle mass has disappeared because of a reduction in the number and size of muscle fibers. Maximum isometric contraction force is 20% lower by the sixth decade and 50% lower by the eighth decade compared to young adults.

The reasons for these changes are not completely understood, but a relative deficiency of growth hormone and a decrease in the routine performance of vigorous muscular work are likely contributing factors. Research is being done to determine if treatment of healthy older persons with growth hormone, exercise, or both can reverse these changes. Encouraging results on the beneficial effects of exercise have already been obtained. Elderly persons who have performed daily weight lifting (eight repetitions at 80% of maximum) using their proximal leg muscles have had a 180% increase in strength after 6 wk of training and have had a marked improvement in tandem gait speed. Studies are being performed to evaluate the long-term benefits of regular weight training and other exercises in the elderly. More specific information is needed to determine the optimal frequency, intensity, and duration for different exercises.

Older persons are also at risk for deconditioning and for an accelerated loss of muscle during any acute illness that restricts mobility, especially if they are on complete bed rest. Some geriatricians estimate that for each day of absolute bed rest, 2 wk of reconditioning are necessary to return to baseline function. When restricted to bed, healthy older persons lose muscle mass and strength at a rate of about 1.5% per day. The greatest deconditioning occurs in the antigravity muscles—those used to sit up, stand up, and pull up—which are essential for performing activities of daily living. Early intervention with physical therapy and an individualized exercise regimen should be included in the care plan for any older person who requires hospitalization for acute illness, especially those restricted to bed.

Despite age-related reductions in muscle strength, healthy older adults have muscle functional ability similar to that of younger adults. Usually, healthy elders can easily climb stairs, rise from a squatting position, walk along a straight line, hop on either foot, and perform typical activities of daily living. However, a significant loss of strength, particularly one that affects mobility, can threaten independence and lead the patient to seek medical help.

AGE–RELATED MUSCULAR SYMPTOMS

Diagnosis

In the elderly, many conditions can produce symptoms that are primarily muscular (see TABLE 76–1). The conditions include lesions of the CNS and peripheral nervous system and abnormalities of neuromuscular transmission and of the muscle fibers themselves.

Other conditions that do not affect muscular function directly may cause symptoms suggestive of muscle disease in the elderly. Such conditions, which include cardiovascular, respiratory, endocrinologic, and other systemic illnesses, account for more than half of muscular complaints. Anxiety or depression with fatigue and lack of motivation for activities of daily living can also limit exercise performance, often without intrinsic muscle weakness. Moreover, rheumatologic diseases (such as degenerative joint disease, rheumatoid arthritis, and polymyalgia rheumatica) may cause muscular symptoms such as as difficulty in walking, unsteadiness with occasional falls, and stiffness with leg pains especially at night. Significant degenerative joint disease can limit mobility by producing structural spinal changes and joint symptoms in the limbs and occasionally by damaging the spinal cord, nerve roots, and peripheral nerves.

TABLE 76–1. CONDITIONS CAUSING MUSCULAR SYMPTOMS IN ELDERLY PATIENTS

Lesions affecting the descending motor pathways	Intracranial lesions	Midline subdural hematoma Subfrontal or interhemispheral neoplasm Communicating hydrocephalus Midline mass lesion in posterior fossa (such as metastatic tumor in cerebellum) Degenerative diseases of the central nervous system
	Spinal cord lesions	Compression of spinal cord secondary to osteoarthritis or disk disease, vertebral collapse (osteopenia vs. neoplasm), epidural metastasis, epidural abscess Anterior horn cell disease caused by amyotrophic lateral sclerosis or postpolio syndrome Radiation myelopathy Lyme disease
Lesions affecting the motor nerve roots	Comprehensive or infiltrative lesions	Spinal stenosis Infiltration of roots by lymphoma or carcinoma Paget's disease
	Inflammatory lesions	Acute inflammatory polyneuritis Chronic inflammatory demyelinating polyneuropathy
Lesions of peripheral nerve motor fibers	Inflammatory or infectious lesions	Acute inflammatory polyneuritis Chronic inflammatory demyelinating polyneuropathy (idiopathic vs. associated with plasma cell disorder producing paraprotein) Diphtheria
	Endocrine disease or lesions caused by toxins	Thyroid disease Heavy metal toxicity (lead, mercury)

(continued)

TABLE 76–1. CONDITIONS CAUSING MUSCULAR SYMPTOMS IN ELDERLY PATIENTS *(Continued)*

Lesions affecting neuromuscular transmission	Autoimmune or neoplasm-associated defects	Myasthenia gravis Myasthenia gravis with thymoma Lambert-Eaton syndrome
	Toxin- or drug-induced transmission disorders	Botulism Aminoglycoside, β-blocker, or lithium toxicity Drug-induced myasthenia gravis (eg, penicillamine)
Abnormality in muscle fiber	Inflammatory or infectious disorders	Dermatomyositis (with or without associated neoplasm) Polymyositis (large number of potential causes) Inclusion body myositis
	Endocrine, electrolyte, or drug-induced disorders	Thyroid disease Vitamin D deficiency with osteomalacia Phosphate or magnesium deficiency Steroid, penicillamine, chloroquine, emetine, clofibrate, ethanol, lovastatin, amiodarone, colchicine, and tryptophan toxicity
	Muscular dystrophies (onset late in life is uncommon)	Myotonic dystrophy Oculopharyngeal dystrophy Scapuloperoneal dystrophy

Lesions of the CNS can produce abnormalities in gait and leg muscle strength that might be misinterpreted as symptoms of peripheral nerve or muscle fiber diseases. The clinical history and physical examination help identify the abnormality (see TABLE 76–2).

Papilledema, unilateral weakness or sensory loss, and a gait disturbance with the head turned or the neck flexed suggest a CNS cause. Patients with central and peripheral nervous system disorders may present with motor symptoms that are often symmetric and limited to the legs.

Patients with **descending motor pathway dysfunction** (eg, midline subdural hematoma or midline posterior fossa mass) frequently have much greater muscle weakness when asked to perform common tasks (functional testing) than when strength is assessed by physical examination (direct muscle strength testing). In contrast, patients with **peripheral nerve and muscle damage** have similar weakness on functional and direct muscle testing.

In patients without significant joint or soft tissue disease, **muscle weakness** is suggested by the inability to walk on the heels and toes, rise from a squatting position, rise from a chair without using the arms, or step onto the seat of a chair. A normal person should be able to extend the knee completely against gravity. A tendency of the knee to remain slightly flexed suggests a weakness of the quadriceps of the thigh, which is often associated with stumbles and falls. The patient should be able to raise outstretched arms above the head easily and to blanch the knuckles with a forceful grip.

Patients with **pathologic fatigue** from a neuromuscular transmission defect (eg, myasthenia gravis) complain of fluctuations in their abilities to perform activities such as chewing, keeping eyes open, speaking, and smiling. Pathologic fatigue is characterized by drooping eyelids when a person fixates on a target, such as a pen or a flashlight, or when a person repeats movements, such as elevating the arms above the head or rising from a chair.

In patients who have no electrolyte or pH disturbance, **muscle aches and cramps** commonly indicate a peripheral nerve disorder and less commonly a primary muscle fiber disturbance. Intense pain, most prominent in proximal muscles in the morning, may indicate polymyalgia rheumatica (see Ch. 74). Pain in localized muscle regions may indicate fibromyalgia. Pain largely restricted to muscle groups and tissue around joints may indicate diffuse arthritic disease with limited muscle function.

Focal muscle wasting indicates an abnormality in either motor nerve or muscle. **Diffuse muscle wasting** can occur after as little as 4 to 6 wk of absolute bed rest, usually with remarkable preservation of muscle strength despite the reduced muscle mass.

In patients with weakness from CNS disease, **tendon reflexes** are typically increased with plantar extensor responses. However, many older people without demonstrable disease lack ankle reflexes. Loss of reflexes with only mild weakness is typical for disease of the peripheral nerve or nerve root, although occasionally cerebellar lesions depress tendon reflexes, suggesting muscle weakness. Loss of reflexes in patients with primary muscle disease often parallels the degree of weakness. Reflexes are usually maintained in disorders of neuromuscular transmission but are frequently lost or hypoactive in patients with Lambert-Eaton syndrome, a disorder of neuromuscular transmission. However, loss of reflexes without any discernible disease is also common in the elderly.

TABLE 76–2. DIFFERENTIATING SELECTED CAUSES OF MUSCULAR SYMPTOMS IN THE ELDERLY

Cause	*Site of Involvement*	*Clinical Features and Diagnostic Tests*					
		Distribution of Weakness	*Sensory Involvement*	*Tendon Reflexes*	*Muscular Atrophy*	*Other Clinical Features*	*Useful Diagnostic Tests*
Chronic subdural hematoma above and between both frontal lobes	Frontal lobes (interhemispheric or subfrontal)	Symmetric leg weakness	None	Normal to slightly increased in legs; variable plantar extensor responses	None	Headache, personality change, drowsiness	MRI or CT scan of head, clotting profile
Metastasis	Midportion of cerebellum	Gait disturbance; often no true weakness	None	Often decreased; variable plantar extensor responses	None	Unsteady gait, headache	MRI or CT scan of head with emphasis on posterior fossa
Chronic spinal cord compression caused by C-5 and C-6 osteoarthritis	Cervical spinal cord	Symmetric or slightly asymmetric weakness in hands and legs	Pain and occasional decrease in pin and touch response in C-6–C-7 nerve root distribution	Decreased in arms and increased in legs; plantar extensor responses	Intrinsic hand muscles	Limited motion of neck, pain with movement, occasional worsening of leg weakness with head flexion or extension	MRI scan of posterior fossa, cervical and upper thoracic spine; X-rays of cervical spine (flexion and extension views)

Amyotrophic lateral sclerosis	Anterior horn cell	Asymmetric or bulbar	None	Variable	Marked, develops early	Fasciculations, cramps, tremor	EMG, nerve conduction
Chronic inflammatory demyelinating polyneuropathy	Peripheral nerve	Symmetric, distal, greater than proximal	Distal dysesthesias and loss of vibration greater than pin and touch	Decreased	Mild to moderate	Muscle aches, trouble using stairs, tripping	Nerve conduction, EMG, nerve biopsy, CSF analysis
Myasthenia gravis	Neuromuscular junction	Extraocular, bulbar, proximal limb muscles	None	Normal	None	Weakness fluctuates, diurnal variation	Edrophonium test, repetitive nerve stimulation, CT scan of chest (thymus), acetylcholine receptor antibody levels
Polymyositis	Skeletal muscle fibers	Symmetric, proximal limb and bulbar muscles	Aching	Parallel strength	Slight	Slowly progressive weakness over weeks to months	Creatine kinase, ESR, EMG, muscle biopsy

MRI = magnetic resonance imaging; CT = computed tomography; EMG = electromyography; CSF = cerebrospinal fluid; ESR = erythrocyte sedimentation rate.

Diagnostic Tests

Serum enzyme measurements: **Creatine kinase** is found primarily in skeletal muscle, heart, and brain with the concentration in skeletal muscle being more than three times that in the heart and brain. Three forms of creatine kinase exist: **MM** (skeletal muscle), **MB** (cardiac muscle), and **BB** (brain). Normal adult skeletal muscle contains about 95% MM and 5% MB. However, regenerating skeletal muscle fibers revert to an embryonic isoenzyme pattern, and MB increases to between 10% and 50%. Therefore, creatine kinase isoenzyme measurements are not useful in diagnosing or monitoring patients with neuromuscular disorders.

Muscle damage significantly elevates the serum creatine kinase concentration (normal < 130 u./L). An elevation of creatine kinase is a much more sensitive determinant of muscle damage than elevation of any other serum enzyme. **Normal exercise,** depending on its intensity and the person's conditioning, elevates creatine kinase levels as much as threefold to eightfold. Levels peak several hours after exercise, and maximum levels persist for 24 to 36 h, partly because of the long plasma half-life of creatine kinase (38 to 118 h). Thus, creatine kinase measurements should be avoided within 48 h of heavy exercise. Creatine kinase levels are also elevated by muscle damage caused by prolonged pressure, which may occur in elderly people who lie immobile on a hard surface.

Creatine kinase elevations occur in many conditions affecting the motor unit (anterior horn cell, motor axon and terminal branches, neuromuscular junctions, and muscle fibers). **Mild creatine kinase elevations** (less than four times the upper limit of the normal range) occur in some healthy persons with a large muscle mass, in families predisposed to malignant hyperthermia, in healthy persons after minor muscle trauma (including intramuscular injections and needle electromyography), and in persons with certain chronic anterior horn cell diseases such as amyotrophic lateral sclerosis and postpolio syndrome. **Moderate to marked creatine kinase elevations** occur in inflammatory myopathies, such as polymyositis and dermatomyositis, and after conditions that produce muscle necrosis, such as hypokalemic myopathy.

Metabolic and endocrine tests: Measurements of serum electrolyte and bicarbonate levels (to evaluate for acidosis or alkalosis) are helpful, particularly if weakness is accompanied by muscle cramps and aching. Hypokalemia, hypophosphatemia, hypocalcemia, and hypermagnesemia can produce muscle weakness. Chronic hypofunction or hyperfunction of the thyroid, adrenal, or parathyroid glands also may produce weakness and should be excluded. Erythrocyte sedimentation rate and other blood studies (eg, antinuclear antibody and rheumatoid factor) can be used to screen for collagen-vascular diseases, and serum and urine immunoelectrophoresis can be used to check for immunoglobulins and Bence-Jones protein in multiple myeloma.

Imaging studies: **Plain x-ray studies** of the spine can identify many rheumatologic conditions, such as chronic osteoarthritis and chronic disk herniation with early lumbosacral spinal canal narrowing, and other conditions that might produce muscular symptoms, such as covert metastatic disease with vertebral collapse. In chronic motor neuropathies, a skeletal survey helps establish the cause, eg, multiple myeloma or osteomalacia.

Although imaging studies of skeletal muscle are not routinely performed, **ultrasonography, computed tomography,** and **magnetic resonance imaging** can quantify muscle atrophy and identify the muscle groups with greater damage before needle biopsy is performed. Ultrasonography also helps identify muscle abscess. **Technetium diphosphonate or pyrophosphate imaging** can demonstrate muscle fiber damage in polymyositis.

Computed tomography and magnetic resonance imaging can also identify lesions in the brain and spinal cord and occasionally in soft tissues and muscle that other studies cannot identify. Examples include lesions producing symmetric dysfunction in the descending motor pathways, thymoma (in myasthenia gravis), or oat cell carcinoma of the lung (in Lambert-Eaton syndrome).

Electrodiagnosis: Nerve conduction assessment, repetitive stimulation, and electromyography are the primary electrodiagnostic tests used to examine the motor unit (see TABLE 76–3).

Nerve conduction assessment uses skin electrodes to stimulate a peripheral nerve at various points and other electrodes to record the motor and sensory action potentials at distal sites, so that nerve conduction velocity can be calculated. In healthy adults, conduction velocities of peripheral nerves typically range from 45 to 75 m/sec. In those with chronic demyelinating polyneuropathies, the velocity may be decreased by $\geq$ 40%.

In **repetitive stimulation testing,** maximal stimuli are applied to the peripheral motor nerve, and the muscle action potential is measured. Usually, the nerve is stimulated at low frequency (3 Hz) before and after a brief period of maximal isometric exercise. An incremental decrease in the action potential amplitude usually indicates a defect in neuromuscular transmission, as occurs in myasthenia gravis. In contrast, Lambert-Eaton syndrome produces an incremental increase with repetitive stimulation.

Electromyography records electrical activity of muscle at rest (when normally there is none) and during mild and strong contraction. With voluntary contraction, more motor unit potentials of increasing amplitude are recruited as the strength of contraction increases.

In neurogenic disorders that damage the motor axon, electromyographic findings depend on the type and duration of the nerve disease. If the damage produces axonal death, **fibrillations** (spontaneous activity

TABLE 76–3. ELECTRODIAGNOSTIC FINDINGS IN LESIONS CAUSING MUSCULAR SYMPTOMS

Electro-diagnostic Test	*Lesion in Descending Motor Pathways*	*Lesion of Lower Motor Neuron*	*Lesion of Neuromuscular Transmission*	*Lesion of Skeletal Muscle*
Nerve conduction	Normal	Often normal; abnormal only with demyelination of large nerve fibers	Normal	Normal
Repetitive stimulation	Normal	Normal	Variable; usually abnormal if stimulated muscle is weak	Normal
Electro-myography	Reduced firing frequency of motor unit potentials	Signs of acute or chronic denervation	Normal or myopathic in very weak muscles	Myopathic or normal

of a single muscle fiber) and **positive waves** (a biphasic action potential initiated by movement of the recording needle, often occurring in an area of damaged, fibrillating, muscle fibers) usually develop in single denervated muscle fibers after 3 wk or more.

Fasciculations (spontaneous activity of part or all of a motor unit) often do not indicate axonal death. Typically, they occur with slowly progressive diseases of the anterior horn cell or nerve roots or in electrolyte disturbances. Many normal persons develop fasciculations, especially after exercise.

Electromyography often distinguishes primary muscle disease from nerve disease. Typically with myopathy, the test shows a normal number of motor unit potentials, often with decreased amplitude, during maximum contraction. With chronic denervation, the test shows a reduced number of motor unit potentials with very high amplitude. However, inflammatory myopathies, such as polymyositis and dermatomyositis (important causes of muscle weakness in the elderly), may produce fibrillations and positive waves identical to those following acute nerve damage.

Muscle biopsy: Muscle biopsy is useful for distinguishing neurogenic from myopathic disease and for diagnosing certain connective tissue diseases, such as polyarteritis nodosa and polymyositis. Muscle biopsy is also useful in diagnosing the muscular dystrophies, congenital myopathies, and specific metabolic diseases of muscle—all of which are rare in the elderly.

Biopsy is not useful for acute generalized weakness or subacute or chronic neurogenic weakness (eg, acute inflammatory polyneuritis, diabetic polyneuropathy) or neuromuscular transmission disease (eg, myasthenia gravis).

Nerve biopsy: More difficult and traumatic than muscle biopsy, nerve biopsy has limited use. It can distinguish segmental demyelination from axonal degeneration and identify inflammatory neuropathies. Nerve biopsy also can establish a specific diagnosis in certain uncommon diseases, such as amyloidosis, sarcoidosis, leprosy, and certain unusual metabolic and hereditary neuropathies. In elderly patients, the indications are very restricted, the most common being the diagnosis of chronic inflammatory demyelinating polyneuropathy.

Muscle mass assessment: This evaluation requires a 3-day meatless diet followed by a 24-h urine collection. The 24-h urinary creatinine measurement, which varies < 10%, correlates directly and reliably with total muscle mass and can be used to determine response to therapy. For persons ages 30 to 50, the range is about 1800 to 1700 mg/24 h; for those ages 60 to 70, 1600 to 1400 mg/24 h; and for those ages 70 to 80, 1400 to 1200 mg/24 h. Serial collections of 24-h urine specimens made weeks to months apart are often helpful in documenting sequential changes in muscle mass.

NEUROMUSCULAR TRANSMISSION DISORDERS

Disorders affecting neuromuscular transmission include myasthenia gravis and Lambert-Eaton syndrome.

MYASTHENIA GRAVIS

Myasthenia gravis is an autoimmune disease in which the number of acetylcholine receptors at the skeletal muscle motor endplate is reduced. This receptor deficiency is caused by circulating antireceptor antibodies that block the acetylcholine binding sites and accelerate the turnover rate for the receptor (its internalization and destruction). The role of the thymus gland is not known, but 66% of patients have thymic hyperplasia, and 10% to 15% have thymoma.

Myasthenia gravis can occur at any age, but peak incidence in women occurs in the third and fourth decades and in men in the sixth and seventh decades. Among the elderly, myasthenia gravis is more common in men.

Symptoms and Signs

Myasthenia gravis is characterized by weakness and fatigability of skeletal muscle. Symptoms typically fluctuate; they are most pronounced at the end of the day and are relieved by rest. Initial symptoms include ptosis, diplopia, or blurred vision (from extraocular muscle involvement) in > 50% of patients; generalized weakness and fatigue in about 10%; and dysphagia, facial weakness, or slurred nasal speech in about 5%. Symptoms remain limited to the extraocular muscles in about 15% of patients and become generalized in 85%, usually within the first year. Symptoms reach maximum severity in the first year in 50% of patients and within 5 yr in almost all patients.

Myasthenic crisis is characterized by the acute onset of respiratory insufficiency, often with difficulty swallowing and speaking, and increased weakness in the arms and legs. Infection, trauma, and certain medications (aminoglycosides, cardiac drugs, antihistamines, and tranquilizers) can precipitate myasthenic crisis in some patients.

Diagnosis

The diagnosis is suspected on the basis of symptoms and confirmed by certain tests. In the **anticholinesterase test,** a double-blind comparison of edrophonium 5 mg IV vs. placebo is carried out while the patient is monitored by an ECG. During the procedure, IV atropine and resuscitative equipment are kept available. **Repetitive stimulation testing** often shows a decremental response 1 to 2 min after exercise. The number of **anti–acetylcholine receptor antibodies** (that block α-bungarotoxin binding sites to the acetylcholine receptor) is often increased, while the numbers of **acetylcholine receptor modulating antibodies** and **antistriational muscle antibodies** are usually normal.

Treatment

First-line therapy is often an **anticholinesterase drug,** such as pyridostigmine bromide at an initial dose of 30 mg orally; the dose should be repeated as necessary at intervals of at least 3 h. The dosage must be individualized. Concomitant use of **ephedrine** 25 mg bid or tid may have a synergistic effect.

In the elderly, the most severe symptoms typically occur in the extraocular and bulbar muscles, which are especially resistant to anticholinesterase treatment; thus additional therapy is usually necessary. **Immunosuppressants** (eg, azathioprine) and **corticosteroids** (eg, prednisone) are the mainstays of long-term management.

Management of myasthenia gravis rarely causes cholinergic crisis, characterized by increasing muscle weakness and increasing cholinergic side effects. If it occurs, treatment consists of withholding medications, intubating the patient, and providing ventilatory support.

LAMBERT–EATON SYNDROME

Lambert-Eaton syndrome is an autoimmune disorder frequently associated with small cell carcinoma of the lung and autoimmune diseases (especially in women and younger patients). It is characterized by diminished release of acetylcholine from the motor nerve terminal. Serum from patients with Lambert-Eaton syndrome contains circulating IgG antibody that blocks the voltage-dependent calcium channels in the terminals of normal motor nerve fibers. Lambert-Eaton syndrome occurs about five times more often in men than in women. Subacute cerebellar degeneration has occurred in both neoplastic and nonneoplastic Lambert-Eaton syndrome.

Symptoms, Signs, and Diagnosis

Patients have muscle fatigue, primarily in the leg and trunk muscles, with little or no muscle atrophy. In contrast to myasthenia gravis, bulbar and extraocular muscles are often unaffected. Paradoxically, repetitive stimulation testing shows a several-fold increase in amplitude (also seen in botulism, hypermagnesemia, and hypocalcemia and with certain antibiotics, typically aminoglycosides). Lambert-Eaton syndrome also produces hyporeflexia; yet muscle contraction for a few seconds before testing temporarily restores normal tendon reflex activity.

About 50% of patients with Lambert-Eaton syndrome have autonomic abnormalities; the most frequent symptom is dry mouth. Impotence, decreased lacrimation and sweating, orthostatic symptoms, and diminished pupillary response to light also occur.

Treatment

As with myasthenia gravis, drugs are used to increase acetylcholine availability and control immune-mediated disease mechanisms. **Guanidine** 10 to 35 mg/kg/day increases acetylcholine availability but causes significant side effects. Initial treatment usually consists of alternate-day therapy with **prednisone** in a moderate dose and **azathioprine** 1.5 to 2 mg/kg/day. **Immune globulin** 2 gm/kg IV given in divided infusions is the treatment of choice for patients refractory to immunosuppressive therapy. **Plasmapheresis** (five or six exchanges) to remove circulating antibodies can also be used in refractory patients.

Elderly patients should be monitored for malignancy for at least 2 to 3 yr after diagnosis. In some patients, neuromuscular transmission improves after neoplasm removal. Patients should also be monitored for the development of other immune-mediated diseases.

INFLAMMATORY MUSCLE DISORDERS

Inflammatory muscle disorders include dermatomyositis, polymyositis, and inclusion body myositis.

DERMATOMYOSITIS

Dermatomyositis is considered an autoimmune, connective tissue disease. Natural history data for late-onset (after age 40) forms are not available. About 10% of patients have a malignancy; breast and lung tumors are the most common, with a disproportionate increase in tumors of the ovary, uterus, and bowel. No consistent relationship exists between tumor discovery and onset of dermatomyositis.

Symptoms, Signs, and Diagnosis

An erythematous skin rash (usually the presenting feature) and muscle weakness are the major clinical signs. Proximal limb muscles are typically weaker than distal muscles. Neck flexors are particularly weakened. Muscles supplied by cranial nerves are typically spared, except for those involved with swallowing. Dysphagia, myalgias, and muscle tenderness occur in about 50% of patients.

Diagnosis is confirmed by the characteristic rash, proximal muscle weakness, elevated blood muscle enzyme levels (especially creatine kinase levels), electromyography findings consistent with muscle inflammation, and histologic evidence of myopathy. The erythrocyte sedimentation rate is frequently elevated.

Treatment

During the acute stages, most patients benefit from bed rest while immunosuppressive therapy is initiated. Usually, **prednisone** is started at 1 to 2 mg/kg/day (60 to 100 mg/day). Another immunosuppressive drug, such as **azathioprine** 2 to 3 mg/kg/day in divided doses, may be administered concomitantly. Long-term management includes physical therapy, frequent monitoring of muscle power, and regular physical activity.

Elderly patients require frequent monitoring for covert neoplasms, especially of the breast and lung. No predictable relationship exists between tumor removal and resolution of myopathy, but some patients have remarkable recoveries.

POLYMYOSITIS

Polymyositis is considered an autoimmune, connective tissue disease, but it may result from various disorders (unidentified foreign protein, viruses, or other illness) that cause slowly progressive myopathy with muscle fiber damage from cytotoxic lymphocytes. Prevalence ranges from 6 per 100,000 to 8 per 100,000; incidence peaks between 45 and 65 yr. It is most common in blacks and women.

Symptoms, Signs, and Diagnosis

Muscle weakness usually occurs in the hips and thighs; it begins as aching pain in about 10% of patients and as tenderness on palpation in another 20%. Distal muscle weakness occurs in only 25%. Muscle atrophy and loss of tendon reflexes are rare in the early stages. Dysphagia occurs eventually in 66% of patients. Cardiac involvement is relatively common, and ECG abnormalities such as atrioventricular conduction defects and bundle branch block occur in about 33% of patients.

The diagnosis is based on typical symptoms and signs, a myopathic pattern on electromyography, typical biopsy findings, and elevated creatine kinase levels. The patient may also have arthralgia, fever, an elevated erythrocyte sedimentation rate, and a polyclonal hypergammaglobulinemia on electrophoresis.

Treatment and Prognosis

Treatment is the same as for dermatomyositis. The overall mortality is about four times that of the general population, with death usually occurring from pulmonary or cardiac complications. Blacks and women have a less favorable prognosis. About 50% of patients recover, and therapy can be discontinued within 5 yr of the onset of symptoms. About 20% have persistent active disease requiring continued therapy. The remaining 30% develop inactive disease with permanent residual muscle weakness.

INCLUSION BODY MYOSITIS

The cause of inclusion body myositis is unknown. The disorder resembles chronic polymyositis, usually occurs in patients > 50 yr, and affects men twice as often as women. Amyloid deposits and cytoplasmic and intranuclear filamentous inclusions of unknown origin are characteristic. Autosomal dominant inheritance accounts for some cases.

Symptoms, Signs, and Diagnosis

Progressive proximal and distal muscle weakness usually develop gradually without pain. Unlike in polymyositis and dermatomyositis, muscle atrophy develops relatively early in inclusion body myositis. Facial muscles are occasionally involved, but extraocular muscles are always spared. Rarely spinal, respiratory, and abdominal muscles are affected. Dysphagia is rare, and cardiac involvement is unknown. Tendon reflexes are normal or increased and become reduced only with marked muscular wasting. Usually, inclusion body myositis progresses slowly, and patients remain ambulatory for many years after symptoms begin. Chronic progressive muscle weakness and nuclear inclusion bodies on muscle biopsy are diagnostic.

Treatment

Immunosuppressive therapy is ineffective. Occasionally, IV infusions of immune globulin give improvement. Supportive care and bracing for occasional foot drop or severe wrist drop are helpful.

ENDOCRINE–INDUCED MUSCLE DISORDERS

Endocrine-induced muscle disorders include corticosteroid myopathy, muscle disorders in hyperthyroidism, muscle disorders in hypothyroidism, muscle weakness associated with osteomalacia, and hypokalemic myopathy. (Muscle weakness may also occur with osteoporosis, but it likely results from disuse atrophy.)

CORTICOSTEROID MYOPATHY

Corticosteroid myopathy results from prolonged corticosteroid therapy, usually given for conditions that also cause muscle weakness such as myasthenia gravis or inflammatory myopathies, or from conditions associated with elevated corticotropin levels such as Cushing's disease.

The incidence of muscle weakness ranges from 2% to 20% in those receiving long-term corticosteroid therapy and from 50% to 80% in those with Cushing's disease.

Symptoms and Signs

Muscle weakness usually begins in the hip girdle, especially the quadriceps, and eventually spreads to nearly all muscles, though the proximal muscles tend to be most affected. In chronic corticosteroid myopathy, muscle wasting is often apparent, though exercise decreases it. Muscles supplied by cranial nerves other than neck flexors are spared. Occasionally, patients experience mild aching in the thigh muscles, but severe pain does not occur. Tendon reflexes remain unchanged, and no fasciculations develop. Patients often complain that they become fatigued more rapidly during activities demanding sudden bursts of power.

Diagnosis and Treatment

Typically, serum creatine kinase and other muscle enzyme levels, electromyography studies, and nerve conduction studies are normal. Muscle biopsy often shows striking atrophy of type 2 fibers. If the patient has inflammatory myopathy, decreasing the corticosteroid dose increases creatine excretion, and muscle weakness worsens.

The treatment of corticosteroid myopathy is empiric. The only certain principles are to reduce the corticosteroid dosage gradually and monitor the patient closely. Complete recovery usually occurs in 2 to 3 mo. To reduce the likelihood of corticosteroid myopathy, many authorities recommend switching to alternate-day corticosteroid administration as soon as feasible.

MUSCLE DISORDERS IN HYPERTHYROIDISM

(See also HYPERTHYROIDISM in Ch. 79)

Hyperthyroidism can cause a subacute proximal myopathy in elderly patients without the prominent tachycardia or other obvious systemic signs seen in younger patients. It can also cause myokymia (continuous quivering or undulating movement of muscle surface and overlying skin), acute bulbar myopathy, ocular myopathy, and, rarely, hypokalemic periodic paralysis.

Symptoms and Signs

Often, the initial symptoms are weakness of proximal limb muscles and increased muscle fatigue. Usually, the shoulder girdle and upper arm muscles are weaker than the leg muscles. In the legs, the iliopsoas muscle may be primarily affected. Muscle atrophy develops relatively early and occasionally is pronounced. More than 15% of patients have prominent muscle twitches, often with increased tendon reflexes, which may mimic those of amyotrophic lateral sclerosis.

Diagnosis and Treatment

The diagnosis is confirmed by thyroid function tests. Serum muscle enzyme levels are normal. Electromyography often demonstrates fasciculations and myopathic features in weak muscles. Muscle biopsy is usually normal.

The euthyroid state should be restored. During the first few weeks of treatment, propranolol 120 to 320 mg/day often is effective in reducing proximal muscle weakness.

The long-term prognosis is good. After the euthyroid state has been maintained for several months, muscle bulk and strength typically return to normal.

MUSCLE DISORDERS IN HYPOTHYROIDISM

(See also HYPOTHYROIDISM in Ch. 79)

Hypothyroidism leads to impaired energy metabolism within the muscle fiber and decreased contractile force. Also, a defect in the repair and replacement of myofibrillar proteins results from reduced protein turnover. Slow muscle contraction and relaxation result from the diminished activity of myosin ATPase and the impaired uptake of calcium by the sarcoplasmic reticulum. Reduced cardiac output results from β-adrenergic hyposensitivity. The pathophysiology responsible for muscle cramps and muscle fiber enlargement is unknown. Deposition of mucopolysaccharides in muscle has been seen inconsistently.

Symptoms and Signs

The primary symptoms are proximal weakness, fatigue, slowed movements, stiffness, myalgias, cramps, and occasionally, enlarged muscles, especially the anterior compartment muscles of the leg. These symptoms develop over weeks to months. Some patients develop pronounced proximal leg muscle weakness and atrophy. Tendon reflexes are slowed with relaxation of the Achilles tendon reflex being markedly prolonged. In about 33% of hypothyroid patients, myoedema (mounding) lasting ≥ 5 sec can be elicited by direct percussion of muscle. A similar response can be seen in malnourished patients.

Complications include increased frequency of carpal and tarsal tunnel syndromes and a distal, symmetric, sensory motor polyneuropathy. Rarely, marked fatigability of hip girdle and trunk muscles results from impaired neuromuscular transmission. Repetitive nerve stimulation mimics Lambert-Eaton syndrome.

Diagnosis

In primary hypothyroidism, the circulating thyroid hormone level is decreased, and the thyroid-stimulating hormone level is increased; in secondary hypothyroidism, a rare disorder, both circulating thyroid hormone and thyroid-stimulating hormone levels are decreased. Usually, muscle enzyme levels, especially creatine kinase levels, are increased several times the normal values. Other laboratory abnormalities typical of hypothyroidism, such as an elevated serum cholesterol level, also occur.

Electrodiagnostic studies may show compression neuropathies. Electromyographic findings are variable; they may show no abnormality or a mixture of neurogenic and myopathic features. Occasionally, evidence of muscle membrane hyperirritability appears. Muscle biopsy may be normal or occasionally show a reduction in the proportion and size of type 2 muscle fibers.

Treatment and Prognosis

Treatment consists of a small initial dose of thyroid hormone, which is gradually increased over a period of weeks. Once the euthyroid state is achieved, elevated thyroid-stimulating hormone levels and serum creatine kinase levels return to normal. Surgery rarely is needed to reverse median or tibial nerve compression. The long-term prognosis is good; however, patients with severe muscle wasting may never recover full muscle strength and bulk.

MUSCLE WEAKNESS ASSOCIATED WITH OSTEOMALACIA

(See also Ch. 73)

Osteomalacia results from vitamin D deficiency. The pathophysiology of the myopathy is unknown.

About 33% of osteomalacia patients have muscle weakness and initially complain of weakness in the pelvic and thigh muscles. Typically, the patient has pain in the back, hip girdle, and legs. Muscle wasting is proportionate to weakness. About 50% of patients have a waddling gait and use Gowers' maneuver to rise from the supine position. About 20% have a marked limp or are unable to walk. Virtually all patients display weakness of pelvic and thigh muscles. Tendon reflexes are normal to brisk, and sensation is normal. No cranial nerve abnormalities occur. Bone pain and tenderness are most prominent in the pelvis, femurs, spine, and ribs. Frequently, collapse of vertebrae occurs, sometimes with skeletal deformities. Occasionally, patients describe total body pain, suggesting a primary psychiatric disorder.

Diagnosis

Osteomalacia is suggested by severe pain, especially in the lower lumbar and hip girdle regions, and muscle weakness. Radiographic abnormalities (eg, pseudofractures, biconcave vertebrae) are found in about 70% of patients with osteomalacia, reduced serum calcium and phosphorus levels in about 40%, and elevated serum alkaline phosphatase activity in > 80%. Urinary calcium excretion is markedly reduced, and serum levels of vitamin D and its metabolites are decreased. The serum creatine kinase level is normal or slightly elevated. Electromyography may show a myopathic pattern; nerve conduction studies are normal. Muscle biopsy findings are normal or indicate nonspecific changes. Bone biopsy is a simple confirmatory procedure. Oral tetracycline can be given before bone biopsy to label the front of mineralization.

Treatment

Initial treatment requires vitamin D IM 10,000 u./day. Once bone pain resolves, vitamin D can be given orally. For most patients, the long-term prognosis is good. However, if marked wasting, especially of the quadriceps muscle of the thigh, has occurred, patients may never regain full strength despite normal serum levels of vitamin D and phosphate.

HYPOKALEMIC MYOPATHY

(See also Ch. 3)

In the elderly, hypokalemia is the most common cause of electrolyte myopathy. A common cause of hypokalemia in this age group is long-term diuretic use. About 20% to 30% of patients treated with starting doses of thiazide diuretics without potassium repletion develop hypokalemia; the percentage increases with high doses. This tendency for hypokalemia is exaggerated in poorer patients, among whom dietary potassium deficiency is common because many foods high in potassium are more expensive.

Hypocalcemia and hypomagnesemia can also produce prominent neuromuscular symptoms including tetany, irritability, myoclonus, and tremor, but they do not typically cause muscle weakness.

Symptoms and Signs

Muscle weakness usually develops slowly over days to weeks with the legs primarily being affected. In severe cases, weakness spreads to the arms, trunk, neck, and occasionally, thoracic and diaphragmatic muscles. Ocular and bulbar muscles are spared.

The underlying cause of the hypokalemia determines the pattern of weakness. For example, patients with diabetic acidosis (in which serum potassium levels fall rapidly over hours) may present with respiratory weakness, and the arms may become weak before the legs. In general, chronic hypokalemic myopathy produces greater weakness of proximal muscles than of distal muscles. Tendon reflexes become hypoactive and then vanish. The patient has no pain or other sensory complaints. In severe cases, **muscle fiber necrosis** with myoglobinuria, muscle pain, tenderness, and muscle swelling can develop.

Diagnosis and Treatment

The serum potassium level is usually < 3 mEq/L. The serum creatine kinase level may be normal or elevated. Nerve conduction velocities are normal.

Conditions associated with hypokalemia include alcoholic myopathy, intestinal potassium wastage, Bartter's syndrome, aldosteronism, and licorice intoxication. Acute hypokalemic paralysis may occur after amphotericin B treatment and with diabetic ketoacidosis, renal tubular acidosis, chronic diarrhea, and most conditions that produce chronic hypokalemia.

Chronic myopathy usually reverses after 1 to 4 wk of potassium replacement therapy. If myoglobinuria and rhabdomyolysis have occurred, treatment should include vigorous hydration and alkalinization of the urine to avoid renal tubular necrosis and renal failure. Depending on the cause of hypokalemia, long-term potassium replacement may be needed.

MYOPATHY CAUSED BY MUSCULAR DYSTROPHIES

The onset of primary muscular dystrophy in elderly patients is extremely rare. However, the two types most likely to present in old age are myotonic dystrophy and oculopharyngeal muscular dystrophy.

MYOTONIC DYSTROPHY

This autosomal dominant, multisystem disorder is caused by an abnormality on chromosome 19.

Symptoms, Signs, and Diagnosis

Usually, distal weakness develops in persons in their 20s and 30s, but with mild forms of the disease, the primary symptoms may be frontal baldness and cataracts occurring late in life. Older patients have minimal muscle weakness with cardiac conduction defects (atrioventricular block, bundle branch block), posterior capsular cataracts, GI hypomotility, and respiratory insufficiency (decreased vital capacity especially when supine) caused by weakness of the respiratory muscles, primarily the diaphragm. Tendon reflexes are depressed, especially in the legs.

Diagnosis is established by DNA testing; specific probes are available. Muscle biopsy findings and mildly to moderately elevated serum creatine kinase levels have secondary value in establishing the diagnosis.

Treatment

Treatment is nonspecific. The goal is to manage complications: respiratory insufficiency; cardiac arrhythmias, particularly conduction block; and GI hypomotility. Surgery can be problematic because patients react with paradoxic rigidity to succinylcholine and other muscle relaxants; nondepolarizing relaxants are recommended. The long-term prognosis depends on the severity of muscle weakness and the presence of complications.

OCULOPHARYNGEAL MUSCULAR DYSTROPHY

Onset of this autosomal dominant disorder usually occurs in the 50s and 60s. Persons develop ptosis that is almost always bilateral. Typically, the patient shows a prominent contraction of the occipitofrontal muscle, and the head is tipped back to compensate visually for the ptosis. Dysphagia for solid foods usually follows extraocular weakness. Palatal mobility is often diminished, and the gag reflex is impaired. Some laryngeal weakness with dysphonia is common. Tendon reflexes may be diminished or even absent. Some patients complain of cramps in calf muscles despite the absence of significant weakness. Years later, the muscles of the limbs, especially of the proximal hip girdle, may become weakened. The diagnosis depends on clinical features and a positive family history. The disease is often confused with myasthenia gravis. There is no specific treatment.

IDIOPATHIC MUSCLE CRAMPS

Idiopathic muscle cramps without significant muscle weakness frequently occur in otherwise healthy middle-aged and elderly patients.

Symptoms, Signs, and Diagnosis

Muscle cramps may develop at rest or with minor exercise. Typically, they occur at night during sleep and affect the calf or foot muscles, causing forceful plantar flexion of the foot or toes. Diagnosis is based on the history and lack of physical signs or disability.

Treatment

Stretching the affected muscles for several minutes before sleep is often an effective preventive measure. Stretching immediately after cramping occurs usually relieves symptoms and almost always is preferable to empiric drug treatments. An effective method for stretching the gastrocnemius and soleus muscles is for the person to stand 3 to 4 ft from a wall while facing it. Then the person leans against the wall with outstretched arms, keeping the heels on the floor, the knees locked, and the body straight. The person should stretch the calves for two or three 1-min intervals with 1-min rest periods between stretches. Such exercises improve muscle and tendon flexibility and can reduce the motor unit activity in the stretched muscles.

Quinine sulfate 200 to 300 mg at bedtime is prescribed, but recent studies show that it is not effective for night cramps. Quinine can also cause bitter taste, tinnitus, flushing, pruritus, and GI disturbances, and it interacts with many other drugs. Calcium supplements (such as calcium gluconate 1 to 2 gm bid) are well tolerated, but their effectiveness is also doubtful. Agents used with quinine and calcium treatment include diphenhydramine 50 to 100 mg at bedtime, magnesium oxide 100 to 200 mg bid, and low doses of benzodiazepines. However, with all these drugs, the toxic effects are likely to outweigh any benefit. Mexiletine 150 mg tid is sometimes effective when increased irritability of the lower motor neuron is suspected. Avoiding caffeine and other sympathetic stimulants may be helpful.

---

77. FOOT PROBLEMS

Foot problems often cause disability and decrease productivity. These problems range from simple ailments (eg, corns or ingrown nails) to serious complications of diabetes mellitus and peripheral vascular disease.

Neglect of the feet throughout a person's active years results in painful conditions later on. Foot disorders begin early in life and are influenced by factors such as heredity, shoe styles and fit, gait patterns, level of activity, terrain, and improper care.

EVALUATION OF THE FOOT

History

The patient's chief concern should be recorded in his own words. The nature of the problem as well as the location, duration, onset, severity, symptoms, and previous treatment should be noted. The patient should indicate which part of the foot is most painful when walking; then the examiner should determine whether or not the same symptoms can be elicited using palpation and range-of-motion testing with the patient at rest. Relevant economic, psychologic, and social factors should be recorded. Self-treatment should also be noted because it is often the precipitating factor in seeking professional help.

An appropriate review of systems should be conducted, and significant findings should be considered in relation to the patient's problem. Often, symptoms and signs of systemic disease are first noted in the feet. When reviewing the history, note especially any of the following conditions and their treatment: diabetes, cardiac disease, arthritis, hypertension, and peripheral vascular disease. Any history of night cramps should also be noted.

Evaluation also requires a consideration of the patient's lifestyle in relation to the presenting problem. The patient's environment and degree of ambulation should be considered. Many geriatric patients may be physically unable to seek appropriate attention for their medical problems. Others may not understand a particular treatment or may be reluctant to stray from old and outdated remedies. Still others may delay seeking professional help for economic reasons.

Physical Examination

Skin and nail evaluation: Many foot problems involve the skin. During inspection, the size and location of any hyperkeratotic lesions or excrescences should be recorded. Changes in long-standing lesions—such as bleeding and discoloration—should be noted, and their significance should be determined, possibly by biopsy. Any bacterial infection, tinea pedis, dry skin, ulcerations, or verrucae should also be recorded.

The toenails should be inspected for signs of hypertrophy and mycotic infection. Missing nails, changes in the color and continuity of the nail plate, and foot odor should be noted.

Vascular evaluation: The feet and legs should be evaluated for trophic changes (eg, loss of hair growth; red, shiny, atrophic skin; and pigmentation changes). The temperature of the feet should be noted, and if claudication is present, appropriate information should be elicited. The pedal pulses (dorsalis pedis and posterior tibial) should be palpated, and any varicosities or edema should be noted. If vascular disease is suspected, Doppler and plethysmographic studies should be performed.

Neurologic evaluation: This part of the physical examination should include motor function testing. The Achilles and superficial plantar reflexes should be elicited, and vibratory sensation should be evaluated, along with sensitivity to pain, temperature, and touch. Muscle-strength testing should be performed, and the results should be recorded with any areas of discomfort noted.

Orthopedic evaluation: One of the most important components of a foot evaluation is observing the patient's gait. Often, this will be the key to determining an effective treatment plan for biomechanical conditions. Postural deformities, physical limitations, and the position of the foot at heel strike and through the gait cycle are identified by watching the patient walk.

The foot has 26 bones, which along with ligaments, tendons, and muscles provide support and mobility. There are 14 phalanges (3 for each of the lesser toes and 2 for the great toe or hallux), 5 metatarsals, and 7 tarsal bones. The talus, or ankle bone, supports the fibula laterally and the tibia medially. It provides the fulcrum around which motion occurs. The talus is seated on the calcaneus, or heel bone.

Motion occurs primarily around the subtalar, or talocalcaneal, joint. This motion occurs in three planes and includes inversion-eversion, abduction-adduction, and dorsiflexion and plantar flexion. A combination of dorsiflexion, abduction, and eversion is commonly referred to as pronation, while a combination of the opposite movements—plantar flexion, adduction, and inversion—is known as supination. The degree of pronation or supination should be determined, especially when corrective devices are being considered.

On inspection, structural foot deformities are obvious. **Hallux valgus (bunion)** is a painful condition involving the first metatarsophalangeal joint. X-rays should be taken and the degree of deformity noted. A **bunionette** is a similar condition involving the fifth metatarsophalangeal joint, in which the fifth toe is maintained in a varus position and the head of the metatarsal becomes prominent laterally. This, too, can be evaluated on x-rays, which should also detect any bone changes (eg, osteoporosis, demineralization, old fractures, or arthritis). Range-of-motion testing and grading should be done for all joints. Any limitations of movement or crepitus should be recorded. Finally, the patient's foot type and shoe style should be noted.

COMMON FOOT PROBLEMS

Elderly persons may suffer from a wide variety of foot problems, including dermatologic problems, nail disorders, orthopedic and structural deformities, complications of systemic disease, arthritis, gout, and neurologic disorders.

DERMATOLOGIC FOOT PROBLEMS

Corns and Calluses

Usually the result of undue friction and pressure around a bony prominence, these common lesions are often associated with improper or tight foot wear. A **corn,** also known as a **clavus** or **heloma,** is *a somewhat conical, concentrated hyperkeratotic lesion most commonly found on the dorsal surface of the proximal interphalangeal joint of the lesser toes.* This joint also becomes contracted in hammer toe syndrome, making it vulnerable to excessive pressure from shoes and stockings. The problem may be complicated by a bunion deformity, in which the great toe deviates laterally, causing a contraction of the second toe. Digital contractures and arthritic changes may also cause lesions to develop on the distal aspect of the toes. The fifth toe is prone to developing a corn because of rotational deformity. If not properly treated, these hard hyperkeratotic lesions can lead to inflammation and infection. A **soft corn,** or **heloma molle,** usually occurs interdigitally and is caused by pressure from adjacent toes. The lesion becomes soft because of accumulated moisture in the web space.

Treatment consists of debriding the lesion and applying aperture or balance padding to redistribute pressure away from the painful area. This may be done with a small 1/8-in. felt pad with a concentric opening placed directly over the lesion. Medicated pads should be avoided because their acid content often destroys tissue, leading to further disability. An emollient skin cream should be used afterward to reduce keratosis. Orthodigital devices, such as tube-shaped foam pads or polyurethane and silicone molds, may be fabricated for the patient who is able to bend over and apply them. Another conservative treatment option is custom-made, molded orthopedic shoes made from casts of the patient's feet to compensate for any bone abnormalities. Such abnormalities should be identified on the prescription for the shoes. (These shoes are commonly called space shoes.)

A **callus,** or **tyloma,** is *a diffuse, circumscribed hyperkeratotic lesion found on the plantar aspect of the foot,* where friction and pressure occur. A callus may also result from weight changes and improper shoe modifications. Symptoms range from generalized burning to severe pinpoint pain. A somewhat similar but more circumscribed lesion is the **intractable plantar keratoma.** This painful lesion is usually found directly under the head of the involved metatarsal. Such lesions may result from plantar declination of the bone or may be associated with arthritic changes or trauma. They must be differentiated from viral **warts,** which look similar. On debridement, warts characteristically reveal areas of pinpoint bleeding.

Treatment of a callus consists of debriding the lesion and applying protective padding such as moleskin, lamb's wool, or polyurethane. An emollient skin cream, preferably one with a urea base, provides dermal hydration. Adhesive padding should be *avoided* in patients with diabetes or peripheral vascular impairment. **Treatment of a wart** consists of paring down the lesion and applying an acidic preparation or performing surgical excision. Excision on the plantar aspect of the foot should be avoided because of subsequent pain and potential scarring.

Orthotic devices should be used when these lesions result from biomechanical factors. X-ray evaluation, as well as clinical examination, provides insight into the cause of the underlying problem. Orthotic devices can be made from various materials, depending on the patient's tolerance; they can be modified if new lesions develop from bony changes associated with arthritis and aging. Compliance is usually good because the devices can be transferred from one pair of shoes to another.

Dryness and Scaling

These problems, often caused by decreased sebaceous gland activity, become more apparent with aging. **Pruritus** may result, and scratching may produce open wounds and inflammation. Pruritus is also common with conditions such as **tinea pedis, contact dermatitis,** and **eczema.** Low doses of oral antihistamines along with a topical corticosteroid should be used until the symptoms subside. Afterward, prophylactic use of a urea-based, emollient skin cream is usually sufficient to control the condition. With contact dermatitis, the causative factor—usually a pair of shoes or stockings or the laundry detergent used to wash the stockings—should be eliminated.

Tinea Pedis

Commonly known as **athlete's foot,** tinea pedis is usually caused by *Trichophyton rubrum, T. mentagrophytes,* or *Epidermophyton floccosum.* Since fungi thrive in a warm, moist environment, hyperhidrosis complicates the condition. Most commonly, tinea pedis appears interdigitally and in the moccasin pattern (the soles, heels, and sides of the feet) typical of *T. rubrum.* Vesicular eruption, fissuring, loss of the epidermis, and secondary bacterial infection may occur. The elderly are especially susceptible to such outbreaks because of changes in the distal tissues resulting from peripheral vascular disease and the aging process. These patients often develop cracks and fissures, which provide a convenient portal of entry for invasive organisms. Tinea resembles **erythrasma,** with which it is often confused. The latter is caused by a gram-positive bacillus and is diagnosed by a coral-red fluorescence when examined under a Wood's light. Erythrasma is treated with oral erythromycin and topical antifungal preparations.

Diagnosis of tinea pedis may be aided by a dermatophyte-testing medium, in which a simple color change indicates fungal infection. Traditional methods of diagnosis include microscopic examination with a potassium hydroxide preparation and a fungal culture.

Treatment of tinea infections consists of soaking the feet in warm water and Epsom salt, then applying a topical antifungal cream, such as clotrimazole or miconazole nitrate. If inflammation and itching occur, a preparation combining clioquinol and hydrocortisone or one combining clotrimazole and betamethasone dipropionate can be used. When edema and bacterial infection occur, the feet should be elevated, ambulation reduced, oral antibiotics given, and frequent clinical observations made.

Griseofulvin is an oral mycostatic agent that relies on an adequate vasculature, which many geriatric patients do not have. Also, certain side effects (eg, urticaria, skin rashes, nausea and vomiting, headache, and fatigue) may preclude its use in frail elderly patients. More severe reactions include paresthesias of the hands and feet, proteinuria, and leukopenia. Patients taking griseofulvin should have routine complete blood counts to exclude leukopenia and liver function tests to exclude liver toxicity.

Psoriasis

This disorder is common in geriatric patients. The characteristic lesion appears on the foot with hyperkeratosis and fissuring. The nails show pitting and subungual hyperkeratosis. Local treatment consists of applying a topical corticosteroid and periodically debriding the nails.

Hyperhidrosis

Excessive sweating of the feet may cause a foul odor (bromhidrosis). Hyperhidrosis may be precipitated or aggravated by tinea pedis, poor pedal hygiene, or metabolic disease. The usual treatment is a 10% formaldehyde solution, frequent sock changes, and routine use of a topical foot powder.

NAIL DISORDERS

The primary function of the nail is to protect the distal phalanges against injury and trauma. Many changes in the nail plate can be attributed to aging and are associated with trauma, dermatologic conditions, and systemic disease.

Onychia and Paronychia

Onychia is *inflammation of the nail matrix;* **paronychia** is *inflammation of the matrix plus the surrounding and deeper structures*. The most common cause of onychia and paronychia is trauma (eg, a direct injury or pressure from new or too-small shoes). Skin diseases (eg, **psoriasis** and **eczema**) are commonly responsible for inflammatory reactions around the nail. Patients with **diabetes mellitus** tend to develop inflammation around the nail bed because of poor circulation and diminished resistance to infection.

Unguis Incarnatus

(Onychocryptosis)

This condition is commonly known as an **ingrown toenail.** The lateral nail edge penetrates the periungual tissue, causing an inflammatory reaction and sometimes secondary bacterial infection. If the infection is not resolved, painful granulation tissue forms, requiring surgical intervention. Faulty footwear and improper nail care are the primary causes.

Treatment consists of removing the ingrown portion of the nail, in some cases by inserting an English anvil pattern nail splitter under the nail plate. Depending on the severity of the condition, local anesthesia may be needed. After the wound is cleaned, a topical antibiotic and a dry, sterile dressing are applied. Warm Epsom salt soaks should be used twice daily, and a new dressing should be applied after each soak. For severe infection, systemic antibiotics should be used.

Onychomycosis

A localized fungal infection of the nail or nail bed, onychomycosis is characterized by degeneration of the nail plate with changes in growth and appearance. The degeneration ranges from simple scaling to actual destruction of the nail's entire architecture. The nail becomes brittle, hypertrophic, and granular. Infection usually progresses from one nail to the next. The thickened nail plate often shows subungual keratosis and debris. The causative agents are usually *Trichophyton rubrum, T. mentagrophytes,* and *E. floccosum,* although candidal infections may also produce onychomycosis. **Diagnosis** may be made with the appropriate dermatophyte-testing technique.

With onychomycosis, repeated microtrauma of the enlarged nail plate from shoe pressure can cause severe discomfort and disability. Antifungal therapy is rarely effective because of the nail matrix involvement. Also, the diminished pedal blood supply in many elderly patients precludes the use of oral antifungal agents. Instead, **treatment** consists of reduction of the nail plates at regular intervals and patient education. Using topical antifungal agents around the nail bed to keep the tissue soft may help.

Onychauxis and Onychogryphosis

Onychauxis is *hypertrophy of the nail plate;* **onychogryphosis** is *longstanding hypertrophy characterized by a curved or hooked nail* (also known as a ram's horn nail). Pressure, including that from bed sheets at night, on such nails may produce severe pain. Because of the severe hypertrophy, the nail may penetrate the adjacent toe, causing inflammation and pain. In a patient with diabetes or peripheral vascular disease, pressure necrosis may result, causing ulceration and gangrene. **Treatment** involves frequent nail cutting or trimming and instruction in proper foot care and hygiene.

When severe nail conditions cause pain and disability, and conservative measures have failed, surgery should be considered. A partial or complete destruction of the nail matrix can be performed simply and effectively, using local anesthesia, usually on an outpatient basis.

ORTHOPEDIC AND STRUCTURAL DEFORMITIES

Heel Pain

A common problem, heel pain begins almost immediately upon weight bearing and either lessens with walking or remains constant. The pain usually occurs around the plantar aspect of the heel and may radiate distally to the arch. Such pain may adversely affect a patient's ability to carry out simple daily tasks or even his entire outlook.

Often, the pain results from gradual age-related atrophy of the fat padding beneath the calcaneus. It also may be due to excessive activity that causes increased pressure and irritation to the area. The most common cause of heel pain is a **heel spur,** in which pain usually results from inflammation caused by the constant pulling of the plantar fascia at its origin in the calcaneus. In most cases, abnormal pronation causes excessive tension on the fascia. Pain in the longitudinal arch *without* concomitant heel pain is known as **plantar fasciitis.**

Treatment for heel pain depends on the nature and extent of bone damage as shown on x-ray. With a heel spur, a shelf of bone may be seen at the base of the calcaneus on a lateral view. Local injections of a corticosteroid and an anesthetic agent should be given weekly until symptoms subside. Typically, this consists of 0.5 to 1 mL of betamethasone sodium phosphate and betamethasone acetate suspension (or other suitable agent) and 1 mL 2% plain lidocaine. The injection should originate at the medial side of the heel and be aimed toward the area of greatest pain.

Plantar strapping can be used in conjunction with corticosteroid and anesthetic therapy to relieve tension on the plantar fascia. A low-dye strapping may be used to control pronation at the subtalar joint. With the foot slightly inverted and perpendicular to the leg, the tape is applied proximal to the fifth metatarsal head and extended around the heel, stopping just proximal to the first metatarsal head. Scaphoid (navicular) padding provides further support and is highly recommended; anchor straps incorporating such padding should be applied around the instep. Strapping should be replaced in about one week during a follow-up evaluation.

Oral nonsteroidal anti-inflammatory drugs **(NSAIDs)** such as piroxicam 20 mg daily or naproxen 500 mg bid, physical therapy such as ultrasound and hydrotherapy, heel cups, and plantar paddings may reduce discomfort in the heel. When the pain has diminished, a biomechanical examination should be performed, and an appropriate orthotic device should be made to compensate for the pronation, alleviate strain on the plantar fascia, and provide adequate support for the heel.

In Haglund's disease, or **"pump bump,"** pain occurs in the posterior portion of the heel. The condition seems to result from pressure on the posterior-superior aspect of the calcaneus, where irritation from the shoe counter or heel strap may produce a bursal sac. With bursitis, aspiration may be needed. Heel lifts raise the heel above the counter, alleviating symptoms. Aperture padding around the bursal sac also relieves pressure. During episodes of acute pain, slippers should be worn. Also, physical therapy, such as ultrasound and hydrotherapy, should be considered. NSAIDs may help ease the discomfort of Haglund's deformity. If conservative therapy fails, surgical excision may be necessary.

Hallux Valgus

Commonly called **bunion,** this is *a condition in which a deviation of the first metatarsophalangeal joint causes the toe to drift laterally, the first metatarsal head protrudes medially, and exostosis may occur.* An adventitious bursa may form at the point of greatest pressure. As the hallux drifts laterally, the second toe may override it, causing a painful dorsal lesion. A hammer toe syndrome may develop, followed by a tyloma beneath the second metatarsal because of contracture of the second toe. Two other conditions involving the first metatarsophalangeal joint are metatarsus primus varus, in which the first metatarsal drifts medially, and hallux rigidus (see ARTHRITIS AND GOUT, below).

Treatment is aimed at relieving pain and providing comfort. Surgical correction is usually the treatment of choice, but the patient's lifestyle and ability to perform self-care should be considered before deciding on surgery. Often, a bunion is irritated by shoe friction and pressure because the foot with the deformity occupies more space than a normal foot. Removing the shoe affords some relief. When the deformity is severe, a bunion-last type shoe or a custom-made, molded shoe should be considered. Until such footwear can be obtained, a cutout should be made in the patient's shoe at the area of greatest pressure. Acute inflammation in the area of the adventitious bursa is usually relieved by injecting a corticosteroid combined with an anesthetic. Oral NSAIDs are also effective in treating symptoms.

Metatarsalgia

A generalized ache or soreness directly below the metatarsal heads, metatarsalgia results from atrophy of the plantar fat pad that supports the metatarsal heads. It may be accompanied by a plantar callus and, if untreated, may lead to anterior metatarsal bursitis or arthritis of the involved metatarsophalangeal joints. **Treatment** consists of redistributing the pressure away from the metatarsal heads. This can be accomplished with an orthopedic shoe, an orthosis, or another device that provides cushioning and shock absorption to this area of the foot.

Hammer Toe Syndrome

In this condition, *the involved toe is in a fixed, contracted position at the proximal interphalangeal joint*. The toe, being higher in the shoe than normal, is exposed to excessive friction, often resulting in a painful heloma. In severe cases, the lesion may become inflamed and ulcerated, leading to secondary bacterial infection and ambulatory disability. **Treatment** consists of removing the irritating shoe and debriding the lesion. Surgical correction, ranging from simple tenotomy to arthroplasty of the digit, should be considered in severe cases.

Morton's Neuroma

This deformity is caused by entrapment of the interdigital nerves as they pass between the metatarsal heads. It characteristically occurs in the third interspace, where the metatarsal heads are in closest proximity, and causes severe, disabling pain. The pain, which may radiate to the toes or legs, requiring shoe removal and foot massage, is pathognomonic. Nonsurgical **treatment** consists of local injections of a long-acting corticosteroid proximal to the site of pain. If symptoms are not alleviated, surgical excision is advised.

Fractures

Because older persons are especially prone to falls and other injuries, foot fractures are common. Ice should be applied immediately to the injured area to reduce inflammation, and analgesics should be given to manage pain. X-rays should be taken to confirm the diagnosis and determine the extent of injury; the dorsoplantar, lateral, and oblique views are helpful. Toe fractures may be treated by splinting the injured toe to an adjacent one to ensure immobilization. Realigning a displaced fracture of the toe requires local anesthesia. More severe fractures, such as those of a metatarsal or tarsal bone, require a plaster or semirigid cast or Unna's boot. With any fracture, walking should be restricted, and crutches may be necessary. Follow-up x-rays should be taken over the next few months to assess healing.

COMPLICATIONS OF SYSTEMIC DISEASE

Peripheral vascular disease and **diabetes mellitus** can lead to major foot problems; thus, an understanding of the nature and consequences of these diseases is essential in planning long-term goals (see Chs. 42 and 80).

Symptoms and Signs

Symptoms of **vascular disease** in the legs and feet include exertional pain, edema, skin color changes, coldness, burning, numbness, loss of hair growth, and ulcerations. With advancing vascular disease, changes in the nails occur, most notably thickening and onychomycosis.

Pain on walking indicates intermittent claudication. Patients exhibit a diagnostic limp if they continue walking after symptoms begin. **Pain on**

rest indicates more advanced arterial disease and tissue ischemia. Poor circulation diminishes the ability to combat infection, and even the slightest cut or bruise may cause ulceration and gangrene.

Patients with **diabetes** have many of the same symptoms as those with peripheral vascular insufficiency. Diabetes affects primarily the small arteries and nerves in the feet, causing paresthesias, motor weakness, numbness, burning, and cramping. Other clinical findings in elderly diabetics include color and temperature changes, dry and scaly skin, and edema that may result from generalized systemic disease or localized infection. Nail changes are similar to those of vascular insufficiency.

Diabetic patients are prone to **ulcer formation,** especially on the weight-bearing surfaces of the foot. Ulcers often lead to infection, osteomyelitis, and gangrene. Diabetic patients may precipitate ulcer formation by using an acidic, over-the-counter, corn remedy, which causes skin sloughing and soft tissue destruction.

Whether an ulcer is neurotrophic or vascular should be determined. A **neurotrophic ulcer** is usually painless, and the patient may not be aware of it. In contrast, a **vascular ulcer** causes extreme pain and is more prone to infection because of the circulatory impairment.

Treatment

Treatment of **vascular sclerotic conditions** consists of using warm soaks and, under close supervision, thermostatically controlled heating elements to dilate the blood vessels. Patients need special care and should be evaluated regularly. They should be taught the importance of their role in prevention and treatment. Many times, simple problems can be resolved if treated early. Daily self-inspection of the feet is strongly advised, especially for patients with neuropathy and an associated lack of feeling.

For an **ulcer,** necrotic tissue should be debrided aseptically to enable viable tissue to heal. Drainage should be cultured and appropriate antibiotic therapy initiated. An enzymatic debriding agent such as collagenase or fibrinolysin with desoxyribonuclease should be applied. Flexible hydroactive dressings are particularly useful on dry wounds and on those with light exudate. These dressings help isolate the lesion from bacterial and other contaminants and are effective in areas such as the heel where constant friction is a problem. The foot should be maintained at rest in a level position, and ambulation should be restricted as much as possible since it may cause further trauma and increase the risk of infection. The patient should be cautioned against cigarette smoking and exposure to temperature extremes. Tissue perfusion may be enhanced by pentoxifylline, a drug that increases the flexibility of red blood cells, thereby decreasing blood viscosity and improving blood flow. Aspirin may also help increase local circulation to ulcerated areas.

After the ulcer heals, shoes should be modified to divert pressure from sensitive areas. This may be done with padding or other protective devices or with an inlay or an accommodative orthotic device.

When an ulcer cannot be managed conservatively, bypass surgery may be indicated to increase circulation to the limb, provided circulation is adequate above and below the occluded area. For a diabetic patient with vascular insufficiency and microangiopathy, early consultation with a vascular surgeon is extremely important to ascertain whether surgery would be beneficial. Plethysmographic and Doppler studies are indicated to evaluate the extent of the damage. X-rays should be taken to rule out osteomyelitis. If gangrene develops, amputation is usually necessary.

ARTHRITIS AND GOUT

The most common condition causing foot pain in older persons is some form of arthritis.

Osteoarthritis

This form of arthritis often involves the ankle and the first metatarsophalangeal joint, where a **hallux rigidus** may occur. Symptoms increase with ambulation and include pain, swelling, stiffness, and weakness at the involved joint. Motion may be limited by exostosis formation, which is thought to be primarily biomechanical. Diagnosis is made by observing the patient's walk and noting decreased motion at the interphalangeal joint of the hallux. Palpation of the first metatarsophalangeal joint reveals stiffness and pain with a pronounced limitation of motion. Once osteoarthritis is established, characteristic x-ray findings include narrowing of the joint space (caused by loss of articular cartilage), osteophyte formation, and increased density of subchondral bone.

Treatment is symptomatic, ranging from NSAID therapy to surgical intervention if marked loss of joint function has occurred. For a hallux rigidus, local infiltration of a corticosteroid with an anesthetic agent may provide symptomatic relief, followed by exercise of the joint and traction of the toe to help increase range of motion. If this approach fails, an appropriate orthotic device should be made with a Morton's extension that cushions motion at the metatarsophalangeal joint to reduce pain during walking.

Rheumatoid Arthritis

In this form of arthritis, progressive stiffening of the joints may lead to deformity and ankylosis. The patient may have morning stiffness, pain on motion, and subcutaneous nodules. Laboratory findings often include an increased erythrocyte sedimentation rate, positive latex fixation test, and hypochromic anemia. X-rays typically show splaying of the forefoot, claw toes, loss of articular cartilage, and bony erosions.

Conservative **treatment** of the rheumatoid foot includes patient education and support. Periods of rest from weight bearing are essential, as are shoe modifications to accommodate painful plantar areas. A custom-made orthopedic shoe is particularly helpful. Local injection of a corticosteroid helps alleviate joint pain, as do oral doses of NSAIDs and analgesics. Several surgical procedures are available and should be considered when conservative therapy provides minimal benefit.

Gout

More common in men than in women, gout is characterized by the deposit of urate crystals **(tophi)** in the synovial membrane and articular cartilage. Typical punched-out lesions may be seen radiographically and are pathognomonic. Diagnosis may be confirmed by microscopic evaluation of aspirated synovial fluid for urate crystals with their characteristic strongly negative birefringence.

The inflammatory response, initiated by the urate crystals, often begins in the great toe and is characterized by increasing joint pain, swelling, erythema, and heat. While other areas, such as the instep or ankle, may be involved, acute gouty arthritis usually seems to affect the first metatarsophalangeal joint. Walking is difficult or impossible—even the bed sheets may become an irritant during the acute attack. Gout-like symptoms may develop after prolonged use of thiazide diuretics. If this occurs, alternative antihypertensive therapy should be considered.

Prevention of gout includes lifestyle changes and drug therapy. Gradual weight reduction should be initiated if necessary, and alcohol in any form should be avoided. Increased fluid intake and uricosuric drugs enhance uric acid excretion. Two such drugs, probenecid and sulfinpyrazone, lower uric acid levels and help prevent tophi formation. These drugs act by blocking the renal tubular resorption of urate. The recommended dosage for probenecid is 0.25 gm bid for 1 wk, followed by 0.5 gm bid; for sulfinpyrazone, it is 100 to 200 mg bid with a gradual increase to 400 mg bid. Allopurinol, a xanthine oxidase inhibitor, decreases uric acid formation. Given at a single daily dose of 300 mg or at a dosage of 100 mg bid or tid, allopurinol helps prevent gout attacks.

Treatment of an attack usually consists of oral colchicine 0.5 to 1.2 mg initially, then 0.5 to 0.6 mg/h until symptoms subside or GI discomfort develops. Because colchicine toxicity can cause death and reduced renal function is common in the elderly (even when serum creatinine concentration is normal), colchicine therapy should be limited to the lowest number of doses that is effective. Paregoric is often used to treat the side effects of colchicine therapy. Indomethacin 50 mg q 6 to 8 h for the first 24 to 72 h, followed by 25 mg tid or qid is also effective for acute gout attacks. Other NSAIDs are effective, too. Analgesics may be used for severe pain.

NEUROLOGIC DISORDERS

Tarsal Tunnel Syndrome

In this disorder, compression of the posterior tibial nerve at the ankle results in severe pain leading to disability and reduced ambulation. Presenting symptoms include burning and discomfort, which may be severe and usually radiate to the toes. Pain increases upon ambulation and is relieved by rest. The condition may be diagnosed by Tinel's sign, distal tingling produced by tapping on the nerve at the site of compression.

Treatment consists of local injections of a corticosteroid (eg, dexamethasone or triamcinolone acetonide) in combination with a local anesthetic. Strapping to alleviate pressure on the nerve should be used with injection therapy. When conservative measures are ineffective, surgical decompression of the nerve should be considered.

Dorsal Cutaneous Nerve Trauma

Pain in the dorsolateral aspect of the foot usually results from pathologic conditions of the intermediate dorsal cutaneous nerve, whereas pain in the dorsomedial aspect may be caused by conditions of the medial dorsal cutaneous nerve. In elderly patients who have undergone bunion surgery, the latter nerve is often injured because of improper surgical technique or entrapment by fibrosis during healing. **Treatment** consists of local corticosteroid injections along with strapping or custom-made shoes. Pressure should be avoided at the site of the nerve injury. When severe fibrosis or entrapment of a nerve is suspected, surgical intervention should be considered.

§3. ORGAN SYSTEMS: METABOLIC AND ENDOCRINE DISORDERS

78. AGE–RELATED ENDOCRINE AND METABOLIC CHANGES

The endocrine and metabolic control systems offer many of the greatest opportunities for preventing disabilities associated with aging. Thyroid disease is common and often undiagnosed, but early detection and treatment can prevent unnecessary disability. Diabetes mellitus is extremely common, and normalizing blood glucose levels reduces its devastating vascular and neurologic complications. Hyperparathyroidism, hyperthyroidism, and hypothyroidism are clinical masqueraders. Early diagnosis by screening for hypercalcemia leads to proper treatment, preventing disability.

Menopause, a normal state of ovarian hormone deficiency, dramatically affects older women, often producing disabling consequences. But estrogen replacement therapy can largely eliminate them. Hypogonadism in older men has been less thoroughly studied, but many cases of male sexual disability can be improved by proper diagnosis and treatment. Furthermore, a growing knowledge of the importance of lipoprotein (particularly cholesterol) metabolism disorders has led to improved prevention and treatment, helping reduce the incidence of atherosclerosis and its consequences.

Changes in Hormone Levels

With aging, many aspects of the endocrine system change. Some endocrine organs and axes become hypoactive, either from diseases or physiologic down-regulation; some change little or not at all; and a few become hyperactive. These diverse and at times striking changes result from changes in hormone production and secretion rates, metabolic clearance rates, and tissue responsiveness or sensitivity (based on changes in hormone receptors or postreceptor mechanisms). Thus, an analysis of observed changes may be extremely complex.

Serum hormone levels reflect the sum of all these changes (see TABLE 78–1). Many changes are interrelated, one often serving as a compensatory response for another. For example, pituitary gonadotropins rise as gonadal hormones decline; insulin rises because of age-associated insulin resistance; and parathormone rises probably because of a fall in serum 1,25-dihydroxycholecalciferol with a resulting decrease in calcium absorption through the intestine.

On the other hand, the rise in vasopressin appears to reflect primary overproduction by the hypothalamoneurohypophysial system. The cause of the striking age-related rise in serum norepinephrine (but not epinephrine) is uncertain; possibilities include decreased numbers of

TABLE 78–1. EFFECTS OF AGE ON SERUM HORMONE LEVELS

Increased Levels	*Normal Levels*	*Decreased Levels*
Atrial natriuretic peptide	Calcitonin	Corticotropin†
Insulin	Cortisol*	Thyroid-stimulating hormone (TSH)‡
Norepinephrine	Epinephrine	Growth hormone
Parathormone	Prolactin	Insulin-like growth factor-1 (IGF-1, somatomedin-C)
Vasopressin	Thyroxine (T_4)	Renin
		Aldosterone
		Triiodothyronine (T_3)

* Mildly increased in some studies.
† May be normal.
‡ May be normal; in about 15% of persons over age 65, TSH is increased because of autoimmune thyroiditis, not because of age.

β-adrenergic receptors, postreceptor resistance, and abnormal baroreceptor function. The cause of the rise in serum atrial natriuretic peptide is also uncertain. Presumably, an expansion of intravascular volume stimulates atrial stretch receptors. The unresolved question is whether the primary event results from physiologic aging changes or subclinical heart failure.

Declining gonadal function and steroidogenesis result in decreases in sex hormone levels (see TABLE 78–2). In women, serum estrogen and progesterone decrease because of menopause. In most men, bioavailable testosterone decreases. In both sexes, androsterone, dehydroepiandrosterone (DHEA), and dehydroepiandrosterone sulfate also decline, reflecting an unexplained failure of the zona reticularis of the adrenal cortex. Although the atrophy of the ovaries and the more gradual atrophy of the testes are not surprising, the causes are unknown.

Clinical Significance of Changes

Knowledge of expected hormonal changes may be clinically useful. For example, the rise in serum insulin due to insulin resistance requires weight loss and exercise to protect the patient from the adverse effects of hyperinsulinemia. The rise in parathormone leads to accelerated bone resorption and, in women, requires calcium supplements and estrogen replacement therapy, both of which suppress bone resorption and parathormone secretion. The rise in vasopressin predisposes the elderly to hyponatremia (hypo-osmolarity, water intoxication). Drug-induced hyponatremia (eg, chlorpropamide) is seen almost exclusively in persons > 60 yr.

TABLE 78–2. EFFECTS OF AGE ON SERUM LEVELS OF STEROIDS AND RELATED HORMONES

Increased Levels	*Normal Levels*	*Decreased Levels*
Elderly women		
Follicle-stimulating hormone Luteinizing hormone Ovarian testosterone*	Total testosterone	Androsterone Dehydroepiandrosterone Dehydroepiandrosterone sulfate Estradiol Estrone Progesterone
Elderly men		
Dihydrotestosterone (DHT)† Follicle-stimulating hormone Luteinizing hormone Free estradiol Free estrone		Androstenedione Androsterone Dehydroepiandrosterone Dehydroepiandrosterone sulfate Testosterone Bioavailable testosterone

* May be normal.

† High in men with benign prostatic hyperplasia (BPH) but tends to be normal in men without BPH.

The high serum level of atrial natriuretic peptide, a potent diuretic, may contribute to nocturia in older people. When the person lies in bed, central intravascular volume rises, triggering a further burst of atrial natriuretic peptide which, in turn, causes sleep-disturbing nocturia. In older people, nocturia does not result primarily from decreased urine volume at each urination but rather from a reversal of the day-night ratio of total urine volume.

The modest declines in triiodothyronine (T_3), thyroid-stimulating hormone, and corticotropin levels have little clinical significance. However, growth hormone (GH) secretion falls markedly with aging, and the response to all stimuli (growth hormone-releasing factor [GHRF], sleep, pyridostigmine, naloxone) is blunted. Consequently, insulin-like growth factor-1 (IGF-1), an important anabolic factor, is subnormal in most older persons and markedly subnormal in about 33% of institutionalized older persons. Administration of human growth hormone is under study for a possible anabolic effect, which might be useful in very old, frail persons. The decrease in renin and aldosterone could result from the same intravascular volume expansion that increases atrial natriuretic peptide levels. In general, renin and atrial natriuretic peptide respond to the same stimuli but in opposite directions.

Although some steps are still unclear, changes in carbohydrate and lipoprotein metabolism are closely correlated. Further, carbohydrate metabolism affects and is affected by changes in fluid and electrolyte balance, acid-base balance, and total energy balance (ie, weight gain or loss). Protein-calorie nutritional status has pervasive effects on metabolic regulatory systems, and hyperinsulinemia secondary to insulin resistance is now thought to predispose elders to hypertension and to increased very-low-density lipoprotein (VLDL) and decreased high-density lipoprotein (HDL) levels.

Some important mysteries remain in the area of endocrine-metabolic interactions. For example, estrogens and progestins profoundly alter lipoprotein and cholesterol metabolism and may affect the rate of atherogenesis. These interrelationships are under study. Except for decreased sexual drive, the effects of male hypogonadism in the elderly are unknown. Along with decreased growth hormone secretion, the decline in testosterone levels may contribute to decreased muscle mass and strength previously thought to result from aging per se. Questions also remain about the cause of impotence in older men. Most evidence points to vascular or neurologic disease; erectile failure does not result from a decrease in testosterone.

79. THE NORMAL AND DISEASED THYROID GLAND

The thyroid gland produces thyroxine (T_4) and triiodothyronine (T_3), hormones essential for life and health. With normal aging, the gland's function changes. More important, the thyroid gland may be affected by two major conditions whose incidences increase with age (hypothyroidism and nodule formation) and one whose incidence remains fairly constant (hyperthyroidism).

THYROID FUNCTION IN NORMAL AGING

With aging, the thyroid gland undergoes moderate atrophy and develops nonspecific histopathologic abnormalities—fibrosis, increasing numbers of colloid nodules, and some lymphocytic infiltration. Correspondingly, its production of T_4 declines by nearly 50% between young adulthood and advanced old age. However, this decline is generally thought to be physiologic compensation for decreased tissue use of the hormone rather than a manifestation of primary thyroid failure. The crucial evidence for this conclusion is that serum T_4 levels remain unchanged with advancing age; if thyroid dysfunction were the major cause of decreased hormone production, serum T_4 levels would fall.

The decrease in T_4 use correlates well with the age-related decline in lean body mass, suggesting that the primary event is shrinkage of metabolically active, protein-rich tissues (muscle, skin, bone, and viscera). This shrinkage may lead to reduced use and catabolism of thyroid hormones and, sequentially, to a subtle rise in thyroid hormone levels, a resulting decrease in thyrotropin **(TSH)** output, a decrease in thyroidal T_3 and T_4 output, and a return of serum T_4 levels to normal. When stimulated by increased TSH, the healthy aged thyroid gland can increase its hormone production normally.

Serum levels of thyroid hormones change very little with age. Serum T_4, free T_4, and free T_4 index (serum T_4 multiplied by an index of protein binding, such as a T_3 resin uptake) remain unchanged. Serum T_3, free T_3, and free T_3 index (serum T_3 multiplied by an index of protein binding) fall slightly with normal aging. The metabolic clearance rate of T_4 decreases, while the metabolic clearance rate of T_3 falls little or not at all. Thus, with a decreased amount of T_4 being metabolized to T_3 daily and an unchanged clearance of T_3, serum T_3 levels must fall. The best estimate is a 10% to 15% decrease; normal ranges for persons $\geq$ 70 yr should be adjusted accordingly.

Because acute and chronic illnesses are more common in older persons, a low serum T_3 level or **euthyroid sick syndrome** is common. Features and variants of this syndrome are low serum T_3; high serum reverse T_3; low serum T_4 and free T_4 index; euthyroid hyperthyroxinemia (high serum T_4, free T_4 index, and free T_4); normal to low free T_4 in the most seriously ill; blunted TSH response to thyrotropin-releasing hormone (TRH); and subnormal serum TSH between 0.02 and 0.4 μU/mL (0.02 and 0.4 mU/L) detectable by third-generation TSH assay.

In population-wide studies, the average serum TSH level rises—a fact that appears to directly contradict the explanation given for the constancy of serum T_4. However, evidence suggests that the rise in TSH reflects the high prevalence of Hashimoto's disease in the elderly. In one study, for example, the rise in the mean serum TSH level was completely eliminated by excluding persons with Hashimoto's disease.

THYROID DISEASE IN THE ELDERLY

The three most important conditions of the thyroid are hypothyroidism, hyperthyroidism, and nodules. The prevalence of overt **hypothyroidism** is 2% to 5% in those > 65 yr. The prevalence rises with age, is much higher in women than in men at all ages, and is always higher in geriatric inpatients (hospital or nursing home) than in elders living in the community. Another 5% to 14% of those $\geq$ 65 yr have mild (subclinical) hypothyroidism. The incidence and prevalence of **hyperthyroidism** remain relatively constant with age, but the etiologic distribution shifts somewhat from Graves' disease toward multinodular and uninodular toxic goiter. The prevalence of overt hyperthyroidism averages about 0.4% and is higher in women and inpatients. The prevalence of **thyroid nodules** increases with age. One study shows that by age 80, 9% of women and 1.5% of men living in the community have one or more palpable thyroid nodules.

HYPOTHYROIDISM

A condition in which the body's tissues are exposed to a subnormal concentration of thyroid hormone.

Etiology

The most common causes of irreversible thyroid failure in adults are Hashimoto's disease (chronic autoimmune thyroiditis), irradiation or surgical removal of the gland, and idiopathic hypothyroidism. Infrequent causes include pituitary and hypothalamic lesions with TSH deficiency, iodine-induced hypothyroidism, antithyroid drugs, and very large amounts of certain natural substances in foods, eg, goitrin in rutabagas, thiocyanate in cabbage, and aminotriazole in cranberries. Transient hypothyroidism may occur after thyroid surgery or treatment with radioactive iodine (^{131}I) or during episodes of subacute thyroiditis.

The treatment of hyperthyroidism and thyroid cancer account for most cases of iatrogenic hypothyroidism. Irradiation with ^{131}I is the most frequent treatment for Graves' disease or a solitary hyperfunctioning adenoma. More than 50% of patients with Graves' disease who receive therapeutic doses of ^{131}I ultimately develop hypothyroidism. On the other hand, patients who have hyperthyroidism associated with nodular goiter rarely develop hypothyroidism when treated with ^{131}I.

Thyroidectomy is the treatment of choice for some cases of hyperthyroidism (certain patients with Graves' disease and most patients with multinodular goiter) and most cases of thyroid cancer. Because the goal of thyroid cancer therapy is usually complete ablation of the gland, hypothyroidism often occurs. Usually, such therapy consists of radical subtotal thyroidectomy followed by large doses of ^{131}I.

Idiopathic hypothyroidism in adults is generally thought to result from undiagnosed Hashimoto's disease. Supporting this theory is the fact that antithyroid antibodies are sometimes detected in the serum, even though antibodies tend to disappear in known chronic thyroiditis when the gland reaches an advanced stage of atrophy. Direct cytologic proof of this theory is lacking because the biopsy or aspiration of an atrophic, nonpalpable gland is unwarranted.

Pathogenesis and Pathophysiology

Hashimoto's disease is an *autoimmune inflammatory process of the thyroid gland*. Four types of thyroid-directed antibodies appear in the serum of patients with the disease, but the mediator of the inflammatory and cytotoxic lesion remains unknown. Inhibitory antibodies that bind to the TSH receptors, displacing TSH, have been identified; they may account for some of the decline in thyroid function. The so-called antimicrosomal antibody is actually an antithyroid peroxidase (anti-TPO) antibody; this antibody may explain the inefficient synthesis of thyroid hormone. As the disorder progresses, histologic evidence of thyroid follicle destruction can be found along with florid lymphocytic infiltration and eosinophilic changes in the cytoplasm of thyroid epithelial cells. In some cases, fibrosis supervenes, and the gland ultimately loses all thyroid epithelium.

Hypothyroidism after ^{131}I therapy is difficult to predict because its pathogenesis is not fully understood. In patients with Graves' disease, pathologic changes associated with Hashimoto's disease often appear concurrently, but the presence of lymphocytic infiltration before ^{131}I therapy is not a good predictor of hypothyroidism afterward. Many cases of hypothyroidism appear in the first year after ^{131}I therapy, but new cases continue appearing at a rate of 2% to 5%/yr over the next 15 to 20 yr. This linear relationship suggests that irradiation produces a delayed effect, with the length of the delay varying widely. This pattern is compatible with accepted principles of radiation biology. Early hypothyroidism appears to be dose related and attributable to acute radiation thyroiditis; later hypothyroidism appears to develop because lower doses cause a failure of DNA replication, so that thyroid cell replacement eventually ceases.

On the other hand, the presence of Hashimoto's disease preoperatively is a good predictor of **hypothyroidism after subtotal thyroidectomy** for Graves' disease. Of course, the size of the remnant left by the surgeon and the integrity of its blood supply also determine the likelihood of hypothyroidism.

The frequency of serum antithyroid antibodies and of clinical or histologic evidence of Hashimoto's disease rises sharply with advancing age, especially in women. Thus, the likelihood of developing hypothyroidism, either spontaneously or after subtotal thyroidectomy, increases with age. Furthermore, DNA in older people is more susceptible to radiation-induced damage and less well repaired, so hypothyroidism following treatment with ^{131}I also increases with age.

Symptoms and Signs

Hypothyroidism in the elderly is a great masquerader. Fewer than 33% of elderly patients with hypothyroidism present with the characteristic symptoms and signs—fatigue, loss of initiative, depression, myalgia, constipation, and dry skin. Even when patients do present with these symptoms and signs, they are commonly attributed to aging. Most elderly persons with hypothyroidism develop nonspecific syndromes, which are common in frail elderly persons—mental confusion, anorexia, weight loss, falling, incontinence, and decreased mobility. Musculoskeletal symptoms, including arthralgias, are frequent, but arthritis is rare. Muscular aches and weakness, often mimicking polymyalgia rheumatica or polymyositis, and an elevated creatine kinase level make the differential diagnosis even more difficult.

The physical examination findings are also difficult to interpret. Puffiness around the eyes and myxedematous facies are difficult to distinguish from normal facial changes associated with aging. Even the most reliable sign, prolonged relaxation time following muscular contraction, may not be detectable because of decreased amplitude or absent reflexes. Occasionally, noninflammatory effusions may occur in the joints and in pleural, pericardial, and peritoneal cavities, adding to the diagnostic confusion.

Laboratory Findings

The diagnosis of hypothyroidism is based on precise, reliable assays of serum TSH and T_4 levels. The serum T_3 level has little value because it is normal in some 33% of patients with hypothyroidism. An **elevated serum TSH level** is extremely sensitive (about 0.99) for the diagnosis of hypothyroidism, and a subnormal serum T_4 level is highly specific. A **subnormal free T_4 index** is even more specific because it corrects for abnormalities in the thyroxine-binding proteins.

Because of its greater sensitivity and adequate specificity, the serum TSH level alone should be measured in patients suspected of having hypothyroidism and in those needing to have it ruled out. A serum TSH level above normal (usually $> 4.5\ \mu U/mL$) indicates hypothyroidism. If the serum TSH level is normal, hypothyroidism is essentially ruled out, and the serum free T_4 index level usually does not need to be measured. If the serum TSH level is above normal, a serum free T_4 index level should be measured to differentiate overt hypothyroidism (subnormal free T_4 index) from mild hypothyroidism (normal free T_4 index).

Mild hypothyroidism (also called compensated hypothyroidism and subclinical hypothyroidism) is associated with a serum TSH level between 4.5 and 15 $\mu U/mL$. Compensated hypothyroidism is an inappropriate term because it implies that serum free T_4 index has been restored to baseline, whereas it may be below baseline but within the normal range. Subclinical hypothyroidism is also inaccurate because some patients have mild symptoms that disappear with thyroid hormone therapy.

Occasionally, an **antithyroid peroxidase assay** is useful because it confirms the presence or absence of Hashimoto's disease. It is particularly useful in predicting a progression from mild to overt hypothyroidism. Although serum cholesterol and creatine kinase levels are elevated in hypothyroidism, these measurements are rarely useful diagnostically; on the other hand, a diagnosis of hypothyroidism may explain abnormal cholesterol and creatine kinase values.

Similarly, a diagnosis of hypothyroidism may explain anemia, hyponatremia, hypoglycemia, and hypercapnia. The anemia is usually mild, with hemoglobin no lower than 9 gm/dL. Typically, it has the characteristics of the anemia of chronic disease, but it may be mildly macrocytic. Because autoimmune diseases tend to coexist, frank pernicious anemia occurs in perhaps 2% of patients with hypothyroidism. Older persons have more circulating antidiuretic hormone (vasopressin) than younger persons and thus a greater susceptibility to hyponatremia. Hypothyroidism accentuates this tendency to excessive water retention without proportionate sodium retention. Hypoglycemia and hypercapnia, manifestations of advanced thyroid deficiency, are frequent findings in myxedema coma.

A key problem in older people is distinguishing hypothyroidism from severe cases of the euthyroid sick syndrome, or detecting hypothyroidism superimposed on the syndrome. Because the serum T_3 level has little bearing on the diagnosis of hypothyroidism, the characteristic low T_3 level in euthyroid sick syndrome is irrelevant. The difficulty arises primarily in the critically ill patient who has the low T_4 syndrome. Free T_4 index and total T_4 are subnormal in euthyroid sick syndrome, partially because the circulating inhibitor of protein binding also inhibits the binding of thyroid hormones to inanimate sites such as resin or charcoal used in the T_3 uptake assay.

In severe euthyroid sick syndrome, even free T_4 by equilibrium dialysis may be subnormal. This finding is often associated with a subnormal serum TSH level and presumably results from suppression of pituitary TSH output, another feature of euthyroid sick syndrome. Another diagnostic problem is that during recovery from the syndrome the serum TSH may rebound to supranormal levels while serum free T_4 and free T_4 index are still slightly subnormal. Thus, the diagnosis of hypothyroidism in the critically ill patient can be made only if the serum TSH level is markedly elevated (> 15 μU/mL) or if the free T_4 measures are markedly subnormal (free $T_4 < 0.6$ ng/dL, free T_4 index < 2 ng/dL); both findings are preferable for this diagnosis. When both serum TSH and free T_4 levels are low, a theoretic possibility of pituitarigenic hypothyroidism exists, but these findings almost always signify the euthyroid sick syndrome.

Diagnosis

The diagnosis of hypothyroidism requires clinical suspicion and reliable laboratory tests appropriately selected and interpreted (see above). The differential diagnosis includes normal aging, euthyroid sick syndrome, depression, the various causes of dementia, idiopathic obesity, Cushing's syndrome, myopathies, neuropathies, various arthritides, fibrositis, myositis, Parkinson's disease, various colonic conditions that cause constipation or ileus, pericarditis, heart failure, cirrhosis, renal disease, and various dermal conditions.

The disorder is so common in the elderly and the diagnosis so difficult to make clinically and so easy to make based on laboratory data that the physician should not hesitate to order blood tests. A recommended policy is that serum TSH be measured in any person > 65 yr undergoing a diagnostic evaluation or a comprehensive geriatric assessment, whether the person is an inpatient, an outpatient, or someone being admitted to a board-and-care residence or nursing home.

Although this policy is not controversial, population-wide screening of the elderly is. Theoretically, such screening would be similar to the highly successful screening programs for neonatal hypothyroidism. All studies, however, have concluded that the prevalence of undiagnosed hypothyroidism, although greater in persons > 65 yr than in younger persons, is still too low to make such screening cost-effective and that diagnoses in the elderly are likely to be made through the patient care system before great harm occurs. On this latter point, the situation differs from that of the newborn.

Treatment

The average replacement dosage is 0.075 to 0.1 mg/day of levothyroxine sodium in patients ≥ 65 yr (in contrast to 0.125 to 0.15 mg/day in younger patients). *Unless the patient is in impending or actual myxedema coma, replacement therapy should be given cautiously,* starting with a dosage of 0.0125 to 0.025 mg/day and increasing at intervals of ≥ 2 wk. The increases should be no more than 0.025 mg/day.

The most serious hazard of early therapy is myocardial infarction, although serious cardiac complications are uncommon. In fact, T_4 therapy for proven hypothyroidism is one of the safest, most effective medical treatments. Still, patients should be monitored closely for angina, dyspnea, arrhythmias, and unusual weakness.

About 1 to 2 mo after reaching a dosage of 0.075 mg/day of levothyroxine sodium, the serum TSH level should be measured, always by a second-generation TSH assay **(sensitive or s-TSH)** capable of detecting < 0.1 μU/mL. If s-TSH is still above normal, the dosage may be increased to 0.1 mg/day. If s-TSH is below normal (< 0.4 μU/mL), the dosage should be lowered.

Serum T_3 and T_4 measurements are usually unnecessary because serum TSH measurements alone reliably detect hypothyroidism or hyperthroidism. However, sometimes the serum TSH level falls slowly. Thus, if the TSH level is still high 1 to 2 mo after reaching a dosage of 0.1 mg/day of levothyroxine sodium in a geriatric patient, the dosage should be maintained for another 2 mo. If the TSH level is still elevated after 2 mo, the dosage should be raised to 0.112 or 0.125 mg/day.

HYPERTHYROIDISM

A condition in which the thyroid gland secretes an inappropriately large amount of thyroid hormones. **Thyrotoxicosis** refers to *an inappropriately large amount of thyroid hormones from any source*.

Incidence and Etiology

Thyrotoxicosis usually results from hyperthyroidism; occasionally, however, it results from excessive ingestion of pharmaceutical thyroid hormone and rarely from an extrathyroidal source, such as an ovarian struma. The causes of hyperthyroidism are Graves' disease, a single hyperfunctioning adenoma, a multinodular goiter, some forms of subacute and chronic thyroiditis, and rarely, a primary TSH-producing pituitary lesion or excessive TSH production caused by pituitary resistance to thyroid hormones.

Although hyperthyroidism may seem uncommon among the elderly, the prevalence actually changes little with age. Graves' disease becomes less common, while hyperthyroidism associated with multinodular goiter becomes more common.

Pathogenesis and Pathophysiology

The common denominator in hyperthyroidism is a loss of normal physiologic regulation of thyroid hormone secretion. In **Graves' disease,** an autoimmune disorder leads to the production of an antibody to the TSH receptor on thyroid follicular cells. This antibody behaves like TSH itself, activating the adenylate cyclase system and thereby stimulating the thyroid cell.

In hyperthyroidism associated with one or more **adenomas,** the responsible area of the thyroid gland is autonomous; ie, it produces and secretes excessive thyroid hormone even though serum TSH is fully suppressed. The cause of this autonomy is unknown, though it is not a thyroid-stimulating antibody. Presumably, the autonomy is intrinsic to the cells of certain adenomas.

In **subacute thyroiditis,** either the granulomatous or lymphocytic type, damaged follicles leak thyroglobulin, T_3, and T_4 into the circulation. Sometimes, the resulting hormone level in the blood causes thyrotoxicosis. In certain cases of **Hashimoto's disease,** a similar leakage may cause thyrotoxicosis, usually of short duration.

In all these conditions characterized by excessive thyroid hormone release independent of TSH control, the pituitary responds normally by shutting down its TSH production. Thus, the hypothalamopituitary sector of the axis is normal; the dysregulation occurs in the immune system or the thyroid gland itself.

A rare cause of hyperthyroidism is a **TSH-secreting adenoma of the pituitary.** Two causes that are even rarer are a **hypothalamic disorder** in which an overproduction of thyrotropin-releasing hormone **(TRH)** leads sequentially to hypersecretion of TSH and thyroid hormones and the **inherited syndrome of pituitary resistance** to thyroid hormones.

Regardless of the cause of hyperthyroidism, the result is supranormal levels of thyroid hormones in T_3-responsive tissues. The various types of hyperthyroidism are characterized by overproduction of T_3 and, to a lesser extent, T_4. In T_3 hyperthyroidism, which accounts for about 5% of hyperthyroidism at all ages, the serum T_4 level is normal despite clinical evidence of hyperthyroidism.

In hyperthyroidism, extrathyroidal tissues convert the excess secreted T_4 to T_3. Thus, a supraphysiologic concentration of T_3 arrives at target tissues and is transported into the nucleus, where it binds to a receptor. The hormone-receptor complex then binds to the promoter region of T_3-responsive genes, leading to an overproduction of enzymes and other proteins that mediate the characteristic actions of T_3.

Symptoms and Signs

Hyperthyroidism in the elderly is even more of a masquerader than hypothyroidism. Older patients have fewer characteristic symptoms of hyperthyroidism than younger patients, and only about 25% of those ≥ 65 yr present with the typical complex of symptoms and signs. One study of patients with hyperthyroidism shows that advanced age is associated with significant decreases in complaints of increased perspiration, heat intolerance, increased appetite, irritability, and thyroid enlargement. Average heart rate and thyroid size also decrease with age.

These age-related changes in the clinical picture cannot be explained precisely, but age and concomitant disease may alter the response of various organs and tissues to excessive thyroid hormones. For example, the response to catecholamines decreases in older persons, possibly because of a decreased number of or affinity for catecholamine receptors. Because catecholamines act synergistically with T_3 in producing many typical symptoms and signs of hyperthyroidism, reduced responsiveness to catecholamines could explain the atypical picture. Another possible factor is the aging of the myocardium, which predisposes it to react unfavorably to thyroid hormones.

However, the study of patients with hyperthyroidism mentioned above also shows that some symptoms and signs are highly sensitive and specific for distinguishing hyperthyroidism from euthyroidism in patients in their 60s and 70s. Although the number of typical symptoms was lower in older patients with hyperthyroidism, thyroid enlargement, weight loss, pulse rate ≥ 90, and fatigue had sensitivities > 0.70; an increased number of bowel movements, lid lag, increased appetite, fine tremor, heat intolerance, and increased sweating had specificities ≥ 0.98. Weight loss and atrial fibrillation were significantly more common in patients in their 60s and 70s.

Common atypical presentations in the elderly may be classified as cardiovascular, GI, neuropsychiatric, and neuromuscular, although aspects of each may exist in a single patient (see TABLE 79–1). **Cardiovascular features** are atrial arrhythmias, heart failure, and angina, which may dominate the clinical picture to the exclusion of the usual features of hyperthyroidism. Because cardiac disease is so common in the elderly, the possibility of underlying hyperthyroidism may not be suspected. The **GI picture** shows a failure to thrive. Features include anorexia, dyspepsia, abdominal distress, rapid weight loss, exhaustion, and bowel disturbances (diarrhea, constipation, or diarrhea alternating with constipation). Thus, GI malignancy is almost always at the top of the differential diagnosis list; hyperthyroidism may not be on it at all.

Neuropsychiatric features include apathy, listlessness, anorexia, marked weight loss, weakness, and mental confusion. The clinical condition, which has been called "apathetic thyroidism," may be classified primarily as depression; often it meets the criteria of the *Diagnostic and Statistical Manual of Mental Disorders*, Fourth Edition **(DSM-IV)**, for that diagnosis. The **neuromuscular type** is characterized by symptoms and signs of proximal and some distal myopathy with severe weakness and usually some weight loss.

TABLE 79–1. CLINICAL FEATURES OF HYPERTHYROIDISM IN THE ELDERLY

Smaller thyroid gland	Less diarrhea
Multinodular goiter	More constipation
Lower incidence of Graves' disease	Less excitability
More arrhythmias	More apathy
Less tachycardia	Less hyperkinesis
More angina	More depression
More heart failure	More arthralgias
Less hyperphagia	More muscular weakness
More anorexia	More hepatomegaly
More weight loss	

Laboratory Findings and Diagnosis

All geriatric patients with chronic symptoms should be tested for hyperthyroidism. However, screening all elderly persons is not justified because too few cases are detected.

The best single test is the s-TSH measurement, for which sensitivity and specificity are both ≥ 0.98. Using this test alone is also the most cost-effective way to detect hyperthyroidism, even though it costs more than a free T_4 assay. A subnormal s-TSH value strongly suggests the diagnosis of hyperthyroidism; an undetectable level (< 0.1 μU/mL by a second-generation assay or preferably < 0.02 μU/mL by a third-generation assay) is almost pathognomonic.

Serum thyroid hormone levels may be measured to confirm the diagnosis or, in the infrequent case in which serum s-TSH is normal but clinical suspicion persists, to establish that the patient is not euthyroid. Many physicians still order serum T_3 and T_4 (or free T_3 index and free T_4 index) measurements in the initial battery of tests, but doing so is wasteful. When considering these tests, the physician should recall that T_3 is more sensitive than T_4 for the diagnosis of hyperthyroidism because it tends to rise earlier and more sharply.

While laboratory testing is essential for diagnosing hyperthyroidism in the elderly, it does not detect every case. Starvation or serious illness (either severe hyperthyroidism per se or concomitant disease) invariably lowers the serum T_3 level, so that it no longer reflects thyroid activity. Thus, a patient with hyperthyroidism may have a normal serum T_3 level. With more serious illness, the T_4 and free T_4 index may also decline into the normal range. An elevated free T_4 (measured by equilibrium dialysis), a supranormal radioiodine uptake test, or an undetectable serum s-TSH usually provides the correct diagnosis.

The diagnosis may also be complicated by transient **euthyroid hyperthyroxinemia** in some patients with acute systemic illness (eg, pneumonia) and in many patients with acute psychiatric illnesses. This condition can be fairly reliably differentiated from hyperthyroidism by a serum s-TSH measurement and most reliably differentiated by repeating thyroid function tests after 2 wk. By that time, serum free T_4 index has generally returned to normal.

In all varieties of euthyroid sick syndrome, a single measurement of serum s-TSH has replaced the more tedious and expensive TRH response test, although the latter still may be useful when findings are particularly puzzling. However, advanced age, depression, or euthyroid sick syndrome may blunt the TRH response test or cause a subnormal s-TSH. The key distinction is that complete absence of response to TRH or an undetectable basal s-TSH is extremely rare in euthyroid sick syndrome, but it is the rule in hyperthyroidism.

Treatment

The treatment of choice for most elderly patients with hyperthyroidism from **Graves' disease** or a **single autonomous nodule** is ^{131}I therapy. It is preferred because of the age-related risks of surgery and the special difficulties of antithyroid drug therapy. In elderly patients with Graves' disease, antithyroid drugs are effective if compliance is good; in those with uninodular toxic goiters, such drugs are slow to work and almost never lead to permanent remission.

In **multinodular toxic goiter,** the response to ^{131}I therapy is often delayed and incomplete. Many doses of ^{131}I may be needed, leaving the patient hyperthyroid many months after the diagnosis. Thus, surgery may be preferred, at least for low-risk patients.

Antithyroid drugs: Giving antithyroid drugs for 2 or 3 mo before administering a therapeutic dose of ^{131}I rapidly restores euthyroidism in Graves' disease. These drugs also deplete the thyroid gland of its store of hormone; thus, the risk of thyrotoxicosis after ^{131}I therapy is minimized because stored hormone cannot be dumped into the blood during acute radiation thyroiditis.

Administration of antithyroid drugs in older persons is the same as in younger persons. **Propylthiouracil** is given initially at 100 to 150 mg orally q 8 h. The dosage is lowered sequentially based on symptoms and signs and serum hormone levels, which are monitored about q 2 mo. Serum s-TSH measurements are most useful. If the therapeutic response is inadequate, the drug dosage may be increased to 300 mg q 8 h.

Methimazole is longer acting than propylthiouracil and therefore can be given as a single daily dose. The initial dosage is 30 to 45 mg/day. Every 1 or 2 mo, the dosage needs to be adjusted, depending on the response. With either methimazole or propylthiouracil, if the patient's course is erratic (eg, the patient slips quickly into hypothyroidism after small increases in dose), the simplest, surest solution is to add a small dose of **levothyroxine sodium,** usually 0.05 mg/day.

Propranolol and other **β-adrenergic blockers** can help manage the symptoms of hyperthyroidism, unless contraindicated because the patient has heart failure. A β-adrenergic blocker may be given along with an antithyroid drug before ^{131}I therapy or surgery. β-Adrenergic blockers do not affect thyroid hormone secretion rates; rather, they blunt the interaction of thyroid hormones with catecholamines. In high doses (eg, propranolol 320 mg/day), the extrathyroidal conversion of T_4 to T_3 is inhibited as well. The dosage must be individualized, but 40 mg tid is typical.

Pharmacologic doses of **inorganic iodide** (Lugol's solution 0.1 to 0.3 mL tid or saturated solution of potassium iodide one drop tid) act by inhibiting the release of thyroid hormones from the gland. Often, iodide's effect is temporary, so it should not be relied on as the sole therapy beyond 10 to 14 days. Iodide administration is still one of the standard methods of preparing a patient for subtotal thyroidectomy, and it may be valuable in thyroid storm.

The cholecystographic contrast materials **ipodate sodium** and **iopanoic acid** are extremely potent inhibitors of the enzyme that converts T_4 to T_3 in extrathyroidal tissues (and probably in the thyroid gland as well). Although not approved in the USA for treating hyperthyroidism, they are extremely effective, lowering the serum T_3 level to the normal range within 48 to 72 h. These inhibitors are useful before and during a thyroid storm as well as in patients with serious complications of thyrotoxicosis, such as heart failure. An appropriate dose of ipodate sodium is 1.0 gm/day orally for short-term use or 0.5 gm/day orally for > 2 wk.

Symptomatic treatment: In thyrotoxic patients with atrial fibrillation, cardioversion should not be attempted until euthyroidism is achieved. Once it is, the atrial rhythm spontaneously reverts to normal in about 2/3 of patients. Psychiatric symptoms in elderly hyperthyroid patients should be treated on a prn basis; they usually clear completely when the patient becomes euthyroid.

THYROID NODULES

Although death from thyroid cancer is extremely rare (1100/yr in the USA, 0.24% of all cancer deaths, and 0.05% of all deaths), the thyroid nodule is a topic of great interest and controversy because of differing opinions about the seriousness of the finding of such a nodule. Most nodules either are benign or behave benignly even if they appear malignant on histologic examination. The 5-yr survival rate for all patients with thyroid cancers is 93%, compared with the average survival of the age-adjusted population. In the elderly, nodules do tend to be more invasive and malignant, but most are still papillary or papillofollicular and have excellent prognoses. Most of the 7% deficit in survival can be accounted for by cases of anaplastic carcinoma and lymphoma, which often present in ways other than asymptomatic thyroid nodules.

The mortality of patients with thyroid nodules may be so low because of an aggressive medical approach to diagnosis and surgical resection. Therefore, these medical practices must be continued.

Symptoms, Signs, and Diagnosis

A nodule may be merely an enlarged lobe, a lobule in a diffuse goiter, or a pyramidal lobe. Nodules may also be regenerating areas after subtotal resection, localized subacute or chronic thyroiditis, cysts, or hemorrhage and calcification in a colloid adenoma. Concern about malignancy is lowest if the dominant nodule is not the only one, if both lobes are abnormal to palpation, or if the history reveals a sudden appearance with pain and tenderness, suggesting hemorrhage into a degenerating colloid adenoma. Radiation-induced cancer has occurred after latent periods as long as 30 to 40 yr. Thus, a history of radiation to the face, neck, or thorax is important.

Hashimoto's disease causes the gland to feel very firm with multiple small nodules. Colloid adenomas may be softer than normal, though their consistency varies from patient to patient. Tenderness suggests hemorrhage into a colloid adenoma. Fluctuation suggests cystic changes, but these are more likely to result from hemorrhage or necrosis of a colloid adenoma than from a simple, water-clear cyst.

Anaplastic carcinoma often has features that clearly suggest malignancy. The patient has a large, growing thyroid mass that has a stony hardness and is irregular, immobile, and fixed to other tissues. Also, the patient may be hoarse.

Evaluation of thyroid nodules remains controversial, regardless of the patient's age. Often, **fine-needle aspiration** is used as the first and only diagnostic study. Results of thyroid function tests are normal except with the relatively uncommon hyperfunctioning nodule. In that case, serum T_4 and T_3 levels are high, and serum s-TSH is subnormal or undetectable. When these findings are obtained, a **radionuclide scan** should be done to prove that the nodule is hot. When thyroid function tests are normal, a radionuclide scan has routinely been used to exclude a functioning lesion, which is almost always benign, and an **ultrasonogram** has been used to identify simple cysts, also usually benign. However, these expensive procedures have a low diagnostic yield because of their extremely poor specificity for malignancy.

Serum thyroglobulin measurement has low specificity. X-rays of microcalcifications, representing psammoma bodies, have low sensitivity but high specificity for the diagnosis of papillary adenocarcinoma.

Treatment

In deciding whether to treat nodules surgically, the physician must consider the higher risk of surgical morbidity in older persons. Cytologic evidence of malignancy or suspicion of malignancy based on the fine-needle aspiration calls for surgery unless concomitant medical conditions absolutely contraindicate it. If the physician has doubts about the cytologic impression (eg, the cytologist can diagnose a follicular neoplasm but usually cannot tell if it is benign or malignant), a better treatment choice is TSH-suppressive therapy with levothyroxine sodium and another fine-needle aspiration in 6 to 12 mo.

If thyroid carcinoma is discovered during surgery, the next step is also controversial. Most physicians recommend a near-total thyroidectomy followed by ^{131}I therapy to ablate the remainder. Then a total-body scan is performed to search for residual tissue capable of capturing ^{131}I. If the results are positive, a therapeutic dose is administered.

However, no evidence shows that this approach is superior to near-total thyroidectomy alone; its alleged advantage derives solely from nonrandomized studies with prominent selection bias. At all times, except when preparing for a scan or a therapeutic dose of ^{131}I, the patient should receive doses of levothyroxine sodium sufficient to reduce the serum TSH level below normal but not to cause symptoms of hyperthyroidism.

80. DIABETES MELLITUS AND OTHER DISORDERS OF CARBOHYDRATE METABOLISM

DIABETES MELLITUS

Diabetes mellitus is *a metabolic syndrome characterized by hyperglycemia and sometimes ketoacidosis;* it results from a lack of or markedly diminished insulin secretion or from ineffective insulin action associated with moderately diminished insulin secretion. Secondary vascular changes include abnormalities in the small vessels (microangiopathy) and large vessels (macroangiopathy). Microangiopathy appears as diabetic retinopathy and nephropathy. Macroangiopathy leads to stroke, myocardial infarction, and peripheral vascular disease. Many peripheral nervous system abnormalities also contribute to the clinical picture of diabetes. Most are due to metabolic changes, although a few may be secondary to vascular changes.

PHYSIOLOGY

The liver produces glucose through two processes: **glycogenolysis,** the breakdown of glycogen that provides about 75% of the glucose after an overnight fast, and **gluconeogenesis,** the synthesis of new glucose from noncarbohydrate precursors delivered to the liver. As the fasting period lengthens, glycogenolysis decreases considerably, and gluconeogenesis becomes the dominant process.

Glucose production is regulated by insulin levels, glucagon levels, and autoregulation. Insulin decreases glucose production; glucagon increases it. Autoregulation is the process by which the glucose level mediates hepatic glucose production independently of external hormonal stimuli. During fasting, insulin levels fall as glucagon levels rise.

But after a meal, the increased plasma glucose level stimulates pancreatic β cells to release insulin, while glucagon production by the α-islet cells is suppressed. The insulin first passes through the liver, where about 50% is degraded. The rest enters the general circulation, where its half-life is about 5 min. Insulin then binds to specific receptors on the cell surfaces of the liver, muscle, and fat tissue, where it may exert an effect for several hours.

Thus, after a meal, hepatic glucose production is markedly suppressed, and glucose enters the tissues. About 25% of the meal's carbohydrate content is stored in the liver, and the rest goes to peripheral tissues—mostly muscle.

In younger persons without diabetes, plasma glucose levels rise 20 to 50 mg/dL immediately after a meal and return to baseline 2 h later. With age, resistance to insulin gradually increases, so that **postprandial plasma glucose** levels rise an additional 5 mg/dL with each decade after the fifth decade. **Fasting plasma glucose** levels rise only 1 to 2 mg/dL in a decade.

Five mechanisms have been proposed to explain aging's effect on carbohydrate metabolism: poor diet, physical inactivity, decreased lean body mass in which to store carbohydrate, impaired insulin secretion, and insulin resistance. Low carbohydrate intake explains only a small part of the problem. Recent studies indicate that older persons who routinely exercise vigorously do not show glucose intolerance—a finding that suggests inactivity plays a large role in age-related glucose intolerance. Although lean body mass diminishes with age, tissue redistribution cannot explain age-related changes in carbohydrate metabolism. Also, insulin secretion in response to glucose does not diminish with age. Almost all studies of the insulin response to various stimuli (oral or IV glucose, amino acids, or tolbutamide) show normal or even increased insulin levels in older people. Although many older people do have a delayed response to oral glucose, the significance of this delay is uncertain.

In contrast, insulin resistance is associated with aging, especially in those ≥ 60 yr who do not exercise regularly. The mechanism, however, remains unclear. The site of insulin resistance probably lies in intracellular pathways of insulin sensitive tissues; ie, defects in insulin binding and receptor function do not explain the resistance.

CLASSIFICATION AND PATHOGENESIS

Diabetes mellitus can be divided into three general categories: type I or insulin-dependent diabetes mellitus, type II or non–insulin-dependent diabetes mellitus, and secondary diabetes mellitus.

Type I or Insulin-Dependent Diabetes Mellitus

Patients with type I diabetes mellitus have certain HLA antigens (DR3 or DR4) and produce autoantibodies against pancreatic islet cells, the insulin molecule, and/or a constituent of islet cells recently identified as the enzyme glutamic acid decarboxylase. These antibodies may be present for years before diabetic symptoms appear.

Type I patients develop ketosis, signifying a virtual absence of effective insulin. Without insulin therapy, they usually progress rapidly to diabetic coma and die.

About 6% of the US population has some form of diabetes, but only 10% of this group has type I diabetes mellitus. Although most of these patients are children and young adults (< 30 yr), the previously used term **juvenile-onset diabetes** is misleading because some adult and elderly patients also have ketosis-prone diabetes. Even patients in their 70s and 80s can present with diabetic ketoacidosis. However, toxic levels of ketone bodies usually accumulate more slowly in the elderly.

Type II or Non–Insulin-Dependent Diabetes

Previously called **adult-onset, maturity-onset,** or **ketosis-resistant diabetes,** type II diabetes mellitus involves relative insulin deficiency and resistance to insulin action. The combination of normal or high insulin levels and hyperglycemia implies insulin resistance. Both increased insulin levels and decreased insulin action have been documented in the two groups at increased risk for type II diabetes—the obese and the elderly.

If pancreatic β-cell reserve is sufficient, hyperinsulinemia preserves normal glucose levels. Eventually, impaired glucose tolerance occurs, although hyperinsulinemia continues. This state of mild glucose intolerance with near-normal fasting blood glucose levels may persist indefinitely. But in patients in whom insulin secretion is subsequently impaired, plasma glucose levels increase to those consistent with diabetes, and plasma insulin levels fall to normal or below. These patients are thought to have an increased genetic susceptibility to decreased β-cell reserve.

Type II diabetes is distinguished by an absence of ketosis, which indicates that the patient has some effective insulin. About 35% of patients with type II diabetes use exogenous insulin. But unlike patients with type I diabetes, they do not need exogenous insulin to sustain life.

Obesity and age are independent risk factors for type II diabetes mellitus. Some 80% to 90% of type II diabetic patients are obese, and the prevalence doubles for every 20% increase over desirable body weight and for each decade after the fourth, regardless of weight. The prevalence in persons ages 65 to 74 is about 15%. An even higher percentage of people beyond the eighth decade may have type II diabetes mellitus. Type II diabetes is more prevalent in certain populations, eg, American Indians, blacks, and those of Hispanic ancestry.

Secondary Diabetes Mellitus

This category includes diabetes mellitus resulting from diseases that destroy the pancreas (eg, hemochromatosis, pancreatitis, and cystic fibrosis), certain endocrine diseases in which excess hormones interfere with insulin action (eg, growth hormone in acromegaly, cortisol in Cushing's syndrome, and catecholamines in pheochromocytoma), and certain drugs that suppress insulin secretion (eg, phenytoin) or inhibit insulin action (eg, estrogens or glucocorticoids).

SYMPTOMS AND SIGNS

As carbohydrate metabolism deteriorates, the postprandial glucose level fails to return to the preprandial level for 3 to 5 h, but symptoms and signs do not appear as long as the plasma glucose level does not exceed the renal threshold. In people with a normal glomerular filtration rate, the plasma glucose level can reach 160 to 180 mg/dL before glucosuria occurs; in older people and those with renal disease, it can be much higher. When **glucosuria** occurs, urine formed after meals tests positive for glucose, while urine formed before meals may test negative. Thus, patients may be only intermittently glucosuric and usually are asymptomatic.

As the metabolic abnormality worsens, regulation of hepatic glucos production becomes impaired, resulting in fasting hyperglycemia an plasma glucose levels exceeding the renal threshold for most or all (the day. Patients have persistent glucosuria but usually have no symı toms, except perhaps fatigue. With further progression, the glucosuria usually causes an osmotic diuresis. Patients experience **polyuria,** which leads to dehydration and **polydipsia.** Because endogenous insulin is increasingly ineffective, the body cannot consume sufficient calories from dietary carbohydrates; thus, weight loss occurs despite **polyphagia. Blurred vision** may result from changes in the ocular lens shape caused by hyperglycemia-induced osmotic changes. Patients may also have an **increased susceptibility to certain infections,** especially fungal (usually candidiasis) and staphylococcal infections.

If hyperglycemia goes unrecognized in a patient who does not have ketoacidosis, especially if the hyperglycemia is associated with another medical stress (such as urosepsis), **hyperosmolar nonketotic syndrome** may be the first indication of diabetes. In this situation, hyperglycemia becomes so profound and prolonged (with glucose levels often exceeding 1000 mg/dL) that the patient develops extreme dehydration and suffers decreased mentation that may progress to coma. Many patients show focal neurologic signs, including seizures, that resolve when normal metabolism is restored.

When excessive ketone bodies accumulate, as happens in elderly persons with type I diabetes, the body's buffer systems cannot neutralize them, and the kidneys cannot excrete them. The excess ketone bodies accumulate in the blood, causing **anorexia** and, occasionally, nausea. Further accumulation depletes body bases, resulting in **ketoacidosis.** If the patient is not treated quickly and correctly, coma and death follow. While most older patients with diabetes never develop ketosis and a few do so over several years, most young ketosis-prone diabetic patients probably progress from normal carbohydrate metabolism to ketoacidosis in only weeks. Almost all have symptoms and signs of uncontrolled diabetes at the time of diagnosis.

DIAGNOSIS

The diagnosis of type II diabetes mellitus is usually made in an asymptomatic patient undergoing screening during a routine physical examination or an evaluation for another medical problem. Elderly patients may experience only vague constitutional symptoms (eg, fatigue or loss of energy), partly because of their increased renal glucose threshold. Occasionally, symptoms or signs of **peripheral neuropathy** may be the initial manifestation. Because diabetes is so common in the elderly, screening, follow-up testing, and treatment are strongly recommended.

Any one of the following is sufficient to diagnose diabetes mellitus: (1) random plasma glucose level ≥ 200 mg/dL with symptoms of uncontrolled diabetes (eg, polyuria, polydipsia), (2) fasting plasma glucose level ≥ 140 mg/dL, or (3) plasma glucose level ≥ 200 mg/dL 2 h after ingesting 75 gm of glucose (oral glucose tolerance test). The glucose tolerance test is rarely needed or advised for the elderly. For whole-blood glucose levels, these values are 10% to 15% lower; ie, 120 mg/dL instead of 140 mg/dL and 180 mg/dL instead of 200 mg/dL. Abnormal values must be confirmed to avoid misdiagnosis from a laboratory error.

The normal fasting plasma glucose level is < 115 mg/dL, and the normal plasma glucose level 2 h after glucose ingestion is < 140 mg/dL. Patients with 2-h levels between normal and diabetic (140–199 mg/dL) have **impaired glucose tolerance** (previously called **chemical, latent, subclinical, borderline,** or **asymptomatic diabetes).** About 10% to 30% of all persons > 65 yr have impaired glucose tolerance. Although these patients do not develop microvascular complications, they are much more prone to the macrovascular complications of stroke, coronary occlusion, and especially peripheral vascular disease than persons with normal glucose levels. Over many years, about 50% of these patients will continue to have impaired glucose tolerance, and 30% will return to normal. Only 20% will develop diabetes mellitus, and they will do so at a rate of only 1% to 5% per year.

TREATMENT

Diabetic therapy has four components: diet, exercise, sulfonylurea agents, and insulin. Type I patients must be treated with insulin. About 35% of type II patients also take insulin, 45% receive sulfonylurea agents, and 20% use diet alone.

Diet

To maintain desirable body weight, the patient should have a balanced, nutritious diet. Patients on fixed insulin regimens have less flexibility with the timing and carbohydrate content of their meals than those not taking insulin. The rate of absorption of insulin depends mainly on the kind and amount given. Insulin's onset and peak action are fairly predictable, so patients should follow their prescribed diet and eat (especially carbohydrates) at appropriate times to avoid hypoglycemia. Patients taking intermediate- or long-acting insulin need a bedtime snack. Those who inject intermediate-acting insulin early in the morning and eat dinner late need a midafternoon snack. Because exercise increases insulin's absorption rate and enhances its effectiveness, patients should ingest enough carbohydrate before exercising to prevent hypoglycemia.

For patients not taking insulin, the timing and content of meals are less important, as long as the number of calories is appropriate. Because 80% to 90% of type II diabetic patients are obese, the number of calories is particularly important.

An appropriate diabetic diet should be ordered; detailed dietary counseling is carried out by a trained dietitian. Ordering the diabetic diet involves three steps (see TABLE 80–1):

1. Determine the patient's desirable body weight.

2. Estimate the appropriate number of total calories.

3. Apportion the calories among carbohydrate, protein, and fat. There are two general kinds of carbohydrates: simple and complex. Simple carbohydrates are monosaccharides such as glucose (dextrose) and fructose (a constituent of honey) and disaccharides such as sucrose (table sugar) and lactose (a constituent of milk). When eaten without other foods, simple carbohydrates may rapidly increase plasma glucose levels in diabetic patients. Complex carbohydrates are long polymers of glucose found in starches such as rice, potatoes, and vegetables.

The amount of carbohydrate is an important determinant in the postprandial rise of glucose levels. However, a low carbohydrate diet usually means an increased fat intake. And because diabetic patients are susceptible to macrovascular disease, lowering cholesterol levels, especially low-density lipoprotein (LDL) cholesterol levels, is important. High fat diets usually include a large percentage of saturated fat, which raises LDL cholesterol levels. Although monounsaturated and polyunsaturated fats do not increase LDL cholesterol levels, substituting them for saturated fat raises two practical considerations.

TABLE 80–1. CONSIDERATIONS IN ORDERING DIABETIC DIETS

1. Determine desirable body weight		
Women	For first 5 ft, allow 100 lb; for each in. > 5 ft, allow 5 lb	
Men	For first 5 ft, allow 106 lb; for each in. > 5 ft, allow 6 lb	
For a large frame, add 10%; for a small frame, subtract 10%		
2. Determine total caloric intake		
To maintain weight		15 kcal/lb or 30 kcal/kg
To lose weight		10 kcal/lb or 20 kcal/kg
To gain weight (also for adolescents and persons who perform increased physical activity)		20 kcal/lb or 40 kcal/kg
For each decade over age 50, decrease total by 10%		
Round off to the nearest 50 kcal. Although the total will differ slightly between calculations based on pounds and those based on kilograms, the difference has little practical importance because neither prescribing nor following diets is precise.		
3. Apportion calories among carbohydrate, protein, and fat*		
Carbohydrate	About 55% of calories	Simple carbohydrates should be eaten with a meal
Protein	About 15% of calories	
Fat	Less than 30% of calories	Saturated, monounsaturated, and polyunsaturated fat should *each* be about 10% of total calories
		Cholesterol < 300 mg/day

* These percentages of carbohydrate, protein, and fat reflect the recommendations of the American Diabetes Association (ADA).

First, few foods contain high levels of unsaturated fats. Avocados, nuts, and olives are high in monounsaturated fats, but these foods are hardly mainstays of balanced diets. To receive a substantial amount of unsaturated fat, patients must cook in selected oils (eg, olive, corn, canola, and certain varieties of safflower and sunflower) or use appropriate salad dressings. Second, since fat contains more than twice as many calories as carbohydrate and protein per gram, it should be limited in the hypocaloric diets of overweight type II diabetic patients. Therefore, a high carbohydrate, low fat diet seems to be the best approach. Recent evidence suggests that a high protein diet may make the patient more susceptible to the eventual development of nephropathy.

The diabetic diet should be as close as possible to the patient's usual diet to improve the chances of compliance. Once the food plan is agreed on, the insulin dose is adjusted to the diet, not vice versa. Recent studies suggest that eating high fiber foods or fiber supplements, such as bran or guar, is associated with lower postprandial and perhaps lower fasting plasma glucose levels. However, the amount of fiber needed often leads to bloating, flatulence, and abdominal cramping, and occasionally to diarrhea. Although most of these symptoms improve or disappear with time, they are unacceptable to many patients. Therefore, high fiber foods should be encouraged, but large amounts of fiber from any source usually will not be tolerated.

The obese patient and the physician must have a realistic expectation for a hypocaloric diet. On average, the caloric intake should be about 500 kcal/day less than the caloric expenditure. Because the catabolism of 1 lb of body fat releases 3500 kcal, it takes about 7 days to lose 1 lb (500 kcal/day × 7 days), resulting in a loss of 52 lb/yr. More important, this approach restructures the patient's eating habits, which is critical for long-term successful dietary treatment of diabetes.

Fortunately, control of diabetes improves after only a slight weight loss. Insulin sensitivity increases when obese patients are in negative caloric balance, which occurs within weeks (long before much of the extra weight is lost). As hyperglycemia lessens, depressed insulin secretion may improve, leading to better control. *The importance and efficacy of weight reduction in obese diabetic patients cannot be overemphasized.*

Lean patients should eat to maintain desirable body weight. Therefore, except for possible recommendations concerning fat intake, dietary changes should be minimized, especially in older persons, whose lifetime eating habits are usually difficult to alter.

Exercise

Regular exercise makes people feel better, benefits the cardiovascular system when sufficiently vigorous and prolonged, and burns additional calories in obese patients (see Ch. 31). However, in patients receiving insulin, moderate to vigorous exercise can lead to hypoglycemia, primarily because absorption from the injection site increases. Patients using intermediate- and long-acting insulin may have hypoglycemia hours after exercising, unless they ingest complex carbohydrates just before or after exercising.

A secondary cause of hypoglycemia during physical activity is the increased use of glucose by muscles. However, if a type I patient has poor control of diabetes before exercising, glucose levels may rise further, and ketosis may develop or worsen. The cause is probably increases in catecholamines, glucagon, and growth hormone opposing the action of insulin, which all occur with vigorous exercise.

Physical training also increases insulin sensitivity (ie, patients respond better to insulin injection or endogenous insulin). However, for this training effect to occur, exercise must be sufficient to lower the resting heart rate, and it must continue. The increased insulin sensitivity disappears within 1 wk of discontinuing the training regimen.

Exercise rarely leads to significant weight loss without a concomitant decrease in caloric intake. For example, walking 1 mi consumes about 100 kcal—the equivalent of two cookies. The same number of calories is used if the patient runs a mile; it simply takes less time. A list of activities and their corresponding caloric expenditures is provided in TABLE 80–2. Although few obese patients undertake, much less sustain, a vigorous exercise program, they should be encouraged to take regular walks as a start.

Sulfonylurea Agents

All sulfonylureas stimulate insulin secretion directly and potentiate the effect of other insulin secretagogues. They also potentiate the action of insulin in peripheral insulin-sensitive tissues (liver, muscle, and fat). Although this effect was initially thought to result from increased insulin binding, evidence now indicates that these agents act on postreceptor processes. Sulfonylureas are ineffective in type I patients and should be used only for type II diabetes.

No single sulfonylurea is considered best. In making a selection, physicians should weigh four criteria: effectiveness, side effects, compliance, and cost. Potency (ie, the amount of drug necessary to achieve the desired results) is clinically irrelevant. Tolbutamide is the least effective drug, followed by acetohexamide. Chlorpropamide, tolazamide, glyburide, and glipizide are equally effective, but *chlorpropamide should not be used in patients > 65 yr because of the risk of hyponatremia and prolonged hypoglycemia.* A patient who does not achieve control with maximum doses of one of the three more effective agents has only about a 10% chance of succeeding with one of the other two. The five sulfonylureas recommended for the elderly and available in the USA are listed in TABLE 80–3.

Side effects: Fewer than 5% of patients taking sulfonylureas have side effects, the most common ones being GI and dermatologic reactions. Chlorpropamide can cause the **alcohol flushing syndrome,** which may occur in 10% to 30% of patients. Chlorpropamide can also cause **hyponatremia** via the **syndrome of inappropriate antidiuretic hormone (SIADH) secretion,** which is more likely to occur in older patients, especially those also receiving thiazide diuretics.

Hypoglycemia can occur with any sulfonylurea, especially in patients with renal insufficiency and those who eat irregularly. Although hypo-

TABLE 80–2. CALORIC EXPENDITURE DURING VARIOUS ACTIVITIES

Activity	*Calories Expended/hour**
Light	**50–199**
Lying down or sleeping	80
Sitting	100
Driving an automobile	120
Standing	140
Performing domestic work	180
Moderate	**200–299**
Walking (2½ mph)	210
Bicycling (5½ mph)	210
Gardening	220
Canoeing (2½ mph)	230
Golfing	250
Lawn mowing (power mower)	250
Lawn mowing (hand mower)	270
Bowling	270
Marked	**300–399**
Fencing	300
Rowing (2½ mph)	300
Swimming (¼ mph)	300
Walking (3¾ mph)	300
Playing badminton	350
Horseback riding (trotting)	350
Square dancing	350
Playing volleyball	350
Roller-skating	350
Playing table tennis	360

(continued)

TABLE 80–2. CALORIC EXPENDITURE DURING VARIOUS ACTIVITIES *(Continued)*

Activity	*Calories Expended/hour**
Vigorous	≥ **400**
Ditch digging (hand shovel)	400
Ice-skating (10 mph)	400
Chopping or sawing wood	400
Playing tennis	420
Climbing hills (100 ft/h)	480
Skiing (10 mph)	490
Playing squash	600
Jogging (6 mph)	600
Playing handball	600
Bicycling (13 mph)	660
Sculling (racing)	840
Running (10 mph)	1000

* Caloric expenditure is shown for a 150-lb person. Expenditure would be slightly lower for lighter persons and slightly higher for heavier persons.

Modified from Biermann J, Toohey B: *The Diabetic's Sports and Exercise Book: How to Play Your Way to Better Health.* Philadelphia, JB Lippincott, 1977, p 241.

glycemia can last several days, regardless of which drug is prescribed, it may last longer with chlorpropamide because of this drug's extensive duration of action. *Because of the duration of all sulfonylurea-induced hypoglycemia, patients with changes in mentation from hypoglycemia must be admitted to the hospital and treated with IV glucose until they can maintain a normal, or raised, glucose level.*

Reversible intrahepatic cholestasis leading to obstructive jaundice is a rare side effect of sulfonylureas, but it is more common with chlorpropamide. These drugs do *not* have deleterious cardiovascular effects, despite the contention of the University Group Diabetes Program study, which was not borne out by further analysis of its data or by six additional studies.

TABLE 80–3. DOSES AND SELECTED CHARACTERISTICS OF SULFONYLUREA AGENTS

Agent	*Tablet Strength (mg)*	*Usual Daily Dose Range (mg)*	*Maximum Daily Dose (mg)*	*Duration of Action (h)*
Tolbutamide	250, 500	500–2000 (divided)	3000	6–12
Acetohexamide	250, 500	250–1500 (single or divided)	1500	12–24
Tolazamide	100, 250, 500	100–750 (single or divided)	1000	12–24
Glyburide*				
micronized (Glynase)	1.5, 3.0	0.75–12.0 (single or divided)	12	12–24
nonmicronized	1.25, 2.5, 5.0	2.5–15.0 (single or divided)	20	12–24
Glipizide	5, 10	5–30 (single or divided)	40	10–24

* Bioavailability data indicate that micronized glyburide (Glynase) is 97% to 100% absorbed; nonmicronized glyburide is 60% to 80% absorbed. Micronized glyburide is clinically as effective as nonmicronized glyburide but *not* more effective.

Indications and dosages: About 75% of type II diabetics have few symptoms or none at all and should be treated first with diet alone. If diet fails (as indicated either by a fasting plasma glucose level ≥ 140 mg/dL or, in those with a fasting plasma glucose level < 140 mg/dL, by a 1- to 2-h postprandial plasma glucose level consistently > 180 mg/dL), tolazamide, glyburide, or glipizide should be given.

Suggested initial doses of the sulfonylureas are listed in TABLE 80–4. Every week or two, plasma glucose responses should be monitored, and the dose should be increased gradually until either the fasting plasma glucose level falls to < 140 mg/dl or the maximum dose is reached. If the latter occurs, the patient should be switched to a maximum dose of one of the other two agents mentioned above. Any response will be evident in several weeks, although the chances of suc-

TABLE 80–4. RECOMMENDED INITIAL DAILY DOSES OF SULFONYLUREA AGENTS

Agent	*Total Dose (mg) if FPG < 180 mg/dL)*	*Total Dose (mg) if FPG > 180 mg/dL*
Tolbutamide	500	1000
Acetohexamide	250	500
Tolazamide	100	250
Glyburide		
micronized (Glynase)	0.75	1.5
nonmicronized	1.25	2.5
Glipizide	2.5	5.0

FPG = fasting plasma glucose

cess are only about 10%. If the fasting plasma glucose level remains ≥ 140 mg/dL, the glycated hemoglobin value may help determine whether to start insulin therapy.

Glycated (glycosylated) hemoglobin is the product of an irreversible, nonenzymatic reaction between blood glucose and hemoglobin. Because the RBC has a 120-day life span, this value reflects average glucose levels over the preceding 2 to 3 mo. Glycated hemoglobin values do not guide day-to-day therapeutic decisions but are used to help decide whether greater efforts are needed to optimize control. Continually elevated glycated hemoglobin values motivate some patients to begin monitoring their blood glucose levels.

If the fasting plasma glucose level falls to < 140 mg/dL in response to diet or was never above 140 mg/dL, the 1- to 2-h postprandial plasma glucose level is used to determine the next step. If the postprandial plasma glucose level exceeds 180 mg/dL, a sulfonylurea agent should be given. The dose should be gradually increased until the postprandial plasma glucose level remains between 140 and 180 mg/dL. Because older patients are more sensitive to sulfonylureas, the dose increments should be smaller than those for younger patients. If the postprandial plasma glucose level falls to < 140 mg/dL, the dose should be reduced, especially if the glycated hemoglobin level is in or close to the normal range. Discontinuing the sulfonylurea may even be possible, especially in an obese patient who loses weight.

In patients taking a sulfonylurea, the blood glucose level is often > 140 mg/dL in the morning, yet < 100 mg/dL in the late afternoon. In such cases, the lower glucose value determines the therapeutic decisions concerning the sulfonylurea dose. If an afternoon snack does not alleviate hypoglycemia before the evening meal, the dose should be reduced, or tolbutamide or acetohexamide (shorter-acting agents) should be substituted for glyburide or glipizide, regardless of what the fasting plasma glucose or postprandial plasma glucose levels were in the morning. Alternatively, the evening dose may be increased and the morning dose may be decreased; however, there are no reports showing the efficacy of this approach.

After several weeks of sulfonylurea therapy, fasting plasma glucose levels of patients fall into one of three categories: > 180 mg/dL, between 140 and 180 mg/dL, and < 140 mg/dL. In patients who are taking the maximum dose of a sulfonylurea and whose fasting plasma glucose levels are > 180 mg/dL, the physician may switch to the maximum dose of another sulfonylurea for several weeks, but this approach rarely works. The better approach is to discontinue the drug and begin insulin therapy. In patients whose fasting plasma glucose levels fall between 140 and 180 mg/dL, maximum doses of sulfonylureas are maintained for 3 mo. Their glycated hemoglobin levels, which are markedly elevated initially, should then reflect their current glycemic status, and the need for insulin therapy can be determined. In patients with fasting plasma glucose levels < 140 mg/dL, postprandial plasma glucose levels should be monitored.

Tolbutamide is inactivated rapidly in the liver and therefore must be taken at least bid and sometimes tid. A reasonable dosage progression is 250 mg bid, 500 mg bid, 500 mg tid, 1 gm bid, 1 gm tid. Tolazamide, glyburide, and glipizide are also degraded to mostly inactive metabolites in the liver but at a slower rate. The first half of a maximum dose of these three drugs is usually taken before breakfast (ie, tolazamide up to 500 mg, nonmicronized glyburide up to 10 mg, micronized glyburide up to 6 mg, and glipizide up to 20 mg), and the second half is taken before dinner. Acetohexamide is also rapidly metabolized by the liver, but the metabolite is 2.5 times as active as the parent compound. One gram of acetohexamide is taken before breakfast, and the other 500 mg is taken before dinner. Generally, these drugs should be taken before meals to enhance compliance; glipizide should be taken 30 min before meals to enhance its effectiveness.

Special considerations: A few drugs potentiate the effects of sulfonylureas by displacing them from serum albumin to which they are bound. The most important of these drugs are the sulfonamides; less important drugs include chloramphenicol, clofibrate, warfarin, phenylbutazone, and oxyphenbutazone. Using two sulfonylureas together is inappropriate because there is no additive benefit.

When insulin fails to control diabetes, adding a sulfonylurea provides either no improvement or only a modest one. The expense of adding a sulfonylurea should be considered, as should the fact that an increased insulin dose may achieve better results.

On the other hand, when a maximum dose of a sulfonylurea fails to control type II diabetes, insulin may be added to the regimen. The maximum sulfonylurea dose should be continued and intermediate (NPH or lente) insulin given at bedtime. The idea is that the insulin lowers the fasting plasma glucose level, and the sulfonylurea maintains the glucose level during the day. This approach can help convince reluctant patients to start taking insulin.

If sulfonylurea therapy fails in obese patients, they should be treated with insulin, although this approach may cause them to gain more weight as control improves if total caloric intake is not reduced. However, a few extra pounds adds little health risk compared with the eventually devastating effects of hyperglycemia.

Insulin

Goals of therapy: Achieving near euglycemia delays, ameliorates, and may prevent the development of retinopathy, nephropathy, and neuropathy regardless of age. However, the closer a diabetic patient gets to euglycemia, the greater the risk of hypoglycemia, so a balance must be struck between the benefits of tight diabetic control and the risks of hypoglycemia. Since many older diabetic patients have coronary artery and cerebrovascular disease, hypoglycemia may pose a greater risk. Therefore, the balance may need to be tipped toward less strict control.

The degree of control that can be achieved is directly related to the amount of self-testing a patient performs. Many patients are unwilling to consistently monitor blood glucose several times a day, but some patients can be persuaded to perform a combination of blood and urine tests. However, when tight control is the objective, urine tests cannot be substituted for blood tests.

The physician should continually encourage patients to monitor blood glucose more frequently, to start such monitoring if they are relying only on urine testing, or to start urine testing if they are not monitoring themselves at all. Diabetes educators and patient support groups often can influence patients to make more vigorous efforts to achieve better diabetic control. Many patients need months to years of persuasion before they monitor themselves appropriately.

For a **urine test,** a first-voided urine sample should be used because it reflects a large part of the period of greatest interest. A positive result is considered unsatisfactory (ie, the target plasma glucose level has been exceeded), while a negative result is considered satisfactory (ie, the target level has been met).

Self-monitoring of blood glucose levels involves obtaining a drop of blood by pricking a finger with a lancet, which is usually inserted into a spring-loaded device. The patient then places the drop of blood on a pad at the end of a reagent strip. In some systems, the blood is left on the pad for a specific length of time and then wiped off. Next, the patient either places the strip in a glucose meter that records the blood glucose value, or the patient compares the color of the strip to a chart. In other systems, the patient places the strip in the meter and places a drop of blood on the strip; after a preset length of time, the machine records the value. With this system, wiping the blood is not necessary. Generally, meters that do not require wiping are easier for older patients to use.

Unfortunately, self-monitoring is expensive. A reagent strip costs about 50 cents, and a meter costs between $50 and $150. If the patient is comparing the strip to a chart, the strips can be cut in half lengthwise without sacrificing accuracy. This visual comparison method has two other advantages. First, it provides a way of double-checking the glucose concentration recorded by the meter. Second, the strips can be kept in a dark, dry environment (such as the vial they come in, which contains a desiccant) and read later by another trained person. However, visual reading is often difficult for older patients, and most now use methods that require neither wiping nor visual comparison.

Ideally, all patients, especially those taking insulin, should test four times a day—before each meal and before a bedtime snack. Many patients cannot or will not test this often, but the more tests, the better the chance of achieving near normal blood glucose levels.

The use of self-monitoring in patients who are not taking insulin is more controversial. Theoretically, one might expect that the results of self-monitoring would enhance patient motivation and compliance, but studies have not confirmed this. However, self-monitoring can help motivated patients to determine which carbohydrate-containing foods are more likely to provoke hyperglycemia.

Suggested levels of diabetic control for patients who need insulin and who use a blood glucose self-monitoring device are listed in TABLE 80–5. The glucose levels correspond to the values represented by the colors on a Chemstrip comparison chart or the values halfway between two colors. (Chemstrip is a type of blood glucose monitoring strip that can be read visually as well as by a meter.) Most people can judge whether the color on the strip is near one shown on a chart or is about halfway between two colors.

Which level of control to select, at least initially, is influenced by the patient's age, the length of time a type I patient has had diabetes, the patient's awareness of hypoglycemic symptoms, and the clinical evidence of autonomic neuropathy.

Level 1 of diabetic control is selected for type I patients who have had diabetes for > 5 yr, any patients who have hypoglycemia without concomitant symptoms, any patients with clinical evidence of autonomic neuropathy, and any patients > 65 yr old who are taking insulin. If preprandial levels of ≤ 180 mg/dL can be achieved without significant hypoglycemia, the goal is cautiously advanced to level 2, except for those > 80 yr old. Because of their life expectancy and the increased danger of hypoglycemia when associated with coronary artery and cerebrovascular disease, these patients are kept at level 1 indefinitely.

TABLE 80–5. LEVELS OF DIABETIC CONTROL

Level 1	Preprandial glucose levels of ≤ 180 mg/dL
Level 2	Preprandial glucose levels of ≤ 150 mg/dL
Level 3	Preprandial glucose levels of ≤ 120 mg/dL
Level 4	1- to 2-h postprandial glucose levels of ≤ 210 mg/dL*
Level 5	1- to 2-h postprandial glucose levels of ≤ 150 mg/dL

* ≤ 200 mg/dL if using a glucose meter; ≤ 210 mg/dL if visually reading Chemstrips.

Level 2 (preprandial levels ≤ 150 mg/dL) is the initial goal for all other groups of patients. Those who have hypoglycemia without premonitory symptoms and those between ages 65 and 80 are maintained at level 2. All other patients who are able to achieve level 2 without significant hypoglycemia are cautiously advanced to level 3 (ie, preprandial levels ≤ 120 mg/dL). Levels 4 and 5 require measuring postprandial blood glucose levels, and unfortunately few patients attempt this.

Under the current, relatively crude system of replacing or supplementing endogenous insulin with exogenous insulin, some episodes of hypoglycemia are almost unavoidable if glucose levels are to approach normal most of the time. Nevertheless, because tight control has such important benefits, patients should be asked to tolerate mild episodes of hypoglycemia two or three times a week. However, if episodes occur more frequently, distress the patient, are not quickly stopped, or most important, are not easily recognized, the insulin dose should be reduced, and the patient must settle for a level of less control.

The symptoms and signs of **hypoglycemia** fall into two categories: autonomic, those caused by increased activity of the autonomic nervous system, and neuroglucopenic, those caused by decreased activity of the central nervous system (see TABLE 80–6). The brain, which has an absolute requirement for glucose, seems to accommodate itself to the prevailing concentration. Thus, when patients with poor glucose control lower their blood glucose levels (eg, from 300 mg/dL to 150 mg/dL), they often experience mild autonomic symptoms. These symptoms invariably disappear after several weeks, and the patients must be encouraged to continue tightening diabetic control. Conversely, type I diabetic patients under tight control have a lower threshold for both hypoglycemic symptoms and the release of counterregulatory hormones. Thus, symptoms and endogenous gluconeogenesis do not occur until more critical levels of hypoglycemia are reached.

TABLE 80–6. SYMPTOMS AND SIGNS OF HYPOGLYCEMIA

Autonomic	*Neuroglucopenic*
Weakness	Headache
Sweating	Hypothermia
Tachycardia	Visual disturbances
Palpitations	Mental dullness
Tremor	Confusion
Nervousness	Amnesia
Irritability	Seizures
Tingling of mouth and fingers	Coma
Hunger	
Nausea (unusual)	
Vomiting (unusual)	

All patients who take insulin should carry with them a source of simple carbohydrate. Almost any candy that contains sugar will do. Alternatively, patients can obtain glucose tablets from pharmacies or diabetes supply stores. If a patient is uncertain whether symptoms result from hypoglycemia, self-monitoring should be performed. However, if symptoms are severe, treatment without documentation is better than no treatment. Most patients ingest more carbohydrate than is needed. Usually, only 10 gm of simple carbohydrate is needed to reverse hypoglycemia. If symptoms do not improve in 10 to 15 min, another 10 gm should be ingested. If several hours will elapse before the next meal, a small snack containing protein and carbohydrate should be eaten. Amino acids from the ingested protein will help replenish hepatic glycogen via gluconeogenesis.

Choice of insulin preparation: The most important criterion for selecting an insulin preparation is the time of its course of action—specifically, the onset, peak, and duration. Estimates of these values are summarized in TABLE 80–7. Responses to insulins vary widely among patients and even in the same patient from day to day. Also, a small number of patients have a delayed response to regular insulin, so that the course of this short-acting agent is similar to that of semilente insulin. Further, adding regular insulin to lente or ultralente insulin in the same syringe delays its onset of action in all patients. Apparently, the excess zinc in the lente series of insulins binds the regular insulin and retards its absorption.

Thus, when combinations of short- and intermediate-acting insulins are used, regular insulin should be added to neutral protamine Hagedorn **(NPH)** insulin. On the other hand, if short- and long-acting insulins are used together, regular insulin should be added to ultralente

TABLE 80–7. APPROXIMATE TIME–ACTIVITY RELATIONSHIPS OF VARIOUS INSULIN PREPARATIONS GIVEN SUBCUTANEOUSLY

Kind of Insulin	*Preparation*	*Onset of Action (h)*	*Peak Action (h)*	*Duration of Action (h)*
Short acting	Regular*	0.5–1	2–4†	4–6
	Semilente	1–2	3–6	8–12
Intermediate acting	NPH	1.5–4	6–16	20–24
	Lente	1–4	6–16	20–24
Long acting	PZI	6–8	14–20	> 32
	Ultralente	6–8	14–20	> 32

NPH = neutral protamine Hagedorn; PZI = protamine zinc insulin.
* Also called crystalline zinc insulin (CZI).
† In some patients, the action of regular insulin may peak later than indicated here (between 4 and 8 h) and last considerably longer. Therefore, adding regular insulin to intermediate-acting insulin may cause afternoon hypoglycemia in these patients.

insulin. Although absorption of the regular insulin is delayed somewhat, the problem would be greater with protamine zinc insulin **(PZI)** suspension because the excess protamine would make little short-acting insulin available until the regular:PZI ratio exceeds approximately 1:1.

Beef insulin is more antigenic than **pork** and **human insulins.** However, titers of IgG antibodies that bind insulin are extremely low with the current purer insulins, and the clinical significance is unknown. In some patients, human insulin has a slightly earlier onset and peak action than beef and pork insulins.

Sensitivity to exogenous insulin can vary over time, even without a recognizable cause (eg, infection, weight change, emotional stress). Therefore, patients need to be monitored, and insulin doses need to be adjusted about monthly, even though office visits will be less frequent, usually every 3 to 6 mo. This requires ongoing communication between physician and patient, a family member, or nursing home personnel. Decisions on changing the insulin dose are based on the results of blood or urine tests and on the degree of diabetic control desired. Some patients can be taught to adjust their own insulin doses based on their glucose self-monitoring results.

TABLE 80–8. PERIODS OF GLUCOSE CONTROL FOR COMPONENTS OF INSULIN REGIMEN AND TIMING OF TESTS REFLECTING CONTROL

Insulin	*Time Injected*	*Period of Control*	*Timing of Test Reflecting Insulin Control*
Regular	Before a meal	Between that meal and either the next one or the bedtime snack (if insulin is taken before evening meal)	Both after the meal before which insulin is injected and before the next meal or bedtime snack (if insulin is taken before evening meal)
NPH	Before breakfast	Between lunch and evening meal	Before evening meal
	Before evening meal or before bedtime	Overnight	Before breakfast
Ultralente	Before breakfast and/or before evening meal	Overnight	Before breakfast

Starting insulin therapy in the hospital: The relationships between types of insulin and periods of control are shown in TABLE 80–8. Lean patients (< 125% desirable body weight) starting therapy on **regimen A or B** (shown in TABLE 80–9) receive 10 u. of NPH in the morning and 4 to 5 u. in the evening. Obese patients (≥ 125% desirable body weight) receive initial doses of 20 u. and 10 u., respectively. The doses are increased gradually until level 1 control (see TABLE 80–5) is achieved before breakfast and the evening meal. Then the need for regular insulin is assessed by evaluating the before-lunch and before-bedtime-snack glucose levels. The initial dose is usually 2 to 4 u. in lean patients and 6 to 8 u. in obese patients. These amounts are gradually increased until level 1 or 2 control is achieved. The initial doses of regular insulin can be started with the NPH insulin to avoid prolonging hospitalization. However, the regular insulin doses are not increased until before-breakfast and before-evening-meal glucose levels of ≤ 180 mg/dL have been achieved.

Further increases in intermediate- and short-acting insulin to attain tighter control should be made at home, not in the hospital. Eating, activity, and emotional patterns usually differ in these settings, and *tight control in the hospital can lead to hypoglycemia at home.*

TABLE 80–9. VARIOUS INSULIN REGIMENS*

Regimen	*Before Breakfast*	*Before Lunch*	*Before Evening Meal*	*At Bedtime*
A	NPH/regular	——	NPH/regular	——
B	NPH/regular	——	Regular	NPH
C	Regular	Regular	NPH/regular	——
D	Regular	Regular	Regular	NPH
E	Ultralente/ regular	Regular	Regular†	——

* Insulin is usually injected 30 min before a meal.

† Either half or the entire ultralente dose may be given before the evening meal, since the long-acting preparation is thought to provide a basal level of insulin with activity affecting mostly the overnight period.

The regimens that use regular insulin before each meal (**C, D, and E** in TABLE 80–9) begin with 4 to 5 u. for lean patients and 8 to 10 u. for obese patients. The initial dose of NPH and ultralente insulin in these regimens is 10 u. for lean patients and 16 u. for obese patients. All doses are then adjusted according to the appropriate tests as summarized in TABLE 80–8.

Changes are made daily, depending on test results. Once target levels are approached, changes are made less frequently: weekly if the patient performs self-tests often enough (two to four times a day) and can be taught algorithms or monthly if the test results have to be reviewed by a physician. In general, insulin should be adjusted—up or down—by about 10% or 4 u., whichever is less.

Considerations for specific regimens: **Regimens A and B** offer the least flexibility in the timing and content of meals; hypoglycemia is most likely to occur if meals are delayed. In **regimens A and C,** the intermediate-acting insulin given before the evening meal may have peak activity in the middle of the night rather than toward morning; increasing the dose may lead to hypoglycemia in the middle of the night. Administering the intermediate-acting insulin before bedtime **(regimens B or D)** should solve this problem.

In **regimens C and D,** if the period between lunch and the evening meal is prolonged (usually > 5 to 7 h), the before-evening-meal blood glucose level may be too high because the effect of the regular insulin given before lunch may have worn off. In **regimen E,** since ultralente insulin starts working 6 to 8 h after injection, hypoglycemia may occur between lunch and the evening meal, especially if the evening meal is late, or before breakfast if ultralente is given in the evening. This is usually not a problem when the dose of long-acting insulin is low (about 10 u.).

Many patients who rely exclusively on self-monitoring of blood glucose levels prefer not to test their urine at all. However, since diabetic ketoacidosis can occur with blood glucose levels < 300 mg/dL, *physicians should teach type 1 patients to test their urine for ketone bodies when they are ill.*

Side effects of insulin therapy: Besides hypoglycemia, insulin therapy has five side effects: a delayed reaction at the injection site (dermal reaction); an immediate reaction at the injection site, often spreading as an urticarial rash to other areas (called systemic or true insulin allergy); clinical insulin resistance; lipoatrophy; and lipohypertrophy.

Local dermal reactions are 2- to 3-cm erythematous, pruritic papules that appear several hours after the injection and gradually disappear over the next several days. They seem to be a delayed sensitivity response to impurities in the insulin preparation. These reactions were fairly common for the first several months of insulin therapy with the older, less pure preparations. Occasionally, these reactions still appear with the newer purer insulin preparations. Invariably, they disappear after several months. If necessary, they can be treated by adding a small amount of an antihistamine or corticosteroid to the insulin injection.

Systemic insulin allergy occurs in < 0.1% of patients who require insulin and is more common with intermittent insulin therapy. Within 10 to 60 min, a large local reaction occurs at the injection site and may quickly spread to a generalized urticarial pattern (about 50%). Like penicillin allergy, insulin allergy is associated with occasional angioneurotic edema or anaphylactic shock, is mediated by IgE antibodies, produces positive skin test results, and is treated by desensitization.

Clinical insulin resistance is *an insulin requirement of > 200 u./day for several days in the absence of infection or diabetic ketoacidosis.* Besides gross obesity, the most common cause is a high titer of IgG (insulin-binding) antibodies. Like systemic insulin allergy, clinical insulin resistance is uncommon (< 0.1% of patients requiring insulin) and more likely with intermittent insulin therapy. Most patients who need insulin generate low titers of IgG antibodies; why a few patients generate high titers is not known. Fortunately, the situation is self-limited, and insulin responses return to normal, usually within 6 mo.

Lipoatrophy, *loss of subcutaneous fat tissue at injection sites,* was much more common with older impure preparations, especially in young females. Lipoatrophy is thought to result from an immune response to impurities in the preparations. Often, it can be successfully treated by injecting the patient's usual dose of a pure insulin preparation into the area, starting at the periphery. Within several weeks, the lipogenic effect of insulin starts to restore the local fat deposits. Paradoxically, however, a patient occasionally develops lipoatrophy when starting to take a pure insulin preparation.

Lipohypertrophy, *an accumulation of subcutaneous fat,* occurs with repeated injections at the same site, presumably because of the local lipogenic effect of insulin. Continued injections at these sites may lead to erratic insulin absorption. Therefore, rotation of injection sites must be encouraged.

HYPEROSMOLAR NONKETOTIC SYNDROME

Hyperosmolar nonketotic syndrome results from a marked deficiency of effective insulin. Although small amounts of circulating insulin can be measured, large amounts of the stress hormones (glucagon, epinephrine, norepinephrine, cortisol, and growth hormone) antagonize insulin's effects. The resulting hyperglycemia causes an osmotic diuresis, leading to dehydration and electrolyte depletion. The absence of significant ketosis implies that the production of free fatty acids via lipolysis is not markedly increased. This is probably because of the restraining effects of the remaining insulin (lipolysis is much more sensitive to insulin than the pathways of carbohydrate metabolism) and an independent inhibition by the markedly increased plasma osmolality.

Because significant ketosis and subsequent acidosis do not develop, patients do not have GI symptoms and thus do not immediately seek medical care. They are often able to tolerate polyuria and polydipsia for weeks. This tolerance leads to severe electrolyte depletion and dehydration until renal plasma flow is sufficiently impaired to allow the glucose levels to become extremely high. Thus, this syndrome is characterized by severe hyperglycemia (> 800 mg/dL) and hyperosmolality (> 340 mOsm/kg) and by profound dehydration without significant ketosis (usually defined as a nitroprusside reaction of < 2+ in a 1:1 dilution of plasma). Plasma osmolality **(Posm)** can be estimated using the following formula:

$$\text{Posm (mOsm/kg)} = 2([\text{Na}] + [\text{K}]) + \frac{[\text{glucose}]}{18} + \frac{\text{BUN}}{2.8}$$

Na and K are given as mEq/L, and glucose and BUN levels, as mg/dL.

TABLE 80–10 presents some important distinctions between the pure syndromes of hyperosmolar nonketotic syndrome and diabetic ketoacidosis. Many older patients have a mixed syndrome with high glucose and osmolality values but a compensated acidosis (ie, with significant ketosis, low P_{CO_2} and HCO_3^- values, but a normal or slightly de-

TABLE 80–10. COMPARISON OF HYPEROSMOLAR NONKETOTIC SYNDROME AND DIABETIC KETOACIDOSIS

Feature	*Hyperosmolar Nonketotic Syndrome*	*Diabetic Ketoacidosis*
Age of patient	Usually > 40 yr	Usually < 40 yr
Duration of symptoms	Usually > 5 days	Usually < 2 days
Glucose*	Usually > 800 mg/dL	Usually < 800 mg/dL
Sodium*	More likely to be normal or high	More likely to be normal or low
Potassium*	High, normal, or low	High, normal, or low
Bicarbonate*	Normal	Low
Ketone bodies	< 2+ in 1:1 dilution of serum or plasma	At least 4+ in 1:1 dilution of serum or plasma
pH	Normal	Low
Serum osmolality	Usually > 350 mOsm/kg	Usually < 350 mOsm/kg
Cerebral edema	Not clinically evident	Occasionally clinically evident
Prognosis	10–20% mortality	3–10% mortality
Subsequent course	Long-term insulin therapy not required in many cases	Long-term insulin therapy required in virtually all cases

* Serum level

creased pH). Conditions associated with hyperosmolar nonketotic syndrome are listed in TABLE 80–11. If this syndrome is not the initial presentation of diabetes, it often occurs when a type II patient has another, often severe, illness.

The **treatment** of hyperosmolar nonketotic syndrome in patients with either the pure form or with a compensated acidosis involves fluid, insulin, and potassium replacement. Adequate fluid replacement is critical for lowering glucose levels, even in patients receiving appropriate insulin therapy. Initial fluid replacement with 0.9% sodium chloride

TABLE 80–11. FACTORS ASSOCIATED WITH ONSET OF HYPEROSMOLAR NONKETOTIC SYNDROME

Conditions	*Drugs*	*Miscellaneous*
Diabetes mellitus*	Diuretic (potassium-depleting)	Burns
Infection	Diazoxide	Hemodialysis
Acute pancreatitis	Phenytoin	Peritoneal dialysis
Pancreatic carcinoma	Propranolol	Hypothermia
Acromegaly	Glucocorticoids	Heatstroke
Cushing's syndrome	Hypertonic sodium bicarbonate	
Thyrotoxicosis		
Subdural hematoma		
Uremia (with vomiting)		

* Initial manifestation without known precipitating cause.

(normal saline) solution or 0.45% sodium chloride (half normal saline) solution should be 500 to 1000 mL/h for at least the first several hours, until intravascular volume is restored. However, *because many older patients have limited cardiac reserve, their lungs must be assessed frequently to avoid overhydration and pulmonary edema* (which, unfortunately, are common with treatment of hyperosmolar nonketotic syndrome). Patients with a history of heart disease may need pulmonary wedge or central venous pressure monitoring.

Low-dose insulin given IM or IV is effective in hyperosmolar nonketotic syndrome, as it is in diabetic ketoacidosis. An initial bolus injection does not improve the response and thus is unnecessary. Doses between 3 and 10 u./h are usually effective. The usual route of administration is IV, which should be continued until the patient can eat; then intermediate-acting insulin can be given subcutaneously.

Even though the total-body depletion of potassium is marked, initial serum levels of potassium may be low, normal, or high. During treatment, however, serum levels invariably decrease, so potassium replacement is needed in all patients (assuming urine flow) but may be started at different times. Often, replacement must be delayed because of the cardiac response to elevated levels of serum potassium.

The **prognosis** is worse for patients with hyperosmolar nonketotic syndrome than for those with diabetic ketoacidosis. Most deaths are related to the severity of the complicating illness, which either causes hyperosmolar nonketotic syndrome or develops because of it. Usually death does not result from the metabolic derangements per se.

TABLE 80–12. FACTORS AFFECTING DIABETES CONTROL IN THE ELDERLY

Altered sense	Neoplasia
Decreased vision	Decreased exercise and mobility
Decreased smell	Drugs
Altered taste perception	Medications (non–potassium-sparing diuretics, glucocorticoids, phenytoin)
Decreased proprioception	Alcohol
Difficulties in food preparation and consumption	Neuropsychiatric problems
Tremor	Bereavement
Arthritis	Depression
Poor dentition	Cognitive impairment and dementia
Alterations in GI function and nutrient absorption	Social factors
Altered recognition of hunger and thirst	Inadequate education
Altered renal and hepatic function	Poor dietary habits
Acute infections	Living alone
	Poverty

Modified from Lipson LG: "Diabetes in the elderly: Diagnosis, pathogenesis and therapy." *American Journal of Medicine* 80(suppl 5A):10–21, 1986; used with permission.

Long-term treatment of patients who recover from hyperosmolar nonketotic syndrome may not include insulin. Unlike the type I diabetic patient who requires continued insulin therapy after recovering from diabetic ketoacidosis, many type II diabetic patients can be treated successfully with sulfonylureas and/or diet after recovering from hyperosmolar nonketotic syndrome.

SPECIAL CHALLENGES IN THE ELDERLY

Diabetes care in the elderly can be particularly difficult because of circumstances associated with aging (see TABLE 80–12). Older patients may have trouble preparing meals because of tremors, osteoarthritis, or affective or cognitive disorders. Depression or bereavement may lead to poor self-care, poor hygiene, anorexia, and noncompliance with medication regimens. Cognitive impairment can also contribute to these problems. Persons with severe dementia may be particularly insensitive to hunger or thirst—the former leading to weight loss, the latter to dehydration and, if uncorrected, hyperosmolar nonketotic syndrome.

Taste perception can change, with bitter or salty tastes becoming more predominant. Many older people are either edentulous or have poorly fitting dentures that interfere with chewing. These factors make it difficult for older diabetic patients to eat appropriate, nutritious meals at regular intervals. This can be particularly dangerous in patients taking insulin and somewhat less dangerous in patients taking sulfonylureas. Because of a diminished sense of thirst, an older person with raised serum osmolality may become severely dehydrated.

Given these factors, care of an elderly diabetic patient is a particular challenge. Because the prevalence is so high in this population, the problem is enormous. These patients should be approached with patience and understanding, and available support systems should be used as much as possible.

81. LIPOPROTEIN DISORDERS

Coronary artery disease (CAD) is to a large degree preventable and controllable and to some degree reversible. The major lipoprotein risk factors that contribute to CAD can be ameliorated by dietary changes, exercise, weight reduction, smoking cessation or reduction, and if needed, drug therapy.

Four major groups of studies provide consistent, strong support for identifying and modifying risk factors in the elderly to prevent and ameliorate major cardiovascular diseases. These groups of studies include prospective epidemiologic population studies, epidemiologic studies showing trends in reduced CAD mortality, controlled clinical trials on lowering lipid levels, and studies of regression of coronary artery atherosclerosis.

Long-term prospective epidemiologic population studies: Studies in persons 65 to 85 yr emphasize the independent relationships of high-density lipoprotein cholesterol **(HDL-C)**, low-density lipoprotein cholesterol **(LDL-C)**, and triglyceride levels; blood pressure; cigarette smoking; and diabetes to CAD. The absolute excess risk of CAD mortality attributable to plasma total cholesterol **(TC)** rises substantially with age; TC levels continue to be associated with an increased risk of CAD into at least the eighth decade for both men and women. The TC:HDL-C ratio accounts for a significant risk gradient associated with CAD in those > 50 yr. Triglyceride levels influence CAD risk at any HDL-C level but influence it significantly only in women. In men and women, CAD risk at any triglyceride level was strongly influenced by the HDL-C level.

In a 10-yr study of men who were 60 to 79 yr and free of CAD on entering the study, the relative risk of CAD mortality in those in the highest quartile for plasma TC level was 1.5 compared with those in the other three quartiles combined. This relative risk did not change greatly with age, ranging from 1.4 in men between ages 60 and 64 to 1.7 in men ages 75 to 79. However, because CAD mortality rose with age, the excess risk for such mortality attributable to elevated plasma cholesterol levels increased between ages 60 and 79 from 2.2 deaths per 1000 person years to 11.3 deaths per 1000 person years. It was concluded that cholesterol lowering might actually produce greater reductions in CAD mortality in elderly men than in middle-aged men. Although the relative risk for CAD mortality associated with high blood TC levels is lower in the elderly than in middle-aged adults, CAD event rates rise with age. Therefore, the number of deaths that could be attributed to high blood TC levels will be greater in the elderly than in middle-aged adults. When compared to relative risk, the excess risk, *the absolute difference in disease rates due to a risk factor,* is an excellent guide to the potential value of treating high blood TC levels, particularly in the elderly.

In the elderly, LDL-C and Lp(a) lipoprotein are major, independent, positive risk factors for carotid artery atherosclerosis and stroke, and HDL-C is a significant independent negative risk factor. A high Lp(a) level is also an independent risk factor for CAD. Because a high Lp(a) level probably has a synergistic effect on the risks of coronary and carotid artery disease, the Lp(a) level should be measured in patients who have had a myocardial infarction, CAD, or stroke and in those with major CAD risk factors. In these persons, aggressive modification of other CAD risk factors is important because Lp(a) levels cannot be lowered by diet and can be lowered only modestly by nicotinic acid therapy.

Epidemiologic studies showing trends in reduced CAD mortality: Over the last 20 yr, striking improvements in the major CAD risk factors and parallel reductions in CAD mortality have taken place. The decline in CAD mortality has involved all geographic regions of the USA, all major sex-race groups, and all age groups over age 35. In the USA, the CAD death rate per 100,000 persons ages 65 to 74 decreased by 28% between 1968 and 1978. For persons ages 75 to 84, the rate decreased by 19%. Reduced intake of dietary saturated fat and reductions in plasma cholesterol have contributed substantially to the decline in CAD mortality since the late 1960s. The drop in CAD mortality is marked in persons in higher socioeconomic classes, who are more likely to participate in preventive medicine programs and who are more likely to modify diet and lifestyle. This trend toward reduced CAD mortality may also be related to improved medical care for persons with acute CAD, to better control of hypertension, and to reduced smoking.

Recent autopsy studies indicate that the extent of coronary atherosclerosis is declining in the USA over time. This is concordant with the observed decline in CAD mortality in all population groups in the USA over the past 20 yr. These data imply that people are reaching old age with less severe atherosclerotic disease; thus, creating regimens designed to stop the progression of atherosclerosis and to induce regression is easier.

Controlled clinical trials on lowering lipid levels and studies of regression of coronary artery atherosclerosis: The Oslo Heart Trial compared patients who used dietary and smoking-reduction interventions with a group who used no interventions. Of necessity, this trial was not a blind study. The intervention group showed a 47% reduction in CAD events.

The Lipid Research Clinics' Coronary Primary Prevention Trial was a multicenter, randomized, double-blind, 7-yr test of the efficacy of lowering cholesterol in 3806 asymptomatic men with primary hypercholesterolemia. At the beginning of the study, the men were 35 to 59 yr and were free of overt CAD. With cholestyramine and dietary intervention, the average decrease in LDL-C levels was 11% more than with placebo, and the average increase in HDL-C levels was 3% more than with placebo. Reduction of plasma TC and LDL-C by diet alone was greater in older persons than in younger persons. A 21% reduction in deaths from CAD was reported along with a 17% reduction in all CAD end points and a 19% reduction in CAD events, neither of which were affected by age at entry into the study.

The Helsinki Heart Trial was a multicenter, randomized, double-blind, 5-yr study of the efficacy of simultaneously raising HDL-C and lowering non–HDL-C levels with gemfibrozil and diet. Studies were carried out in 4081 asymptomatic men ages 40 to 55 yr with non–HDL-C ≥ 200 mg/dL. About half of the men received gemfibrozil 1200 mg; the other half received a placebo. Gemfibrozil increased HDL-C by 11% and reduced TC by 10%, LDL-C by 11%, and triglycerides by 35% from baseline levels. In the gemfibrozil group, the cumulative rate of cardiac end points at 5 yr was 27.3 per 1000 compared with 41.4 per 1000 in the placebo group, a reduction of 34% ($p < 0.02$). The reduction in CAD risk could be attributed to both decreased LDL-C and increased HDL-C levels.

Randomized controlled trials in patients who have had a myocardial infarction or who have hemodynamically significant coronary artery stenosis (and who therefore, like the elderly, have advanced coronary atherosclerosis) have shown significant reductions in nonfatal CAD end points and reductions in both CAD and all-cause mortality.

Nine major controlled clinical trials that predominantly focused on secondary CAD prevention have been completed. These trials, most of which used changes in coronary artery atherosclerosis as their primary end points, used a wide variety of interventions to modify lipoprotein levels: extremely low fat, vegetarian diets; reduced saturated fat and cholesterol diets; nicotinic acid; cholestyramine; colestipol plus nicotinic acid; colestipol plus lovastatin; and ileal bypass. These studies have shown that a reduction in plasma TC and LDL-C and an elevation in HDL-C can reduce nonfatal and fatal CAD events by up to 75% (with a range of 25% to 75%). The coronary artery angiographic trials suggested that reductions in LDL-C or increases in HDL-C can reduce progression and induce regression of atherosclerosis in 16% to 82% of patients. Four of the studies suggested that benefits to women were at least as great as those to men, if not greater. Although the therapeutic interventions were primarily done in middle-aged men, age at entry to the controlled trials did not appear to be a significant variable with regard to the likelihood of regression, cessation, or progression of atherosclerosis.

A variety of interventions that lower LDL-C and triglycerides and/or increase HDL-C have been shown to stop progression of and/or induce regression of femoral and carotid artery atherosclerosis.

Concern has been raised about a possible increase in all-cause mortality in those treated with cholesterol-lowering drugs in controlled clinical trials. Pooling data from available controlled clinical trials reveals a trend toward reduced all-cause mortality in patients with established CAD. In the cholesterol-lowering trial using ileal bypass, which had a 10-yr follow-up, not only was CAD morbidity and mortality reduced, but so was all-cause mortality. Although more data must be collected prospectively about the relationships of cholesterol lowering, changes in plasma cholesterol, and low plasma cholesterol to all-cause mortality, available data suggest that cholesterol lowering with diet and drugs probably reduces all-cause mortality along with CAD mortality.

Factors Affecting Lipoprotein Cholesterol Levels

Blood lipoprotein levels are potently influenced by age, sex, menopause, race, obesity, diet, physical activity, alcohol, cigarette smoking, and heredity. Understanding the influence of these factors is important in understanding the pathophysiology, treatment, and prevention of CAD.

Age: In men, mean levels of plasma TC increase until about age 70, then decline. In women, they increase more gradually, and at about age 55 to 60, TC levels exceed those in men. Particularly in women, the age-associated increase in plasma TC results primarily from the increase in LDL-C levels and much less from the small increase in very low-density lipoprotein cholesterol **(VLDL-C)** levels. In men, mean levels of HDL-C increase after age 55, but at some point they level off; in women, they decrease after age 65 until they reach a point about 10 mg/dL higher than those in men.

Postmenopausal estrogens: The lower rates of CAD in premenopausal women compared with those in men may be related to their lower plasma LDL-C and higher HDL-C levels, which result in part from endogenous estrogens. When women undergo menopause, they lose this protection against CAD: LDL-C and Lp(a) levels rise and HDL-C levels fall. Women who undergo surgical or early natural menopause lose this protection earlier than most women.

Postmenopausal women given unopposed estrogen replacement therapy have lower LDL-C and higher HDL-C levels, which produce a substantial decrease in the LDL-C:HDL-C ratio. Such therapy also lowers Lp(a) levels. In epidemiologic studies using unopposed estrogen therapy, the risk of cardiovascular death is reduced. The practice of adding progestins to reduce the risk of endometrial hyperplasia and endometrial and breast cancer probably does not have a significant adverse effect on plasma lipoprotein levels. Fasting plasma triglyceride levels should be measured before initiating estrogen replacement therapy (with or without progestins) because estrogens substantially elevate triglyceride levels in women with preexisting hypertriglyceridemia, often to levels that can cause lethal pancreatitis. Estrogen replacement therapy (with or without progestins) is contraindicated in women with familial hypertriglyceridemia whose triglyceride level is > 300 mg/dL after modifying diet and alcohol intake.

Genetics: Coronary artery disease is rare and life expectancy prolonged in persons with familial hyperalphalipoproteinemia with primary and familial elevation of HDL-C levels (> 75 mg/dL) and in those with familial hypobetalipoproteinemia with hereditary depression of LDL-C levels (< 100 mg/dL). Conversely, in **progeria** (a premature aging syndrome), moderate elevation of plasma TC and LDL-C levels and marked depression of HDL-C levels have been reported. Moreover, in total lipodystrophy and Cockayne's syndrome (two other premature aging syndromes), very low HDL-C levels are common. For a discussion of the familial hyperlipoproteinemias, see below.

CLASSIFICATION AND ETIOLOGY

Previously, qualitative electrophoretic lipoprotein phenotyping and measurements of TC and LDL-C levels were used to differentiate the types of lipoprotein disorders. Today, measurements of lipoprotein cholesterol and triglyceride levels are used. However, the two systems are parallel and supplementary (see TABLE 81–1).

Most persons with a lipoprotein disorder have hypercholesterolemia with raised LDL-C levels (type II hyperlipoproteinemia), hypertriglyceridemia (primarily type IV or V), hypoalphalipoproteinemia, and/or high Lp(a) levels. Persons who have type II hyperlipoproteinemia have elevated LDL-C levels, often with moderately elevated triglyceride and modestly reduced HDL-C levels. Those who have hypertriglyceridemia with elevated VLDL-C levels (type IV or V) usually have low HDL-C and normal or low LDL-C levels. When triglycerides are markedly elevated (usually > 1000 mg/dL), chylomicrons are usually present (type I). Persons with hypoalphalipoproteinemia (bottom decile for HDL-C level) often have normal TC and LDL-C levels and normal to modestly elevated triglyceride levels. Persons with high Lp(a) levels may or may not have other risk factors for CAD. However, patients with familial hypercholesterolemia have higher mean Lp(a) levels than persons with normal cholesterol levels.

TABLE 81–1. LIPOPROTEIN DISORDERS

Disorder	*Lipoprotein Abnormality*	*Typical Lipoprotein Levels (mg/dL)*	*History and Clinical Findings*	*Primary Mode of Inheritance; Estimated Prevalence*
Type I Hyperlipoproteinemia	High TG, primarily chylomicrons	TC 150-400 TG 1,000-15,000 HDL-C $\leq$ 35	Typically presents in childhood Recurrent abdominal pain Pancreatitis Eruptive xanthomas Hepatosplenomegaly Lipemia retinalis	Recessive; 1/1,000,000 (?)
Type IIA Hyperlipoproteinemia	High TC, LDL-C, with normal TG	TC 250-1000 TG 50-200 LDL-C $\geq$ 160	Severe premature atherosclerosis MI, angina§,** Tenosynovitis (achilles, patellar) Periorbital xanthelasma* Tendinous xanthomas‡ Tuberous xanthomas†,‡ Arcus juvenilis corneae	Dominant; 1/200–1/500
Type IIB Hyperlipoproteinemia	High TC, LDL-C, with high TG	TC 250-1000 TG 200-400 LDL-C $\geq$ 160	Severe premature atherosclerosis MI, angina§,** Tenosynovitis (achilles, patellar) Periorbital xanthelasma* Tendinous xanthomas‡ Tuberous xanthomas†,‡ Arcus juvenilis corneae	

Type III Hyperlipoproteinemia	High TC, high TG, high IDL (beta migrating VLDL)	TC 200-800 TG 300-1400 HDL-C ≤ 40	Severe premature atherosclerosis MI, stroke, peripheral vascular disease, claudication, carotid obstruction§,** Glucose intolerance* Hyperuricemia* Essential hypertension Obesity Palmar-planar xanthomas*,‡ Tuberous xanthomas*,‡ Tendinous xanthomas†,‡	Recessive; 1/1000 (?)
Type IV Hyperlipoproteinemia	High TG, VLDL TG, and TC	TC 150-350 TG 300-800 HDL-C ≤ 40	Premature atherosclerosis MI, stroke§,** Glucose intolerance Hyperuricemia Obesity Essential hypertension Periorbital xanthelasma*	Dominant; 1/200
Type V Hyperlipoproteinemia	High TG, VLDL TG, and chylomicron TG	TC 200-800 TG 800–10,000 HDL-C ≤ 35	Premature atherosclerosis MI, stroke§,** Abdominal pain Pancreatitis Glucose intolerance Hyperuricemia Essential hypertension Obesity Eruptive xanthomas* Hepatosplenomegaly Peripheral sensory neuropathy	Dominant; 1/1000 (?)

(continued)

TABLE 81–1. LIPOPROTEIN DISORDERS *(Continued)*

Disorder	*Lipoprotein Abnormality*	*Typical Lipoprotein Levels (mg/dL)*	*History and Clinical Findings*	*Primary Mode of Inheritance; Estimated Prevalence*
Hypoalphalipoproteinemia	Low HDL-C with normal TC and TG	HDL-C ≤ 35 TG < 250 TC < 250	Severe premature atherosclerosis MI, stroke§,** Hyperuricemia Glucose intolerance Essential hypertension Obesity	Dominant; 1/200
High Lp(a) levels	High Lp(a)	Lp(a) 20–30 borderline high > 30 high	Severe premature atherosclerosis, stroke, peripheral vascular disease	
Hyperalphalipoproteinemia	High HDL-C	HDL-C ≥ 75 TG < 250 TC < 250		
Hypobetalipoproteinemia	Low LDL-C	LDL-C ≤ 100 TG < 250		

TG = triglycerides; TC = total cholesterol; LDL-C = low-density lipoprotein cholesterol; IDL = intermediate-density lipoproteins; VLDL = very low-density lipoproteins; HDL-C = high-density lipoprotein cholesterol; MI = myocardial infarction.

Findings are common unless otherwise noted.

* Occasional

† When present, these physical findings are almost always diagnostic of familial hyperlipidemia

‡ Rare

§ Often in patient *and* common in first-degree relatives

** Premature cardiovascular disease in patient and, commonly, in first-degree relatives

The three dominantly transmitted, familial lipoprotein disorders—types II, IV, and V hyperlipoproteinemia—are common. Each type is estimated to affect about 1 per 200 to 1 per 500 persons. Type II hyperlipoproteinemia and hypoalphalipoproteinemia may not be as prevalent in the elderly as in the general population. They are associated with higher mortality rates than other lipoprotein disorders, so persons with these disorders are less likely to survive to old age.

Most physicians never see a patient with type I familial hyperlipoproteinemia (chylomicronemia). However, type V hyperlipoproteinemia (chylomicronemia with increased VLDL triglyceride levels) is more common, though not nearly as common as type II hyperlipoproteinemia and hypertriglyceridemia.

The genes for type III hyperlipoproteinemia appear to be relatively common, but clinical cases occur in only an estimated 1% of those with the genes. In type III familial hyperlipoproteinemia, the basic metabolic defect involves an abnormality in apolipoprotein E, which causes reduced clearance of the E-rich intermediate-density lipoproteins in the liver. The apolipoprotein E defect, while apparently *necessary* for the expression of the type III phenotype, is not *sufficient* by itself. However, the additional necessary factors are as yet poorly understood.

Secondary causes of hyperlipoproteinemia are shown in TABLE 81–2.

DIAGNOSIS

In 1993, the National Cholesterol Education Program **(NCEP)** updated its guidelines for identifying elevated TC and LDL-C levels; it also identified HDL-C levels < 35 mg/dL with significantly increased CAD risk and ≥ 60 mg/dL with significantly decreased risk (see TABLE 81–3). The new NCEP guidelines are useful in screening young and elderly patients.

Hypercholesterolemia Screening

No single cholesterol value should be used to classify a patient clinically. Values may vary significantly from day to day; persons having a high initial value often have a considerably lower value on the second measurement, a phenomenon known as *regression toward the mean*. If a lipoprotein cholesterol abnormality is found on the first screening test, preferably at least two subsequent evaluations should be performed (see FIGS. 81–1, 81–2, and 81–3).

Epidemiologic data indicate that applying NCEP guidelines to the elderly might require subsequent evaluations in up to 70% of patients and therapy in a substantial percentage of them.

In the elderly, a *full lipid profile* should be obtained, not just a plasma TC level. Otherwise, up to 25% of patients may be misclassified and inappropriately advised about their risk of CAD. In many of these patients, the predominant cause of the elevated TC level is an elevated HDL-C level, *not* an elevated LDL-C level; therefore, their risk of CAD

TABLE 81–2. SECONDARY CAUSES OF LIPOPROTEIN DISORDERS

High TC, LDL-C Levels	*High TG, Low HDL-C Levels*
Diseases	
Poorly controlled diabetes	Poorly controlled diabetes
Hypothyroidism	Alcoholic hepatitis, alcoholism
Obstructive liver disease*	Severe metabolic stress (MI, cerebrovascular accident)
Nephrotic syndrome*	Hypothyroidism
Uremia*	Obstructive liver disease, acute hepatitis*
Orthostatic proteinuria	Nephrotic syndrome*
Dysproteinemias (myeloma, Waldenström's macroglobulinemia)†	Uremia (with or without dialysis)
Acute intermittent porphyria†	Dysproteinemias, systemic lupus erythematosus†
Anorexia nervosa†	Glycogen storage disease†
Cushing's syndrome†	Idiopathic hypercalcemia†
	Chlorinated hydrocarbon exposure*
Diet	
Excess dietary saturated fat, cholesterol	Excess alcohol (may elevate both TG and HDL-C)
Drugs	
Corticosteroids	Corticosteroids
Androgenic steroids	Estrogens, oral contraceptives
Progestins	Synthetic vitamin A compounds (for acne)
Thiazide diuretics	β-Blockers
	Androgenic steroids (low HDL-C)
	Nicotine (low HDL-C)
	Zinc (low HDL-C)

TC = total cholesterol; LDL-C = low-density lipoprotein cholesterol; TG = triglycerides; HDL-C = high-density lipoprotein cholesterol; MI = myocardial infarction
* Occasional
† Rare

is decreased, not increased. Moreover, many patients with CAD have normal TC and triglyceride levels but an HDL-C level below the 10th percentile; persons with this lipid profile are at *very high risk* for CAD.

Total cholesterol and, to a lesser degree, HDL-C measurements are not significantly affected by eating, whereas triglyceride levels are sensitive to food and can be accurately measured only after a fast. Screening should include at least TC and HDL-C levels, which can be obtained

TABLE 81–3. RISK STATUS BASED ON PRESENCE OF CAD RISK FACTORS OTHER THAN LDL CHOLESTEROL*

Positive risk factors	Age Men ≥ 45 yr Women ≥ 55 yr or premature menopause without estrogen replacement therapy Family history of premature CAD (definite myocardial infarction or sudden death before age 55 in father or other male first-degree relative or before age 65 in mother or other female first-degree relative) Current cigarette smoker Hypertension (blood pressure ≥ 140/90 mm Hg† or current antihypertensive therapy) Low HDL cholesterol (< 35 mg/dL†) Diabetes mellitus
Negative risk factors‡	High HDL cholesterol (≥ 60 mg/dL)

*High risk, defined as a net of two or more coronary artery disease (CAD) risk factors, leads to more vigorous intervention, shown in FIGS. 81–1 and 81–2. Age is treated as a risk factor because rates of CAD are higher in the elderly than in the young and higher in men than in women of the same age. Obesity is not listed as a risk factor because it operates through other risk factors that are included (hypertension, hyperlipidemia, decreased high-density lipoprotein [HDL] cholesterol, and diabetes mellitus), but it should be considered a target for intervention. Physical inactivity is similarly not listed as a risk factor, but it too should be considered a target for intervention, and physical activity is recommended for everyone. High risk due to coronary or peripheral atherosclerosis is addressed directly in FIG. 81–3.

†Confirmed by measurements on several occasions.

‡If the HDL cholesterol level is ≥ 60 mg/dL, subtract one risk factor (because high HDL cholesterol levels decrease CAD risk).

Modified from Grundy SM, Bilheimer D, Chait A, et al: "Summary of the Second Report of the National Cholesterol Education Program (NCEP) Expert Panel on Detection, Evaluation, and Treatment of High Blood Cholesterol in Adults (Adult Treatment Panel II)." *The Journal of the American Medical Association* 269(23):3015–3023, 1993.

without having the patient fast. A definitive screening test requires a 12-h fast and measures TC, triglyceride, and HDL-C levels; if the triglyceride level is < 400 mg/dL, LDL-C levels can be calculated.

Physicians should determine whether the laboratories they use follow a national standardization program because those that do not follow it tend to report higher cholesterol levels and are less accurate in measuring TC and HDL-C levels. An actual difference of 5
HDL-C level significantly affects a patient's risk of CAD.

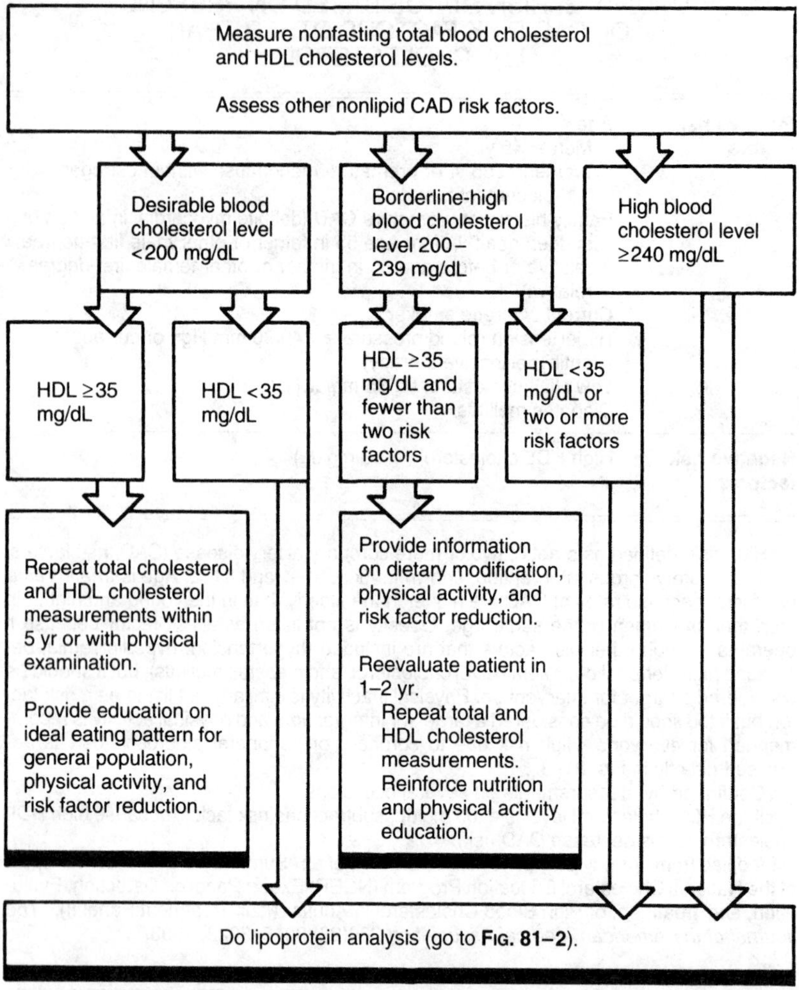

FIG. 81–1. Primary prevention in adults without evidence of coronary artery disease (CAD); initial classification is based on total cholesterol and high-density lipoprotein (HDL) cholesterol levels. (From Grundy SM, Bilheimer D, Chait A, et al: "Summary of the Second Report of the National Cholesterol Education Program (NCEP) Expert Panel on Detection, Evaluation, and Treatment of High Blood Cholesterol in Adults (Adult Treatment Panel II)." *The Journal of the American Medical Association* 269(23):3015–3023, 1993.)

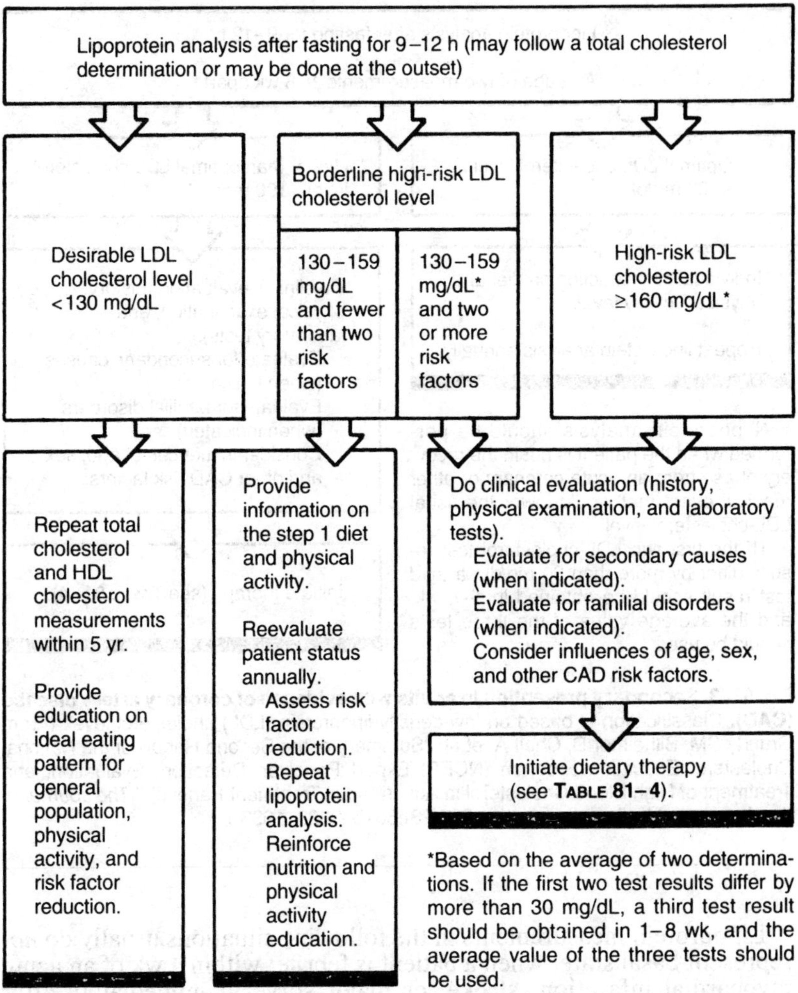

FIG. 81–2. Primary prevention in adults without evidence of coronary artery disease (CAD); subsequent classification is based on low-density lipoprotein (LDL) cholesterol level. (From Grundy SM, Bilheimer D, Chait A, et al: "Summary of the Second Report of the National Cholesterol Education Program (NCEP) Expert Panel on Detection, Evaluation, and Treatment of High Blood Cholesterol in Adults (Adult Treatment Panel II)." *The Journal of the American Medical Association* 269(23):3015–3023, 1993.)

Lipoprotein analysis after fasting for 9–12 h*

Average of two measurements 1–8 wk apart†

↓

Optimal LDL cholesterol level ≤100 mg/dL	Higher than optimal LDL cholesterol level >100 mg/dL
↓	↓
Individualize instruction on diet and physical activity level. Repeat lipoprotein analysis annually.	Do clinical evaluation (history, physical examination, and laboratory tests). Evaluate for secondary causes (when indicated). Evaluate for familial disorders (when indicated). Consider influences of age, sex, and other CAD risk factors.
	↓
	Initiate therapy (see **Table 81–4**).

*Lipoprotein analysis should be performed when the patient is not in the recovery phase from an acute coronary or other medical event that would lower the usual LDL-cholesterol level.

†If the first two LDL-cholesterol test results differ by more than 30 mg/dL, a third test result should be obtained in 1–8 wk, and the average value of the three tests should be used.

Fig. 81–3. Secondary prevention in adults with evidence of coronary artery disease (CAD). Classification is based on low-density lipoprotein (LDL) cholesterol level. (From Grundy SM, Bilheimer D, Chait A, et al: "Summary of the Second Report of the National Cholesterol Education Program (NCEP) Expert Panel on Detection, Evaluation, and Treatment of High Blood Cholesterol in Adults (Adult Treatment Panel II)." *The Journal of the American Medical Association* 269(23):3015–3023, 1993.)

Lipoprotein measurements in the following situations usually do *not* represent basal state: when a patient is febrile; within 4 wk of an acute myocardial infarction, stroke, or major surgery; immediately after acute excessive alcohol intake; during any major infection; when diabetes mellitus is severely out of control (fasting blood glucose level > 250 mg/dL, glycosylated hemoglobin > 9%); or during deliberate rapid weight loss.

After finding an abnormal lipoprotein cholesterol level and confirming it with two subsequent evaluations, the physician should distinguish between primary or familial lipoprotein disorders and secondary lipoprotein disorders.

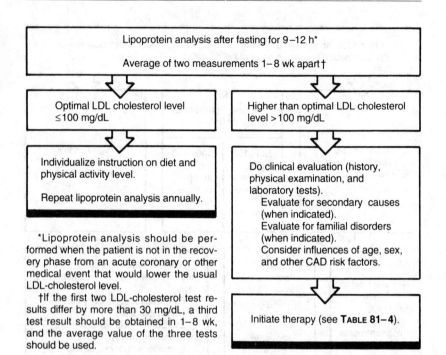

Primary and Familial Lipoprotein Disorders

Any geriatric patient who sustained a myocardial infarction or stroke before age 60 should be assessed for primary and familial lipoprotein disorders. (Primary and familial lipoprotein disorders are not synonymous, but they are usually congruent.) If secondary causes can be ruled out, the disorder is usually one of the common familial hyperlipoproteinemias. The physician should identify other first-degree family members with lipoprotein disorders.

The most common familial hyperlipoproteinemias are transmitted as autosomal dominant traits; thus, on average half of the offspring (themselves adults) are similarly affected, and all offspring should be screened.

Certain characteristic findings—such as tendinous, tuberous, and palmar-planar xanthomas and arcus juvenilis corneae—are diagnostically useful. Obesity (with or without concurrent essential hypertension), glucose intolerance, and hyperuricemia should alert the physician to the likelihood of a concurrent primary hypertriglyceridemia or hypoalphalipoproteinemia.

Secondary Lipoprotein Disorders

Even in patients with well-defined familial lipoprotein disorders, secondary disorders are common and may exacerbate the expression of the primary disorder, particularly in severe hypertriglyceridemia (see TABLE 81–2). Thus all newly diagnosed patients should undergo a thorough physical examination and a drug, occupational, family, dietary, and alcohol-intake history. The following laboratory tests also should be performed: T_4, TSH, BUN or creatinine, and fasting blood glucose measurements; urinalysis; and liver function tests. Covert hypothyroidism (with normal T_4 and elevated TSH levels) is a relatively common cause of elevated TC and LDL-C levels and is associated with an increased risk for premature myocardial infarction.

The most common cause of secondary hypercholesterolemia is probably a diet high in saturated fat or cholesterol, whether or not a polygenic tendency for hypercholesterolemia exists.

In older persons, the most common causes of secondary hypertriglyceridemia are excessive alcohol intake, exogenous estrogen supplementation, poorly controlled diabetes, uremia, corticosteroid use, and β-blocker use. Isolated low HDL-C levels with normal plasma triglyceride levels may result from smoking, androgenic steroid use, severe restriction of physical activity, or morbid obesity.

TREATMENT

The NCEP guidelines recommend that persons in the top quintile for plasma TC levels and those with LDL-C levels ≥ 160 mg/dL (> 100 mg/dL if they have evidence of CAD or other atheromatous disease) should be treated.

TABLE 81–4. TREATMENT DECISIONS BASED ON LDL CHOLESTEROL LEVEL

Patient Category	*Initiation Level*	*Goal*
Dietary treatment		
Without CAD and with fewer than two risk factors	≥ 160 mg/dL	< 160 mg/dL
Without CAD and with two or more risk factors	≥ 130 mg/dL	< 130 mg/dL
With CAD	> 100 mg/dL	≤ 100 mg/dL
Drug treatment		
Without CAD and with fewer than two risk factors	≥ 190 mg/dL	< 160 mg/dL
Without CAD and with two or more risk factors	≥ 160 mg/dL	< 130 mg/dL
With CAD	≥ 130 mg/dL	≤ 100 mg/dL

LDL = low-density lipoprotein; CAD = coronary artery disease

From Grundy SM, Bilheimer D, Chait A, et al: "Summary of the Second Report of the National Cholesterol Education Program (NCEP) Expert Panel on Detection, Evaluation, and Treatment of High Blood Cholesterol in Adults (Adult Treatment Panel II)." *The Journal of the American Medical Association* 269(23):3015–3023, 1993.

Treatment should always begin with dietary changes. The LDL-C levels at which treatment with diet and drugs should begin are shown in TABLE 81–4.

Additional clinical guidelines are as follows:

1. Decisions should not be based primarily on the patient's age. Many elderly patients are physiologically and mentally much younger than their chronologic age.

2. Consideration should be given to the presence of other life-limiting conditions. In patients with other diseases that limit life expectancy to ≤ 1 yr, aggressive lipid-lowering therapies probably should not be initiated.

3. Long-term negative effects of lipid-lowering therapy need not be a source of undue concern because the duration of therapy is shorter in the elderly than in the young. Moreover, some short-term benefits may be realized almost immediately: Major LDL-C lowering can lead to increased endothelial cell production of nitrous oxide (a potent vasodilator) and can reduce platelet aggregation, and major triglyceride lowering sharply decreases plasminogen activator inhibitor and increases fibrinolysis. Often, within 1 to 2 yr of therapy, atherosclerotic lesion

progression and regression can be affected. Also, elderly patients appear to tolerate lipid-lowering agents as well as younger patients do, and efficacy and side effects are comparable.

4. Asymptomatic patients who are at risk should be treated. Patients who have clinical, electrocardiographic, or radiographic evidence of coronary, femoral, or carotid atherosclerosis should be aggressively treated.

The targets for dietary treatment of hypercholesterolemia should be to reduce TC and LDL-C levels to those recommended in NCEP guidelines and to reduce triglycerides to < 500 mg/dL (to avoid pancreatitis). Because a high triglyceride level is a potent independent risk factor in postmenopausal women, lowering the level to < 250 mg/dL is probably valuable in these patients. Levels of HDL-C should be elevated to > 35 mg/dL and preferably to 40 mg/dL. Diets and most drugs that lower LDL-C levels do not substantially alter Lp(a) lipoprotein levels.

Dietary Treatment

High LDL-C levels: The American Heart Association's three-phase diet has been simplified to a two-step diet by the NCEP (see TABLE 81–5). The NCEP recommends the step 1 diet for high-risk persons. If a person with clinical evidence of atherosclerosis already follows the equivalent of a step 1 diet (as many Americans do), the person should begin the step 2 diet. Achieving adequate calorie and protein intake can be difficult in the elderly, so the diet must be modified cautiously. However, the step 1 dietary guidelines and the practical approach shown in TABLE 81–6 should be safe for older adults, including diabetic patients.

The full effects of dietary therapy at any step may not be achieved for 8 to 12 wk; the patient should not advance to the next step unless the therapeutic goal has not been reached in this time. Weight loss helps reduce TC, triglyceride, and LDL-C levels but is at least as difficult in older people as in younger ones.

Hypertriglyceridemia: For patients with hypertriglyceridemia, low HDL-C levels, and an increased risk of CAD, dietary interventions are important. The major objective of dietary treatment is to raise HDL-C levels, though treatment that lowers the triglyceride level alone may be valuable in women > 50 yr. When the triglyceride level is > 1000 mg/dL, a sharp reduction in total fat intake (to < 30 gm/day) helps prevent triglyceride-induced pancreatitis. Goals of dietary interventions are as follows:

Lose weight using a low-fat diet. In most overweight patients, including those with primary and familial hypertriglyceridemia, triglyceride levels drop sharply with only modest weight loss. A patient usually does not need to reach ideal body weight or even to lose more than 5 to 10 kg to bring triglycerides within normal range.

Reduce alcohol intake to three or fewer drinks per week. If triglyceride levels are ≥ 500 mg/dL, alcohol consumption should be discontinued.

TABLE 81–5. STEPWISE APPROACHES TO DIETARY TREATMENT OF HYPERCHOLESTEROLEMIA

American Heart Association Diet				*National Cholesterol Education Program Diet*		
Nutrient	*Phase I*	*Phase II*	*Phase III*	*Nutrient*	*Step 1*	*Step 2*
Total fat (% of total calories)	30%	25%	20%	**Total fat** (% of total calories)	< 30%	< 30%
Saturated (% of total calories)	10%	8%	7%	Saturated fatty acids (% of total calories)	< 10%	< 7%
Polyunsaturated (% of total calories)	10%	8%	7%	Polyunsaturated fatty acids (% of total calories)	Up to 10%	Up to 10%
Monounsaturated (% of total calories)	10%	8%	7%	Monounsaturated fatty acids (% of total calories)	10–15%	10–15%
Carbohydrate (% of total calories)	55%	60%	65%	**Carbohydrates** (% of total calories)	50–60%	50–60%
Protein (% of total calories)	15%	15%	15%	**Protein** (% of total calories)	10–20%	10–20%
Cholesterol (mg/day)	< 300	200–250	100–150	**Cholesterol** (mg/day)	< 300	< 200
				Total calories	To achieve and maintain desirable weight	To achieve and maintain desirable weight

TABLE 81–6. PRACTICAL APPROACH TO A LOW–CHOLESTEROL, LOW–SATURATED FAT DIET

Reduce Intake of:	*Choose:*	*Use Substitutes:*
Meats and meat products Fatty cuts of beef, lamb, pork, spareribs, organ meats, regular cold cuts, sausage, hot dogs	Fish, chicken and turkey (without the skin), lean cuts of beef, lamb, pork, veal	Cold cuts prepared from processed turkey, except those containing organ meats
Dairy products Whole milk (4% fat), evaporated or condensed whole milk, cream, half-and-half, most nondairy creamers, whipped toppings	Skim or 1% fat milk Buttermilk	Polyunsaturated based cream substitutes
Whole milk yogurt, whole milk cottage cheese (4% fat), all natural cheeses (blue, Roquefort, Camembert, cheddar, Swiss), cream cheese, sour cream, ice cream	Nonfat (0% fat) or low-fat yogurt; low-fat cottage cheese (1%, 2%); low-fat cheeses (should be labeled no more than 2-6 gm fat/oz)	Sherbet, sorbet, frozen low-fat yogurt made from skim milk and no eggs
Butter Eggs (< 3/wk)	Margarines made from liquid vegetable oils and packaged in tub or squeeze bottle	Egg substitutes; egg whites (2 whole egg whites = 1 egg in recipes); cholesterol-free egg substitutes
Commercial baked goods Pies, cakes, doughnuts, croissants, pastries, muffins, biscuits, high-fat crackers, high-fat cookies, egg noodles, breads in which eggs are a major ingredient	Homemade bread goods using unsaturated oils, angel food cake, low-fat cookies, crackers, pretzels Rice, pasta Whole-grain breads and cereals (oatmeal, bran, rye, multigrain)*	Pastries made with polyunsaturated or monounsaturated oils, egg substitutes, or egg whites
Saturated fats and oils, dressings Chocolate, butter, coconut oil, palm oil, kernel oil, lard, bacon	Unsaturated vegetable oils: corn, olive, rapeseed, safflower, sesame, soybean, sunflower	Cocoa powder, carob

(continued)

TABLE 81–6. PRACTICAL APPROACH TO A LOW–CHOLESTEROL, LOW–SATURATED FAT DIET *(Continued)*

Reduce Intake of:	*Choose:*	*Use Substitutes:*
Saturated fats and oils, dressings *(continued)*		
Butter, butter-margarine mixture	Margarine made from liquid vegetable oils and packaged in tub or squeeze bottle	Diet margarine made from liquid oils
Dressing made with egg yolk	Mayonnaise, salad dressings made with liquid oils, as above	Low-fat diet dressings made with liquid oils
Coconut	Seeds and nuts*	
Vegetables prepared in butter, saturated fats, cream, or sauces with saturated fat	Fresh, frozen, canned, dried fruits or vegetables*	

* Fruits, vegetables, grains, seeds, and nuts contain no cholesterol, and most contain no saturated fat.

Reduce the intake of total fat, saturated fat, and cholesterol, using step 2 of the NCEP diet or phase III of the American Heart Association diet. In persons who have triglyceride levels ≥ 1000 mg/dL with mixed elevations of chylomicron and VLDL triglyceride or the much rarer primary hyperchylomicronemia, total fat intake should be restricted to 10% to 20% of total calories. This rigid low-fat diet is instituted primarily to prevent triglyceride-induced pancreatitis. Also, the sharp decrease in VLDL-C levels and the increase in HDL-C levels may help protect persons who have chylomicronemia and increased VLDL triglyceride levels from severe premature CAD. Weight loss is crucial in obese persons. In patients with severe hypertriglyceridemia, estrogen use is contraindicated.

Type III hyperlipoproteinemia: For persons with type III hyperlipidemia who are overweight, the *single* most important strategy is weight reduction. Patients should reduce intake not only of total fat, saturated fat, and cholesterol but also of dietary sucrose.

Hypoalphalipoproteinemia: The only consistently effective dietary intervention is weight loss, which may raise HDL-C levels. Other methods of raising HDL-C levels include supplementation with omega-3–rich fish oils (4 to 12 gm/day), smoking reduction, and supervised aerobic physical activity (up to five 30-min periods per week). At least initially, exercise should be supervised by a physician (see also Ch. 31).

Drug Therapy

Drug therapy should be used for patients who have persistent primary or familial hyperlipoproteinemias when diet therapy is insufficient (see TABLE 81–7).

TABLE 81–7. DRUG THERAPY FOR HYPERLIPIDEMIA

Agent	*Indications*	*Usual Dosage*	*Adverse Effects*
Cholestyramine†‡	High LDL-C Type II hyperlipoproteinemia Do not use as a single agent if TG is ≥ 300 mg/dL after diet therapy	8–24 gm resin (2–4 packets or scoops) daily in 3 or 4 divided doses; many patients respond to 8 gm/day*	Constipation (common) and other GI symptoms; increased VLDL (and TG); binds other drugs; may augment or reduce warfarin's effect; rarely (reversibly) elevates liver enzymes
Colestipol (in conjunction with nicotinic acid)‡	High LDL-C Type II hyperlipoproteinemia	10–30 gm resin (2–6 packets or scoops) daily in 3 or 4 divided doses; many patients respond to 10 gm/day*	Same as above
Nicotinic acid† (in conjunction with colestipol).‡ Use fast-acting only, not slow-release versions	High LDL-C with high TG High TG type II hyperlipoproteinemia, especially IIB (used with resins because of synergistic action) Isolated low HDL-C	2–6 gm daily in 3 or 4 divided doses; take with meals to minimize flushing§	Cutaneous flushing and pruritus; GI symptoms, ulcer, gastritis; frequent liver function abnormality; impaired glucose tolerance; hyperuricemia. Adverse effects are common.

(continued)

TABLE 81–7. DRUG THERAPY FOR HYPERLIPIDEMIA *(Continued)*

Agent	*Indications*	*Usual Dosage*	*Adverse Effects*
Nicotinic acid† (in conjunction with colestipol).‡ Use fast-acting only, not slow-release versions *(continued)*	Type III hyperlipoproteinemia (if other therapies fail) Type IV hyperlipoproteinemia (if other therapies fail) Type V hyperlipoproteinemia (if other therapies fail)		Because of increased risk of myositis and hepatotoxicity, do not use concurrently with lovastatin, pravastatin, simvastatin, or fluvastatin, if possible
Probucol††	High LDL-C Type II hyperlipoproteinemia (use with resin to further reduce LDL-C)	500 mg bid	Minor GI symptoms; HDL-C lowered as much as or more than LDL-C; rarely, foul-smelling sweat; prolonged QT interval
Gemfibrozil†	High TG Low HDL-C High LDL-C with high TG Type IV hyperlipoproteinemia Type III hyperlipoproteinemia Type V hyperlipoproteinemia	600 mg bid; maximum dose 1.5 gm/day**	Minor GI symptoms; rash, eosinophilia, anemia; increased gallstones; rarely, muscle cramps, aches (myositis); myositis more common if patient has uremia or is receiving lovastatin, pravastatin, simvastatin, fluvastatin, or cyclosporine. Adverse effects are rare overall.
Omega-3 fatty acids††	High TG that does not respond optimally to gemfibrozil or nicotinic acid	4–15 gm/day	Fishy taste after belching; diarrhea. Adverse effects are rare overall.

(continued)

TABLE 81–7. DRUG THERAPY FOR HYPERLIPIDEMIA *(Continued)*

Agent	*Indications*	*Usual Dosage*	*Adverse Effects*
Lovastatin†‡ (alone and in conjunction with bile acid-binding resins)	High LDL-C Type IIB hyperlipoproteinemia	20–80 mg/day. At 20–40 mg dose, give in evening; at 60–80 mg, give in divided doses (AM and PM)	Liver function test abnormalities; myalgia (myositis). Adverse effects are rare overall.
Pravastatin†	High LDL-C Type IIB hyperlipo-proteinemia	10–40 mg/day; give at bedtime	Liver function test abnormalities; myalgia (myositis); headache. Adverse effects are rare overall.
Simvastatin†	High LDL-C Type IIB hyperlipo-proteinemia	5–40 mg/day; give at bedtime	Liver function test abnormalities; myalgia (myositis). Adverse effects are rare overall.
Fluvastatin††	High LDL-C Type IIB hyperlipo-proteinemia	20–40 mg/day; give at bedtime	Liver function test abnormalities, dyspepsia, myalgia (myositis). Adverse effects are rare overall.
Cholestyramine and nicotinic acid	LDL-C higher than target using single-drug therapy	8–24 gm resin and 2–6 gm nicotinic acid	Same as individual drugs
Colestipol and nicotinic acid	LDL-C higher than target using single-drug therapy	10–30 gm resin and 2–6 gm nicotinic acid	Same as individual drugs
Cholestyramine and lovastatin or **pravastatin** or **simvastatin** or **fluvastatin**	LDL-C higher than target using single-drug therapy	8–24 gm resin and 20–80 mg lovastatin or 10–40 mg pravastatin or 10–40 mg simvastatin or 20–40 mg fluvastatin	Same as individual drugs

(continued)

TABLE 81–7. DRUG THERAPY FOR HYPERLIPIDEMIA *(Continued)*

Agent	*Indications*	*Usual Dosage*	*Adverse Effects*
Colestipol and lovastatin or **pravastatin** or **simvastatin** or **fluvastatin**	LDL-C higher than target using single-drug therapy	10–30 gm resin and 20–80 mg lovastatin or 10–40 mg pravastatin or 10–40 mg simvastatin or 20–40 mg fluvastatin	Same as individual drugs
Probucol and cholestyramine or **colestipol**	LDL-C higher than target and HDL-C lower than target using single-drug therapy	1 gm probucol and 8–30 gm resin	Less constipation than with resin alone; less diarrhea than with probucol alone; HDL-C higher than with probucol alone
Gemfibrozil and cholestyramine or **colestipol**	LDL-C at target, TG higher than 250 mg/dL, and HDL-C lower than 35 mg/dL or TG and HDL-C at target *and* LDL-C higher than target after gemfibrozil therapy	1200 mg gemfibrozil and 8–30 gm resin	Same as individual drugs
Lovastatin and gemfibrozil	LDL-C at target, TG higher than 250 mg/dL, and HDL-C lower than 35 mg/dL or TG and HDL-C at target *and* LDL-C higher than target after gemfibrozil therapy	20–80 mg lovastatin and 1200 mg gemfibrozil	Myositis or increased CK is much more common than with either drug alone. Do not use combination therapy if creatinine is > 2 mg/dL or if patient is taking cyclosporine.

(continued)

TABLE 81–7. DRUG THERAPY FOR HYPERLIPIDEMIA *(Continued)*

Agent	*Indications*	*Usual Dosage*	*Adverse Effects*
Pravastatin and gemfibrozil	LDL-C at target, TG higher than 250 mg/dL, and HDL-C lower than 35 mg/dL or TG and HDL-C at target *and* LDL-C higher than target after gemfibrozil therapy	10–40 mg pravastatin and 1200 mg gemfibrozil	Myositis or increased CK is much more common than with either drug alone. Do not use combination therapy if creatinine is > 2 mg/dL or if patient is taking cyclosporine.

LDL-C = low-density lipoprotein cholesterol, TG = triglycerides, HDL-C = high-density lipoprotein cholesterol, CAD = coronary artery disease, VLDL = very low-density lipoproteins, CK = creatine kinase

* Always start with small doses (2 packs or 2 scoops per day); gradually increase dose prn.

† CAD event rate reduction proved by controlled clinical trials.

‡ Cessation of progression of coronary artery atherosclerosis and/or regression of lesions proved by controlled clinical trials.

§ Always start with small dose (500 mg/day); gradually increase dose by 500-mg increments.

** Reduce dose if uremia is present.

†† CAD event rate reduction not yet proved.

Bile acid–binding resins: Drug therapy to lower LDL-C levels can begin with nonabsorbable bile acid–binding resins, such as **cholestyramine** and **colestipol,** which interrupt the normal enterohepatic circulation of bile acids and indirectly increase the liver's catabolism of LDL-C through increased LDL-receptor synthesis by hepatocytes. A small dose (8 to 10 gm/day) should be used initially, particularly in the elderly, and the dose should be adjusted based on the effect on LDL-C levels. The most common side effect is constipation, which can usually be avoided by eating dried fruit (eg, prunes, raisins, apricots) or using stool softeners. Because resins are not systemically absorbed, they have essentially no systemic side effects (aside from rare, mild, reversible changes in liver enzymes) and have been shown to be safe and effective in reducing CAD morbidity and mortality.

Bile acid–binding resins can augment warfarin's effects; if the two drugs are taken within a short time, the resins can also bind warfarin. Thus, resins should be used cautiously, if at all, with warfarin-like anticoagulants. The resins should *not* be given concurrently with exogenous thyroid hormones, sex steroids, prednisone, or digoxin, all of which may be bound in the intestine by resins. These drugs should be given at least 2 h before the first resin dose of the day.

In persons whose primary defect is high LDL-C levels and whose triglyceride levels are < 250 mg/dL, the bile acid–binding resins are effective and safe. However, such therapy may raise triglyceride levels. Either nicotinic acid or gemfibrozil (1200 mg/day) and a bile acid–binding resin should be considered, particularly in patients with elevated LDL-C and triglyceride levels whose triglyceride level rises to > 300 mg/dL during resin therapy. Alternatively, an HMG-CoA reductase inhibitor can be used.

The bile acid–binding resins are probably contraindicated as single drug therapy in patients with high LDL-C levels and marked hypertriglyceridemia (triglycerides > 300 mg/dL) and in those with severe hemorrhoids or a history of bowel resection or severe constipation. In such patients, pravastatin or simvastatin may be the drug of choice. If the triglyceride level remains > 300 mg/dL and the patient is either at high risk or has had an atherosclerotic event, gemfibrozil may be added.

Nicotinic acid: Although nicotinic acid can be used as a first-line drug, it is usually given with the resins when they fail to reduce LDL-C levels sufficiently. Nicotinic acid inhibits secretion of VLDL from the liver, reducing VLDL-C and LDL-C levels. It reduces the incidence of recurrent myocardial infarction and mortality from all causes.

The initial dose is 250 mg bid. The frequency of administration and the total daily dose should be increased slowly at about weekly intervals, as necessary. Generally, an initial dosage of 1.5 to 2 gm/day is required. Every 6 to 8 wk, liver function tests; blood glucose, uric acid, and LDL-C measurements; and stool tests for occult blood should be performed.

Nicotinic acid's side effects are frequent, bothersome, and often severe, although flushing and tachycardia may be reduced by taking aspirin 150 to 300 mg simultaneously. Besides the side effects listed in TABLE 81–7, nicotinic acid very rarely produces toxic amblyopia. Hepatotoxicity appears to be more frequent and more severe when the slow-release forms of nicotinic acid are used; thus, the fast-release forms are preferable.

HMG-CoA reductase inhibitors: The HMG-CoA reductase inhibitors (lovastatin, pravastatin, simvastatin, and fluvastatin) block intracellular cholesterol biosynthesis, forcing the cell to synthesize more LDL receptors, which increases the catabolism of LDL-C.

In clinical trials, side effects of these drugs have been relatively rare and are usually transient; they include myalgia, dyspepsia, skin rashes, headaches, fatigue, and constipation. Despite an initial concern that these drugs might increase the risk of cataract formation, subsequent studies have not borne this out. Also relatively rare, the major biochemical changes include **increases in liver enzymes** (particularly transaminases) and in creatine kinase levels with myositis. Thus, liver function tests and creatine kinase measurements should be performed before treatment, every 6 wk for the first 3 mo, every 8 wk for the rest of the first year, and at 3- to 6-mo intervals thereafter. The current convention is *not* to discontinue the HMG-CoA reductase inhibitor unless the liver enzyme elevations exceed three times the upper limit of normal.

Erythromycin and its derivatives should never be given concurrently with an HMG-CoA reductase inhibitor because of the increased risk of hepatotoxicity. Myositis is particularly common in persons receiving an HMG-CoA reductase inhibitor and cyclosporine. Reportedly, the concurrent use of these drugs also produces **rhabdomyolysis** and **myoglobinuria.** Thus, the concurrent use of these drugs should be restricted to special situations in which other cholesterol-lowering regimens are ineffective, and patients taking this drug combination should be closely monitored. HMG-CoA reductase inhibitors can be effectively combined with resins, but they probably should *not be used concurrently with niacin because of increased risk of myositis and hepatotoxicity.*

If the long-term safety of the HMG-CoA reductase inhibitors can be established, they will probably become the cholesterol-lowering drugs of choice because they are easy to administer and effective in reducing LDL-C levels.

Lovastatin generally should be started at 20 mg/day and taken with the evening meal. The dose can be increased to 40 mg/day, then to 60 mg/day taken as a single evening dose. When the dose reaches 80 mg/day, the drug can be taken twice a day. Lovastatin alone usually reduces LDL-C levels 25% to 40%, may reduce the triglyceride level 5% to 20%, and increases HDL-C levels 5% to 10%.

Pravastatin 10 to 40 mg/day usually reduces LDL-C levels 22% to 34%, reduces triglyceride levels 15% to 24%, and increases HDL-C levels 6% to 12%. The initial dose is 10 mg at bedtime; this is increased as necessary. Occasionally, in patients whose predominant disorder is hypertriglyceridemia and who do not tolerate or do not respond to gemfibrozil, nicotinic acid, or omega-3 fatty acids, pravastatin 40 mg may be effective, although it is not primarily a triglyceride-lowering drug.

Simvastatin 5 to 40 mg/day usually reduces LDL-C levels 22% to 40%, reduces triglyceride levels 6% to 20%, and increases HDL-C levels 8% to 13%. The initial dose is usually 5 mg at bedtime; the dose is increased as necessary. Simvastatin does not undergo significant renal excretion; therefore, renal disease is not usually a reason to modify the dosage. However, for those with severe renal impairment, therapy should begin with the lowest possible dose and be closely monitored.

Fluvastatin 20 to 40 mg/day usually lowers LDL-C levels 20% to 25% and produces small but statistically significant increases in HDL-C levels and correspondingly small decreases in triglyceride levels. The increases in HDL-C levels and the decreases in LDL-C levels are larger in women.

Gemfibrozil: This is the drug of choice for treating hypertriglyceridemia and hypoalphalipoproteinemia in the elderly. A fibric acid derivative, gemfibrozil increases the hydrolysis of VLDL triglycerides and the syntheses of HDL-C and apolipoprotein A-I. It decreases LDL-C and triglyceride levels and has been shown to reduce CAD morbidity and mortality in appropriate patients. Gemfibrozil therapy should be considered in patients with elevated triglyceride levels (> 300 mg/dL), low HDL-C levels (< 35 mg/dL), and moderately high LDL-C levels (< 190 mg/dL). Well tolerated by most patients, gemfibrozil rarely causes gastrointestinal upset or myositis, although the latter is more common when the drug is given to those with poor renal function. Such patients, especially if they are also receiving cyclosporine, should be given a reduced dose.

Combined gemfibrozil–HMG-CoA reductase inhibitor therapy: When patients do not respond adequately to a single drug, two drugs are often required to lower LDL-C, raise HDL-C, and lower triglycerides to optimal target levels (< 130 mg/dL, > 35 mg/dL, and < 200 mg/dL, respectively). Patients at highest risk for CAD often have combined hyperlipidemia, usually with high TC, high triglyceride, and low HDL-C levels, which are often maintained even after major dietary, weight, and exercise modification. When patients with combined hyperlipidemia are treated with gemfibrozil alone, triglyceride levels usually can be normalized and HDL-C levels often (but not always) can be elevated > 35 mg/dL, but TC and LDL-C levels may not be adequately lowered and often increase. On the other hand, when the same patients are treated with lovastatin, pravastatin, or simvastatin alone, LDL-C levels can usually be normalized, but triglyceride levels often remain high, and HDL-C levels often remain low (< 35 mg/dL). *Therefore, those at highest risk, particularly if they have had a CAD event, may require two-drug therapy,* eg, gemfibrozil and lovastatin or gemfibrozil and pravastatin.

Because myopathy, rhabdomyolysis, myoglobinuria, and renal injury have been reported in patients taking gemfibrozil and lovastatin, the following guidelines are strongly recommended:

1. Two-drug therapy should be used primarily in secondary prevention. It may also be used in primary prevention for very high-risk patients who have other major CAD risk factors and who do not respond optimally to one-drug therapy.
2. It should not be used in patients with substantially reduced creatinine clearance rates because of the increased risk of myopathy.
3. It should not be used concurrently with cyclosporine or nicotinic acid because of the increased risk of myopathy.

4. It should be used in *reliable* patients who are well informed about the possibility of myositis and are prepared to discontinue therapy at the onset of myositic symptoms. Patients must have a phone number they can call 24 hours a day to report any muscle pain, tenderness, or weakness.

5. Patients should have baseline and follow-up creatine kinase and liver function tests every 6 to 8 wk.

6. Patients should take gemfibrozil 1.2 gm/day and initially lovastatin 20 mg/day or pravastatin 10 mg/day. The dose of the HMG-CoA reductase inhibitor should be adjusted to the smallest amount that will reduce LDL-C levels to the target range.

7. Ideally, follow-up should be conducted by physicians at a lipid therapy center who are experienced in using each drug.

There is little experience using simvastatin or fluvastatin, but the starting dose for simvastatin is 10 mg, and the starting dose for fluvastatin is 20 mg. The other guidelines should be followed.

Probucol: Another cholesterol-lowering drug, probucol is considered a second-choice agent by the NCEP guidelines. Probucol therapy usually reduces LDL-C levels about 8% to 15%, but it also reduces HDL-C levels by as much as 25%. Probucol appears to increase the rate of LDL-C catabolism, probably through nonreceptor-mediated pathways. A recent hypothesis is that the antioxidant effect of probucol might reduce atherosclerosis by reducing the atherogenic effect of oxidized LDL-C. No extensive, placebo-controlled, double-blind, long-term clinical studies assessing the effect of probucol on the risk of CAD are yet available. Currently, the role of probucol in treating patients with high LDL-C levels is uncertain because the drug reduces HDL-C levels; yet xanthoma regression has been reported as HDL-C levels decrease.

Generally, probucol is well tolerated; diarrhea is the most common side effect. The drug prolongs the QT interval and is probably *contraindicated* in patients with ventricular irritability and an initially prolonged QT interval and in those taking other drugs that prolong the QT interval. The combination of probucol and resins is effective, with less reduction in the HDL-C level than with probucol alone and much less constipation than with resins alone.

Omega-3 fatty acids: Recently, these fish oils have been used to lower triglyceride levels, usually in dosages < 15 gm/day. These agents are not useful as cholesterol-lowering drugs; in patients with hypertriglyceridemia, omega-3 fatty acids may elevate HDL-C levels 10% to 15%. Available over the counter, the fish oils may increase the hydrolysis of VLDL triglyceride. At much higher dosages (usually > 50 gm/day), they may be associated with thrombocytopenia and increased bleeding time; such dosages are almost never used clinically. In those rare cases when doses > 20 gm/day are used, platelet counts and bleeding time should be monitored. At such doses, fish oils may also interfere with glucose control in diabetics. Very few controlled, long-term clinical studies exist showing the lipid-lowering effectiveness or side effects of these agents; however, in short-term trials, doses of ≤ 15 gm/day appear to be safe.

Therapy for isolated low HDL-C levels: Treating an elderly patient who has isolated low HDL-C levels (usually well below 35 mg/dL) with a TC level < 200 mg/dL, and a triglyceride level < 250 mg/dL provides a particularly difficult therapeutic challenge. If lifestyle changes (weight loss, increased aerobic exercise, cessation of cigarette smoking) do not increase HDL-C levels, and particularly if the patient has already sustained an atherosclerotic event or is at high risk because of primary hypoalphalipoproteinemia and other associated risk factors, drug intervention is warranted. However, no clinical trial data exist on the best mode of therapeutic intervention. Particularly if the Lp(a) lipoprotein level is also high, nicotinic acid 1.5 to 6.0 gm/day or gemfibrozil 1.2 to 1.5 gm/day may be effective. If nicotinic acid and gemfibrozil are ineffective or cannot be tolerated, lovastatin, pravastatin, simvastatin, or fluvastatin may be given with a goal of lowering the TC level to < 160 mg/dL or the LDL-C level to < 100 mg/dL. Although the HDL-C level is usually not changed, the ratio of TC:HDL-C is usually very substantially decreased.

82. DISORDERS OF MINERAL METABOLISM

Increasingly, disorders of mineral metabolism are occurring among the elderly. Disorders of calcium metabolism include bone diseases, eg, osteoporosis, osteomalacia, and Paget's disease (see Ch. 73), and disorders of calcium regulation resulting in hypocalcemia or hypercalcemia. Other disorders of mineral metabolism include hypophosphatemia, hyperphosphatemia, hypomagnesemia, and hypermagnesemia.

DISORDERS OF CALCIUM METABOLISM

The normal serum calcium level ranges between 8.8 and 10.4 mg/dL. About 45% of total blood calcium is bound to serum proteins; 5% is complexed with anions, such as phosphate, bicarbonate, and citrate; and only 50% is ionized. The ionized fraction affects cellular function and is normally maintained between 4.8 and 5.2 mg/dL. The proportion of ionized calcium to total calcium is affected not only by the amount of protein (particularly albumin) and anion bound to ionized calcium but also by the blood pH. Acidosis decreases protein binding; alkalosis increases it. Moreover, the interaction between ionized calcium and the cell membrane is affected by the pH. Thus, at the same level of ionized calcium, alkalosis can precipitate tetany, and acidosis can prevent it. Changes in potassium and magnesium levels can also alter the response to calcium.

Although most hospital laboratories still routinely measure only total serum calcium, measurement of ionized calcium is increasingly available. An ionized calcium measurement is more precise and appropriate because the value is unaffected by changes in bound calcium. Many elderly patients may have a normal total serum calcium level yet have an abnormally high ionized calcium level because the albumin level is low. Therefore, if the ionized calcium level cannot be measured, a total calcium measurement and an albumin determination should be obtained simultaneously, and the total calcium value should be corrected to compensate for any albumin deficit. This can be done by adding 0.8 mg/dL to the total calcium value for each 1 gm/dL decrease in albumin below normal (4 gm/dL). Thus, a patient with a total calcium measurement of 10.4 mg/dL and a serum albumin measurement of 2.5 gm/dL would have a deficit of about 1.2 mg/dL of protein-bound calcium (0.8 mg/dL × 1.5 gm/dL albumin deficit) and a corrected total serum calcium of 11.6 mg/dL, which is clearly abnormal. Often, a low total serum calcium value is simply the result of a decreased serum albumin level. Because hypoalbuminemia is common in the elderly, particularly in chronically ill and malnourished patients, this correction is particularly important.

In interpreting any abnormality of serum calcium concentration, the physician should also assess acid-base balance and potassium and magnesium levels. Measuring the serum phosphate level is important not only for the diagnosis but also because changes in phosphate can alter serum calcium, as discussed below.

Calcium Regulation

The serum ionized calcium concentration is maintained at a constancy, with variations in an individual usually $< 5\%$ at different times of day and under different dietary conditions. This constancy results from a complex interaction among three major calcium-regulating hormones: parathyroid hormone, 1,25-dihydroxycholecalciferol (calcitriol), and calcitonin. Other systemic growth regulators, such as glucocorticoids and thyroid hormones, can also affect calcium regulation. Moreover, important local factors—such as prostaglandins, interleukins, and growth-stimulating factors—act on bone. The physiologic roles of these factors are unknown, but they have been implicated as the cause of hypercalcemia in malignancy.

Parathyroid hormone (PTH): The most important regulator of serum calcium, PTH is an 84–amino acid, single-chain polypeptide secreted by the parathyroid glands. Although the biologically active portion of the PTH molecule is in the first 30 or so amino acids at the N-terminal, the active circulating form is probably the intact 1-84 molecule. This molecule is cleaved in the liver and kidneys and has a short half-life.

Some of the N-terminal fragments may circulate and may be biologically active, but the number appears to be small. The C-terminal fragments are biologically inactive but have a longer half-life.

An increasing serum calcium concentration produces a rapid decrease in PTH secretion **(proportional control).** Prolonged hypercalcemia can result in atrophy of the parathyroid glands. More important, prolonged hypocalcemia can result in massive hyperplasia **(integral control).** These integral responses are slow; when the hypocalcemic stimulus is removed, hyperplasia persists and may produce rebound hypercalcemia. This phenomenon is termed **tertiary hyperparathyroidism,** and some authorities suggest that the glands become autonomous. However, in most situations, they are simply slow to involute.

The PTH increases serum calcium concentration by at least four actions: increased resorption from bone; increased distal renal tubular reabsorption of calcium; stimulation of 1,25-dihydroxycholecalciferol production in the kidney, which increases intestinal absorption of calcium; and decreased renal tubular reabsorption of phosphate. The reduction in the serum phosphate concentration may enhance the bone-resorptive response to PTH and prevent redeposition of the calcium mobilized from bone.

The effects of PTH on **bone formation** are complex. The hormone can inhibit collagen synthesis by osteoblasts, but when given intermittently in low doses, it produces an anabolic effect that has been used to treat osteoporosis. In patients who have a vitamin D or magnesium deficiency, the bone-resorptive effect of PTH is blunted. In those with a vitamin D deficiency, this blunted effect may result from decreased mineralized bone surfaces, according to some studies. Osteoclasts, which resorb bone and release calcium into the extracellular fluid under PTH stimulation, cannot act on unmineralized bone surfaces.

The effects of PTH on the **kidney** appear to be mediated at least partially by the stimulation of adenylate cyclase and an increased cyclic adenosine monophosphate **(cAMP)** concentration. Although PTH also increases cAMP in bone, the role of this mediator in bone resorption is not clear. The increase in cAMP occurs in osteoblasts, which may be the major target cells for PTH, with bone resorption produced indirectly by the release of a mediator from osteoblasts. Although osteoclastic bone resorption usually increases only when the size and number of osteoclasts increase, rapid changes in their activity have been observed after PTH administration. These changes include an expansion of the ruffled border, the bone-resorbing apparatus that secretes hydrogen ions and lysosomal enzymes onto the bone surface, removing both mineral and matrix from bone.

The level of PTH needed to maintain a normal serum calcium level seems to increase with age, presumably because of a relative calcium deficiency in the elderly. With aging, the intrinsic capacity of the intestine to absorb calcium decreases, and the response to 1,25-dihydroxycholecalciferol is blunted. Moreover, PTH-mediated renal synthesis of 1,25-dihydroxycholecalciferol may be impaired because renal mass is reduced. No evidence indicates that the increased tubular reabsorption of calcium, the decreased tubular reabsorption of phosphate, or the stimulation of bone resorption by PTH is impaired in the elderly. In fact, the catabolic effects of PTH on bone may be enhanced.

In the parathyroid glands of the elderly, the proportion of mitochondria-rich oxyphil cells increases, while the capacity to secrete PTH is sustained. The increase in serum immunoreactive PTH concentration with age may be relatively greater for assays that measure the C-terminal inactive metabolite of PTH, which is normally excreted by the kidneys and thus retained as renal function decreases. However, increased PTH with age is also seen with immunoassays that measure the whole molecule and with bioassays.

1,25-Dihydroxycholecalciferol (calcitriol): The synthesis and activation of the second important calcium regulator, 1,25-dihydroxycholecalciferol, is complex. First, 7-dehydrocholesterol is converted to vitamin D_3 in the skin under the influence of ultraviolet radiation. Vitamin D is then hydroxylated in the liver to a circulating form, 25-hydroxycholecalciferol, which is tightly bound to a vitamin D–binding protein. Finally, it is converted to the active hormone, 1,25-dihydroxycholecalciferol, in the kidneys.

The production of 1,25-dihydroxycholecalciferol is stimulated by low blood calcium or phosphate levels and inhibited by high blood calcium or phosphate levels. The effect of low calcium levels is mediated mainly through PTH. The concentration of 1,25-dihydroxycholecalciferol in the blood is 16 to 40 pg/mL, and 99% is bound to vitamin D–binding protein. The concentration of 25-hydroxycholecalciferol is much higher, 8 to 40 ng/mL, and it is even more tightly bound to vitamin D–binding protein. The serum also contains another renal oxidation product, 24,25-dihydroxycholecalciferol, the precise function of which is not known, although it may simply be an inactivation product.

The major effect of physiologic concentrations of 1,25-dihydroxycholecalciferol is to enhance the intestinal absorption of calcium. These concentrations may also promote the synthesis of calcium-binding and transport proteins in many cells since vitamin D–dependent proteins and receptors for this hormone are found in most tissues. High concentrations of 1,25-dihydroxycholecalciferol have a catabolic effect on bone, stimulating bone resorption and inhibiting formation. These effects are probably important only when a marked deficiency in calcium or phosphate intake occurs. In these circumstances, 1,25-dihydroxycholecalciferol levels increase, making more calcium and phosphate available for the needs of soft tissues and for vital bone remodeling (eg, fracture repair). Through an additional loop in calcium regulation, 1,25-dihydroxycholecalciferol directly inhibits PTH synthesis and secretion. The absence of this feedback may be important in the increased PTH levels seen with aging and renal failure.

Although 1,25-dihydroxycholecalciferol synthesis and response to either PTH or low serum calcium are impaired in older persons, serum levels are usually within normal limits, except in those with severe renal disease or vitamin D deficiency. Serum 25-hydroxycholecalciferol levels tend to decrease with age, probably mainly because of decreased intake or decreased sun exposure. Levels are normal in older persons who take vitamin D supplements.

Calcitonin: The least important of the calcium-regulating hormones in man, calcitonin is a 32–amino acid peptide secreted in response to hypercalcemia. It reduces serum calcium by decreasing bone resorption. Calcitonin acts directly on osteoclasts, stimulating cAMP production and causing cell contraction, loss of ruffled borders, and decreased resorptive activity. It is secreted by parafollicular (or C) cells, which have migrated to the thyroid gland from the ultimobranchial body.

After thyroid ablation, patients may have low calcitonin levels but maintain a normal serum calcium level. Similarly, patients with medullary carcinoma of the thyroid, who produce excessive calcitonin, can still maintain normal serum calcium concentration and bone remodeling.

HYPOCALCEMIA

A corrected serum calcium level < 8.8 mg/dL or an ionized calcium level < 4.8 mg/dL.

Etiology and Pathogenesis

A decreased serum calcium level is common among chronically ill, elderly patients. However, most of these patients have a normal corrected calcium level or a normal ionized calcium level with a low serum albumin level. **Vitamin D and calcium deficiencies** are common causes of hypocalcemia in the elderly. Other causes are shown in TABLE 82–1. In many cases, hypocalcemia results from several abnormalities.

Primary hypoparathyroidism: In the elderly, primary hypoparathyroidism (hypoparathyroidism caused by loss of parathyroid tissue or secretion) occurs most often from **surgical damage** to the parathyroid glands. Common after thyroid and parathyroid surgery, transient hypoparathyroidism presumably results from damage to the parathyroid glands or to their blood supply, prior suppression of normal parathyroid tissue in both hyperparathyroidism and hyperthyroidism, and the hungry-bone syndrome, in which increased bone formation and mineralization result in the rapid removal of calcium from the circulation. Permanent hypoparathyroidism is most common after a complete thyroidectomy for cancer; however, this complication occurs infrequently when experienced head and neck surgeons perform the operation.

TABLE 82–1. CAUSES OF HYPOCALCEMIA

Primary hypoparathyroidism	Surgical (transient or permanent) Idiopathic (autoimmune) Severe hypomagnesemia Infiltrative (hemochromatosis or malignancy)
Relative hypoparathyroidism	Inhibition of bone resorption (calcitonin, plicamycin, bisphosphonates) Hyperphosphatemia Pancreatitis Osteoblastic metastases
PTH resistance	Pseudohypoparathyroidism
Osteomalacia and rickets	Vitamin D deficiency Vitamin D resistance
False hypocalcemia	Decreased serum albumin

Idiopathic hypoparathyroidism can be isolated or familial and may be associated with autoimmune failure of multiple endocrine glands. Metabolic or infiltrative damage to the parathyroid glands can occur in hemochromatosis and malignancy. Antiparathyroid antibodies that inhibit glandular function have been detected in some patients, particularly those with multiple endocrine failure.

Severe hypomagnesemia is associated with hypocalcemia and impaired PTH secretion. The synthesis of PTH is not impaired. After an infusion of magnesium, hormone synthesis improves, and PTH is rapidly released. However, the serum calcium level responds more slowly; this slower response has been attributed to end-organ resistance, particularly of bone. **Hypermagnesemia** may also inhibit PTH secretion, but it is not a clinically important cause of hypocalcemia (see also DISORDERS OF MAGNESIUM METABOLISM, below).

Relative hypoparathyroidism: This abnormality occurs when calcium's entry into the extracellular fluid is so diminished or its exit so accelerated that an increase in PTH secretion cannot compensate. **Inhibitors of bone resorption,** particularly plicamycin and other cytotoxic agents, can produce hypocalcemia. These drugs may also impair parathyroid gland function. Calcitonin can produce transient hypocalcemia in patients with high bone turnover (eg, those with Paget's disease).

Phosphate excess can develop from a variety of causes. Rapid cell breakdown in rhabdomyolysis or during chemotherapy for leukemia or lymphoma, phosphate retention in acute renal failure and shock, and excessive administration of phosphate either IV or by enema can cause a marked reduction in serum calcium and accompanying tetany. *Phos-*

phate excess is particularly dangerous because it not only reduces the serum calcium level but also results in the deposition of calcium and phosphate in soft tissue, damaging the kidneys, blood vessels, and lungs.

In **acute pancreatitis,** hypocalcemia has been attributed to a sequestration of calcium by fatty acid salts in the retroperitoneal space and occasionally by chylous ascites in the peritoneal cavity. Most patients with a low total serum calcium concentration and pancreatitis have a normal ionized calcium concentration and a low serum albumin concentration.

True hypocalcemia is rare in patients with **osteoblastic metastases** and presumably is related to rapid mineralization, which exceeds calcium entry from intestinal absorption or bone resorption. Most patients with a low total serum calcium concentration and osteoblastic metastases have a normal ionized calcium concentration and a low serum albumin concentration.

PTH resistance: Hormonal resistance has been clearly delineated in several syndromes of **pseudohypoparathyroidism.** In pseudohypoparathyroidism type 1A, a defect in PTH response results from a reduction in the amount of the guanine nucleotide regulatory protein, which links the PTH receptor with adenylate cyclase. This defect is usually associated with other abnormalities, such as short metacarpals, short stature, and mental retardation, in **Albright's hereditary osteodystrophy.** Patients with this condition do not respond to a PTH injection with the expected increase in renal cAMP excretion and phosphate clearance. Other patients with pseudohypoparathyroidism do not show a deficiency in the guanine nucleotide regulatory protein and may have postreceptor abnormalities or a circulating inhibitor of PTH.

Symptoms and Signs

Mild hypocalcemia may be asymptomatic or may be accompanied by nonspecific CNS symptoms. Chronic hypocalcemia is associated with an increased incidence of cataracts and calcification of the basal ganglia. Associated endocrine syndromes and chronic candidiasis occur in some patients with multiple endocrine failure. A patient with chronic hypocalcemia may also present with mild diffuse brain disease mimicking depression, dementia, or psychosis.

When hypocalcemia is severe or when an associated alkalosis increases neuromuscular irritability, **tetany** develops. Tetany is characterized by paresthesias, particularly around the mouth, and muscle spasms, particularly of the hands, feet, and face. Without concurrent alkalosis, tetany usually does not occur until the serum calcium level is < 7 mg/dL or the ionized calcium level is < 3 mg/dL. Patients who do not have tetany may still have latent neuromuscular irritability, which can be demonstrated by provocative tests for Chvostek's sign and Trousseau's sign. **Chvostek's sign** is a *contraction of the facial muscles elicited by tapping the facial nerve*. (It can occur in normal patients.) **Trousseau's sign** is *carpopedal spasm caused by a reduction of the* *blood supply to the hand* when a tourniquet applied to the arm for 3 to 5 min exerts pressure that is higher than systolic blood pressure. The **ECG** can also help diagnostically because it shows a prolonged QT interval in hypocalcemia.

Laboratory Findings and Diagnosis

A low corrected total calcium or ionized calcium level cannot be assessed adequately without concomitant measurements of phosphate, magnesium, potassium, and bicarbonate levels as well as renal function tests. When the serum calcium level is low, the serum phosphate level is usually high. This inversion occurs even in severe vitamin D deficiency, when phosphate reserves are low, possibly because of a physicochemical effect on exchangeable calcium and phosphate in the skeleton. However, mild hypocalcemia can occur with hypophosphatemia, not only in patients with vitamin D deficiency but also in those who have both magnesium and phosphate depletion.

The differential diagnosis is usually easy when hypocalcemia is caused by vitamin D deficiency, pancreatic disease, or renal failure. The distinction between primary hypoparathyroidism and pseudohypoparathyroidism can be made by measuring immunoreactive PTH concentration; PTH is high only in pseudohypoparathyroidism. The response to PTH administration is also helpful. Human synthetic amino N-terminal 1-34 PTH (teriparatide acetate) has been used investigationally for this purpose and is available for diagnostic use.

Treatment

Immediate treatment of **tetany** consists of an IV infusion of calcium. This treatment is effective even when the major precipitating cause is alkalosis or a magnesium or potassium abnormality; however, with hypomagnesemic hypocalcemia the response is short-lived, and magnesium must also be administered. Usually, 10% calcium gluconate is given IV over a few minutes; subsequently, more calcium gluconate may be added to a continuous IV drip. A large amount may be needed if there is a substantial sink in the skeleton (a large amount of unmineralized osteoid), as occurs especially in some postoperative patients with primary or secondary hyperparathyroidism. A 10-mL calcium gluconate ampule contains only 90 mg calcium, and the skeleton contains 600 to 1000 gm. If a large amount of unmineralized osteoid exists, several grams of calcium may be needed during repletion. The dose is determined by closely monitoring serum calcium concentration.

The treatment of **hypocalcemia lasting more than 1 day** has been considerably altered by the availability of 1,25-dihydroxycholecalciferol as **calcitriol.** Calcitriol 0.5 to 2.0 μg/day orally is usually given in divided doses at 12-h intervals because of its relatively short half-life. Calcitriol together with oral calcium supplements (1 to 2 gm/day of elemental calcium) can rapidly increase the serum calcium level in most patients. Thus, if after thyroid or parathyroid surgery, the serum calcium level remains low despite calcium administration, symptomatic hypocalcemia can usually be avoided by administering calcitriol.

Although calcitriol is expensive, it has several advantages over other agents. It is rapidly absorbed, does not require further metabolism to become active, and is rapidly cleared. One serious problem with vitamin D therapy is toxicity, ie, severe symptomatic hypercalcemia. A dose of calcitriol only slightly greater than the physiologic replacement dose can cause hypercalcemia and hypercalciuria; however, these effects are transient, disappearing rapidly when the drug is discontinued. Still, the serum calcium level should be monitored in patients receiving calcitriol. With **vitamin D** itself or with **25-hydroxycholecalciferol,** the margin of safety is greater, but these agents require further metabolism to become active, and toxicity is prolonged, particularly when long-term therapy with large amounts of vitamin D produces accumulations in liver and adipose tissue.

In the past, **dihydrotachysterol,** a pseudo 1-hydroxylated analog of vitamin D, was used in renal failure and vitamin D–resistant syndromes, but calcitriol appears to be more effective and reliable. Calcitriol is also effective for **chronic hypocalcemia in primary hypoparathyroidism and pseudohypoparathyroidism;** it can be combined with a calcium supplement (1 to 2 gm/day of elemental calcium). When hypomagnesemia occurs with calcium, potassium, and phosphate deficiencies, correcting the hypomagnesemia makes treating the other deficiencies easier.

A **thiazide diuretic** or **chlorthalidone** has been used in some patients to increase phosphate excretion and decrease calcium excretion. **Hypocalcemia from phosphate excess** can be avoided by decreasing phosphate intake or by using aluminum hydroxide gel or large doses of calcium carbonate, which bind phosphate in the intestine and reduce its absorption.

HYPERCALCEMIA

A corrected serum calcium level > 10.4 mg/dL or an ionized calcium level > 5.2 mg/dL.

Etiology and Pathogenesis

In most cases, excessive bone resorption is the primary pathogenetic factor, but often increased intestinal absorption or renal tubular reabsorption of calcium also contributes to hypercalcemia. Compared with a low total serum calcium concentration from hypoalbuminemia, a high serum calcium concentration from increased protein-bound calcium (with a normal ionized calcium value) is less common and usually drug related. **False hypercalcemia** can occur when hemoconcentration results from diuretic therapy or prolonged hemostasis or when a rare case of myeloma occurs in which the immunoglobulin is atypical and strongly binds calcium. Hypercalcemia from **increased protein binding** can occur early in diuretic therapy, particularly with thiazides and amiloride, which not only causes hemoconcentration but also de-

TABLE 82–2. CAUSES OF HYPERCALCEMIA

Increased bone resorption	Primary hyperparathyroidism Persistent secondary (or tertiary) hyperparathyroidism Metastatic malignancy Hematologic malignancy Humoral hypercalcemia of malignancy Immobilization Hyperthyroidism
Increased intestinal absorption	Vitamin D toxicity Milk-alkali syndrome Sarcoidosis and other granulomas
Miscellaneous	Familial benign hypocalciuric hypercalcemia Addison's disease Acute renal failure (recovery phase)
False hypercalcemia	Hemoconcentration Increased calcium-binding proteins or anions

creases urinary calcium excretion. Compensation usually occurs; sustained hypercalcemia during diuretic therapy usually results from primary hyperparathyroidism (see TABLE 82–2).

Dividing hypercalcemia into mild and severe forms is clinically useful. A prolonged, mild elevation in serum calcium almost always results from primary hyperparathyroidism, though it may also result from hyperthyroidism, sarcoidosis, or familial benign hypocalciuric hypercalcemia. Acute, severe symptomatic hypercalcemia most often results from malignancy, although it may also result from any of the other causes, particularly with a vicious circle of dehydration, producing increasing serum calcium with further fluid loss and decreased capacity for renal calcium excretion.

Increased bone resorption: Common among the elderly, **primary hyperparathyroidism** has an increased incidence among postmenopausal women, perhaps because of the loss of an opposing effect of estrogen on PTH-stimulated bone resorption. At least 80% of patients with primary hyperparathyroidism have a single parathyroid adenoma. The others have multiple adenomas or pluriglandular hyperplasia. Primary hyperplasia often occurs in association with other endocrine neoplasms in two multiple endocrine neoplasia syndromes. In type 1, pancreatic, parathyroid, and pituitary tumors occur. In type 2, hyperparathyroidism is associated with medullary carcinoma of the thyroid and pheochromocytoma.

Generally, **secondary hyperparathyroidism** results when parathyroid hyperplasia develops from prolonged calcium deficiency, so it is ordinarily associated with low or normal serum calcium levels. However, patients with marked secondary hyperplasia can develop hypercalcemia under certain circumstances, eg, when chronic renal failure is associated with phosphate depletion or aluminum intoxication or after renal transplantation **(tertiary hyperparathyroidism).** Hypercalcemia can also occur after recovery from acute renal failure associated with rhabdomyolysis, probably due to the release of calcium previously deposited with phosphate in soft tissues.

Several different pathogenetic mechanisms can produce hypercalcemia of malignancy. **Metastatic bone involvement** with a local increase in resorption is the most common. This condition probably does not result from direct osteolysis by the tumor but from the local release of resorbing factors either from the tumor cells themselves or from adjacent hematopoietic or bone cells stimulated by the tumor. This syndrome often occurs in breast cancer.

Hematologic malignancies frequently cause hypercalcemia. In multiple myeloma, an osteoclast activating factor released by the myeloma cells has been implicated. This osteoclast activating factor represents several different bone-resorbing cytokines, including interleukin-1 and tumor necrosis factors α and β. Interleukin-6, which is not as potent a stimulator of bone resorption, probably enhances the effects of interleukin-1 and tumor necrosis factors. Myeloma cells and other lymphomas produce these factors. Some hematologic malignancies can also produce parathyroid hormone–related protein (PTHrP). This factor is so named because it has some homology to PTH, although it is chemically distinct, and because it acts on the PTH receptor. Parathyroid hormone–related protein is produced by many tumors, particularly squamous cell tumors, and is a normal product of keratinocytes. Its physiologic role is not known. Some lymphomas produce hypercalcemia by excessive conversion of 25-hydroxycholecalciferol to 1,25-dihydroxycholecalciferol, which also occurs in sarcoidosis and other granulomas.

In **humoral hypercalcemia of malignancy,** a circulating substance produced by a tumor acts on bone and probably on the kidneys to increase the serum calcium concentration. Humoral hypercalcemia of malignancy is most commonly seen with squamous cell tumors, renal tumors, and hepatomas. Rarely, the factor is prostaglandin E_2; more often, it is parathyroid hormone–related protein. Evidence also indicates that a transforming growth factor of either the α or β type can be produced by tumors and stimulate bone resorption.

Immobilization can produce hypercalcemia in persons with rapid bone turnover. In the elderly, rapid remodeling is rare except in Paget's disease. **Hyperthyroidism** directly increases bone resorption but usually causes only a modest increase in the serum calcium concentration.

Increased intestinal absorption: Vitamin D intoxication, milk-alkali syndrome, and sarcoidosis are major causes of hypercalcemia in which intestinal absorption plays an important role. **Massive doses of vitamin D** can produce prolonged hypercalcemia; the metabolites 25-hydroxycholecalciferol and 1,25-dihydroxycholecalciferol have a more transient hypercalcemic effect. **Milk-alkali syndrome** is probably the combined result of a defective barrier to intestinal calcium absorption and decreased renal function associated with nephrocalcinosis. **Sarcoidosis** and other granulomatous diseases (tuberculosis, histoplasmosis, and foreign-body granulomas) produce hypercalcemia by excessive, unregulated synthesis of 1,25-dihydroxycholecalciferol by activated macrophages.

Other causes of hypercalcemia: **Familial benign hypocalciuric hypercalcemia** is important because it may be mistaken for primary hyperparathyroidism, resulting in inappropriate parathyroid surgery. The PTH values may be only modestly elevated in familial benign hypocalciuric hypercalcemia, and the hallmark of the syndrome, low urinary calcium excretion, can also occur in elderly patients with primary hyperparathyroidism. Serum calcium measurements in other family members may be needed to confirm the diagnosis.

Hypercalcemia can also occur in **Addison's disease,** probably due to a combination of increased bone resorption and hemoconcentration.

Symptoms and Signs

Most patients with hyperparathyroidism do not have characteristic symptoms, and usually the disorder is detected by routine measurement of serum calcium. However, elderly patients with primary hyperthyroidism may have many symptoms and signs, including hypertension, muscular weakness, irritability, mild GI disturbances, renal colic, bone cysts, and decreased bone mass. Surgical extirpation can reverse some of these symptoms and signs; however, hypertension and CNS symptoms commonly persist after surgery.

Hypercalciuria and nephrolithiasis can be asymptomatic. After hypercalciuria and hypercalcemia are reversed, moderate or severe renal impairment may progress. The development of nephrocalcinosis produces irreversible damage. Although symptomatic cystic bone lesions are rare, mild degrees of osteitis fibrosa cystica with subperiosteal bone resorption in the hands and a salt-and-pepper–like appearance of the skull can be observed radiologically. Patients with primary hyperparathyroidism usually lose cortical bone mass in the appendicular skeleton, although trabecular bone mass in the spine may be relatively well preserved. With hyperparathyroidism, the risk of fracture (especially in the extremities) is probably increased, but data are limited.

Severe hypercalcemia from any cause is associated with progressive dehydration due to direct inhibition of renal tubular reabsorption of sodium and water and decreased fluid intake due to anorexia, nausea, and vomiting. Occasionally, patients with mild primary hyperparathyroidism develop severe hypercalcemia because of an intercurrent illness that causes dehydration. When the serum calcium concentration exceeds 12 mg/dL, mental confusion can occur. As the patient becomes increasingly dehydrated, the calcium concentration may increase, resulting in coma and death. *Calcium concentrations > 16 mg/dL are life-threatening and constitute a medical emergency.*

Laboratory Findings and Diagnosis

In primary hyperparathyroidism, the serum calcium concentration is elevated, and the phosphate concentration is low. Tubular reabsorption of calcium is increased, and tubular reabsorption of phosphate is decreased. Because the filtered load of calcium is also increased, calcium excretion is usually high, although it rarely exceeds 500 mg/24 h. Some elderly patients with mild chronic primary hyperparathyroidism and minimal serum calcium elevation have a low rate of urinary calcium excretion. Urine and serum calcium and phosphate levels may be the same in primary hyperparathyroidism and hypercalcemia of malignancy; thus these measurements are not useful in differential diagnosis.

Sustained mild hypercalcemia over several years strongly indicates primary hyperparathyroidism, although occasionally such hypercalcemia can occur in sarcoidosis. On the other hand, a rapid onset of hypercalcemia, especially with anemia, weight loss, and hypoalbuminemia, suggests malignancy. Serum protein electrophoresis, thyroid function tests, and a chest x-ray should be obtained in all cases. Additional tests for specific malignant disorders should be performed when appropriate. Because mild hyperchloremic acidosis can occur in hyperparathyroidism, the chloride:phosphate ratio may be used as a diagnostic indicator. Hyperchloremia is useful diagnostically because it is less likely to occur in other forms of hypercalcemia.

In vitamin D toxicity, milk-alkali syndrome, and thyrotoxicosis, the serum phosphate level is usually normal or elevated. Vitamin D toxicity can be detected by measuring the serum 25-hydroxycholecalciferol concentration. Measuring 1,25-dihydroxycholecalciferol, which is elevated in primary hyperparathyroidism, sarcoidosis, and occasionally in hematopoietic malignancies, is not generally useful.

Measuring circulating immunoreactive PTH has become increasingly useful in the differential diagnosis of hypercalcemia. Currently available assays show that most patients with primary hyperparathyroidism have elevated PTH values, and most patients with malignancy have low PTH values, although occasionally overlap occurs. Patients with vitamin D intoxication, milk-alkali syndrome, and sarcoidosis also have low PTH values.

In the elderly, interpretation of PTH assays is complicated because levels normally increase slightly with age. Moreover, older patients often have impaired renal function and therefore accumulate the C-terminal fragments of PTH, which are measured in most immunoassays. Thus, an immunoradiometric assay, which detects only intact PTH, is a better discriminator.

Coexisting hyperparathyroidism and malignancy are not rare in elderly patients. Thus, such signs of malignancy as hypoalbuminemia, anemia, and weight loss may be present.

Nephrogenous cAMP has been used as a biologic marker of PTH action. However, it is not helpful in differentiating hyperparathyroidism from humoral hypercalcemia of malignancy, which is also associated with increased cAMP excretion.

Localization of a parathyroid adenoma, although not strictly diagnostic, may help to avoid prolonged surgical exploration and permit the use of local anesthesia. The thallium-technetium digital subtraction scan is the most useful test for this purpose. However, false-positive results often occur with a multinodular goiter, which is common in older patients. Therefore, localization studies are usually not recommended preoperatively except in high-risk patients. However, neck exploration should always be undertaken by an experienced surgeon knowledgeable in parathyroid anatomy.

Treatment

Treatment depends on the serum calcium level, the onset of hypercalcemia, the severity of associated symptoms, and the underlying cause. In patients with serum calcium levels > 12 mg/dL, especially if the onset is recent, immediate efforts should be made to reduce levels while diagnostic studies are undertaken.

Because dehydration and impaired renal function often contribute to hypercalcemia, the first step is rehydration. Extracellular fluid volume should be expanded with IV 0.9% sodium chloride solution. Because elderly patients may have difficulty handling large fluid loads, furosemide may also be needed. This diuretic increases urinary calcium and sodium excretion but should be given only if necessary to prevent or treat fluid overload. Effective reduction of serum calcium with furosemide requires large doses (80 to 100 mg IV q 2 h), which can produce recurrent dehydration or hypotension in the elderly. Rarely, hemodialysis is used to treat severe hypercalcemia that does not respond to other therapy.

Hypercalcemia can produce potassium loss, which may be aggravated by saline loading. Therefore, serum potassium levels should be monitored, and potassium should be replaced as necessary. Hypophosphatemia is usually not a problem, but when the serum inorganic phosphate concentration is < 1 mg/dL, IV phosphate replacement may be appropriate. *Except under these circumstances, IV phosphate therapy should be avoided, particularly in the presence of hypercalcemia.* Intravenous phosphate therapy should be closely monitored, and it should be stopped when serum phosphate levels reach the normal range or when any decrease in renal function occurs. Intravenous phosphate can cause irreversible damage because calcium phosphate salts may be deposited in the tissues of the kidneys, blood vessels, and lungs. Hypophosphatemia is discussed below.

Calcitonin rapidly lowers serum calcium, although usually not to normal levels. The main disadvantage is that its effects are short-lived. Despite continued administration of calcitonin, escape from its effects occurs in 48 to 72 h in most patients. This escape may represent down-regulation of calcitonin receptors or postreceptor desensitization. **Prednisone** 20 to 40 mg/day reduces hypercalcemia in patients with vitamin D intoxication and sarcoidosis and in some patients with hypercalcemia of malignancy. Using calcitonin and prednisone together may produce a greater, more prolonged effect than using either one alone. Rarely, patients with prostaglandin-dependent hypercalcemia respond to nonsteroidal anti-inflammatory drugs (eg, indomethacin). However, because these drugs can further impair renal function, particularly in patients who are dehydrated or have renal damage, they should probably be avoided.

Patients with **hypercalcemia of metastatic malignancy, humoral hypercalcemia of malignancy,** or **any type of hypercalcemia in which the serum calcium level remains markedly elevated after hydration** require additional therapy. Usually, the best way to reduce the serum calcium level is to inhibit bone resorption. Until recently, the most widely used drug for this purpose was plicamycin, but bisphosphonates are now available. These drugs are as effective as plicamycin in inhibiting bone resorption but are less toxic. The most potent bisphosphonate available in the USA is **pamidronate.** When given in a single infusion of 60 mg in 1000 mL of 0.9% sodium chloride over 2 to 4 h, pamidronate can reduce serum calcium levels in most patients in 2 to 3 days; repeated infusions may be required. Often, the reduction in serum calcium is long-lasting. Pamidronate is relatively safe, although transient fever often occurs on the day after the infusion, and large doses may inhibit bone resorption so much that hypocalcemia develops. Also available for IV infusion, **etidronate** must be given in larger doses (7.5 mg/kg in 250 mL of 0.9% sodium chloride solution daily for 3 to 6 days) and is probably somewhat less effective. **Plicamycin** and **gallium nitrate** are effective inhibitors of bone resorption in hypercalcemia of malignancy, but they are more likely to produce toxic side effects than are the bisphosphonates.

The treatment for **primary hyperparathyroidism** is usually surgery, although some patients with mild asymptomatic hypercalcemia may not be candidates and should be treated conservatively. Otherwise, surgical exploration of the neck should be considered as soon as the diagnosis is made. Age alone is not a contraindication to surgery. When performed by a skilled head and neck surgeon, the operation is well tolerated even in patients > 80 yr and often produces a substantial improvement in health. Although elderly patients can tolerate parathyroid surgery, they often develop rebound hypocalcemia after adenoma removal, probably from a combination of suppression of the remaining parathyroid glands and the hungry-bone syndrome. Vigorous treatment with calcitriol as well as IV and oral calcium should be instituted early to avoid tetany.

If surgery is contraindicated, refused, or delayed, the most important treatment goal for mild hypercalcemia is to avoid dehydration. Long-term therapy with oral phosphate has been used, but it often produces diarrhea and may further impair renal function. Small oral doses of elemental phosphate (1 to 1.5 gm/day) should be considered for patients who have low serum phosphate levels.

Postmenopausal women with hyperparathyroidism generally have low bone mass, presumably due to excessive resorption. Treatment with **estrogens** (and progestins to prevent endometrial hyperplasia) decreases serum calcium levels and urinary calcium and hydroxyproline excretion, suggesting that bone resorption has been decreased.

DISORDERS OF PHOSPHATE METABOLISM

Serum phosphate levels vary much more than serum calcium levels. The normal range is 2.5 to 4.5 mg/dL of inorganic phosphate. While 80% of the body's phosphate is stored in bone as hydroxyapatite, the remaining 20% is largely organic. Nucleic acids, nucleotides, phospholipids, and phosphoproteins are vital to energy metabolism, membrane function, and cell regulation.

HYPOPHOSPHATEMIA

A serum concentration of inorganic phosphorus < 2.5 mg/dL.

Etiology

Phosphate depletion can result from poor intake, impaired intestinal absorption, or excessive renal loss. Mild hypophosphatemia is common, probably resulting from both decreased intake and impaired intestinal absorption. The age-related increase in parathyroid function might also lower the renal threshold for tubular reabsorption of phosphate. **Severe hypophosphatemia,** *serum levels < 1.5 mg/dL,* usually results from prolonged, severe decreased dietary intake and impaired absorption. Vomiting, acidosis, and alcoholic ketoacidosis may also contribute to hypophosphatemia. Aluminum hydroxide antacids, renal dialysis, and a rapid recovery of renal function after acute renal failure or transplantation are other important causes of phosphate loss. Serum phosphate concentrations may also be extremely low with relatively mild degrees of intracellular phosphate depletion when extracellular phosphate rapidly shifts into the cells. This shift usually occurs when insulin and glucose are administered together in the treatment of diabetes.

Treatment

Because IV phosphate can cause hypocalcemia and soft tissue calcification and because many elderly patients have impaired renal function and do not handle phosphate loads well, *IV phosphate must be administered cautiously, even when serum concentrations are extremely low*. Patients with severe phosphate depletion often have depleted levels of other ions as well, particularly potassium and magnesium; determining which abnormality is causing the symptoms can be difficult. However, patients with extremely low phosphate levels and evidence of impaired CNS function and muscular weakness should be given IV sodium phosphate; those who also have a potassium depletion should be given potassium phosphate. Serum calcium, inorganic phosphate, potassium, and magnesium levels should be monitored.

Oral phosphate supplements are usually unnecessary in patients whose diet is adequate. However, in hypophosphatemic patients who also have hypercalcemia, these supplements may lower the serum calcium concentration. Elderly patients have difficulty taking more than 1 to 2 gm/day of oral phosphate, even when administered in divided doses, because of diarrhea.

HYPERPHOSPHATEMIA

A serum concentration of inorganic phosphorus > 4.5 mg/dL.

Etiology

Hyperphosphatemia occurs most commonly in chronic renal failure (see also Ch. 63). In rare cases of severe hyperphosphatemia, patients undergo rapid cell lysis with release of phosphate. This condition can occur during chemotherapy in patients with leukemia or other tumors. Excessive intake of phosphate rarely causes hyperphosphatemia, partly because a high phosphate concentration leads to diarrhea and partly because renal excretion is so efficient. Hyperphosphatemia caused by the administration of large volumes of phosphate-containing enemas has been reported. If the serum phosphate concentration is extremely high, deposition of calcium phosphate salts in bone and soft tissue occurs, and the serum calcium concentration may fall to low levels, producing tetany.

Treatment

When renal function is normal and hydration is well maintained, hyperphosphatemia is usually transient. If tetany occurs, IV calcium may need to be given, but *excessive administration in the presence of a high phosphate concentration can cause deposition of calcium phosphate salts and lead to kidney, blood vessel, and lung damage*. In chronic renal failure, hyperphosphatemia can be controlled by a low phosphate intake and calcium or aluminum salts, which bind phosphate.

DISORDERS OF MAGNESIUM METABOLISM

Magnesium, a cation abundant in the body, is distributed almost equally between bone and soft tissue. Unlike serum calcium concentration, serum magnesium concentration is not tightly regulated and can vary considerably with diet and changes in cellular uptake. The normal serum magnesium level is 1.9 to 2.5 mg/dL (1.6 to 2.2 mEq/L). About 20% to 30% of serum magnesium is bound to plasma proteins, and some competition may occur between calcium and magnesium for protein binding.

Evidence of primary regulation of serum magnesium is scant, but high concentrations can inhibit PTH secretion, presumably acting at the same sites as extracellular calcium. Low magnesium concentrations may stimulate PTH secretion transiently; however, when a marked depletion occurs (< 0.9 mg/dL), PTH secretion may be impaired, and hypocalcemia can develop. Magnesium in bone probably exists largely on the surface of hydroxyapatite crystals and can slow crystal growth. Intracellular magnesium is needed for many enzyme activities, particularly those involving nucleotide phosphate metabolism, and it plays a vital role in DNA, RNA, and protein synthesis. Maintaining normal serum magnesium concentration depends mainly on dietary intake, but usually renal and intestinal mechanisms can effectively conserve magnesium. With a magnesium-deficient diet, both renal and fecal magnesium excretion fall rapidly to low levels.

HYPOMAGNESEMIA

Serum magnesium concentration < 1.9 mg/dL (1.6 mEq/L).

Common in elderly patients, mild to moderate hypomagnesemia is probably not an accurate reflection of intracellular or bone stores, which can be maintained for long periods after serum concentrations begin to fall. Nevertheless, hypomagnesemia is a warning sign that depletion may develop. Renal losses can occur in many conditions, including aldosterone excess, diuretic therapy, and diabetes mellitus. A few patients develop severe magnesium depletion because of a primary defect in renal tubular reabsorption of magnesium. Alcoholism and malabsorption syndromes associated with steatorrhea frequently cause magnesium depletion. Serum magnesium concentrations fall rapidly in some patients after removal of parathyroid adenomas, presumably because of a rapid uptake in bone.

Symptoms and Signs

The symptoms and signs of magnesium depletion are nonspecific. Neuromuscular irritability and muscle weakness are common. Because hypomagnesemia is frequently associated with low serum concentrations of calcium, potassium, and phosphate, attributing particular symptoms or signs to magnesium depletion is difficult.

Treatment

When possible, magnesium depletion should be avoided by maintaining adequate dietary intake. Mild hypomagnesemia can usually be reversed with a magnesium-rich diet. If magnesium depletion has been prolonged or if parathyroid and cell functions are likely to be impaired, 50% magnesium sulfate (4 mEq/mL) 2.5 mL IM can be given. For patients at high risk for hypotension, a smaller dose should be given. Magnesium sulfate can be given IV but only as a more dilute solution (≤ 10%) and at a rate not exceeding 1 mEq/min.

Magnesium salts are powerful laxatives, and depletion often occurs in persons with GI disorders, so magnesium replacement by the oral route is difficult. Small amounts of oral magnesium hydroxide or magnesium chloride can be used, but some patients require magnesium sulfate IM at regular intervals to prevent deficiency.

When hypomagnesemia occurs with calcium, potassium, and phosphate deficiencies, correcting the hypomagnesemia makes treating the other deficiencies easier.

HYPERMAGNESEMIA

Serum magnesium concentration > 2.5 mg/dL (2.2 mEq/L).

Hypermagnesemia is rare except in renal failure or after parenteral magnesium administration. It can depress CNS and cardiac functions. Occasionally, hypermagnesemia is an indication for dialysis.

83. MENOPAUSE AND OVARIAN HORMONE THERAPY

MENOPAUSE

The permanent cessation of menses.

Menopause occurs when the dwindling number of ovarian follicles lose their ability to respond to stimulation by gonadotropic hormones and when estrogen levels fall. After 1 yr without menses, a woman generally is considered to have passed the menopause. Menopause may be confirmed, if necessary, by demonstrating an elevated level of **serum**

follicle-stimulating hormone. A low level of serum estradiol is not diagnostic because premenopausal women often have low levels during menses.

The average age at which menopause occurs is 51 yr. This is not influenced by prolonged periods of hypothalamic amenorrhea, number of pregnancies, or oral contraceptive use. Although the average age at menopause has probably not changed since antiquity, the average life expectancy of women in the USA has increased, which means that 1/3 of their lifetime is postmenopausal. Thus, management of menopause-related problems is becoming increasingly important.

Menopause is associated with several effects; vasomotor flushes, or hot flashes, are perhaps the most well known. Other effects include osteoporosis, genital atrophy, and atherosclerosis. Osteoporosis is discussed in Ch. 73.

VASOMOTOR FLUSHES

(Hot Flashes)

A **hot flash** is *the subjective sensation of intense warmth in the upper body, typically lasting 4 min but ranging from 30 sec to 5 min.* A hot flash may follow a prodrome of palpitations or a sensation of pressure within the head and can be accompanied by weakness, faintness, or vertigo. Hot flashes frequently awaken patients from sleep, causing insomnia and fatigue and leading, in turn, to other symptoms (eg, irritability, impaired memory, poor concentration).

A **vasomotor flush,** the objective counterpart of this phenomenon, is *a visible ascending flush of the thorax, neck, and face, followed by profuse sweating.* An increase in skin perfusion occurs about 1½ min before the subjective sensation and 6 min before the peak increase in skin temperature. This increase in skin blood flow releases heat, causes a simultaneous fall in core temperature, and is followed 6 min later by a peak in serum levels of luteinizing hormone.

Incidence

About 80% of menopausal women complain of hot flashes. Of these women, 85% are symptomatic for > 1 yr, and 25% to 50% are symptomatic for up to 5 yr. Hot flashes become less frequent and less intense with age, unlike the other sequelae of menopause, which progress over time.

Pathogenesis

Hot flashes result from the withdrawal of estrogen, when a woman experiences either natural or surgical menopause or when exogenous estrogen is discontinued. The ovary does not usually stop functioning at one particular moment—typically, its function waxes and wanes over a number of years. Flashes occur when estrogen secretion declines, but they stop when estrogen secretion increases. Hypoestrogenemia per se does not cause hot flashes. For example, women with Turner's syndrome, who are hypoestrogenemic, do not have hot flashes unless exogenous estrogen is withdrawn. Similarly, men with prostate cancer develop hot flashes if their estrogen treatment is discontinued.

The phenomenon of hot flashes can occur without an intact pituitary, since a total hypophysectomy does not prevent it. Presumably, estrogen influences central neurotransmitters that regulate the thermoregulatory center in the hypothalamus. Estrogen withdrawal alters these neurotransmitters, causing thermoregulatory instability. Adjacent hypothalamic centers that control luteinizing hormone release are also stimulated, resulting in peaks of serum luteinizing hormone levels.

Diagnosis and Treatment

A thorough history and physical examination should be sufficient to diagnose menopausal hot flashes and exclude other conditions (eg, thyrotoxicosis, carcinoid, pheochromocytoma).

Optimal treatment of hot flashes is with **hormone replacement therapy.** The use of estrogens and progestins is discussed under HORMONE REPLACEMENT REGIMENS, below.

Clonidine, a centrally acting α-adrenergic agonist-antagonist, is 30% to 40% effective at reducing hot flashes. A proposed mechanism is that the drug may inhibit the binding of norepinephrine to neuronal receptors in the hypothalamus; norepinephrine release may be the event that initiates hot flashes. The initial dose of clonidine is 0.1 mg bid, which may be increased to 0.2 mg bid if no adverse effects occur and hot flashes persist. Clonidine has a high incidence of side effects (eg, postural dizziness and blurred vision), but it is better tolerated by hypertensive patients, who may be the best candidates for this treatment.

Self-management techniques may help a patient control the associated effects of hot flashes. For example, aerobic exercise, relaxation techniques, meditation, massage, and yoga may reduce stress, fatigue, and depression.

GENITAL ATROPHY

Atrophy of estrogen-dependent genitourinary tissue.

Pathogenesis

The tissues of the lower vagina, labia, urethra, and bladder trigone are of common embryonic origin derived from the urogenital sinus; all are estrogen dependent. With the loss of estrogen at menopause, the vaginal walls become pale (because of diminished vascularity) and thin (usually only three or four cells thick). The epithelial cells contain less glycogen, which before menopause had been metabolized by lactobacilli to create an acidic pH, thereby protecting the vagina from bacterial overgrowth. Loss of this protective mechanism leaves the thin, friable tissue vulnerable to ulceration and infection. The vagina also loses its rugae, becoming shorter and inelastic.

Symptoms and Signs

Patients may complain of symptoms secondary to vaginal dryness, such as dyspareunia and vaginismus, which may lead to diminished libido. These symptoms are less likely if intercourse continues regularly; periods of abstinence are more likely to be associated with stenosis and subsequent discomfort during sexual activity. Patients may also have symptoms secondary to vaginal ulceration and infection, such as vaginal discharge, burning, itching, or bleeding.

The urethra and the bladder trigone undergo atrophic changes similar to those of the vagina. Dysuria, urgency, frequency, and suprapubic pain may occur even without infection, possibly because the markedly thin urethral mucosa may allow urine to come in close contact with sensory nerves. In addition, with menopause, the loss of resistance to urinary flow by thick, well-vascularized urethral mucosa may contribute to stress incontinence. Loss of estrogens may also affect the muscles that are responsible for maintaining continence.

Diagnosis

The diagnosis of **atrophic vaginitis** may be made by visual examination of the vaginal tissue, but any atypical lesions should undergo biopsy. If a discharge is present, cultures for such pathogens as *Neisseria gonorrhoeae, Chlamydia, Trichomonas,* and *Gardnerella (Hemophilus vaginalis)* should be obtained. If *Candida* is found, the patient should undergo screening for diabetes, since the low glycogen content of unestrogenized vaginal epithelial cells ordinarily will not support this organism's growth. Atrophy may be confirmed by a vaginal cell maturation index, using scrapings from the lateral vaginal wall at the level of the cervix. The exfoliated cells are classified by degree of maturation; a small proportion of superficial cells indicates a high degree of vaginal atrophy.

The diagnosis of **atrophic urethritis and trigonitis** is confirmed when vaginal atrophy is present and urinary symptoms (eg, urgency, frequency, dysuria, suprapubic pain) occur without infection. Urethroscopy reveals a pale, atrophic urethra.

Treatment

Estrogen is the only effective therapy for genital atrophy. The dose required is generally less than that needed for hot flashes or osteoporosis; thus, treatment for those conditions should improve genital atrophy. If genital atrophy is the only indication for estrogen treatment, daily use of an oral or vaginal estrogen preparation for a minimum of 2 to 12 wk is required to reverse the atrophic changes; intermittent therapy, two to three times a week, should then be prescribed. Usual daily **oral doses** are as follows: conjugated estrogens 0.3 or 0.625 mg; estropipate 0.625 or 1.25 mg; or micronized estradiol-17β 1 or 2 mg. **Vaginal estrogens** are given as conjugated estrogens 0.625 mg or micronized estradiol-17β 0.1 mg. Although the vaginal cream preparations exert a local effect, they are rapidly absorbed systemically. Thus, the addition of a progestational agent is advised for patients with an intact uterus to prevent endometrial hyperplasia (see ESTROGENS and PROGESTINS, below). **Transdermal estradiol** 50 μg/24 h twice weekly is also effective.

If estrogens are contraindicated, synthetic mucopolysaccharides or water-soluble lubricants may relieve dyspareunia. Vaginal stenosis may be improved by using graduated vaginal dilators.

Wearing cotton underwear can help prevent infections by allowing moisture to evaporate from the vaginal area. Women who are susceptible to vaginal infection should not wear tight-fitting clothes.

ATHEROSCLEROSIS

Although there is no direct evidence that estrogen prevents atherogenesis, the following findings suggest that estrogens may have some benefit in reducing cardiovascular disease: (1) In all age groups, women have a lower incidence of cardiovascular disease than do men; (2) women who undergo a premature surgical menopause and do not take estrogens are twice as likely to have cardiovascular disease as are age-matched premenopausal controls; (3) postmenopausal women who use estrogens have a significantly lower incidence of cardiovascular disease compared with those who do not; and (4) women with coronary artery disease detected by angiography have a higher survival rate if they are estrogen users. However, healthier women may also be more likely to seek and be prescribed estrogens by their physicians.

The loss of estrogen at menopause is associated with a 6% decline in HDL cholesterol levels and a 5% rise in LDL cholesterol levels, which may explain the higher cardiovascular disease rate among postmenopausal women compared with premenopausal women. Similarly, the lower incidence of cardiovascular disease among postmenopausal women who take estrogen may be explained in part by the resultant 15% to 19% decrease in LDL cholesterol levels and the 16% to 18% increase in HDL cholesterol levels.

The lipid effects of oral estrogens are thought to be the result of a direct action on the liver after intestinal absorption, since vaginal and transdermal estrogens do not similarly affect lipoproteins. One exception is subcutaneous estradiol implants 50 to 100 mg, which favorably alter serum lipid levels, perhaps because of the supraphysiologic levels of estradiol initially released.

OVARIAN HORMONE THERAPY

Insufficient data are available to indicate that all postmenopausal women should receive estrogen replacement therapy. For that reason, the benefits and risks (see below) as they pertain to each patient should be reviewed with the patient in detail. Ultimately, she must decide whether to receive therapy and give informed consent.

Before hormonal therapy is initiated, the patient must be evaluated with a thorough history and physical examination including blood pressure, breast, and pelvic examinations and Papanicolaou (Pap) test. Mammography should be performed (and repeated annually after age 50) so that estrogens are not inadvertently prescribed for a patient with preexisting subclinical breast cancer.

An endometrial biopsy should be considered if the patient has a history of abnormal vaginal bleeding, is at increased risk for preexisting endometrial hyperplasia, has heavy bleeding, or receives estrogen therapy and bleeds at any time other than immediately following withdrawal of progestin. Biopsy may be accomplished by vabra aspiration or, if adequate tissue cannot be obtained, by fractional dilatation and curettage (D & C). A patient who is to receive unopposed estrogens for an extended time should have an endometrial biopsy before starting therapy and annually thereafter, regardless of whether she bleeds.

ESTROGENS

Pharmacology

Nonsynthetic (natural) estrogens: Nonsynthetic estrogens may be administered by oral, vaginal, transdermal, or subcutaneous routes. The most commonly prescribed nonsynthetic oral estrogens are **conjugated estrogens** 0.625 mg; **estropipate** 1.25 mg; and **micronized estradiol-17β** 1 mg. At these doses, the mean peak serum estradiol level ranges from 30 to 40 pg/mL, similar to that of the premenopausal early follicular phase; the estrone level ranges from 150 to 250 pg/mL. These doses are generally effective in relieving menopausal symptoms (eg, hot flashes) and preventing osteoporosis. In general, conjugated estrogens are twice as potent as estrone preparations because they have a prolonged action, in part as a result of their storage in and slow release from adipose tissue. Moreover, conjugated estrogens contain equine estrogens, which are quite potent.

Orally administered estradiol is rapidly converted in the intestinal mucosa to estrone, which is then presented to the liver, where 30% of an initial dose is conjugated with glucuronide on the first pass. These conjugates undergo rapid renal and biliary excretion. The biliary conjugates are hydrolyzed by the intestinal flora, allowing 80% to be reabsorbed and returned to the liver. Estrogen may then be reconjugated and excreted, or it may enter the systemic circulation.

This enterohepatic circulation contributes to the prolonged effect of orally administered estrogens. Thus, patients with altered gut flora (eg, because of antibiotic therapy) may not sufficiently hydrolyze these conjugates, thereby preventing reabsorption, and may need higher doses for a therapeutic effect. Also, patients chronically maintained on phenytoin have enhanced glucuronidation and therefore excrete estrogens more rapidly; they too may need higher doses.

Since the concentration of estrogen after oral ingestion is four to five times higher in the portal than in the general circulation, more estrogen is presented to hepatocytes than to cells of other organs. Thus, the liver is more profoundly affected by estrogens given orally than by those given parenterally. Although many of these actions on the liver may be deleterious (eg, stimulating renin-substrate and coagulation factors), some effects may be beneficial (eg, increasing HDL cholesterol levels and decreasing LDL cholesterol levels).

Parenteral estrogens may be given vaginally, transdermally, or subcutaneously. **Vaginal estrogens** are absorbed and enter the systemic circulation, achieving 1/4 the circulatory level of an equal oral dose. However, vaginal estrogens exert a potent local effect: a dose of 0.3 mg conjugated estrogens given vaginally produces the same degree of epithelial maturation as does a dose of 1.25 mg given orally. The continued use of vaginal estrogen leads to higher blood levels because of enhanced transfer across a healthier, better vascularized epithelium.

Subdermal estradiol pellets 25 mg are effective but have a variable life span of 3 to 6 mo and are difficult to remove. **Transdermal estradiol patches** 50 µg/24 h applied twice weekly provide constant serum levels of 60 pg/mL estradiol and 50 pg/mL estrone, which are usually adequate to reduce menopausal symptoms and prevent osteoporosis.

Synthetic estrogens: Synthetic estrogens are chemical derivatives of estradiol and are 100 times more potent, on a per-weight basis, than are natural estrogens in stimulating the production of hepatic proteins. Since the minimal dose for therapeutic effect exceeds the lowest dose that markedly elevates hepatic globulins (5 µg), synthetic estrogens are *not* routinely recommended for postmenopausal use.

Adverse Effects

Estrogens may cause nausea, mastalgia, headache, and mood changes. Discussed below are the more serious risks including endometrial, ovarian, and breast neoplasia; gallbladder and thromboembolic disease; hypertension; and effects on glucose tolerance.

Endometrial neoplasia: Unopposed estrogen use (ie, without the addition of a progestin) may induce endometrial hyperplasia and, potentially, adenocarcinoma. The risk of endometrial cancer appears to increase two- to fourfold, from 1/1000 women per year to 4/1000 women per year, and is related to both the dose and the duration (minimum, 1 to 2 yr) of unopposed estrogen therapy. Reducing the dose or using the drug cyclically will *not* provide adequate protection.

Concomitant use of progestins is advised in a patient with an intact uterus. Progestins can both prevent and reverse hyperplasia. Their use reduces the incidence of endometrial cancer to below that of women not receiving hormonal therapy. The duration of progestin use is important; although administration for 7 days per month significantly reduces the incidence of hyperplasia, administration for 10 to 13 days offers greater protection.

Endometrial carcinoma associated with estrogen use has an excellent prognosis, since it is generally low grade and less apt to have invaded the myometrium. The adjusted 5-yr survival rate is 94%, possibly because of earlier diagnosis.

Ovarian neoplasia: Estrogen replacement therapy may increase the risk of endometrioid cancer of the ovary (which accounts for 10% to 20% of all ovarian malignancies), but this association has *not* been conclusively established. Whether progestin use will reduce the risk, if it indeed exists, is unknown.

Breast neoplasia: Estrogen use may theoretically increase the risk of breast cancer, since (1) breast tumors can be estrogen sensitive, (2) estrogens can induce mammary tumors in rodents, and (3) women with prolonged endogenous estrogen exposure (eg, early menarche, late menopause, nulliparity) are at increased risk for breast malignancies. However, an association between estrogen replacement therapy and breast cancer has not been found, except for a possible modest increase in risk with long-term use (ie, > 10 yr). Nonetheless, women at particularly high risk for breast cancer may decline estrogen treatment for menopause. (High risk for osteoporosis represents a different risk:benefit consideration.) The American Cancer Society advises annual mammography for all women ≥ 50 yr of age, but such examinations are usually recommended starting at age 40 for women who take estrogens.

Whether the addition of a progestin may protect the breast, as it does the endometrium, is unsubstantiated. The mitotic activity of the breast increases during the luteal phase when maximum progestin secretion occurs (peak endometrial mitosis occurs during the follicular phase when progesterone secretion is minimal). Moreover, progestins induce mammary ductal growth in rodents. No evidence exists that progestins reduce the risk of breast cancer, and they may adversely affect lipoproteins. Therefore, *the use of progestins in women without an intact uterus is unnecessary and possibly detrimental.*

Gallbladder disease: During the first year of use, oral estrogen replacement therapy increases the risk of cholelithiasis by 20%. Cholelithiasis probably occurs because estrogens increase the hepatic excretion of LDL cholesterol as well as reduce the amount of chenodeoxycholic acid in bile, which keeps cholesterol in solution.

Thromboembolic disease: Oral contraceptives, particularly those with the highest estrogen content, are associated with thromboembolic disease. This effect appears to be dose related; controlled epidemiologic studies of postmenopausal estrogen replacement at physiologic doses show no increase in thrombosis.

Hypertension: Estrogen replacement therapy modestly lowers blood pressure in some women, but it induces or exacerbates hypertension in others. Oral estrogens may increase the hepatic production of renin substrate or may stimulate the production of an aberrant form. In either case, associated elevation in blood pressure is usually reversible when estrogen therapy is discontinued. Moreover, estrogen replacement is not associated with an increased risk of stroke.

Glucose tolerance: Although oral contraceptives are associated with impaired carbohydrate metabolism, the lower doses used for estrogen replacement therapy have not been linked to impaired glucose tolerance. Postmenopausal women with diabetes who take estrogen show either no change or an improvement in their disease, evidenced by lower glucose levels or reduced insulin requirements. Estrogen appears to increase the binding of insulin to its receptor. Moreover, animal models have shown that experimentally induced hyperglycemia improves with estrogen therapy.

Contraindications

Absolute contraindications to postmenopausal estrogen replacement are known or suspected active endometrial or breast cancer, undiagnosed genital bleeding, acute liver disease, and either active thromboembolic disease or a history of estrogen-related thromboembolic disease.

Relative contraindications include chronic liver dysfunction (the liver's impaired ability to metabolize estrogen leads to excessive serum estrogen levels, which may be compensated for by using smaller or less frequent doses); preexisting symptomatic uterine leiomyomata or active endometriosis (estrogen use may prevent the postmenopausal involution of these conditions); poorly controlled hypertension; history of thromboembolic disease; and acute intermittent porphyria (estrogens are known to precipitate attacks).

PROGESTINS

Postmenopausal progestins are primarily used to reduce the risk of endometrial hyperstimulation caused by estrogen replacement therapy. For patients who are not candidates for estrogen replacement, progestins may relieve hot flashes or provide prophylaxis against osteoporosis.

Pharmacology

Progesterone and its derivatives are well absorbed when given vaginally, rectally, or intramuscularly. Although oral administration is convenient and common, the drug's highly variable degree of absorption after oral administration, with as much as a threefold difference among patients, leads to variable clinical effects. For this reason, a progestin dose that is adequate for one patient may be excessive for another. After absorption, oral progestins reach the liver in high concentration, where they may greatly affect the hepatic metabolism of serum lipoproteins. These progestins are then rapidly metabolized by the liver to desoxycorticosterone.

Medroxyprogesterone acetate, the most commonly used progestin in the USA, is effective against endometrial hyperplasia and has only minor effects on serum lipid levels. Patients unable to tolerate the usual 10-mg oral dose may be given 5 mg. In most cases, the 5-mg dose offers similar protection against hyperplasia, except in patients who absorb the drug poorly. The IM depot formulation is well absorbed but has a highly variable duration of action and often causes irregular vaginal bleeding. The usual dose is 50 to 150 mg IM every 1 to 3 mo; the 50-mg dose is usually adequate to relieve hot flashes, while the 150-mg dose may be as effective as 0.625 mg conjugated estrogens in reducing urinary calcium loss.

Megestrol acetate is effective in suppressing hot flashes. Daily oral doses of 40 to 80 mg are required, since this agent has $1/4$ to $1/8$ the potency of medroxyprogesterone acetate on a per-weight basis. **Micronized progesterone** 200 to 300 mg orally is also active against endometrial hyperplasia and does not significantly alter serum lipid levels.

19-Nortestosterone derivatives are the progestins used in oral contraceptives; they have partial androgenic properties and an adverse effect on serum lipid levels. **Norethindrone (norethisterone)** was initially used in doses of 2.5 to 5 mg, but recent studies have shown that 1 mg (as used in low-dose oral contraceptives) is equally effective against endometrial hyperplasia but has much less impact on lipid levels. **D,L-Norgestrel,** known for its more potent androgenic properties, was used in a 0.5-mg dose, but a dose of 0.15 mg appears equally effective. Only the L isomer is biologically active, so 0.15 mg D,L-norgestrel is equivalent to 0.075 mg levonorgestrel. The effect of this dose on lipid levels is unknown.

Adverse Effects

Progestins may produce abdominal bloating, mastalgia, headache, mood changes, and acne. All progestins, but particularly the 19-nortestosterone derivatives, also adversely affect serum lipid levels, decreasing HDL cholesterol and increasing LDL cholesterol in a dose-dependent manner. Thus, the risk of developing cardiovascular disease may outweigh the benefit of preventing endometrial cancer. Since the protective activity of progestins on the endometrium appears related more to the duration of use (ie, 13 out of 25 days) than to the dose, the minimal effective dose should be used. For medroxyprogesterone acetate, the minimal effective dose is 10 mg, and for norethindrone, 1 mg; both these doses have minimal effects on serum lipid levels. Since progestins have not been proved to protect against breast cancer and may adversely affect lipoproteins, thus predisposing to cardiovascular disease, *these agents are not recommended for women without an intact uterus* who are receiving estrogens.

HORMONE REPLACEMENT REGIMENS

The most common schedule of oral hormone replacement therapy in the USA is cyclic, with conjugated estrogens 0.625 mg given daily and medroxyprogesterone acetate 10 mg given on days 1 through 13 each month. On this regimen, many patients have withdrawal bleeding between days 11 and 18. The schedule may be modified by substituting another estrogen for conjugated estrogens or another progestin for medroxyprogesterone acetate.

To avoid withdrawal bleeding, continuous rather than cyclic treatment has been used. Conjugated estrogens 0.625 or 1.25 mg as needed to control symptoms are given continuously with medroxyprogesterone acetate 5 mg/day. Most women have irregular vaginal bleeding for the first 2 to 3 mo, but amenorrhea usually occurs within 1 yr. Medroxyprogesterone acetate can be reduced to 2.5 mg/day after several months, although higher doses are usually required with the higher dose of estrogen. If the higher dose leads to unacceptable abdominal bloating and mastalgia, norethindrone 0.35 to 1.05 mg/day can be given instead of medroxyprogesterone acetate.

INF
NEU

§3. ORGAN SYSTEMS: INFECTIOUS DISEASE

NEUROLOGIC DISORDERS

§3. ORGAN SYSTEMS: INFECTIOUS DISEASE

84. NORMAL CHANGES IN HOST DEFENSE

Infectious diseases occur more often and are usually more severe in elderly than in younger adults, probably because aging affects host defenses. **Immune senescence,** as well as the time lapse between primary exposure and rechallenge with pathogens, diminishes the vigor of the immune response. Aging and age-related disorders not only increase the susceptibility to infection but also depress the vigor of immune responses. Many chronic disorders that are common in the elderly also increase susceptibility to infection (eg, chronic obstructive pulmonary disease, cancer, diabetes mellitus). In addition, the potential for exposure to pathogens is greater in hospitals and nursing homes. Thus, understanding the changes in host resistance that occur with age is essential to the care of older patients.

OVERVIEW OF THE IMMUNE SYSTEM

The immune system comprises several cell types, which form a network of interacting elements. Together, these elements generate **cell-mediated immunity** (T lymphocytes, or T cells), **humoral immunity** (B lymphocytes, or B cells), and **nonspecific immunity** (monocytes and polymorphonuclear neutrophil leukocytes).

Monocytes, macrophages, Langerhans' cells, and dendritic cells—collectively called **antigen-presenting cells**—are the first cells to interact with microbial pathogens and other antigens. They take up and process antigen into small peptides, which then become complexed with major histocompatibility complex **(MHC)** class I or II molecules. The antigen peptide–MHC complex is transported to the surface of the antigen-presenting cell and is ready for "presentation" to T cells. T cells can recognize antigen peptides only when they are on the surface of other cells (although virally infected cells are targeted by cytotoxic T cells) with MHC class I or II molecules. The antigen peptide–MHC complex activates T cells.

Helper or inducer T cells (which proliferate in response to antigen both in vivo and in vitro) recognize antigen that is associated with MHC class II molecules, which are expressed primarily on antigen-presenting cells. Helper cells can be distinguished from other T cells by the CD4 surface marker. Conversely, **suppressor or cytotoxic T cells** usually recognize antigen that is associated with MHC class I molecules, which are expressed on all nucleated cells. These T cells can be distinguished by the CD8 surface marker. Suppressor T cells down-regulate the immune response, maintain tolerance to "self," and counterbalance the action of helper T cells. Other T cells, **large granular lymphocytes,** have natural killer activity.

Cytokines play an important role in the response to antigen. Macrophages and other antigen-presenting cells secrete **interleukin-1 (IL-1),** which induces fever and inflammation and increases the permeability of blood vessels. IL-1 facilitates the activation of T cells, which in turn secrete **interleukin-2 (IL-2).** IL-2 supports the proliferation of T cells and the secretion of other lymphokines (including γ-interferon), which further activate macrophages and IL-4 and IL-6, which stimulate B-cell growth and, therefore, the production of antibody.

Although some antigens can activate B cells to produce antibodies in the absence of T cells, most B cells require the help of T cells and their products for full activation to antibody secretion. Regulation of the immune system depends on the balance between helper and suppressor T cells. *In old age, T-cell function declines, resulting in diminution of cell-mediated immunity, humoral immunity, and self-tolerance.* These changes lead to a decline in the response to foreign antigens and the emergence of more autoantibodies but not autoimmune diseases (which peak in middle age).

CELL–MEDIATED IMMUNITY

The thymus plays an important role in cell-mediated immunity because it is the site where T-cell precursors from the bone marrow mature and differentiate. T cells that recognize antigens and have *moderate* affinity for self MHC molecules expand in number (positive selection) in the thymus and enter the circulation. Most T cells that have *too high* an affinity for self MHC molecules are negatively selected and are deleted within the thymus. Negative selection is not complete, and peripheral mechanisms also contribute to self-tolerance.

The thymus gland involutes in middle age. The loss of thymic mass begins at about age 30 and continues until age 50, at which time only 5% to 10% of thymic mass remains. Most investigators have found that the total number of T and B cells in circulation changes little with age. However, modest changes occur in T-cell subsets: helper (CD4+) cells increase in number, while suppressor (CD8+) cells decrease in number. The percentage of immature T cells in the thymus and in the blood also increases, as the thymus loses its capacity to induce differentiation of T-cell precursors. Other changes with age include a decrease in the number of germinal centers in lymph nodes and an increase in the number of plasma cells and lymphocytes in bone marrow.

While aging does not affect the number of T cells in the blood, only about 1/5 to 1/2 of an older person's T cells respond to **mitogen.** Those cells that do respond demonstrate an impaired ability to divide sequentially in culture. Yet, older and younger persons have the same number of and affinity to mitogen receptors on the cells. Furthermore, the generation of a **cytoplasmic factor** that stimulates DNA synthesis by isolated nuclei is comparable in younger and older persons, although nuclei isolated from the lymphocytes of older donors show an impaired response to this cytoplasmic factor. Thus it appears that the proliferative defect is due to the failure of the nucleus to synthesize DNA, even though many of the cell surface and cytoplasmic events after activation proceed normally in lymphocytes from older persons.

The decline in T-cell function leads to a deficiency in cell-mediated immunity. About 25% of healthy older persons have a marked decline, 50% have a moderate decline, and 25% have no decline. Evidence that cell-mediated immunity can lose its **functional capacity** is shown in the diminished hypersensitivity response to common skin-testing antigens (eg, *Candida,* mumps, and purified protein derivative of tuberculin). Further evidence of delayed hypersensitivity is seen in the lymphocyte transfer test. In this model of the graft-vs.-host reaction, the functional capacity of lymphocytes injected into the skin is assayed. Lymphocytes from older donors are less capable of inducing a reaction than are lymphocytes from younger donors.

Lymphocytes from elderly persons sensitized to *Mycobacterium tuberculosis* and to the influenza and varicella-zoster viruses show an impaired proliferative response to these antigens, compared with lymphocytes from sensitized younger persons. This observation may help explain why infections with these pathogens are usually more severe in older persons. The elderly are at increased risk of developing **reactivation tuberculosis.** Reactivation of the dormant bacterium correlates with the presence of other diseases or with the institution of immunosuppressive therapy, which may accentuate the decline in cell-mediated immunity. Similarly, reactivation of **varicella-zoster virus** (causing **shingles**) is more common in healthy older persons than in younger persons.

HUMORAL IMMUNITY

Changes in humoral immunity result primarily from impaired T-cell function; changes in B-cell function appear to be secondary. The *total concentration* of immunoglobulins in serum changes little with age, although modest changes in the *distribution* of immunoglobulin classes are reported: The serum concentrations of IgA and IgG tend to increase, while those of IgM and IgD decrease.

A **diminished antibody response** to influenza, parainfluenza, pneumococcus, and tetanus vaccines has been demonstrated in older persons; the maximal antibody response requires a larger dose of antigen and is maintained for shorter periods. Also, the class of immunoglobulin produced in response to antigen changes—relatively more IgM and relatively less IgG.

Despite a diminished antibody response to foreign antigens, **autoantibodies** are found more frequently in the serum of older persons. This phenomenon is not associated with an increased incidence of autoimmune disorders, but it reflects dysregulation of the immune system. One class of autoantibodies, autoanti-idiotypes, may directly inhibit the antibody response to foreign antigens.

Findings of monoclonal immunoglobulins not associated with malignant myeloma increase dramatically with age. About 2% of persons > 70 yr of age and (in one study) 19% of those > 95 yr of age have **monoclonal gammopathy of uncertain significance** (benign monoclonal gammopathy), in contrast to < 0.1% of persons < 50 yr of age. **Chronic lymphocytic leukemia,** a disease restricted almost exclusively to elderly patients, also results from the clonal expansion of B cells, specifically B cells that express the CD5 cell surface antigen.

INFLAMMATION AND NONSPECIFIC IMMUNITY

Inflammation, one of the earliest responses to injury and infection, is characterized by increased local blood flow, increased permeability of blood vessels, and rapid mobilization of polymorphonuclear neutrophil leukocytes **(PMNs).** This line of defense is mediated by various substances, including catecholamines, histamine, serotonin, and prostaglandins. Chemotaxis and opsonization, which stimulate specific immune responses, are coordinated by the clotting, kinin, and complement systems.

In general, the inflammatory and nonspecific immune defenses decrease moderately, if at all, with age. Yet the serum complement components C3 and properdin may increase. Studies show that macrophages from young and old mice have comparable ability to phagocytose antigen, support T-cell proliferation, and secrete lymphokines. However, studies of older persons show that the capacity of PMNs to migrate and kill *Candida albicans* in vitro is impaired.

Authorities once thought that the febrile response and leukocytosis—but not the relative increase in immature PMNs and PMN precursors (the shift to the left)—were diminished in older patients. However, it now appears that, as with local inflammatory responses, disease burden accounts for the impaired nonspecific inflammatory response to infectious disease. The clinical response to infection is also blunted in younger patients with severe multisystem illness; thus, the accumulation of diseases, not the passage of years, impairs nonspecific immunity in some elderly persons. Some specific pathologic conditions impede host defenses: For example, the hyperglycemia of diabetes mellitus impairs PMN function, and vascular disease reduces blood flow, compromising resistance to local infection and wound healing.

EFFECTS OF INFECTIOUS DISEASE

Risk Factors

Many clinical factors contribute to the higher incidence and increased severity of infections in the elderly. The elderly are more often hospitalized or placed in nursing homes, where the risk of **nosocomial infection** is high. In these settings, the elderly are frequently exposed to antimicrobial therapy and are at risk for infection with *Clostridium difficile* and difficult-to-treat microbes, such as methicillin-resistant *Staphylococcus aureus* and resistant gram-negative bacteria. Outbreaks of tuberculosis, *Escherichia coli* 0157:H7 infections, *Salmonella* infections, and influenza are more likely to occur in institutions.

Pathologic conditions that accompany aging are also major risk factors for infection. Valvular disease (including sclerotic heart valves), metabolic diseases (such as diabetes mellitus), neurologic disease, chronic respiratory disease, and urologic disease (including prostatic hypertrophy) increase a person's susceptibility to infection. In addition, prosthetic joints, artificial heart valves, pacemakers, and other implanted devices, which are more common in the elderly, are associated with a higher rate of infections.

The risk of infection also increases in persons who lack access to medications or whose nutrition is inadequate. Social isolation, death of a spouse, and loss of functional independence are sources of **psychologic stress,** which may also compromise host resistance.

Dissemination of Infection

Not only are the elderly more susceptible to infection, they are also less able to keep infections from spreading (eg, bacteremia). For example, **erysipelas,** a rapidly spreading group A β-hemolytic streptococcal infection of the dermis, occurs more often in infants and older persons than in the rest of the population. The skin of older persons is characterized by thinning, loss of Langerhans' cells (skin tissue macrophages), and diminished blood supply in some areas. This decrease in local defense facilitates the development of aggressive infections. **Gram-negative bacteremia** without an obvious primary site of infection develops more often in older patients (although the urinary tract is a common source).

Prophylaxis

All elderly persons should receive vaccination with tetanus toxoid, pneumococcal vaccine, and annual influenza vaccine if they are not contraindicated (see Ch. 85). However, aging impairs the immune response to vaccines. In one study, 40% of healthy older persons did not develop protective immunity after influenza vaccination compared with only 5% of younger adults. Developing more potent vaccines and using adjuvants that enhance the immune response are currently being investigated.

Adequate nutrition is necessary for maximal host resistance. Correcting nutritional deficiency or giving therapeutic doses of nutritional supplements may improve host defenses. For example, zinc sulfate and vitamin E have been reported to enhance immune function in the elderly.

Recognition and treatment of diseases such as diabetes mellitus, heart failure, thyroid disease, and occult malignancy reduce the risk and severity of infections. Structural abnormalities that increase risk should be corrected whenever possible. For example, prostatectomy or other treatments for urinary obstruction can improve urine flow and decrease the amount of residual urine, thereby reducing the incidence of urinary tract infections. Orthopedic procedures that enhance mobility and improve the quality of life can secondarily improve host resistance.

Good **infection control measures** are required in institutional settings. Health care workers should wash their hands after each patient contact, receive annual influenza vaccination, and be accorded appropriate sick leave to reduce the chance that they will transmit infections to the institutionalized population.

SPECIFIC INFECTIONS

Age-associated changes in the respiratory, urinary, and gastrointestinal tracts of elderly persons put them at increased risk of infection.

RESPIRATORY TRACT INFECTIONS

Normally, fibronectin (a high-molecular-weight glycoprotein) binds to bacteria and blocks the sites on the microbial cell surface that allow bacteria to adhere to buccal epithelium. During illness, salivary protease activity increases, destroying fibronectin and facilitating colonization of the oropharynx by coliform bacteria. Gram-negative bacterial colonization occurs in about 3% of healthy younger persons and about 6% of healthy elderly persons. The incidence increases with disability and illness, so that the rate in hospitalized patients > 65 yr of age approaches 40%.

In addition, an impaired cough reflex and reduced clearance of respiratory tract secretions become more common with age. Aspiration and alteration of microbial flora, which also increase with age, can overwhelm the defenses of the lower respiratory tract, leading to pneumonia. Microbes that reach the alveoli activate macrophages and T cells, which then initiate local inflammatory and immune responses. The decline in T-cell function may contribute to a diminished immune response in the alveoli and, consequently, to the increased severity of pneumonia in older persons (see PNEUMONIA in Ch. 46).

The elderly are also more susceptible to severe influenza, in part because of an impaired immune response to the virus (see Ch. 47). Infection with influenza destroys ciliated epithelial cells of the respiratory tract and depresses mucociliary clearance, leading to increased mortality in the elderly. Complications, including both secondary bacterial infections (eg, with *Streptococcus pneumoniae* or *Staphylococcus aureus*) and noninfectious processes, usually cardiovascular or respiratory in origin, are common.

Immunization with influenza and pneumococcal vaccines is recommended for persons > 65 yr of age, although the vaccines' efficacy may be reduced in elderly persons.

Urinary Tract Infections

Adherence of bacteria to urogenital epithelial cells increases in women with frequent urinary tract infections, and urine loses bacteriostatic properties in some elderly persons. Conditions that enhance bacterial growth include glycosuria (which accompanies diabetes mellitus) and renal function disorders that reduce the ability to concentrate and acidify urine.

Age-related prostatism in men leads to incomplete bladder emptying and thus to urinary stasis. Elderly persons are often subjected to instrumentation of the urinary tract, which may introduce bacteria and lead to colonization and subsequent infection.

Gastrointestinal Tract Infections

Age-related changes in the GI tract compromise its resistance to infection. Achlorhydria allows the stomach and upper small intestine to be colonized by coliform bacteria, which puts patients who aspirate gastric contents at increased risk for gram-negative pneumonia. Elderly patients are also more susceptible to *Salmonella* infections because of the higher pH level of the upper GI tract and possibly because of diminished IgA production. In addition, GI diseases common in old age facilitate the development of infection. Gallstones can cause local obstruction, cholecystitis, and cholangitis. Colonic obstruction and diverticular disease can lead to life-threatening systemic infection.

85. VACCINES AND IMMUNIZATION

The principal target of immunization efforts in the USA has been children. Less attention has been paid to immunization of adults, particularly the elderly. For example, all persons > 65 yr old should receive influenza vaccine, but only 15% to 30% actually do receive it in any given year (see Influenza Vaccine, below). With the recognition that the immunizations recommended for older adults have been neglected or inappropriately administered, interest in adult immunization, particularly with influenza and pneumococcal vaccines, has been renewed.

GENERAL PRINCIPLES

Immunization is either active or passive. **Active immunization** is usually carried out in anticipation of exposure to a disease; how much protection is conferred depends on the recipient's immune response. The immunizing agents are vaccines or toxoids. **Vaccines** consist of either whole killed bacterial cells, wholly or partially purified bacterial proteins or polysaccharides, inactivated viruses or purified viral proteins, or live attenuated viruses. **Toxoids** consist of bacterial toxins that have been modified to render them nontoxic, although they retain the ability to induce production of antitoxin antibodies.

Passive immunization, which does not provoke an immune response, is used when exposure to a disease has recently occurred or is anticipated. It is accomplished by administering **immune globulins,** usually of human but sometimes of animal origin. Specific hyperimmune globulin preparations are derived from donor pools preselected for a high level of antibody against a specific disease (eg, tetanus, rabies, hepatitis B, or varicella zoster). Immune or hyperimmune globulins derived from humans have a high degree of safety. Since 1985, all human plasma entering a donor pool has been screened for antibody to human immunodeficiency virus. Furthermore, the purification process used to prepare immune globulins excludes HIV. Use of immune globulins of equine origin (eg, botulism antitoxin and several antivenins) should be preceded by an intradermal test dose to determine if the patient is allergic or hypersensitive to horse serum. Serum sickness is a late, dose-related complication of equine globulin products.

In addition to specific immunogens, vaccines and toxoids contain other substances that could cause allergic or other adverse reactions. The suspending fluid may contain minute amounts of protein or other components of the biologic system in which the immunogen was produced (eg, egg antigens or antigens derived from the cells in which vaccine viruses were grown). Preservatives, stabilizers, or antibiotics used in viral cell cultures may also be present in minute amounts. Adjuvants, usually consisting of aluminum salts, are sometimes added to enhance the immune response. Such adjuvants are believed to be harmless when injected IM, but if given subcutaneously, they may produce granulomatous inflammation or even necrosis.

Immunization of older persons should be based on risk-benefit considerations. In general, known hypersensitivity to a vaccine component is a *contraindication* to using that vaccine. A very small number of people are allergic to eggs, and some vaccines, including influenza vaccine, are prepared in eggs. Hypersensitivity to an antibiotic used in culture media is another possible but infrequent risk; for example, penicillin is not currently used in preparing any vaccine.

The immunologic response to most vaccines decreases in the elderly; whether age per se is the major attenuating factor or whether underlying disease (which is more prevalent in the elderly) affects the immunologic response is not clear. For example, elderly nursing home residents produce much lower levels of antibody to the influenza vaccine than do young adults. A similar response occurs with pneumococcal vaccine. Nonetheless, response is sufficient for conferring protection in most elderly persons.

In general, immunologically compromised persons should not be given live attenuated virus vaccines because of the risk of vaccine-induced disease. Patients who have received immune or hyperimmune globulins within the preceding 3 mo should not receive live attenuated virus vaccines because the administered antibody may interfere with the subclinical infection, which is the desired response to the vaccine.

A number of vaccines may be given together without loss of efficacy. For example, influenza and pneumococcal vaccines may be administered concurrently but at separate sites. TABLE 85–1 lists the active im-

TABLE 85–1. AGENTS COMMONLY USED FOR ACTIVE IMMUNIZATION

Agent	*Type of Preparation*	*Dosage Schedule*	*Comments*
For general use			
Tetanus and diphtheria toxoids	Bacterial toxoids	IM q 10 yr at mid-decade birthday	Also used in wound management and for diphtheria contacts
Influenza virus vaccine, trivalent	Inactivated virus	IM annually	Indicated for all persons > 65 yr of age and for those at any age with chronic disease
Pneumococcal polysaccharide vaccine	23-valent, purified capsular polysaccharides	IM once in a lifetime	Indicated for all persons > 65 yr of age and for those at high risk (eg, those with asplenia)
For selective use			
Poliomyelitis vaccine	Live attenuated virus (oral polio vaccine)	3 doses orally	Used for booster doses in adults, if needed in special circumstances; *not* to be used for primary immunization of adults

(continued)

TABLE 85–1. AGENTS COMMONLY USED FOR ACTIVE IMMUNIZATION *(Continued)*

Agent	*Type of Preparation*	*Dosage Schedule*	*Comments*
For selective use *(continued)*			
Poliomyelitis vaccine *(continued)*	Inactivated virus (enhanced-potency inactivated polio vaccine)	3 doses s.c.	Used for primary immunization of adults, if needed
Hepatitis B vaccine	Purified HBsAG, produced in yeast	3 doses IM	Indicated for persons at risk, especially health care workers, homosexual men, IV drug abusers, sexual contacts of HBsAG carriers, persons with prolonged residence where the disease is highly endemic
Rabies vaccine	Inactivated virus, grown in human diploid cells	5 doses IM for postexposure prophylaxis	Preexposure prophylaxis in special circumstances (3 doses)
Meningococcal vaccine	Purified polysaccharides, serogroups A, C, Y, W-135	IM once	Used for outbreak control and in persons at increased risk
Typhoid vaccine	Whole killed *Salmonella typhi*	2 doses s.c. 4 wk apart; booster doses at 3-yr intervals	Indicated only for travelers to areas where the disease is known to be endemic
	Live attenuated *Salmonella typhi*	Enteric-coated tablet orally every other day for 4 doses	Indicated only for travelers to areas where the disease is known to be endemic
Cholera vaccine	Whole killed *Vibrio cholerae*	2 doses IM 4 wk apart; booster doses at 6-mo intervals	Indicated only for travelers to countries requiring cholera vaccination
Yellow fever vaccine	Attenuated live virus	Single dose s.c. and booster doses at 10-yr intervals	Indicated only for travelers to areas where the disease is endemic

TABLE 85–2. AGENTS USED FOR PASSIVE IMMUNIZATION

Disease	*Agent*	*Comments*
Hepatitis A	Immune globulin	For susceptible contacts; outbreak control
Hepatitis B	Hepatitis B immune globulin	For exposed susceptibles; begin active immunization with hepatitis B vaccine
Rabies	Rabies immune globulin	For postexposure prophylaxis; begin active immunization with rabies vaccine
Tetanus	Tetanus immune globulin	For management of tetanus-prone wounds
Varicella zoster	Varicella-zoster immune globulin	For use in immunocompromised, exposed susceptibles; may modify but not prevent disease
Botulism	Botulism antitoxin	For treatment of botulism

Note: Equine antivenins directed against coral snake, pit viper (including rattlesnake), and black widow spider venins are also available.

munizing agents recommended for general or selective use in elderly patients. TABLE 85–2 summarizes the preparations of immune globulins that are sometimes indicated for older adults.

GENERAL IMMUNIZATIONS

The immunizations recommended for general use include tetanus and diphtheria toxoids, influenza vaccine, and pneumococcal vaccine. All persons > 65 yr old should be adequately protected against these diseases.

TETANUS AND DIPHTHERIA TOXOIDS

Tetanus and diphtheria toxoids for adult use **(Td)** consist of formalinized toxoids derived from tetanus and diphtheria toxins. This product differs from the vaccine used in children (diphtheria, tetanus, pertussis [DTP]) in that Td contains no pertussis antigen and a reduced dose of diphtheria toxoid to minimize reactions. Tetanus toxoid alone is recommended for persons who have had adverse reactions to the diphtheria component in Td.

Persons who have been primarily immunized previously in adult life or as children need booster doses at 10-yr intervals to maintain adequate immunity. Pediatric immunization schedules generally end with a preschool booster dose of these antigens; therefore, subsequent booster doses might be given at the mid-decade birthday (eg, 15, 25, 35, 45, 55, etc), which is a convenient recall date. If a person probably was not primarily immunized, two IM doses of Td should be given a month apart, followed by the usual schedule of booster doses at 10-yr intervals.

Whether booster doses of Td are needed every 10 yr during all of adult life is controversial. Most cases of tetanus and diphtheria in the USA in recent years have occurred in persons who never completed the primary immunization series. Some serologic data suggest that once primary immunization is complete and the first 10-yr booster dose has been given at age 15, a single midlife booster dose at age 50 or 55 may be sufficient to maintain adequate immunity throughout life. However, serologic surveys carried out in the past 10 yr indicate that > ½ of persons > 60 yr of age did not have protective levels of antitoxin antibodies against either tetanus or diphtheria. The CDC Advisory Committee on Immunization Practices continues to recommend booster doses of Td every 10 yr. Booster doses have few contraindications; the major one is a neurologic or severe hypersensitivity reaction after a previous dose.

In trauma management, an additional dose of Td is recommended only when the patient has a contaminated or severe puncture wound, and then only if > 5 yr have elapsed since the last dose. The Td product is preferred to tetanus toxoid alone because it provides an economical and convenient means of enhancing diphtheria immunity.

INFLUENZA VACCINE

Influenza vaccine contains inactivated whole influenza viruses or subunit components. To prepare a split-virus, or subunit, vaccine, the viral envelope is disrupted with organic solvents and the viral products are subsequently purified and concentrated. The composition of influenza vaccines often changes from year to year because of the continuing antigenic drift of influenza viruses. Changes in the vaccine are based on the specific immunologic characteristics of the influenza viruses that have recently circulated in the USA and elsewhere in the world. The vaccine is given annually because the antigenic composition is updated regularly and because the immunity induced is relatively short-lived.

Since 1976, the influenza vaccine has been a trivalent product containing the two influenza A strains predominant during recent influenza seasons (H1N1 and H3N2), as well as an influenza B strain. Some vaccine recipients developed Guillain-Barré syndrome after the swine influenza vaccination program in 1976. The risk of Guillain-Barré syndrome associated with swine influenza immunization at that time was about one case per 100,000 persons vaccinated. Since the swine influenza antigen was removed from influenza vaccines, no subsequent association with Guillain-Barré syndrome has been noted.

Influenza outbreaks in the USA have the greatest impact on elderly persons, who account for > 80% of all influenza-related deaths. About 90% of these deaths occur in persons with recognized underlying high-risk conditions (eg, those with chronic pulmonary, cardiac, renal, or metabolic diseases), but some deaths also occur in apparently healthy older adults.

The vaccine should be given annually to all adults who have high-risk conditions and to all adults > 65 yr old. In young adults, influenza vaccines have a protective effect of about 75% to 80% against the influenza virus. The efficacy declines with age, even with annual immunization, but the vaccine is still effective in reducing the severity of illness, protecting against serious complicating bacterial pneumonia, and reducing mortality.

A recently developed live attenuated influenza A vaccine given intranasally has shown promising results in older persons. The use of nonimmunogenic drugs in preventing influenza is discussed in Ch. 47.

PNEUMOCOCCAL VACCINE

The pneumococcal vaccine contains 25 μg each of 23 individual polysaccharides, derived from the 23 pneumococcal capsular types that account for most bacteremic pneumococcal infections in the USA. All adults > 65 yr old should receive pneumococcal vaccine. Other indications for this vaccine include sickle cell disease, splenic dysfunction or anatomic asplenia (eg, surgical splenectomy), leukemia, Hodgkin's disease, lymphoma, multiple myeloma, chronic renal failure, nephrotic syndrome, systemic lupus erythematosus, and chronic diseases associated with increased risk of pneumococcal disease (eg, diabetes mellitus and chronic cardiopulmonary disease) regardless of the patient's age. While the indications for pneumococcal vaccine are similar to those for influenza vaccine, pneumococcal vaccine need be given only once in a lifetime rather than annually. If vaccination status is uncertain, the vaccine should be readministered. Local reactions may occur if the dose is duplicative, especially if the previous dose was given within 5 yr.

Pneumococcal vaccine has not been used to maximum advantage in the USA. Fewer than 20% of adults > 65 yr old have actually been immunized with pneumococcal vaccine. Of patients with serious pneumococcal infections who were hospitalized at least once within 5 yr of the illness, ≤ 33% received pneumococcal vaccine. One survey found that > 50% of physicians gave pneumococcal vaccine only to patients with cardiopulmonary disease and not to otherwise healthy elderly patients.

The reason why the vaccine has not been more widely used probably relates to conflicting evidence of efficacy in earlier vaccine products and to differing perceptions about the importance of pneumococci in causing pneumonia, bacteremia, and death, particularly in the elderly. Evidence now shows that the vaccine is 70% to 75% effective in the healthy elderly but less effective in patients with significant underlying disease such as cardiopulmonary disease or malignancy. Immunization not only helps decrease the incidence of disease, but also may reduce pneumococcal sepsis and mortality in those who contract pneumonia (see also PNEUMONIA in Ch. 46).

The attack rate of invasive pneumococcal infection begins to increase at about age 55 and rises even more sharply at age 65. Blacks and native Americans not only are more likely to have underlying high-risk conditions at any age but also are more susceptible to invasive pneumococcal infection. Thus, all persons between ages 50 and 55, and particularly blacks and native Americans, should be assessed for high-risk conditions that indicate the need for pneumococcal vaccine. All persons not previously immunized should receive pneumococcal vaccine at age 65. Consideration should also be given to immunizing healthy adults at an earlier age (eg, 55 yr) before significant underlying disease develops and when a more brisk immune response can be expected.

SELECTED IMMUNIZATIONS

Immunizations available for selective use include poliovirus, hepatitis B, rabies, meningococcal, typhoid, cholera, and yellow fever vaccines. The indications vary with each vaccine (see also TABLE 85–1).

POLIOVIRUS VACCINE

Routine polio vaccination of elderly adults who have not been primarily immunized is no longer necessary, since the risk of poliomyelitis in the USA is extremely low. Poliomyelitis vaccination should be considered only for elderly adults who plan international travel with prolonged exposure in an area where the disease is endemic.

Two types of poliovirus vaccine are currently available in the USA: live oral polio vaccine and enhanced-potency inactivated polio vaccine administered subcutaneously. Persons who were primarily immunized with either oral polio vaccine or enhanced-potency inactivated polio vaccine need only a booster dose of enhanced-potency inactivated polio vaccine. Oral polio vaccine is the most widely used, but it is not recommended for primary immunization of adults. If primary immunization is necessary, enhanced-potency inactivated polio vaccine is recommended.

HEPATITIS B VACCINE

The first vaccine against hepatitis B consisted of purified, inactivated hepatitis B surface antigen **(HBsAg)**, derived from plasma obtained from chronic carriers of HBsAg. Current hepatitis B vaccines, first introduced in 1987, are derived from yeast cells that have been genetically coded to synthesize large amounts of HBsAg. These vaccines have replaced the plasma-derived hepatitis B vaccine.

Major target populations for whom the vaccine is recommended include homosexual men, IV drug abusers, certain institutionalized populations, household or sexual contacts of chronic hepatitis carriers, and health care personnel who are exposed to blood or blood-contaminated body fluids. Under most circumstances, elderly adults should receive hepatitis B vaccine only if they are traveling to areas where the disease is endemic and they may be exposed. The vaccine is administered IM in the deltoid region in three doses, the second dose 1 mo after the first, and the third dose 6 mo later.

RABIES VACCINE

Rabies vaccines available today are prepared from inactivated viruses grown in diploid-cell cultures. These vaccines represent a substantial improvement over those available before 1980. They have a high degree of efficacy both in preventing rabies after exposure and in providing preexposure prophylaxis against rabies in certain populations.

Preexposure rabies immunization should be considered for persons at high risk (eg, veterinarians, animal handlers, persons with occupations or hobbies resulting in unavoidable exposure to potentially rabid animals, and laboratory workers who work with wild rabies virus). For preexposure immunization, three injections of the vaccine are required, the second 1 wk after the initial dose and the third 3 or 4 wk later. Booster doses are recommended every 2 yr in persons at continuing risk for exposure. If a person who has received preexposure immunization is subsequently bitten by an animal known or believed to be rabid, two 1-mL doses of the vaccine are administered, one immediately and the other 3 days later. Human rabies immune globulin need not be given to such patients.

For persons who have not received preexposure prophylaxis, exposure to animals known to be or suspected of harboring the rabies virus entails a different postexposure prophylaxis procedure. In this case, five 1-mL doses of rabies vaccine are given IM. The initial dose is given as soon as possible after exposure, with the additional doses given on days 3, 7, 14, and 28. Postexposure rabies prophylaxis in this case should also include one dose of human rabies immune globulin (consisting of antirabies globulin concentrated from the plasma of hyperimmunized donors), administered at the time of the first dose of rabies vaccine to provide passive antirabies antibodies until the vaccine response is established. The recommended dose of 20 IU/kg should be divided, with about 50% of the dose injected in the area around the wound and the rest administered IM. The recommended dose of human rabies immune globulin results in very little, if any, attenuation of the host's immunologic response to rabies vaccine.

Any decision to provide postexposure rabies prophylaxis should take into account the animal species involved, the circumstances of the bite or other exposure, the vaccination status of the exposed person, and the presence of rabies in the region. Local or state public health officials should be consulted if questions arise about the need for rabies prophylaxis. In some jurisdictions, any animal bite is reportable to the responsible government agency.

MENINGOCOCCAL VACCINE

The meningococcal vaccine—quadrivalent A, C, Y, and W-135—that is licensed for use in the USA consists of purified capsular polysaccharides that induce specific serogroup immunity. It is highly effective in preventing meningococcal disease caused by these serogroups in about 90% of susceptible adults. Only a single 0.5-mL IM dose is required, and the immunity is believed to be long-lived.

Elderly adults should be considered for meningococcal immunization only if they are traveling to areas where meningococcal disease is known to be highly endemic or epidemic. In local epidemics or household cases, prophylaxis with rifampin (600 mg q 12 h for four doses) may be given to those intimately exposed.

TYPHOID VACCINE

The routine administration of typhoid vaccine is no longer recommended in the USA. The vaccine also should not be administered routinely to victims of natural disasters, such as earthquakes and floods. Typhoid vaccine should be considered for elderly adults traveling to areas where the disease is known to be endemic.

Two types of typhoid vaccine are available in the USA. The killed vaccine for parenteral use has been available for many years. An oral vaccine containing live attenuated typhoid bacilli has recently become available. The dosage schedule for the oral vaccine calls for one enteric-coated capsule to be taken four times on alternate days, 1 h before a meal. The oral vaccine is more expensive than the parenteral vaccine, but it causes fewer adverse reactions. The two products are about equally effective. Live oral typhoid vaccine should not be given to immunocompromised patients.

CHOLERA VACCINE

Cholera vaccine is marginally effective, and immunity lasts for little more than 6 mo. It is recommended only for travelers to countries that require cholera vaccination for entry.

YELLOW FEVER VACCINE

Yellow fever vaccine is recommended only for people traveling to areas where the disease is endemic. Because this vaccine contains live attenuated virus, it should be used cautiously in elderly adults. If a person has underlying immunocompromising disease, a letter from the physician outlining the medical contraindications to the vaccine will usually suffice to obtain an entry waiver to countries that require the vaccine.

FUTURE TRENDS

A number of additional vaccines are under development and may be licensed for use in the USA within the next 10 yr. New or improved versions of standard vaccines will continue to be introduced, and standard techniques will be used to develop bacterial or viral component vaccines or live attenuated virus vaccines. Examples include hepatitis A vaccine and live attenuated varicella vaccine, both currently under investigation. The varicella vaccine may be particularly important in the elderly if it can be shown to reduce the risk of shingles.

Hepatitis B vaccine represents the first major use of recombinant DNA technology for vaccine development. Further use of such technology may lead to the development of vaccines effective against meningococci of serogroup B, respiratory syncytial virus, enteric viruses, cytomegalovirus, and malaria. Vaccines directed against human immunodeficiency virus infection are under vigorous study.

Few, if any, of these anticipated developments will be appropriate for widespread use in elderly adults. Emphasis will continue to be placed on more extensive use of diphtheria and tetanus toxoids, influenza vaccine, and pneumococcal vaccine.

86. ANTIMICROBIAL AGENTS

PHARMACOKINETICS AND CHOICE OF AGENT

The use of antimicrobials in the elderly is not fundamentally different from that in younger adults. However, the etiology and severity of infection are often different in the elderly, requiring prescribers to alter their choice of agents. Additionally, age-related changes in pharmacokinetics often force a change in the dose, frequency, and route of administration of antimicrobials, especially in the frailest elderly persons.

Pharmacokinetics

Usually, young healthy male volunteers are tested for determining the pharmacokinetics of new drugs. However, elderly bodies handle many drugs differently than younger bodies do, including some antimicrobials. For example, peak plasma concentrations of ciprofloxacin, a fluorinated 4-quinolone derivative, are about twice as high in elderly, sick patients as in young volunteers receiving the same dose. Since 4-quinolones seem to have dose-dependent side effects, such differences may be of considerable clinical importance. General aspects of geriatric clinical pharmacology are discussed in Ch. 21; issues specific to antimicrobial agents are discussed below.

Absorption: Aging results in decreased gastric acid, prolonged gastric emptying, and decreased small-bowel motility. The effects of these changes on drug absorption have not been thoroughly investigated; theoretically, they could either increase or decrease it, although generally drug absorption is not altered in the elderly.

Distribution: An elderly person has about 29% less lean body mass than does a younger adult. As a result, water-soluble antimicrobial agents (eg, aminoglycosides, penicillins, cephalosporins, and amphotericin B) reach higher concentrations in plasma and tissue fluid. Conversely, given the relatively high percentage of fat in the elderly, fat-soluble antimicrobials (eg, chloramphenicol, doxycycline, and fluconazole) achieve lower concentrations in plasma and tissue.

Since most infections are localized to peripheral body sites, adequate concentrations of an anti-infective agent at the site of infection are crucial. Although some newer antibiotics (eg, macrolides such as clarithromycin and azithromycin) achieve rather low plasma concentrations, their intracellular concentrations are up to 40 times higher and may persist for several days, allowing long dosing intervals and short treatment times.

Protein binding: With few exceptions, antimicrobial agents bind to albumin in plasma to some extent. The bound portion cannot penetrate microorganisms and thus lacks antimicrobial effect. It is also unable to pass freely to extravascular compartments. In most cases, protein binding is rapidly reversible, and the drug may be displaced from the albumin by highly bound drugs or substances such as bilirubin. Displacement may have clinical consequences. The sulfonamides are the only antimicrobials that are highly bound and likely to displace other drugs and bilirubin.

Plasma albumin concentration decreases somewhat with age. While this is probably of little importance, disease-related changes in protein binding can cause antimicrobials to be displaced from albumin, resulting in higher concentrations of free drug. In uremia, hypoalbuminemia gives the same result; more free drug may also lead to more rapid elimination.

Elimination: Metabolism and biliary excretion of antimicrobials seem to be relatively constant with aging. A possible exception is the decreased first-pass metabolism of some drugs (eg, ciprofloxacin), which leads to increased plasma concentrations. Since aging is associated with reduced kidney function, renally excreted antimicrobials (notably aminoglycosides) may have markedly altered pharmacokinetics in the elderly, especially if renal excretion is the only mode of elimination. The plasma half-life of such drugs is longer in older than in younger adults. The increase in plasma half-life is normally moderate in patients with a creatinine clearance > 30 mL/min. Lower clearances result in drastic increases in the plasma half-life, with considerable risk of drug accumulation and adverse reactions. Serum creatinine level is not a reliable indicator of kidney function in older patients; therefore, creatinine clearance should be estimated with a nomogram or a formula that takes into account age, sex, weight, and serum creatinine level (see the creatinine clearance formula under Drug Doses in Ch. 63).

Choice of Agent

The increased risk for certain infections, especially nosocomial infections, should be considered when choosing an antimicrobial for an elderly patient. In patients with symptoms and signs of septicemia, empiric treatment must be correct because mortality can be very high. In contrast, early treatment does not affect the mortality rates for some infections. For example, the mortality rates for pneumococcal septicemia did not vary during the first 5 days of hospitalization when patients who received no antibiotics were compared with those who received benzylpenicillin (in studies done in the 1950s). Afterward, however, mortality was almost nonexistent among the treated patients, while 80% of the untreated patients died.

ANTIBIOTICS

The groups of antibiotics discussed below include the aminoglycosides, β-lactams (penicillins, cephalosporins, monobactams, carbapenems), macrolides and azalides, nitroimidazoles, polymyxins, quinolones, sulfonamides and trimethoprim, and tetracyclines, as well as miscellaneous antibiotics.

AMINOGLYCOSIDES

Aminoglycosides irreversibly inhibit bacterial protein synthesis and are rapidly bactericidal against staphylococci and gram-negative aerobic bacteria, including *Pseudomonas* spp. The most important aminoglycosides are amikacin, gentamicin, neomycin, netilmicin, and tobramycin. Neomycin is used topically for some ear, eye, and skin infections, or orally for hepatic coma or for selective decontamination of the large bowel before colorectal surgery. Streptomycin is still used for tuberculosis and occasionally for endocarditis. Amikacin, gentamicin, netilmicin, and tobramycin differ in resistance to bacterial aminoglycoside-inactivating enzymes; amikacin and netilmicin are most resistant.

Pharmacokinetics: Aminoglycosides are not absorbed from the GI tract. The drugs are excreted renally, and since they are not protein bound or metabolized, the excretion closely follows that of creatinine. Aminoglycosides are reabsorbed and accumulate in the renal tubules. Because the drugs have a narrow therapeutic spectrum, antibacterial levels in peripheral compartments are difficult to achieve. In persons with normal renal function, the plasma half-life is about 2 h. It increases with reduced renal function and is about 4, 9, 18, and 29 h in patients with creatinine clearances of 70, 35, 18, and 9 mL/min, respectively. Thus, it is essential to adjust the dose in proportion to the estimated or measured creatinine clearance.

Side effects and interactions: Aminoglycosides reduce glomerular filtration and may cause tubular necrosis at toxic levels. As a consequence of **nephrotoxicity,** the half-life increases during therapy; if doses are not reduced, the drug may accumulate, increasing the risk of **ototoxicity.** Nephrotoxicity is reversible in most patients; however, those who receive repeated aminoglycoside treatments may develop persistent hypokalemia. On the other hand, ototoxicity is often irreversible, and its risk increases with age. It may affect the vestibular or the cochlear branch of the eighth cranial nerve and can be unilateral or bilateral. Because renal function is reduced with age, overdosing is more difficult to avoid in the elderly. Ototoxicity is related to serum levels at the end-of-dose period, which should not exceed 2 mg/L of gentamicin, netilmicin, or tobramycin or 10 mg/L of amikacin.

In general, the use of aminoglycosides should be restricted because effective and safer alternatives are now available. *Serum concentration monitoring is strongly recommended in all patients receiving aminoglycosides but especially in the elderly.* Trough levels should be drawn within 30 min before the next dose, while peak levels should be obtained 30 min after the end of an infusion or 1 h after an IM injection. The second sample ensures that therapeutic concentrations have been achieved and may not have to be repeated during treatment. Concentration monitoring should begin on the second treatment day and should be repeated at least twice weekly.

The four most important aminoglycosides (amikacin, gentamicin, netilmicin, and tobramycin) have no clinically significant differences in risk of nephrotoxicity and ototoxicity or auditory vs. vestibular toxicity. Establishing a causal relationship between a drug and an ototoxic reaction requires a pretreatment audiogram, often difficult and impractical in an older patient with a severe systemic infection. The risk of nephrotoxicity and ototoxicity is increased in patients receiving cisplatin or methotrexate, in whom aminoglycosides should be avoided.

β–LACTAM ANTIBIOTICS

All β-lactams inhibit the final step in bacterial cell wall synthesis by binding to enzymes that catalyze the process. These drugs are bactericidal, although there may be significant differences between bacteriostatic and bactericidal concentrations. Resistance to β-lactam antibiotics is due to production of β-lactamases, to alterations of the bacterial cell wall rendering it impermeable to the drugs, or to alterations of the penicillin-binding enzymes.

PENICILLINS

Benzylpenicillin

(Penicillin G)

Penicillin G is active against gram-positive bacteria (eg, β-hemolytic and α-hemolytic streptococci and *Streptococcus pneumoniae*). The latter has become less susceptible or more resistant to penicillin during the late 1980s and early 1990s. Enterococci are less susceptible, and *Enterococcus faecium* may be resistant. Most strains of *Staphylococcus aureus* and coagulase-negative staphylococci (eg, *S. epidermidis*) are resistant. Of the gram-negative bacteria, *Neisseria meningitidis* is highly susceptible. *Hemophilus influenzae* is somewhat susceptible if it is not encapsulated (most strains infecting the elderly lack a capsule). Many gram-negative and most gram-positive anaerobes are sensitive, but *Bacteroides* spp are often resistant because they produce β-lactamase. Spirochetes (eg, *Treponema pallidum* and *Borrelia burgdorferi*) are sensitive to penicillin G.

Pharmacokinetics: Penicillin G is acid labile and should be administered parenterally. It is excreted renally, with a serum half-life of about 1 h in patients with normal renal function. Doses should be adjusted in patients with severe renal impairment (creatinine clearance < 30 mL/min).

Indications: Penicillin G is indicated in borreliosis and in infections caused by streptococci (eg, endocarditis, erysipelas, and pneumococcal pneumonia or meningitis) and meningococci. For treatment of streptococcal endocarditis, penicillin G is combined with an aminoglycoside to obtain synergistic antibacterial activity.

Side effects and interactions: Penicillin G has a high degree of safety, although hypersensitivity reactions occur in about 5% of patients. Anaphylactoid reactions are rare, especially in the elderly. All IgE-mediated reactions contraindicate further use of any penicillin. Drug fever and hematologic reactions (neutropenia, thrombocytopenia, and anemia) may occur in prolonged treatment with high doses (eg, for endocarditis). Such reactions are rapidly reversible if treatment is discontinued. Neurotoxicity may develop if patients with renal failure are given high doses.

Phenoxymethyl Penicillin
(Penicillin V)

The antibacterial spectrum and activity of penicillin V are identical to those of penicillin G. Penicillin V is acid resistant and thus can be given orally. About 50% of the dose is absorbed but is reduced by food. Penicillin V is a first-line antibiotic for oral treatment of infections caused by β-hemolytic streptococci or pneumococci.

Penicillinase-Resistant Penicillins
This group includes cloxacillin, dicloxacillin, floxacillin (not available in the USA), methicillin, nafcillin, and oxacillin. The antibacterial spectrum includes all penicillin G–susceptible organisms and penicillinase-producing staphylococci. Resistance (to methicillin) is relatively uncommon in *S. aureus* but is common in coagulase–negative staphylococci (eg, *S. epidermidis*).

Pharmacokinetics: Methicillin and nafcillin are not absorbed orally and must be given parenterally. Dicloxacillin and floxacillin are the preferred oral agents. The protein binding of oxacillin, cloxacillin, floxacillin, and dicloxacillin is > 90%, leading to slow penetration of peripheral compartments. Therapeutic concentrations cannot be achieved in CSF. The drugs are excreted renally, with a half-life ≤ 1 h. Half-life increases in renal failure, but since the drugs are also metabolized in the liver, it rarely exceeds 4 h.

Indications: These penicillins are used to treat staphylococcal infections. Because their antibacterial spectrum is otherwise similar to that of penicillin G, they are effective in treating staphylococcal and β-hemolytic streptococcal infections (eg, soft tissue infections).

Aminopenicillins: Ampicillin and Amoxicillin

These penicillins are more active than penicillin G against gram-negative aerobes (eg, *Escherichia coli, Proteus mirabilis,* and *H. influenzae*) and against enterococci. Because they are hydrolyzed by β-lactamases, penicillinase-producing staphylococci are resistant.

Pharmacokinetics: These drugs can be given orally and are excreted renally; the half-life is about 1 h. The bioavailability of amoxicillin and ester-bound ampicillin is higher (> 90%) than that of ampicillin (about 60%).

Indications: Because ≥ 15% of *E. coli* strains are resistant to ampicillin and amoxicillin, these antibiotics have limited value in treating urinary tract infections; they are indicated mainly for *H. influenzae* or enterococcal infections.

Side effects and interactions: Ampicillin and amoxicillin cause skin rashes more often than do penicillins G and V. A morbilliform rash is occasionally seen in patients with viral infections or leukemia 10 to 12 days after therapy starts. More rashes have been reported when ampicillin is combined with allopurinol. Diarrhea is common with oral ampicillin; therefore, an ampicillin ester or amoxicillin should be used.

Antipseudomonal Penicillins

Azlocillin, carbenicillin, mezlocillin, piperacillin, and ticarcillin are β-lactamase sensitive. Their antibacterial spectrums, while similar to those of ampicillin, also include gram-negative aerobes such as *Enterobacter* and *Pseudomonas* spp. The most active are azlocillin and piperacillin. All are poorly absorbed from the GI tract and must be given parenterally. The sodium salt of the indanyl ester of carbenicillin may be given orally. Pharmacokinetics are similar to those of penicillin G.

Antipseudomonal penicillins are indicated in patients with severe infections known or believed to be caused by *Pseudomonas* spp. For infections outside the urinary tract, they should be combined with an aminoglycoside to avoid emergence of resistance. Side effects are similar to those of ampicillin. Bleeding complications have been reported, especially with carbenicillin and ticarcillin, when used in high doses; in most cases, the cause seems to be platelet dysfunction. With high doses of carbenicillin, patients who have severe renal impairment may develop hypernatremia.

Combinations of Penicillins and β-Lactamase Inhibitors

Several β-lactams have very poor antibacterial activity but have a high affinity to β-lactamases and inhibit them. When these β-lactams are combined with a penicillin, the antibacterial spectrum of the penicillin expands to include β-lactamase–producing bacteria such as *S. aureus* and *Bacteroides* spp. The clinically useful β-lactamase inhibitors are clavulanic acid (combined with ampicillin or ticarcillin) and sulbactam (combined with amoxicillin). Tazobactam (not available in the USA) combined with piperacillin increases the activity of piperacillin against the above-mentioned species but not against *P. aeruginosa*.

Pharmacokinetics: The β-lactamase inhibitors have kinetics very similar to those of penicillins.

Indications and side effects: Combinations of penicillins and β-lactamase inhibitors are used in lower respiratory tract, urinary tract, and soft tissue infections that are known or suspected to be caused by β-lactamase–producing bacteria. The side effects are the same as those of penicillins, but upper GI symptoms (eg, vomiting) are more common.

CEPHALOSPORINS

Traditionally, the cephalosporins are divided into generations based on their antibacterial spectrums. This classification is largely artificial, and some derivatives fall between generations.

First-Generation Injectable Cephalosporins

First-generation cephalosporins include the older cephalosporins: cefazolin, cephradine, cephalexin, cefadroxil, cephapirin, cephaloridine, and cephalothin. They are active against gram-positive aerobes (including penicillinase-producing staphylococci but excluding enterococci) and against *Escherichia coli, Klebsiella* spp, and some *Proteus* spp. Methicillin-resistant staphylococci, enterococci, and *Listeria monocytogenes* resist these cephalosporins as well as others. All first-generation cephalosporins are sensitive to hydrolysis by cephalosporinase-type β-lactamases.

Pharmacokinetics: All first-generation cephalosporins are eliminated renally, with half-lives between 0.7 (cephalothin) and 2.0 h (cefazolin). Cephalothin is metabolized in the liver by deacetylation to about 40% active drug.

Indications: These antibiotics are indicated for community-acquired, especially gram-positive, infections. They are also given prophylactically in the perioperative period. In many countries, they have been replaced by newer, cephalosporinase-resistant derivatives.

Side effects: *Cephaloridine, no longer available in the USA, is nephrotoxic and should not be used.* The others share a high degree of safety. Hypersensitivity reactions occur less often than with penicillins. The risk of cross-reaction between cephalosporins and penicillins is about 3% to 7%, and caution is recommended in patients with a history of anaphylactoid reactions to a penicillin.

Second-Generation Injectable Cephalosporins and Cephamycins

The two most important second-generation cephalosporins are cefuroxime and cefamandole. While cefuroxime has a spectrum of activity similar to that of cefamandole, it demonstrates somewhat better resistance to β-lactamases. While the antibacterial spectrum is similar to that of first-generation agents, it includes more strains because of enhanced β-lactamase stability. Second-generation cephalosporins are also active against *Hemophilus influenzae,* but enterococci and methicillin-resistant staphylococci resist them.

The cephamycins (eg, cefoxitin, cefotetan, cefmetazole) differ from the cephalosporins in that they have a methoxy group at the seventh position in the nucleus. This moiety confers such a high degree of β-lactamase stability that the cephamycins are resistant to the β-lactamase produced by *Bacteroides fragilis, Serratia marcescens,* and *Neisseria gonorrhoeae.*

Pharmacokinetics: These antibiotics are poorly absorbed from the GI tract and must be given parenterally. They are not metabolized, and—with the exception of cefotetan, which is partly eliminated in bile—they are excreted renally. The half-life is about 1 h for second-generation cephalosporins and cefoxitin and 3.5 h for cefotetan.

Indications: Second-generation cephalosporins are used to treat community-acquired infections, especially when a mixed gram-positive and gram-negative cause is suspected or when the patient is allergic to penicillin. The main role of the cephamycins is prophylaxis in abdominal and gynecologic surgery. Cefuroxime is also used to treat bacterial meningitis.

Side effects and interactions: Cefuroxime and cefoxitin have a high degree of safety. Cefamandole, cefmetazole, and cefotetan have a 3-methylthiotetrazole side chain, which leads to hypoprothrombinemia (reversible with vitamin K), especially in the elderly. As with the penicillins, prolonged treatment with high doses of injectable cephalosporins may cause fever or hematologic reactions. In the elderly especially, diarrhea may be caused by the cytotoxin of *Clostridium difficile,* leading to colitis or pseudomembranous colitis. Hypersensitivity reactions are rare, and a cross-allergenicity with penicillins is doubtful.

Like other β-lactams, these antibiotics (especially cefoxitin) may be potent inducers of β-lactamase. Combinations of certain β-lactam agents have been found to be antagonistic, especially against *Pseudomonas aeruginosa* and *Enterobacter* spp.

Third-Generation Injectable Cephalosporins and Cephamycins

This rapidly growing group of antibiotics includes cefoperazone, cefotaxime, ceftazidime, ceftizoxime, ceftriaxone, moxalactam (latamoxef), cefmenoxime, cefpirome, and cefepime; the last three are not available in the USA. Cefoperazone and moxalactam are cephamycins; the others are cephalosporins. They are highly resistant to cephalosporinases. All are susceptible to hydrolysis by the extended-spectrum cephalosporinases found in Enterobacteriaceae, especially *Klebsiella* spp. In addition to activity against organisms covered by the second-generation cephalosporins, they are active against most strains of *Proteus, Enterobacter,* and *Serratia* spp. Ceftazidime has the highest activity against *Pseudomonas* spp, although cefpirome and cefepime also have some activity against those species. Moxalactam and cefoperazone have high activity against anaerobes, while the others show varying, generally low, activity. Gram-positive organisms other than enterococci and methicillin-resistant staphylococci are susceptible.

Pharmacokinetics: The pharmacokinetics of these antibiotics differ considerably. They are not absorbed after oral administration. Cefotaxime is metabolized by deacetylation in the liver to a considerably less active compound. Cefotaxime, cefpirome, ceftizoxime, and moxalactam are excreted only renally, with serum half-lives of 1 to 2.5 h. Cefmenoxime, cefoperazone, and ceftriaxone (the latter two are highly protein bound) are also excreted in bile, leading to high fecal concentrations of active drug. Their half-lives vary from 1.5 h for cefmenoxime to 8 h for ceftriaxone, which can be given once daily, making it particularly useful in the nursing home or home care setting.

Indications: Third-generation cephalosporins and cephamycins are indicated for nosocomial infections caused by susceptible gram-negative or gram-positive pathogens (eg, urosepsis and pneumonia). Except for ceftazidime, cefpirome, and cefepime, they should not be used when *Pseudomonas* is the verified or suspected pathogen. Cefoperazone and moxalactam may be used for infections caused by mixed aerobic-anaerobic bacteria. The efficacy of cefotaxime and ceftriaxone in bacterial meningitis caused by pathogens other than *L. monocytogenes* is well documented. Ceftriaxone's effectiveness has also been documented for treating borreliosis. Ceftazidime has been used successfully as empiric monotherapy in febrile neutropenic patients.

Side effects and interactions: Biliary-excreted derivatives tend to disturb the normal fecal flora, leading commonly to *C. difficile* cytotoxin–induced diarrhea or colitis in the elderly. Cefoperazone and moxalactam have a 3-methylthiotetrazole side chain and may cause hypoprothrombinemia, which has been reported mainly in elderly patients. Other side effects are rare.

Oral Cephalosporins

Older oral cephalosporins (eg, cefaclor, cefadroxil, cephradine, and cephalexin) and some newer ones (eg, loracarbef) have a relatively narrow antibacterial spectrum. Newer derivatives have improved antibacterial activity and can be classified as second-generation (eg, cefuroxime axetil) or third-generation (eg, cefpodoxime proxetil, ceftibuten, and cefixime) cephalosporins. NOTE: *Cefpodoxime proxetil is not available in the USA*. All second- and third-generation oral cephalosporins are highly active against *H. influenzae* and *Moraxella catarrhalis*. Cefixime and ceftibuten lack activity against staphylococci. The activity of ceftibuten against pneumococci is borderline, and none of the drugs are active against *Pseudomonas* spp.

Pharmacokinetics: These drugs are eliminated renally, and their half-lives are generally from 0.8 to 2.0 h. Some of them, especially cefuroxime axetil, are better absorbed when taken with food.

Indications: Oral cephalosporins are used mainly for treating patients with urinary tract infections and those allergic to penicillins. The second- and third-generation derivatives may also be suitable for follow-up therapy after parenteral treatment with a cephalosporin. Patients requiring suspensions for oral treatment of staphylococcal infections should be given a cephalosporin rather than penicillinase-resistant penicillins, which have a very bitter taste.

Side effects: The poorly absorbed derivatives markedly alter the normal fecal flora, possibly resulting in diarrhea that may be due to *C. difficile* cytotoxin; they may select methicillin-resistant staphylococci if used frequently in hospitalized patients. Oral cephalosporins are otherwise generally safe, with side effects that occur about as often as those seen with penicillins.

MONOBACTAMS

Monobactams are β-lactams with a simple nuclear structure. Only one, **aztreonam,** is in clinical use. It is active only against gram-negative aerobes (with activity similar to that of ceftazidime). Gram-positive organisms and anaerobes are naturally resistant, since aztreonam has no affinity for their penicillin-binding proteins.

Pharmacokinetics: Aztreonam is not absorbed orally and must be administered parenterally. It is excreted renally, with a half-life of about 2 h; the half-life is increased in patients with renal failure. About 30% of the dose is metabolized.

Indications: Aztreonam is indicated in nosocomial infections caused by gram-negative aerobes. In lower respiratory tract, skin, and soft tissue infections, it should be combined with an antibiotic active against gram-positive bacteria. An important indication for aztreonam is hypersensitivity, including anaphylactoid reactions, to other β-lactam antibiotics.

Side effects: Aztreonam's safety compares with that of an injectable, renally excreted cephalosporin lacking a 3-methylthiotetrazole side chain. No cross-allergenicity with other β-lactams has been demonstrated.

CARBAPENEMS

Carbapenems (thienamycins) are β-lactams with an exceptionally broad antibacterial spectrum. The group includes imipenem and meropenem, the latter being under development. Carbapenems are active against all bacteria except *Pseudomonas maltophilia, Streptococcus faecium,* group JK corynebacteria, methicillin-resistant staphylococci, and most strains of *P. cepacia*. Emergence of resistance (seen mainly in *P. aeruginosa*) is unique in that there is no cross-resistance with other β-lactams. Zinc-containing β-lactamases (seen mostly in *P. maltophilia*) hydrolyze carbapenems, while other β-lactamases are inactive.

Pharmacokinetics: Carbapenems have complicated pharmacokinetics. They are not absorbed from the GI tract and must be given parenterally. About 30% of the imipenem dose is metabolized; the metabolites and the parent compounds are excreted renally. In heavy metabolizers, urine concentrations are low and fall rapidly below inhibitory levels for some bacteria, mainly *Pseudomonas* and *Proteus* spp. To avoid renal metabolism and nephrotoxicity, imipenem is combined in a 1:1 ratio with cilastatin, an inhibitor of dehydropeptidase I. The half-life of both carbapenems is about 1 h.

Indications and side effects: Imipenem is indicated for treatment of infections caused by mixed aerobic-anaerobic flora (eg, intra-abdominal infections), for empiric treatment of serious nosocomial infections (eg, septicemia), and for empiric monotherapy in febrile neutropenic patients. Imipenem and cilastatin have high degrees of safety. Nausea and seizures may develop if large doses are administered rapidly. However, neurotoxicity is rare if dosage recommendations are followed.

MACROLIDES AND AZALIDES

The macrolide group of antibiotics is growing rapidly and includes, among others, clarithromycin, erythromycin, roxithromycin (not available in the USA), spiramycin, and troleandomycin. The azalide group, with azithromycin as its first member, has similar chemical properties. These antibiotics inhibit bacterial protein synthesis and are bacteriostatic.

They are all active against gram-positive bacteria (eg, streptococci, staphylococci, and *Listeria monocytogenes*), a few gram-negative aerobic species (eg, *Moraxella catarrhalis, Legionella* spp, and *Campylobacter* spp), *Mycoplasma pneumoniae,* and *Chlamydia* spp. Azithromycin is also active against genitourinary pathogens including *Chlamydia trachomatis*. Gram-negative anaerobes commonly resist both macrolides and azalides. Emergence of resistance is common in staphylococci, especially in hospital environments. Up to 40% of group A β-hemolytic streptococci are resistant to these antibiotics. Clarithromycin and azithromycin have considerable activity against atypical mycobacteria, including the *Mycobacterium avium-intracellulare* complex. Clarithromycin and roxithromycin are active against *Toxoplasma gondii*.

Pharmacokinetics: Erythromycin base is acid labile and cannot be absorbed orally unless it is enteric coated. Erythromycin salts are more acid stable. Erythromycin can also be given parenterally. Some of these antibiotics, especially azithromycin and clarithromycin, achieve very high intracellular concentrations (eg, in macrophages) and are released slowly as active drug from such cells. Macrolides and azalides are eliminated by hepatic metabolism and biliary excretion. Serum half-lives vary from 1 h to > 12 h.

Indications: In the elderly, macrolides are used mainly for treating *Mycoplasma, Chlamydia, Legionella,* and *Campylobacter* infections. In hypersensitive patients with streptococcal infections, they may replace penicillin G or V. Clarithromycin may be used with other tuberculostatic agents in patients with atypical mycobacterial infections.

Side effects and interactions: Oral macrolides and azalides frequently cause upper GI side effects (eg, nausea and vomiting). Reversible hearing defects have been reported with erythromycin, and erythromycin estolate may cause cholestatic hepatitis. Several of the newer compounds are metabolized via the cytochrome P-450 system and may therefore interact with other drugs (eg, astemizole and terfenadine) metabolized in the liver.

NITROIMIDAZOLES

The nitroimidazoles include, among others, metronidazole and tinidazole (not available in the USA). Metronidazole was developed to treat protozoal infections (trichomoniasis, giardiasis, and amebiasis) but was found to be bactericidal against obligate anaerobic bacteria (eg, *Clostridium* spp and *Bacillus fragilis*). These drugs are not active against aerobes or microaerophiles, including the so-called anaerobic streptococci (which are not obligate anaerobes). Since anaerobic infections are often mixed, nitroimidazoles should be combined with an antibiotic active against aerobes (eg, an aminoglycoside or a cephalosporin) for systemic bacterial infections. In the elderly, an important use is oral treatment of diarrhea caused by *Clostridium difficile*.

Pharmacokinetics: These drugs are rapidly and completely absorbed when given orally but can also be given rectally or parenterally. They penetrate abscesses and peripheral compartments well, including the CSF and brain. Renal elimination follows hepatic metabolism. The half-life is about 4 h for metronidazole and 12 h for tinidazole.

Side effects and interactions: Nitroimidazoles cause few serious adverse reactions. A metallic taste is common with metronidazole. Neuritis may develop with overdosage, and nausea is common at high doses. If taken with alcohol, metronidazole may provoke a disulfiram-like reaction.

Cimetidine reduces plasma clearance of metronidazole by about 30%, leading to risk of overdose. Phenobarbital can induce hepatic enzymes that metabolize metronidazole, leading to reduced levels of active drug. Metronidazole increases the effect of warfarin. If coadministered with metronidazole, disulfiram has an increased effect. These interactions are also likely to occur with tinidazole.

POLYMYXINS

Polymyxins (polymyxin B, colistin) are bactericidal polypeptide antibiotics that interact with phospholipids in the bacterial cytoplasmic membrane. The derivatives discussed here are active exclusively against gram-negative aerobes, including *Pseudomonas* spp, and resistance is uncommon.

Pharmacokinetics: Polymyxins are used only parenterally or topically. They are not metabolized and are excreted renally, with half-lives heavily dependent on renal function (4 h for polymyxin B and 3 h for colistin in patients with normal renal function). Doses must be reduced if renal function is even only slightly impaired.

Indications and side effects: Polymyxins are indicated mainly for infections caused by multiresistant strains of *Pseudomonas* spp. Polymyxins may cause neurotoxicity, nephrotoxicity, and hypersensitivity reactions, especially if doses are high. For these reasons, *use should be restricted,* especially in elderly persons, who usually have reduced renal function. Effective and safer alternatives are now available.

QUINOLONES

Quinolone antibiotics are synthetic carboxylic acids that inhibit DNA gyrase (topoisomerase II). This enzyme supercoils DNA in the bacterial chromosome and plasmids, giving quinolones a rapid bactericidal effect. The older quinolones are nonfluorinated (eg, nalidixic acid, cinoxacin, and pipemidic acid [not available in the USA]); the large and rapidly growing group of newer derivatives are fluorinated (eg, ciprofloxacin, enoxacin, lomefloxacin, norfloxacin, ofloxacin, and pefloxacin [not available in the USA]). Nonfluorinated quinolones are active only against gram-negative aerobic bacteria, excluding *Pseudomonas* spp. Fluorinated quinolones are also effective against *Pseudomonas* spp and against many gram-positive species, as well as mycoplasmas (ofloxacin) and chlamydiae (ofloxacin).

Pharmacokinetics: All quinolones are available in oral forms; ofloxacin, ciprofloxacin, and pefloxacin can also be given parenterally. They are variably metabolized. The drugs are eliminated renally and by transintestinal secretion (passing from the bloodstream to the intestinal lumen). The half-lives vary from 1.5 to > 4 h.

Indications: The older, nonfluorinated derivatives have no advantages over the fluorinated quinolones. The latter, and especially ciprofloxacin, which has the best antipseudomonal activity, offers an oral alternative for infections caused by multiresistant gram-negative aerobes, such as *P. aeruginosa.* All fluorinated derivatives can be used to treat and provide prophylaxis against urinary tract infections and enteric bacterial infections. Although they are commonly used for prophylaxis in neutropenic patients, this is likely to lead to more quinolone-resistant gram-positive organisms. Ofloxacin is currently the only quinolone documented as effective for community-acquired pneumonia caused by *H. influenzae* or *S. pneumoniae,* acute urethral syndrome, and chlamydial infections.

Side effects and interactions: All quinolones may cause nonspecific neurologic side effects, such as dizziness, headache, dimmed vision, and paresthesia, which are dose dependent, reversible, and rare after oral administration. Phototoxicity occurs with some derivatives (eg, nalidixic acid and lomefloxacin). Nausea and vomiting may occur after oral or IV administration. Arthralgia has been reported in few cases.

Nalidixic acid, which is > 90% bound to plasma protein, can displace coumarin derivatives from albumin, increasing the risk of bleeding. Fluorinated quinolones are less bound to albumin. Ciprofloxacin, pefloxacin, and especially enoxacin interact with theophylline, which may result in adverse theophylline reactions. Antacids reduce absorption of quinolones.

SULFONAMIDES AND TRIMETHOPRIM

Most bacteria (excluding enterococci) require *p*-aminobenzoic acid (PABA) to begin folic acid synthesis. Sulfonamides compete with PABA to induce a bacteriostatic effect. They are active against streptococci other than enterococci (which are naturally resistant) and some aerobic gram-negative bacilli. Trimethoprim and some other antimicrobial agents (eg, pyrimethamine) inhibit dihydrofolic acid reductase, thereby interfering with tetrahydrofolic acid synthesis. Trimethoprim is also bacteriostatic and active against gram-negative and gram-positive aerobes (including enterococci, which tend to become rapidly resistant).

When sulfonamides and trimethoprim are combined, they are often synergistic, making the combination bactericidal. The most common combination is trimethoprim and sulfamethoxazole **(TMP-SMX)** in a 1:5 ratio, which is also active against *Pneumocystis carinii*. Development of resistance to sulfonamides is common; resistance to TMP-SMX has also increased, especially in developing countries.

Pharmacokinetics: The sulfonamides are classified as those with short half-lives (≤ 8 h), those with intermediate half-lives (8 to 16 h), and those with long half-lives (> 16 h). Oral absorption and protein binding vary. Elimination is by renal excretion, and the derivatives are variably metabolized. Trimethoprim has a half-life of about 10 h.

Indications: Given their side effects (see below), the sulfonamides and TMP-SMX should be used restrictively in the elderly. Trimethoprim has a broader antibacterial spectrum than the sulfonamides, causes fewer serious side effects, and can treat or prevent urinary tract infections. TMP-SMX is indicated in acute exacerbations of chronic bronchitis and in some serious systemic infections (eg, enteric fever, paratyphoid, and *P. carinii* infections).

Side effects and interactions: Sulfonamides frequently cause skin rashes. Febrile mucocutaneous syndromes occur rarely; such reactions are, however, more common in adolescents and young adults than in the elderly. If these agents are given for > 7 days, toxic hepatitis may develop. Dose-related, generally reversible hematologic reactions (neutropenia, thrombocytopenia, pancytopenia) can occur, especially in older persons who have received high doses for ≥ 10 days. Side effects of trimethoprim alone usually are mild and reversible. Rarely a serious meningitis appears, especially in patients with Sjögren's syndrome. If used for prolonged periods, trimethoprim (alone or in TMP-SMX) may cause folic acid deficiency, preventable by administering folinic acid.

Sulfonamides may increase the activity of highly protein-bound drugs. Trimethoprim and especially TMP-SMX interact with phenytoin and coumarin derivatives, increasing the risk of toxic reactions. If combined with cyclosporine, TMP-SMX may increase its nephrotoxicity.

TETRACYCLINES

Tetracyclines are bacteriostatic and inhibit protein synthesis in aerobic and anaerobic bacteria, rickettsiae, mycoplasmas, chlamydiae, and some protozoa. The various derivatives (eg, tetracycline, chlortetracycline, oxytetracycline, methacycline, minocycline, and doxycycline) do not differ markedly in antimicrobial spectrum. Resistance is common and often plasmid mediated (ie, transferable between bacterial cells).

Pharmacokinetics: The main differences among the various tetracyclines are pharmacokinetic. All are absorbed after oral administration, doxycycline and minocycline more efficiently than the others. Penetration of peripheral compartments is good, especially for doxycycline and minocycline. The different drugs are eliminated by liver metabolism and by renal and biliary excretion (followed by enteric reabsorption) with half-lives of about 10 h for most, 15 h for minocycline, and 18 h for doxycycline. However, renal elimination is low for doxycycline and negligible for minocycline.

Indications: In elderly persons, tetracyclines are used to treat pneumonia caused by *Mycoplasma* or *Chlamydia* spp and exacerbations of chronic bronchitis. Their value in sinusitis is doubtful. They are also used to treat many skin disorders, including rosacea.

Side effects and interactions: In the elderly, the most important side effects are diarrhea, *Candida* overgrowth, and induction of resistance in the normal flora. Phototoxic reactions may also occur. Nephrotoxicity occurs rarely with older tetracyclines but not with doxycycline and minocycline. Bleeding diathesis may develop from a reduction in vitamin K–producing bacteria in the gut.

Because chelates bind to metal ions, coadministration with antacids reduces absorption of tetracyclines. Dairy products also reduce absorption of most tetracyclines. Carbamazepine, phenytoin, and barbiturates induce liver metabolism of the tetracyclines, leading to a reduced half-life. Demeclocycline can cause diabetes insipidus.

OTHER ANTIBIOTICS

Chloramphenicol

Chloramphenicol is a broad-spectrum, bacteriostatic antibiotic active against a wide range of gram-positive and gram-negative aerobic and anaerobic species. Resistance to chloramphenicol is often plasmid mediated and varies in frequency, depending on the extent of usage. In most Western countries, resistance is rare.

Pharmacokinetics: Chloramphenicol is rapidly and almost completely absorbed from the GI tract and can be administered orally or IV. It should not be administered IM because of the risk of erratic absorption. It penetrates all peripheral sites well, including CSF and brain, and is eliminated by hepatic metabolism. The half-life is 2 to 3 h.

Indications: Because of its side effects, systemic chloramphenicol is generally reserved for life-threatening infections, mainly purulent meningitis, brain abscesses, and enteric fever.

Side effects and interactions: One patient in every 5,000 to 100,000 who receive chloramphenicol develops a dose-independent aplastic anemia with pancytopenia; the mortality rate is > 50%. Though this reaction usually occurs shortly after treatment, it can occur up to 6 mo later. Reversible dose-dependent bone marrow toxicity may develop if large doses (total dose > 25 gm) are given for prolonged periods. The hematologic side effects do not occur with topical preparations (eg, ophthalmic ointment).

Chloramphenicol interacts with several other drugs. It reduces the metabolism of phenytoin. This interaction is important, since patients with intracerebral infections often receive both drugs. Chloramphenicol also inhibits the metabolism of tolbutamide, with risk of hypoglycemia, and of dicumarol, with risk of hypoprothrombinemia.

Clindamycin and Lincomycin

Clindamycin and lincomycin, collectively known as lincosamides, inhibit bacterial protein synthesis and are active against most anaerobes (including *Bacillus fragilis*) and gram-positive (not gram-negative) aerobes. The aerobic spectrum includes streptococci (not enterococci) and staphylococci. Clindamycin is also active against the protozoan *Toxoplasma gondii*.

Pharmacokinetics: Lincomycin is slowly and incompletely absorbed from the GI tract, whereas clindamycin is well absorbed. Both drugs can be administered orally or IV. Reports that lincomycin penetrates bone better than does clindamycin have not been confirmed. Both drugs are eliminated by hepatic metabolism and by biliary and renal excretion. The half-life is about 4 h for lincomycin and about 2.5 h for clindamycin.

Indications and side effects: With its superior antibacterial spectrum and pharmacokinetic properties, clindamycin should be preferred over lincomycin. It is indicated for anaerobic and staphylococcal infections and as a second-line drug for treating toxoplasmosis. Antibiotic-associated diarrhea, colitis, or pseudomembranous colitis caused by the cytotoxin of *Clostridium difficile* is relatively common, more so in elderly than in younger patients.

Ethambutol

Ethambutol is active only against species of *Mycobacterium,* mainly *M. tuberculosis* and *M. bovis*. Atypical mycobacteria (eg, *M. avium, M. intracellulare*) are resistant to ethambutol alone, but ethambutol combined with other tuberculostatic agents may have synergistic effects. Mutation to resistance is common with ethambutol, as it is with other tuberculostatic agents. Ethambutol should be combined with other tuberculostatic agents to minimize the risk of resistance.

Pharmacokinetics: Ethambutol is given orally. It penetrates the CSF, where therapeutic concentrations are achieved. It is eliminated renally and is only moderately metabolized. The half-life is about 4 h.

Side effects: Optic neuritis, usually reversible when treatment is stopped, has been reported with high doses. Patients should have baseline and monthly ophthalmologic examinations.

Nitrofurantoin

Nitrofurantoin is active against gram-negative and gram-positive urinary tract pathogens and is used primarily to treat or provide prophylaxis against bacterial cystitis. It is not indicated for renal cortical or perinephric abscesses. It is well absorbed when given orally and is not administered parenterally. It is excreted unchanged in urine, and its half-life is about 20 min. The dose should be reduced in those with renal impairment.

Side effects: Nausea and vomiting may occur; skin reactions are more common in the elderly. Toxic hepatitis may develop if high doses are given for a prolonged duration. Nitrofurantoin causes the urine to become brown, and patients should be warned about this side effect. The most severe adverse effect is the development of interstitial pulmonary infiltrates, which cause dyspnea and may result in pulmonary fibrosis if the antibiotic is not discontinued. Lung reactions, reported primarily in elderly women, are associated with high doses for > 10 days. Deaths have occurred, mainly in patients with concomitant cardiac decompensation.

Isoniazid

Isoniazid is a tuberculostatic agent active only against *M. tuberculosis* and *M. bovis*.

Pharmacokinetics: Isoniazid is rapidly absorbed after oral administration; it can also be given parenterally. It penetrates peripheral compartments well, including the CSF, and is metabolized by the liver. The rate of metabolism varies among individuals. Two genetic populations have been identified: fast acetylators, in whom the drug has a half-life of about 1 h, and slow acetylators, in whom the drug has a half-life of 2.5 to 3 h. About 35% of whites and 80% of Orientals are fast acetylators; about 50% of blacks and whites are slow acetylators. Both parent compound and metabolites are excreted renally.

Indications, side effects, and interactions: Isoniazid should generally be combined with other tuberculostatic agents (eg, rifampin, ethambutol, or pyrazinamide) to avoid emergence of resistance. Isoniazid is given alone as prophylaxis in tuberculin-positive persons at high risk of developing active tuberculosis (eg, those with renal failure, diabetes mellitus, immunosuppression). Adverse effects are dose dependent; neuritis, the most common, is preventable by administering pyridoxine. Because of the genetic differences in rate of metabolism, serum concentration monitoring should be considered.

Isoniazid interacts with several other drugs. Antacids reduce its absorption. In slow acetylators, the metabolism of phenytoin, phenobarbital, and carbamazepine may be inhibited, with subsequent drug accumulation. Isoniazid-induced hepatotoxicity is idiosyncratic, but the incidence of hepatitis increases with age. Daily alcohol consumption and alcoholic liver disease increase the risk of developing isoniazid-induced hepatitis.

Rifampin and Rifabutin

Rifampin and rifabutin (ansamycin), which is a derivative of rifampin, are bactericidal and inhibit RNA synthesis in aerobic bacteria, including mycobacteria. Rifampin is important in the treatment of tuberculosis and is combined with other tuberculostatic agents (eg, isoniazid, ethambutol, pyrazinamide). Rifampin is also used for treating infections caused by methicillin-resistant staphylococci. Resistance develops rapidly. Rifabutin is more active than rifampin only against atypical mycobacteria, especially the *M. avium-intracellulare* complex. It is also approved for prophylaxis against infections with atypical mycobacteria in patients with severe immune deficiencies.

Pharmacokinetics: Rifampin and rifabutin are highly lipid soluble and are rapidly absorbed when given orally. Rifampin can also be given parenterally. Tissue penetration is good. It is eliminated by hepatic metabolism and biliary excretion of metabolites. Its half-life is about 2 h.

Side effects and interactions: The main adverse effect of rifampin is hepatotoxicity, and liver function should be monitored during therapy. Because of its hepatic metabolism, rifampin may interact with many other drugs. It may even induce enzymes that increase its own metabolism. Enzyme induction can occur when rifampin is combined with any of the following drugs: digitoxin, cyclosporine, coumarin derivatives, quinidine, theophylline, disopyramide, mexiletine, metoprolol, propranolol, verapamil, sulfasalazine, dapsone, chloramphenicol, glucocorticoids, tolbutamide, chlorpropamide, and diazepam. The same adverse effects and interactions occur with rifabutin.

Vancomycin and Teicoplanin

Vancomycin and teicoplanin are polypeptide antibiotics active against gram-positive aerobes and anaerobes, including methicillin-resistant staphylococci, enterococci, and *C. difficile*. Resistance has been reported in enterococci, but not yet in staphylococci. The drugs are not absorbed orally. They are eliminated renally, with half-lives of 2 to 4 h. Penetration of CSF is poor. The dose should be adjusted in patients with renal impairment, and serum concentration should be monitored.

These drugs are indicated for serious gram-positive infections caused by enterococci or methicillin-resistant staphylococci. Vancomycin is also given orally to treat *C. difficile*–induced diarrhea and colitis, although oral metronidazole is almost as effective, is much less expensive, and carries less risk of selecting resistant enterococci. A topical form is used to treat peritonitis in patients on chronic ambulatory peritoneal dialysis. If infused rapidly, vancomycin may cause "red-neck syndrome." Allergic reactions, mainly rashes, have been reported with both drugs. Nephrotoxicity and ototoxicity can occur with vancomycin; serum concentrations should be monitored.

ANTIFUNGAL DRUGS

The antifungal agents discussed below include amphotericin B and nystatin, flucytosine, and the imidazoles (ketoconazole and fluconazole).

AMPHOTERICIN B AND NYSTATIN

Amphotericin B and nystatin are polyene macrolides that interact with sterol metabolism in the cytoplasmic membrane of many fungi. The antifungal spectrum is wide and includes *Candida* spp, *Aspergillus fumigatus, Cryptococcus neoformans, Coccidioides immitis, Histoplasma capsulatum,* and *Blastomyces* spp. No resistance among these species has been reported.

Pharmacokinetics: Both amphotericin B and nystatin are nonabsorbable and are applied topically for treatment of and prophylaxis against *Candida* infections in the mouth, GI tract, and vagina. Amphotericin B is also given by slow IV infusion for systemic infections. It is highly protein bound, and its mode of excretion is only partly known. Doses are not reduced in patients with renal failure.

Side effects: Amphotericin B frequently causes adverse reactions. Fever, chills, and nausea are common with infusion, and the dose should be increased slowly over 3 to 5 days. Coadministration of corticosteroids or antiemetics may be necessary. Nephrotoxicity commonly develops, and renal function must be monitored in all patients. Although amphotericin B is commonly given in a bladder irrigation for treatment of candidal cystitis, this use is not approved by the FDA. Treatment is associated with minimal toxicity.

FLUCYTOSINE

Flucytosine (5-fluorocytosine) is active mainly against *Candida* spp and *C. neoformans*. When entering the fungal cell, flucytosine is deaminated to 5-fluorouracil, which disrupts RNA synthesis. Development of resistance is common, especially if the drug is used topically or in systemic doses that are too low.

Pharmacokinetics: Flucytosine is well absorbed orally and can also be infused IV. It penetrates peripheral compartments well, including the CSF. The drug is not metabolized; it is eliminated renally, with a half-life of 2.5 to 4 h. The dose should be reduced in patients with renal failure. Serum concentrations should be monitored to avoid overdosage, which increases the risk of toxicity, or underdosage, which increases the risk of resistance.

Indications and side effects: Flucytosine is indicated for systemic *Candida* infections caused by susceptible strains. In these infections, it can be given alone or combined with low doses of amphotericin B. Flucytosine is also given for cryptococcal meningitis, always combined with full doses of amphotericin B. Topical use should be avoided because of the risk of resistance. Flucytosine causes few side effects when given in recommended doses. If overdosage occurs (serum concentrations > 100 mg/L), 5-fluorouracil may be found in serum and may depress the bone marrow.

IMIDAZOLES

The imidazole (azole) group of antifungal agents includes, among others, ketoconazole and fluconazole. They inhibit ergosterol synthesis and interfere with formation of the cytoplasmic membrane in fungal cells. The effect is fungistatic. Species susceptible to imidazoles are *Candida, Cryptococcus, Coccidioides, Blastomyces, Histoplasma, Trichophyton,* and *Epidermophyton*. Resistance may occur.

Pharmacokinetics: Ketoconazole is administered topically or orally, while fluconazole also can be given parenterally. Ketoconazole's absorption from the GI tract is moderate; fluconazole's is high. Elimination is by liver metabolism, and the half-lives are 8 and 30 h for ketoconazole and fluconazole, respectively.

Indications: Imidazoles are indicated for mucocutaneous *Candida* infections, and fluconazole is also given for cryptococcal meningitis. They are used prophylactically against systemic candidiasis in immunosuppressed patients and topically for treatment of fungal nailbed infections.

Side effects and interactions: When applied topically, the imidazoles cause few adverse reactions. Systemic use may lead to hepatic toxicity, manifested in most cases by elevated liver transaminases. Endocrine disorders (eg, gynecomastia and reduced libido) have been reported with ketoconazole.

The imidazoles interact with many drugs. Cimetidine, ranitidine, and antacids reduce the absorption of ketoconazole. Severe interactions have been described between cyclosporine and ketoconazole; in transplant patients, the blood levels of cyclosporine increased twentyfold, resulting in nephrotoxicity when the two drugs were given together. Metabolic interactions can occur between ketoconazole and rifampin, isoniazid, and methylprednisolone, resulting in increased metabolism of the first two and decreased metabolism of the last. Fluconazole inhibits the metabolism of tolbutamide, warfarin, cyclosporine, and phenytoin.

ANTIVIRAL DRUGS

The antiviral drugs discussed below include acyclovir, amantadine, rimantadine, foscarnet, and ganciclovir. Zidovudine is discussed in Ch. 87.

ACYCLOVIR

Acyclovir acts specifically on herpes simplex virus and varicella zoster virus. Other herpesviruses lack the specific thymidine kinase that activates acyclovir and are naturally resistant to it. Resistance also occurs in herpes simplex virus and may present a clinical problem in severely immunocompromised patients (eg, those with AIDS).

Pharmacokinetics: Acyclovir can be given orally or IV. It penetrates peripheral compartments well, including CSF and the brain. It is not metabolized and is excreted renally, with a half-life of about 3 h.

Indications: Acyclovir is indicated for prophylaxis against and early (within 48 h of symptom onset) treatment of infections caused by herpes simplex and varicella zoster viruses. It is given IV for treatment of severe infections (eg, herpes simplex virus encephalitis and disseminated herpes zoster). Higher doses are required for varicella zoster virus infections.

Side effects: When given orally, acyclovir causes few adverse reactions; when given IV, it may cause thrombophlebitis. If infusions are rapid, BUN and serum creatinine levels may increase markedly.

AMANTADINE AND RIMANTADINE

These synthetic amines inhibit the uncoating of influenza A virus nucleic acid and thus viral replication. Resistance occurs in some strains. Both drugs, especially amantadine, are well absorbed and are excreted in the urine, with a half-life of 14 h for amantadine and about 30 h for rimantadine. Amantadine is not metabolized, while rimantadine undergoes hepatic metabolism.

These agents are indicated for prophylaxis against and *early* (within 24 h of symptom onset) treatment of influenza A infections in elderly patients, especially those with underlying diseases (eg, severe cardiac decompensation and lung disorders) that may worsen the course of an influenza A infection. Amantadine prophylaxis should be considered when influenza A outbreaks occur in nursing homes and other institutions (see Ch. 47). Amantadine may cause neurotoxicity, especially neuritis and, rarely, seizures. Both drugs have anticholinergic effects.

FOSCARNET

Foscarnet inhibits the virus-encoded DNA polymerase in herpesviruses (eg, herpes simplex virus, varicella zoster virus, Epstein-Barr virus, and cytomegalovirus) and human immunodeficiency virus (HIV). The exact mode of action is unknown.

Pharmacokinetics: Foscarnet is not absorbed orally and must be infused IV. It achieves therapeutic concentrations in CSF and probably also in the brain. Elimination is by renal excretion, with a half-life of 1 to 8 days.

Indications: Foscarnet is indicated mainly for systemic cytomegalovirus infections (eg, retinitis and esophagitis). It is also a second-line drug for HIV infections.

Side effects and interactions: Foscarnet is nephrotoxic, and about 50% of patients develop increased serum creatinine and BUN levels.

Increased serum calcium is common. Nephrotoxic drugs (eg, aminoglycosides and cyclosporine) may potentiate the nephrotoxicity of foscarnet.

GANCICLOVIR

Ganciclovir is a nucleoside analog that inhibits viral DNA synthesis in herpesviruses, including herpes simplex virus, varicella zoster virus, cytomegalovirus, and Epstein-Barr virus. It is indicated for severe cytomegalovirus infections (eg, retinitis and esophagitis).

Pharmacokinetics: Ganciclovir is not absorbed when administered orally and must be given IV. It is well distributed and achieves therapeutic concentrations in CSF and the brain. Elimination is by metabolism and renal excretion, with a half-life of 2 to 6 h. Doses need not be reduced in patients with renal impairment, since such patients metabolize ganciclovir faster.

Side effects and interactions: Ganciclovir depresses the bone marrow and may cause anemia, neutropenia, or thrombocytopenia. Fever is common during ganciclovir treatment. Drugs that reduce renal excretion (eg, probenecid) may increase ganciclovir's elimination time.

87. HUMAN IMMUNODEFICIENCY VIRUS INFECTION

Human immunodeficiency virus **(HIV)** is a retrovirus responsible for the acquired immunodeficiency syndrome **(AIDS).** Retroviruses contain an enzyme called reverse transcriptase that converts viral RNA into a proviral DNA copy that becomes integrated into the host cell DNA. HIV infects a major subset of T cells defined phenotypically by the T4 or CD4 transmembrane glycoprotein and functionally as helper/inducer cells. Much of the immune system dysfunction in AIDS appears to be explained by the loss of these critically important helper T cells. As a result of the loss, HIV-infected patients are vulnerable to life-threatening opportunistic infections such as *Pneumocystis carinii* pneumonia, cryptococcal meningitis, candidiasis, cytomegalovirus infection, and encephalitis.

Epidemiology

Few epidemiologic data exist regarding the incidence of HIV infection in older populations. A rough estimate is that 10% of AIDS cases occur in those ≥ 50 yr old and that 4% of cases occur in those > 70 yr old.

Greater attention needs to be paid to the risks of HIV transmission and how to disseminate information on prevention to middle-aged and elderly persons. Despite a dramatic decrease in the incidence of transfusion-related HIV transmission, the blood screening process is not foolproof. Heterosexual transmission, which is bidirectional (men can infect women and women can infect men) during intercourse, is increasingly common worldwide. However, homosexual and bisexual men constitute the largest group of AIDS cases among older persons. Most older people remain sexually active, yet little is known about their sexual behavior. Elderly persons trying to begin new relationships must now contend with AIDS along with the many other psychologic and social barriers facing them (see Ch. 68).

AIDS poses a profound challenge to long-term care facilities and home care agencies. Geriatricians face a complex array of clinical problems when caring for older AIDS patients. In addition, nursing homes and other long-term care facilities are confronting the challenges of caring for younger AIDS patients because many younger patients have no other options for care. Geriatricians will be looked to for leadership as these facilities cope with this new patient population and its attendant needs.

Diagnosis

Early diagnosis of HIV infection allows treatment that may delay progression of AIDS. However, detection of HIV-related illnesses may be delayed in the older patient if symptoms are vague and are attributed to diseases that are common in old age. Such may be the case especially when fatigue, weight loss, low-grade fevers, and diarrhea are the initial complaints. Other unexplained clinical or laboratory findings (such as decreases in white blood cell counts, anemia, recurrent fever, or unusually rapidly progressive dementia) or therapeutic failures (such as in treating presumed bacterial pneumonia) also necessitate having an extended differential diagnosis that includes AIDS.

The standard serologic tests used to detect antibodies to HIV include the enzyme-linked immunosorbent assay (ELISA) and the Western blot test. HIV antigenemia may occur for weeks or months before HIV antibodies become detectable. The p24 antigen is a marker for viral replication and may be present in the early stages of infection. Polymerase chain reaction is a highly sensitive gene amplification technique that may be clinically useful in identifying patients with latent infection or no detectable antibody to HIV.

Serologic testing for HIV antibodies may be warranted in the workup of newly demented patients who have risk factors for HIV infection or whose dementia has a rapid or atypical clinical course. It may also be warranted in the evaluation of elderly persons who develop Kaposi's sarcoma. Kaposi's sarcoma can occur in elderly persons without HIV infection, but the disease progresses very slowly and is virtually never a cause of death (see Kaposi's Sarcoma under TUMORS in Ch. 101).

Pneumocystis carinii pneumonia (in 57% of cases) and candidal esophagitis (in 15% of cases) predominate as AIDS-defining diagnoses in the elderly, as they do in younger populations. When atypical pneumonia occurs in elderly persons at risk for HIV infection, pneumocystis pneumonia should be considered. The clinical manifestations of cryptococcal meningitis may be quite subtle with few, if any, symptoms. Headache and lethargy may be the only complaints, and meningeal signs are found in < 1/3 of patients.

Clinicians too often avoid taking a sexual history when interviewing elderly patients. Yet, the sexual history helps define those at highest risk. Homosexual men, heterosexual men who frequent prostitutes, and heterosexual men and women with multiple sexual partners should be considered candidates for HIV screening. Additionally, elders who use illicit IV drugs should undergo screening.

Prognosis and Treatment

Elderly patients with HIV infection progress more rapidly to symptomatic disease and have poorer survival rates than do younger patients. After the diagnosis of AIDS, the median survival of older people (> 59 yr) is 6 mo (30% have a 1-yr survival).

The prophylaxis and treatment of HIV-related disease are in flux. A multidisciplinary care approach is recommended for managing the myriad medical, psychosocial, and functional problems faced by the elderly AIDS patient.

Zidovudine (AZT) is currently the drug most widely used to treat HIV infection. It is a nucleoside analog with a high affinity for the reverse transcriptase in HIV, which leads to inhibition of the synthesis of the DNA copy of the HIV RNA genome. Resistance to zidovudine emerges regularly after 20 to 50 wk of treatment. Other HIV-active nucleoside analogs (eg, **dideoxyinosine** and **dideoxycytidine**) can then be used.

Zidovudine often causes dose-dependent bone marrow toxicity (eg, anemia, thrombocytopenia, or neutropenia). Current recommendations do not include altering doses in elderly persons whose renal function is normal for their age. Early in treatment, headache and nausea are common. In general, drugs for HIV-related disease carry greater risks of toxicity in older patients.

In AIDS patients with cryptococcal meningitis, initial therapy should consist of amphotericin B for about 2 wk; whether flucytosine should be added during this initial 2-wk period is under study. For patients who improve, therapy can then be changed to fluconazole 400 mg/day to complete a 10-wk course. Lifelong therapy consisting of fluconazole 200 mg/day is necessary to prevent relapse.

§3. ORGAN SYSTEMS: NEUROLOGIC DISORDERS

88. NORMAL AGING AND PATTERNS OF NEUROLOGIC DISEASE

Neurologic diseases encountered in old age fall into three categories. First are those that occur nearly exclusively in the elderly—the degenerative and cerebrovascular disorders. Degenerative disorders encompass those in which the cause is unknown; some diseases (eg, familial Alzheimer's disease) may be classified differently as more is learned about them. Second are disorders that occur at any age but have different implications, manifestations, treatment, and prognosis in the elderly. For example, seizures occurring for the first time in the elderly are more likely than those occurring in the young to be the result of some identifiable structural abnormality. Third are diseases that more typically occur in younger persons such as muscular dystrophy, demyelinating disease, and migraine. When they occur in late life, the cause may be unusual or the diagnosis may be incorrect.

Neurologic disorders are common in the elderly. The most serious, usually stroke or dementia, account for more than half of all disabilities requiring supervision in a nursing home. Acute conditions such as delirium are also common and serious, but they may be treatable. Yet, even less severe and potentially treatable neurologic conditions, such as movement disorders, are burdensome for the elderly and their caregivers. Neurologic diseases often rob elders of independence, productivity, drive, and personality.

New modes of therapy can successfully prevent or ameliorate some neurologic disorders. The incidence of cerebrovascular disease has decreased markedly in the USA, largely because of detection and treatment of hypertension. Advances in the treatment of Parkinson's disease have helped tens of thousands of people. The second most common type of dementia in the elderly, vascular (multi-infarct) dementia, is now more easily detectable with new imaging techniques, and this dementia may be prevented or ameliorated with appropriate treatment of hypertension and diabetes.

Noninvasive means of visualizing the nervous system are providing more knowledge about many neurologic diseases, and advances in research techniques have been applied extensively to diseases of the nervous system. For example, advances in molecular biology have been used to identify sites on three chromosomes associated with familial Alzheimer's disease. Genetic mutations that result in overproduction of amyloid, which may be a factor in Alzheimer's disease, have also been identified. Other so-called degenerative diseases afflicting the elderly (eg, motor neuronal disorders, Huntington's chorea, spinocerebellar degeneration) are now clearly established as genetic disorders.

AGING AND THE NERVOUS SYSTEM

Unlike cells in other organ systems, cells in the nervous system cannot reproduce. For example, damaged cells in liver, lung, or bowel may regenerate in part, but brain cells disappear if they become atrophied or injured. New cells cannot be produced, and damaged cells usually wither and die.

The number of nerve cells decreases with normal aging. In some areas (eg, brain stem nuclei) the cell loss is minimal, while in others (eg, the hippocampus) the loss is profound. Overall, brain weight gradually declines (about 10%) from the second or third decade to the age of 90. Compared with the entire intracranial contents, the area of the cerebral ventricles may enlarge on cross section three to four times from the third decade until the ninth decade. The clinical implications of these changes are difficult to judge, since brain weight and ventricular size are not well correlated with intelligence. Also, severe dementia may exist in those whose ventricular size may be normal for their age.

Other changes in the brain include deposition of the aging pigment **lipofuscin** in nerve cells, deposition of **amyloid** in blood vessels and cells, and appearance of **senile plaques** and, less frequently, **neurofibrillary tangles.** Although plaques and tangles are the hallmark of Alzheimer's disease, they also appear in the brains of older people without clinical evidence of dementia (albeit in lesser numbers). This finding has led to the idea that Alzheimer's disease is actually accelerated aging. However, the recent demonstration of genetic linkages in many patients with this disorder makes that argument less tenable.

Changes in neurotransmitter systems, particularly the dopaminergic and less so the cholinergic system, occur with aging. For example, levels of choline acetylase, cholinergic receptors, γ-aminobutyric acid, serotonin, and catecholamines are lower. While the significance of these reduced levels is not completely understood, abnormally low levels of some enzymes and neurotransmitters may be associated with functional changes (eg, low choline acetyltransferase levels in Alzheimer's disease or low dopamine levels in Parkinson's disease). Conversely, the activity of other enzymes, such as monoamine oxidase, may increase. Inhibitors of monoamine oxidase may forestall the onset of disability in patients with Parkinson's disease.

Certain properties of the brain may mitigate these adverse changes. First is a property called **redundancy,** ie, many more nerve cells exist than are needed. For example, diabetes insipidus (which arises from a lack of antidiuretic hormone) does not appear until > 85% to 90% of the nerve cells in the supraoptic and paraventricular nuclei have been destroyed. Furthermore, hydrocephalic patients who have only a thin cerebral cortical mantle may still have normal intelligence. The number of cells required for certain functions is not known, so the extent of redundancy is difficult to estimate.

Second, **compensatory mechanisms** may appear if the brain is damaged. For example, when speech centers in the dominant hemisphere are damaged, the nondominant hemisphere may compensate and speech function may gradually return. Large areas of the cerebellum may be destroyed by injury, vascular disease, or tumor, and recovery is often seen as other motor systems take over. Compensatory mechanisms are more effective in the higher centers, so that the spinal cord, for example, has less ability than the brain to compensate after injury. In addition, myelinated peripheral nerves regenerate slowly. Although few functional changes are noted in peripheral nerves with aging, conduction times do decrease.

Finally, **more plasticity at the nerve cell level** probably exists than was previously recognized. Recent studies have shown two simultaneous processes: a gradual deterioration and dying off of nerve cells, and compensatory lengthening and an increasing number of dendrites in the remaining nerve cells. Possible new connections in the dendritic tree may make up for fewer cells. This process is normal with aging, but evidence of attempts at plasticity in the dendritic tree also occur in Alzheimer's disease, perhaps a biological attempt to preserve function.

Both the negative and positive aspects of these changes are affected by external factors. Older people, particularly those with some degree of brain disease, are especially susceptible to the actions of drugs. Sleeping medications, which may be effective and safe for most people, may make an older person confused or delirious. Stress, from either medical illness or psychologic factors, can produce delirium, and depression can produce a dementia-like syndrome.

In persons who do not have brain disease, intellectual performance tends to be maintained at least into the 80s. However, performing tasks may take longer, which indicates some slowing in central processing. Verbal skills are well maintained into the 70s, as is particularly noted in the preservation of the vocabulary store. Other subtle changes in mentation occur normally, including more difficulty in learning (especially languages) and noncritical forgetfulness.

NEUROLOGIC EVALUATION

The assumption that deterioration of or changes in the nervous system are a *normal* consequence of aging is usually false. When neurologic dysfunction occurs, thorough evaluation is warranted; treatment may be needed and possible.

Nonneurologic diseases may complicate the neurologic evaluation of elderly patients. For example, a patient with hemiplegia often develops periarthritis of the shoulder, which may interfere with assessing arm strength. A patient's diminished hearing and sight may impede assessment of apraxias and neurologic causes of vision loss. Depression may confuse the mental status examination and makes diagnosing dementia difficult. A low educational level, an inability to read, or a different cultural perspective (eg, those who were born in a foreign country or whose native language is not English) may skew mental status testing (see Ch. 89). Also, few standard neurologic tests are available for evaluating the aged, partly because of a lack of interest in this population and also because of the difficulty in obtaining satisfactory control populations for testing. As a result of some large-scale longitudinal studies, normal behavior and intelligence standards are now being established for older persons.

The neurologic examination is no different for an elderly person than for any other adult. It is organized in the same orderly fashion, which every physician has developed through experience. However, certain findings, which are more common in the elderly, may confound examiners who are unfamiliar with these variations. The clinician must then decide whether to dismiss them or whether to suspect a neurologic lesion. The following are some of the variations seen with aging.

The **pupil** of the eye is often small in older people. The pupillary light reflex may be sluggish, and the pupillary miotic response to near vision may be diminished. Upward gaze and, to a lesser extent, downward gaze are slightly limited. The smooth pursuit movements in tracking a moving finger may appear more jerky and irregular. **Bell's phenomenon** (reflex upward movement of the eyes on closure) is absent in some elderly patients.

When checking the **motor system,** the clinician must remember that elderly people, particularly women, often appear weak on routine testing; ie, it is easy to overpower sustained contraction of the extremities. If the weakness appears to be symmetric and is not troublesome to the patient, then it is most likely normal. **Tone,** measured by flexing and extending the arm at the elbow, may be increased slightly, but arm movements should not be jerky or demonstrate cogwheel rigidity. Greatly increased tone may be an early sign of parkinsonism. **Motor reaction time** decreases with age, partly because of slower conduction of signals along the peripheral nerves. A reduction in motor coordination is due to changes in central mechanisms.

Except for the Achilles tendon jerk, which may be diminished or absent in the elderly, the **muscle stretch reflexes** (deep tendon reflexes) usually show no changes with aging. The change in the Achilles tendon response is likely the result of less elasticity in the tendon coupled with slowed nerve conduction. **Muscle atrophy,** or at least the loss of muscle bulk, is normal in the elderly unless accompanied by loss of function. The small muscles in the hand are particularly affected.

The **sensory examination** is usually within normal limits. However, a loss of vibratory sensation below the knees is common and is usually not accompanied by loss of proprioception, as tested by perception of joint position. Loss of vibratory sensation has been attributed to small-vessel changes in the posterior column of the spinal cord. However, joint position sense, which presumably uses a similar pathway, is preserved.

In many elderly persons, **gait** is short-stepped and guarded, and it has been characterized as being like walking on a slippery floor. This is likely due to a combination of factors such as slight sensory loss, mild midline cerebellar atrophy, and a decreased ability to rapidly integrate the efferent and afferent functions of the postural system because of nerve cell loss.

Pathologic reflexes such as a snout reflex, palmomental reflex, and Babinski's reflex are not normal in aging. Babinski's reflex is usually caused by cervical cord compression from arthritic changes; often it is not accompanied by other signs.

Signs elicited at the neurologic examination must be considered in light of the patient's age, history, and other findings. Any finding that is symmetric and is unaccompanied by other neurologic signs or complaints should be recorded but considered a variant of aging. Patients should be reevaluated periodically to note changes, development of asymmetry, or new complaints.

89. MENTAL STATUS EXAMINATION

The part of the medical examination that assesses the appearance, speech, mood, fears, perceptions and beliefs, and cognitive state of patients.

Cognitive impairment and psychiatric symptoms are relatively common in the elderly. Recognizing them is important because they are often curable or treatable. In addition, mental status assessment may be needed for elderly patients to establish their legal competence for making a will, for giving informed consent for procedures, or for managing their own care. A change in mental status may indicate acute medical illness.

Unlike the medical history that addresses distressing mental experiences or behaviors that occurred in the past, the mental status examination assesses the patient's mental capacity at the time of the evaluation. The medical history and the manner in which it is recounted can give clues to current mental status, but an examination is needed to determine and document it.

Quantified versions of the mental status examination can be used in screening for cognitive or emotional disorders of elderly persons in the community or in clinics and for assessing response to treatment. Even in its quantified versions, the mental status examination—like the physical examination—does not provide a diagnosis. Diagnosing requires integrating all information including the history, physical and mental status examinations, and laboratory tests.

CLINICAL ASSESSMENT

Approach to the Patient

The mental status examination begins by explaining why the evaluation is needed and by requesting the patient's permission and cooperation. For example, say: "I would like to ask you some questions about your feelings, your thinking, and your memory, as a routine part of the examination. Is that all right with you?"

The examination is conducted supportively, but direct questions must be asked to elicit specific information. For example, when inquiring about hallucinations, ask: "Do you hear voices?" The examiner's response to the patient's description of abnormal mental phenomena should be calmly sympathetic but not surprised or disbelieving: "That must have been frightening for you." If the patient's reply is ambiguous or positive, further questioning is needed to determine whether the phenomenon is really present. If a patient reports hearing voices, continue: "Do you hear them when you don't see the person who is talking? Do you hear them through your ears or are they in your thoughts? Do you hear them as clearly as you hear me now?"

Similarly, the cognitive examination should be conducted sympathetically. Incorrect responses should not be pointed out or corrected. If the patient cannot answer, go on to the next question after being sure that the question was heard and attended to. This avoids emotional responses to failure, catastrophic reactions that in themselves can worsen cognitive performance.

Always begin the examination by observing the patient's appearance and attention. If the patient's responsiveness or facial expression suggests possible cognitive impairment (either dementia or delirium), begin by examining the cognitive state (see below). Otherwise, proceed with the examination in the following order.

Appearance and Attention

Observe the patient's clothing and grooming for signs of social neglect or inability to dress, perhaps because of apraxia. Look for hearing aids and glasses, and ascertain that the patient hears and sees well enough to respond to the requirements of examination. Note any gait disturbance as the patient walks to the examining room; a patient in bed should be gotten up to walk if possible. Observe facial expression, responsiveness, and attentiveness.

Attention is *the capacity to focus and sustain perception.* Patients may report an inability to concentrate on reading and calculating. Attention can be evaluated by asking the patient to subtract 7 from 100 and to keep subtracting 7 from the remainder. Persons with little education can be asked to count backward from 20 or to recite the months of the year backward. The capacity to *shift* attention can be assessed by asking the patient to count to 10, then say the alphabet from A to J, and finally, to combine the two tasks—alternating between numbers and letters (1, A, 2, B, . . .).

Most cerebral diseases and metabolic disorders affect attention. Brain lesions of the frontostriatal system, parietal cortex, and basal ganglia, as well as the syndromes associated with dementia, delirium, developmental disorders, depression, mania, and schizophrenia, are associated with inattention.

Speech

Listen for whether the patient speaks rapidly, as in mania, or slowly, as in depression or dementia; whether the speech is clear or is slurred, as in dysarthria secondary to stroke or parkinsonism; and whether the patient has trouble naming objects or uses jargon, as in aphasia due to stroke or Alzheimer's disease. Early in dementia, speech may be vacuous—grammatically correct but having little content—and the patient may fail to answer questions directly.

Mood

Ask about mood: "How are your spirits?" or "How is your mood?" Also inquire about whether the patient feels depressed, hopeless, worthless, or guilty: "Do you feel that you are a good person?" or "Do you feel guilty about things you've done?" If the mood appears elevated, ascertain whether the patient is overly optimistic: "How does the future look?" or overconfident: "Do you feel you have unusual talents or abilities?" At this point, ask about mood-associated disturbances of energy, appetite, or sleep. Some elderly patients who are depressed have a sense of dread or impending doom. Some who have depressed moods also feel apathetic, and they may exhibit irritability that is not directed at anything or anyone in particular (see also Ch. 95).

Ask depressed patients directly about suicidal thoughts and intentions, since suicide rates are high, particularly in physically impaired elderly men who are living alone. The examiner need not be concerned that asking about suicide will put the thought into the patient's mind. For example, say: "Do you ever feel that life is not worth living? Have you thought of harming yourself?" If the patient reports suicidal thoughts, ask about plans: "Have you made a plan as to how you would do it?" Psychiatric referral is indicated for patients with suicidal thoughts, and immediate hospitalization is warranted for those with plans.

Depression may be associated with somatic complaints of pain and tiredness and also with panic attacks (shortness of breath, palpitations, sweating), phobias, and obsessions.

Several brief rating scales can aid in the quantified assessment of mood. For patients with normal cognition, a self-rated questionnaire such as the General Health Questionnaire can be used to assess emotional distress, including depression and anxiety. For patients with cognitive impairment, the examiner can complete the Hamilton Depression Scale (see TABLE 95–3), based on the interview with the patient.

Fears

Assess the patient for signs of **phobias,** which are *irrational fears of particular places, things, or situations, causing the person to avoid the provoking stimulus*. For example, the patient may stay at home because he fears open spaces or riding in cars. He may avoid high buildings because he fears elevators or small spaces. Many elderly women become confined to their homes because they have agoraphobia.

Perceptions and Beliefs

Evaluate the patient for abnormal perceptions and beliefs: obsessions and compulsions, delusions, and hallucinations. Obsessions and compulsions are usually seen in the elderly in association with severe depression. **Obsessions** are *recurrent, unwanted ideas* that the patient cannot resist thinking about, even though they may seem unreasonable. Common obsessions center around cleanliness or the thought that some action (eg, putting money in the bank) has been left undone. **Compulsions** are *repeated, unwanted behaviors,* such as handwashing or repeated checking. Compulsions are often a response to an obsession, but sometimes there is no clear connection. These behaviors are elicited by asking: "Do you have thoughts that keep coming to your mind? Do you have trouble getting them out of your mind? Are the thoughts reasonable, or do they sometimes seem silly? Are there things you have to do (such as wash your hands) over and over, more than you need to?"

Delusions are *false, fixed, idiosyncratic ideas*. Documenting delusions often requires interviewing a reliable informant. Delusions may be elicited by asking: "Are people treating you kindly?" or "Is anyone trying to harm you?" Delusions of harm, harassment, or food poisoning may be seen in schizophrenia with onset in late life, sometimes referred to as paraphrenia. Depressed persons may have delusions of poverty or fatal illness. They may believe that their bad behavior will result in harm to others. Patients with dementia may have delusions of persecution (eg, believing that someone is stealing from them) or delusions of misidentification (eg, believing that their family members are strangers or that persons long dead are alive). Delusions should be distinguished from overvalued ideas (emotionally laden preoccupations or hobbies that override other activities or concerns) and from culturally determined suspicions or religious beliefs.

Hallucinations are *false visual, auditory, olfactory, or tactile perceptions*. Hallucinations are elicited by asking: "Do you see (hear, smell, feel) things that other people do not? Are there voices around you? Is there one voice or more than one? What do they say?" Hallucinations, particularly visual and tactile ones, are prominent in delirium. Auditory hallucinations may occur in dementia and late-life schizophrenia. Simple hallucinations, such as hearing one's name called, may occur in late-life depression.

Cognitive State

Evaluate the patient's **cognition,** or *capacity to think and understand the world*. Cognition is related to intelligence; it also depends on alertness and is impaired by drowsiness, stupor, coma, depression, or brain diseases such as Alzheimer's disease or stroke. The clinical assessment of cognition should include evaluating attention, memory, and language functions (see below).

QUANTITATIVE ASSESSMENT

A quantified measurement of cognition ensures a systematic, standardized assessment and allows monitoring of the patient's progress over time. Serial measurements should be carried out in any elderly patient being treated with medications, since many drugs can cause delirium or subtle changes in cognition. Quantified measurements are also useful for screening community or clinic populations for cognitive impairment.

The Mini–Mental State Examination (**MMSE**—see FIG. 89–1) can be used as a screening test or as a diagnostic aid in the clinical examination. The items of the MMSE were selected to sample important cognitive domains. A physician uses the tool not to make a specific diagnosis but rather to document general cognitive impairment, which needs further evaluation. The MMSE is a valid screening tool for cognitive disorders in community and hospital settings. Scores lower than 24 out of a possible 30 suggest delirium or dementia and can also reflect severe depression. However, some persons with no diagnosable cognitive or emotional disorder have low scores. In general, such persons have less education, are in poorer physical health, and are taking more medications than those with higher scores. Race and sex do not appear to influence scores.

The components of the MMSE include orientation, registration, attention and calculation, recall, and language. Attention is affected in persons with delirium, depression, or subcortical disorders, as well as in those with Alzheimer's disease. Although memory is affected in many of the over-85 population, normally even the oldest old should be able to recall at least two of three objects. Those who complain of memory loss but are able to recall three objects should be evaluated for depression.

Language function is briefly surveyed by requiring the person to name objects, repeat a phrase, follow an oral command, and read and write a sentence. These functions are affected by focal disease of the left hemisphere, as may occur in stroke or when the left hemisphere is affected by Alzheimer's disease. The capacity to perform learned motor functions, or praxis, is evaluated by asking the patient to draw pentagons. Apraxia is brought on by lesions of the parietal lobes, particularly the right lobe, which may be damaged by stroke or Alzheimer's disease.

	Score	*Points*
Orientation		
1. What is the		
Year?	_____	1
Season?	_____	1
Date?	_____	1
Day?	_____	1
Month?	_____	1
2. Where are we		
State?	_____	1
County?	_____	1
Town/city?	_____	1
Floor?	_____	1
Address/name of building?	_____	1
Registration		
3. Name three objects, taking one second to say each. Then ask the patient all three after you have said them. Repeat the answers until the patient learns all three.	_____	3
Attention and Calculation		
4. Ask for serial sevens. Give one point for each correct answer. Stop after five answers. Alternative: Spell *world* backward.	_____	5
Recall		
5. Ask for names of three objects learned in question 3. Give one point for each correct answer.	_____	3

	Score	*Points*
Language		
6. Point to a pencil and a watch. Have the patient name them as you point.	_____	2
7. Have the patient repeat "No ifs, ands, or buts."	_____	1
8. Have the patient follow a three-stage command: "Take the paper in your right hand. Fold the paper in half. Put the paper on the floor."	_____	3
9. Have the patient read and obey the following: "Close your eyes."	_____	1
10. Have the patient write a sentence of his or her own choice. (The sentence should contain a subject and an object and should make sense. Ignore spelling errors when scoring.)	_____	1
11. Enlarge the design printed below to 1 to 5 cm per side and have the patient copy it. (Give one point if all the sides and angles are preserved and if the intersecting sides form a quadrangle.)	_____	1
Total	_____	30

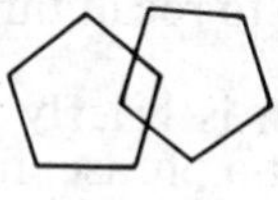

FIG. 89–1. Mini–Mental State Examination form. (Modified from Crum RM, Anthony JC, Bassett SS, Folstein MF: "Population-based norms for the mini-mental state examination by age and educational level," *Journal of the American Medical Association* 269(18):2386–2391, 1993. Copyright 1993, American Medical Association.)

Patients with cognitive disorders often suffer from behavioral abnormalities, including insomnia, anorexia, wandering, incontinence, and violence, that require physician management. These behaviors can be assessed by a number of validated scales, including the Nursing Home Behavior Problem Scale, the Psychogeriatric Dependency Rating Scale, the Sandoz Clinical Assessment–Geriatrics (SCAG), and the Nurses Observation Scale for Inpatient Evaluation (NOSIE).

Abnormalities of mental state often contribute to lack of capacity to perform tasks of daily living, make a will, or sign contracts. Although legal competency can be determined only by the court, physicians and nurses are often asked to submit evidence about mental capacities (see COMPETENCE AND DECISIONAL CAPACITY in Ch. 108). Each of these states of capacity must be examined directly, since the mental status examination can predict capacity only in extreme cases. Capacity to make clinical decisions can be assessed by the Hopkins Competency Assessment Test, but in general, standard methods for measuring capacity have not yet been developed.

90. COGNITIVE FAILURE: DELIRIUM AND DEMENTIA

(See also Chs. 9 and 89)

Syndromes that affect cognitive, physical, or behavioral functions and are associated with an acute or chronic CNS disorder.

An estimated 4 to 5 million Americans (about 2% of all ages and 15% of those over age 65) have some form and degree of cognitive failure. The most common syndrome is **dementia** and the second most common is **delirium** (sometimes called **acute confusional state**). Other forms of cognitive decline in the elderly include the **amnestic syndromes,** which are rare. All of these terms refer to dysfunction or loss of **cognitive functions,** the processes by which knowledge is acquired, retained, and used.

In the elderly, disorders that affect cognition are not only common but devastating. Because most of these disorders are chronic, irreversible, and progressive, they loom among the most terrifying diseases to the elderly and their families. Yet, not all disorders that produce cognitive impairment are irreversible, and some require prompt treatment to successfully prevent brain damage. Therefore, recognizing cognitive decline and determining its cause are essential.

Loss of cognitive function is a form of **brain failure,** and syndromes of brain failure resemble other major organ failure syndromes. When brain failure is recognized, some immediate therapeutic efforts may be instituted, but the critical task is to try to determine the cause. However, recognition of brain failure, like recognition of cardiac or pulmo-

TABLE 90–1. DIFFERENCES BETWEEN DELIRIUM AND DEMENTIA*

Delirium	*Dementia*
Rapid in onset	Develops slowly
Fluctuating course	Slowly progressive course
Potentially reversible	Not reversible
Profoundly affects attention	Profoundly affects memory
Focal cognitive deficits	Global cognitive deficits
Usually caused by systemic medical illness or drugs	Usually caused by Alzheimer's disease or lacunar infarcts
Requires immediate medical evaluation and treatment	Does not require immediate medical evaluation and treatment

* These differences generally hold true and are helpful diagnostically, but exceptions are not rare. For example, traumatic brain injury occurs suddenly but may result in severe, permanent dementia; hypothyroidism may produce the slowly progressive picture of dementia but be completely reversible with treatment.

nary failure, does not immediately indicate whether the condition is reversible or to what degree the failing organ can compensate. Thus, recovery is usually presumed possible until proved otherwise.

Traditionally, cognitive change in the elderly has been classified as delirium or dementia. Although delirium and dementia have distinct characteristics, distinguishing between them can be difficult. Because no laboratory test can reliably establish a definitive cause of cognitive failure, evaluation is usually based on the history and physical examination. A knowledge of baseline function is essential for determining the extent of change and the rate at which it has occurred.

Of greatest clinical importance is avoiding the common clinical error of mistaking delirium for dementia in a sick older patient. The evaluation of dementia can be slow and prolonged because the cause is rarely immediately life-threatening. Conversely, because delirium is usually caused by an acute illness or drug toxicity, patients worsen rapidly and are at risk for death unless they are quickly diagnosed and treated.

The differences between delirium and dementia are listed in TABLE 90–1. Delirium is rapid in onset; dementia develops slowly, although dementia caused by anoxia may occur acutely. Delirium primarily affects the ability to attend. In the early stages of dementia, memory rather than attention is affected, although attention may be severely impaired in the late stages. Because delirium is often caused by toxic or metabolic factors that impair brain cell function and because dementia is usually caused by damage or loss of brain cells, delirium is often regarded as potentially reversible and dementia as permanent. Therefore, the permanence of cognitive decline is probably the clearest way to distinguish these two conditions. Although most people with delirium recover fully, an unknown number never do. In addition, a small number of persons with dementia have a reversible cause and do recover. Thus, differentiation is not always clear, and the features of the two syndromes sometimes overlap. The diagnosis of dementia should not be applied until all appropriate treatments have been tried and several months have passed to allow for recovery.

DELIRIUM
(Acute Confusional State)

A clinical state characterized by fluctuating disturbances in cognition, mood, attention, arousal, and self-awareness, which arises acutely either without prior intellectual impairment or superimposed on chronic intellectual impairment.

The terms delirium and acute confusional state are confusing and are used differently by different experts. Some practitioners use the terms delirium and acute confusional state synonymously; others use delirium to refer to a subset of confused people who demonstrate hyperactivity. Still other clinicians use delirium to refer to full-blown confusion and the term confusional state to refer to mild disorientation (see also Ch. 9).

Criteria for the diagnosis of delirium are listed in TABLE 90–2. A person who is less alert (clouding of consciousness) and has difficulty paying attention will have difficulty accurately perceiving and interpreting data from the environment, may misinterpret factual information or have illusions, and will have difficulty acquiring or remembering new information. With difficulty receiving, perceiving, interpreting, and remembering things, the person will not reason logically, will have difficulty manipulating symbolic data (eg, performing arithmetic or explaining proverbs), will become very anxious and agitated or withdraw from the environment, will become less active and involved, and may think in paranoid and delusional ways.

Etiology

Many conditions can cause delirium. Initially, the causes can be classified as either primary brain diseases **(organic brain disease)** or diseases that occur primarily elsewhere in the body but affect the brain, usually through associated toxic or metabolic changes (such as dehydration and electrolyte disorders caused by excessive diuresis or poor

TABLE 90–2. DIAGNOSTIC CRITERIA FOR DELIRIUM

Reduced ability to maintain attention to external stimuli (eg, questions must be repeated because patient's attention wanders) and to appropriately shift attention to new external stimuli (eg, patient persists in answering previous question)

Disorganized thinking, indicated by rambling, irrelevant, or incoherent speech

At least two of the following:

1. Reduced level of consciousness (eg, difficulty staying awake during examination)
2. Perceptual disturbances (ie, misinterpretations, illusions, or hallucinations)
3. Disturbance of sleep-wake cycle, with insomnia or daytime sleepiness
4. Increased or decreased psychomotor activity
5. Disorientation to time, place, or person
6. Memory impairment (eg, inability to learn new material, such as memorizing the names of several unrelated objects to be repeated after 5 min, or to remember past events, such as history of current episode of illness)

Clinical features develop over a short period of time (usually hours to days) and tend to fluctuate during the course of a day

One of the following:

1. Evidence from the history, physical examination, or laboratory tests of a specific organic factor judged to be causally related to the disturbance
2. If no such evidence is found, an organic cause can be presumed if the disturbance cannot be explained by any nonorganic mental disorder (eg, a manic episode to explain agitation and sleep disturbance)

Modified from American Psychiatric Association: *Diagnostic and Statistical Manual of Mental Disorders,* Third Edition, Revised (DSM-III-R). Washington, DC, American Psychiatric Association, 1987, p. 103; used with permission. *Note*: The DSM-IV (1994) lists separate criteria for delirium by cause.

intake of fluids during acute illness). The causes of delirium can be further categorized as **metabolic or toxic, structural,** or **infectious.** In each case, the cerebral hemispheres or the arousal mechanisms of the reticular activating system of the brain stem become physiologically impaired.

Metabolic or toxic causes: Virtually any metabolic disorder can cause delirium in the elderly. Some of the more important metabolic and toxic causes of delirium are listed in TABLE 90–3.

TABLE 90–3. METABOLIC AND TOXIC CAUSES OF DELIRIUM

Cause	*Explanation*
Electrolyte imbalances Hyperkalemia Hypokalemia Metabolic acidosis	Nutritional deficiencies or renal or hepatic failure is often the precipitating cause
Chronic endocrine abnormalities Hypothyroidism Hyperthyroidism Hyperparathyroidism	Confusion brought on by hyperparathyroidism is often the result of hypercalcemia
Anoxia	—
Transient ischemia	—
Hypoglycemia	Confusion can often occur in a patient with poorly managed diabetes
Postictal state	—
Postconcussion	Can occur without concurrent evidence of intracranial bleeding
Drugs with anticholinergic properties Antihistamines (eg, diphenhydramine) Antiemetics Antispasmodics Tricyclic antidepressants Antipsychotics Antiparkinsonian drugs Muscle relaxants	—
Other drugs Benzodiazepines Alcohol Narcotics Other CNS depressants Digoxin Cimetidine Antihypertensives	Alcohol, narcotics, and other CNS depressants can cause confusion, particularly when used with anticholinergic drugs or benzodiazepines

Structural causes: Structural lesions that can precipitate delirium include vascular occlusion and cerebral infarction, subarachnoid hemorrhage, and cerebral hemorrhage. Primary or metastatic brain tumors, subdural hematomas, or brain abscesses may also lead to delirium. Because each cause requires a different therapeutic approach, prompt and accurate differentiation is imperative. Most structural lesions may be detected by CT or MRI, and many lesions produce focal neurologic signs observable on physical examination.

Infectious causes: Delirium caused by acute meningitis or encephalitis can often be diagnosed clinically; fever usually but not always accompanies a systemic infection (see Ch. 92). However, for treatment to succeed, antibiotic therapy and supportive measures must be instituted before the causative organism has been identified. Slower-developing embolic abscesses or opportunistic infections are more difficult to diagnose clinically and, in some cases, require brain biopsies for proper evaluation.

Infections outside the CNS can also cause delirium, especially in the frail elderly, although the reasons are not clearly understood. Pneumonia, even without impaired oxygenation; urinary tract infections; sepsis; and fever from viral infections can produce confusion. Treating the infection usually normalizes mental status, although full recovery may take weeks.

Symptoms and Signs

The clinical picture of delirium varies widely and often changes rapidly. The severity and progression of the following symptoms may vary markedly from patient to patient and in the same patient at different times, even within several minutes.

The most prominent manifestation is a clouding of consciousness accompanied by disorientation to time, place, or person. Confusion regarding day-to-day events, daily routines, and individual roles is common. The ability to pay attention is poor. Changes in personality and affect are common, with symptoms of dizziness, irritability, inappropriate behavior, fearfulness, excessive energy, or even frankly psychotic features such as hallucinations or paranoia. Some persons become quiet, withdrawn, or apathetic, whereas others become agitated or hyperactive; physical restlessness is often expressed by pacing. A person may display contradictory emotions within a short time span. Thinking becomes disorganized, and speech is often disordered, with prominent slurring, rapidity, neologisms, aphasic errors, or chaotic patterns. Normal patterns of sleeping and eating are usually grossly distorted.

Diagnosis

A rapid medical evaluation is imperative because delirium has a grave prognosis and the underlying condition is often treatable. According to some estimates, 18% of hospitalized elderly persons with delirium die, and hospitalization is twice as long for those who develop confusion as for those who do not.

If the cause is unknown, the evaluation should include a detailed history (including information from as many relatives or caregivers as possible), physical examination, and mental status examination. Family members and friends usually report that the patient's recent behavioral changes are alarming and out of character. The time course for these changes is rarely more than hours or days. Getting reliable information about the patient's baseline cognitive status is essential.

Laboratory tests should include SMA-12/60 (Sequential Multiple Analyzer) tests, CBC with differential, VDRL test, urinalysis with culture, blood cultures, thyroid function tests, and a toxicology screen. *If a CNS infection is suspected, the CSF should be examined as soon as possible.* If the cause is still undetermined, further evaluation with a chest x-ray, CT brain scan, or an electroencephalogram is indicated.

Treatment

Many symptoms are reversible when the underlying cause is identified quickly and managed properly, particularly if the cause is an infection, an iatrogenic factor, drug toxicity, or an electrolyte imbalance. Avoiding anticholinergic anesthetic adjuvants and reducing the use of psychoactives and narcotics have been shown to reduce the risk of developing delirium after surgery. Consultation with the anesthesiologist before surgery, especially for patients with underlying dementia, is critical.

In addition to specific treatment of causes, several general principles can help in management. First, fluids and nutrition should be given, since the patient often is unwilling or physically unable to maintain a balanced intake. For the patient suspected of alcohol use or withdrawal, nutrition should include multivitamins, especially thiamine. Second, the environment should be as quiet and calm as possible, preferably with low lighting but avoiding total darkness. Staff and family members should reassure the patient, reinforce orientation, and explain proceedings at every opportunity. Third, *additional drugs should be avoided unless needed to reverse the underlying condition.* However, sometimes agitation must be treated symptomatically, particularly when it threatens the well-being of the patient, a caregiver, or staff. Restraints used judiciously can help prevent the patient from pulling out IV and other lines. Restraints should be applied by someone trained in their use, released at least every 2 h to prevent injury, and discontinued as soon as possible.

Few scientific data are available to guide the choice of drugs to treat delirium. Low doses of haloperidol (as little as 0.25 mg) or thioridazine (5 mg) can help in managing the delirious geriatric patient, although larger doses (haloperidol 2 to 5 mg or thioridazine 10 to 20 mg) are often needed. Short- or intermediate-acting benzodiazepines (eg, alprazolam, triazolam) can also control agitation over the short term; these too should be used in the smallest effective dose. Whenever possible, the physician responsible for overall care, rather than one who is on call at night or on weekends, should choose and monitor drug therapy. All psychoactive medications should be reduced and then eliminated as soon as possible so that recovery can be assessed.

Despite excellent medical care, some delirious patients never fully recover. Although the exact proportion is not known, it appears to be higher than previously thought. However, cognitive status may continue to improve slowly for several months.

DEMENTIA

A deterioration of intellectual function and other cognitive skills, leading to a decline in the ability to perform activities of daily living.

Criteria for the diagnosis of dementia are given in TABLE 90–4. Although new memory retention decreases with age, other cognitive functions remain relatively intact. Therefore, dementia represents a marked change from the normal level of functioning. Dementia is a common disorder, affecting > 15% of persons > 65 yr old and as many as 50% of persons > 80 yr old. It accounts for more than half of nursing home admissions and is the condition most feared by aging adults.

Traditionally, dementia has been classified as Alzheimer's or non-Alzheimer's type. TABLE 90–5 lists the known causes of dementia.

Dementia is sometimes categorized as reversible or irreversible, according to its cause, although this complicates the distinction between dementia and delirium. Clinical criteria that distinguish delirium from dementia traditionally do not overlap—in particular, dementia is regarded as a chronic, slowly progressive, irreversible disorder and delirium is regarded as acute in onset and reversible with treatment. However, as discussed above, some overlap of the two syndromes does exist. A patient may have insidious hypothyroidism with slowly progressing symptoms of cognitive loss—a perfect picture of dementia—that may be completely reversed by thyroid replacement therapy. Conversely, a person who experiences brain anoxia from a myocardial infarction may become acutely disoriented, poorly attentive, and globally impaired but never recover. Therefore, it may be easier and perhaps more correct to categorize disorders that produce cognitive impairment from which the brain recovers as delirium and those from which the brain does not recover as dementia.

Reversible dementia is also a term commonly used to describe patients who become depressed and confused but who regain their mental competence when the depression is treated—a condition sometimes called **pseudodementia.** While depression alone may mimic dementia, the stress of being depressed together with the adverse impact of depression on the ability to concentrate and think appears to cause decompensation (failure) of cognitive function in persons who already have little cerebral reserve. The onset may be sudden or slow, the

TABLE 90–4. DIAGNOSTIC CRITERIA FOR DEMENTIA

Demonstrable evidence of impairment in short- and long-term memory. Impairment in short-term memory (inability to learn new information) may be indicated by inability to memorize the names of 3 objects and repeat them after 5 min. Long-term memory impairment (inability to remember information that was known in the past) may be indicated by inability to remember past personal information (eg, what happened yesterday, birthplace, occupation) or facts of common knowledge (eg, past presidents, well-known dates)

At least one of the following:

1. Impairment in abstract thinking, indicated by inability to find similarities and differences between related words, difficulty in defining words and concepts, and other similar tasks
2. Impaired judgment, indicated by inability to make reasonable plans to deal with interpersonal, family, or job-related problems and issues
3. Other disturbances of higher cortical function, such as aphasia (disorder of language), apraxia (inability to carry out motor activities despite intact comprehension and motor function), agnosia (failure to recognize or identify objects despite intact sensory function), and constructional difficulty (eg, inability to copy three-dimensional figures, assemble blocks, or arrange sticks in specific designs)
4. Personality change, ie, alteration or accentuation of premorbid traits

The disturbances described above significantly interfere with work or usual social activities or relationships

Signs and symptoms do not occur exclusively during the course of delirium

One of the following:

1. Evidence from the history, physical examination, or laboratory tests of a specific organic factor judged to be causally related to the disturbance
2. If no such evidence is found, an organic cause can be presumed if the disturbance cannot be explained by any nonorganic mental disorder (eg, major depression accounting for cognitive impairment)

Modified from American Psychiatric Association: *Diagnostic and Statistical Manual of Mental Disorders, Third Edition, Revised (DSM-III-R)*. Washington, DC, American Psychiatric Association, 1987, p. 107; used with permission. *Note*: The DSM-IV (1994) lists separate criteria for dementia by type or cause.

course may be fluctuating or progressive, and a patient's recovery may be full or partial. When depression and cognitive blunting appear in an older person, dementia and treatable depression usually coexist. Treatment of depression transiently improves, but does not restore, cognitive losses.

TABLE 90–5. CAUSES OF DEMENTIA

Metabolic-Toxic	*Structural*	*Infectious*
Anoxia Pernicious anemia Pellagra Folic acid deficiency Hypothyroidism Bromide intoxication Hypoglycemia Hypercalcemia associated with hyperparathyroidism Organ system failure Hepatic encephalopathy Uremic encephalopathy Respiratory encephalopathy Chronic drug-alcohol-nutritional abuse	Alzheimer's disease Vascular disease Multi-infarct dementia Binswanger's dementia Huntington's chorea Multiple sclerosis Pick's disease Cerebellar degeneration Parkinson's disease Wilson's disease Amyotrophic lateral sclerosis Progressive multifocal leukoencephalopathy Progressive supranuclear palsy Brain tumor Irradiation to frontal lobes Surgery Normal-pressure hydrocephalus Brain trauma Chronic subdural hematoma Dementia pugilistica	Neurosyphilis (general paresis) Tuberculous and fungal meningitis Viral encephalitis Human immunodeficiency virus (HIV)–related disorders Creutzfeldt-Jakob disease Gerstmann-Sträussler syndrome

ALZHEIMER'S DISEASE

(Senile Dementia of the Alzheimer Type)

A progressive neuropsychiatric disease, found sometimes in middle-aged and more often in older adults, that affects brain matter and is characterized by the inexorable loss of cognitive function as well as by affective and behavioral disturbances.

Epidemiology

Alzheimer's disease was first described in a 51-yr-old woman, in whom the disease was called presenile dementia because of her young age. Alzheimer's disease and presenile dementia have similar neuropathologic and clinical features, and the term presenile dementia has generally been abandoned.

Alzheimer's disease is a major public health issue. Four million Americans have Alzheimer's disease, at an annual cost of about $90 billion, including medical and nursing home care, social services, lost productivity, and early death. It accounts for > 50% of the dementias in the elderly. About 60% of people in long-term care facilities have Alzheimer's disease, and 20% of patients with Parkinson's disease develop it. Multi-infarct dementia and Alzheimer's disease coexist in about 15% of cases.

Alzheimer's disease is the fourth or fifth leading cause of death in Americans > 65 yr old. It is about twice as common in women as in men (perhaps because women live longer, but female sex may be a risk factor).

Etiology

Alzheimer's disease is thought to be familial (genetic) in about 20% of cases and sporadic in 80%. However, markers pointing to the locus of a gene involved in Alzheimer's disease have been found on chromosomes 14, 19, and 21 in both sporadic and familial cases. These findings support the epidemiologic observation that the disease has an autosomal dominant genetic pattern with low but variable late-life penetrance. Retrospective studies of the genetic aspects of Alzheimer's disease are difficult to undertake because family members may not have lived long enough for the disease to be expressed. As more is understood about the factors that regulate gene expression, it may be possible to postpone or prevent the disease.

The causative role of infectious agents and environmental contaminants, including slow viruses and metals (eg, aluminum), has been suspected but not yet substantiated. However, environmental factors are the focus of active investigation.

Pathogenesis

Alzheimer's disease appears to result from a degenerative process characterized by **loss of cells** from the cerebral cortex, hippocampus, and subcortical structures, including selective cell loss in the nucleus basalis of Meynert. Loss of cells in the locus ceruleus and nucleus raphis dorsalis also occurs. Cerebral glucose use is reduced in some areas of the brain (parietal lobe and temporal cortices in early-stage disease, prefrontal cortex in late-stage disease), as determined by positron emission tomography; whether this reduction precedes or follows cell death is not known. The microvasculature may also be affected, as seen in angiophilic angiopathy.

The role of **amyloid** in the pathogenesis of Alzheimer's disease is controversial. Ongoing research is trying to determine if amyloid is a toxic cause of cognitive decline or a biologic reaction and secondary phenomenon. Neuritic or **senile plaques** (composed of neurites, astrocytes, and glial cells surrounding an amyloid core) and **neurofibrillary tangles** (comprising paired helical filaments) play an important role in the pathogenesis of Alzheimer's disease. Although senile plaques and neurofibrillary tangles occur with normal aging, they are much more prevalent in persons with Alzheimer's disease.

Specific **protein abnormalities** are found in patients with Alzheimer's disease, and choline acetyltransferase is markedly reduced, which decreases the availability of acetylcholine. The levels of somatostatin, corticotropin-releasing factor, and other neurotransmitters are also significantly reduced. Thus, patients with Alzheimer's disease have multiple neurotransmitter deficiencies. Normal aging has been associated with decrements in some neurotransmitters as well as with some of the neuropathologic findings in Alzheimer's disease. Therefore, the question has arisen: is the disease the result of an acceleration of normal aging changes? Most patients with Down syndrome who live long enough develop Alzheimer's disease (usually after age 40) and exhibit the same senile plaques and neurofibrillary tangles.

Compelling data show that **apolipoprotein E4 (apoE4),** known primarily for its role in cholesterol transport, is closely associated with Alzheimer's disease. Of the other alleles or variants of apolipoprotein E, apoE2 is poorly associated with Alzheimer's disease and may actually have a protective effect against the disease; indeed, one French group speculates that apoE2 may be a marker for a longevity gene. However, apoE4 appears to mark susceptibility to the development of Alzheimer's disease. Because apoE4 binds to beta-amyloid, a protein important in the disease's development, apoE4 may play a central role in causing Alzheimer's disease as well as being a marker for it.

Symptoms and Signs

Alzheimer's disease can be subdivided according to clinical stage. *However, patients vary greatly, and disease progression often is not as orderly as the following description implies*. In addition, the disease progresses gradually; the course is not rapid or fulminating. The patient's condition steadily declines, although sometimes symptoms seem to plateau for a time.

The **early stage** is characterized by loss of recent memory, inability to learn and retain new information, language problems (especially word finding), mood swings, and personality changes. Patients may have progressive difficulty performing activities of daily living (eg, balancing their checkbook, finding their way around, or remembering where they put things). Abstract thinking or proper judgment may be diminished. Patients may respond to loss of control and memory with irritability, hostility, and agitation. Some patients may have isolated aphasia or visuospatial difficulties. Although the early stage may not compromise sociability, families may report strange behavior (eg, the patient gets lost on the way to the store or forgets the name of a recent dinner guest), accompanied by the onset of emotional lability.

A patient in the **intermediate stage** of Alzheimer's disease is completely unable to learn and recall new information. Memory of remote events is affected but not totally lost. The patient may require assistance with bathing, eating, dressing, or toileting. Behavioral disorganization may be characterized by wandering, agitation, hostility, uncooperativeness, or physical aggressiveness. At this stage, the patient has lost all sense of time and place because normal environmental and social cues are used ineffectively. Patients often get lost, sometimes to the point of being unable to find their own bedroom or bathroom. Although they remain ambulatory, they are at significant risk for falls or accidents secondary to confusion.

In the **severe or terminal stage,** a patient is unable to walk, is totally incontinent, and is unable to perform any activity of daily living. Recent and remote memory is completely lost. Patients may be unable to swallow and eat and are at risk for malnutrition, pneumonia (especially from aspiration), and pressure necrosis of the skin. Placement in a long-term care facility often becomes necessary because they are totally dependent on their caregivers. Eventually, patients become mute and cannot relate any symptoms to the physician. For this reason and because elderly patients often have no febrile or leukocytic response to infection, the clinician must rely on experience and acumen whenever a patient looks ill.

Motor or other focal neurologic features occur very late in the disease, although the incidence of seizures is increased at all stages. The **end stage** of Alzheimer's disease is coma and death, usually from infection.

Complications

Complications may be categorized as behavioral, psychiatric, and metabolic. **Behavioral complications** include hostility, agitation, wandering, and uncooperativeness (see Ch. 10). Common **psychiatric complications** include depression, anxiety, and paranoid reactions. True psychosis (paranoia, delusions, and hallucinations) probably occurs in about 10% of persons with Alzheimer's disease. In addition, perhaps 80% of family members or caregivers develop depression over time. **Metabolic problems** (eg, dehydration, infection, and drug toxicity) can worsen cognitive impairment and make management of the patient more difficult. **Other complications** include falls, incontinence, and confusion at dusk, a phenomenon known as sundowning (see SLEEP DISORDERS ASSOCIATED WITH DEMENTIA in Ch. 11). Additionally, the drugs used to treat Alzheimer's disease (especially antipsychotics for behavior disorders) can cause movement disorders, orthostatic hypotension, constipation, urinary retention, glaucoma, seizures, and worsened confusion. These complications put the patient at risk for premature institutionalization and should be treated, since many can be controlled or reversed.

Diagnosis

The diagnosis is usually based on the history, physical examination, laboratory tests, and the exclusion of other causes of dementia. Definitive diagnosis can be made only from brain tissue obtained at biopsy, which is not ordinarily performed.

The clinician should differentiate the early-stage cognitive deficit from **benign senescent forgetfulness.** Persons with benign senescent forgetfulness simply learn and recall new information slowly; if they are given extra time for such tasks, their intellectual performance is adequate. People who have this condition and who are concerned about having early Alzheimer's disease should be reassured that a decrease in learning speed and recall is part of normal aging.

The essential features of dementia are impairment of short-term and long-term memory and of abstract thinking and judgment as well as other disturbances of higher cortical function or personality change. The progression of cognitive impairment clinically confirms the diagnosis; ie, patients with Alzheimer's disease do not improve. A report from the National Institute of Neurological Disorders and Stroke and the Alzheimer's Association lists the following criteria for the probable diagnosis of Alzheimer's disease, although these criteria are tentative and subject to change: (1) dementia established by clinical examination; documented by the Mini–Mental State Examination, Blessed Dementia Scale, or a similar examination; and confirmed by neuropsychologic tests; (2) deficits in two or more areas of cognition; (3) progressive worsening of memory and other cognitive functions; (4) no disturbance of consciousness; (5) onset between ages 40 and 90 yr, most often after age 65; and (6) no systemic disorders or brain diseases that could account for the progressive deficits in memory and cognition. Before stricter diagnostic criteria were imposed, Alzheimer's disease was misdiagnosed up to 50% of the time.

The basic evaluation should include a CBC, electrolyte panel measurements, SMA-12/60 (Sequential Multiple Analyzer) tests, thyroid function tests, folate and vitamin B_{12} levels, VDRL test, and urinalysis; ECG and chest x-ray may be useful in some patients. Assessment tools such as the Hachinski Ischemic Score can be used to differentiate multi-infarct dementia from Alzheimer's disease (see NON-ALZHEIMER'S DEMENTIAS, below). A CT or MRI scan should be done when the history suggests a mass, when focal neurologic signs exist, or when the dementia is of brief duration to rule out tumors, infarcts, subdural hematoma, and normal-pressure hydrocephalus. Magnetic resonance imaging is more sensitive than CT for detecting small infarcts and mass lesions. Positron emission tomography remains primarily a research technique. A lumbar puncture is rarely needed but should be considered if a chronic infection is suspected as the cause of cognitive impairment. While no diagnostic measures for Alzheimer's disease are currently available, several potential markers (eg, apolipoprotein E4, or apoE4) are being tested. ApoE4 can be identified in the blood, making it likely that a blood test will become available to help diagnose Alzheimer's disease and identify those at risk of developing it. Also, recent data suggest that persons with Alzheimer's disease have a strong pupillary response to very dilute anticholinergic eyedrops.

A diagnosis of Alzheimer's disease should be made only when all causes of dementia have been excluded. The **differential diagnosis** of Alzheimer's disease includes multi-infarct dementia; the dementia associated with Parkinson's disease; viral diseases such as Creutzfeldt-Jakob disease and AIDS; Lyme disease; kuru; cerebral vasculitis; end-stage multiple sclerosis; progressive multifocal leukoencephalopathy;

metabolic, endocrine, and nutritional dementias (including hypothyroidism or hyperthyroidism); adverse and long-term drug reactions; dementia associated with alcoholism; and dementia pugilistica (see NON-ALZHEIMER'S DEMENTIAS, below).

Depression, the most common psychiatric problem in the elderly, closely mimics early-stage Alzheimer's disease and coexists in about 20% of cases; therefore, depression should be considered in patients who present with cognitive impairment.

Prognosis and Treatment

Cognitive decline is inevitable, but the rate of progression is unpredictable. Survival ranges from 2 to 20 yr, with an average of 7 yr.

Although Alzheimer's disease is not curable, treatment is essential, since a person's capability for self-care and adaptation depends on CNS function. The level of impairment progresses differently, and most interventions are directed at complications that can emerge quickly, resulting in failure to manage self-care, medical problems, and poor nutrition. The physician should be alert for treatable medical problems, help maintain the patient's nutrition, and monitor drug use. Minimizing disability (eg, diminished cognitive function superimposed on Alzheimer's disease by drug toxicity or coexisting treatable diseases such as heart failure or infection) is a critical component of care.

While some **drugs** that enhance cholinergic neurotransmission, such as tacrine, are somewhat helpful for some patients, their effects are rarely substantial. A trial of tacrine starting with 10 mg qid and increasing up to 40 mg qid may be considered. Liver function must be monitored. The drug can also cause blood pressure changes, vertigo, convulsions, paresthesias, conjunctivitis, pharyngitis, nervousness, and sweating. The drug should be continued for several months to assess its effectiveness.

Many drugs adversely affect the CNS, increasing confusion and lethargy. Drug-drug interactions may also produce unwanted side effects. Antidepressants, antihistamines, and antipsychotics should be avoided or prescribed judiciously, since their anticholinergic activity can worsen the symptoms of Alzheimer's disease. If an antidepressant is needed, drugs without anticholinergic activity such as trazodone, fluoxetine, or sertraline usually should be used rather than tricyclic antidepressants.

Drugs are generally unnecessary in the early stage, because behavioral disorganization has not yet occurred. **Cueing and scheduling** may help the patient maintain function. The patient's environment should be simplified, defined, and familiar; isolation and understimulation should be avoided. The environment should also be safe and secure; for example, signal systems can be installed to monitor those who tend to wander. **Other treatment** includes orientation therapy (eg, familiarization with digital clocks and calendars), exercise to reduce restlessness, occupational and music therapy, group therapy (reminiscence therapy and socialization activities), and family counseling. Persons with Alzheimer's disease should remain as active as possible; families should include them in activities but avoid those activities that cause anxiety or confusion.

Patients and family members often deny the severity or existence of cognitive deficits or become overwhelmed by them. The physician should help the family understand that although the disease is progressive in nature, many of the complicating factors can be controlled. Team members (social worker, nutritionist, nurse, home health aide, and others) can assist in providing counseling and support to patients and their caregivers. The stress of caring for a person with Alzheimer's disease can adversely affect the physical and emotional health of family members, resulting in compromised care. Day-care centers and nursing homes may provide respite for family caregivers and socialization for persons with Alzheimer's disease (see RESPITE CARE in Ch. 25). However, day care may not be possible if the patient develops paranoia, depression, or agitation that requires the use of psychoactive drugs.

Severely ill persons may require care in a nursing home, particularly a home that has a special unit for Alzheimer's patients. The patient's wishes should be clarified before he is incapacitated. Financial and legal arrangements (eg, durable power of attorney, durable power of attorney for health care) should be made in the early stage of the illness (see also Chs. 108 and 109).

NON–ALZHEIMER'S DEMENTIAS

The non-Alzheimer's dementias include multi-infarct dementia, Binswanger's dementia or subcortical arteriosclerotic encephalopathy, the dementia associated with Parkinson's disease and Huntington's disease, Pick's disease, the frontal lobe dementia syndromes, normal-pressure hydrocephalus, subdural hematoma, progressive multifocal leukoencephalopathy, the dementia associated with progressive supranuclear palsy, and the dementias associated with infections (eg, Creutzfeldt-Jakob disease, Gerstmann-Sträussler's syndrome, and the acquired immunodeficiency syndrome).

A patient with non-Alzheimer's dementia can present similarly to one with Alzheimer's disease. Sometimes, specific impairment occurs in areas of higher function, including speech (aphasia), motor activity (apraxia), interpretation of sensory input (agnosia), judgment, short-term memory, personality, and behavior. These changes may produce agitation, anxiety, depression, apathy, irritability, or superficial euphoria (see also Ch. 10).

Personal habits or interests may be altered dramatically or stopped entirely without explanation. In contrast to the cognitive and behavioral changes of Alzheimer's dementia, these changes can occur suddenly and do not necessarily progress. Gait abnormalities, seizures, incontinence, muscle abnormalities, or other medical symptoms may be part of the non-Alzheimer dementia syndrome and can occur early in the course of the illness.

Etiology and Classification

The causes of non-Alzheimer's dementia, like those of delirium, can be categorized as metabolic or toxic, structural or intrinsic, and infectious.

Metabolic or toxic causes: If not corrected, some of the metabolic or toxic causes of delirium (eg, chronic anoxia associated with severe chronic obstructive pulmonary disease) can result in dementia. The more profound acute anoxia that accompanies cardiac arrest, anesthesia accidents, or carbon monoxide poisoning can also result in permanent brain damage and dementia, occasionally with myoclonus.

Conditions resulting from nutritional and vitamin deficiencies (eg, pernicious anemia or pellagra) can cause a chronic memory disorder. Liver or kidney failure is also associated with intellectual impairments and dementia-like syndromes. A patient with full-blown hepatic or uremic encephalopathy usually presents with a change in consciousness as well as with asterixis or myoclonus, but subclinical variations of these conditions may mimic dementia. The hypercalcemia associated with hyperparathyroidism can also cause decreased intellectual performance. Severe and frequent hypoglycemia can lead to a progressive dementia, especially if the patient has brittle diabetes and a history of poorly controlled serum glucose. Less predictably, some cognitive impairment can follow major cardiac surgery (even without documented hypoxia or hypotension) or repeated bilateral electroconvulsive therapy for depression.

Structural or intrinsic cause: Most of the non-Alzheimer's dementias have structural or intrinsic causes. The most common diagnosis is **multi-infarct dementia,** the dementia associated with cerebrovascular disease (see CHRONIC CEREBROVASCULAR LESIONS in Ch. 91). In this condition, small strokes, called lacunae, destroy enough brain tissue to impair function. Multi-infarct dementia occurs more often in people with hypertension but can generally be avoided with control of blood pressure. Some degree of multi-infarct dementia is found in up to 20% of autopsies.

The symptoms of multi-infarct dementia are sometimes similar to those of Alzheimer's disease, and the two diseases may be difficult to distinguish. An assessment insstrument such as the Hachinski Ischemic Score (see TABLE 90–6) may be helpful. Early onset (age <75 yr); male sex; history of cigarette smoking, previous strokes, diabetes, heart disease, or hypertension; and the presence of focal neurologic deficits or an intermittent course of clinical progression may help differentiate multi-infarct dementia from Alzheimer's disease. The results of laboratory tests, including CT or MRI scan, also can support the

TABLE 90–6. HACHINSKI ISCHEMIC SCORE FOR MULTI–INFARCT DEMENTIA

	*Possible Score**	*Patient's Score*
1. Abrupt onset of symptoms	0 or 2	______
2. Stepwise deterioration	0 or 1	______
3. Fluctuating course	0 or 2	______
4. Nocturnal confusion	0 or 1	______
5. Relative preservation of personality	0 or 1	______
6. Depression	0 or 1	______
7. Somatic complaints	0 or 1	______
8. Emotional incontinence	0 or 1	______
9. History or presence of hypertension	0 or 1	______
10. History of strokes	0 or 2	______
11. Evidence of associated atherosclerosis	0 or 1	______
12. Focal neurologic symptoms	0 or 2	______
13. Focal neurologic signs	0 or 2	______
	Total	______
Total score (items 1–13):	7 points suggests multi-infarct or mixed dementia	
Modified score (without scoring items 3, 4, 6, 11):	4 points suggests multi-infarct or mixed dementia	

* Items 1, 3, 10, 12, and 13 are of primary importance and are weighted with 2 points. Do not assign one point to any of these categories. Score only with either 0 or full 2-point value.

Modified from Hachinski VC, Iliff LD, Phil M, et al: "Cerebral blood flow in dementia." *Archives of Neurology* 32:632–637, 1975. Copyright 1975, American Medical Association.

diagnosis of multi-infarct dementia, but no diagnostic method is foolproof. Even at autopsy, definitive diagnosis is sometimes impossible because the two diseases share some neuropathologic characteristics.

Binswanger's dementia or **subcortical arteriosclerotic encephalopathy** involves multiple infarcts in hemispheric white matter associated with severe hypertension and systemic vascular disease. Although clinically similar to multi-infarct dementia, Binswanger's dementia may be characterized by more focal neurologic symptoms associated with acute strokes and a more rapid course of deterioration.

More than 25% of patients with **Parkinson's disease** have dementia; some estimates of the incidence are as high as 80%. At autopsy, patients with Parkinson's disease may have some of the neuropathologic brain findings and many of the biochemical changes seen in patients with Alzheimer's disease. A less severe, subcortical dementia is also associated with Parkinson's disease. The diagnosis is further confusing because patients with Alzheimer's disease often demonstrate progressive symptoms of parkinsonism. The clinical diagnosis is usually based on whether the motor signs were present before or after the cognitive decline. Also, tremor is uncommon in Alzheimer's disease.

Patients with **Huntington's chorea** may also present with symptoms of dementia, but the diagnosis is usually clarified by the family history, younger age at onset, and the disease's characteristic motor abnormalities.

Pick's disease is a less common form of dementia, involving the frontal and temporal regions of the cortex. Patients have prominent apathy and memory disturbances; they may show increased carelessness, poor personal hygiene, and decreased attention span. Pick's disease is often confused with Alzheimer's disease. While the clinical presentation and CT findings in Pick's disease can be quite distinctive, absolute diagnosis is possible only at autopsy. The **Klüver-Bucy syndrome** can be seen early in the course of Pick's disease, with emotional blunting, hypersexual activity, hyperorality (bulimia and sucking and smacking of lips), and visual agnosias.

As in Pick's disease, **frontal lobe dementia syndromes** may be the result of intrinsic pathology, but these dementia syndromes may may also be caused by a primary or metastatic tumor, previous surgical manipulation, or irradiation to the brain, which results in residual intellectual damage. Repeated head trauma (as in **dementia pugilistica,** which occurs in professional fighters) can also lead to a frontal lobe dementia syndrome, but again the history aids in diagnosis.

Normal-pressure hydrocephalus is characterized by a triad of symptoms: progressive dementia, incontinence, and a gait disturbance that is sometimes described as magnetic because the feet appear to be stuck to the floor. The onset of normal-pressure hydrocephalus can be insidious. The disease is more common in men and has occasionally been associated with meningitis, subarachnoid hemorrhage, head injury, or neurosurgical interventions. It may result from scarring of arachnoid villi over convexities of the brain, which results in slowed absorption of CSF with ventricular dilatation and frontal lobe signs. The laboratory diagnosis is based on the finding of high-normal CSF pressure with brain imaging evidence of ventricular dilatation and wide cerebral sulci without widening of the subarachnoid space. The results of treatment with CSF shunting are inconsistent. The dementia is sometimes reversible, and some experts recommend a therapeutic lumbar puncture to remove about 50 mL of CSF. Gait and cognition should be monitored for several days.

Subdural hematoma can cause a change in mental status, producing coma, delirium, or a dementia syndrome. Cognitive changes may begin any time after blood begins to accumulate and can progress rapidly or slowly, according to the size and location of the hematoma. This chronic syndrome may resemble vascular dementia, with focal neurologic signs along with the cognitive changes. Removing the hematoma may restore function or prevent further losses; however, some experts believe that after hematomas have exerted pressure on the brain for long periods of time, perhaps a year or more, removing them does little to improve cognitive function.

Progressive multifocal leukoencephalopathy may be present in immunocompromised patients or in those with concurrent debilitating diseases (eg, tuberculosis, lymphoma, sarcoidosis). The dementia is usually accompanied by many systemic and CNS symptoms, including hemiparesis, ataxia, blindness, and behavioral alterations. The dementia associated with **progressive supranuclear palsy** is commonly preceded by other neurologic symptoms, eg, pseudobulbar palsy, dystonic axial rigidity, supranuclear ophthalmoplegia, and dysarthria.

Infectious causes: The most well-known infectious cause of dementia is **Creutzfeldt-Jakob disease,** in which memory deficits, electroencephalographic changes, and myoclonus are prominent. The infectious agent is a slow virus that causes a characteristic spongiform encephalopathy quite different from that of Alzheimer's disease. However, Creutzfeldt-Jakob disease may share some characteristics of the frontal lobe dementia syndromes. Patients are often apathetic, are personally unkempt, and display psychomotor retardation. Motor symptoms, incontinence, and seizures may develop later in the disease's course. The onset of illness is usually in the fifth or sixth decade. The course is more rapid than that of Alzheimer's disease and usually lasts from 6 to 24 mo.

Patients with **Gerstmann-Sträussler's syndrome,** another dementia with an infectious cause, typically present with ataxia, followed later by cognitive decline.

General paresis, once a common cause of dementia in Western societies occurring as a late sequela of syphilis, is still prevalent in developing countries. In addition to intellectual decline, tremors and pupillary changes can occur. The CSF should be tested using the fluorescent treponemal antibody (FTA) test, since the VDRL test is not adequate. A positive finding for syphilis establishes the diagnosis.

Patients with **acquired immunodeficiency syndrome** can also develop dementia. This dementia may be caused by the human immunodeficiency virus, by the virus that causes progressive multifocal leukoencephalopathy, or by a variety of other opportunistic infectious agents, including fungi, bacteria, viruses, or protozoa that can be identified at autopsy.

Diagnosis

Regardless of the cause, non-Alzheimer's dementias have no pathognomonic marker; diagnosis is made clinically. However, certain clinical features help distinguish these other forms of dementia from Alzheimer's disease. The general assessment includes many of the tests previously listed for the evaluation of delirium and Alzheimer's disease (see above).

Special attention must be paid to the possibility of a psychiatric condition. Acute or subacute cognitive failure, a common manifestation of depression in people who were previously functioning normally (especially elderly persons), may be difficult to differentiate from dementia. Depression associated with dementia (sometimes called **pseudodementia)** may make this differentiation more difficult. Neuropsychologic test batteries may help in distinguishing the various dementias but are not unequivocal. Often, only the clinical course and response to treatments (including the use of antidepressants) confirm these conditions.

Prognosis and Treatment

Dementia is usually considered irreversible, progressive, and incurable. Yet, certain conditions that cause chronic cognitive decline are treatable or at least partially reversible. Even when intellectual function cannot be restored, simple supportive measures (eg, frequent orientation reinforcement, a bright and cheerful environment, a minimum of new stimulation, and regular low-stress activities) can be of great help. If daily routines can be simplified and the caregivers' expectations reduced without the patient sensing a total loss of self-control or personal dignity, the patient may actually show some improvement.

Functioning can often be further improved by eliminating or strictly limiting drugs with CNS activity. However, antidepressants may help patients who develop clinical depression. In this case, the lowest effective dose should be used, since dementia patients appear to be particularly sensitive to the anticholinergic effects of some drugs and may react with increased confusion. No evidence exists that cholinergic-enhancing drugs benefit patients with non-Alzheimer's dementias.

Once the medical evaluation is completed and a course of treatment is established, most responsibility falls on the family; the stresses are tremendous. Although curative therapy is rarely available, the clinician can still be of great help to the families. By recognizing the early symptoms of caregiver burnout and guiding families to the appropriate social agencies, the clinician can support the family and thereby enhance the patient's overall care.

AMNESTIC SYNDROMES

A seemingly contradictory state in which a patient can perform some complex tasks learned previously but cannot remember other simple tasks or learn new material despite repeated efforts.

Etiology and Classification

Amnestic syndromes can be associated with bilateral cerebral infarctions, severe head trauma involving bilateral brain lesions, chronic or acute brain anoxia, nutritional deficiencies, encephalitis, large subdural hematomas, bilateral brain tumors, postoperative brain lesions, subarachnoid hemorrhage, status epilepticus, and certain medications. Certain areas of the limbic system are central to memory formation and retrieval, but other brain areas also play an important role. Combinations of injuries to the cerebral hemispheres, hippocampus, amygdala, thalamus, hypothalamus, or other subcortical regions can lead to any of a series of memory disturbances, including amnesia.

In **Korsakoff's psychosis,** perhaps the best known of the amnestic syndromes, recent memory is severely impaired. This disorder is often associated with chronic alcoholism, which leads to protracted thiamine deficiency and pathologic involvement of the maxillary bodies and other areas of the cerebral cortex.

Transient global amnesia is probably associated with ischemic episodes in an otherwise intellectually intact person. Functioning generally returns to normal within minutes to hours after the attack. This amnesia is different from that following a seizure, in which the electroencephalogram may show an underlying abnormality after or between episodes.

Another clinically important entity is **psychogenic amnesia,** which is associated with acute psychologic stress (eg, posttraumatic stress disorder) or with a more chronic process (eg, depression). Memory is often so impaired that the diagnosis may be confusing (ie, the amnesia may mimic pseudodementia), especially in the elderly. Depressed patients who have received a course of electroconvulsive therapy often report retrograde amnesia, even after full recovery from the depression. More commonly, mild amnesia is reported by patients taking short-acting or long-acting benzodiazepines or anticholinergic drugs (eg, scopolamine, atropine, or benztropine).

Symptoms and Signs

Memory may be lost for past events **(retrograde amnesia)** or current events **(anterograde amnesia).** Patients may attempt to camouflage their memory deficits by **confabulation,** replacing lost circumstances with imaginary ones, often formulated on the spur of the moment and replaced with yet another explanation at the next examination. When accurate details are not immediately available, the clinician may be misled by the patient's confabulation; many casual observers are also deceived by it. Because confabulation requires language and social skills, it is far more common in patients with amnesias than in those with progressive dementias, in whom other cognitive functions are more impaired or lost.

Other symptoms associated with amnesia include intrusiveness and emotional changes ranging from apathy to mild euphoria. Patients often lack insight into either their memory losses or their personality changes and may deny them when they are pointed out. Emotional symptoms and memory difficulties develop either acutely or slowly over time, depending on the underlying cause.

Diagnosis

Because an amnesia can develop acutely and herald further neurologic and intellectual damage, a rapid and thorough evaluation is indicated. The memory deficit is usually more discrete than in delirium, and usually neither clouding of consciousness nor marked impairment of attention accompanies amnesia. In addition, the amnesias commonly lack the pervasive impairments of other intellectual functions seen in the progressive dementias. Cognitive function may remain intact except for the memory deficit.

Unless the patient has an acute medical emergency, which would usually be discovered by routine examination and the laboratory evaluations outlined previously (see DELIRIUM, above), neuropsychologic tests are indicated to pinpoint the focal nature of the amnesia and to distinguish the condition from a dementia syndrome. Confabulation can be uncovered by knowledge of the patient's history or by consultation with staff or family members about a specific experience.

Prognosis and Treatment

Not all amnesias are permanent. In transient global amnesia, memory problems may last 6 to 36 h, then resolve fully without residual damage other than memory loss for the period of time encompassing the amnesia. Korsakoff's psychosis can sometimes be slowed or even partially reversed if alcohol is discontinued permanently and the nutritional deficiencies are corrected. However, amnesias associated with bilateral brain lesions or severe subarachnoid hemorrhages are rarely reversible.

As with delirium, the treatment of amnesia depends on the underlying cause. For example, for patients experiencing transient ischemic attacks, treating the associated hypertension or atherosclerosis may help prevent future episodes. Although not always immediately responsive to treatment, some amnesias resolve slowly over months or years after the underlying problem is corrected.

91. CEREBROVASCULAR DISEASE

(Stroke)

A heterogeneous category of illness that describes brain injury, usually sudden, caused by vascular disease.

Epidemiology

Stroke is the third leading cause of death in the USA and in most other industrialized countries. Each year about 500,000 Americans have a stroke and about 150,000 die. At any one time, there are about 2,000,000 stroke survivors in the USA. Stroke incidence and stroke deaths increase with age, especially after 65 (see TABLE 91–1). The prevalence of cerebrovascular disease in the USA is generally higher in men and blacks (see FIG. 91–1).

More impressive than the mortality rates are the ways in which stroke changes the survivors' quality of life. Many patients are impaired in their ability to walk, see, and feel. In some cases, they cannot speak or otherwise communicate, read, recall, or think as well as they could before the stroke. Daily functions in the workplace, home, and community may be affected.

Classification

The two major categories of stroke are brain hemorrhage and brain ischemia. **Brain hemorrhage** can be subdivided into **subarachnoid hemorrhage,** *bleeding into the spaces and spinal fluid around the brain,* and **intracerebral hemorrhage,** *bleeding directly into the brain.* These different patterns of hemorrhage have different causes, symptoms and signs, outcomes, and treatments. In intracerebral hemorrhage, bleeding injures tissue by local pressure effects; the blood destroys tissue, interrupting important brain pathways. Subarachnoid hemorrhage suddenly increases the pressure within the cranium, impairs the drainage of spinal fluid, and irritates the arteries at the base of the brain. Subarachnoid hemorrhage is less common than intracerebral hemorrhage after age 60, probably because arteriovenous malformations and saccular aneurysms are less likely to be life threatening, the dangerous ones having ruptured in younger life. Each type of hemorrhage accounts for about 10% of all strokes but for a much higher percentage of stroke deaths.

Brain ischemia, *injury to brain tissue caused by an inadequate supply of blood and nutrients,* accounts for about 80% of strokes. Ischemic strokes can be subclassified as (1) atherostenosis of the large arteries (carotid and vertebral) in the neck and within the cranium; (2) occlusions of the small penetrating arteries deep within the brain; (3) embolism arising from the heart or great vessels; and (4) general circulatory failure, or systemic hypoperfusion, caused by shock, poor cardiac output, or hypotension. These different subgroups of ischemia have varied causes, symptoms and signs, prognoses, and treatments. Penetrating artery occlusive disease, cerebral hemorrhage, and cerebral embolism

TABLE 91–1. STROKE DEATH RATES PER 100,000 POPULATION BY AGE, RACE, AND SEX IN THE USA, 1983

	Age (yr)					
Race and Sex	*35–44*	*45–54*	*55–64*	*65–74*	*75–84*	*> 84*
White	5.6	18.0	49.1	167.6	643.5	1950.9
Men	5.5	19.1	56.5	197.1	714.8	1862.9
Women	5.6	16.9	42.6	144.6	602.0	1986.5
Black	22.0	64.0	143.0	341.5	807.4	1570.7
Men	24.3	74.1	163.8	388.0	844.1	1479.4
Women	20.1	55.7	126.0	308.4	786.7	1603.1

Adapted from Caplan LR: "Stroke in African-Americans." *Stroke* 22:558–560, 1991; reproduced with permission. Copyright 1991 American Heart Association.

increase in frequency during old age, probably because of the increased prevalence of hypertension, cardiac disease, and arrhythmias (eg, atrial fibrillation) and the effects of age on the cerebral vessels.

General Principles of Evaluation

Since the 1950s, most texts and the nomenclature have emphasized the temporal features of stroke. The terms **transient ischemic attacks (TIAs), stroke in progress, reversible ischemic neurologic deficit (RIND),** and **completed stroke** describe only the time course of ischemia and not the cause. The physician needs to address the cause to develop a treatment plan.

The following questions should be answered, generally in the order suggested: Based on the classification of hemorrhage and ischemia noted above, what is the type and subtype of stroke? How severe is the brain damage? Is there tissue at risk for further damage? What is the nature and severity of the patient's neurologic signs? Can and should the patient be treated in other than just a supportive way? Are there limits to acceptable and potentially effective treatment? What personal, family, medical, social, economic, and community resources could help the patient cope with and adapt to disability?

The extent of brain damage is determined by the severity of neurologic abnormalities and the findings in brain-imaging studies. To assess the tissue at risk for further damage, the physician must know the cause

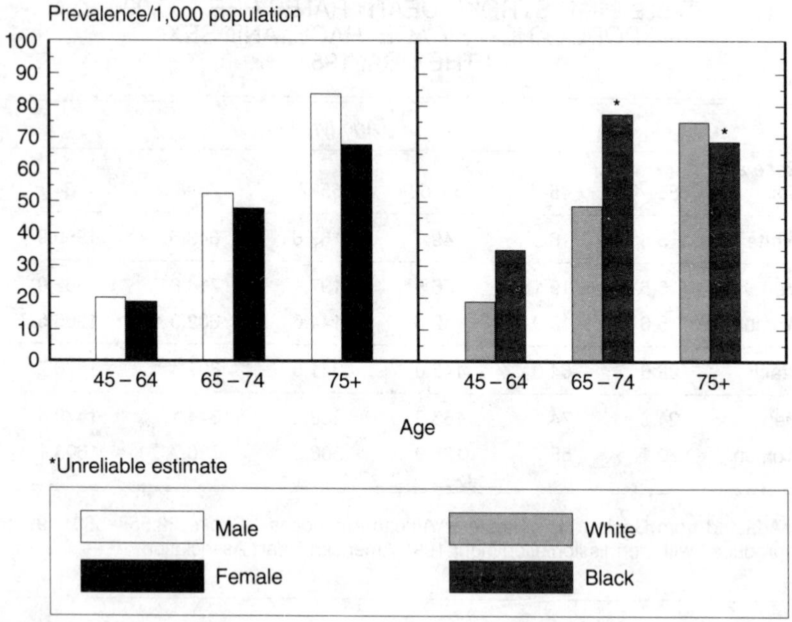

FIG. 91–1. Prevalence of cerebrovascular disease by age, sex, and race in the USA, 1987. Prevalence is higher in men than in women at any age. It is much higher in blacks than in whites up to age 75, but it may be higher in whites after age 75. (From *Morbidity and Mortality Chartbook on Cardiovascular, Lung, and Blood Diseases/1990.* National Heart, Lung, and Blood Institute, U.S. Department of Health and Human Services, 1990.)

as well as the vessels and arterial territory involved. For example, a patient with a sudden hemiparesis may have symptoms due to a tiny infarct because it occurred in the internal capsule where the total blood supply to a single penetrating lenticulostriate artery was blocked. Blockage may have been from hyaline material because of long-standing hypertension. Another patient with weakness of one arm may have an occlusion in a much larger vessel, such as the contralateral internal carotid artery in the neck. A patient with unilateral paralysis caused by penetrating artery disease is at little immediate risk of having the condition worsen, but that patient will be at risk for further penetrating artery occlusions unless the cause of the disease—hypertension—is effectively treated. A patient with carotid artery occlusion is at immediate risk of having the condition seriously worsen. Further, a patient with a peripheral cerebral hemispheric infarct caused by an embolus from a clot within a left ventricular aneurysm is in imminent danger of brain damage from further embolization to other cerebral arteries.

Prophylaxis

Preventing stroke is clearly preferred to treating it, yet preventive measures are often overlooked. Besides treating a stroke, the physician should recommend general health practices for preventing additional strokes as well as progressive vascular disease. These recommendations apply to all geriatric patients and include controlling hypertension; treating cardiac disorders, coronary artery disease, heart failure, and arrhythmias; measuring blood lipid levels and treating hyperlipidemia; forcefully admonishing the patient to stop smoking, to avoid recreational drugs (such as amphetamines, cocaine, heroin), and to use alcohol only in moderation; encouraging regular exercise; warning the patient to avoid overeating, undereating, and exhaustion; and treating hematologic problems (eg, anemia, polycythemia, and bleeding diathesis).

TIAs are a warning sign of impending stroke, and all prospective studies show dramatically increased stroke risk in patients who have had one or more TIA. Thus, detection of TIAs is essential; their presence should trigger a search for their cause. Prospective studies of patients with stenosis of the internal carotid artery in the neck, detected by noninvasive techniques, show a low rate of stroke ($< 2\%$) without preceding TIAs.

Most patients know little or nothing about the anatomy and physiology of the nervous system or the afferent and efferent connections of the brain, limbs, and senses. They attribute numbness and weakness of the limbs and dimness of vision to peripheral parts rather than to the CNS. Patients must be asked specific questions such as the following: Have you had temporary prickling or loss of feeling in your arms or legs? Have you had a temporary limp or other walking problem? Have you ever felt like you had a shade or curtain come over one of your eyes? Recent headaches can indicate occlusive disease and should be diagnostically pursued, as described later.

A TIA is not a homogeneous entity but rather a *symptom* of heterogeneous vascular, cardiac, and hematologic problems. No single treatment is effective for all, and a delay in diagnosis can be disastrous if the patient has a disabling stroke. Patients who have had TIAs should *not* simply be given an aspirin a day, but instead they should be assessed for the specific cause.

General Principles of Treatment

In some patients, a severe stroke results in an extremely poor quality of life; in some, no treatment is likely to help. Stroke patients may have other serious diseases (eg, cancer, incapacitating heart or lung disease, dementia) that affect treatment decisions. Nevertheless, all stroke patients deserve humane supportive care. Advance directives, written by the patient before the stroke, can guide the physician on what kind of support to provide (eg, hydration, nutrition, treatment of infections).

Clearly, aggressive treatment is not warranted in all cases. Certain treatments may be contraindicated (eg, anticoagulants in patients with severe hypertension or gastrointestinal bleeding), but others may be appropriate. Although some treatments (eg, anticoagulants, vascular or brain surgery) have higher risks and complication rates in the elderly, age alone is never an absolute contraindication to treatment.

Stroke is a complex disease. If expertise and technology to care for the stroke patient are not available locally, patients with potential for recovery should be transferred to a center with special facilities. Similarly, rehabilitation is best performed in special centers. Success in retraining and adapting to neurologic handicaps depends on the nature of the underlying anatomic abnormality (ie, what part of the brain is injured) rather than on the cause of the injury. Visual field defects, aphasia, spatial disorientation, paralysis, and gait ataxia all require very different rehabilitation and adjustment strategies (see STROKE REHABILITATION in Ch. 29).

Recovery depends as much, if not more, on the personal and socioeconomic circumstances of the stroke victim as on the injury itself. The patient's physical and mental health and capabilities before the stroke are important predictors of subsequent ability to cope and work toward recovery. If no one is at home to help the patient, recovery is extremely difficult. Social and economic factors also influence recovery: a patient who lives on the first floor; can drive a car or has access to a driver; has nearby shopping, recreational, and medical facilities; and can afford rehabilitation equipment and therapists is much more likely to return to an active, useful life than someone without these resources. Acute depression, which is a common complication, or a history of chronic or recurrent depression can also impede recovery.

HEMORRHAGIC STROKE

Cerebrovascular disorders caused by bleeding into brain tissue or meningeal spaces.

SUBARACHNOID HEMORRHAGE

The most common causes of subarachnoid hemorrhage are cerebral aneurysms, arteriovenous malformations, bleeding diatheses, head trauma, and amyloid angiopathy. Patients rarely develop symptoms from arteriovenous malformations later in life without having had symptoms of bleeding or epilepsy when younger. Aneurysms do occur in the elderly, but they are slightly more common in younger persons. The most common bleeding disorder leading to subarachnoid hemorrhage in the elderly is iatrogenic, a result of prescribing warfarin and other anticoagulants.

Head trauma is common in the elderly because of the increased tendency to fall. The patient is often confused or amnesic after the fall and cannot provide a clear account of the event. Thus, head injury is often not diagnosed: the physician incorrectly attributes the blood found in CSF at lumbar puncture to a spontaneous subarachnoid hemorrhage that caused the fall and confusion, rather than considering the fall to be the initial event. Such trauma victims are often needlessly subjected to angiography to seek out aneurysms.

Amyloid angiopathy is a degenerative hyalinization of the arteries in the brain and subarachnoid spaces that can cause subarachnoid and intracerebral hemorrhage. Patients often have multiple, recurrent bleeding episodes and may be demented because Alzheimer-like changes in the cortex often coexist.

Symptoms, Signs, and Diagnosis

Patients with subarachnoid hemorrhage invariably have headache. Head pain often begins suddenly, usually while the patient is physically active, and becomes severe almost immediately. The pain is usually diffuse, but at times it is most severe at the back of the head and neck and may radiate down the back in a sciatic pattern. Nausea and vomiting are common, caused by a sudden increase in intracranial pressure. Usually patients are unable to perform any activity, and they often become restless, agitated, and confused.

Unlike persons with intracerebral hemorrhage or ischemic stroke, those with subarachnoid hemorrhage are generally not paralyzed and often do not have important focal neurologic signs. Blood is usually released quickly into the subarachnoid space at arterial pressure and becomes widely dispersed around the brain and spinal cord. Thus, focal neurologic signs (eg, hemiparesis, hemisensory loss, hemianopia) are usually absent because most patients with subarachnoid hemorrhage do not have localized collections of blood within the brain. Focal signs can develop later because of vasoconstriction and delayed ischemia.

On examination, the most apparent abnormality is usually changes in level of consciousness—restlessness, delirium, sleepiness, stupor, or coma. Stiff neck, difficulty in concentration, and impairment of short-term memory and of extensor plantar reflexes are also common.

The most important **diagnostic tests** are CT, lumbar puncture, and cerebral angiography. Within the first 24 to 48 h of bleeding, unenhanced CT scans are likely to show blood as hyperdensity within the cisterns, between the cerebral gyri, and in the ventricles. Small subarachnoid hemorrhages and those occurring days before may not be visible. However, CT can also show small contusions, subdural hematomas, and skull fractures; sometimes an aneurysm can be visualized on an enhanced scan. Restlessness and agitation interfere with the patient's ability to cooperate for a cranial CT scan and thus may compromise quality.

All patients with symptomatic subarachnoid hemorrhage have grossly visible blood-stained CSF under increased pressure when lumbar puncture is performed within a few days of the hemorrhage. In patients with severe unexplained headache, a CT scan usually should be performed before lumbar puncture. However, if the patient has no focal neurologic signs or papilledema and can walk normally, a spinal tap can be safely performed without CT to exclude a subarachnoid hemorrhage or meningitis. Subarachnoid blood and vascular malformations can also be seen on MRI scans. Magnetic resonance angiography is a useful screening test for large aneurysms, but standard catheter angiography is currently the definitive test for determining location, size, and morphologic characteristics of aneurysms. When the diagnosis of subarachnoid hemorrhage is confirmed, angiography is usually delayed until the patient is relatively fit for surgery.

The most common **complications** are cardiac arrhythmias, hydrocephalus, delayed vasoconstriction (so-called spasm), and rebleeding. The hemorrhage can induce vasoconstriction of cerebral arteries beginning ≥ 48 h afterward; vasoconstriction can continue for ≥ 1 wk. Vasoconstriction from spasm can also follow surgical manipulation of the vessels, especially if blood is released into the subarachnoid space during or after surgery. Large hemorrhages, or those with thick focal collections of blood, are particularly likely to be complicated by spasm and delayed cerebral ischemia.

Headache, decreased alertness, and focal neurologic signs (eg, hemiparesis) are the most common findings in patients with spasm. The major differential diagnostic consideration is rebleeding. In patients with spasm, CT scans show no new bleeding and may reveal a hypodense area of cerebral infarction. Rebleeding is manifested by a sudden increase in headache intensity, decreased alertness, and new blood on CT scan or lumbar puncture. Angiography not only defines the aneurysm but shows general or focal vasoconstriction.

Treatment

Treatment of subarachnoid hemorrhage depends on the cause. When the hemorrhage is caused by an aneurysm or arteriovenous malformation, the aim is to clip or coat the involved vessels before the next episode of bleeding because mortality increases greatly with each episode. When the hemorrhage results from the use of warfarin, hypoprothrombinemia must be quickly reversed with vitamin K. Patients with subarachnoid hemorrhage due to head trauma should be quickly evaluated and treated surgically, if indicated.

All patients with subarachnoid hemorrhage should be monitored in a quiet room. Dehydration should be avoided, since it can lead to decreased cerebral blood flow. Although increased systemic blood pressure may be precipitated by the sudden increase in intracranial pressure, severe hypertension should be controlled. Increased intracranial pressure causes an increase in venous pressure in the brain and dural venous sinuses; the systemic blood pressure must exceed this elevated venous pressure if the brain is to be perfused. Corticosteroids in doses equivalent to prednisone 60 to 100 mg/day help control increased intracranial pressure and brain swelling. When spasm of a cerebral vessel is suspected, both nimodipine and hypervolemic therapy should be considered.

INTRACEREBRAL HEMORRHAGE

Hypertension and coexisting degenerative changes due to aging increase susceptibility to intracerebral hemorrhage in the elderly. Usually, bleeding into the brain arises from small arteries or arterioles. Bleeding diatheses, especially warfarin-induced hypoprothrombinemia, pose a great risk because the bleeding is more gradual and progressive, more often resulting in death than other causes of intracerebral hemorrhage.

Amyloid angiopathy accounts for up to 20% of intracerebral hemorrhage in patients > 70 yr of age. Special stains are needed to detect the congophilic changes in the blood vessels of surgical or postmortem specimens. Aneurysms and arteriovenous malformations are uncommon causes. Occasionally, bleeding occurs into a previously unsuspected brain tumor, especially if it is metastatic.

Symptoms, Signs, and Diagnosis

The earliest symptoms of intracerebral hemorrhage result from the loss of function subserved by the brain region in which the bleeding occurs. For example, bleeding into the left putamen and internal capsule causes right limb paralysis; hemorrhage in the right occipital lobe causes a left visual field defect; and cerebellar hemorrhage causes coordination deficits. The hemorrhage may expand within minutes, or at most a few hours, and acts like a solid mass, increasing intracranial contents and pressure and causing headache, vomiting, and decreased alertness. If the hemorrhage remains small, symptoms of increased intracranial pressure may not occur. Nearly 50% of patients with small to moderate intracerebral hemorrhages do not have headache and remain alert. This is especially true in the elderly, because previous atrophy in the brain provides additional space to accommodate the extra contents.

On examination, signs of focal abnormality of brain function are apparent. The most important neurologic signs of hypertensive intracerebral hemorrhage at the most common locations are listed in TABLE 91–2: putamenal hemorrhages account for about 35% of cases; lobar hemorrhages, about 25%; and thalamic hemorrhages, about 20%. Caudate, pontine, and cerebellar locations each account for about 7%.

Warfarin-induced hemorrhages tend to occur in the lobes of the cerebrum and the cerebellum, begin more insidiously, and progress more gradually. Amyloid angiopathy hemorrhages are almost always lobar. Traumatic hematomas are usually multiple; they are located on the surface of the brain, especially the orbital frontal lobes and tips of the temporal lobes, sites that are close to the rough bony ridges at the base of the skull.

Diagnosis of intracerebral hemorrhage has been revolutionized by CT. Hematomas appear as white, hyperdense, well-circumscribed lesions;

TABLE 91–2. NEUROLOGIC SIGNS OF HYPERTENSIVE INTRACEREBRAL HEMORRHAGE AT COMMON LOCATIONS

Location	*Signs*
Putamen	Contralateral hemiparesis, hemisensory loss, and at times hemianopia; conjugate deviation of eyes to side of hemorrhage; normal pupil size and reaction
Left	Aphasia
Right	Left visual neglect
Thalamus	Contralateral hemisensory loss with slight hemiparesis or hemiataxia; eyes deviated down or down and in; reduced vertical gaze; small, poorly reactive pupils
Caudate nucleus	Contralateral slight transient hemiparesis; restlessness and confusion; occasionally, ipsilateral Horner's syndrome
Lobe	
Frontal	Decreased spontaneity; contralateral Babinski's sign
Parietal	Contralateral hemisensory loss and hemineglect
Left	Reading and writing deficits; aphasia
Temporal	Agitation and upper quadrantanopia contralaterally
Left	Wernicke's fluent aphasia
Occipital	Contralateral hemianopia
Pons	Quadriparesis; reduced alertness; no horizontal gaze; small reactive pupils. (Some pontine hemorrhages affect the tegmentum or base unilaterally, causing a hemiparesis and crossed cranial nerve signs)
Cerebellum	Gait ataxia; vomiting; sometimes, ipsilateral conjugate gaze paresis or 6th nerve palsy

their location and size, drainage into the ventricles or onto the surface, and shifts of intracranial contents are accurately portrayed. In addition, CT scans can show an unsuspected tumor or vascular malformation adjacent to the hematoma. If the patient is anemic, the hematoma may appear to be hypodense or have a fluid level.

Hemorrhages can also be visualized by MRI, which can better reveal the extent and dissection of the hemorrhage in the coronal and sagittal planes. Both MRI and magnetic resonance angiography can show vascular malformations. Separation of hemorrhage and ischemia is less obvious on MRI than on CT and requires an analysis of the differences in

TABLE 91–3. TREATMENT OF INCREASED INTRACRANIAL PRESSURE

Medical	*Surgical*
Intubation and mechanical hyperventilation	Drainage of hematoma or large infarct
Dexamethasone 10 mg IV or IM initially, then 4 mg IM, IV, or po q 6 h	Ventricular drainage or shunt
Mannitol 1–2 gm/kg over 10–20 min initially, then 50–300 mg/kg IV q 6 h	Excision of bleeding arteriovenous malformation or tumor
Glycerin (glycerol) 1–5 gm/kg po q 6 h	Repair of aneurysm

T1 and T2 weighted images. Old hemosiderin from old hemorrhages is also detected by MRI.

Clinical Course and Treatment

Treatment of intracerebral hemorrhage depends on cause, location, and amount of bleeding. Patients with large hemorrhages usually die before treatment can be initiated. Those with small hemorrhages, which are self-contained and have self-limited clinical courses, require little treatment except prophylactic measures (eg, controlling hypertension to prevent a recurrent hemorrhage). Although hypertension should be controlled, blood pressure should not be reduced to normal levels, as this could compromise cerebral perfusion. Corticosteroids and osmotic agents, such as mannitol and glycerol, may help control increased intracranial pressure (see TABLE 91–3). Moderate-sized (2 to 4 cm) hematomas are the most important to treat, especially if the patient's condition is worsening.

Progression of the intracerebral hemorrhage is usually manifested by a decrease in consciousness and an increase in focal neurologic signs. For example, on admission, a patient with a right putamenal hemorrhage has left hemiparesis and conjugate deviation of the eyes to the right. The left plantar reflex is extensor, and the pupils are normal. If the hematoma expands or the region surrounding the hematoma becomes edematous, the right plantar reflex may become extensor, the eyes may not move horizontally in either direction, the right pupil may become dilated and fixed, and stupor may develop. Without aggressive treatment, patients whose condition worsens in this manner while under medical observation have a high mortality rate. Surgical drainage of an expanding hematoma can be lifesaving because it decompresses the brain and decreases intracranial pressure. However, because surgical drainage substitutes a cavity for the hematoma, it does not diminish the extent of paralysis or other focal abnormalities. For these reasons, neurologic examination should be repeated frequently in persons with new intracerebral hemorrhages.

Thalamic and pontine hematomas are not accessible surgically. Surgical decompression is most feasible for cerebellar hemorrhages and lobar hematomas near the brain surface. An example is the case of a vigorous hypertensive man of 82 yr who presented with headache, left hemianopia, and decreased alertness. A CT scan showed a right temporal lobe hemorrhage about 4 cm at its greatest diameter. The man gradually became stuporous and developed bilateral extensor plantar reflexes. His physicians struggled with the decision of whether to drain the hematoma surgically, fearful that he might be severely disabled and become a permanent burden to his family and society. Because this man had previously been vigorous and had a supportive family with ample resources and optimism, surgical drainage was performed. He was left with only a nondisabling visual field defect and lived for another 10 yr, surviving to dance at his granddaughter's wedding.

With recent advances, some hematomas can be drained stereotaxically, using a burr hole, rather than by performing a craniotomy.

ISCHEMIC STROKE

Cerebrovascular disorder caused by insufficient cerebral circulation.

Except when caused by systemic hypotension, which usually begins abruptly, ischemic stroke generally begins with transient ischemic attacks **(TIAs)** and has a fluctuating, stepwise, or progressive clinical course. Ischemia is caused by an impediment to blood flow, almost always in the form of a narrowed or occluded artery leading to a local brain region. Arterial occlusion triggers a chain of events: some tend to increase the ischemia and worsen the neurologic deficit, and others (ie, compensatory body reactions) act to confine the area of ischemia and the deficit (see TABLE 91–4). During the first week after ischemia begins, a thrombus gradually adheres to the arterial wall and becomes organized, diminishing the early tendency of the loosely attached clot to embolize or propagate distally. Similarly, the collateral circulation needs time to become established and stabilized.

During the relatively unstable period of a few days to 2 wk after occlusion, any decrease in cerebral perfusion should be avoided. Blood pressure should not be lowered unless it is ≥ 170/110 mm Hg. Cardiac output should be maximized. Hypovolemia, a frequent problem in the stroke patient who may not eat and drink enough, should be avoided. Since the simple act of sitting or standing may worsen the ischemia early in its course, patients should be watched closely and blood pressure should be checked when they first sit or stand. Patients whose neurologic signs fluctuate or worsen usually should remain supine to maximize cerebral blood flow until the instability passes.

TABLE 91–4. INSTABILITY AFTER A VASCULAR OCCLUSION

Factors Promoting Deficit	*Factors Limiting Deficit*
Regional cerebral blood flow in territory supplied by the occluded artery is reduced	Reduced pressure and tissue acidosis stimulate opening of collateral arteries
Local stagnant flow and activation of clotting factors enlarge the clot	Collateral arteries dramatically increase flow in the supply area of the occluded artery
Clot propagates distally	Fibrinolytic systems are activated
Loosely adherent clot embolizes, blocking distal arteries	Emboli break up and pass distally

LARGE VESSEL ATHEROSTENOSIS

Atherosclerosis is a generalized process. In whites, atherosclerosis of the cerebrovascular bed is most common at the origins of the internal carotid artery and the vertebral artery in the neck and at the intracranial basilar artery. The large intracranial arteries (anterior, middle, and posterior cerebral arteries) and their superficial convexal artery branches are affected much less often.

Atherosclerosis of the extracranial internal carotid and vertebral arteries is twice as common in white men as in white women; it correlates highly with coronary and peripheral vascular occlusive disease and hyperlipidemia. A history of angina pectoris, prior myocardial infarction, or leg claudication in a patient with a TIA strongly suggests a diagnosis of extracranial atherostenosis.

Atherostenosis of the neck arteries is less common in blacks and in persons of Japanese or Chinese descent than in whites, but the major intracranial arteries are more predisposed to stenosis. In these populations, intracranial artery stenosis does not correlate epidemiologically with coronary or peripheral vascular disease or hyperlipidemia, occurs at a younger age than does extracranial disease, and does not have a strong male preponderance. Diabetic patients and persons with hypertension also have a high prevalence of intracranial disease.

Symptoms and Signs

The most common presenting symptom is at least one TIA, which is often brief but may recur for weeks or months if untreated. Some patients present with sudden-onset stroke, probably caused by the embolization of intra-arterial clot or plaque material originating in regions of extracranial atherostenosis and traveling distally to block intracranial recipient arteries. Headache is also common and is probably caused by the dilatation of collateral arterial channels. Specific symptoms and signs relate to the anatomy of the involved artery and the area it supplies.

Internal carotid artery in the neck: The first branch of the internal carotid artery is the ophthalmic artery, which arises intracranially and supplies the optic nerve, retina, and iris. Transient decreases in arterial flow cause attacks of transient monocular blindness, or **amaurosis fugax,** on the side of the lesion. These attacks are usually described as being like a shade falling or a curtain moving across the eye from the side. Transient monocular blindness episodes are usually brief, lasting 30 sec to a few minutes. Some attacks are precipitated by sudden standing or bending or by exposure to bright natural light.

Patients with carotid artery disease often have attacks of hemispheric ischemia characterized by weakness or numbness of the contralateral limbs or the opposite part of the face. The hand and arm are involved more often than the face or leg. The attacks vary; the hand may be involved in one spell, the leg in another, and the arm and leg in a third. Aphasia is common when the left internal carotid artery is involved.

When spells of transient monocular blindness and attacks of numbness or weakness of the opposite limbs occur, the physician can be confident that the diagnosis is internal carotid artery disease within the neck or within the carotid siphon before the ophthalmic artery branch. Plaque disease and stenosis are most severe at the origin of the internal carotid artery, where it branches from the common carotid artery. TABLE 91–5 lists some signs of internal carotid artery atherostenosis.

Subclavian artery: Atherostenosis usually affects the subclavian arteries proximal to the origins of the vertebral artery branches. The left side is stenosed more often than the right. The most common symptoms involve the ischemic arm, which often aches, is cool, and becomes fatigued easily on exercise. The radial pulse on the ischemic side is usually weak or delayed, and the blood pressure is lower than in the opposite arm. At times a bruit is audible in the supraclavicular fossa. Much more common than stroke, TIAs related to subclavian artery disease are characterized by temporary dizziness, blurred vision, diplopia, or staggering; sometimes they are provoked by exercising the ischemic arm. Patients with subclavian artery atherostenosis usually do well, unless they use the ischemic arm vigorously in sports (eg, golf), and treatment is usually not indicated.

Vertebral artery: Typical characteristics of TIAs related to vertebral artery disease in the neck are evanescent dizziness, vertigo, diplopia, or blurred vision. The clinical findings are identical to those in subclavian disease, except that the arm is not ischemic and the pulses and blood pressures in the upper limbs are equal. Sometimes, patients with a vertebral artery occlusion in the neck present with a sudden poste-

TABLE 91–5. SIGNS OF INTERNAL CAROTID ARTERY ATHEROSTENOSIS IPSILATERAL TO THE VASCULAR LESION

Neck	Bruit best heard with stethoscope bell—long, focal, high-pitched
Face	Increased pulses in facial, preauricular, and superficial temporal arteries when CCA is normal and ECA acts as collateral vessel; decreased pulses in facial, preauricular, and superficial temporal arteries when CCA or ICA and ECA are stenosed
	Increased ABC pulses: A—angular, near medial corner of eye; B—brow, laterally; C—cheek
	Coolness in supraorbital region
	Reversal of blood flow in frontal artery
Eyes	Iris: Red speckling (rubeosis iridis); fixed, dilated, or irregular pupil; Horner's syndrome
	Retina: White retinal infarcts; Hollenhorst plaques—bright refringent cholesterol crystals usually at bifurcations of retinal arteries; decreased caliber of retinal arteries; asymmetric hypertensive retinopathy—less prominent on side of stenosis; central venous retinopathy—engorged veins, microaneurysms, small-clot hemorrhages, sometimes papilledema

CCA = common carotid artery; ECA = external carotid artery; ICA = internal carotid artery.

rior circulation stroke; the ischemia is caused by blockage of the intracranial vertebral artery or the posterior cerebral artery or its branches resulting from embolic material originating in the proximal vertebral artery. A similar situation occurs with thrombosis originating in the internal carotid artery. The most frequent site of vertebral artery atherostenosis is the origin and first few centimeters of the vessel. The distal portion of the vertebral artery in the neck is vulnerable to tearing or dissection during neck trauma, sudden movement, or manipulation.

Intracranial carotid artery and middle and anterior cerebral artery branches: When stenosis affects the intracranial carotid artery proximal to the ophthalmic artery branch, the syndrome is similar to that of internal carotid artery origin, but no neck bruit is heard and noninvasive studies of the internal carotid artery are normal. Stenosis of the intracranial carotid beyond the ophthalmic artery origin is accompanied by spells of hemispheric ischemia presenting as lateralized weakness, sensory loss, or visual neglect, but transient monocular blindness

TABLE 91–6. SYMPTOMS AND SIGNS OF LATERAL MEDULLARY ISCHEMIA

Symptoms	*Signs*
Ipsilateral	
Jabbing pain in eye or face	Decreased pain and temperature sense along trigeminal distribution
Lid droop; decreased facial sweating	Horner's syndrome
Dizziness and feelings of motion	Nystagmus
Hoarseness and dysphagia	Decreased movement of ipsilateral palate, pharynx, and vocal cord
Incoordination of arm and leg	Incoordination, tremor, and rebound of arm and leg
Contralateral	
Difficulty telling temperature over arms and legs	Decreased pain and temperature sense over limbs and trunk
General	
Walking imbalance	Gait ataxia
Difficulty sitting or standing	Falls to side when sitting or standing Tachycardia Labile blood pressure

does not occur. Also lacking are signs and noninvasive evidence of decreased ophthalmic artery flow. Aphasia is common in left hemispheric ischemia, and defective drawing and copying ability and left visual neglect are common with lesions of the right hemisphere.

Middle cerebral artery disease usually is most severe in the proximal segment or the upper trunk branch. Anterior cerebral artery disease is less common than middle cerebral artery disease and usually affects the proximal portions of the artery.

Middle cerebral artery disease usually causes weakness and numbness of the contralateral limbs, trunk, and especially the face. When the left middle cerebral artery is affected, aphasia usually occurs; with right middle cerebral artery disease, the patient has visual-spatial dysfunction and left-sided neglect (lack of attention to all activity on the left side). Anterior cerebral artery disease causes weakness and numbness of the contralateral lower extremity. At times, the patient may lack spontaneity, be disinterested, and suffer from incontinence. In the in-

TABLE 91–7. SYMPTOMS AND SIGNS OF BASILAR ARTERY ATHEROSTENOSIS

Symptoms	Diplopia Dysphagia Dizziness Dysarthria Bilateral leg or leg and arm weakness Crossed weakness—one side of face, opposite side of body and limbs Bilateral numbness Deafness or tinnitus Occipital headache
Signs	Palsies of extraocular movement (3rd, 4th, and 6th cranial nerves) Internuclear ophthalmoplegia Nystagmus—horizontal or vertical Bilateral bulbar weakness (face, lips, palate, pharynx, tongue) Crossed 6th or 7th cranial nerve paralysis and hemiparesis Decreased hearing Pseudobulbar palsy Quadriparesis Bilateral extensor plantar reflexes Gait ataxia Limb ataxia Stupor Locked-in syndrome Bilateral decreased position sense in limbs

tracranial internal carotid artery siphon and disease of the middle and anterior cerebral arteries, stroke is more common than TIA. The stroke is caused primarily by hemodynamic insufficiency, with poor perfusion of the affected vascular territories, and is often gradually progressive.

Intracranial vertebral artery: Occlusion or severe stenosis of the intracranial vertebral artery blocks flow through the posterior inferior cerebellar artery branch, causing ischemia of the lateral medulla and cerebellum. The most common symptoms and signs of lateral medullary ischemia are listed in TABLE 91–6. Cerebellar ischemia is manifested by staggering gait, ataxia, sensations of disequilibrium, and nausea. Large cerebellar infarcts can cause pressure on the posterior cranial fossa and coma from compression of the brain stem; this potentially fatal complication is treated with surgical decompression of the lesion and removal of infarcted tissue.

Basilar artery: The most common symptoms and signs of basilar artery atherostenosis are listed in TABLE 91–7. Basilar artery occlusion is potentially fatal unless collateral circulation occurs. The basilar artery supplies the pons; the region most vulnerable to ischemia is the base of the pons, which the long motor tracts pass through. Ischemia causes bilateral weakness of the trunk and limbs with exaggerated reflexes and extensor plantar signs. Sometimes premonitory spells of dizziness and diplopia occur, especially when the occlusion begins in the vertebral artery and spreads to the basilar artery.

Posterior cerebral arteries: The cardinal symptoms and signs of posterior cerebral artery atherostenosis relate to the visual fields. Patients may have transient attacks of hemianopia or scotomata, and the hemianopia often develops suddenly. Loss of memory, alexia, and an agitated delirium also occur when the lesion is large and includes the posterior cerebral artery's temporal lobe territory.

Laboratory Findings and Diagnosis

Sometimes occlusions are caused by hematologic abnormalities, either alone or superimposed upon a stenotic lumen. Polycythemia and thrombocytosis are major causes of vascular occlusion. A hypercoagulable state can complicate cancer and other systemic illnesses. A CBC count, prothrombin time test, and platelet count should be performed routinely in every patient with TIA or stroke.

Both **CT and MRI** can be useful in delineating the affected vascular territory when an infarct is present. Negative results give hope that the ischemia is reversible, whereas a large infarct carries a poor prognosis for recovery. The distribution of infarction yields clues to the likely location of the vascular lesion. Carotid occlusion often causes infarction near the border zones between the anterior and the middle cerebral arteries, between the middle and the posterior cerebral arteries, or in the deep white matter. A small zone of infarction in the central part of the middle cerebral artery territory suggests a small superficial branch embolic infarct arising from the heart or the internal carotid artery. Both CT and MRI also can show zones of edema and shifts of intracranial contents.

B-mode ultrasound images of the internal carotid and vertebral artery origins in the neck have a high sensitivity and specificity for showing severe occlusive lesions. **Color-flow Doppler ultrasonography** also accurately shows occlusive lesions of the neck arteries. **Transcranial Doppler ultrasonography** provides useful information about flow velocities in the major intracranial basal arteries; it can show whether occlusive extracranial lesions reduce intracranial flow and can detect severe occlusive disease within the major intracranial arteries. **Magnetic resonance angiography,** a new technology, can also screen for extracranial and intracranial occlusive disease and aneurysms. The combination of extracranial and intracranial ultrasonography and magnetic resonance angiography is very effective in showing most important large artery occlusive lesions.

Angiography remains the definitive test for imaging the extracranial and intracranial arteries and veins. With small amounts of contrast material, computer-generated images provide high-resolution pictures.

Two commonly cited principles of angiography are not universally applicable to geriatric patients. They are (1) that angiography is warranted only if surgery is planned or considered, and (2) that all four major arteries and the aortic arch must be visualized for diagnosis. Angiography is needed when the diagnosis is unclear despite clinical, imaging, and noninvasive testing. However, for many patients, ultrasound testing and magnetic resonance angiography now provide sufficient information to preclude angiography. For others, the results of these tests make it possible to limit standard angiography to one or two vessels.

Angiography has definite risks (stroke, injury to the artery in which the catheter is placed, allergic reactions—a combined morbidity and mortality rate of about 1%), but they can be minimized by using the smallest amount of dye and the least number of injections needed for accurate diagnosis. The expertise of the angiographer and the information supplied by the responsible clinician are vital to these decisions. The angiographer should begin by injecting the artery most likely to harbor the lesion. When sufficient information is obtained to determine treatment, no further angiography should be performed.

Treatment

Treatment based on accurate diagnosis is more rational than empiric guesswork. Some medical treatments (eg, use of anticoagulants) are potentially risky, especially when unwarranted. Choice of treatment depends on the location and severity of the occlusion. There are five principal, specific treatment alternatives: surgical endarterectomy, warfarin, aspirin or other platelet antiaggregates, heparin, and surgical bypass of an occlusive lesion. General treatment considerations are discussed at the beginning of this chapter. In choosing among the specific treatments, the following guidelines are suggested:

1. Endarterectomy is the procedure of choice if the vessel is seriously stenotic (ie, the residual lumen is <2 mm) and surgically accessible, and the patient has not already had a severe stroke in the area of brain tissue supplied by the vessel.

2. Warfarin should be used when the vascular lesion is severely stenotic and inaccessible (eg, internal carotid artery siphon or middle cerebral artery), or the patient is not a candidate for or refuses surgery. The prothrombin time should be kept at about 1.5 times the control value. Warfarin is most effective in preventing "red clots" composed of erythrocytes and thrombin, which might be expected to form in regions of very reduced flow (eg, very stenotic arteries, veins, or dilated cardiac chambers).

3. Aspirin is prescribed if the vascular lesion is not severely stenotic. The optimal dose is as yet undetermined; 1.3 gm/day in divided doses (eg, 325 mg qid or 650 mg bid) has been effective in trials, although a dose of 300 to 325 mg/day is probably just as effective. Theoretically, a dose as low as 100 mg/day might work as well, if not better. Ticlopidine, another drug that affects platelet aggregation and function, is given in a dose of 500 mg/day to patients who cannot take aspirin. Patients taking ticlopidine should be monitored for leukopenia. Aspirin and other platelet antiaggregates should prevent "white clots" composed of fibrin-platelet clumps that form in fast-moving streams on irregular surfaces (eg, craggy plaques in nonstenosed arteries). Dipyridamole alone has not been shown to be effective.

4. Heparin is prescribed for short-term (2 to 3 wk) treatment in patients with complete occlusion of large arteries. This prevents propagation and embolization of clot until the loosely adherent thrombus becomes organized on the vascular wall and collateral circulation is well established. Heparin may also be used when the neurologic signs are fluctuating, the occluding lesion is undefined, and more definitive information is not yet available. Heparin should be given in a continuous IV infusion, keeping the activated partial thromboplastin time at 1.5 to 2 times the control value. Warfarin should be administered 2 to 4 days after beginning heparin treatment. When warfarin is initiated for this indication, it is usually continued for 1 to 3 mo.

5. The indications for extracranial-intracranial bypass surgery are undetermined. A controlled randomized international study concluded that the procedure is no better than medical therapy for most patients with an inaccessible occlusive vascular lesion in the anterior circulation. Bypass might be considered for isolated, well-studied patients refractory to medical treatment.

PENETRATING ARTERY DISEASE

The small arteries that penetrate deeper brain structures (eg, the basal gray nuclei, internal capsule, thalamus, and pons) are especially susceptible to degenerative changes caused by hypertension. Medial hypertrophy, fibrinoid changes, and lipohyalinosis gradually narrow the lumens of these arteries, impeding blood flow. Patients with fibrinoid degeneration and lipohyalinosis of penetrating arteries are invariably hypertensive or have a history of hypertension. Plaques within arteries, blocking or extending into the orifices of penetrating arteries, and microatheromas are more common in diabetic patients.

When a penetrating artery becomes occluded and flow is sufficiently diminished, a small, deep infarct called a **lacuna** results. The lesions are < 2 cm at their greatest diameter and affect only deeper structures. At times, microatheromas or microdissections occlude the origins of the penetrating arteries, causing infarcts in identical distributions. Lacunae are relatively more common in the posterior circulation and increase in frequency with age. Race and sex do not appear to be correlated with lacunar infarcts.

Symptoms and Signs

Because the lesions are small and deep, patients do not have symptoms related to vasodilation or increased intracranial pressure (eg, headache, vomiting, or decreased alertness). The clinical syndrome develops over a short period—usually < 1 wk. Though less common in penetrating artery disease than in large artery atherostenosis, TIAs are characteristic and brief, usually lasting no longer than a few days. Symptoms of brain dysfunction relate to the ischemic region. The most common patterns are unilateral weakness of the face, arm, and leg and unilateral paresthesias of the face, trunk, and limbs. Multiple lacunae may lead to dementia and parkinsonism.

Physical examination discloses that abnormalities are limited to dysfunction of deep structures. When lacunae are located deep in the cerebral hemisphere, weakness or numbness should not be accompanied by hemianopia, visual field loss or neglect, or abnormal cognitive function or behavior. When the brain stem is involved, the signs are seldom if ever limited to dysfunction of tegmental structures (cranial nerve nuclei and eye movements). Common lacunar syndromes are listed in TABLE 91–8; pure motor hemiparesis and pure sensory stroke are by far the most common.

Diagnosis

Diagnosis depends on a combination of epidemiologic features, symptoms and signs, and laboratory findings. In a typical example, the patient has a history of hypertension, rapidly evolving clinical symptoms and signs typical of one of the lacunar syndromes (see TABLE 91–8), and CT or MRI evidence of lacunae or no relevant lesion. With this combination of findings, no further testing is needed. Lacunar infarction ordinarily is not diagnosed in patients with no history of hypertension or diabetes.

Lacunae may not show on CT or MRI. When these imaging techniques show superficial infarcts that could account for the symptoms, the diagnosis of lacunar infarction is excluded. Electroencephalograms are rarely helpful, usually showing normal function or minor symmetric abnormalities. Angiography is usually not indicated in patients with typical lacunar infarcts. Hypertension, the cause of lacunae, often leads to coexisting atherostenosis of larger arteries; thus, in patients with typical lacunae, vascular narrowing is often found during noninvasive testing or angiography.

TABLE 91–8. ACUTE LACUNAR SYNDROMES

Pure motor hemiparesis	Unilateral weakness of face, arm, and leg, usually with exaggerated reflexes and Babinski's sign; dysarthria may be present but dysphasia and other cognitive and behavioral abnormalities are lacking
Pure sensory stroke	Unilateral paresthesias, dysesthesias, or numbness of face, arm, leg, and trunk; no accompanying weakness, ataxia, hemianopia, or cognitive or behavioral abnormalities
Sensorimotor stroke	Unilateral numbness and weakness of face and limbs without cognitive, visual, or behavioral abnormalities
Dysarthria–clumsy hand syndrome	Slurred speech; facial and tongue weakness with ipsilateral clumsiness of the hand; increased reflexes and Babinski's sign may be present
Ataxic hemiparesis	Unilateral combined ataxia and weakness with exaggerated reflexes in arm and/or leg and Babinski's sign
Pure dysarthria	Dysarthria, sometimes with dysphagia without other findings
Hemiparkinsonism or hemidystonia	Unilateral abnormal posture, tone, and movement
Sensory stroke limited to the face	Like pure sensory stroke but limited to the face
Hemiataxia	Unilateral incoordination, often with abnormal gait

Treatment

Hypertension should be controlled when the patient is no longer vulnerable to ischemia. For the first 1 to (at most) 3 wk, changes in position, blood pressure, blood volume, and blood flow can increase the ischemic deficit. Deep penetrating arteries are end vessels, and any decrease in flow through adjacent arteries can enlarge the infarct. Only when blood pressure is in the so-called malignant range (> 200/120 mm Hg) should it be immediately lowered. Blood glucose should be controlled in diabetic patients. Phlebotomy is important in patients with a hematocrit > 45%. A high hematocrit causes increased blood viscosity and makes the patient susceptible to lacunar infarction as well as to large artery occlusion. All stroke patients who smoke should be encouraged to stop.

TABLE 91–9. COMMON CARDIAC SOURCES OF CEREBRAL EMBOLIZATION

Valvular disease or condition	Rheumatic valvulitis Prosthetic heart valves Calcific aortic stenosis Mitral annulus calcification Nonbacterial thrombotic (marasmic) endocarditis Bacterial and fungal endocarditis
Myocardial ischemia	Acute infarction Ventricular aneurysms Akinetic zones Mural thrombi
Arrhythmias	Atrial fibrillation Sick sinus syndrome
Lesions within cardiac chambers	Myocarditis Cardiomyopathy Sarcoidosis Amyloidosis

CEREBRAL EMBOLIZATION

Emboli can arise from the aortic arch or from plaques or dissections in the proximal portions of the large extracranial and intracranial arteries, in which case the epidemiologic and clinical findings will be the same as those discussed under LARGE VESSEL ATHEROSTENOSIS, above.

The heart is also frequently a source of emboli, especially in the elderly. Newer cardiac diagnostic tests and brain imaging techniques have led to more cases of cerebral embolization being identified than in the past. The most common cardiac sources of cerebral embolization are listed in TABLE 91–9. Most important are all varieties of valvular disease, myocardial ischemia, and atrial fibrillation. As many as 5% of persons > 70 yr of age have atrial fibrillation, making this a common risk factor for emboli.

Symptoms and Signs

Neurologic symptoms usually begin abruptly, often while the patient is awake and active. Most often the deficit is maximal at or near onset, because the sudden blockage of a distal artery does not allow adequate time for collateral circulation to be established. Emboli do pass distally; when this occurs, the deficit may worsen or improve. Stepwise worsening usually occurs within 48 h. When angiography is performed > 2 days after the onset of symptoms, emboli are usually no longer visible in the intracranial arteries. In the anterior circulation, emboli most often reach branches of the anterior and middle cerebral arteries. In the posterior circulation, the recipient site is most often the long circumferential cerebellar arteries and branches of the posterior cerebral arteries. When the embolus causes a large infarct, headache and decreased alertness are common. Neurologic signs are identical to those discussed under LARGE VESSEL ATHEROSTENOSIS, above.

Laboratory Findings and Diagnosis

Both **CT** and **MRI** usually reveal superficial, slice-of-pie–shaped infarcts in the cerebral hemisphere or cerebellum in the territories of the anterior cerebral, middle cerebral, posterior cerebral, and cerebellar arteries. There may be many scattered infarcts, some unexpected, in different vascular territories. **Ultrasonography** and **magnetic resonance angiography** reveal embolic sources within the proximal extracranial arteries. **Angiography** shows abrupt distal cutoff of intracranial branch arteries without underlying local atherostenosis, filling defects in the form of thromboemboli, and proximal regions of atherostenosis.

An **ECG** may be useful to detect myocardial ischemia, chamber hypertrophy, or arrhythmias. **Echocardiography** is especially useful, demonstrating valvular disease, regions of decreased contractility, tumors such as myxomas, and chamber enlargement. Paradoxic embolism can be studied by introducing saline IV and using Doppler ultrasonography to detect the passage of bubbles through septal defects during echocardiography. **Transesophageal echocardiography** is especially sensitive for detecting atrial disease, septal defects, and patent foramen ovales. It can also demonstrate ulcerative protruding atheromas in the ascending aorta, another important source of embolism. **Holter monitoring** can detect intermittent arrhythmias. **Radionuclide cardiac scans** can corroborate regions of ischemic damage and abnormal function.

Treatment

Treatment depends on the nature of the embolic source; treating proximal atherostenotic embolic sources has already been discussed in the section on atherostenosis, above. Specific medical treatment may be available for the cardiac abnormality (eg, antiarrhythmic agents or coronary vasodilators for ischemia). Some cardiac lesions require surgical correction.

Anticoagulants are usually indicated when the patient is vulnerable to further emboli. In some patients (eg, those with recent myocardial infarction or reversible arrhythmia), this risk is transient; in others (eg, those with intractable atrial fibrillation), it is lifelong. Heparin may be given in a constant infusion, controlled to keep the activated partial thromboplastin time at 1.5 to 2 times the control value. Heparin is gradually replaced with warfarin for long-term therapy, keeping the prothrombin time at about 1.3 to 1.5 times control (equivalent to an INR

[International Normalized Ratio] of 2 to 3). The risk of intracranial bleeding has been described above, especially in elderly patients with large infarcts, hypertension, and excessive anticoagulation.

Anticoagulants are contraindicated if the infarct is large; they are also contraindicated if the patient is hypertensive, unless blood pressure can be reduced without increasing the neurologic deficit. Doses of anticoagulants should be conservative, with monitoring of the activated partial thromboplastin time and prothrombin time and observation for early signs of systemic bleeding.

In patients with artificial valves who develop new emboli while taking warfarin, the addition of dipyridamole in a dose of 75 mg orally q 6 h may be helpful. The risk:benefit ratio of prophylactic anticoagulation in patients with potential cardiac embolic sources, such as atrial fibrillation, is being investigated. The dipyridamole-warfarin combination may produce less bleeding than aspirin-warfarin, but dipyridamole sometimes causes orthostatic hypotension.

SYSTEMIC HYPOPERFUSION

Cerebral ischemia can be caused by circulatory failure; the heart is unable to pump adequate amounts of blood and nutrients to the brain. Acute myocardial infarction, cardiac arrest, and life-threatening ventricular arrhythmias are the most common causes. Less often, pulmonary embolism, acute gastrointestinal or systemic bleeding, or shock is responsible.

Symptoms, Signs, and Diagnosis

Most often, the patient is pale, sweating, and hypotensive when first examined. Neurologic dysfunction is usually abrupt in onset and follows systemic symptoms related to the underlying disorder. The most prominent findings are decreased alertness and symmetric depression of hemispheric functions. When ischemia is severe, the brain stem may not function normally and brain stem reflexes (pupillary, corneal, doll's eye, pharyngeal) may be absent. Bilateral weakness or decorticate or decerebrate rigidity indicates that the motor system is involved. In some patients, the arms are most severely affected, with relative sparing of the face and legs, a distribution described as "a man in a barrel." When poor cerebral perfusion has been severe or prolonged, the patient is usually comatose. Loss of brain stem reflexes for > 24 h carries a poor prognosis, as does persistent coma. When stupor lightens, patients may show deficits in visual function and memory. A CT scan is usually normal during the acute period in all but the most severely affected, but electroencephalograms usually show severe bilateral slowing.

Treatment is directed at the underlying cardiac or systemic process.

CHRONIC CEREBROVASCULAR LESIONS
(Multi-infarct Dementia)

Although many lay people attribute intellectual loss in late life to "hardening of the arteries," there is absolutely no evidence that cerebrovascular disease plays any etiologic role in Alzheimer's disease, the most common cause of dementia in the elderly.

Control zones for basic daily functions (eg, the ability to move, feel, see, eat, speak, and excrete waste) are strategically located in the middle of the main arterial supply areas. Other functions (eg, the ability to calculate, plan, discipline, and read) are more dependent on associative cortical areas, which are generally located between zones of arterial supply. Intoxicants, metabolic disorders, and degenerative diseases readily affect higher functions, while cerebrovascular disease tends to disrupt basic functions. Vascular disease "bites the soma and licks the mind," whereas degenerative and toxic-metabolic diseases waste the intellect while sparing somatic functions until late in their course. However, patients with cerebrovascular disease do become demented when brain damage is severe.

Most patients with chronic vascular dementia have (1) high risk factors for stroke (eg, hypertension, diabetes, coronary or peripheral vascular occlusive disease, cardiac disease, or hyperlipidemia); (2) a history of transient ischemic attacks or sudden-onset neurologic deficits (strokes); and (3) abnormal, often asymmetric neurologic signs (eg, weakness, sensory loss, exaggerated reflexes, Babinski's sign, visual field defects, pseudobulbar palsy, incontinence).

There are three major **subcategories of vascular dementia:** large-artery thromboembolism, état lacunaire (the lacunar state), and subcortical arteriosclerotic encephalopathy (Binswanger's dementia). In **large-artery thromboembolism,** multiple large-vessel occlusions or cardiogenic emboli cause cerebral damage. A CT scan shows areas of damage in superficial cerebral arterial territories. In **état lacunaire,** deep cerebral and brain stem structures are decimated by multiple lacunae, which give the brain a Swiss-cheese–like appearance at necropsy or on CT. The volume of white matter is reduced, with resulting ventricular enlargement. Patients have a plethora of pyramidal and extrapyramidal signs and pseudobulbar palsy. They look stiff, exhibit parkinsonian signs, and walk slowly. In **subcortical arteriosclerotic encephalopathy,** damage to broad areas of the cerebral and cerebellar white matter and basal gray matter results from hypertension and partial occlusions of many deep-penetrating arteries. Both CT and MRI show periventricular and white matter abnormalities, which include hypodensities and periventricular lucencies without zones of cortical infarction.

Treatment of vascular dementia depends entirely on control of risk factors and specific therapy aimed at the cause of the individual stroke (see also NON-ALZHEIMER'S DEMENTIAS in Ch. 90). L-Dopa may help control some of the parkinsonian symptoms.

STROKE COMPLICATIONS

At times, the complications of stroke are more devastating than the stroke itself. A patient's relatives often say that the person was doing well until "complications set in." Stroke seems to activate the body's clotting system, leading to venous thromboembolism and myocardial infarction during the acute period or during convalescence from the stroke. At times, it is difficult to know whether the myocardial or cerebral ischemia came first.

In elderly patients aggressive diagnostic tests, invasive medical and surgical therapies, and prolonged bed rest often take a heavy toll on spirit and vigor. Pneumonia, limb contractures, pressure sores, and depression are particularly common and must be prevented or at least treated when they appear. Antidepressants are particularly effective in treating the depression associated with stroke.

The following strategies may help prevent and treat stroke complications: (1) Prescribe tight elastic or air-filled support stockings and frequent active and passive leg motion. (2) Turn patients in bed frequently, and pay special attention to pressure sites. (3) Maintain adequate fluid intake and nutrition. (4) Administer small doses of heparin (5000 u.) s.c. q 8 to 12 h (so-called miniheparin) to prevent thromboembolism, when not contraindicated. (5) Encourage early ambulation (as soon as the patient's signs become stable), always with close monitoring by nurses and doctors. (6) Pay attention to pulmonary hygiene. Stopping smoking, encouraging deep breathing, and providing respiratory therapy are important. (7) Watch closely for infectious complications, especially pneumonia, urinary tract infections, and skin infections; treat them early. (8) Avoid overdistention of the urinary bladder, preferably without using an indwelling catheter. (9) Early during hospitalization for acute disease, begin rehabilitation strategies, including active and passive exercises, full range-of-motion movement, and teaching patients about their functional disabilities. (10) Emphasize risk factor control early: stopping smoking, losing weight, controlling diet, etc. (11) Maintain a positive outlook; all members of the health care team should emphasize regaining a good, active life. Do not emphasize returning to previous, normal function since that may not be possible, but many patients can lead an active life despite residual handicaps. Many patients concentrate so much on regaining normal arm or hand function that they lose sight of the fact they can resume nearly all other previous activities despite the loss of hand dexterity. (12) Prepare the family early and continuously for the patient's return home. Family members should be instructed on the patient's needs and any necessary changes in the home. When returning home is not feasible, starting early to search for a suitable alternative is important. (13) Continue the preventive measures and treatments begun at the acute-care hospital when the patient is transferred to a rehabilitation facility or to home. Stroke support groups and contact with persons who have overcome similar stroke handicaps are often valuable to the patient.

92. MENINGITIS

The annual incidence of bacterial meningitis in the elderly is 15 cases per 100,000. The elderly account for about 10% of all meningitis cases; yet, > 50% of the deaths occur in those > 60 yr of age. Mortality is high (53% to 79%), in part because elderly patients are often debilitated and have coexisting illnesses. Delays in diagnosis and infection with more problematic organisms also contribute to the high mortality rate.

Etiology

Bacterial meningitis: Although the mechanism of infection is the same in older as in younger persons, the bacteriology differs somewhat. About 55% of cases are caused by *Streptococcus pneumoniae,* generally as a sequela of bacteremia from pneumonia, otitis media, or basilar skull fracture. The nasopharynx is the usual site of entry for *Neisseria meningitidis,* which is responsible for about 15% of cases. *Listeria monocytogenes* accounts for 10% of cases, is associated with very high mortality, and causes infections more frequently during the summer. Although persons with *L. monocytogenes* meningitis often have coexisting diseases affecting cellular immunity or are chronic users of corticosteroids, elderly persons who are apparently healthy also show increased susceptibility to this organism. Gram-negative aerobic bacilli (8% of cases) cause meningitis through bacteremia from pneumonia, decubitus ulcers, osteomyelitis, urosepsis, head trauma, or neurosurgery.

Staphylococcus aureus (responsible for about 5% of meningitis cases) is isolated more frequently in hospitalized patients, particularly those who have had endocarditis, pneumonia, or neurosurgery. *S. epidermidis* is the most common cause of CSF shunt infections. Organisms less often associated with meningitis include *Hemophilus influenzae* (as protective antibody levels decrease with age), various streptococcal species, and anaerobic organisms. The latter may be associated with head and neck malignancy, upper respiratory tract infections, or neurosurgery.

Other causes of meningitis: Viral (aseptic) meningitis is less common in older than in younger persons, whereas meningitis from *Mycobacterium tuberculosis* is seen more often in the elderly than in younger HIV-negative populations. Infection with other pathogens (eg, the fungus *Cryptococcus neoformans*) may occur when immunosuppressive drugs are used or when cell-mediated immunity is depressed because of malignancy or HIV infection.

Symptoms and Signs

Fever, headache, meningeal irritation (meningismus), and cerebral dysfunction occur in > 85% of adults with **bacterial meningitis.** The meningismus may be subtle, marked, or accompanied by Kernig's or Brudzinski's sign (elicited in only about 50% of patients). Cerebral dysfunction is manifested by confusion, delirium, or a declining level of consciousness. Cranial nerve palsies and focal neurologic deficits develop in only about 10% to 20% of adults, seizures in about 30%. Because papilledema occurs initially in < 1% of cases, its presence should suggest an alternative diagnosis (eg, an intracranial mass lesion). With disease progression, patients may develop signs of increased intracranial pressure, including coma, hypertension, bradycardia, and palsy of cranial nerve III; these findings suggest a poor prognosis.

Certain symptoms and signs may suggest the cause of acute bacterial meningitis. About 50% of adults with meningococcemia, with or without meningitis, present with a prominent rash located principally on the extremities. The rash is initially erythematous and macular but quickly evolves into a petechial phase, with new lesions appearing even during the physical examination. Rhinorrhea or otorrhea may be seen in patients with basilar skull fracture and leakage of CSF; pneumococcus is the most common cause of meningitis in such cases. A persistent dural defect commonly accounts for recurrent bacterial meningitis. *L. monocytogenes* is more likely than other organisms to cause seizures and focal neurologic deficits early in the course of meningitis, leading to ataxia, cranial nerve palsies, or nystagmus secondary to rhombencephalitis.

Some elderly patients with acute bacterial meningitis, especially those with underlying conditions such as diabetes or cardiopulmonary disease, may not have typical symptoms and signs but rather an insidious presentation with lethargy or obtundation, variable signs of meningeal irritation, and no fever. Therefore, all elderly patients who present with altered mental status that has no clear cause should be considered candidates for CSF examination to exclude meningitis.

The clinical presentation of **tuberculous meningitis** is quite variable. The presentation is usually indolent, with an insidious prodrome characterized by malaise, lassitude, low-grade fever, intermittent headache, and personality changes. Within 2 to 3 wk, a meningitic phase develops with protracted headache, meningismus, vomiting, and confusion. Focal neurologic signs usually consist of unilateral or, less commonly, bilateral cranial nerve palsies. Hemiparesis is a result of ischemic infarction of the cerebral circulation, most commonly the middle cerebral artery.

The presentation of **cryptococcal meningitis** in the elderly is usually not associated with AIDS, as it is in younger persons. The clinical presentation is typically subacute, with headache the most frequent complaint; fever, meningismus, and personality changes may also occur. Seizures and focal neurologic deficits are rare.

Diagnosis

The definitive diagnosis of **acute bacterial meningitis** rests on CSF examination. The opening pressure is elevated in virtually all patients. The number of WBCs in the CSF is usually 1000 to 5000/μL, with a range of < 100 to > 10,000/μL. Most patients have a predominance of neutrophils, although about 10% have a predominance of lymphocytes. The glucose concentration is usually low, with a CSF:serum glucose ratio of < 0.31 in about 70% of patients. The protein concentration is virtually always elevated, presumably because the blood-brain barrier is disrupted. Gram stain of CSF is positive in about 60% to 90% of cases. Specific bacterial antigen tests (eg, counterimmunoelectrophoresis or latex agglutination) should also be performed. The sensitivity of these tests ranges from 56% to 100%, although specificity is high. However, a negative result does not rule out the diagnosis of acute bacterial meningitis.

In **tuberculous meningitis,** pleocytosis is moderate, with the number of cells exceeding 500/μL in only about 20% of cases. While neutrophils may predominate initially, conversion to a lymphocyte predominance occurs over several weeks. However, in patients who are receiving antituberculous drugs, predominance may shift from lymphocytes to neutrophils on subsequent CSF examinations, the so-called therapeutic paradox of tuberculous meningitis. The CSF glucose concentrations are usually moderately depressed, and protein concentrations are elevated in most cases. Identifying tubercle bacilli by acid-fast CSF smears is difficult (< 25% are positive), although subsequent high-volume specimens may increase the yield. Cultures of CSF are negative in almost 20% of patients. None of the newer rapid diagnostic tests under development for tuberculous meningitis are available for routine clinical use.

Most patients with acute **cryptococcal meningitis** have a CSF pleocytosis ranging from 20 to 500/μL, usually with < 50% neutrophils. However, severely immunocompromised patients may have very low WBC counts. India ink preparations of CSF are positive in 50% to 75% of patients, and this test should be performed on CSF samples whenever infection is suspected. The cryptococcal polysaccharide antigen test is positive in 86% of patients with cryptococcal meningitis.

Treatment

If acute bacterial meningitis is suspected, a lumbar puncture should be performed to determine whether results of routine CSF tests are consistent with the diagnosis. If results of Gram stain or rapid bacterial antigen tests are negative, the patient should immediately receive empiric antimicrobial therapy based on age and underlying disease status.

A patient with focal neurologic signs or papilledema should have a CT scan without delay before the lumbar puncture to exclude an intracranial mass lesion. However, empiric antimicrobial therapy should be initiated immediately, *before the CT scan and lumbar puncture,* because of the high morbidity and mortality rates in patients with bacterial meningitis in whom therapy is delayed.

Because *S. pneumoniae, N. meningitidis,* and *L. monocytogenes* are the likely infecting microorganisms in patients > 50 yr old and enteric gram-negative bacilli are possible although less likely pathogens, empiric therapy should consist of ampicillin plus a third-generation cephalosporin (either cefotaxime or ceftriaxone), pending culture results. In postneurosurgical patients, the empiric regimen of choice is vancomycin plus ceftazidime to cover the possibility of infection by staphylococci and gram-negative bacilli (including *Pseudomonas aeruginosa*). Once an infecting microorganism is identified, antimicrobial therapy should be modified for optimal treatment (see TABLE 92–1). Recommended doses are shown in TABLE 92–2.

TABLE 92–1. ANTIMICROBIAL THERAPY FOR BACTERIAL MENINGITIS

Organism	*Standard Therapy*	*Alternative Therapies*
Streptococcus pneumoniae		
Penicillin-sensitive*	Penicillin G or ampicillin	Third-generation cephalosporin, vancomycin, or chloramphenicol
Penicillin-resistant		
Intermediate†	Third-generation cephalosporin§	Vancomycin or chloramphenicol
High‡	Vancomycin**	
Neisseria meningitidis	Penicillin G or ampicillin	Third-generation cephalosporin§ or chloramphenicol
Hemophilus influenzae		
ß-Lactamase–negative	Ampicillin	Third-generation cephalosporin§ or chloramphenicol
ß-Lactamase–positive	Third-generation cephalosporin§	Aztreonam
Enterobacteriaceae	Third-generation cephalosporin§	Aztreonam

(continued)

TABLE 92–1. ANTIMICROBIAL THERAPY FOR BACTERIAL MENINGITIS *(Continued)*

Organism	*Standard Therapy*	*Alternative Therapies*
Pseudomonas aeruginosa	Ceftazidime††	Aztreonam or fluoroquinolone‡‡
Streptococcus agalactiae	Ampicillin or penicillin G††	Third-generation cephalosporin§ or vancomycin
Listeria monocytogenes	Ampicillin or penicillin G††	Trimethoprim-sulfamethoxazole
Staphylococcus aureus		
Methicillin-sensitive	Nafcillin or oxacillin	Vancomycin
Methicillin-resistant	Vancomycin	Trimethoprim-sulfamethoxazole
Staphylococcus epidermidis	Vancomycin**	——

Modified from Tunkel AR, Wispelwey B, Scheld WM: "Bacterial meningitis: Recent advances in pathophysiology and treatment." *Annals of Internal Medicine* 112: 610–623, 1990; used with permission.

* Minimum inhibitory concentration (MIC) to penicillin ≤ 0.06 μg/mL.
† MIC to penicillin ranges from 0.1 to 1.0 μg/mL.
‡ MIC to penicillin ≥ 1 μg/mL.
§ Cefotaxime or ceftriaxone.
** Addition of rifampin should be considered.
†† Addition of an aminoglycoside should be considered.
‡‡ Effectiveness in bacterial meningitis has not been clearly documented.

Tuberculous meningitis is treated with isoniazid, rifampin, and pyrazinamide. Ethambutol or streptomycin is added if drug resistance is suspected. Adjunctive corticosteroid therapy should be given to patients with extreme neurologic compromise, impending herniation, or impending or established spinal block. Some authorities also give corticosteroids to patients with CT evidence of either hydrocephalus or basilar meningeal inflammation. Prednisone 1 mg/kg/day, tapered over 1 mo, is usually recommended, although varying doses of dexamethasone or hydrocortisone are also used.

Cryptococcal meningitis is treated with amphotericin B (0.3 mg/kg/day) plus flucytosine (150 mg/kg/day in four divided doses) for 4 to 6 wk. However, some authorities do not recommend adding flucytosine because of the high incidence (about 38%) of adverse effects,

TABLE 92–2. RECOMMENDED DOSES OF ANTIMICROBIAL AGENTS FOR BACTERIAL MENINGITIS*

Antimicrobial Agent	*Total Daily Dose*	*Dosing Interval (h)*
Amikacin†	15 mg/kg	8
Ampicillin	12 gm	4
Aztreonam	6–8 gm	6–8
Cefotaxime	8–12 gm	4–6
Ceftazidime	6 gm	8
Ceftriaxone	4 gm	12
Chloramphenicol	4–6 gm‡	6
Ciprofloxacin	800 mg	12
Gentamicin†	3–5 mg/kg	8
Nafcillin	9–12 gm	4
Oxacillin	9–12 gm	4
Penicillin G	24 million u.	4
Rifampin	600 mg	24
Tobramycin†	3–5 mg/kg	8
Trimethoprim-sulfamethoxazole	10 mg/kg§	12
Vancomycin	2–3 gm	8–12

Modified from Tunkel AR, Wispelwey B, Scheld WM: "Bacterial meningitis: Recent advances in pathophysiology and treatment." *Annals of Internal Medicine* 112:610–623, 1990; used with permission.

* All drugs are given IV. Patients are assumed to have normal renal and hepatic function.

† Aminoglycosides should not be used to treat meningitis but may have synergistic effects against certain organisms when combined with other agents (see Table 92–1).

‡ Higher dose used for pneumococcal meningitis.

§ Dose based on trimethoprim component.

particularly pancytopenia. If flucytosine is used, serum concentrations should be monitored and maintained between 50 and 100 μg/mL. If flucytosine is not used, the dose of amphotericin B should be increased to 0.5 to 0.7 mg/kg/day.

93. MOVEMENT DISORDERS

Movement disorders comprise a complex group of diseases and conditions that may cause involuntary movements (dyskinesias), abnormal muscle tone (dystonias), or postural disturbances. Specific movement disorders include tremor, chorea, athetosis, akathisia, hemiballismus, and myoclonus. Syndromes in which movement disorders are a major component of a generalized disease include parkinsonism, progressive supranuclear palsy, and the Shy-Drager syndrome.

Movement disorders are distinguished by their clinical characteristics, which include age and rapidity of onset, family history of genetic movement disorders, coexisting conditions that might contribute to the movement disorder, extent of symptoms (whether localized or generalized), the body parts affected, and specific characteristics of the abnormal movements and associated symptoms and signs.

Extrapyramidal disorders arise outside the cerebellum and pyramidal tract. Much is known about their clinical aspects, but fundamental anatomic, physiologic, and pathogenetic bases are poorly understood. However, information on biochemical alterations in the basal ganglia helps in understanding the mechanisms by which symptoms occur and suggests a rational approach to treatment.

The most prominent biochemical feature of the basal ganglia is a high content of putative neurotransmitters, notably acetylcholine, dopamine, and γ-aminobutyric acid. Substrates and enzyme systems for their production and degradation are found within the basal ganglia. Some neurotransmitters are produced in the part of the basal ganglia in which their actions occur; others are transported by connecting axons from their production site to another area, where their actions occur. For example, dopamine is produced in the pars compacta of the substantia nigra and is transported via a neuronal tract—the nigrostriatal pathway—to the caudate nucleus and putamen, where it acts.

Normal function appears to depend on an exquisite balance between the various neurotransmitters—which may be viewed neurophysiologically as either **inhibitory** (dopamine and γ-aminobutyric acid) or **excitatory** (acetylcholine). Disturbances in production, transport, action, or degradation result in symptoms specific to the part of the brain in which the neurotransmitter acts. In general, dopamine deficiency facilitates cholinergic hyperactivity, leading to hypokinetic rigid disorders such as parkinsonism. Dopamine hyperactivity, cholinergic hypoactivity, or both result in the hyperkinesia encountered in such disorders as the choreas. Current treatment focuses on agents that can reestablish neurotransmitter balance by promoting the release, enhancing the production, preventing the degradation, or simulating the effects at receptor sites of the specific neurotransmitters involved.

PARKINSONISM
(Paralysis Agitans)

A syndrome characterized by tremor, muscular rigidity, akinesia, and loss of postural reflexes.

Parkinsonism, one of the most frequently encountered disorders of the basal ganglia, is a prominent cause of disability in those > 50 yr of age. Its prevalence is estimated at about one million cases in the USA; 50,000 new cases occur each year. The incidence increases with age, peaking at about 75 yr. While < 1% of those < 50 yr develop parkinsonism, the incidence exceeds 2% in those > 50 yr. The estimated overall lifetime risk is 2.5% among whites. Though similar data are unavailable for blacks and Orientals, prevalence rates in both groups are lower than those in whites.

Classification and Etiology

The constellation of symptoms described below occurs in both primary parkinsonism **(Parkinson's disease)** and secondary parkinsonism **(Parkinson's syndrome).**

Primary parkinsonism: When no cause can be distinguished, the condition is designated as primary parkinsonism. Most cases of parkinsonism belong in this category. The disease most frequently appears between the ages of 50 and 79 yr, but the incidence declines beyond the eighth decade. A rare juvenile form has been described in persons < 30 yr of age. The disease affects both sexes and all races. No evidence exists to indicate a hereditary factor, although a familial incidence is claimed by some authorities.

Secondary parkinsonism: Secondary parkinsonism is distinguished from primary parkinsonism by having a known cause. In many conditions, the most common of which are listed in TABLE 93–1 and discussed briefly below, a parkinsonian syndrome is the predominant clinical manifestation.

The parkinsonian syndrome is occasionally seen during the acute phase of several types of **viral encephalitis,** although permanent extrapyramidal residua are rare. The exception is the parkinsonian syndrome that developed after the epidemic of encephalitis lethargica from 1915 to 1926; sporadic cases still occur occasionally.

TABLE 93–1. CAUSES OF SECONDARY PARKINSONISM

Infections
- Viral encephalitis

Atherosclerosis of cerebral vessels

Drugs and toxins
- Antipsychotics
- Reserpine
- Metoclopramide
- Methyldopa
- Meperidine analog (MPTP)
- Carbon monoxide
- Manganese

Metabolic disorders
- Parathyroid dysfunction
- Anoxia

Tumors

Head trauma

Degenerative disorders
- Parkinson's dementia complex (occurs only in Guam)
- Striatonigral degeneration
- Progressive supranuclear palsy
- Olivopontocerebellar atrophy
- Parkinsonism with autonomic dystrophy (Shy-Drager syndrome, multisystem atrophy)

Cerebral atherosclerosis with multi-infarcts of the cerebrum produces parkinsonism. Typically, akinesia and gait disturbances occur and are more properly classified as pseudoparkinsonism. These symptoms rarely respond to therapeutic measures effective for Parkinson's disease. Parkinsonism has been reported after **carbon monoxide poisoning.** Usually occupationally related, **chronic manganese intoxication** produces a parkinsonian syndrome accompanied by dystonia and mental changes.

Parkinsonism may appear as a **side effect of drugs** that deplete or block the action of cerebral monoamines, most commonly various antipsychotic drugs such as the phenothiazines and butyrophenones. Metoclopramide and some antihypertensive agents (eg, reserpine and methyldopa) may also induce parkinsonism. Some reactions are dose dependent; others are related to individual susceptibility (eg, risk increases with age and in women). Once the drugs are withdrawn, symptoms usually disappear within a few days, although occasionally they persist for months or even years; sometimes symptoms begin or worsen when the drugs are stopped. A meperidine analog, MPTP (1-methyl-4-phenyl-1,2,3,6-tetrahydropyridine), occasionally injected by IV drug abusers, can induce irreversible parkinsonism.

Hypoparathyroidism is associated with calcification of the basal ganglia, which produces parkinsonism (rarely) as well as chorea and athetosis. A CT scan may demonstrate small calcium deposits in the basal ganglia. Patients with **brain tumors** near the basal ganglia may present with hemiparkinsonism, ie, parkinsonian symptoms restricted to one side of the body. Frontal lobe tumors occasionally produce gait and movement abnormalities that mimic parkinsonism. Other disorders that may be confused with parkinsonism include **myxedema, normal-pressure hydrocephalus, hepatic encephalopathy,** and **depression.**

A parkinsonian syndrome may occur to varying degrees in several so-called **degenerative diseases of unknown cause** that involve multiple areas of the CNS (eg, progressive supranuclear palsy, olivopontocerebellar atrophy, and the Shy-Drager syndrome).

Pathophysiology

Primary and secondary parkinsonism do not seem to differ in pathophysiology or even in pathogenetic mechanisms for symptom production. Striatal dopamine deficiency is common to all types of parkinsonism. Invariably in primary parkinsonism, cell loss is noted in the substantia nigra in association with formation of an intracellular inclusion body—the **Lewy body.** In secondary parkinsonism, there may be loss of substantia nigra cells, impairment of the nigral striatal pathway, or loss of striatal cellular elements, but Lewy bodies do not form. The loss of nigral cells with destruction of the nigrostriatal pathway results in the decreased level of striatal dopamine.

The cause of the selective nigral cell destruction is unknown; however, several pathogenetic mechanisms have been suggested. The most acceptable, though not proved, concerns cellular damage by the oxidative production of toxic free radicals. It is postulated that a relative excess of free radicals develops in nigral cells caused by oxidative stress, leading to increased oxidative degradation of dopamine and the accumulation of toxic metabolic products. The factors that cause oxidative stress are not known. Yet, its effect can be counteracted by inhibiting monoamine oxidase (MAO), thereby limiting the catabolism of dopamine and accumulation of toxic metabolic products. Selegiline (L-deprenyl), a selective MAO-B inhibitor, may protect the brain cells involved in Parkinson's disease. This agent is discussed under Treatment, below.

Symptoms and Signs

The disease begins insidiously; any of its cardinal manifestations may appear alone or in combination. The most common initial symptom is **tremor,** usually in one hand or sometimes in both and involving the fingers in a pill-rolling motion. The tremor is present at rest **(resting tremor),** may be accentuated by posture, and usually decreases with active, purposeful movement. It disappears with sleep. The tremor is rhythmic, low in frequency, generally low in amplitude (alternately affecting flexor and extensor muscles), and may involve upper or lower limbs, lips, tongue, or head.

Muscular rigidity is usually readily evident on passive movement of a limb. Passive movement may demonstrate a smooth resistance (like trying to bend a lead pipe—**lead-pipe rigidity**), sometimes with superimposed ratchet-like jerks **(cogwheel phenomenon).** The patient may be slow to initiate movement **(bradykinesia)** and while carrying out routine tasks may find his volitional movement suddenly and unexpectedly halted; the patient may be unable to follow through to complete the action. Bradykinesia is especially evident in writing and feeding and can be striking when the patient attempts to walk and finds that his feet are suddenly "frozen to the ground." However, bradykinesia may not be present at the onset of the disease. Rapidly alternating movements are very difficult to perform.

Gait becomes shuffled with short steps, and the arms fail to swing. The steps may inadvertently quicken, and the patient may break into a run to keep from falling (festination). **Postural abnormalities** are evident in the erect and sitting positions; an erect posture is not readily assumed or maintained. The head tends to fall forward on the trunk, and the body falls forward or backward unless supported. The tendency to fall forward **(propulsion)** or backward **(retropulsion)** results from the loss of postural reflexes. Bradykinesia prevents the patient from stopping the fall, by either taking a step or moving the arms. Kyphotic deformity of the spine, causing a stooped posture, is a hallmark of the disease, a result of altered striatal activity with imbalance between right and left.

The face can become masklike, with lack of expression and diminished eye blinking. Blepharospasm can be readily induced when the frontal muscle is tapped (Meyerson's sign). Micrographia and difficulty with activities of daily living (eg, tying shoes) often develop. Speech becomes slow and monotonous. The patient has difficulty swallowing and tends to drool. The skin has an oily quality and may be afflicted with seborrheic dermatitis.

Mood abnormalities, usually depression or anxiety, are common and may be the heralding symptoms. Sometimes bradykinesia and decreased facial expression make a person appear depressed, even when mood is unaffected. Although intellectual impairment does occur, whether it is intrinsic to the disease or associated with a superimposed but unrelated dementing illness is controversial.

Although parkinsonism is invariably progressive, the rates at which symptoms develop and disability ensues are extremely variable. Sometimes the disease progresses rapidly, and patients become disabled within 5 yr. More often, the course is slower and more protracted, and patients remain functional for many years.

Diagnosis

Parkinsonism is diagnosed on the basis of the symptoms and signs. Early signs include infrequent blinking and lack of facial expression, loss of voice volume, poverty of movement, impaired postural reflexes, and the characteristic gait abnormality. About 30% of patients may not have tremor initially, and it often becomes less prominent as the disease progresses; this should not obscure the diagnosis. Rigidity of some degree usually develops, and its absence makes the diagnosis of parkinsonism suspect.

Patients with essential tremor, which is the disorder most commonly confused with parkinsonism, have animated facies, normal rates of movement, normal muscle tone, and no gait impairment (see ESSENTIAL TREMOR, below). Furthermore, essential tremor occurs as an action tremor rather than a resting tremor, which is most common in parkinsonism. Parkinsonism may be more difficult to distinguish in elderly persons with reduced spontaneity of movement, short-stepped (rheumatic) gait, and mild depression or dementia.

No specific laboratory test can confirm the diagnosis of parkinsonism. Routine blood, spinal fluid, and urine tests yield normal results. The disturbance in cerebral dopamine metabolism may result in decreased CSF levels of homovanillic acid; however, this finding is not reliable in confirming the diagnosis and testing is not recommended. The EEG is usually normal, although diffuse slowing may be present and sleep recordings may be abnormal. Neither CT nor MRI scan of the head shows abnormalities in primary parkinsonism but may be helpful in diagnosing some of the secondary forms. When a treatable cause is suspected, a CT or MRI scan should generally be performed.

Treatment

No curative therapy is available for primary parkinsonism or for most cases of secondary parkinsonism. The major exception is secondary parkinsonism resulting from drugs. Almost all other cases require lifelong treatment with drugs directed primarily at symptom control. *Treatment programs should be individualized,* using as a guide the type and severity of symptoms, the degree of functional impairment, any associated disease processes, and the expected benefits and risks of available drugs. This caution applies especially to the elderly, who have reduced tolerance for dopaminergic and anticholinergic agents, the mainstays of parkinsonism therapy (see also Antiparkinsonian Drugs in Ch. 21).

Patients with symptoms of recent onset, especially if tremor predominates and functional impairment is mild, are best treated with drugs that centrally inhibit cholinergic activity. However, anticholinergics are often poorly tolerated by the elderly, producing sedation, confusion, urinary retention, dry mouth, blurred vision, and orthostatic hypotension. They are contraindicated in persons with glaucoma, benign prostatic hypertrophy, and dementia. **Diphenhydramine,** an antihistamine with anticholinergic action, in a dose of 25 mg tid may suffice.

More effective but more toxic is **trihexyphenidyl** 2 mg 3 to 5 times/day; it should be administered cautiously and usually below the optimal dosage.

Amantadine, another useful drug, is generally prescribed at 100 mg bid. Amantadine's mode of action in the treatment of parkinsonism is unknown, but its mild anticholinergic effects appear to play only a small part. It may promote dopamine release in the corpus striatum or may reduce dopamine reuptake.

Selegiline (an MAO-B inhibitor) in doses of 5 mg bid may be used in an early stage to prevent or slow disease progression. The drug inhibits oxidative metabolism of dopamine. Trials indicate that selegiline can delay the need for additional antiparkinsonian agents. However, whether selegiline slows the disease or just suppresses symptoms is controversial. The drug is generally well tolerated with few side effects. Although chemically related to other MAO inhibitors, selegiline does not require dietary restrictions.

Patients with fully established parkinsonian symptoms that impair motor function should be treated with drugs capable of replenishing or activating striatal dopaminergic effects. There are as many recent studies supporting delayed use of dopaminergic agents as there are those that promote early use. Most experts believe that treatment should not be instituted until symptoms cause functional impairment. In so doing, the risk of late side effects of dopaminergic agents, which can be most distressing, is delayed.

The best way to accomplish dopamine replacement is to use **levodopa combined with carbidopa.** Levodopa is converted to dopamine in both the CNS and the periphery. To reduce peripheral conversion, levodopa is combined with carbidopa (a peripheral decarboxylator inhibitor), which does not cross the blood-brain barrier.

Treatment usually begins with a half tablet of the 25:100 combination (ie, 25 mg carbidopa to 100 mg levodopa) bid or tid. After 1 wk, the dose can be increased to a full tablet tid if needed and if side effects are tolerable. After several weeks, the dose can be increased again. Side effects may be peripheral—such as flushing, abdominal cramping, and anorexia—in which case increasing the amount of carbidopa may be helpful, or they may be central—such as anxiety, nightmares, confusion, and hypotension—in which case decreasing the dose of levodopa may be necessary. A controlled-release form (50:200) may reduce side effects but generally requires a slightly higher total daily dose.

Levodopa-carbidopa is often given in combination with other drugs, although these other drugs may occasionally be used as single therapies. A cautious induction period with each is required. **Bromocriptine** is begun with 1.25 mg/day and gradually increased by 2.5-mg increments every 2 days to a total daily dose of 10 to 15 mg. **Pergolide** is begun at 0.05 mg/day with increments of 0.05 mg every 2 or 3 days until a daily dose of 1 to 3 mg is reached. Selegiline, amantadine, and anticholinergic agents may also be administered with levodopa-carbidopa. TABLE 93–2 lists the most commonly used antiparkinsonian drugs and their major side effects.

TABLE 93–2. COMMONLY USED ANTIPARKINSONIAN DRUGS

Drug	*Starting Dose*	*Average Daily Dose*	*Total Daily Dose Range*	*Major Side Effects*
Carbidopa-levodopa 25/100 mg	12.5/50 mg tid	25/100 mg qid	75/100 to 150/600 mg	Nausea, anorexia, confusion, psychotic disturbances, nightmares, dyskinesia
Carbidopa-levodopa controlled release 50/200 mg	25/100 mg bid	50/200 mg qid	150/600 to 300/1200 mg	Same as above
Bromocriptine	1.25 mg/day	2.5 mg qid	10 to 15 mg	Nausea, vomiting, confusion, hallucinations, hypotension, dyskinesia
Pergolide	0.05 mg/day	0.25 mg qid	1 to 3 mg	Nausea, vomiting, confusion, hallucinations, hypotension, dyskinesia
Amantadine	100 mg/day	100 mg bid	100 to 200 mg	Confusional state, urinary retention, elevated intraocular pressure, levido reticularis
Selegiline	5 mg/day	5 mg bid	5 to 10 mg	Nausea, headache, insomnia, confusional state
Trihexyphenidyl	1 mg bid	2 mg tid	6 to 12 mg	Dry mucous membranes, increase in intraocular pressure, urinary retention, confusional state, cognitive impairment, hyperthermia

A new approach to replenishing the dopamine deficit by **transplantation or grafting of fetal nigral cells** to the corpus striatum shows promise. Nigral cells harvested from aborted fetuses are stereotactically inserted in the striatum, particularly the putamen, of patients with Parkinson's disease. These cells appear to remain viable, to form neural connections, and to be capable of producing dopamine. Because selection criteria have been strict (eg, limiting participation in studies to only those who have developed difficulties with pharmacotherapy), the usefulness of this approach cannot yet be fully assessed.

PROGRESSIVE SUPRANUCLEAR PALSY

(Steele-Richardson-Olszewski Syndrome)

A rare disorder characterized by parkinsonian symptoms, pseudobulbar signs, vertical-gaze palsy, and subcortical dementia.

About 4% of patients with parkinsonism actually have the clinical manifestations of progressive supranuclear palsy. Onset usually occurs during or after the sixth decade, but some patients develop signs of the disorder in their fifth decade. The pathogenesis is unknown. Evidence of a transmissible cause is lacking, and familial cases have not been reported. There is no ethnic or racial predilection, although men are more often affected. The disease usually progresses rapidly, with marked incapacity occurring within 2 to 3 yr and death within 10 yr, generally due to intercurrent infection.

Pathologic examination shows degenerative changes in the brain stem and diencephalon and nuclear masses in the cerebellum. Other findings include nerve cell loss, neurofibrillary tangles, granulovacuolar degeneration, gliosis, and occasionally, perivascular cuffing.

Symptoms, Signs, and Diagnosis

The clinical manifestations of progressive supranuclear palsy include progressive impairment of voluntary gaze of supranuclear origin, with vertical-gaze palsy (downward more than upward) being most prominent. Other ophthalmologic symptoms include blurred vision, diplopia, photophobia, burning, tearing, and retraction of the upper lids leading to a staring, astonishment-like appearance. Other findings are gait unsteadiness with falling (usually backward), dysarthria, dysphagia, rigidity, bradykinesia, hypomimia (lack of facial expression and movement), and hyperactive neck extension. Tremor is not prominent. Depression or subcortical dementia is common later in the course; sleep disturbances (insomnia or hyposomnia), agitation, irritability, apathy, slowed thinking, and pseudobulbar affect are also seen.

Mild to moderate atrophy of the midbrain, the cerebellum, and occasionally, the cerebral hemispheres may be seen on CT or MRI scan.

Routine laboratory studies are not affected, except for an occasional increase in CSF protein level. The EEG often shows nonspecific abnormalities early in the disease course, but with progression, bifrontal nonrhythmic bursts of delta activity may be seen.

Treatment

No fully effective treatment is available. Although dopaminergic agents can control the parkinsonian symptoms, they have no effect on the ocular motor difficulty and tend to accentuate the behavioral abnormalities.

SHY–DRAGER SYNDROME

A multisystem degenerative disease with involvement of the central (preganglionic) autonomic, cerebellar, basal ganglia, pyramidal, and spinal motor neurons.

The major feature differentiating Shy-Drager syndrome from parkinsonism is autonomic derangement. The mean age of onset is 55 yr (range, 37 to 75 yr). A male predominance is noted, with a 2:1 or 3:1 ratio. No genetic predisposition has been shown, and familial incidence has been reported in only one case. The pathogenesis of the disease is unknown. About 11% of patients with severe orthostatic hypotension have this syndrome. The disease is progressive, and death occurs 7 to 10 yr after the onset of neurologic symptoms. Cardiac arrhythmias, aspiration, sleep apnea, and pulmonary emboli are common causes of death.

Symptoms, Signs, and Diagnosis

The major manifestation is autonomic insufficiency with wide swings in blood pressure but no change in pulse rate. Patients complain of dizziness, syncope, or light-headedness on standing; postexertional weakness; gait unsteadiness; or dimming of vision. Impaired temperature control, reduced sweating, sphincter disturbance with urinary or fecal incontinence, diarrhea, constipation, nocturnal diuresis, impotence, iridic atrophy, impaired eye movements, Horner's syndrome, anisocoria, nystagmus, and abnormal convergence may also occur.

Central neuron degeneration is manifested by parkinsonian features, intention tremor, ataxia, dysarthria, and in some cases, corticobulbar and corticospinal tract signs. Anterior horn cell degeneration leads to wasting and fasciculation of distal muscles. Intellectual and emotional function is preserved until late in the disease course. Laboratory studies are usually normal, with some nonspecific EEG abnormalities. The electromyogram may show anterior horn cell involvement.

Treatment

Nonpharmacologic treatment of the autonomic dysfunction includes avoiding extreme heat, alcohol, large meals, getting up rapidly, and excessive straining at stool. Compressive clothing and stockings, increased salt and fluid intake, and sleeping in a reverse Trendelenburg position may ameliorate some of the orthostatic symptoms. Drugs that are sometimes useful in treating the orthostatic hypotension include indomethacin, midodrine, propranolol, and pindolol. Additionally, fludrocortisone, starting at doses of 0.1 mg/day, can be used to expand the plasma volume.

TREMOR

Essential tremor (most specifically senile tremor), cerebellar tremor, and neuropathic tremor are the tremors occurring most often in the elderly.

ESSENTIAL TREMOR

(Familial Tremor; Senile Tremor)

An exaggeration of normal, alternating muscle contractions, often referred to as shaking, involving the hands, head, or face, or all three areas.

Essential tremor refers to sporadic cases, while **familial tremor** refers to cases with an associated family history. **Senile tremor** refers to cases in which essential tremor begins in old age; yet, despite its name, senile tremor is not a normal concomitant of aging. Most patients develop the tremor in the seventh decade. It occurs equally in men and women but is more prevalent in whites than in blacks.

Senile tremor most often involves the upper limbs and head. At first, it occurs only with voluntary movements; later, it becomes more constant and even occurs at rest. There is no associated weakness or alteration in muscle tone. The cause is unknown; however, since senile tremor has both cerebellar and extrapyramidal features (in that it occurs both at rest and with movement), degeneration of some critical pathway linking these systems is assumed.

Senile tremor can be embarrassing, even debilitating. It can make speech unsteady, make carrying objects difficult, make eating uncomfortable, and ultimately lead to social isolation. Anxiety may exacerbate it.

Tremor often does not respond to treatment in the elderly as well as it does in younger adults. Alcohol suppresses the tremor, and many patients discover this on their own. In an effort to decrease the tremor, patients may abuse alcohol. However, small amounts used occasionally may be appropriate therapy. β-Blocking agents such as propranolol 20 mg tid or nadolol 20 to 40 mg/day may help, but side effects may limit the dose. The anticonvulsant primidone at 50 to 100 mg qid is sometimes helpful. In severe cases, sedatives and acetazolamide can be tried.

Most patients with senile tremor do not require pharmacologic treatment. Rather, they need reassurance that the tremor does not indicate parkinsonism or other disease. (For the differences between essential tremor and parkinsonism, see Diagnosis under PARKINSONISM, above.) Helpful hints for daily living activities—such as holding objects close to the body so as not to drop them, placing napkins between cups and saucers to keep them from rattling, not eating soup in public, and avoiding uncomfortable or awkward positions—can reduce embarrassment and help those with tremor adjust to what is likely to be a lifelong problem.

CEREBELLAR TREMOR

Elderly patients with cerebellar disease may have both a postural and a characteristic tremor that is readily demonstrated on finger-nose or heel-shin testing. The tremor results from lesions of the lateral dentate nucleus of the cerebellum or its projections. The tremor frequency is 3 to 5 Hz. It may vary in amplitude and have a coarse side-to-side component. It tends to increase when the limbs maintain an outstretched position but is not evident during sleep or with complete relaxation. In contrast, cerebellar ataxia consists of irregular, uncoordinated, and nonpatterned movements.

Titubation is *a rocking back and forth movement with a rotating or side-to-side component* that occurs with midline cerebellar disease (of the vermis cerebelli). There is no effective treatment for cerebellar tremor.

NEUROPATHIC TREMOR

Although rare, neuropathic tremor may be a manifestation of peripheral neuropathy due to porphyria, diabetes, alcohol abuse, uremia, amyloidosis, vincristine therapy, or relapsing polyneuropathy. The mechanism is unclear, but the tremor may result from an imbalance in the sensory input to the motor neuron pool. Alternatively, it may be an enhancement of physiologic tremor by weakened muscle or impaired stretch reflexes. This tremor is not responsive to propranolol or any other therapy.

OTHER TREMORS

The tremor seen in **alcohol withdrawal** is rapid and coarse, involves the entire body, and is characteristically abolished or diminished by a drink of alcohol. A permanent tremor of different quality (more generalized and akin to tremulousness) may be seen in chronic alcoholism. The pathophysiology is unknown. **Narcotic withdrawal,** although uncommon in the elderly, may be manifested by a fine tremor of the facial muscles and fingers.

Drugs may induce tremor, especially in the elderly, in whom drug tolerance is reduced and polypharmacy is common. Tremor-inducing drugs include theophylline, tricyclic antidepressants, terbutaline, metaproterenol, valproic acid, lithium, and some antipsychotics. In addition, caffeine may induce tremor. **Poisoning** with methyl bromide or with heavy metals such as mercury, arsenic, or bismuth can also cause tremor.

Metabolic encephalopathy due to liver failure, uremia, or respiratory acidosis may cause **asterixis,** which is characterized by irregular flapping movements of the outstretched hands. **The tremor of hyperthyroidism** is fine, regular, and rapid; it is usually confined to the outstretched hands and fingers.

These tremors should be treated by attending to the underlying cause.

THE CHOREAS

Disease entities that, although wholly unrelated etiologically, are manifested primarily by choreiform movements—rapid, highly complex, involuntary jerky movements.

In some choreas, close relationships to infectious processes are found; other choreas are genetic. The conditions associated with chorea in the elderly are shown in TABLE 93–3.

Pathologic changes have been found in various parts of the basal ganglia, many of which influence the motor system via the globus pallidus. It is postulated that choreiform movements result when impaired afferent connections cause a loss of inhibition of the pallidum.

Choreiform movements sometimes occur as an isolated symptom in persons > 60 yr of age and are then called **senile chorea.** Involuntary complex movements of the face, mouth, and tongue may occur alone or with unilateral or bilateral limb movements. Senile chorea probably has several causes, and some cases may be a variant of Huntington's cho-

TABLE 93–3. CONDITIONS ASSOCIATED WITH CHOREA

CNS infections	Encephalitis lethargica (von Economo's disease) Meningoencephalitis secondary to viral infection Parenchymatous neurosyphilis
Autoimmune disorders	Systemic lupus erythematosus (SLE) Henoch-Schönlein purpura Rheumatoid arthritis Periarteritis nodosa Serum sickness reaction to tetanus antitoxin Lyme disease
Metabolic disorders	Thyrotoxicosis Hypo- and hyperparathyroidism Hypocalcemia
Drug intoxications	Atropine poisoning and other anticholinergic intoxications Anticonvulsants Amphetamines Levodopa Lithium Phenothiazine and related antipsychotic drugs Isoniazid
Genetic disorders	Huntington's chorea Acute intermittent porphyria Wilson's disease Acanthocytosis Olivopontocerebellar atrophy, dominant form

Miscellaneous disorders	Pick's disease
	Alzheimer's disease
	Senile chorea
	Benign familial chorea
	Polycythemia
	Beriberi
	Cerebrovascular disease
	  Arteriosclerotic vascular disease
	  Meningovascular syphilis
	Brain tumor, primary or metastatic
	Trauma; subdural hematoma

rea. Neither mental disturbance nor family history of Huntington's chorea is associated with senile chorea. Symptoms often come on abruptly, are usually unilateral, and show little if any progression.

DYSTONIAS

Movement disorders characterized by intense, irregular, sustained torsion spasms of the musculature, resulting in marked abnormalities of bodily posture.

Dystonic movements may involve one or more body sites or may be generalized, involving all the limbs and trunk simultaneously. The pathophysiology and underlying morbid anatomy are unknown.

Many conditions, such as tumors or arteriovenous malformations of the brain, cause dystonia; as a rule, these conditions produce focal dystonic movements or postures that more frequently affect the upper limbs, particularly the hand. *When focal dystonia is encountered in an adult, a complete evaluation should be undertaken to determine the cause.*

Specific Dystonias

Spasmodic torticollis: In spasmodic torticollis, involuntary activity of the sternocleidomastoid, trapezius, and scalene muscles results in sustained contractions leading to slow, twisting, turning movements of the head **(torticollis)** or, less often, forward flexion **(anterocollis)** or forceful extension **(retrocollis).** In some instances, the torticollis is one of various extrapyramidal disorders that occur after viral encephalitis.

The disorder can occur at any age but most often appears in the third to sixth decades. The course varies: in some patients, it is transitory and remits after a few months; in others, it is relentlessly progressive and leads to incapacity.

Cranial dystonias: Blepharospasm, oromandibular dystonia, and laryngeal and pharyngeal dystonia are cranial dystonias. They occur in adult life, usually in the fifth or sixth decade; their cause is unknown; and they are resistant to most therapies. Each is characterized by intermittent spasms of selected groups of muscles, which markedly interfere with function. **Blepharospasm** is involuntary spasm of the orbicular muscle of the eye, causing forceful closure of the eyes. Oromandibular and orofacial dystonias are involuntary spasms of the facial muscles, jaw muscles, tongue, and platysma, which cause arrhythmic movements. These dystonias may be provoked by attempts to talk or eat.

Spastic dysphonia: In spastic dysphonia, adductor muscles of the larynx are spasmodic. Speech is tight and constricted, with the smooth flow of words broken up into an irregular pattern. This differs from voice tremor, in which the speech is normally regular but broken up by a tremor pattern. If the vocal cord and abductor muscle are dystonic, a breathy dysphonia is produced, with the patient running out of words when speaking.

Tardive dystonia: In tardive dystonia, dystonic movements are caused by antipsychotic drugs (see also TARDIVE DYSKINESIA AND AKATHISIA, below). The face and neck are most often affected, but the entire body may be involved. However, abnormal involuntary movements tend to remain focal in older patients.

Treatment

Treatment of dystonias is difficult. High doses of anticholinergic drugs may be effective, but their side effects in older patients often preclude their use. Some patients may benefit from baclofen, bromocriptine, carbamazepine, clonazepam, diazepam, reserpine, or tetrabenazine. More recently, control of focal dystonia has been accomplished with botulinum toxin type A. Injection of this agent into the affected muscle produces graded but temporary weakness and relief of dystonic symptoms. It has been most effective in cases of torticollis, blepharospasm, and laryngeal dystonia. Unfortunately, the benefit is rarely permanent, and additional injections every few months are necessary.

TARDIVE DYSKINESIA AND AKATHISIA

Tardive dyskinesia: *A syndrome of persistent, stereotyped, repetitive abnormal involuntary movements associated with chronic exposure to antipsychotic drugs, which bind with and block the dopamine receptor.* Higher doses and prolonged treatment increase the likelihood of inducing the movements. Abnormal involuntary movements typically start while taking the medication and may worsen when reducing the dose or discontinuing the drug. Reinstituting the drug may alleviate the symptoms. The cause is related to dopamine receptor supersensitivity. The prevalence of tardive dyskinesia increases with age and is more common in elderly women. The incidence in the elderly is about four times that in young adults.

Classic oral tardive dyskinesia involves tongue movements and chewing, lip puckering, and lip smacking that differ from choreiform movements in that they are repetitive and predictable. Tardive dyskinesia and tardive akathisia are other expressions of this disorder.

Tardive akathisia: *A subjective state of motor restlessness or an aversion to being still.* Vocal, truncal, and limb movements become stereotyped and repetitive. Repeatedly rubbing or stroking parts of the body, crossing and uncrossing the arms or legs, picking at clothes, pacing, marching in place, swinging the legs, and moaning, grunting, or shouting are all manifestations of tardive akathisia.

Akathisia is usually caused by drugs, especially antipsychotics and tricyclic antidepressants. It is frequently misdiagnosed as agitation, which too often leads prescribers to increase the dose of the very medication that has caused the problem.

Treatment

Treatment of tardive dyskinesia and akathisia includes, if possible, discontinuing the drug that caused the disorder. Orobuccal dyskinesia, if significant, can be treated with reserpine at a dose of 0.25 mg/day and gradually increased to an average dose of 5.0 mg/day, although response is not always good. Akathisia can also be treated with reserpine, but discontinuing the drug causing the symptom is usually all that is needed. Opioids, propranolol, and benzodiazepines are rarely helpful.

HEMIBALLISMUS

A violent, involuntary movement that occurs with destructive lesions of the contralateral subthalamic nucleus (the corpus Luysii).

The abnormal movements of hemiballismus occur when at least 20% of the corpus Luysii is destroyed. However, the substantia nigra, pyramidal tract, and red nucleus must be intact. Although a variety of pathologic processes (eg, metastatic tumors, cysts, and infectious diseases) can be underlying causes, most cases result from vascular lesions, either hemorrhagic or occlusive. Consequently, these movements occur in older patients, sometimes after a transitory hemiparesis from a stroke.

As the neurologic signs of the stroke clear or some time later, the ballistic movements begin. They do not occur during sleep, are localized to one side of the body, and involve the limbs in a forceful throwing movement, a result of almost continuous activity of the proximal musculature. The arm and leg may be equally involved, but involvement of one is usually more prominent. The neck, tongue, or face may also be affected.

Initially, the violence of these movements may exhaust and incapacitate the patient to such an extent that death ensues. However, the initial intensity usually decreases gradually so that the movements become tolerable and can be somewhat suppressed or briefly interrupted by voluntary action. In about 6 to 8 wk, the movements stop spontaneously, particularly when the cause of hemiballismus was an occlusive vascular lesion. When tumor provokes hemiballismus, movements persist.

Treatment is not very effective, but haloperidol may be tried for postsynaptic blockade. Valproic acid and reserpine have also helped some patients. Surgical measures, such as thalamotomy, are indicated only in life-threatening cases. In fact, hemiballismus has occurred after attempted thalamotomy for other extrapyramidal disorders, when poor localization led to inadvertent destruction of the corpus Luysii.

MYOCLONUS

Sudden, brief, involuntary single or repetitive contractions of a muscle or group of muscles.

Myoclonus can vary in amplitude, frequency, and distribution. The muscle jerks may be induced by sudden noise, movement, light, or visual threat; they are caused by muscular contractions (positive myoclonus) or inhibitions (negative myoclonus) arising from hyperexcitable neurons in the spinal cord, medial reticular formation, or cerebral cortex.

Myoclonus can be classified according to cause. In the elderly, the major causes are related to the dementias, metabolic or toxic encephalopathies, or focal CNS damage. Additional causes are listed in TABLE 93–4.

Myoclonus can be an early feature of **Creutzfeldt-Jakob disease** (subacute spongiform encephalopathy). The myoclonus can be elicited by a stimulus or can occur spontaneously and is associated with a periodic synchronous discharge on the EEG. In the later stages of **Alzheimer's disease,** patients may exhibit myoclonus. The event is shorter and more focal than that in Creutzfeldt-Jakob disease and can be seen at rest, with voluntary activity, or with stimulation. Myoclonus following a **hypoxic insult** is usually precipitated by voluntary motor action. Associated cerebellar ataxia, dysarthria, postural lapses, gait disturbances, and grand mal seizures may occur.

Metabolic derangements, including uremia, hypercapnia, hepatic failure, hypoglycemia, hyponatremia, and need for chronic hemodialysis, may be complicated by multifocal, asymmetric, stimulus-sensitive myoclonus. Facial or proximal limb muscles are predominantly involved. If the metabolic abnormality persists, generalized myoclonic jerks and, ultimately, seizures may occur.

Nocturnal leg myoclonus is an uncommon condition in which myoclonus occurs generally at night and affects only the legs. It affects mostly elderly persons, and it appears to be an isolated condition with a benign, but sometimes annoying, course. Nocturnal leg myoclonus does not respond to quinine therapy.

Chronic levodopa treatment in some parkinsonian patients can induce myoclonus, characterized by single, abrupt, symmetric jerks of the arms and legs usually during sleep, drowsiness, or at rest. A reduction in dose can alleviate the frequency and severity of the myoclonus. **Toxic doses** of some drugs, such as tricyclic antidepressants, valproic acid, lithium, carbamazepine, phenytoin, antihistamines, and MAO inhibitors, can also induce myoclonus. High-dose penicillin or cephalosporin infusion can induce nonrhythmic, asymmetric, and stimulus-sensitive myoclonus.

TABLE 93–4. CAUSES OF MYOCLONUS

Dementias	Creutzfeldt-Jakob disease Alzheimer's disease
Metabolic disorders or conditions	Hepatic failure Renal failure Chronic hemodialysis Hyponatremia Hypoglycemia Nonketotic hyperglycemia
Toxic encephalopathies	Drugs, including levodopa Bismuth Heavy-metal poisons Methyl bromide, DDT
Physical encephalopathies	Posthypoxia Posttrauma Heatstroke Electric shock
Degeneration of the basal ganglia	Wilson's disease Torsion dystonia Progressive supranuclear palsy Huntington's chorea Parkinson's disease
Viral encephalopathies	Subacute sclerosing panencephalitis Encephalitis lethargica Herpes simplex encephalitis Postinfectious encephalitis

Treatment: Drugs that may alleviate the myoclonus are clonazepam, valproic acid, carbamazepine, levodopa, estrogens, 5-hydroxytryptophan, and piracetam, although most often it is safest to give no treatment.

§3. ORGAN SYSTEMS: PSYCHIATRIC DISORDERS

SKIN DISORDERS

§3. ORGAN SYSTEMS: PSYCHIATRIC DISORDERS

94. NORMAL CHANGES OF AGING AND PATTERNS OF PSYCHIATRIC DISEASE

Failure to differentiate disease-related psychiatric changes from manifestations of normal aging has blurred the understanding of mental function in healthy older adults. Many decrements in capacity or performance viewed as age related—particularly those associated with cognition and behavior—actually reflect modifiable consequences of illness.

NORMAL CHANGES OF AGING

Changes in Cognition

A longitudinal study of cognitive capacity in a cohort of men followed from 1919 to 1961 described increments in verbal ability and total intellectual performance from age 20 to age 50, although mathematical ability declined slightly. From 50 to 60 yr of age, scores of intellect showed little change. These studies were among the first to raise serious doubts about the presumed normal decline in mental ability with aging, which had been inferred from earlier cross-sectional research.

A 12-yr longitudinal study of older men (median age, 71 yr) conducted by the National Institute of Mental Health examined a broad range of variables. Physical and psychiatric disease was absent or minimal; the goal was to separate the impact of aging from that of illness. As these healthy men moved from their 70s to their 80s, various intellectual functions declined while others improved. For example, quality of cognitive operations, draw-a-person exercises, and sentence completions declined, while vocabulary and picture arrangement ability improved. This suggests that older persons may have difficulty with activities requiring a quick reaction time or a high degree of precision, although they maintain the ability to understand their situation and learn from new experiences.

Moreover, men who developed arteriosclerotic cardiovascular disease had significantly greater decrements in intellectual performance than those who remained healthy. Therefore, significant changes in intellectual performance should not be dismissed as normal consequences of aging but should be evaluated as potentially modifiable manifestations of disease (psychiatric as well as general medical). For example, both depression and hypothyroidism are treatable problems that can be covert and cause cognitive impairment.

Changes in Behavior and Personality

Corresponding to the stereotype of inevitable intellectual decline with aging are stereotypes of regressive behavior and increasing inflexibility of personality traits. However, these are more a sign of psychiatric disturbance than a manifestation of aging. Consider the issue of cautiousness. Research shows that the elderly are more cautious than younger adults about risk taking when the payoff is predictable and constant. If the size of the payoff depends on the degree of risk, however, older persons are no more cautious than younger persons.

Anxiety can result in cautiousness, causing delays in decision making and reactions. In other words, excessive cautiousness in the elderly may signal underlying anxiety or a related clinical disorder. However, it is entirely appropriate for a frail or disabled older person to be more careful in general. A maladaptive overcautiousness resulting from anxiety must be distinguished from an appropriate, adaptive response to reality.

If older adults appear to be more rigid than younger adults, then cohort differences (ie, generational differences that stem from having grown up during different historic periods)—and not age differences—are more likely involved. Research shows not only that personalities remain stable with aging but also that behavioral and psychologic adaptiveness continues and does not normally give way to regression or rigidity. If certain behaviors or traits become increasingly exaggerated, maladaptive, and unmodifiable, neurosis rather than normal aging may be to blame. Treatment rather than acceptance is in order.

PATTERNS OF PSYCHIATRIC DISEASE

Epidemiology

The high frequency of mental health problems in the elderly is significant; they impact mental status and emotional states and potentially influence the course of physical illness. Epidemiologic studies since the 1950s have documented a 15% to 25% prevalence of serious mental disorders in those ≥ 65 yr old. More than 25% of state mental hospital patients in the USA (> 50% in the United Kingdom) are ≥ 65 yr of age.

Psychiatric problems are a primary or secondary diagnosis in 70% to 80% of nursing home residents; one study identified 94% of nursing home residents as having mental disorders, according to criteria in the *Diagnostic and Statistical Manual of Mental Disorders,* Fourth Edition (DSM-IV). Because of improved general medical care in the community, patients admitted to nursing homes tend to be sicker, both mentally and physically, than in the past. However, mental disorders, particularly organic disorders, have always been prevalent in nursing home patients.

Organic disorders (most commonly, Alzheimer's disease) affect about 10% of those ≥ 65 yr old—the rate is considerably higher (at least 25%) in those ≥ 85 yr old. Significant symptoms of depression have been described in 15% of community-dwelling elderly persons, and of schizophrenia, in 0.5% to 1.0%. The prevalence of alcohol abuse is difficult to determine but is considered to be high, conservatively estimated at 2% to 5%. Suicide occurs more often in elderly men than in any other age group (see Suicide, below).

Discrepancies in the prevalence rates of depression in the elderly may be explained by noting that different classifications of depression are often compared. Lower prevalence figures typically take into account only primary depressions, ie, those occurring without physical disorders or drug side effects. Secondary depressions accompany or result from somatic illness or adverse drug effects. The elderly are at greater risk than other age groups for secondary depressions because they have more physical illness and the highest rate of drug use. For example, one study found that 24% of 406 elderly men seen for physical disorders in a primary care setting complained of clinically significant depressive symptoms; other studies report even higher frequencies of depressive symptoms in such persons. Thus, higher prevalence figures are more accurate because they include both primary and secondary depressions.

Symptoms and Signs

Psychiatric symptoms that develop in later life are often dismissed as normal manifestations of aging. Even schizophrenia-like symptoms may be dismissed as eccentricity or misdiagnosed as senility. Treatment cannot be planned if a problem is not acknowledged and identified.

Memory and intellectual difficulties: Significant changes in intellectual functioning are no longer readily dismissed, given the heightened awareness of Alzheimer's disease. But the degree to which depression, anxiety, and other psychiatric disorders can interfere with cognition is still underappreciated. **Pseudodementia** (eg, depression or psychosis mimicking dementia) is an extreme form of such interference.

Change in sleep pattern (see also Ch. 11): Complaints of diminished sleep time are often met with assurances that it is a normal part of aging. However, such a change should be viewed clinically as a group characteristic that does not apply to all individuals. Not all studies have found that total sleep time is reduced in later life. Furthermore, the reduction is typically gradual; a change in sleep pattern should not be taken for granted, especially if it is of recent onset. An older person who reports noticeable reduction in sleep time (not just sleeping less at night because of daytime naps) should be evaluated.

Besides signaling potential medical (eg, musculoskeletal, genitourinary, cardiac) problems, changes in sleep pattern can be a hallmark of psychiatric disorders. Early morning awakening may be an important clue to an underlying depression; difficulty in falling asleep or restless sleep with frequent awakenings may signal an anxiety disorder.

Change in sexual interest or capacity (see also Chs. 68 and 69): As a group, healthy older men and women with a history of normal sexual activity and current opportunity retain an interest and capacity for sexual experience, although individuals may be exceptions. Significant changes, particularly of recent onset, call for diagnostic assessment with a focus on medical and surgical factors, drug side effects, and psychiatric causes. Medical problems and drug side effects affect the sexual function of men more than women, since these factors can interfere with erectile and ejaculatory capacity.

Common medical causes of erectile dysfunction include atherosclerosis (especially in diabetic patients), hypothyroidism, malnutrition, and Parkinson's disease. Among possible drug causes, alcohol consumption should be considered; alcohol in high amounts not only serves as a depressant, thereby negatively influencing sexual interest, but also can interfere with erectile and ejaculatory capacity. Depression or anxiety in both men and women can lower motivation for romantic involvement and diminish sexual satisfaction. Regardless of the cause, many sexual problems can be ameliorated or eliminated with proper intervention.

Fear of death: Research shows that while the elderly often think about death, they fear death less than do other age groups. Thinking or talking about death is not the same as fearing or dreading it. Thoughts or conversations about death are naturally more common in the elderly, since they more likely have peers and relatives who have died or are dying. Dread of death is uncommon in persons who are not dying or experiencing some major loss, although reports show a normal and common dread of death in middle-aged persons, who may suddenly perceive how little time is left. At this stage, people find themselves confronting an existential awareness of their own mortality; with further aging, they adapt to this realization.

A terminal illness, an underlying depression, or other emotional conflict—not the awareness of aging itself—predisposes certain elderly persons to death anxiety. In these cases, confronting mortality is different; a terminal illness brings an awareness of dying that can lead to despondency. Eventually, most people come to terms with their fate and can reasonably accept their condition. Depression at any age clouds a person's thinking and often increases thoughts about death. A noticeable and persistent uneasiness about death may signal underlying depression that could benefit from treatment. Evaluation is all the more important given the high rate of suicide in the elderly and the role of depression as a major risk factor.

TABLE 94–1. RISK FACTORS FOR SUICIDE

Age > 55 yr	Persistence of low mood toward the end of depressive illness, even though energy has returned
Male sex	History of drug or alcohol abuse
Painful or disabling physical illness	History of prior suicide attempts
Solitary living situation	Family history of suicide
Debt, decreased income, or poverty	Suicidal preoccupation and talk
Bereavement	Well-defined plans for suicide
Depression, especially associated with agitation, excessive guilt, self-reproach, and insomnia	

From Blazer DG, Bachar JR, Manton KG: "Suicide in late-life: Review and commentary." *Journal of the American Geriatrics Society* 34:519-525 © 1986 American Geriatrics Society.

Suicide

Depression is one of the most common risk factors for suicide. Other risk factors are outlined in TABLE 94–1. While suicide rates among those 18 to 24 yr of age increased significantly from 1970 to 1980, the highest rates in the USA occur in those ≥ 65 yr old (see TABLE 94–2). Moreover, since 1980 the suicide rate for the elderly has been slowly rising; in 1986 it was 21.6 per 100,000—a 25% increase since 1980. The differences are most striking among white men. Suicide is nearly 25% more common in white men 65 to 74 yr of age and > 70% more common in those 75 to 84 yr old, compared with those 18 to 24 yr of age. Furthermore, different cohorts appear to have different suicide rates in old age as well as during other phases of life. The relative size of the birth cohort may be a factor; for example, the baby boom cohort has a high risk of suicide.

Some recent data suggest that the elderly do not seek or respond to offers of help designed to prevent suicide as well as do younger patients. Also, elderly persons make fewer suicide gestures and more often succeed at suicide attempts.

In addition to direct or overt suicidal acts, suicidal behavior can be indirect or covert, making the assessment of suicide potential difficult. An example of covert suicidal behavior is provided below, under the paradigms for examining interactions between mental and physical health factors.

Atypical Presentations

Just as infection may have an atypical presentation in the elderly (eg, without fever or elevated WBC count), psychiatric illness may be manifested in atypical forms (eg, vague physical decline and multiple somatic complaints).

TABLE 94–2. PERCENTAGE OF SUICIDES PER 100,000 POPULATION BY AGE AND SEX (1979–1980)

Age (yr)	*Male (%)*	*Female (%)*
5–14	0.6	0.2
15–24	20.2	4.3
25–34	25.0	7.1
35–44	22.5	8.5
45–54	22.5	9.4
55–64	24.5	8.4
65–74	30.4	6.5
75–84	42.3	5.5
85+	50.6	5.5

From Blazer DG, Bachar JR, Manton KG: "Suicide in late-life: Review and commentary." *Journal of the American Geriatrics Society* 34:519-525 © 1986 American Geriatrics Society.

In later life, **vague physical decline** does not always indicate physiologic aging or the subtle progression of underlying physical illness. Rather, psychosocial factors may aggravate medical problems, at times precipitating a latent physical disorder. The nature and rate of physical decline, under the influence of depression, can reflect the will to live or die. For example, a patient whose overall health is deteriorating because of heart failure may be suffering from despair and loss of hope and may decide to stop taking medication. Covert suicidal behavior can be missed.

Depressed older persons have many concerns about their bodies. In one study of depressed patients > 60 yr old, somatic concerns were found in > 60% of both men and women. Physical symptoms and **multiple somatic complaints** require diligent medical attention, including a search for underlying psychogenic factors.

Depression can lead to social withdrawal or isolation, which is a greater risk in the elderly. Energy previously invested in interpersonal interactions may turn inward, with an exaggerated focus on self and magnification of every ache and pain. Isolated older people may be reluctant to get into conflicts, fearing that an expression of true feelings will drive away the few people to whom they can relate. Anger turned inward may manifest itself as physical instead of emotional pain. In addition, because the elderly are at increased risk for diverse losses (eg, loss of spouse, economic status, physical health, overall independence), they often suffer from diminished self-esteem and depression. A loss of control over one's life may be so disturbing that it may result in physical symptoms that represent maladaptive efforts to control others, gain attention, or signal for help.

Interactions Between Mental and Physical Health

The impact of mental health on the overall course of physical health and illness is increasingly recognized. A growing body of scientific data corroborates the adverse effects of mental health problems on physical illness in later life; impaired immune function and increased prevalence of physical illness, doctor visits, and medication usage have been reported as a consequence of prolonged depression. As a corollary, mental health interventions may have a positive effect on general medical and surgical problems; psychiatric consultation significantly reduces length of stay and improves clinical outcome in hospitalized elderly cardiac and surgical patients.

Many elderly persons who are able to live in the community have the same degree of physical disability as those in nursing homes. What accounts for the difference? Clearly, the availability of family members or other types of social support works in their favor. However, a coexisting psychiatric disorder can destroy a person's capacity to maintain independence, and this phenomenon is significantly underappreciated and often overlooked.

The influence of cognitive, affective, and behavioral problems on the course of overall health in later life is a public health issue of enormous proportions. For example, if a frail older person who is taking drugs for various physical ailments is also suffering from depression or psychosis, that person's ability to think clearly enough to manage the drugs may become so impaired that overall health status may be at serious risk.

There are, of course, many ways in which mental and physical health interact to affect overall health; the paradigms that follow reflect the potential magnitude of public health problems brought about by such an interplay.

The impact of psychologic stress on physical health; example: anxiety → GI symptoms. Accurate diagnosis of GI symptoms can be very difficult. Research shows that psychologic problems may have led to physical discomfort in as many as five of nine elderly persons with GI complaints.

The effect of physical disorder on psychiatric disturbance; example: hearing loss → onset of delusions. More than 25% of elderly persons have impaired hearing; a sensory-deprivation phenomenon may cause psychotic symptoms in some vulnerable individuals.

The interplay of coexisting physical and mental disorders; example: heart failure + depression → further cardiac decline. Cardiac disorder and depression are two of the most common health problems in the elderly. A covert depression can bring about indirect suicidal behavior, as when the patient fails to follow a proper drug schedule; this could cause cardiac function to deteriorate further.

The impact of psychosocial factors on the clinical course of physical health problems; example: diabetic patient with infected foot, living alone → increased risk of gangrene. More than two in five older women and one in seven older men live alone. Having no one to help with medical management and follow-up puts those with chronic illnesses at risk for complications and poorer outcome.

Is the problem mental or physical? Making the correct diagnosis can be especially challenging when differentiating psychologic from physical causes. Consider GI complaints, which are subject to conflicting stereotypes. One stereotype holds that most GI complaints in the elderly are of psychogenic origin—a psychosomatic explanation. The opposing stereotype holds that if one looks hard enough, a physical basis for most GI symptoms will be found in older patients.

To evaluate these views, 300 patients older than 65 yr with GI complaints were followed comprehensively for at least 1 yr after their initial visit to the outpatient department of a medical center. Final diagnoses were as follows: 10%, GI malignancy; 8%, gallbladder disease; 6%, duodenal ulcer; 3%, gastric ulcer; 3%, diverticulosis of the colon; 14%, a wide variety of organic problems; and 56%, GI distress of a purely psychogenic nature. The physical problems of these last patients included irritable colon, spastic colitis, gastritis, heartburn, nausea, diarrhea, constipation, and other psychophysiologic disorders.

In short, the study revealed that both psychogenic (56%) and physical (44%) factors play major roles in patients with GI problems. Thus, the primary care physician or psychiatrist must *simultaneously* perform comprehensive general medical and psychiatric examinations when evaluating GI complaints.

TREATMENT CONSIDERATIONS FOR PSYCHIATRIC DISEASE

After differentiating illness from aging and evaluating the interplay between psychiatric and physical factors, the process of treatment planning begins. Physicians today have access to improved psychotherapeutic, psychopharmacologic, and social interventions. However, with chronic mental illness, as with chronic physical illness, both remissions and exacerbations can occur.

Psychotherapy

Many question the place of psychotherapy in geriatric medicine, but its efficacy has been demonstrated in numerous older patients, especially those with reactive depression, in whom psychosocially induced stress is prominent.

As the average life expectancy increases, time is less likely to be considered an obstacle to psychotherapy. A 65-yr-old may live another 20 yr—ample time to undergo treatment and reap its benefits. Studies show that the elderly are less resistant to unpleasant insights compared with younger patients, thus increasing the opportunity for conflict resolution. Moreover, today's elderly persons are considerably more receptive to psychiatric intervention than were previous cohorts.

Pharmacotherapy

After cardiovascular drugs, psychoactive drugs are the most frequently prescribed for older patients. Psychoactive drugs include antidepressants; anxiolytics; antipsychotics (neuroleptics); hypnotics; certain muscle relaxants, anticonvulsants, and antiparkinsonian drugs; lithium (for the mania of bipolar depressive disorders); and drugs that are claimed to enhance cognitive function (primarily memory).

The same dose of a psychoactive drug usually takes longer to work, remains in the body longer, and may produce a greater effect in an older person than it would in a younger person. Thus, the advice generally has been to "start low, go slow," ie, to begin with a reduced dosage and to increase it gradually, if necessary. Attention should also be paid to potential interactions with other medications (see also Ch. 21).

There are four areas of pharmacokinetics (how the body handles the drug)—**absorption, distribution, metabolism,** and **excretion**—and one area of pharmacodynamics (how the drug affects the body)—**CNS sensitivity**—of interest in managing treatment with psychoactive agents.

Absorption: Most oral psychoactive drugs are absorbed through the intestinal mucosa. Although aging does not significantly alter absorption, other prescribed or over-the-counter drugs can interfere with how efficiently or quickly psychoactive drugs are absorbed. Consequently, more attention must be directed to the timing of psychoactive drug administration (eg, when antacids are taken at the same time as diazepam, they may delay diazepam's absorption and the time it takes to reach peak plasma concentration).

Distribution: With aging, body fat tends to increase, while lean body mass (muscle) and total body water diminish. Most psychoactive drugs (eg, long-acting benzodiazepines) are lipid (fat) soluble; lithium is an example of a water-soluble drug. The greater proportion of fat results in increased storage of lipid-soluble psychoactive agents, increasing the likelihood that a routine dose will accumulate to toxic levels. Women have proportionately more body fat than do men and are at even greater risk. The risk can be minimized by reducing the dose or frequency of administration. While a therapeutic effect may take longer to be realized, the slower onset increases safety. Similarly, because body water decreases with aging, less lithium is needed in older than in younger adults to achieve comparable therapeutic effects. For example, an initial dose of lithium in older persons is 75 to 300 mg orally bid, compared with an initial dose in other adults of 300 mg tid or qid.

Metabolism: Except for lithium, most psychoactive drugs are metabolized by the liver. With aging, altered hepatic enzyme activity may slow metabolism of some drugs. In such cases, the drug remains available and active in the body for a longer period, leading to an increased risk of accumulation and toxicity unless the dosage is also reduced.

Age-related differences in hepatic metabolism may be clinically important. For example, anxiolytics such as diazepam and chlordiazepoxide are generally metabolized three times more slowly in older than in younger persons. The increased volume of distribution for these agents in the elderly may be an additional contributing factor. Conversely, oxazepam, temazepam, and lorazepam (ie, those with half-lives < 24 h) undergo metabolic transformation by glucuronidation. Their clearance rates are unaltered by the aging process. Therefore, they are the preferred anxiolytics for elderly patients. However, rapidly metabolized drugs must often be taken more frequently, which can create a problem in patients with memory impairment. For such patients, a drug taken once a day may be preferable. This is an issue of clinical judgment—balancing the risks and benefits, but emphasizing the *individual* involved.

Excretion: Whereas liver metabolism is the primary mechanism for deactivating lipid-soluble psychoactive agents, renal excretion is the primary pathway for water-soluble lithium. Since renal function is reduced with aging, excretion of lithium takes longer, putting the patient at risk for accumulation unless dosage is adjusted.

CNS sensitivity: Increased sensitivity of CNS receptors may also explain why the dosage of psychoactive drugs may need to be reduced to achieve therapeutic benefit in the elderly. Prescribing the same dosage as for younger patients puts the elderly patient at risk for adverse effects.

Choice of psychoactive drug: Each psychoactive drug category offers a choice of several agents, all with typically similar efficacy. The choice of agent for an elderly patient is often determined by efforts to avoid side effects. For example, tricyclic antidepressants vary in the degree to which they induce anticholinergic effects—untoward reactions that can aggravate glaucoma, urologic dysfunction, or memory impairment. Desipramine and nortriptyline have the lowest anticholinergic potential and are the tricyclics typically selected for elderly patients.

The choice of drug may also depend on whether the patient has other medical problems. For example, all antipsychotic agents have the potential to lower blood pressure. If a schizophrenic patient has episodes of hypotension, an antipsychotic that is less likely to lower blood pressure may be a better choice. Unfortunately, a drug that is less likely to cause one type of side effect may be more likely to cause another. Thus, geriatric psychoactive drug therapy involves making trade-offs within the broader benefit-vs.-risk framework.

95. DEPRESSION

Depression is one of the most common psychiatric disorders of older adults. When measured by traditional scales, the prevalence of clinically significant depressive symptoms among older persons in the community ranges between 8% and 15%, and among institutionalized elderly, about 30%. On the other hand, major depression occurs less often in later life than at other times. The risk for suicide, however, is higher for elderly white men than for any other age, sex, or racial group (see Ch. 94).

These findings, which have surprised both clinicians and epidemiologists, probably reflect a cohort effect: the current cohort between the ages of 70 and 90 yr have had fewer severe depressive disorders in adult life than cohorts that preceded them. Nevertheless, considering that the total older population has increased, the number of cases of depression has not fallen appreciably. Furthermore, the number of cases should increase substantially over the next 20 to 30 yr as younger cohorts, who have a higher prevalence of depression earlier in life, advance in age.

Symptoms and Signs

The clinical manifestations of depression are outlined in TABLE 95–1. However, depression is best understood as a group of disorders that vary in severity. Many elderly persons suffer from **chronic** and **persistent dysphoria** (*restlessness or malaise*). The symptoms do not meet the criteria for dysthymic disorder (see below); rather, affected persons report a depressed mood with generally few accompanying symptoms. The dysphoric elderly have been labeled "the worried well," as they rarely require or benefit from traditional modes of therapy.

Some older persons suffer from a chronic, persistent, and moderately severe **dysthymic disorder.** According to the fourth edition of the *Diagnostic and Statistical Manual of Mental Disorders* (DSM-IV), diagnostic criteria include depressed mood and three additional symptoms, eg, sleep problems, decreased appetite, suicidal ideation, and lethargy. Symptoms must persist for at least 2 yr, but they are not severe enough to constitute a major depressive episode.

TABLE 95–1. CLINICAL MANIFESTATIONS OF DEPRESSION IN LATE LIFE

Mood	Depressed, irritable, or anxious (however, the patient may smile or deny subjective mood change and instead complain of pain or other somatic distress) Crying spells (however, the patient may complain of inability to cry or to experience emotions)
Associated psychologic manifestations	Lack of self-confidence; low self-esteem; self-reproach Poor concentration and memory Reduction in gratification; loss of interest in usual activities; loss of attachments; social withdrawal Negative expectations; hopelessness; helplessness; increased dependency Recurrent thoughts of death Suicidal thoughts (rare but serious when present)
Somatic manifestations	Psychomotor retardation; fatigue Agitation Anorexia and weight loss Insomnia
Psychotic symptoms	Delusions of worthlessness and sinfulness Delusions of ill health (nihilistic, somatic, or hypochondriacal) Delusions of poverty Depressive hallucinations in the auditory, visual, and (rarely) olfactory spheres

Other elderly persons report a brief period (usually lasting a few days) of severe symptoms that usually can be explained by obvious difficulties in adjustment or by bereavement. For example, adjusting to a severe or ultimately fatal chronic illness and losing a spouse are among the more common causes of such symptoms. Affected persons recover with time or when the stressor is removed.

Elderly persons may have other depressive disorders that are not well codified in DSM-IV. Episodes of **brief depression,** quite common in older adults, involve moderately severe depressive symptoms that are consistent with DSM-IV criteria except for their duration (2 wk). Although the symptoms have no clear cause and resolve spontaneously, affected patients may experience these brief episodes in increasingly rapid cycles. Other persons have episodes of **minor depression** that meet the criteria for dysthymic disorder, except that the asymptomatic periods last for months and, therefore, 2 yr of persistent symptoms are never reported.

Some elderly persons have frank **major depression** with or without melancholia. The core symptoms of major depression include dysphoric mood plus at least four of the following symptoms: sleep disturbance (usually decreased sleep), appetite disturbance, weight loss, psychomotor retardation, suicidal ideation, poor concentration, feelings of guilt, and lack of interest in usual activities. **Melancholic depression** exists if these symptoms are predominated by a total lack of interest in the environment, diurnal variation, and psychomotor agitation or retardation. Sometimes major depression is characterized predominantly by psychotic thinking, especially delusions of illness or guilt over past actions, thoughts, or events. Generally, the symptoms are similar in older and younger populations, although older adults have relatively more psychotic symptoms and less self-deprecation and guilt. Psychotic depression is relatively more prevalent in late life than in midlife.

Diagnosis

The diagnosis of depression hinges on a thorough history and physical examination. A review of presenting symptoms against the patient's lifestyle and previous medical and psychiatric history usually permits an accurate diagnosis. The Yesavage Geriatric Depression Scale (see TABLE 95–2) and the Hamilton Depression Scale (see TABLE 95–3) are useful assessment instruments. Although depression scales are used clinically, they are particularly useful in research. *They should not replace a thorough evaluation and interaction between patient and family.* If the patient is retarded or uncommunicative, obtaining a history from family members or other informants is essential. Physical examination must include a complete neurologic evaluation. Frontal lobe signs (eg, the palmomental reflex) help differentiate some dementias from depression.

Laboratory tests serve an adjunctive role in the evaluation of depressed patients. Although not diagnostic, the dexamethasone suppression test may help identify the specific depressive subtype. A positive test result (ie, a post-dexamethasone cortisol level of > 5 µg/dL) is suggestive of endogenous or melancholic depression. Polysomnography, when available, can help identify melancholia as well. Decreased sleep time with shortened rapid eye movement latency provides diagnostic support. A slightly low thyroxine (T_4) level and an elevated thyroid-stimulating hormone (TSH) level are common during a depressive episode.

Differential Diagnosis

The differential diagnosis of major depression includes the many medical and psychiatric illnesses that may present as depression in later life. For example, an idiopathic primary sleep disorder, while mimicking the sleep difficulties found in depression, can result in a reactive (secondary) depressive affect owing to **sleep deprivation.** During the early stages of primary degenerative or multi-infarct **dementia,** a depressive affect may predominate. *Major depression and dementia of-*

TABLE 95–2. YESAVAGE GERIATRIC DEPRESSION SCALE*

1. Are you basically satisfied with your life?	Yes	No
2. Have you dropped many of your activities and interests?	Yes	No
3. Do you feel that your life is empty?	Yes	No
4. Do you often get bored?	Yes	No
5. Are you in good spirits most of the time?	Yes	No
6. Are you afraid that something bad is going to happen to you?	Yes	No
7. Do you feel happy most of the time?	Yes	No
8. Do you often feel helpless?	Yes	No
9. Do you prefer to stay at home rather than go out and do new things?	Yes	No
10. Do you feel you have more problems with memory than most?	Yes	No
11. Do you think it is wonderful to be alive now?	Yes	No
12. Do you feel pretty worthless the way you are now?	Yes	No
13. Do you feel full of energy?	Yes	No
14. Do you feel that your situation is hopeless?	Yes	No
15. Do you think that most people are better off than you are?	Yes	No

Score: ___/15 "No" to questions 1,5,7,11,13	Normal	3±2
"Yes" to other questions	Mildly depressed	7±3
	Very depressed	12±2

* This is the short form.

Adapted from Sheikh JI, Yesavage JA: "Geriatric depression scale (GDS): Recent evidence and development of a shorter version," in *Clinical Gerontology: A Guide to Assessment and Intervention*, edited by TL Brink. Binghamton, NY, Haworth Press, 1986, pp 165–173.

ten coexist, with the usual course entailing remission of the depressive symptoms but persistence or worsening of the cognitive deficit (see DEMENTIA in Ch. 90). Patients with major depression may also present with many symptoms of cognitive impairment **(pseudodementia** or reversible dementia). Pseudodementia may differ from true dementia in the rapidity of onset and the exaggeration (vs. the minimalization) of symptoms. Yet therapy is the only true test of whether the memory problems result from depression only. Some evidence suggests that actual dementia is more likely to follow the depressive episode in older patients who have major depression with cognitive impairment than in those who have major depression without cognitive impairment.

Hypochondriacal symptoms are also often associated with a depressive affect (see Ch. 97). The gradual onset of the syndrome, coupled with the patient's lack of apparent distress, helps confirm the diagnosis of hypochondriasis. Patients with certain **physical illnesses** (eg, hypothyroidism and occult malignancy, especially pancreatic carcinoma) frequently present with depressive symptoms. Depression secondary to pharmacologic treatment of hypertension is also often encountered.

TABLE 95–3. HAMILTON DEPRESSION SCALE*

Item†	*Cue*	*Score*‡
Depressed mood (sad, hopeless, helpless, worthless)	**0**—Absent **1**—Indicates these feelings only on questioning **2**—Spontaneously reports these feelings **3**—Communicates feelings nonverbally (ie, through facial expression, posture, voice, and tendency to weep) **4**—Patient reports VIRTUALLY ONLY these feelings in spontaneous verbal and nonverbal communication	
Feelings of guilt	**0**—Absent **1**—Self-reproach; feels he has let people down **2**—Has ideas of guilt or ruminates over past errors or sinful deeds **3**—Feels present illness is a punishment; has delusions of guilt **4**—Hears accusatory or denunciatory voices, experiences threatening visual hallucinations, or both	
Suicidal ideation	**0**—Absent **1**—Feels life is not worth living **2**—Wishes he were dead or has thoughts of possible death **3**—Expresses suicidal ideas or makes gesture **4**—Attempts suicide (any serious attempt rates 4)	

(continued)

TABLE 95–3. HAMILTON DEPRESSION SCALE* *(Continued)*

Item†	*Cue*	*Score‡*
Insomnia—early	**0**—No difficulty falling asleep **1**—Complains of occasional difficulty falling asleep (ie, takes > 30 min) **2**—Complains of nightly difficulty falling asleep	
Insomnia—middle	**0**—No difficulty **1**—Complains of being restless and disturbed during the night **2**—Wakes during the night (any getting out of bed, except to void, rates 2)	
Insomnia—late	**0**—No difficulty **1**—Wakes in early hours of the morning but goes back to sleep **2**—Is unable to fall asleep again after getting out of bed	
Work and activities	**0**—No difficulty **1**—Thoughts and feelings of incapacity, fatigue, or weakness related to work or hobbies **2**—Loss of interest in hobbies or work—either directly reported by patient, or indirectly indicated by being listless or indecisive (feels he has to push self to work or perform activities) **3**—Decrease in actual time spent in activities or decrease in productivity. In hospital, patient spending < 3 h/day in activities (hospital job or hobbies) exclusive of ward chores rates 3 **4**—Stopped working because of present illness. In hospital, patient engaging in no activities except ward chores or failing to perform ward chores unassisted rates 4	
Retardation (slowness of thought and speech, impaired ability to concentrate, decreased motor activity	**0**—Normal speech and thought **1**—Slight retardation at interview **2**—Obvious retardation at interview **3**—Interview difficult **4**—Complete stupor	
Agitation	**0**—None **1**—"Plays with" hands, hair, etc **2**—Wrings hands, bites nails or lips, pulls hair	

(continued)

TABLE 95–3. HAMILTON DEPRESSION SCALE* *(Continued)*

Item†	*Cue*		*Score‡*
Anxiety—psychic	**0**—No difficulty **1**—Shows subjective tension and irritability **2**—Worries about minor matters **3**—Shows apprehension in face or speech **4**—Expresses fears without questioning		
Anxiety—somatic	**0**—Absent **1**—Mild **2**—Moderate **3**—Severe **4**—Incapacitating	Demonstrates physiologic concomitants of anxiety, such as *Gastrointestinal:* dry mouth, flatulence, indigestion, diarrhea, cramps, belching *Cardiovascular:* palpitations, headaches *Respiratory:* hyperventilation, sighing *Other:* Urinary frequency Sweating	
Somatic symptoms—gastrointestinal	**0**—None **1**—Has loss of appetite but eats without staff encouragement; has heavy feelings in abdomen **2**—Has difficulty eating without staff urging; requests or requires laxatives or medication for bowels or medication for GI symptoms		
Somatic symptoms—general	**0**—None **1**—Has heaviness in limbs, back, or head; backaches, headache, muscle aches; loss of energy and fatigability **2**—Any clear-cut symptom rates 2		
Loss of libido	**0**—No loss **1**—Mild loss **2**—Severe loss		
Hypochondriasis	**0**—Not present **1**—Self-absorbed (bodily) **2**—Preoccupied with health **3**—Voices frequent complaints, requests for help, etc **4**—Has hypochondriacal delusions		

(continued)

TABLE 95–3. HAMILTON DEPRESSION SCALE*
(Continued)

Item†	*Cue*	*Score*‡
Weight loss	**0**—None **1**—Probable weight loss associated with present illness **2**—Definite (according to patient) weight loss	
Insight (score 0 if the patient is not depressed)	**0**—Acknowledges being depressed and ill **1**—Acknowledges illness but attributes cause to bad food, climate, overwork, virus, need for rest, etc **2**—Denies being ill	
	Total score	______

* The value of the ratings depends entirely on the interviewer's skill and experience. Questions should be directed to the patient's condition in the last few days or week.

† For each item, select the cue that best characterizes the patient and enter corresponding score.

‡ A score of ≥ 16 indicates significant depressive symptoms. A reduction of the score by 50% indicates significant response to therapy.

Adapted from Hamilton M: "Development of a rating scale for primary depressive illness." *British Journal of Social and Clinical Psychology* 6:278-296, 1967; used with permission.

Treatment

Treatment of the major melancholic depressions is primarily **pharmacologic.** Discovery of the tricyclic antidepressants in the late 1950s (first imipramine, then amitriptyline) marked a milestone. Although many antidepressants have been developed since then, the newer agents are only marginally more effective. Choosing a drug depends primarily on which one produces fewer or less severe side effects rather than on any unique therapeutic property. Older adults have difficulty tolerating the anticholinergic effects of tricyclic antidepressants or the postural hypotension they are likely to induce. Nortriptyline has relatively few cardiovascular and anticholinergic side effects and has been used increasingly for late-life depression. Desipramine and doxepin are also widely used. Monoamine oxidase inhibitors are used less often because they are no more effective than other drugs and because their use can precipitate significant side effects, especially agitation.

Usual starting doses in otherwise healthy elderly persons are 1/3 to 1/2 of the usual adult doses. This dosing schedule is used to assess the patient's tolerability. The dose is usually divided to promote tolerance of side effects. If possible, the entire dose should be given at bedtime to avoid daytime drowsiness. Doses should be titrated upward slowly (eg, weekly) and *not* every 3 to 5 days, which is the case for younger adults. For example, the daily starting dose for amitriptyline is 30 to 40 mg/day; for nortriptyline, 10 mg at bedtime and then increased by 10 mg/wk to a maximum of 60 mg; for desipramine, 10 mg every morning, noontime, and at bedtime and increased by 10 mg/wk to a maximum of 150 mg; and for doxepin, 30 to 40 mg. Although the dose can be increased gradually, the maintenance dose is usually lower than that required in midlife. Some drugs (eg, amitriptyline, nortriptyline, and desipramine) can be monitored effectively by plasma levels. A significant response usually occurs in 2 to 3 wk, and a total response in 5 to 6 wk. Sleep improves immediately. In recurrent unipolar and bipolar disorders, lithium carbonate 300 to 900 mg/day may be prescribed prophylactically.

Selective serotonin reuptake inhibitors—fluoxetine and sertraline—are now widely prescribed for major depression. Although they are no more effective than the tricyclic antidepressants, they have significantly fewer side effects. The dose should be lowered in older adults, usually to 10 mg/day for fluoxetine and 50 mg every other day for sertraline. Agitation, a common side effect with these drugs, can be especially troublesome for older depressed patients.

Adjuncts may augment the response to antidepressants. For example, low-dose lithium may augment the tricyclic antidepressants, and carbamazepine may reduce the tendency to cycle in and out of depressive episodes.

Some severely depressed patients respond only to **electroconvulsive therapy (ECT).** Typically included are patients who have previously responded to ECT, who demonstrate significant psychotic symptoms or self-destructive behavior, or who do not tolerate or respond to antidepressants. For persons with the most severe depressions, in whom food and fluid intake is markedly reduced, ECT is the treatment of choice after rehydration has been undertaken. ECT is safest when performed with multiple-channel monitoring (EEG, ECG, blood pressure, pulse, and respiratory function) under the supervision of an anesthetist or anesthesiologist and a psychiatrist. Improvement with ECT in elderly persons who do not respond to antidepressant drugs reaches 80% in most studies, which is the same as in younger patients.

The acute amnesia that accompanies ECT is often most disturbing to the older patient who is already preoccupied with cognitive and somatic functioning. Although some memory loss can persist after ECT, the nature and extent of this problem remain to be elucidated.

Psychotherapy also is often effective in treating depression. Common sense and numerous empiric studies suggest that psychotherapy is most effective for nonmelancholic depression, although it may be beneficial even for severe depression. Behavioral and cognitive therapies are considered more effective than nondirected or analytically oriented therapies. Specifically these therapies may help reintegrate the patient into his social environment after a severe depression and may help prevent a relapse. Therefore, psychotherapy is often used in conjunction with pharmacotherapy and ECT. Initial efficacy may be as great in inpatients as in outpatients. Finally, psychotherapy may be especially valuable in preventing relapses of episodic depression.

Treatment of medically ill or hospitalized patients: Some people respond to acute or chronic physical illness by developing psychiatric problems, such as a **major mood disorder** or an **adjustment disorder with depression.** Support and psychotherapy (eg, formal intervention with family and patient to discuss the illness) are often helpful. Small doses of tricyclic antidepressants can be a helpful therapeutic adjunct, especially for sleep problems, but side effects often make their long-term use hazardous. For patients who are dying, similar techniques can be used; however, not every dying patient needs psychologic or psychiatric treatment (see Ch. 19).

Pharmacotherapy for medically ill persons who have a **major depressive disorder** requires special attention. Tricyclic antidepressants and selective serotonin uptake inhibitors (although the latter are of less concern) can cause cardiac side effects in patients with heart disease or unstable blood pressure (eg, a tendency toward orthostatic hypotension). Both classes of drugs are reasonably safe when used properly in persons without serious heart disease. The dilemma, of course, is that a patient with a major depressive disorder will not thrive until the depression is substantially reduced. The inability to respond to rehabilitative efforts and the patient's and family's fear of chronic invalidism become proportionately greater with longer hospitalization. Patients with depression often view themselves as hopeless; their hopelessness spreads to the medical staff, who may pay less attention to them. Modifying the patient's environment may help, but the depression itself also needs to be treated, usually with pharmacotherapy.

Usually, ECT is limited to patients who have resisted pharmacotherapy or who have psychotic symptoms. When proper attention is given to its relative contraindications, ECT given under optimal conditions can be the fastest and most efficient form of antidepressive treatment.

96. ANXIETY DISORDERS

The American Psychiatric Association's *Diagnostic and Statistical Manual of Mental Disorders,* Fourth Edition (DSM-IV) delineates three broad categories of anxiety disorders: phobic disorders, posttraumatic stress disorder, and anxiety states.

Although **phobic disorders** affect some older adults, the more severe phobias (eg, agoraphobia and social phobia) begin early and are more common in children and younger adults. There are few data regarding their course through adulthood into late life.

Posttraumatic stress disorder is a relatively new diagnostic entity, even though the adverse impact of severe stress during childhood or young adulthood on future psychologic functioning has long been recognized. Most research and therapy directed toward posttraumatic stress disorder are derived from stress syndromes associated with war experiences and sexual abuse. Onset generally occurs in childhood or young adulthood; little is known about its continuance into late life.

In contrast, **anxiety states** are common in later life. Up to 5% of community-based older adults experience symptoms of **generalized anxiety disorder,** making it one of the more common psychiatric problems in the elderly. **Obsessive-compulsive disorder,** another anxiety state, is also common in later life, although severe symptoms (eg, compulsive handwashing) are not usually prominent (see Perceptions and Beliefs in Ch. 89). **Panic disorder** often begins in late adolescence or early adulthood, and the symptoms generally recede by later life. Some older adults report episodes of panic, but these are usually less severe than those occurring earlier and are often complicated by depressive symptoms or physical illness (eg, postural hypotension).

Diagnosis

To establish the diagnosis of generalized anxiety, the patient must manifest symptoms from at least three of four DSM-IV categories: (1) **motor tension** (shakiness, jumpiness, trembling, inability to relax); (2) **autonomic hyperactivity** (sweating, palpitations, dry mouth, dizziness, hot or cold spells, frequent urination, or diarrhea); (3) **apprehensive expectation** (worry or anticipation of personal misfortune); and (4) **vigilance and scanning** (distractibility, poor concentration, insomnia, edginess). These symptoms should persist at least 6 mo to qualify for diagnosis.

A number of medical conditions are mistaken for generalized anxiety disorder because patients present with symptoms of anxiety. Hyperthyroidism with an atypical presentation can be missed unless thyroid function is tested. Cardiac arrhythmias that produce palpitations and shortness of breath are common in later life and may resemble a generalized anxiety disorder with periodic exacerbations and remissions. Patients with pulmonary emboli or pulmonary edema may also present with shortness of breath and a feeling of anxiety.

History taking will help rule out other possible causes of anxiety. For example, episodic anxiety may resemble panic disorder, but further questioning may reveal possible postural hypotension, which can be verified by checking blood pressure with the patient sitting and standing. Other older adults with anxiety symptoms may suffer from hypoglycemia, which can be confirmed by a 5-h glucose tolerance test.

Drugs may contribute to anxiety states. Caffeine is a frequent offender, as are over-the-counter sympathomimetic drugs (eg, ephedrine). Anticholinergic agents may subtly impair memory, thereby producing secondary anxiety. Withdrawal from certain drugs, especially alcohol, anxiolytic agents, and sedative-hypnotics, may result in anxiety symptoms.

Other psychiatric disorders may be associated with anxiety. Delirium (acute organic brain syndrome) is often coupled with moderately severe anxiety and agitation, especially if the patient is in unfamiliar surroundings. Major depression also may be associated with anxiety and agitation. In some cases, agitation (ie, the inability to remain still) may resemble anxiety. However, the agitated older adult does not always report the sense of impending doom and dread that characterizes depressive anxiety. The elderly frequently complain of fear and anxiety that border on panic in the early morning, especially if they awaken in the dark when others in the house are asleep. These symptoms tend to remit as the day progresses. Hypochondriasis may be accompanied by moderately severe generalized anxiety, although the anxiety is usually intermittent and less severe than in other psychiatric disorders (see Ch. 97).

Possibly the most common cause of comorbid anxiety in the elderly is Alzheimer's disease. Early signs of cognitive dysfunction and memory loss in socially active persons often lead to generalized anxiety, with periodic episodes of panic; this in turn contributes to social withdrawal and isolation. The severe and traumatic behavioral changes that result from this anxiety syndrome frequently mask the underlying dementia.

Occasionally, the anxiety reported by patients is actually fear (possibly appropriate). The syndrome may exhibit itself only in situations that threaten security. For example, some elderly persons fear being mugged while walking along the street, losing their way to the doctor's office or some other destination, or driving on busy highways. When such stressful experiences are avoided, these persons rarely complain of anxiety and, therefore, do not truly suffer from generalized anxiety disorder.

Treatment

Successful management of generalized anxiety disorder requires a strong physician-patient relationship, counseling, family support, appropriate medication, and of course, an accurate diagnosis. Once the diagnosis is made, the physician can correct potential organic causes; eg, if postural hypotension contributes to a sense of panic, an effort should be made to withdraw nonessential drugs that may contribute to hypotension.

Appropriate intervention for coexisting psychiatric disorders may alleviate symptoms of anxiety. For example, treating major depression with an antidepressant is usually sufficient to eliminate any associated anxiety and agitation. Providing a more structured environment for the mildly to moderately demented patient may alleviate the associated anxiety. If residual anxiety persists, however, the decision to prescribe an anxiolytic drug must be predicated on (1) the suitability of the pharmacologic agent for generalized anxiety and (2) the possibility of drug interactions between other therapeutic agents and the anxiolytic.

Pharmacologic treatment, a major component of the management plan for generalized anxiety, is often the source of difficulties for both patient and clinician. In general, older adults respond satisfactorily but not exceptionally to anxiolytic drugs. Most patients experience relief but not elimination of tension and agitation, and many symptoms persist. In addition, elderly persons often complain of the side effects associated with anxiolytics.

Unless a tricyclic antidepressant or monoamine oxidase inhibitor is prescribed for panic disorder, the **drugs of choice** are the benzodiazepines. In general, elderly persons respond better to shorter-acting agents (eg, alprazolam or oxazepam) than to longer-acting ones (eg, diazepam). Occasionally, the shorter-acting agents may produce a rebound anxiety effect before the next dose is given. In such cases, a longer-acting agent may be preferred. The dosage is usually lower than for younger patients (eg, alprazolam 0.125 mg [half of a 0.25-mg tablet] orally bid or tid). Unless only one or two doses are taken daily, establishing a fixed dosage schedule is better than prescribing the medication as needed. The initial dose for buspirone is 5 mg tid. Divided doses of 10 mg bid or tid are commonly given. Buspirone is an alternative to a potentially addicting drug such as a benzodiazepine. However, buspirone will not bring about subjective improvement as quickly; its anxiolytic effect is usually observed after about 2 wk of continuous therapy. Persons who have responded to benzodiazepines usually do not respond to substitution with buspirone.

Discontinuing benzodiazepines is easier if prescribers make it clear from the outset that treatment is for only a brief period (eg, up to 4 to 6 wk). Once benzodiazepines are used continuously for an extended time, discontinuance is difficult. Nevertheless, periodic efforts should be made to withdraw the drug or at least to reduce the dose. Shorter-acting benzodiazepines should be discontinued gradually.

Patients should be monitored closely for development of **side effects** such as drowsiness, ataxia, slurred speech, impaired coordination, sleep disturbances, and depressive symptoms. Poor concentration and memory loss also may result from anxiolytics. Drug discontinuance is essential for controlling these side effects, even if the patient must be hospitalized to effect withdrawal.

Antipsychotic agents (neuroleptics) should not be prescribed for generalized anxiety, except when symptoms are secondary to delusions or other signs of psychosis. Such drugs may produce side effects (eg, tremulousness, restlessness and agitation, especially akathisia) that can complicate the symptoms of generalized anxiety. The most serious side effect, however, is tardive dyskinesia, which is usually irreversible.

In addition to personal support, direct **psychotherapeutic approaches** are sometimes useful in alleviating generalized anxiety. Unfortunately, intensive psychotherapy is not as successful as might be hoped, and psychoanalysis has little to recommend it. Short-term, insight-oriented therapy, however, may be of some benefit, particularly if the elderly patient suffers from anxiety secondary to bereavement. Grief may be related to loss of a loved one, or it may be associated with a sudden decline in physical health and loss of control over one's environment. Supportive psychotherapy may be an important adjunct in treating generalized anxiety in isolated and physically impaired older adults, whereas structured cognitive therapy has shown some benefit in alleviating panic attacks (in young adults). If anxiety is associated with specific phobias and panic, behavioral therapy may be indicated.

Biofeedback may enable selected older patients to develop some control over symptoms of anxiety. Other patients may benefit from simple instruction in relaxation therapy. In addition, a paced exercise program can be especially helpful in those sensing loss of control over other areas of life.

97. HYPOCHONDRIASIS

Hypochondriasis is a somatoform psychiatric disorder because it is characterized by physical symptoms. Patients have a morbid anxiety about health, usually with symptoms that cannot be attributed to organic disease. Many such complaints are successfully managed by intermittent care. Psychogenic pain disorder, which typically arises in mid-life, may persist into later years, although pain generally remits somewhat with aging (see PSYCHOGENIC PAIN in Ch. 12). Chronic low back pain may be common in later life, but older patients are less likely to seek treatment in pain-management clinics than are younger patients. Of the various somatoform disorders, hypochondriasis is the one most relevant to the elderly; as many as 15% report subjectively perceived physical impairment to be greater than actual impairment.

Symptoms, Signs, and Diagnosis

The hypochondriacal patient misinterprets clinically insignificant physical symptoms or sensations as reflections of a disease state and becomes preoccupied with them. A thorough physical and laboratory evaluation produces no evidence of an organic disease that might account for the nature or perceived severity of the complaints. Despite medical reassurance, the patient's fears or beliefs about the existence of disease persist, causing impaired social, occupational, and even recreational functioning.

Hypochondriasis can be the sole disorder afflicting an older adult, although symptoms suggesting hypochondriasis may be seen in those suffering from depression, anxiety disorders, dementia, and even a schizophrenia-like illness. To meet DSM-IV (*Diagnostic and Statistical Manual of Mental Disorders, Fourth Edition*) criteria for hypochondriasis, however, the somatic complaints must not be secondary to any of these disorders.

History taking: The duration of the patient's symptoms, their pattern (continuous or episodic), and any past history of medical or psychiatric illness must be determined. Because the hypochondriacal patient is prone to prescription drug abuse, a current and past medication history is essential.

Mental status evaluation: Social functioning and self-care capacity should be assessed to determine the extent to which the symptoms interfere with the patient's usual daily activities. A mental status examination allows for assessment of affect and degree of suffering or discomfort secondary to the physical symptoms (see Ch. 89). Because interference with functioning may be secondary to somatic preoccupation, repeated evaluations (especially for an inpatient) are indicated. Given the association of hypochondriacal complaints with suicide, suicidal ideation should be investigated during the interview. Persons with depressive symptoms (including suicidal thoughts) and somatic complaints are more likely to attempt suicide than are persons with depressive symptoms only (see Suicide in Ch. 94).

Physical examination: A complete physical evaluation is important during the initial visit. Blood pressure, both sitting and standing, must also be measured. Neurologic evaluation should include a thorough sensory examination of areas where pain is reported, plus an assessment of possible frontal lobe signs, especially if the patient shows evidence of a dementing illness. Pelvic and rectal examinations should be performed when relevant. Requests for more detailed physical examination should be deferred whenever possible unless clearly indicated. Follow-up visits include a brief physical examination (see under Treatment, below).

Laboratory evaluation: Laboratory tests should be kept to a minimum. Routine screening tests (eg, blood chemistry, hematocrit, and urinalysis) are sufficient unless specific historical and physical findings indicate a need for additional data. A medical record review and firm reassurance help prevent the ordering, and especially the duplication, of expensive tests and procedures such as MRI. This can be difficult when the patient insists that symptoms persist or are worse. Many primary care physicians deal with this issue by referring the patient to a subspecialist, but referrals should be done with care and at least preceded by a discussion with that physician. For many reasons, subspecialists tend to order or reorder technologically sophisticated studies, but they may refrain if given a clear view of the problem beforehand.

Differential Diagnosis

The distinction between hypochondriasis and **depression** can usually be made by observing the patient over time and obtaining adequate historical information. Several distinctions exist. Despite reporting numerous symptoms, the hypochondriacal patient does not appear to suffer as severely as the depressed patient. Furthermore, the depressed patient usually directs hostility inward, whereas the hypochondriacal patient directs it outward. Although both types of patient may withdraw socially, acute withdrawal is usually more pronounced in the depressed patient (see Ch. 95).

Depressed older patients, especially those whose depression began late in life, retrospectively report having had far fewer somatic symptoms in mid-life (except if clearly associated with a physical disorder) than do hypochondriacal patients. Depressive episodes (and their associated physical symptoms) also tend to be episodic, whereas symptoms associated with hypochondriasis are more persistent. Additionally, depressed patients sometimes seem to tolerate the side effects of antidepressant drugs better than do hypochondriacal patients.

The older adult with mild to moderate **dementia** may present with somatic symptoms. However, these problems are usually episodic, unlike the persistent nature of hypochondriacal complaints. Furthermore, the poor performance of hypochondriacal patients on the mental status examination is usually related to somatic preoccupation and, therefore, may improve with repeated testing (as does the performance of depressed patients during recovery), in contrast to the consistently poor performance of demented persons. Also, hostility is much less common in demented patients than in those suffering from hypochondriasis.

Treatment

Hypochondriacs should be recognized as being ill, insofar as they truly experience either real or imagined pain and discomfort. Despite the frustration such patients often provoke, empathy from the clinician is essential to developing a therapeutic relationship. It is also essential to developing a consistent treatment plan. Treatment is often very difficult even in expert hands and may not succeed either in relieving symptoms or in holding the patient's confidence. Therefore, physicians should not be too hard on themselves if they are not succeeding.

The most important treatment element is a comfortable, long-term doctor-patient relationship. Physicians will better serve hypochondriacal patients and alleviate undue strain on the health care system if they are committed to working with them rather than referring them indiscriminately to many specialists. A structured approach to these patients renders their care less troublesome than is usually imagined.

Physicians should agree to see hypochondriacal patients regularly. It may be necessary initially to schedule an appointment every other week, but usually the number of visits can be reduced to ≤ 12/yr. A specified amount of time, usually about 20 min, should be allotted per visit, and if possible, appointments should be begun and terminated promptly. Such regular visits can meet the patient's need to be heard and to have control over his life.

One useful approach is to come to an agreement to differ. The physician expresses confidence that no sinister disease exists, and his confidence is supportive despite the patient's insistence that he is wrong. Sometimes the converse is helpful. For example, the physician may say: "No one can be omniscient and I may be wrong, but I am trying to help you so let's work together rather than argue." The objective is to match the patient's needs. Often even very skillful physicians are defeated; however, many unpromising patients can be managed supportively.

During the visit, the physician should obtain an interval history and perform a brief (5-min) physical examination. The physical examination, albeit brief, is central to the physician-patient relationship, a relationship that is essential if the hypochondriacal patient is to be managed effectively. This examination usually includes determination of sitting and standing blood pressure, pulse rate, cardiac auscultation, and abdominal palpation. During the remainder of the visit, the patient should be encouraged to discuss personal and social issues that go beyond physical concerns.

Physicians should avoid venturing a diagnosis or prognosis. Although hypochondriacal patients seek an answer to their problems, they rarely accept a diagnosis, either somatic or psychiatric. Most have consulted many other physicians and either praise or criticize them to the current physician, who must avoid defending or criticizing these colleagues. Instead, the patient's attention should be focused on his own frustrations, anxieties, and fears.

Promises to cure the patient's illness must also be avoided, since they are unrealistic. The hypochondriacal patient is chronically ill and improves only gradually. When therapeutic promises are not kept, both the patient and the physician become frustrated. At such times, it is tempting to refer the patient elsewhere. Referrals should be made reluctantly, as they expose the patient to unnecessary costs and the risks of tests and treatments by specialists who do not know the patient as well as the primary care physician.

If specific psychologic issues emerge in the course of management, hypochondriacal patients may be referred for individual psychotherapy. These referrals do not replace management by the primary care physician, however, especially since hypochondriacs do not respond to relief from an emotional problem with dramatic improvement in somatic complaints.

The physician should avoid statements such as "It is all in your head." Hypochondriacs rarely benefit from such interpretations, even if they recognize some truth in them. Such comments are likely to topple an already unsteady therapeutic relationship.

Pharmacotherapy: Drug use must be carefully monitored. Hypochondriacal patients are often already taking many pharmacotherapeutic agents when they arrive at the next physician's office. Immediate withdrawal of these drugs is usually impossible. Rather, the physician should begin with small adjustments (eg, slowly decreasing the dose of drugs to which tolerance can develop). Hypochondriacal patients are usually receptive to withdrawal if the physician remains firm in the conviction to eliminate these drugs and is willing to withdraw them gradually. Whenever possible, potentially addicting hypnotics, anxiolytics, and analgesics should be avoided. Rather, low doses of sedating antidepressants (eg, amitriptyline 25 mg orally at bedtime) can be prescribed for sleep, and nonnarcotic analgesics can be used to relieve pain.

If drugs are a major contributing factor to dysfunction, hospitalization may be necessary to achieve withdrawal. Antidepressants and anxiolytics should be reserved for specific symptoms that are targeted for improvement. If the drugs are ineffective, they should be discontinued promptly.

Therapeutic adjuncts: A number of therapeutic adjuncts are available for managing the elderly hypochondriacal patient. An exercise program, physical therapy, and massage may be very effective for patients with poor health habits (eg, lack of exercise and its attendant adverse effects on muscles and joints). Physical therapy for the hospitalized patient breaks the routine of the sick and passive person. If pain and tension are primary complaints, biofeedback may be especially helpful. For the homebound patient, nutritional programs (eg, Meals on Wheels or lunch programs at senior centers) can break the cycle of social isolation.

98. SCHIZOPHRENIA AND SCHIZOPHRENIFORM DISORDERS

Suspiciousness, persecutory ideation, and paranoid delusions are frequently seen in cognitively impaired or emotionally distressed older adults. Between 2% and 5% of elderly persons in the community exhibit excessive suspiciousness and persecutory ideations. As many as 4% to 5% have delusions and hallucinations, and these symptoms are often disabling. Nevertheless, the prevalence of schizophrenia, as defined by the American Psychiatric Association's *Diagnostic and Statistical Manual of Mental Disorders,* Fourth Edition (DSM-IV), is $< 1\%$ in later life.

Although current nomenclature does not help in the differential diagnosis of schizophrenia-like symptoms in the elderly, investigators and clinicians who have worked with older adults generally agree upon five relatively distinct syndromes: (1) abnormal suspiciousness, (2) transitional paranoid reactions, (3) late-life paraphrenia (*severe paranoid illness without deterioration of other cognitive or affective processes*) or paranoia associated with late-onset schizophrenia, (4) persistence of early-onset schizophrenia, and (5) acute paranoid reactions secondary to affective illness.

Symptoms, Signs, and Diagnosis

Most older adults who exhibit **abnormal suspiciousness** do not have contact with mental health professionals. However, they frequently have medical problems and are often seen by a primary care physician or geriatrician. These patients may have vague complaints of external forces controlling their lives. Occasionally, these beliefs become focal, often directed at their children; eg, they believe that their children have deserted them or have plotted to obtain control of their finances or property. Perception of a loss of control, coupled with an inability to evaluate the social milieu, favors the development of such suspiciousness.

Physicians also encounter **suspiciousness associated with memory loss and attention deficits.** Institutionalized persons suffering from dementia are often suspicious of both family and staff. Their accusations are usually disjointed, unfocused, and unaccompanied by sustained emotional distress. Common complaints concern objects being stolen, medicines being swapped, and attendants misbehaving. Symptoms derive from the patient's inability to organize environmental stimuli and comprehend the often confusing activities of the hospital or long-term care facility. It is unknown whether an underlying paranoid personality contributes to excessive paranoid behavior in persons with dementia. Physicians must remember, however, that older persons at times are mistreated in long-term care facilities, and suspiciousness may be grounded in fact.

Transitional paranoid reactions are narrow, focal, and situational. They are usually manifested in women who live alone and believe in plots against them. The focus of hallucinations and delusional thinking usually moves gradually from outside the home to inside it, from complaints of noises in the basement and attic to reports of physical abuse or molestation. Hence, a transition can be observed from external threats to violations of property and person. Social isolation and perceptional difficulties contribute to transitional paranoia.

Paraphrenia is not universally accepted as a distinct syndrome. Those who distinguish the syndrome emphasize that the condition is primary and not secondary to an affective illness or to an organic mental disorder. In addition, the gross disturbances of affect, volition, and function characterizing schizophrenia are not prominent. Nevertheless, paranoid delusions and hallucinations are almost invariably present. Late-life paraphrenia may be chronic, but deterioration to the extent observed in schizophrenia or Alzheimer's disease is not characteristic. The boundaries blur not only between late-life paraphrenia and classic paranoid schizophrenia but also between the transitional paranoid state and paraphrenia.

Persons suffering from late-onset paraphrenia often report plots against them, focusing once again on family members. In contrast to mild suspiciousness, these plots are persistent, extreme, and elaborate. No cognitive impairment is noted. Although the paraphrenic patient is physically independent (diet and hygiene are rarely compromised), social functioning and cooperation with health care staff members are greatly impaired. Such persons rarely speak for long without referring to the symptoms of concern.

No clear association has been established between late-onset paraphrenia and the female sex, social isolation, or a distinct personality type. Nevertheless, paraphrenic patients usually *are* female, live alone, and have shown evidence of difficult social interactions earlier in life. In contrast to schizophrenic patients, however, these persons are warm, friendly, and trusting, especially when interviewed in their own homes and not threatened with the diagnosis of a psychiatric disorder. Paraphrenic patients tend to have hearing problems, but the relationship between hearing impairment and paraphrenia is not nearly as strong as some authorities contend.

Early-onset schizophrenia may persist into late life. Typically the symptoms become less acute, yet social functioning continues to deteriorate gradually over time. Acute paranoid thinking may accompany a severe major depression or an acute manic episode. Treating the mood disorder usually eliminates the paranoid thinking in these patients.

Treatment

The physician caring for the paranoid older adult must establish a trusting and supportive relationship. Displays of respect, a willingness to listen to complaints and fears, and availability by telephone are essential. Most elderly persons do not abuse telephone privileges and are generally willing to wait for the physician to return a call.

The physician should not—at least initially—confront the patient with the lack of reason and false assumptions inherent in paranoid ideation. Such a confrontation is of no value and may disrupt the therapeutic relationship. On the other hand, the physician must not deceive the patient by pretending to agree with the paranoid beliefs. Rather, an interest should be expressed in wanting to understand what is troubling the patient and in working together despite any disagreement over the source of the problem. A desirable goal is to develop a level of confidence that permits an examination of the patient's beliefs.

The physician must also establish a relationship with key persons in the patient's social environment. Family members are often the first to notice a deterioration in the patient's condition and, therefore, the first to contact the physician when a problem arises. Police officers, neighbors, and pharmacists also can serve as valuable allies. By understanding the paranoid behavior, they can contact the physician or family when appropriate and not overreact. However, physicians clearly must maintain standards of privilege and confidentiality when talking to family, neighbors, and friends.

Pharmacotherapy: Effective management also requires antipsychotic drug therapy. Initial dosages may range from 10 to 25 mg/day of thioridazine, 2 to 4 mg/day of thiothixene, or 1 to 3 mg/day of haloperidol.

Daily doses may be increased significantly (eg, thioridazine 50 to 100 mg), but the lower doses usually suffice except in the most acute cases. The drugs may be given once daily (at bedtime) in less severe cases.

The choice of agent is determined by the side effects the physician wishes to avoid. Thioridazine is especially troublesome in patients with postural hypotension, whereas haloperidol may create significant problems in those inclined to develop parkinsonian symptoms. Agents that are less likely to produce parkinsonian side effects are thought to also be less provocative of tardive dyskinesia. In treatment-resistant and severely psychotic persons, clozapine is a possible choice. To date, there has been little cumulative experience with clozapine in older persons, although there is evidence that the incidence of agranulocytosis is higher in older patients.

Most elderly persons are willing to take an antipsychotic drug if told that the drug will help to improve sleep and alleviate anxiety. Compliance is often problematic but less so in later life than earlier. Even paranoid persons usually trust their physicians and are willing to adhere to therapy. If objections occur, the family may be able to help. A strong objection to medication or other interventions may suggest the need for hospitalization if symptoms are severe.

99. ALCOHOL ABUSE AND DEPENDENCE

As the older population increases in number, more adults are at risk for developing significant alcohol-related problems. Alcohol problems are also likely to be more prevalent with the aging of currently middle-aged persons, whose alcohol use throughout adult life has been greater than that of previous cohorts. The prevalence of alcohol abuse and dependence in persons > 65 yr of age ranges from 2% to 5% for men and about 1% for women. These figures are lower than those for younger persons, who are less inclined to abstain from alcohol than are the elderly (> 50% of older men and women reported abstinence in a national survey). However, the risk factors for alcohol-related disorders are similar in both populations: genetic predisposition, male sex, limited education, low income, and a history of psychiatric disorders, especially depression.

Concern about alcohol consumption in the elderly relates not to changing patterns of use but to physiologic changes that accompany aging and pose problems if alcohol is consumed regularly. Given the relatively complete absorption of alcohol, the smaller volume of distribution, and increased organ dysfunction, older adults who drink alcohol regularly are subject to more toxic effects.

Secondary Physical and Psychiatric Problems

Malnutrition may result from chronic alcohol use, especially in heavy drinkers. **Cirrhosis** is one of the eight leading causes of death in the over-65 population. The chronic alcoholic whose hepatic function is compromised may also develop **osteomalacia** because of compromised vitamin D metabolism. Alcohol abuse can contribute to the development of **cardiomyopathies** and **atrophic gastritis.** Probably the most frequent and serious problem, however, is the associated **decline in cognitive status.** Acute alcohol abuse is associated with a variety of neuropsychologic and cognitive defects. Chronic alcohol abuse may lead to a remarkable decline in memory and information processing, although intelligence remains relatively unaffected. The cumulative effect of these physical and cognitive changes is marked impairment in most persons who survive beyond middle age.

The central clinical problem in the older alcoholic patient is the potential for **addiction and tolerance** to alcohol, with concomitant **withdrawal symptoms.** The relatively "quiet" use of alcohol over many years desensitizes the individual and his family to these problems, and the addiction may not be recognized. Interactions with other agents, especially benzodiazepines, may lead to CNS depression and are of major clinical concern. Typically, addiction becomes evident when the older patient is in a setting where alcohol is not readily available. The patient exhibits increased anxiety, sleep problems, nausea, and weakness, secondary to a lower blood-alcohol level. Without intervention, anxiety and agitation progress to a tremulous state within 1 to 2 days, followed by more severe symptoms, including hallucinations and withdrawal seizures (ie, delirium tremens) in some cases.

Diagnosis

The diagnostic assessment hinges on a thorough **history.** Specific information about drinking behavior obtained initially from the patient should be supplemented with information from family members, preferably from at least two generations. Unfortunately, some older alcoholics have little or no social network (eg, the so-called skid-row alcoholic), and historical information is limited.

Initial questions include what kind of alcohol is consumed and how often the patient drinks (ie, continually or in binges). While tolerance for binges decreases with age, guilt or concern about drinking also becomes less common. Patients may not recognize a connection between new symptoms and decades-long drinking habits.

If evidence of cognitive abnormalities emerges on the **mental status examination,** additional assessment is indicated. Every effort must be made to keep the patient abstinent for 2 to 3 wk before conducting a detailed psychologic evaluation. Even when scores reveal little or no impairment, this evaluation provides a baseline for monitoring future changes in mental status (see Ch. 89).

Psychiatric symptoms that may accompany alcohol abuse should be reviewed in detail. For example, major depression and alcohol abuse frequently coincide. Paranoid ideation involving relatives or friends is not uncommon in the elderly alcoholic. Suicidal ideation should be documented, given the increased risk of suicide in elderly alcoholics (see Suicide in Ch. 94).

During the **physical examination,** the physician should screen for medical problems that may aggravate the effects of alcohol abuse or vice versa. Direct signs of alcoholism, such as neglect of personal hygiene, should be noted. A detailed neurologic examination should be performed, especially evaluation of peripheral neuropathy. Traditional signs of chronic alcohol abuse (eg, flushing, injected conjunctiva, tremors, bruises, hepatomegaly, and malnutrition) may be indistinguishable from normal signs of aging or poor general health. A stool guaiac test for occult blood is essential.

Laboratory evaluation should include standard liver function studies (LDH, AST [SGOT], ALT [SGPT], and alkaline phosphatase). Because fluid and electrolyte imbalance is common in the chronic alcoholic, blood chemistry studies, particularly glucose and magnesium, are important. A CBC may reveal a low hematocrit, low hemoglobin, and reticulocytosis, suggesting chronic blood loss or marrow suppression. The electrocardiogram may suggest cardiomyopathy, which may be associated with arrhythmias, especially atrial fibrillation.

Treatment

The greatest treatment challenge is detoxifying older patients who have coexisting medical problems. These patients are usually recognized without difficulty and must be treated in the hospital. Stupor, coma, or serious medical complications are clear indications for hospitalization. Uncomplicated intoxication may be managed in an outpatient setting.

Fluid and electrolyte therapy: Initial treatment of severe intoxication focuses on restoring fluid and electrolyte balance during withdrawal from chronic alcohol use. Although some patients show evidence of delirium tremens, most are stuporous secondary to alcohol intake. Complaints of thirst and dry mucous membranes may suggest dehydration, when in fact the drying may result from exhaled alcohol. To avoid overhydration, the physician should administer 500 to 1000 mL 0.45% sodium chloride solution while awaiting results of blood chemistry studies. If the patient suffers from severe cirrhosis of the liver, the physician should await laboratory tests and tailor therapy accordingly. Glucose solutions should be *avoided* because the older alcoholic may have been subsisting on a high carbohydrate diet as well as on alcohol. In such cases, stress from glucose can produce clinically significant hyperglycemia.

For the treatment of chronic alcoholism, diet must be supplemented with oral multi-vitamins containing folic acid and thiamine 100 mg/day. Chronic alcoholics also may suffer from magnesium and iron deficiency. Treatment of magnesium deficiency requires oral elemental magnesium 240 mg/day or bid. The major side effect is diarrhea. Ferrous sulfate 325 mg/day may supplement this therapy.

Pharmacotherapy: After fluid and electrolyte therapy is begun, the physician should give medications that are cross-tolerant with alcohol. For treatment of alcohol withdrawal, chlordiazepoxide was once preferred because of its relatively extended half-life and cross-tolerance with alcohol. However, **diazepam** is the current drug of choice, given its high therapeutic:toxic effects ratio. For day 1, the patient can be given diazepam 10 mg IV, then 5 mg IV every 5 min until calm (or 20 mg orally, then 20 mg orally every 2 h until calm). The dose may be tapered over the next several days as follows: day 2, 10 mg, 5 mg, 10 mg; day 3, 5 mg tid; day 4, 5 mg bid. Another schedule is to give diazepam 5 to 20 mg orally divided into four equally spaced doses and to reduce the dose by 20% each day. Adequate dosing is confirmed by the cessation of delirium, agitation, and hallucinations without excessive sedation.

Although hospitalization is usually necessary, outpatient withdrawal is possible if no major medical problems exist, if the patient is not severely intoxicated, and if symptoms are monitored daily by the physician and responsible family members. The physician must maintain close contact with the family, and the family must be reliable in administering the benzodiazepine. The starting dose can usually be at the lower end of the range, but the physician must be available by phone during the first 72 h to titrate the dose if necessary.

Following detoxification and withdrawal, treatment focuses on the long-term goal of abstinence. Therapeutic support on the part of the physician and family, who offer encouragement, helps the patient to maintain abstinence. Prophylactic **disulfiram** is also used to help maintain abstinence. This drug should be prescribed only in healthy patients, and a contract must be established between the physician, the patient, and usually one family member. All must agree that the family member is responsible for giving disulfiram, the patient for taking it, and the physician for prescribing it. If a family member is not available, the local hospital emergency department can provide the disulfiram each day.

Therapeutic adjuncts: Self-help groups provide essential long-term support for abstinence. **Alcoholics Anonymous** has proved to be the most effective of these groups in encouraging ongoing abstinence. Older persons, however, frequently resist participating in the program, partly because they continue to deny the problem or believe they can correct it alone. The self-sufficient attitude of many older adults reinforces this negative view of support groups. In addition, membership in Alcoholics Anonymous is usually dominated by young and middle-aged adults. Nevertheless, if the patient can be encouraged to participate in such groups, the chance for success is improved markedly.

100. GERIATRIC PSYCHIATRIC CONSULTATION SERVICES

Geriatric psychiatrists usually serve as consultants rather than as primary care physicians. Because only a small number of physicians specialize in geriatric psychiatry, elderly persons often receive psychiatric care from general psychiatrists.

THE CONSULTATION

A psychiatric consultation begins with a request stating the reason for the consultation and the type of advice being sought. The psychiatrist's objectives are encompassed in the elements listed in TABLE 100–1. The psychiatrist may find discrepancy between the initial question and the underlying problem; if so, he will help redefine and reframe the question while respecting and addressing the referring physician's initial request. The psychiatrist also attempts to address the concerns and agendas of family members, caregivers, case managers, and unit staff.

The psychiatrist may provide the consultation alone or as part of a psychiatric team, the size and exact nature of which vary in different settings. Few studies have been done on the comparable value of these consultations. More research is needed to determine appropriate referral criteria, find ways to identify patients at risk, improve the quality

TABLE 100–1. ELEMENTS OF A GERIATRIC PSYCHIATRIC CONSULTATION

Identification of patient and referral source; reason for consultation	Mental status examination, Mini Mental State score, and depression rating scale
History of the problem with previous treatments	Physical examination
Psychiatric review of systems	Laboratory data
Past psychiatric history and treatments	Assessment with differential diagnosis
Family history	Recommendations: forensic issues, diagnostic workup, medications, psychotherapy, behavior or environmental management, disposition, and follow-up as needed
Past medical history, current medical problems, medications, allergies	
Developmental and social history; assessment of social support	
Functional assessment	

and efficacy of consultations, and devise strategies to maximize compliance with recommendations while always remaining conscious of the costs of these services.

Because of financial and other constraints, many hospitalized elders do not obtain comprehensive psychiatric consultation services and adequate postdischarge follow-up care. Medicare reimburses psychiatric consultations on a one-time basis. Limited reimbursement is available for follow-up visits, which are usually billed as medical psychotherapy. Reimbursement is even less adequate for psychiatrists working in nursing homes, but several proposed policy changes that would provide reasonable payments for such services are under consideration.

HOSPITAL CONSULTATIONS

In the hospitalized elderly, the prevalence of psychiatric problems is reported to range from 27% to 55%, rates that are significantly higher than those found in the community-dwelling elderly. The medically ill elderly are often referred for agitation and competency assessment. Other common requests involve assessment of depression, anxiety, psychosis, and organic mental disorders or help with medical management, treatment compliance, and psychiatric follow-up. The request may be limited, involving transfer of a patient to a psychiatric unit or help with arranging psychiatric follow-up, or it may involve a comprehensive assessment with detailed recommendations for treatment and follow-up.

Medically ill elderly patients are referred for psychiatric evaluation less often than their younger counterparts, and treatment for their psychiatric problems is usually provided by primary care physicians rather than mental health specialists. The elderly often view a consulting psychiatrist with guardedness, because their generation attached a greater stigma to mental illness than do younger generations. Older patients may fear that a psychiatric consultation means someone "thinks they are crazy or wants to put them away."

Overall, less attention is paid to the psychiatric needs of the medically ill elderly than to those of younger persons, possibly because many primary care physicians consider cognitive dysfunction and behavioral abnormalities a normal part of aging. Primary care physicians may overlook psychiatric problems because acute medical problems demand a higher priority, because they are uncomfortable with treating such problems, or because they believe that treatment will be ineffective. Other factors contributing to the neglect of psychiatric problems include financial concerns, patient refusal of treatment, and a belief that services of other mental health professionals are more readily available, are less expensive, or carry less stigma than those of psychiatrists.

Psychiatric consultation is often requested when a question of **competency** arises—particularly when a patient's wishes conflict with the advice of doctors or family members. However, consultation should usually be reserved for cases that pose a real problem for the primary care physician. When consulted, psychiatrists find that patients lack the capacity to make decisions in about 75% of cases. Although the consultant can offer an opinion on **capacity,** competency is a legal question that can be determined only by a court (see COMPETENCE AND DECISIONAL CAPACITY in Ch. 108). Additionally, the consultant should clarify the specific area of capacity in question because capacity may be partial.

The psychiatric consultant can help define the causes of **adjustment problems** and can outline strategies to help the patient cope more effectively. The hospital environment presents many psychologic challenges to the medically ill elderly, including the loss of a familiar environment, the necessity of sharing a room with other patients, frequent interruptions by ever-changing staff, diminished distinction between day and night, and multiple tests and procedures that the patient may not understand. This situation can be frightening and overwhelming, even for those with considerable coping skills and social support. The stresses of hospitalization may be further aggravated by the haste with which patients are now treated and discharged from hospitals. Furthermore, in tertiary care hospitals, patients often are treated by teams of subspecialists, making it difficult for patients to know who their principal physician is.

Additional stresses include the loss of autonomy and independence and the recent loss of a loved one. Such stressful situations can lead to regression, maladaptive behaviors, or adjustment disorders with various emotional and behavioral manifestations.

Depression, psychosis, and acute confusion can occur in medically ill elders, either as part of the medical illness or in addition to it. Psychiatric consultation in these situations can help explore the reasons behind the psychiatric illness and can recommend treatment, both pharmacologic and nonpharmacologic.

The most effective consultation services appear to be those involving high-risk patients likely to benefit from psychiatric intervention, such as patients with hip fractures. In one study, psychiatric screening on admission of patients with hip fractures resulted in earlier discharge and significant cost savings; in another study, psychiatric consultations were associated with an average of 12 fewer hospital days and twice the number of home discharges compared with nursing home placements.

NURSING HOME CONSULTATIONS

While most literature on geriatric consultation-liaison psychiatry focuses on consultations in general hospitals, such consultations can occur in all medical service settings.

Psychiatric disorders are quite prevalent (estimates range from 75% to 95%) in nursing home patients, in whom behavior disorders associated with dementia and depression are particularly common. The Omnibus Reconciliation Act of 1987 (OBRA 87) mandates psychiatric assessment of nursing home patients, but its impact on consultation psychiatry services has not been well studied. Most primary care physicians are not trained in the assessment and management of psychiatric and behavioral problems associated with depression and dementia, although some physicians are. Furthermore, the time required for thorough evaluation and treatment is rarely available to primary care physicians. Thus, despite the OBRA 87 mandates and the high prevalence of psychiatric disorders, only a minority of elderly long-term care residents who need psychiatric assessment and treatment actually receive it.

RECOMMENDATIONS AND INTERVENTIONS

The **written report** of a consultation focuses on data pertinent to the case and should be concise and easily understood by nonpsychiatric colleagues. The report can be in the form of a problem list that includes the questions asked, the major psychiatric syndromes detected along with a differential diagnosis, recommendations for further diagnostic evaluation, and suggestions for management, disposition, and follow-up. *Recommendations should be specific* (eg, specific drug doses and possible side effects) and should clearly state who will be responsible for the proposed interventions. Whenever possible, the consultant should provide answers to the questions asked, and other important issues and unstated questions should be addressed as well.

Direct communication with the referring physician, other team members, the patient, and family members is often as important as the written report. This interaction can clarify any remaining questions about the purpose of the consultation or the consultant's recommendations and can improve compliance with proposed treatment.

The consulting psychiatrist may recommend and coordinate additional diagnostic evaluations to sort out a complicated differential diagnosis or to rule out organic causes of psychiatric symptoms. For example, agitation can result from underlying medical problems such as hypoxia, withdrawal states, and pain.

If **psychoactive medications** are warranted, a geriatric psychiatrist often can help with the complex task of properly prescribing these medications in the medically ill elderly. Altered pharmacokinetics in the elderly can be exaggerated by medical illness, which can further reduce lean body mass and renal or hepatic clearance, thus affecting drug dosing (see Ch. 21 and Pharmacotherapy in Ch. 94). The psychiatrist can help the referring physician follow target symptoms, monitor the patient for emergence of side effects, and recommend drug and dosage adjustments.

The psychiatrist may call attention to drugs that can cause or worsen psychiatric problems or have undesirable interactions with psychoactive medications. Of the 25 drugs most commonly prescribed for the elderly, 10 have anticholinergic side effects that could impair memory and attention span even in normal persons. Patients with organic mental syndromes may be particularly susceptible to cognitive impairment from benzodiazepines and anticholinergic drugs or to the extrapyramidal side effects of antipsychotics. A primary care physician has to weigh medical necessity against the probability that a drug may be affecting mental status.

As part of the consultation, the psychiatrist may recommend ongoing **psychotherapy.** This therapy may be provided by the psychiatric team or by other health professionals, including social workers. Literature on the effectiveness of psychotherapy in the elderly is limited, but most clinicians agree that it helps many hospitalized elderly patients. Supportive individual psychotherapy can minimize the patient's distress and maximize a sense of autonomy, control, and self-esteem by building on remaining strengths and adaptive skills. The consultant addresses such issues, helping the patient to grieve and adjust to losses and to understand the psychologic meaning of the illness and the hospitalization. Consultants can teach patients about their illnesses and help them cope with intellectual deficits. At other times, psychotherapy may involve the family or staff, helping them deal with emotions such as anger, guilt, frustration, and helplessness. Techniques such as **cognitive** or **interpersonal therapy** can also be useful.

Treatment may include **behavior management** and **environmental modification.** Frequent reorientation and reassurance is provided by visits from family members or friends, by having familiar objects in the patient's room, and by reducing noise, light, interruptions, and other disturbances in an intensive care setting. The consultant may direct the unit staff in generating a behavior management program for particularly difficult patients.

The psychiatric consultant should comment on plans for the patient's ultimate **disposition and follow-up.** Disposition requires knowledge about the various services and placements available to the elderly such as retirement communities, nursing homes, Meals-on-Wheels programs, homemaker services, visiting nurses, outpatient and day-care programs, and supportive services for caregivers. Discharge planners and social workers are especially helpful. Patients and families may need help in negotiating the difficult task of placing a patient in a care setting outside the home.

Psychiatric follow-up during the patient's hospitalization ensures maximum benefit from the consultation; postdischarge follow-up can also be an important predictor of the consultation's long-term effectiveness. High relapse rates have been attributed to ineffective follow-up. Ideally, the consulting psychiatrist arranges for psychiatric follow-up on an outpatient basis or makes a home visit. If the psychiatric or behavioral symptoms are severe, a transfer to an inpatient psychiatric unit may be indicated for further evaluation and treatment.

§3. ORGAN SYSTEMS: SKIN DISORDERS

101. SKIN CHANGES AND DISORDERS

Many changes occur in the skin and skin appendages of elderly persons. Some changes result from the aging process itself; others result from the cumulative effects of exposure to sunlight or other environmental factors.

NORMAL CHANGES OF AGING

Age-related structural and functional changes in skin are summarized in TABLE 101–1. Age-related changes in hair and nails are discussed below.

Hair Changes

Hair begins turning gray in about 50% of persons by age 50.

Frontotemporal hair loss (androgenic alopecia) in men begins in the second or third decade; by the seventh decade, 80% of men are substantially bald. In women, the same pattern of hair loss may occur after menopause, although it is rarely pronounced.

Diffuse alopecia normally occurs in both sexes with advancing age; however, it can also result from iron deficiency or hypothyroidism, so these conditions should be excluded when indicated. Certain drugs (especially anabolic steroids and antimetabolites), chronic renal failure, hypoproteinemia, and severe inflammatory skin disease such as erythroderma can also cause diffuse alopecia.

Hair loss with scarring is relatively rare and not associated with aging but with disease. It can be caused by deep bacterial or fungal infections; granulomatous disorders such as sarcoidosis, tuberculosis, or syphilis; and inflammatory disorders such as lichen planus and cutaneous lupus erythematosus. **Cicatricial pemphigoid** is a chronic bullous eruption that affects mucous membranes and sometimes the scalp. Biopsy of the scalp is usually necessary to make these diagnoses.

Hirsutism, excessive or unwanted hair, is also common after the fifth decade, especially in women, presumably as a result of the altered estrogen-androgen balance in hormonally sensitive hair follicles. In women, the most common complaint is the appearance of scattered terminal hairs in the beard area. Men may note increased hairs in the eyebrows, nares, or ears.

TABLE 101–1. STRUCTURAL AND FUNCTIONAL SKIN CHANGES

Structural Changes	*Functional Changes*
Epidermis	Altered skin permeability
Flattening of dermal-epidermal junction	Decreased inflammatory responsiveness
Variation in size, shape, and staining properties of keratinocytes	Decreased immunologic responsiveness
Decreased number of Langerhans' cells	Decreased thermoregulation
Decreased number of melanocytes	Impaired wound healing
Dermis	Decreased sweating and sebum production
Decreased thickness	Decreased elasticity
Decreased cellularity and vascularity	Decreased vitamin D production
Degeneration of elastin fibers	Impaired sensory perception
Appendages	
Decreased number and distorted structure of sweat glands	
Decreased number and distorted structure of specialized nerve endings	
Loss of hair bulb melanocytes and decreased number of hair follicles	

Treatment: Topical minoxidil solution can be used to treat physiologic age-associated hair loss. When applied daily to bald areas, it stimulates regrowth in 25% to 30% of patients, particularly in those who begin treatment early. However, cosmetically significant regrowth occurs in < 10%, and even these patients usually begin to lose hair again within 1 yr. Hair transplantation can be performed by several techniques, including one in which punch grafts from the occipital areas are transplanted to the bald temporal areas. The cosmetic results of this procedure can be enhanced by scalp reduction. Hair loss from endocrine, metabolic, inflammatory, or nutritional disorders can be fully reversed by correcting the underlying disorder.

Unwanted hairs can be repeatedly plucked or cut. Alternatively, the follicle can be permanently destroyed by electrolysis.

Nail Changes

The thickness, shape, color, and growth rate of the nails change with age, reflecting changes in the supporting nail bed and germative matrix. They become dry and brittle and flat or concave instead of convex, often with longitudinal ridging. The color may vary from yellow to gray. Occasionally, the nails become grossly thickened and distorted, a condition known as **onychogryphosis.**

Treatment: No effective treatment exists for these nail changes. For the patient's safety and comfort, a podiatrist should trim thickened toenails with an electric drill and burrs or a carbon dioxide laser. Wearing gloves while doing housework and laundry protects brittle fingernails. Nails should be kept short, and use of nail polish remover, which dehydrates the nail, should be minimized. Evaluation by an experienced examiner can determine treatable conditions, such as fungal infections.

PHOTOAGING

In elderly Americans, most changes in the skin's appearance are the result of chronic ultraviolet irradiation from sunlight and thus occur on commonly exposed areas. This process, known as photoaging, differs clinically, histologically, and physiologically from intrinsic aging, although most patients and many physicians fail to make the distinction. Older people whose pigmentation or lifestyle protects them from sun damage often look younger than their chronologic age.

Some geriatric skin diseases, such as skin cancer, occur almost exclusively in photoaged skin. Others occur without environmental influence or in intertriginous areas, where skin-skin apposition leads to compromised barrier function.

Symptoms and signs: Photoaged skin is characterized by fine and coarse wrinkling, irregular mottled pigmentation, lentigines (brown macules), roughness, sallowness, and telangiectasia. Poorly defined rough, red dysplastic areas called **actinic keratoses** are associated with more severe damage and a higher risk of skin cancer (see below). The overall picture may be hypertrophic or atrophic, depending on the patient's complexion and the severity of sun damage. Slowly resolving purpura (Bateman's or senile purpura) and depigmented stellate pseudoscars on the extremities also indicate photoaging. Cigarette smoking exacerbates the coarse wrinkling of photoaging.

Histologically, photoaged skin shows epidermal dysplasia and atypia, decreased Langerhans' cells, and striking dermal elastosis (deposits of abnormal elastic fibers), among other changes. Also, greater than normal losses of immunologic and inflammatory responsiveness occur.

Prevention: Because photoaging damage is cumulative, preventive measures are most successful if begun during childhood. However, evidence strongly suggests that avoiding sun exposure and regularly using sunscreens, even after marked actinic damage, achieves considerable clinical improvement.

Patients should be encouraged to apply sunscreen before going out, as part of their daily routine. Sunscreens with a sun protection factor (SPF) ≥ 15 should be applied liberally over all exposed areas and reapplied after swimming or washing. Patients should especially avoid going outdoors unprotected when ultraviolet irradiation is strongest, around midday. Because sunscreens also block ultraviolet-induced vitamin D formation in the skin, elderly patients should be advised to consume dairy products or vitamin D supplements to safeguard against osteomalacia.

Treatment: Topical **tretinoin** (all-*trans*-retinoic acid) is useful in treating photoaging. Improvements in global appearance, fine and coarse wrinkling, roughness, mottled hyperpigmentation, and lentigines have been repeatedly demonstrated within 4 to 6 mo. New capillary formation, collagen synthesis, and anchoring fibril formation; regularization of epidermal melanin distribution; and the disappearance of premalignant actinic keratoses have also been reported.

Initial treatment consists of applying tretinoin cream 0.05% once daily at bedtime. The patient should be warned that mild erythema and peeling **(retinoid dermatitis)** will occur, although older adult skin is usually less prone to this problem than younger adult skin. If necessary, the regimen can be changed to every other day until tolerance improves. After 8 to 12 mo, a maintenance regimen of 1 to 3 applications a week may be instituted. Surgical treatment of photoaging, which includes collagen injections, chemical peels, rhytidectomy (face-lift), and various forms of laser surgery, may be performed by a dermatologist or plastic surgeon. Before undergoing such elective surgery, elderly patients should be carefully screened for cardiovascular, renal, and pulmonary diseases that might increase the risk of complications. These patients should also be advised that their healing time for procedures such as dermabrasion and chemical peels will tend to be longer than that for younger adults.

COMMON SKIN DISORDERS

Many common skin conditions affect younger and older adults equally. However, the prevalence of certain inflammatory diseases, infections, and neoplasms of the skin increases with age. The disorders discussed in this chapter occur usually, but not exclusively, in the elderly.

Management Principles

The patient with a skin disorder should be questioned about topical home remedies, such as alcohol, and other products, such as detergents, that may be causing or exacerbating the skin condition. Also, the physician should ascertain the patient's concept of the condition and expectation for therapy.

Management of skin conditions must be tailored to the patient's physical capabilities and circumstances. Many elderly patients are capable of only limited movements because of neurologic impairment or

TABLE 101–2. TOPICAL DERMATOLOGIC FORMULATIONS

Formulation	*Indications and Advantages*	*Disadvantages*
Ointments	Appropriate for dry, scaly, irritated skin; soothing, moisturizing, usually deliver active agent efficiently	May be greasy, promote maceration of weepy or intertriginous lesions
Creams	Appropriate for intertriginous areas; often cosmetically appealing to patient	May cause drying or irritation, especially to broken skin; contain preservatives that may cause allergic sensitization
Lotions	Appropriate for exudative lesions because powder is suspended in an evaporating base; easy to apply to hairy areas	——
Powders	Appropriate for moist lesions and intertriginous or difficult-to-reach areas	May be applied unevenly; may not remain at application site
Soaks and compresses	Appropriate for highly exudative lesions; similar to lotions but cause more drying	To avoid overdrying as lesions improve, patients must substitute a cream or lotion or discontinue therapy

arthritis; often they do not have help applying topical treatments. Regimens that are virtually trouble free for younger patients, such as using oil in bath water, may be dangerous for the elderly.

Because 25% to 50% of elderly patients fail to take prescribed medications and about 60% make medication errors, physicians should ensure that prescribed treatment regimens are as simple as possible. The elderly are two to three times more likely to experience adverse reactions to antihistamines and corticosteroids, drugs frequently used to treat skin disorders. These drugs should be prescribed reluctantly and always with clear, written instructions.

Most dermatologic agents are applied topically, and the choice of a base for the active agent is important (see TABLE 101–2). **Ointments,** *greasy preparations containing little water,* are most useful for treating conditions in which the skin is dry, scaly, or thickened. These agents rarely irritate the skin but may macerate intertriginous areas. **Creams,** *semisolid emulsions of water in oil,* are more cosmetically appealing than ointments because they vanish when rubbed into the skin. Because they dry the skin, they are useful in treating exudative conditions, but they may irritate dry or inflamed skin. Most creams contain stabilizers or preservatives that can induce allergic sensitization when applied to broken skin. **Lotions,** usually *suspensions of fine powder in an aqueous base,* are useful in cooling and drying the skin, especially when acute inflammation or oozing is present. **Powders,** *minute porous particles that may contain an active medication,* absorb moisture from weepy or intertriginous skin. Often, powders are easier to apply than ointments, creams, or lotions. **Soaks or compresses**—consisting of *gauze or other soft material soaked in water, saline, aluminum acetate, or magnesium sulfate solution*—are useful in soothing and drying weeping lesions.

PRURITUS AND XEROSIS

Pruritus

(Itching)

Itching is a common complaint among the elderly. Patients with this complaint should be examined for inconspicuous primary skin lesions such as candidal dermatoses. Systemic disorders associated with generalized pruritus without primary skin lesions include liver and renal disease, iron deficiency anemia, lymphomas, leukemias, polycythemia vera, and parasitosis (usually of the GI tract). Some drugs (eg, barbiturates) can also cause itching. Disorders rarely associated with itching include diabetes mellitus, hyperthyroidism, and solid malignancies.

In research studies, an underlying disorder can be identified in up to 50% of patients with generalized pruritus. However, in most elderly patients, dry skin is more likely to cause pruritus than is an underlying condition.

Diagnosis and treatment: The elderly patient with pruritus who has no obvious skin disease should be examined for clinical clues to systemic disorders, such as lymphadenopathy, hepatosplenomegaly, jaundice, and anemia. Appropriate laboratory tests include a complete blood count; erythrocyte sedimentation rate; electrolyte, urea, and thyroid-stimulating hormone levels; and liver function tests. Urine should be tested for glucose, and if indicated by history or examination, stool should be tested for blood, ova, and parasites. When itching begins suddenly and is severe and unrelenting, an underlying disease should be strongly suspected, and laboratory evaluation should be thorough.

All patients complaining of pruritus should be treated for dry skin because even mild dryness can exacerbate itching, no matter what the cause. Patients should also be advised to avoid very hot baths or showers, as well as irritants such as harsh detergents and alcohol. Antihistamines and major tranquilizers are often prescribed, but they may pose dangers to the elderly and rarely produce a benefit that justifies the risk.

Xerosis

(Dry Skin)

Dry skin is a common cause of pruritus in the elderly. Symptoms are often worst in the winter, when central heating decreases humidity indoors and skin is exposed to cold and wind outdoors.

The skin is scaly, especially over the lower legs, forearms, and hands. The stratum corneum epidermidis may be compromised by fissures or excoriations, allowing environmental irritants to penetrate the skin and progressively worsen the condition, adding inflammation to dryness. This complication of xerosis is called **erythema craquelé** or **asteatotic eczema.**

Treatment: Patients should be advised to keep the air in their home as humid as possible. They should bathe only once a day and avoid using strong soaps, rubbing alcohol, detergents, and other drying agents whenever possible. Patients should also avoid placing potentially irritating materials (such as wool) next to the skin.

Emollients should be applied frequently and liberally, especially after bathing when the skin is still moist. Many lubricating agents are available, ranging from cosmetically elegant lotions to greasy ointments. White petrolatum (petroleum jelly) is an inexpensive and effective lubricant. Creams containing urea or lactic acid help remove scale, keep the skin hydrated, and prevent symptoms. Patients should avoid scented moisturizers because the perfume may irritate dry skin.

A low-potency topical corticosteroid ointment, such as 1% or 2.5% hydrocortisone, is useful in treating inflamed dry skin (see TABLE 101–3). It should be applied to affected areas after a bath or shower and at bedtime. Prolonged use should be discouraged because of systemic absorption.

DERMATITIS

(Eczema)

Often used interchangeably or in combination, the terms **eczema** and **dermatitis** indicate *superficial inflammation of the skin due to irritant exposure, allergic sensitization (delayed hypersensitivity), genetically determined factors, or idiopathic factors.* Pruritus, erythema, and edema progress to vesiculation, oozing, crusting, and scaling. Eventually, the skin may become thickened or lichenified with prominent markings from repeated rubbing or scratching.

Dermatitis of unknown cause is common in the elderly. The patient complains of pruritus; the skin is often excoriated, and papules and lichenified areas may be seen. Frequently, the skin is dry with fine scaling.

TABLE 101–3. RELATIVE POTENCIES OF REPRESENTATIVE TOPICAL CORTICOSTEROID PREPARATIONS*

Potency	*Compound*	*Formulation*
I. Very high	Clobetasol proprionate	Cream or ointment 0.05%
	Halobetasol proprionate	Cream or ointment 0.05%†
II. High	Betamethasone dipropionate	Cream or ointment 0.05%
	Betamethasone valerate	Ointment 0.1%
	Fluocinolone acetonide	Cream 0.02%
	Halcinonide	Cream or ointment 0.1%
III. Medium	Betamethasone valerate	Cream 0.1%
	Fluocinolone acetonide	Cream or ointment 0.025%
	Hydrocortisone valerate	Cream or ointment 0.2%
	Triamcinolone acetonide	Cream, ointment, or lotion 0.1% or 0.025%
IV. Low	Hydrocortisone	Cream, ointment, or lotion 2.5% or 1.0%

* Many equally effective compounds and formulations are not listed.
† Ointments are more potent than creams containing the same corticosteroid in the same concentration.

Treatment: Patients should avoid any practice or product that might irritate the skin, such as excessive use of soaps and detergents. Clothing made of nonirritating fabrics such as cotton should be worn. An emollient should be used liberally, especially after bathing (see Xerosis, above).

A medium-potency corticosteroid ointment should be applied to affected areas tid to help relieve pruritus and control inflammation. If the skin remains dry, an emollient should be applied between applications of the ointment. Once symptoms are alleviated, topical corticosteroid use can be reduced or even discontinued, but use of an emollient should continue.

An antihistamine may reduce pruritus and help the patient sleep. However, in the elderly these agents must be used cautiously because they sometimes produce paradoxical agitation and are strongly anticholinergic. Phototherapy with ultraviolet light in the 290- to 320-nm range (UV-B) or photochemotherapy with PUVA (psoralens plus UV-A) is sometimes effective; however, it is often inconvenient for the patient because supervised treatments at the phototherapy facility are required two or three times a week for several weeks. Therefore, it is not usually considered a treatment option until all others have failed.

Seborrheic Dermatitis

A scaly, erythematous eruption affecting the central part of the face, eyebrows, eyelids, nasolabial folds, postauricular and beard areas, scalp, and body flexures. The central chest and interscapular areas can also be affected. Seborrheic dermatitis affecting the eyelids causes blepharitis and sometimes associated conjunctivitis. Despite its name, seborrheic dermatitis appears to have nothing to do with sebum.

Treatment: **Seborrheic dermatitis of the scalp** can be effectively treated with various shampoos. Active ingredients include sulfur, zinc pyrithione, salicylic acid and sulfur, and tar. The scalp should be shampooed frequently, daily if necessary, and the product left in contact with the scalp for the recommended interval, usually 5 min. If shampooing is inconvenient or physically impossible, the patient can use topical corticosteroid lotions instead. Applied to the scalp bid, such lotions are helpful in severe cases. Hydrocortisone 1% lotion is often sufficient, but many fluorinated corticosteroid preparations are available as well.

Seborrheic dermatitis of the face and trunk is usually effectively treated with hydrocortisone 1% cream applied bid or tid. Preparations containing sulfur or salicylic acid are also helpful.

Seborrheic blepharitis can be treated with hydrocortisone 1% cream. If associated conjunctivitis requires intraocular administration of a corticosteroid ointment or suspension, an ophthalmologist may need to monitor intraocular pressure.

Irritant Contact Dermatitis

The most common form of contact dermatitis, this condition results from skin contact with strong chemicals or other irritants. Although the elderly have a less pronounced inflammatory response to most irritants than do younger patients, chronic irritant dermatitis occurs frequently in the elderly. The reason may be that their slower, muted cutaneous reactions make the contactant less obvious, so exposure continues.

Allergic Contact Dermatitis

Patients may develop delayed, cell-mediated hypersensitivity to many substances that touch the skin. Although older persons are less readily sensitized to experimental allergens, such as dinitrochlorobenzene, they can develop allergic contact dermatitis. Common sensitizers include nickel (found in jewelry), chromates (used in tanning leather), wool fats (particularly lanolin, which is found in many moisturizers and skin creams), rubber additives, topical antibiotics (typically, neomycin), and topical anesthetics such as benzocaine and lidocaine. Eczema at the contact site may be acute, with vesiculation and edema, or more often chronic, with scaling and erythema.

Diagnosis and treatment: If contact dermatitis is suspected but the causative agent is unknown, the patient should be referred to a dermatologist. A detailed history and thorough examination may help identify the agent. If necessary, a **patch test** can be performed. This involves applying a battery of standard potential allergens and other substances the patient uses (eg, cosmetics) to the skin on the back. These test patches are left in place for 48 h; the skin is examined 20 min after the patches have been removed and 4 days later. A positive reaction is indicated by erythema, edema, and often vesiculation appearing 2 to 4 days after the patch application and persisting for several days. In the elderly, clinical changes may not be apparent until 4 days after the patch application.

Once the agent has been identified, it should be avoided as much as possible. All documented cutaneous allergies should be noted on the patient's chart because systemic exposure (eg, via prescription drugs) to chemically related compounds may result in systemic allergic reactions.

Acute eczema with blistering should be treated with soaks of aluminum acetate (Burow's solution) in a 1:20 dilution qid for 15 to 20 min. Once blistering subsides, topical corticosteroid creams or lotions can be applied. For chronic eczema, the patient should use an emollient frequently and apply a medium-potency corticosteroid ointment tid.

Stasis Dermatitis

(Gravitational Eczema; Varicose Eczema)

Inflammation caused by venous hypertension in the lower leg. Stasis dermatitis usually coexists with edema, hemosiderin pigmentation, and dilatation of superficial venules around the ankles. The cause is unknown, but the condition is exacerbated by edema, contact dermatitis from medications, and scratching.

Treatment: The patient should wear properly fitted support stockings or firm bandages to control the edema and should rest with the leg elevated as much as possible. A low-potency topical corticosteroid (eg, hydrocortisone 1% ointment) may help relieve itching. Any possible contact allergen (eg, neomycin ointment) should be avoided.

Exfoliative Dermatitis

(Erythroderma)

A generalized, severe dermatitis. The most common causes of erythroderma are specific dermatoses (such as eczema and psoriasis), drug-induced eruptions (from allopurinol, gold, hydantoin, or sulfonamides), and underlying malignancy (lymphoma or leukemia). Erythema develops and rapidly becomes generalized, often leading to rigors because of uncontrolled cutaneous heat loss. The skin also becomes scaly and thick. (However, it does not lift off in sheets, leaving denuded areas, as in staphylococcal scalded skin syndrome and toxic epidermal necrolysis.) Extensive scaling occurs, and lymphadenopathy often develops. In severe cases, the hair and nails may be shed.

Treatment: *Severe exfoliative dermatitis is a life-threatening condition, and the patient should be admitted to the hospital.* Significant amounts of heat, fluid, and protein are lost through the skin, and elderly patients are at substantial risk of secondary cardiac or renal failure. The patient should be kept in a warm room to minimize heat loss, and core temperature should be monitored. The patient should receive oral or IV fluid replacement; positive fluid balance is essential. A topical emollient (eg, petrolatum ointment) should be used liberally and frequently. If a drug is the suspected cause, it should be discontinued. Systemic prednisone 40 to 60 mg/day should be given early; when erythroderma has been suppressed, the dosage can be tapered gradually.

Nummular Dermatitis
(Discoid Eczema)

Intensely itchy, annular, scaly patches that appear on the limbs first, then become widespread. Discoid or nummular (coin-shaped) eczema occurs in middle-aged and elderly patients. There is no apparent precipitating cause.

Lichen Simplex Chronicus
(Neurodermatitis)

A localized pruritic condition resulting from repeated scratching. It is common in the elderly. The patient complains of itching, and the affected sites are readily accessible for scratching, eg, the lateral aspect of the ankle, dorsum of the foot, shin, back of the neck, forearm, and elbows. The affected sites are well circumscribed and thickened, and have accentuated surface markings.

Treatment: A high-potency topical corticosteroid is often needed to control symptoms. When symptoms improve, the potency can be reduced. Intralesional corticosteroids, such as triamcinolone 5 mg/mL (2 to 5 mg total dose), are often helpful for more troublesome lesions. Tar-containing preparations may also relieve symptoms.

Lesions at some sites, such as the forearms and legs, can be covered for a week at a time with an **Unna's boot** (a firm paste bandage). This treatment helps break the itch-scratch cycle, producing considerable improvement after 1 wk. Phototherapy may alleviate symptoms when other treatments fail.

Idiopathic Hand Eczema

Persistent erythema, vesiculation, and scaling of the palms or lateral digits without an obvious precipitating factor. Skin scrapings should be examined for mycelia to exclude a fungal infection. If contact dermatitis is suspected, patch testing should be performed.

Treatment: The patient should be advised to wear gloves whenever possible, especially when performing household tasks, to avoid exacerbation by irritants. An emollient should be used liberally and frequently. A medium- to high-potency topical corticosteroid ointment may help. Wearing plastic or rubber gloves overnight greatly enhances corticosteroid absorption and may be necessary in severe cases.

SCALING PAPULAR DISEASE

Psoriasis

A disorder characterized by well-defined, erythematous plaques covered with a silvery scale. Although psoriasis may appear on any area of the body, the usual sites are the extensor surfaces (especially knees and elbows), scalp, and buttocks. Psoriatic lesions often appear at sites of trauma such as surgical scars or scratch marks **(Koebner's phenomenon).** Nail involvement produces pitting, thickening, discoloration, and onycholysis (separation of the distal edge of the nail plate from the nail bed).

About 3% of persons over age 60 develop the condition. A detailed drug history should be taken since many drugs, especially β-blockers, can exacerbate psoriasis.

Psoriatic arthritis occurs in a small percentage of older persons with psoriasis and typically produces fusiform swelling and tenderness of the distal interphalangeal joints. Other types of arthritis can also occur: monarthritis, sacroiliitis, and a seronegative arthritis that is otherwise indistinguishable from rheumatoid arthritis. **Exfoliative dermatitis** can occur with psoriasis (see above). **Pustular psoriasis,** a rare variant, is characterized by sterile pustules; they may be localized to the hands and feet or may become generalized.

Treatment: The extent of psoriasis and the patient's mobility determine the treatment. Applying topical preparations tid is often impractical for those whose motion is limited by neurologic impairment or arthritis.

Coal tar ointments (1% to 5%) are effective but messy, can stain clothing, and have an unpleasant odor. More cosmetically acceptable formulations are now available.

Anthralin cream or paste can be effective for thick, scaly plaques, but it must be applied carefully because it can irritate normal skin. (The paste is not available commercially.) The patient also should be warned that anthralin stains clothing and skin. There are two methods of treatment. Lower-strength anthralin cream (0.1% increasing to 0.4%) can be applied to psoriatic plaques at night and removed in the morning, or short-contact anthralin cream (0.4% to 1%) can be applied to psoriatic plaques for 20 min and then removed. If the skin does not become irritated, treatment time is gradually increased.

Topical corticosteroids may be used alone or with coal tar or anthralin. They are especially effective when used under an occlusive dressing. Initial short-term use of a potent topical steroid ointment, such as betamethasone dipropionate 0.05% or triamcinolone acetonide 0.1%, may be needed. As the psoriatic plaques respond to treatment, the ointment strength should be reduced until only lubricants are used. For small, localized lesions, flurandrenolide-impregnated tape can be applied and left on overnight. Topical steroids should be used cautiously to avoid long-term side effects (atrophy, striae, telangiectasia). Systemic corticosteroids should not be used, in part because their withdrawal may cause a recurrence of psoriasis.

Mild scalp involvement can be treated with a **tar-based shampoo** (see Seborrheic Dermatitis, above). For thick scaling, **keratolytic gel** can be applied at night and covered with an occlusive wrap. The gel can be washed out with a tar-based shampoo the next morning, and a steroid solution or gel can be applied to the scalp for the rest of the day. Resistant scalp patches can be injected with **triamcinolone acetonide suspension** 2.5 mg/mL.

Phototherapy with ultraviolet B (UV-B) light in a whole-body treatment cabinet three times a week is highly effective. Phototherapy avoids the side effects associated with frequent topical treatments, and it treats the entire skin surface, thus discouraging new lesions. Regular sun exposure is often as helpful, but it requires a favorable climate and appropriate sunbathing facilities.

Photochemotherapy with PUVA (psoralens plus UV-A) is useful for severe, widespread psoriasis. A photoactive drug, usually methoxsalen 0.6 mg/kg, is taken orally 2 h before treatment. The patient is then exposed to UV-A light at a dosage based on the skin type or on the experimentally determined minimum phototoxic dose. Lesions usually disappear after 20 to 25 treatments. Maintenance treatment every 2 wk is often necessary to prevent flare-ups.

Methotrexate may be used in patients unresponsive to other treatments. This antimetabolite interferes with DNA synthesis and is especially useful in widespread pustular psoriasis, exfoliative psoriasis, and disabling psoriatic arthritis. In elderly patients who have disabling psoriasis and are unable to use topical agents, methotrexate dosages as low as 2.5 or 5 mg/wk can control the disease completely. Close supervision by a dermatologist is recommended. Blood counts and hepatic and renal function must be monitored.

BULLOUS DISORDERS

Bullous Pemphigoid

A chronic, bullous eruption occurring predominantly in elderly persons and characterized by tense bullae on normal or erythematous skin. Pruritus often develops before blistering. Bullae may be localized or generalized, and mucous membranes are involved in about 50% of cases. The disease tends to abate and recur. Men and women are equally affected.

Diagnosis: Histologic examination reveals subepidermal bullae. Immunofluorescent staining reveals deposits of complement (C3) in all patients and immunoglobulin (IgG) along the dermal-epidermal junction in lesional and perilesional skin in many patients. Autoantibodies directed against a protein on the basal surface of keratinocytes, the bullous pemphigoid antigen, cause the blisters to form and can be detected in the serum of about 45% of patients with active disease.

The differential diagnosis includes pemphigus vulgaris, dermatitis herpetiformis, erythema multiforme, benign mucosal pemphigoid, and drug-induced eruptions.

Prognosis: Bullous pemphigoid is chronic. Before the introduction of corticosteroids, the disseminated disease was fatal in about 33% of patients due to sepsis. Once the condition is controlled with corticosteroids, patients often go into prolonged remission, allowing tapering of the dose and discontinuance of drugs.

Treatment: Mild, localized bullous pemphigoid can often be controlled with potent topical corticosteroids; widespread bullous pemphigoid may require hospitalization until the epidermal barrier is restored. Systemic prednisone 40 to 60 mg/day is needed to control severe disease. High-dose corticosteroid therapy in elderly patients requires close monitoring. Before therapy, an evaluation for quiescent tuberculosis including a chest x-ray should be performed. During therapy, elderly patients should be monitored for steroid-induced diabetes and other complications, including upper GI bleeding, fluid retention, hypertension, and confusion.

After the skin lesions have resolved, the corticosteroid dosage should be decreased to about half the initial dose over 1 mo, and then tapered more gradually. The total dose can be given every morning or every other morning to minimize adrenal suppression. Patients should be observed for signs of recurrence as the prednisone dosage is reduced. Topical or intralesional corticosteroids may be used for recalcitrant lesions as a supplement to oral therapy.

After several months of systemic treatment, about 50% of patients with bullous pemphigoid have complete remission and then require no medication.

Because of the risks of prolonged corticosteroid therapy in the elderly, an immunosuppressive agent is usually given concomitantly for its steroid-sparing effect; eg, azathioprine 50 to 150 mg/day, methotrexate 25 to 35 mg/wk orally or IM, or cyclophosphamide 2 to 3 mg/kg/day initially, followed by a maintenance dose of 100 mg/day. Because immunosuppressants require 6 to 8 wk to become effective, the steroid dosage cannot be reduced immediately. Side effects of immunosuppressants include bone marrow depression and hepatotoxicity.

Pemphigus Vulgaris

A rare, potentially life-threatening condition characterized by intraepidermal bullae on the skin or mucous membranes. Although the incidence is highest among middle-aged persons, many patients are elderly.

Symptoms, signs, and diagnosis: Pemphigus is characterized by flaccid bullae that rupture easily and leave superficial erosions on the trunk, limbs, and mucous membranes. The surrounding skin looks normal. Many patients present with mouth pain; oral lesions may dominate the clinical picture, especially early in the disease process. Blistering can progress from localized to generalized, and patients are at high risk for secondary infection and sepsis.

Often, applying a lateral force to the skin causes the overlying epidermis to shear off **(Nikolsky's sign).** Histologic examination shows an intraepidermal blister; immunofluorescent staining reveals intercellular deposits of complement and immunoglobulin directed against the glycoprotein that forms the intercellular cement.

Differential diagnosis includes bullous pemphigoid, benign mucous membrane pemphigoid, toxic epidermal necrolysis, drug-induced eruptions, and erythema multiforme.

Prognosis: Before the advent of corticosteroids, the disease was always fatal with a mean survival of about 1 yr. The mortality rate is now about 25%, with death usually resulting from complications of therapy. Long-term follow-up and prolonged treatment are required.

Treatment: Usually, prednisone 60 to 100 mg/day is needed to control the disease. Widespread pemphigus may require hospitalization until the epidermal barrier is restored. High-dose corticosteroid therapy in elderly patients requires close monitoring. (Appropriate precautions are given under Bullous Pemphigoid, above.)

After the skin lesions have resolved, the corticosteroid dosage should be decreased to about half the initial dose over 1 mo, and then tapered more gradually. The total dose can be given every morning or every other morning to minimize adrenal suppression. As the dosage of prednisone is reduced, the patient should be observed for signs of recurrence. Topical or intralesional corticosteroids may be used for recalcitrant lesions as a supplement to oral therapy. Remission may last many months or indefinitely, but some patients require lifelong treatment.

Because of the risks of prolonged corticosteroid therapy in the elderly, the dose should be tapered and the medication discontinued whenever possible. Often, recurrences can be well managed with early intralesional injections alone. If necessary, immunosuppressive agents may be given instead of or concomitantly with corticosteroids for their steroid-sparing effect (see Bullous Pemphigoid, above).

ULCERS

Decubitus Ulcers

(Pressure Sores)

Decubitus ulcers are discussed in detail in Ch. 14.

Venous Ulcers

Venous ulcers are a major cause of morbidity in elderly patients. Causes of the condition include incompetent superficial veins and perforators, as well as postphlebitic syndrome. These factors result in persistent venous hypertension and a corresponding rise in capillary pressure with fibrinogen leakage into the tissues. Pericapillary fibrin cuffs form, limiting the diffusion of oxygen and other nutrients to the skin, predisposing it to ulcers.

Symptoms and signs: Venous ulcers commonly occur on the medial or lateral aspect of the legs. Edema, hyperpigmentation (from hemosiderin deposits), eczematous changes, and induration often occur in the surrounding skin. Distinctive scars composed of sharply demarcated, sclerotic, atrophic, white plaques **(atrophie blanche)** stippled with telangiectasia and surrounded by hyperpigmentation are commonly found in patients with venous insufficiency.

All patients with venous ulcers should be evaluated for systemic disorders such as heart failure, hypoalbuminemia, neuropathy, diabetes mellitus, arterial insufficiency, and nutritional deficiencies, which may contribute to the condition.

Treatment: Reducing edema is the major element in therapy for venous insufficiency. The patient should be advised to elevate the affected limb whenever possible, especially when lying in bed or sitting. Compression stockings and graduated pressure bandages or Unna's boot, applied from toe to knee, effectively reduce limb edema. Diuretics usually are not helpful and may be dangerous.

Ulcer dressings should be kept as simple as possible. Frequent applications of wet-to-dry dressings with normal saline may help remove debris. If the wound is infected with *Pseudomonas* (which often produces a fruity smell), frequent applications of compresses with acetic acid 5% reduce the bacterial count.

Systemic antibiotics do not enhance healing unless cellulitis is present. If signs of cellulitis (erythema, swelling, warmth, and streaking) do develop around the ulcer, the patient should be given penicillin V 250 to 500 mg qid or dicloxacillin 250 to 500 mg qid for 7 to 10 days. If the patient is allergic to penicillin, erythromycin can be substituted.

Patients with venous ulcers and stasis dermatitis are at risk for developing allergic contact dermatitis from topical antibiotics or other potential sensitizers applied to the broken skin surface. Chronic, low-grade, delayed hypersensitivity reactions may impede ulcer healing and increase local pruritus and edema. Neomycin ointment, wood alcohols, and balsam of Peru are among the most commonly implicated allergens. When an allergy is suspected, topical therapy should be discontinued for at least 2 wk, and the ulcer should be treated with wet-to-dry saline compresses. If possible, patch testing should be performed.

Patients with very deep or nonhealing ulcers may require surgical intervention. Split-thickness skin grafts or pinch grafts may reduce healing time significantly. In the elderly, however, postoperative immobilization increases the risk of deep venous thrombosis and may slow healing of the graft site. Hydrocolloid and biologic dressings, including cultured allogeneic epithelial sheets, improve healing in chronic venous ulcers.

INFECTIONS

The age-related decline in immune function is reflected in a higher incidence of certain chronic skin infections, such as tinea pedis. The compromised tissue perfusion and slower healing of aging skin may explain the increased tendency toward bacterial superinfection of wounds in older persons.

Bacterial Infections

Impetigo

A superficial skin infection caused by staphylococci or streptococci. Vesicles or pustules in the early stages break down to form golden brown crusts that often adhere to the underlying skin. If the infection is extensive, malaise, fever, and lymphadenopathy may occur. Impetigo often develops as a secondary infection in conditions characterized by breaks in the skin that allow microbes to penetrate (eg, eczema, senile pruritus, pediculosis, nodular prurigo, and herpes zoster).

Treatment: Single or localized lesions should be soaked for 10 min in a drying agent such as Burow's solution (aluminum acetate 5%). Extensive lesions require systemic antibiotics to reduce the risk of glomerulonephritis and prevent impetigo from spreading. A skin swab should be taken for microbial culture and sensitivity assays.

Patients with **streptococcal pyoderma** should be treated with penicillin V 250 to 500 mg orally qid for 10 days. If patient compliance is unlikely, long-acting penicillin G benzathine 1.2 million u. IM may be necessary. If the patient is allergic to penicillin, erythromycin 250 to 500 mg orally qid can be given. Patients with **staphylococcal pyoderma** should receive dicloxacillin 250 to 500 mg orally qid for 10 days.

Staphylococcal Scalded Skin Syndrome
(Ritter's Disease)

A severe, extensive bullous condition caused by a staphylococcal skin infection, in which the epithelium lifts off in sheets leaving large denuded areas. Although generally a disease of young children, the condition is increasingly appearing in immunocompromised adults. In elderly patients, staphylococci usually invade the skin and the blood, and death usually results from septicemia.

Toxic epidermal necrolysis, an adverse drug reaction that can produce an identical clinical picture, must be considered in the differential diagnosis. Both these conditions are life threatening and require hospitalization. To differentiate between staphylococcal scalded skin syndrome and toxic epidermal necrolysis, the examiner observes a frozen section from a skin scraping or biopsy to determine the level of cleavage. In staphylococcal scalded skin syndrome, cleavage occurs within the epidermis just below the granular layer. In toxic epidermal necrolysis, subepidermal blister formation occurs with basal cell damage. Differentiation is important because staphylococcal scalded skin syndrome must be treated immediately with penicillinase-resistant antistaphylococcal antibiotics.

Treatment: Therapy is the same as for severe burns, beginning with immediate fluid and electrolyte replacement. A systemic antibiotic (eg, IV oxacillin) should also be given promptly. The source of infection may be difficult to isolate, but culture specimens should be taken from the skin, blood, nares, and any other suspected sites. Silver sulfadiazine cream may help prevent cutaneous superinfection with gram-negative bacteria. Even with treatment, the prognosis is poor.

Erysipelas

A superficial infection of the skin caused by group A or group C hemolytic streptococci. The organisms may enter the skin through minor cuts, wounds, or insect bites.

The affected area may be red and swollen. The lesions have well-defined margins that advance as the infection spreads. Vesicles or bullae may be present, and in the elderly, hemorrhage may occur. Fever, malaise, and lymphadenopathy may also develop.

Treatment: Penicillin V or erythromycin 250 to 500 mg orally qid should be given for 2 wk. Because the infection continues to spread during the first 12 to 24 h of oral therapy, patients with facial lesions often require hospitalization and IV antibiotics to prevent cavernous sinus thrombosis.

Cellulitis

A deep infection of the skin, most frequently caused by group A streptococci and occasionally by gram-negative organisms. In the elderly, cellulitis most commonly occurs as a complication of an open wound, such as a venous ulcer. However, it also develops in intact, edematous skin, especially in the legs. Erythema, tenderness, swelling, warmth, and lymphadenopathy may be present.

Treatment: Penicillin or erythromycin 250 to 500 mg orally qid should be given for 2 wk. If the lesion is large or near a vital structure or if the patient has fever, diabetes mellitus, or peripheral vascular disease or cannot be closely monitored, initial IV therapy is recommended. In some patients, cellulitis responds slowly to antibiotics, and prolonged treatment is needed.

FUNGAL INFECTIONS

Chronic fungal infections are common in the elderly; the age-related decrease in cutaneous immunologic response may be partly responsible.

Tinea Pedis

(Athlete's Foot)

Tinea pedis is discussed in Ch. 77.

Tinea Unguium

A fungal infection of the nails (more often the toenails than the fingernails), usually caused by Trichophyton rubrum *or* T. mentagrophytes. The nails may become grossly thickened and so enlarged that wearing shoes becomes painful.

Treatment: Treatment is prolonged and rarely warranted. Fingernails may be treated with griseofulvin 500 to 1000 mg/day for 6 to 9 mo; toenails require 12 to 18 mo of such therapy. The overall cure rate is 40% to 70%. Although fingernails are more likely to respond to treatment than toenails, recurrence within 1 yr is common; recurrence in toenails is nearly 100%. Available topical antifungals are fungistatic and do not penetrate the nail plate in sufficient concentration to eradicate infection. Fungicidal agents now under investigation offer the prospect of effective topical therapy for tinea unguium. In elderly patients whose main problem is discomfort, conservative management including periodic trimming by a podiatrist may be the most practical approach.

Tinea Cruris

A cutaneous fungal infection of the groin that commonly affects the elderly. Predisposing factors include clothing made of synthetic fabrics that do not breathe, obesity, and immobility.

The patient usually complains of itching, and examination may reveal scaly erythematous areas with well-defined margins. Maceration, lichenification, and secondary candidal or bacterial infection are common. Diagnosis requires microscopic examination of a specimen prepared with potassium hydroxide (KOH) solution.

Treatment: Miconazole 2% or clotrimazole 1% cream should be used bid or tid. Affected areas should be kept as clean and as dry as possible, using cotton between the toes and talc-based powders.

Tinea Incognito

(Steroid-Modified Tinea)

A fungal infection in which clinical manifestations are modified by topical or systemic corticosteroids. When treated with topical corticosteroids, fungal infections appear to improve: inflammation subsides and scaling decreases. But attempts to discontinue the agent result in flare-ups. Prolonged use of corticosteroids can cause striae, atrophy, and telangiectasia to develop with the original dermatitis. Specimens prepared with KOH solution are floridly positive.

Treatment: A topical antifungal agent should be used. If a potent topical corticosteroid has been used, the number of applications may need to be gradually reduced to minimize the rebound flushing and fixed vasodilation seen in steroid-dependent skin.

YEAST INFECTIONS

Candidiasis

An infection caused by the yeast Candida albicans, *which thrives in warm, moist areas such as the groin, the axilla, and the submammary region.* Diabetic and immunosuppressed patients, as well as those receiving systemic antibiotic therapy, are at increased risk. The organism may be carried asymptomatically in the bowel, mouth, and vagina, causing treated sites to become reinfected.

Candidal vulvovaginitis is manifested by pruritus vulvae, vulvar erythema and edema, and a creamy vaginal discharge. Patients with these signs should be tested for glycosuria because diabetes strongly predisposes patients to candidal infections.

Oral candidiasis (thrush) is characterized by creamy white plaques on the tongue or buccal mucosa, which can be easily scraped off.

Perlèche (angular cheilitis) is *a mixed bacterial and candidal infection of the corners of the mouth.* The skin appears moist, cracked, and fissured. Predisposing factors include deep folds at the corners of the mouth, poorly fitting dentures, and retention of saliva and food particles in the affected areas.

Treatment: For **vulvitis,** miconazole 2% or clotrimazole 1% cream can be applied tid. For **vulvovaginitis,** a 100-mg clotrimazole vaginal insert can be applied once a day for 7 days. Nystatin vaginal suppositories can also be used (2 tablets of 100,000 u. each inserted high into the vagina every night for 14 nights). Nystatin cream should then be applied to the labia, perineum, and perineal area, after which the hands should be washed thoroughly.

For **oral candidiasis** or **perlèche,** either nystatin or amphotericin B, available as mouthwashes and lozenges, can be used qid. Dentures should be soaked in nystatin suspension because they are invariably contaminated with *C. albicans.* Miconazole 2% or nystatin cream tid for 1 wk usually produces rapid improvement.

Intertrigo

A dermatitis, usually caused by maceration and exposure to irritants, occurring between two folds of skin—eg, between the buttocks, the thighs, or the scrotum and the thigh. Intertrigo often appears as moist, red, and sometimes scaly and pruritic areas in the flexures. Intense itching or soreness may develop from the groin to the perineum, in the inner thighs, and in the intergluteal cleft. Contributing factors include obesity, poor personal hygiene, and clothing made of synthetic fabrics that do not breathe.

Intertrigo may mimic or coexist with a candidal superinfection. *Candida* often produces so-called satellite lesions—small vesicles at the periphery of the lesion. Examination of a scraping prepared with KOH solution may reveal the characteristic budding yeasts and pseudohyphae.

Treatment: Affected areas should be kept as dry as possible. Topical antifungal creams (eg, clotrimazole 1% or miconazole 2%) should be applied tid if *Candida* is suspected. Nystatin cream, another anticandidal agent, is not effective against dermatophytes and therefore should be used only when there is no suspicion of tinea infection. If inflammation is severe, a low-potency, topical corticosteroid cream (eg, hydrocortisone 1%) can be applied tid. Some available commercial preparations combine an antifungal agent and a topical corticosteroid cream, such as clotrimazole and betamethasone diproprionate cream.

Viral Infections

Herpes Zoster

(Shingles)

An acute eruption caused by a reactivation of latent varicella virus in the dorsal root ganglia of a partially immune host. Herpes zoster may occur at any age, but the peak incidence occurs between ages 50 and 70, and the age-specific incidence increases throughout life. Zoster usually affects otherwise healthy people, but immunosuppressed patients are at higher risk. The increased frequency among older persons may be explained partially by a decrease in cellular immune response to varicella-zoster antigen, which is undetectable in up to 30% of previously immune, healthy persons > 60 yr. Other factors that predispose persons to a reactivation of varicella virus include immunosuppressive drugs, corticosteroids, malignancy, local irradiation, trauma, and surgery. Herpes zoster recurs in about 6% of cases, usually at the same site as the initial episode.

The major difference between herpes zoster in the elderly and in young adults is the incidence of postherpetic neuralgia, which increases sharply with age to about 40% in those ≥ 60 yr. The duration and severity of discomfort increase even more markedly with age than the incidence does. Other complications include encephalitis, ophthalmic disease, motor neuropathies, Guillain-Barré syndrome, and urinary retention.

Symptoms and signs: The patient may develop prodromal symptoms of chills, fever, malaise, GI disturbance, and paresthesia or pain along the affected dermatome. The distribution of dermatomal zoster infections is 50% to 60% thoracic, 10% to 20% trigeminal, 10% to 20% cervical, 5% to 10% lumbar, and < 5% sacral. Rarely, prodromal symptoms persist for 5 to 7 days, leading to a variety of misdiagnoses from herniated disk to acute abdomen. Usually, red papules appear along a dermatome within 3 days. These eruptions rapidly develop into grouped vesicles, which vary in size, may be hemorrhagic, and may be extremely painful. After about 5 days, the vesicles begin to dry and form scabs; gradual healing occurs over the next 2 to 4 wk. Persistent hyperpigmentation or true scarring may result, particularly in the elderly.

In about 50% of patients with uncomplicated herpes zoster, some vesicles appear outside the affected area. However, *if widespread severe dissemination occurs, an underlying lymphoma or other cause of immunodeficiency should be suspected.*

Ophthalmic herpes zoster results from involvement of the ophthalmic division of the trigeminal nerve. Conjunctivitis, iridocyclitis, and keratitis may occur. In such cases, an ophthalmologic consultation should be sought. Lesions on the tip of the nose indicate involvement of the nasociliary and ophthalmic nerves. The risk of postherpetic neuralgia is greater than with involvement of other dermatomes.

Geniculate neuralgia (Ramsay Hunt syndrome) results from involvement of the geniculate ganglion. Facial paralysis (usually temporary) occurs, pain develops in the ear on the affected side, and taste is lost in the anterior two thirds of the tongue. Vesicles appear on the soft palate, fauces, and external auditory meatus on the affected side. Consultation with a neurologist is advisable.

Diagnosis: The finding of multinucleate giant cells on a cytologic smear or biopsy of a vesicle confirms the diagnosis. Although not commonly needed, electron microscopy and vesicle fluid culture can also identify the virus. However, false-negative results are common with vesicle fluid culture.

Treatment: A systemic corticosteroid (eg, prednisone 40 to 60 mg/day), started within a week of the eruption, appears to reduce acute symptoms and the risk of postherpetic neuralgia in elderly patients. Corticosteroids are the treatment of choice in patients with geniculate neuralgia (Ramsay Hunt syndrome).

If the patient is seen within 3 days of the onset of the eruption, oral or IV acyclovir is appropriate. This drug inhibits the development of new vesicles and decreases the duration of viral shedding and discomfort. Acyclovir also appears to decrease the risk of postherpetic neuralgia. The recommended oral dosage is 800 mg 5 times daily for 10 days. The IV dosage is 5 mg/kg q 8 h for 5 days.

Analgesia is usually needed, as well. Simple analgesics, such as acetaminophen or aspirin given q 4 h or nonsteroidal anti-inflammatory drugs may be sufficient, but some patients require more potent medication. However, opioids should be avoided if possible, especially in the elderly, because of the increased risks of adverse reactions and medication errors.

Topical treatment consists of soaking the affected areas in Burow's solution (aluminum acetate 5%), diluted 1:20 to 1:40, to remove vesicle crusts, decrease oozing, and dry and soothe the skin. Gauze dressings are soaked in the solution, applied to the affected areas, and loosely bandaged. The dressings are changed q 2 to 3 h. If impetigo develops, systemic antibiotics should be given (see BACTERIAL INFECTIONS, above).

Until dry crusts appear, herpes zoster lesions contain infectious viral particles. A person who has never had varicella may develop it after direct contact with the lesions or with moist, contaminated dressings. Usually, only young children are susceptible. However, because varicella virus is teratogenic in early fetal development, pregnant women should avoid contact with zoster patients. Severely immunocompromised patients should also avoid exposure. Ordinarily, isolating zoster patients from casual contact with other adults is not necessary, however.

PARASITIC INFECTIONS

Scabies

An eruption caused by a mite, Sarcoptes scabiei. The female mite burrows into the skin and deposits eggs, which hatch into larvae in a few days. Scabies is easily transmitted by skin-to-skin contact and can be rapidly spread between residents of the same household, nursing home, or institution. Infestation is usually present for weeks before the patient becomes allergically sensitized to the insects and develops itching.

Symptoms and signs: Eventually the patient experiences intense pruritus, which usually worsens at night. On examination, the skin is usually excoriated. The characteristic sign is the burrow—a linear ridge with a vesicle at one end—where the mite is usually found. Burrows are common in the interdigital webs, the flexor aspects of the wrists, the axillae, the umbilicus, around the nipples, and on the genitalia. Erythematous papules or nodules in the same areas are also common.

In the elderly, scabies may present less typically, especially if untreated for a long time. The condition may mimic eczema or exfoliative dermatitis because widespread thick crusted lesions are present. The patient may have erythroderma and generalized lymphadenopathy.

Diagnosis and treatment: A mite at the end of a burrow can sometimes be excavated with a needle or a scalpel blade, placed in a drop of mineral oil, and detected under a microscope. However, even in long-term cases with widespread excoriations, few mites are present, and they may be impossible to find. Therefore, treatment is usually based on a presumptive diagnosis.

A lotion or cream containing lindane 1% should be applied to the entire body from the neck down. All patients need help applying the medication and must understand that *all* areas must be covered. After 24 h, the patient should bathe; all clothes and bed linens should be machine-laundered in hot water or dry-cleaned.

A second application of the cream or lotion, also left on the body for 24 h, should be made 7 days later to kill any newly hatched larvae. Itching, which results from allergic sensitization and not from viable organisms, may not subside until 1 to 2 wk after treatment. However, itching can be effectively treated with topical corticosteroids or, in severe cases, with a tapering course of oral corticosteroids.

All household members and close personal contacts should also be treated. In a nursing home, *all* clinical staff, patients, and their household contacts should be treated on the assumption that some infested persons are still asymptomatic.

Pediculosis
(Lice)

Lice may infest the head *(Pediculus humanus capitis),* the body *(P. humanus corporis),* or the genital area *(Phthirus pubis).* Elderly people who have poor personal hygiene or who live in an overcrowded environment are at risk for head and body lice.

Pediculosis capitis is spread by personal contact or by sharing hairbrushes and head wear. The patient develops severe scalp itching, often with secondary eczematous changes and impetiginization. Cervical lymphadenopathy may occur. Examination reveals small gray-white nits (ova) on the hair shafts. Unlike scales, they cannot be easily removed. Adult lice are not usually found.

Pediculosis corporis produces intense generalized itching. The patient frequently develops eczematous changes, severe excoriations, and a secondary bacterial infection. Lice or nits may be found in the seams of the patient's clothing.

Pediculosis pubis is usually spread by sexual contact but can be transferred by clothing or towels. The base of pubic hairs should be carefully searched for lice and their eggs. Sometimes, dark brown particles (louse excreta) may be seen on underclothes.

Treatment: **For head lice,** shampoo containing lindane 1% is applied to the scalp, left in place for 4 min, and rinsed off. The patient should then comb the hair with a fine-tooth comb. The procedure should be repeated in 10 days to destroy any remaining nits. Combs and brushes should be soaked in the shampoo for 1 h.

For body lice, the patient's clothing should be boiled, dry-cleaned, or machine washed with hot water. The seams of the clothing should be pressed with a hot iron. Alternatively, the clothing can be disinfected with an insecticidal powder such as DDT 10% or malathion 1%. Because lice do not remain on the host after feeding, the patient's skin requires therapy only for irritation and pruritus.

For pubic lice, 1% lindane shampoo is applied to the pubic area for 4 min, then rinsed off. This treatment should be repeated in 10 days.

DRUG–INDUCED ERUPTIONS

The most common drug-induced skin eruption is a fairly symmetric maculopapular, pruritic rash. Eruptions typically appear 1 to 10 days after the patient starts taking the drug and last until about 14 days after the patient stops taking it.

The drugs that most commonly cause skin eruptions include penicillins, sulfonamides, gold, phenylbutazone, and gentamicin. However, any oral medication, including OTC preparations and sporadically used drugs, can cause eruptions.

Erythema Multiforme

An inflammatory eruption characterized by symmetric erythematous, edematous, or bullous lesions of the skin or mucous membranes. In about 50% of cases, the cause is unknown. In the others, the disorder appears to be a hypersensitivity reaction that can be triggered by almost any drug and many infections, particularly herpes simplex.

The severity varies from characteristic target lesions with a red periphery and cyanotic center appearing in groups on the limbs to extensive erosion of the skin with bullae on the mucous membranes in the mouth, pharynx, anogenital region, and conjunctiva **(Stevens-Johnson syndrome).** Corneal ulceration is common in those with severe conditions.

Treatment: All suspected causative agents should be removed, when possible. Localized eruptions should be treated symptomatically. Patients with severe conditions require hospitalization so fluid balance and ophthalmologic, renal, and pulmonary statuses can be monitored. The use of systemic corticosteroids is controversial and should not be a routine practice. If herpes simplex precedes recurrent severe erythema multiforme, a regimen of acyclovir 200 mg orally 5 times/day beginning with the herpetic prodrome may prevent attacks.

Toxic Epidermal Necrolysis

(Lyell's Syndrome)

A severe condition that begins with general malaise, skin tenderness, and erythema and rapidly progresses to skin blistering and erosion. Applying a lateral force to the skin causes the overlying epidermis to shear off **(Nikolsky's sign).** The cause in about 33% of cases is a drug—

most commonly a sulfonamide, barbiturate, NSAID, penicillin, or hydantoin. *Toxic epidermal necrolysis is a life-threatening condition with a high mortality rate*.

Treatment: The patient should be managed in a burn unit, and possible causative agents should be removed. All denuded areas of the dermis should be covered with an antibacterial agent, such as silver sulfadiazine cream. When possible, the area should be covered with a biologic dressing, such as a pigskin xenograft. Meticulous eye care with close supervision by an ophthalmologist is necessary. Use of systemic corticosteroids is common, but it has not been proved to influence the course of the disease and does increase the risk of sepsis.

TUMORS

Elderly persons may have benign skin tumors (such as seborrheic keratoses, acrochordons, and keratoacanthomas), premalignant tumors (such as actinic keratoses and Bowen's disease), and malignant tumors (such as basal cell carcinoma, squamous cell carcinoma, Kaposi's sarcoma, cutaneous T-cell lymphoma, lentigo maligna melanoma, nodular melanoma, and superficial spreading melanoma).

BENIGN TUMORS

The association of benign tumors with aging is obvious to most patients, and health care professionals must understand the psychologic impact of these lesions. Such lesions must be distinguished from malignant tumors.

Seborrheic Keratoses
(Seborrheic Warts)

These waxy, raised, verrucous lesions vary in color from flesh tone to black and in size from barely perceptible papules to large plaques. Often, they look as though they were pasted or stuck onto the skin. **Dermatosis papulosa nigra** is a variant of seborrheic keratoses occurring exclusively in blacks, in which the face is studded with numerous small, dark, sometimes pedunculated papules.

One treatment option is curettage and light cautery. Another option is freezing with liquid nitrogen for 15 to 20 sec. Sometimes, light freezing of seborrheic keratoses before curettage makes them easier to remove.

Acrochordons
(Skin Tags)

These lesions are commonly found on the neck, axillae, and trunk of middle-aged and elderly people. Flesh colored or pigmented, the lesions are soft and often pedunculated. They may be removed with sharp scissors or a scalpel or by electrocauterization, usually without requiring anesthesia.

Keratoacanthomas

These rapidly enlarging nodules have a smooth outline and a central keratin plug. Left untreated, they usually resolve spontaneously but may leave a scar. Although keratoacanthomas are benign, most authorities believe they should be managed as a well-differentiated squamous cell carcinoma, primarily because they are difficult to differentiate from it. The tumor is usually removed by curettage and cautery or by excision.

PREMALIGNANT CONDITIONS

Actinic Keratoses

These scaly, sandpaper-like patches appear on sun-exposed areas. Although actinic keratosis may evolve into squamous cell carcinoma, the latent period is long, and the squamous cell carcinoma usually grows very slowly and has little metastatic potential. Nevertheless, patients with multiple lesions anywhere on their exposed skin should be screened every 6 to 12 mo for skin cancer. Patients should also be advised to avoid sun exposure and to use a high-potency sunscreen (SPF 15) when outside.

Treatment: Avoidance of sun exposure leads to regression of early actinic keratoses and may be sufficient therapy for patients with mild disease. Cryotherapy with liquid nitrogen for 10 to 15 sec or curettage and light cautery may be used for individual lesions if the patient does not have too many. Topical 5-fluorouracil **(5-FU)** 1% or 2% solution or 1% cream can also be used, especially for multiple lesions. Stronger concentrations of 5-FU cream (5%) can be applied to lesions on the trunk. The cream or solution should be applied once or twice a day. When applying it, the patient must be careful to avoid the eyes and mucous membranes.

The patient must be told to follow the directions in the package circular for 5-FU exactly and never to leave it on longer than directed. Also, the patient should be informed that treatment with 5-FU produces progressive erythema and burning and, after 2 to 4 wk, ulceration followed by reepithelialization over another 2 wk. Treatment should be discontinued once ulceration occurs. Complete healing usually occurs within 2 mo, and the patient has far fewer lesions for months to years thereafter.

Pain and burning sensations may be decreased, especially on sensitive areas such as the face, by first applying a 1% or 2% 5-FU solution, then 15 to 20 min later applying a medium-potency corticosteroid cream. Tretinoin cream can be combined with 5-FU, especially if the lesions appear on more resistant areas such as the limbs or trunk. Masoprocol may be used as an alternative to 5-FU.

Bowen's Disease

Bowen's disease (squamous cell carcinoma in situ) presents as a persistent, erythematous, scaly plaque with well-defined margins. It can occur anywhere on the skin or mucous membranes. The patient may have a history of arsenic exposure (either medicinal or occupational). Multiple lesions are associated with an increased incidence of internal malignancies and mandate close follow-up.

Treatment: Excision, cryotherapy with liquid nitrogen for 15 to 20 sec, or curettage and cautery may be used. Topical 5-FU, applied as for actinic keratoses, is another option.

MALIGNANT TUMORS

Basal and squamous cell carcinomas are the most common malignant skin tumors. Environmental exposure to ultraviolet light is the major risk factor, although ionizing radiation and chemical carcinogens are also predisposing factors.

Basal Cell Carcinoma

The typical basal cell carcinoma or rodent ulcer has a pearly appearance, rolled edges, and telangiectasia on its surface. More than 90% of these lesions appear on the head and neck. Some are superficial; others are multicentric, appearing as a scaly plaque with a raised pearly edge. Pigmented basal cell carcinomas are sometimes mistaken for malignant melanoma. If not detected and treated early, the carcinoma may invade deep tissues and destroy bone and cartilage, especially around the eyes, nose, and ears. However, basal cell carcinomas rarely metastasize.

Treatment: The size of the carcinoma, depth of invasion, and the patient's history determine the best treatment. All basal cell carcinomas should be confirmed histologically by biopsy, preferably before starting therapy. A 3-mm punch biopsy is generally adequate.

Curettage and cauterization can be used to treat small tumors. The procedure should be performed at least twice to ensure complete removal. Cryotherapy is also effective in treating small lesions. Usually, two freeze-thaw cycles are used.

Surgical excision can be performed with primary closure or a split-thickness skin graft, if necessary, to cover the defect. **Mohs' surgery** can be used for large, recurrent, or high-risk carcinomas. With this micrographically controlled technique of staged excision, the entire tissue margins are examined histologically as surgery proceeds, ensuring complete tumor removal and sparing the maximum amount of uninvolved tissues. **Radiotherapy** can be used when surgery might be undesirable and when carcinoma has recurred following surgery.

Topical 5-FU can be used to treat superficial basal cell carcinomas under extraordinary circumstances, such as when the patient has many tumors. Recurrence rates following 5-FU treatment are high.

All patients with basal cell carcinoma should be closely followed for recurrence and new lesions for at least 5 yr. Patients stand a 33% chance of developing a new carcinoma annually.

Squamous Cell Carcinoma

These tumors usually occur in sun-damaged skin, although up to 25% occur in sites of chronic inflammation, persistent ulceration (eg, longstanding lupus vulgaris or chronic venous ulcers), and radiodermatitis. Fair-skinned people, who have less protection from melanin, have a higher incidence of squamous cell carcinoma. The earliest signs are usually erythema and induration. The overlying epidermis may be scaly or hyperkeratotic. In more advanced lesions, ulceration usually occurs.

Lesions of the vermilion border of the lip, the pinna, and the genitalia are more likely to metastasize than those found elsewhere, such as on the face and limbs.

Treatment: The diagnosis must be confirmed by biopsy. A 3-mm punch biopsy is usually adequate, provided representative viable tissue is obtained. Well-differentiated tumors are generally treated surgically or by local destructive measures, while poorly differentiated tumors are treated by radiotherapy. Although radiotherapy may be more suitable for elderly patients who cannot tolerate anesthesia, it usually entails multiple treatments, which may present problems for persons with limited mobility.

Surgical excision can be used to treat small, well-differentiated tumors. At least 5 mm of tissue beyond the tumor borders must be excised. Squamous cell carcinomas that recur in sites previously treated with another modality (eg, radiotherapy) can also be excised surgically.

Cryotherapy, which does not require anesthesia, can also be used to treat small tumors. The tumor, together with a margin of normal tissue, should be frozen; two freeze-thaw cycles should be used. Although cryotherapy is useful in fair-skinned patients with multiple small lesions, healing can be prolonged in elderly patients.

Radiotherapy is generally used for poorly differentiated tumors of the head and neck and for tumors that recur after surgery. Although the cosmetic results of radiotherapy may be inferior to those of surgery, radiotherapy may be preferable for elderly patients in whom surgery is contraindicated. Radiotherapy is not used to treat tumors on the dorsa of the hand because it may leave friable scars.

Kaposi's Sarcoma

Typically, Kaposi's sarcoma appears as an indolent tumor in elderly patients of Central European origin, especially men of Jewish or Italian ancestry. One or more purple or dark blue macules slowly enlarge to become nodules or ulcers. On histologic examination, the tumor cells are endothelial; proliferating vessels and connective tissue cells are also present. **The lymphadenopathic form of Kaposi's sarcoma,** an aggressive tumor with a poor prognosis, is associated with acquired immunodeficiency syndrome (AIDS) and is not seen in non–HIV-infected patients.

Simple excision or radiotherapy can be performed if the lesions are symptomatic. In the elderly, this tumor grows slowly.

Cutaneous T-Cell Lymphoma

Cutaneous T-cell lymphoma is a rare cutaneous malignancy, previously called mycosis fungoides because of the fungating or mushroom-like tumors of the advanced disease. Caused by a subset of T lymphocytes that normally migrate to the skin, the disease begins as poorly defined eczematous or psoriasiform patches that evolve into plaques and finally tumors or diffuse erythroderma **(Sézary syndrome)** as the number of malignant cells increases. Internal organs become involved late, apparently reflecting the loss of the lymphocytes' original preference for skin because of progressive anaplasia.

Clinical presentations are highly variable, and frequently patients are misdiagnosed for many years as having one or more benign dermatoses. Cutaneous T-cell lymphoma should be suspected when an older patient has lesions with several distinct morphologies (eg, some infiltrated and some atrophic) or with an asymmetric distribution. Diagnosis is confirmed by biopsy, although early lesions may not contain enough atypical lymphocytes to exclude a nonspecific benign dermatitis. Definitive diagnosis may require multiple biopsies over time.

Treatment: No therapy has been proved to cure cutaneous T-cell lymphoma or to prolong survival, although advocates of aggressive early chemotherapy have made these claims. Most authorities prefer to use the least toxic modality that provides acceptable relief. Lesions in the patch and plaques stages often respond to topical corticosteroid creams or ointments or to phototherapy with ultraviolet B (UV-B) or psoralens with ultraviolet A (PUVA). More advanced disease may respond to photopheresis, a treatment in which the patient's lymphocytes are subjected to PUVA therapy extracorporeally, then reinfused, perhaps stimulating an immune rejection of the abnormal T cells. Topical nitrogen mustard therapy, electron beam irradiation, and a wide variety of combination cancer chemotherapy regimens are also used, producing temporary and sometimes prolonged improvement or even remission. Ultimately, however, unless death from another cause supervenes, cutaneous T-cell lymphoma becomes unresponsive to therapy and the patient succumbs, often from sepsis, the direct consequence of the compromised cutaneous barrier.

Melanomas

Lentigo Maligna and Lentigo Maligna Melanoma

Lentigo maligna (Hutchinson's freckle) is *a premalignant pigmented macular lesion, often > 1 cm in diameter with an irregular border.* The lesion appears predominantly on sun-exposed areas (most commonly, the cheeks and forehead). Pigmentation is characteristically varied, with brown, black, red, and white areas often found in a single lesion. Lentigo maligna gradually enlarges and becomes more irregularly pigmented over time.

In patients with lentigo maligna, the risk of developing melanoma by age 75 yr is about 1.2%. The development of nodules signifies invasion and conversion to lentigo maligna melanoma. This form of melanoma is relatively indolent; however, deeply invasive, neglected lesions have the same poor prognosis as other forms of melanoma of equal thickness. Lentigo maligna melanoma accounts for 5% to 10% of all melanomas, and the mean age at diagnosis is 67 yr.

The patient with lentigo maligna can be followed regularly to detect changes (eg, irregular pigmentation, nodularity, or bleeding) that may signify malignant transformation. Some authorities suggest cryotherapy or argon laser therapy to decrease the number of abnormal melanocytes and theoretically reduce the risk of developing melanoma. However, high recurrence rates for lentigo maligna are associated with both cryotherapy and argon laser therapy.

A biopsy is necessary to confirm the diagnosis of lentigo maligna melanoma. If a nodule is present, it should be included in the specimen. Multiple biopsies, either simultaneous or sequential, are often indicated.

Traditional treatment of lentigo maligna melanoma consists of a wide local excision, often requiring a skin flap or split-thickness skin graft to repair the defect.

Nodular Melanoma

Nodular melanoma accounts for about 15% of all melanomas and is more common in the elderly than in the young. The lesions are small, darkly pigmented papules that often enlarge rapidly. Rarely, the melanoma may be amelanotic and therefore pink.

Whenever melanoma is suspected, a deep excisional or incisional biopsy should be performed. An experienced dermatopathologist should perform the histologic interpretation, and confirmed cases should be referred immediately to a dermatologist or other physician experienced in melanoma management.

Treatment recommendations depend on the risk category, which is best determined by a dermatopathologist. If possible, low-risk lesions are excised with 1- to 2-cm margins, and intermediate- to high-risk lesions are excised with 3-cm margins and at least 1 cm of underlying subcutaneous fat. Removing all palpably enlarged lymph nodes has also been recommended, but prophylactic lymphadenectomy of clinically normal nodes appears to have no benefit.

Follow-up is essential; patients should be seen every 6 or 12 mo for life. The prognosis for patients with any type of melanoma depends primarily on the depth of invasion, not on the histologic type (see TABLE 101–4).

TABLE 101–4. PROGNOSIS FOR PATIENTS WITH MELANOMA (ALL TYPES)

*Melanoma Depth**	*Prognosis*
< 0.85 mm	Highly curable; 99% of patients disease free at 8 yr
0.85 – 1.69 mm	Low risk of metastasis; 93% of patients disease free at 8 yr
1.70 – 3.64 mm	Moderate risk of metastasis; 67% of patients disease free at 8 yr
> 3.65 mm	High risk of metastasis; 35% of patients disease free at 8 yr

* Measured from skin surface to point of deepest tumor invasion as evaluated in vertical cross sections.

Superficial Spreading Melanoma

This lesion accounts for about 60% of all melanomas and is the most common form in the elderly. Although the overall incidence of this melanoma peaks in middle age, its age-specific incidence increases through the eighth decade. This type of melanoma appears as a pigmented plaque with an irregular border and variable pigmentation. Like all melanomas, it is usually asymptomatic. Itching and bleeding are associated with advanced lesions.

As with nodular melanoma, treatment recommendations depend on the risk category.

§3. ORGAN SYSTEMS: EYE DISORDERS

EAR, NOSE, AND THROAT DISORDERS

§3. ORGAN SYSTEMS: EYE DISORDERS

102. OPHTHALMOLOGIC DISORDERS

ANATOMY AND PHYSIOLOGY OF THE AGING EYE

Evaluation of the symptoms and signs associated with disorders of the aging eye and visual axis must be based on an understanding of anatomy and physiology. FIG. 102–1 depicts the structures that undergo anatomic or physiologic changes with aging.

OCULAR STRUCTURES

Conjunctiva

The conjunctiva is the thin mucous membrane covering the sclera. Its goblet cells produce mucin, essential for lubricating eyelid movement and providing a protective layer to slow evaporation of the tear film. With aging, the number of mucous cells decreases, either as a result of **keratitis sicca** (with or without Sjögren's syndrome) or nonspecifically. These changes contribute to **dry eye syndrome,** manifested by a scratchy sensation and chronic irritation, often with increased redness from conjunctival vascular dilation (see also Lacrimal Gland and Tear Drainage, below). Diagnosis is confirmed by examining the cornea with slit-lamp biomicroscopy, and treatment usually consists of methylcellulose eyedrops (artificial tears) or a variation of them.

The conjunctiva can also undergo metaplasia and hyperplasia. This may lead to tissue accumulation at the nasal or temporal junction of the sclera and cornea, called a **pinguecula.** Connective tissue that grows, vascularizes, and invades the cornea is called a **pterygium** (see FIG. 102–2). If a pterygium continues to grow and reaches the center of the cornea, it can interfere with vision. Pterygia usually occur in people who spend a lot of time outdoors, especially in dusty and windy environments. Frequently occurring in women, pingueculae may be a cosmetic problem, but they rarely require removal; however, pterygia should be followed, and at first evidence of corneal involvement, surgical excision should be considered.

Sclera

The sclera is seen more clearly when the overlying conjunctiva is thinning. **Arcus senilis,** a deposit of calcium and cholesterol salts appearing as a gray-white ring at the edge of the iris, is a common finding in those > 60 yr. Usually, this sign is not associated with systemic disease, although rarely it is linked to systemic hyperlipoproteinemia.

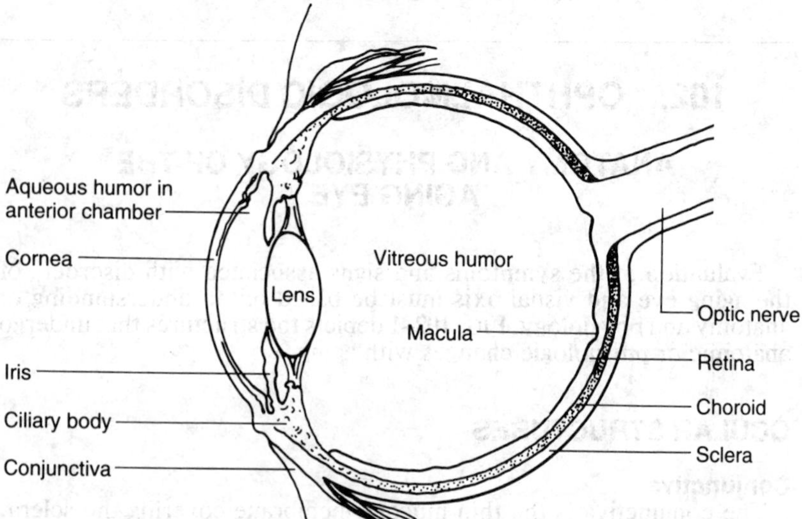

FIG. 102–1. Structures of the eye that undergo anatomic or physiologic changes with aging.

Cornea

Arcus senilis usually occurs in the cornea, 1 to 2 mm inside the limbus, but it will not progress to interference with vision. The major age-related change of the cornea is degeneration of the endothelial cells lining its inner surface. Progressive degeneration can eventually result in failure to keep the cornea free of extracellular fluid. The resulting corneal edema and accompanying hazy appearance interferes with vision and may require corneal transplantation. The hazy appearance of the cornea requires referral to an ophthalmologist.

Iris

The iris contains two sets of muscles that regulate pupillary size and reaction to light. With age, the pupil becomes smaller, reacts more sluggishly to light, and dilates more slowly in the dark. Thus, elderly persons may complain that objects are not as bright (a smaller pupil allows less light to enter the eye), that they are dazzled when going outdoors (slow pupillary constriction), and that they experience difficulty when going from a brightly lit environment to a darker one (slow pupillary dilation). If visual acuity is normal, only reassurance is needed.

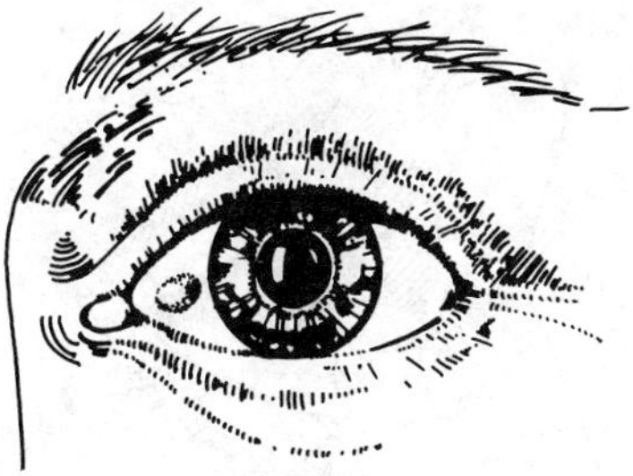

FIG. 102–2. Pinguecula and pterygium. Tissue accumulation at the nasal or temporal junction of the sclera and cornea is called a pinguecula. Connective tissue that becomes vascularized and invades the cornea is called a pterygium.

Relative pupillary size and reaction to light can be evaluated in a dimly lit room by shining a penlight obliquely into each eye and observing constriction of the pupil in the illuminated eye and the contralateral eye. Because pupillary diameter decreases with age, the direct and consensual reactions to light tend to be reduced. If the pupillary response is sluggish or absent, the patient may be taking medication that causes pupillary constriction or dilation.

Retina

Ophthalmoscopy of the retina is difficult in elderly patients because of their small pupils, eye movement, and opacities, but providing a target to stare at may help. Such an examination provides the only opportunity to directly visualize a cranial nerve (optic nerve), the portion of the retina responsible for the highest level of visual acuity (the macula), and blood vessels (retinal artery and vein and capillary bed). Recognizing age-related changes in these structures is important.

The **optic nerve** tends to have less distinct margins and may appear slightly paler because of a loss of capillaries from small-vessel disease secondary to atherosclerosis. The **macula,** which in young people usually has a bright central foveal light reflex, may not have any foveal reflex. Also, yellowish-white spots **(drusen)** often appear in the macular area, and some disruption may occur in the pigmentation pattern (see AGE-RELATED MACULOPATHY, below). Unless these macular changes are accompanied by a distortion of objects or a frank decrease in visual acuity unexplained by other causes, they are not clinically important. The arteries also demonstrate atherosclerotic changes, including slight narrowing and an increased light reflex from thickened vessel walls. The veins may show marked venous indentation (nicking) at the arteriovenous crossings with slight proximal distention. In general, the retina, which glistens in younger people, becomes duller with aging.

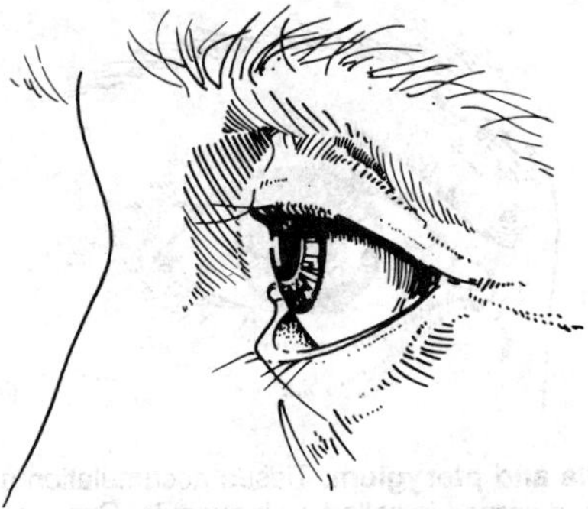

FIG. 102–3. Ectropion of the lower lid margin means that the punctum of the medial lower lid no longer touches the eyeball and tears cannot drain properly from the conjunctival sac into the lacrimal duct.

EXTRAOCULAR STRUCTURES

Lids

With age, the lid margins (especially the lower one) can fall away from the eyeball **(ectropion).** This usually results from decreased strength of the orbicular muscles of the eyes, which squeeze the lids shut. If the lower lid margin no longer touches the eyeball, the punctum of the medial lower lid no longer touches it either, and tears cannot drain properly from the conjunctival sac into the lacrimal sac (see FIG. 102–3). Thus, patients complain of excess tear production and tears draining onto the face (see also Lacrimal Gland and Tear Drainage, below).

With decreased action of the orbicular muscles, the lids may not close completely during sleep, resulting in corneal drying and secondary abrasion, redness, and irritation **(superficial punctate keratitis).** Spasm of the orbicular muscle of the eye may cause the lid margin (especially the lower one) to turn in **(entropion),** bringing the eyelashes in contact with the eyeball and allowing them to rub it with each blink, resulting in chronic irritation. Over time, corneal and conjunctival scarring may result if this condition **(trichiasis)** is not corrected surgically.

For unknown reasons, some people have bilateral intermittent or constant severe spasms of the orbicular muscles of the eyes, so that the eyelids are shut tightly for periods varying from seconds to minutes. This **blepharospasm** can incapacitate a person and often must be treated by partial surgical denervation of the orbicular muscles. More

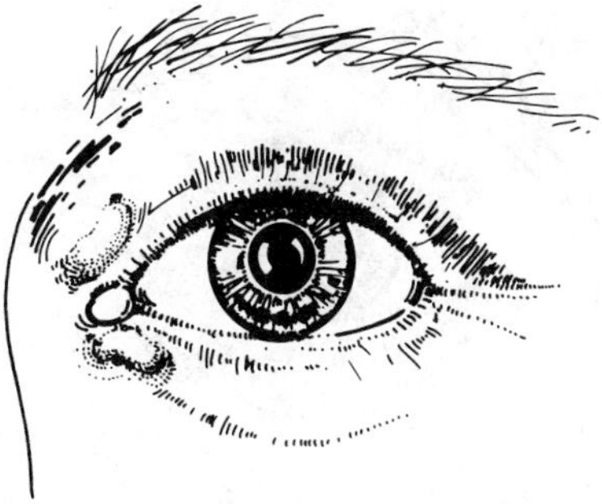

FIG. 102–4. Xanthelasma (a slightly raised, yellowish, well-circumscribed plaque) typically appears along the nasal aspect of one or both eyelids. In some persons, these plaques accompany lipid disorders.

recently, small amounts of botulinus toxin injected into the orbicular muscle of the eye have been used with some success, but a controlled clinical trial has not yet been conducted.

The upper lid also contains a levator muscle, which holds it against the pull of gravity. Decreased muscle tone can result in a slight **lid droop** and thus a decrease in the palpebral fissure (the distance between the margins of the upper and lower lids).

Loss of skin turgor with atrophy and loss of elasticity may cause the skin of the upper lid to hang below the lid margin. Excision of the excess skin is indicated only if vision is disturbed.

A protrusion of fat through the orbital fascia, which forms a septum between the lid and orbital contents, can cause localized or diffuse swelling of the eyelid. The fat can be palpated, and surgical repair of the septum is based on cosmetic considerations.

Seborrheic dermatitis usually begins in childhood but often becomes more severe in old age. The signs are dilated blood vessels at the lid margins, a loss of lashes, and scaling at the base of the remaining lashes. Chronic conjunctivitis often occurs. The most severe cases of blepharitis occur in patients with rosacea. Treatment consists of cleaning the eyelid margin, shampooing the scalp frequently, and if indicated, applying an antibiotic ointment.

With age, many lesions, including **xanthelasma,** may appear on the lids, often at the nasal aspect; these are rarely clinically significant, although they may be associated with hyperlipidemia (see FIG. 102–4). **Squamous cell carcinoma** and, to a much greater extent, **basal cell carcinoma** are, of course, significant (see FIG. 102–5).

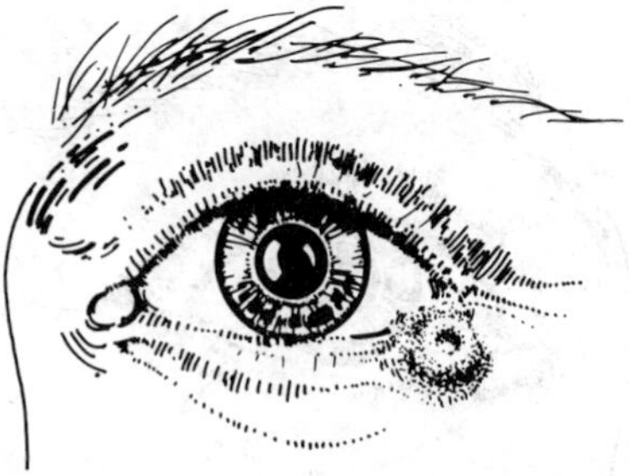

FIG. 102–5. Basal cell carcinoma occurring near the eye usually involves the lower lid. It appears as a papule with a pearly border and a depressed or ulcerated center.

Lacrimal Gland and Tear Drainage

Abnormalities of the lacrimal system may result in either decreased tear production or an overflow of tears because of faulty drainage. Tear production by the lacrimal gland may decrease with age, with fewer tears available to keep the surface of the eye (especially the cornea) well moistened. This incipient **dry eye** condition may result in a chronic foreign-body sensation and is exacerbated by orbicular muscle weakness that produces incomplete lid closure during sleep. Artificial tears should be used. If disease, such as Sjögren's syndrome, involves the lacrimal gland, more aggressive surgical intervention (eg, partial tarsorrhaphy) may be indicated.

Severe tearing (with an overflow of tears) is a frequent complaint. It usually represents a loss of contact between the lacrimal punctum and the eyeball, causing tears to roll down the face instead of draining properly from the conjunctival sac into the lacrimal system (see Lids, above). The condition worsens in cold weather, when tear production increases. The patient should be reassured that excess tearing is preferable to a dry eye condition and that it is not a cause for concern. The patient should be advised to use a handkerchief as necessary. If severe ectropion is causing excess tearing and recurrent low-grade inflammation, surgical correction is indicated.

Occasionally, excessive tearing occurs when the punctum becomes occluded by inflammation from chronic recurrent bacterial infection, a condition known as **dacryocystitis** (see FIG. 102–6).

Tear production can be measured with the **Schirmer test** by suspending a 20-mm strip of filter paper from the lower conjunctival sac for 5 min. If $\geq$ 10 mm is wet, tear production is adequate; if $<$ 10 mm is wet and the patient complains of a scratchy or foreign-body sensation, referral to an ophthalmologist is indicated. If the patient complains of excess tears and the punctum of the lower lid is not in contact with the eyeball, referral is also indicated.

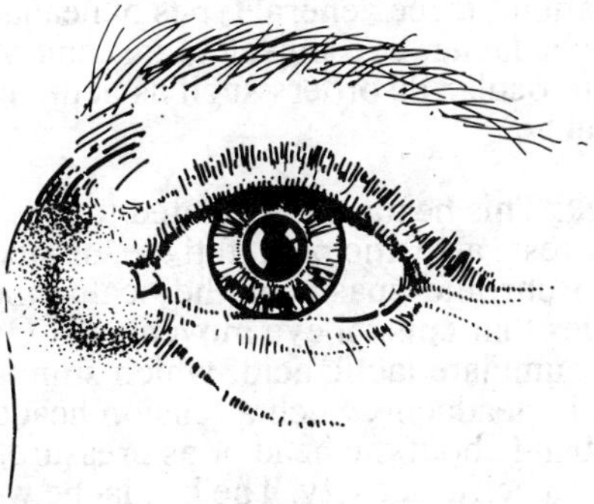

FIG. 102–6. Dacryocystitis from a chronic, recurrent bacterial infection occludes the punctum, resulting in excessive tearing. Swelling between the lower lid and nose suggests dacryocystitis. Pressure on the sac expresses material through the punctum.

Orbit

With age, the loss of periorbital fat often causes the eyeball to sink into the orbit **(enophthalmos).** Although asymptomatic, enophthalmos often poses a cosmetic problem and may require surgery.

SYMPTOMS AND SIGNS ASSOCIATED WITH AGING

The symptoms and signs associated with aging may be divided into two groups: those related to eye comfort (foreign-body sensation and headache) and those related to vision (glare, haziness, flashing lights, moving spots, and refractive changes).

EFFECTS ON EYE COMFORT

Foreign-Body Sensation

A false foreign-body sensation may be related to a dry eye condition, entropion, chronic fatigue of the eye muscles from lack of sleep, poor health, a latent eye muscle imbalance, or excessive close vision (eg, reading when extremely tired). However, a true foreign body must be ruled out.

Headache

In the elderly patient, three general types of headaches can be distinguished: tension headache, eye muscle pain, and vascular headache. Patients with acute ocular disorders such as acute glaucoma may also complain of headache.

Tension headache: This headache is related to any cause of increased muscle tone, eg, stress, arthritic pain, fatigue, or anxiety. These conditions may lead to chronic spasm of the scalp, the face, or the six extraocular muscles that control eye movements. Over time, the spasmodic muscles accumulate lactic acid, which stimulates local pain receptors, resulting in headache. Such a tension headache is usually described as a tight band about the head or as pressure, and in most cases can be related to a specific activity. The headache worsens if the activity continues and is often relieved by muscle relaxants or analgesics. Occasionally, however, the pain is truly debilitating.

Eye muscle pain: This type of headache often presents as a brow ache, first occurring on awakening, especially if the patient was reading or watching television late the previous night. The pain can be a throbbing, dull ache localized behind one or both eyes or across the brow or the entire forehead. It may affect either side of the head. Other symptoms include redness, burning, and tearing, especially after prolonged close-range work or reading at night when fatigued.

A major cause of this type of headache is a tendency for the eyes to turn outward with aging **(exophoria).** This results from a gradual decrease in the tone of the medial rectus muscles, which turn the eyes inward when reading or focusing on objects within 1 to 10 ft.

Exophoria is diagnosed by asking the patient to look through reading glasses at a flashlight about 1 ft away while alternately covering each eye, never allowing both to see the light simultaneously. Each eye is observed as soon as it is uncovered. If the eye moves inward to look at the light, it must have drifted outward while it was covered, suggesting exophoria.

Headache associated with exophoria can often be prevented by resting more, doing close-range work early in the day, or increasing the contractile tone of the medial rectus muscles through muscle exercise therapy.

Vascular headache: In the elderly, a vascular headache may result from temporal arteritis or a migraine. When a headache has a recent onset and is associated with hip-girdle pain, jaw claudication, fatigue, or visual changes, the physician should suspect **temporal arteritis** and obtain an erythrocyte sedimentation rate. If the erythrocyte sedimentation rate is elevated or if suspicion is high before the test results are known, prednisone 60 mg/day should be initiated, and a temporal artery biopsy should be obtained as soon as possible (see also Ch. 74).

Migraine headaches may occur at any age but do not commonly begin in later life. The headache is often preceded by an aura of flashing bright lights in a vertical zigzag or picket-fence configuration, either to the far left or far right of both visual fields, and is always bilateral. This aura may be followed by severe, pounding, relentless pain on the opposite side of the head. The pain is exacerbated by bright lights or movement and eased by lying down in the dark. The aura is caused by marked cerebral vasoconstriction involving vessels of the visual cortex, and the pain results from marked secondary vasodilation (with associated stretching of perivascular nerve endings).

Prophylaxis with a β-blocker or calcium channel blocker may prevent the attack by blocking vasoconstriction. Effective **treatment** consists of taking ergotamine at the onset of the aura to abort the attack by maintaining vasoconstriction. Once headache supervenes, analgesics and rest are indicated. An injection of sumatriptan may ameliorate the symptoms.

EFFECTS ON VISION

Glare

Decreased visual perception related to glare is a frequent complaint. As the eye ages, changes in the lens and vitreous increase the scattering of light in the ocular media. Lens opacities at the periphery, though not directly interfering with vision, can also increase the scattering of light passing through the lens, especially at night or in dim light, because the pupil is slightly dilated. Thus, it is not unusual for the elderly patient to complain about the glare of oncoming headlights while driving at night. As long as visual acuity is normal, the patient should just be advised to curtail driving at night or avoid looking directly at oncoming headlights.

Decreased visual perception from daytime glare is also common. With aging, opacities may appear in various portions of the lens, such as the nucleus and cortex. Such opacities may interfere little with visual acuity, but opacities in the central cortex region just beneath the posterior lens capsule **(posterior subcapsular lens opacities)** tend to scatter light to a greater extent. This occurs because these opacities are closer to the focal point of the lens through which all light must pass on the way to the retina. Although these opacities may eventually increase in size or density and interfere with visual acuity **(posterior subcapsular cataract),** their earliest manifestation is the scattering of light and increased glare, especially in bright light.

Some temporary relief may result from mild dilation of the pupil with mydriatic drops and from sunglasses that allow the patient to see around the opacity. However, these measures should be used only under appropriate ophthalmologic care. Early nuclear opacities may actually improve close vision in the elderly. Cataracts are discussed further below.

Haziness, Flashing Lights, and Moving Spots

Decreased visual perception due to opacities in the ocular media are most often attributed to vitreous floaters or to Moore's lightning streaks. The vitreous humor is a gelatinous-like material that fills the back of the eye between the posterior surface of the lens and the anterior surface of the retina. The vitreous is normally clear, but with age, discrete opacities or structural changes leading to a general haziness may develop. With an ophthalmoscope, an examiner may be able to distinguish between lens opacities (best seen with a +10 lens) and vitreous opacities (best seen with a +2 lens). Although these changes are not serious, they may upset the patient, and an explanation and reassurance are necessary.

The vitreous is firmly attached to the most anterior peripheral portion of the retina and posteriorly at the optic nerve. With age, the vitreous undergoes liquefaction, and as a result, eye movements produce intermittent tension at the vitreous attachment to the retina. This tugging stimulates the peripheral retina mechanically, causing vertically oriented flashing lights, almost always in the far temporal visual field. Unlike the aura in migraine, these flashing lights occur in only one eye at a time. If they are not accompanied by decreased vision or other changes in visual function, they usually need no further evaluation. *However, if they persist and the feeling of a veil over the eye or a decrease in the visual field occurs, the patient should be referred immediately for an ophthalmologic examination to exclude retinal detachment.*

In nearsighted (myopic) patients and in many others in their late 50s and early 60s, opacities appear as lines, spots, webs, and clusters of dots moving slowly across the field of vision. Usually, they move more rapidly with eye movements and become stationary when the eye is not moving. These opacities represent bits of vitreous that have coalesced or vitreous that has broken off from its attachment to the peripheral or central portion of the retina and now floats freely in the vitreous cavity **(floaters).** Floaters may also occur in uveitis. This symptom is annoying but usually has no clinical importance. If, after appropriate examination, the patient is reassured and encouraged to ignore the floaters, they gradually become less noticeable. However, a shower of opacities, often accompanied by flashing lights in the peripheral visual field, requires a referral to rule out retinal detachment.

Refractive Changes

Presbyopia, *loss of accommodation,* is a universal age-related change in lens physiology beginning in the 50s. When a person wishes to see an object closer than 1 or 2 ft ($1/3$ to $2/3$ m), the lens must increase its thickness to provide additional refractive power to focus the light from the near object on the retina. With presbyopia, the lens cannot make this accommodation.

If a person is farsighted **(hyperopic),** presbyopia tends to occur at an earlier age. Usually, a nearsighted **(myopic)** person with presbyopia can read small print by removing the glasses and holding the print close.

Presbyopia is corrected in both nearsighted and farsighted persons with either separate reading glasses or bifocal glasses. Since accommodation is lost progressively from about ages 45 to 65, the reading lens must be changed every 2 or 3 yr.

Refractive changes resulting from **cataracts** are discussed below.

DIAGNOSTIC PROCEDURES

Persons > 65 yr should visit an ophthalmologist once a year. The diagnostic tests that may be used to detect ophthalmologic disorders include a visual acuity examination, visual field examination, and ophthalmoscopy.

VISUAL ACUITY EXAMINATION

A well-illuminated visual acuity chart set at 20 ft is used to test distance vision; a reading card with various print sizes is used to test near vision. (The chart is placed at 10 ft if a mirror is used.) Patients who cannot read the 20/40 line on the chart even while wearing distance eyeglasses should look through a pinhole (the opening made by a pin pushed through a piece of thin cardboard). If the patient needs glasses or a new prescription, acuity should improve to at least 20/30 when the pinhole is used. If acuity does not improve, the patient has a nonrefractive problem and should be referred to an ophthalmologist immediately.

Near vision can also be tested by asking the patient to read ordinary newsprint. If the patient cannot, yet has good distance vision, only a change in reading glasses is indicated.

VISUAL FIELD EXAMINATION

With the confrontational method of assessing the visual fields, the examiner and patient face each other and look at each other's eyes. The examiner swings his outstretched arm in a circle and determines if the patient can detect a moving finger. This method may detect gross visual field defects, but in view of the clinical importance of such defects, a definitive determination should be done quantitatively by a person experienced in visual field examination.

OPHTHALMOSCOPY

Ophthalmoscopy of the lens, vitreous, and retina is best accomplished through a pupil dilated at least 6 mm in diameter. Dilation is achieved by instilling a phenylephrine 2.5% ophthalmic solution, one drop in each eye twice, 10 min apart. If the anterior chamber is very shallow and the patient is prone to develop angle-closure glaucoma, dilation with phenylephrine 2.5% may precipitate an attack. Although this is rare, the patient should be informed that intraocular pressure may rise, causing discomfort, and may require immediate treatment that is very successful in curing the underlying condition. The advantages of thoroughly examining the retina far outweigh the risks of a rare attack of angle-closure glaucoma, which can be treated if diagnosed early.

At first, a + 10 diopter (blue number) lens should be used in the viewing aperture; the pupillary space should be filled with a bright red reflex from the blood-filled choroid beneath the retina. If dark areas block this red reflex, opacities are present in the cornea, lens, or vitreous. If these opacities interfere with visualizing the retina, they can also interfere with the patient's vision, suggesting decreased visual acuity. If opacities are not present, the examiner should slowly focus on the retina by progressively decreasing the lens power until details of the retinal blood vessels come into view.

The posterior retina should be scanned slowly until the optic nerve head is seen. The examiner should record the color (it should be pink), the size of the optic cup as a fraction of the optic nerve head diameter, and most important, the presence of a flat rim of optic nerve surrounding the cup. If this rim slopes down to the cup or if it is notched, glaucoma should be suspected. Comparing the right and left optic nerves is important because asymmetrical optic cup sizes can indicate damage from elevated intraocular pressure.

Next, the examiner should move temporally across the retina about 2 or 3 mm to examine the macular area and the adjacent posterior retina. Diabetic and hypertensive retinopathy and other vascular changes most often occur in these areas. Also, lesions of the macular area, especially age-related maculopathy, can cause decreased vision. Finally, the branches of the central retinal artery and vein should be examined for changes in caliber and for adjacent hemorrhages, exudates, and microaneurysms. Any such changes should prompt referral for definitive diagnosis.

AGE-RELATED EYE DISEASES

Eye disorders commonly affecting elderly persons include cataract, glaucoma, diabetic retinopathy, age-related maculopathy, and certain vascular disorders. An elderly person may also experience certain miscellaneous conditions, such as acute double vision, diabetic ophthalmoplegia, intracranial tumor, and myasthenia gravis.

CATARACT

An opacity of the lens that reduces visual acuity to 20/30 or less.

The lens is normally clear until after age 40, when nonspecific opacities may appear. Because age is the major risk factor for developing cataract, almost anyone who lives long enough will develop it. Other risk factors include smoking, poor nutrition, corticosteroid therapy, a history of atopic dermatitis, and exposure to ultraviolet light (as occurs in sunny climates). The cause of cataract is thought to be oxidative damage to the lens proteins that reduces solubility; eventually insoluble opacities form in otherwise transparent tissue.

Types of Cataract

Cataracts are categorized according to their location within the lens. The four types are cortical, nuclear, posterior subcapsular, and any combination of two or more of these locations. Idiopathic posterior subcapsular cataract usually occurs at an earlier age and probably has a genetic basis. However, corticosteroids should be ruled out as a cause.

Symptoms and Signs

When lens opacities first develop, especially in the nucleus, visual acuity is relatively unaffected, but the refractive index, and thus the refractive power, of the lens increases; that is, the lens shifts toward myopia. This increased refractive power can partially compensate for the loss in accommodation, temporarily correcting presbyopia. Thus, in a person aged 60 to 70, early nuclear lens changes may induce myopia and allow the person to read again without glasses. This condition is referred to as **second sight.**

An early symptom of posterior subcapsular cataract may be glare from bright lights at night or even during the day—the result of light rays being scattered by the opacities (see Glare, above). Over time, however, the lens opacities progress and eventually interfere with vision so that reading becomes difficult even with glasses. The hallmark of all cataracts is painless, progressive loss of vision, but the rate of loss is nonlinear and variable. Both near and far visual acuity should be tested.

Lens opacities can be seen easily by observing the red reflex of the retina and choroid with the ophthalmoscope, using a +10 diopter lens in the viewing aperture. Any lens opacity will show in silhouette as a black area.

Treatment

Cataract surgery involves removing the lens. Removing the entire lens, including its capsule, is called an **intracapsular cataract extraction.** Removing the central portion of the anterior capsule and aspirating the contents of the lens, so that an intact posterior lens capsule remains is termed an **extracapsular cataract extraction.** The latter procedure is more common because it allows for the placement of a posterior chamber intraocular lens.

In 1992, about 1.5 million cataract extractions were performed in the USA, and about 95% of them involved an intraocular lens. In most cases, the lens was placed behind the iris—ie, in the posterior chamber. In a small percentage of cases, the lens was placed in the anterior chamber. Posterior chamber placement is considered safer and results in fewer postoperative complications, but anterior chamber placement is easier to perform. The number of anterior chamber intraocular lens placements is expected to decrease even further. In some cases, the ophthalmologist advises against using an intraocular lens, and correction can be accomplished with glasses or contact lenses. However, the glasses are very thick, and elderly persons often have difficulty inserting and removing contact lenses.

Cataract surgery is an elective procedure, requiring justification that the potential benefits outweigh the possible complications and discomfort. The decision is primarily the patient's. If the patient cannot perform at work, read, drive a car, or watch television, and the surgeon is confident that successful surgery will result in vision of 20/30 or better, surgery should be considered. Waiting until the cataract matures is no longer considered valid. Surgery can be performed at any stage of cataract maturation; the decision should be based on the degree of the patient's visual disability. If, despite decreased vision, the patient can perform all desired activities, surgery can be postponed.

If the patient has associated eye disease, cataract extraction should be approached cautiously. Age-related maculopathy, severe diabetic retinopathy, and other retinal diseases jeopardize the prospect for successful cataract extraction. Surgery should be deferred until there is a reasonable prospect that the result will be acceptable to the patient.

Rarely, an advanced cataract may swell, and the capsule may become leaky. Lens material leaking into the anterior chamber may cause secondary glaucoma, which can be readily diagnosed and successfully treated by surgical removal of the cataract.

Most cataract surgery is performed using local anesthesia. However, special consideration should be given to patients with severe respiratory or cardiovascular difficulties that may preclude their lying supine for the 30 to 60 min necessary for preoperative preparation and surgery.

Complication rates are low. **Major complications** resulting from surgery include faulty wound closure with aqueous humor leakage, prolapse of the iris into the corneal wound, and intractable secondary glaucoma. The most serious complication is explosive choroidal hemorrhage, which can cause blindness. Inflammation of the eye **(endophthalmitis),** another serious complication, is usually noted 24 to 48 h after surgery. Immediate hospitalization and aggressive treatment with

IV antibiotics and corticosteroids are needed to prevent possible loss of the eye. Fortunately, this complication is rare, occurring in about 1 in 5000 cases. Cataract surgery is one of the most successful surgical procedures; about 95% of postoperative patients have excellent vision.

GLAUCOMA

Disorders characterized by increased intraocular pressure that can lead to irreversible damage to the optic nerve and impaired vision. The glaucomas account for about 10% of all cases of blindness in the USA.

ANGLE-CLOSURE GLAUCOMA
(Narrow-Angle Glaucoma)

Angle-closure glaucoma accounts for only about 10% of glaucomas in the USA, but it is the only type that can be cured. It appears to be more prevalent among Orientals, especially Chinese.

The anterior chamber of the eye is bounded anteriorly by the cornea and posteriorly by the lens and iris. A major risk factor for angle-closure glaucoma is an anatomically shallow anterior chamber, especially at the periphery. The chamber becomes even more shallow with advancing age because the lens continues to thicken throughout life, moving the iris forward. Farsighted persons tend to have smaller eyes and thus may be predisposed to this type of glaucoma in later life. The potential for angle closure is suspected on slit-lamp examination and best assessed by gonioscopic examination of the angle structures using special corneal contact lenses.

Elevated intraocular pressure occurs when the base of the iris is pushed forward, sealing off the trabecular meshwork of the outflow channels. Aqueous humor, which is continuously produced in the eye, circulates through the anterior chamber before leaving through the outflow channels in the anterior chamber angle. When these channels are sealed off, intraocular pressure increases to levels as high as 50 to 60 mm Hg in a matter of hours. (The upper limit of the normal range is 20 mm Hg.)

Symptoms, Signs, and Diagnosis

Angle-closure glaucoma usually presents in one eye, although the other eye is likely to be affected. The rapid rise in intraocular pressure is accompanied by redness and pain in or around the eye, severe headache, nausea, vomiting, and blurred vision. Before experiencing blurred vision, patients often see halos around lights. This results from corneal edema.

In an acute glaucoma attack, the eye is tender and feels firmer than the other eye. As intraocular pressure continues to rise, nausea and vomiting can become so severe that an acute abdomen may be suspected. Within 48 to 72 h, depending on the pressure elevation, vision may be irreversibly damaged. *Thus, an attack of angle-closure glaucoma constitutes an emergency requiring immediate referral to an ophthalmologist.*

Treatment

When an ophthalmologist is not available, emergency measures include local instillation of one drop of 2% to 4% pilocarpine every 5 min four to six times or oral administration of 250 mg of acetazolamide or 40 mL of 50% glycerin (ie, 1.0 to 1.5 gm/kg). Immediate hospitalization and referral are indicated.

Although intraocular pressure can usually be reduced with drugs, surgical intervention (laser iridotomy) is the only cure. A small opening is made at the base of the iris to allow the pressure to equalize on both sides and to prevent the iris from obstructing the outflow channels. Other procedures are available, but laser iridotomy can be performed in the ophthalmologist's office in only a few minutes. If surgery is performed before permanent adhesions develop between the iris and outflow channels (within the first 24 h), cure is likely, and further attacks will be prevented.

OPEN-ANGLE GLAUCOMA

Open-angle glaucoma accounts for about 80% of glaucomas in the USA. Unlike angle-closure glaucoma, this type of glaucoma is asymptomatic until very late. It causes a gradual loss of visual fields over years, affects both eyes simultaneously, and occurs about six times more often in blacks, who rarely have angle-closure glaucoma. Although it cannot be cured, open-angle glaucoma can usually be controlled with topical and systemic therapy.

Symptoms, Signs, and Diagnosis

Onset is insidious and usually asymptomatic. The patient may not even notice the progressive loss of visual fields until late in the course of the disease. Routine intraocular pressure monitoring and ophthalmoscopic examination of the optic nerve head may detect open-angle glaucoma in the absence of symptoms. Diagnosis is based on an anatomically normal anterior chamber angle and outflow channels (as viewed by gonioscopy), increased resistance to aqueous humor outflow (as measured by tonography), and a loss of peripheral vision (as measured by quantitative perimetry).

Although in open-angle glaucoma, the intraocular pressure usually is > 21 mm Hg, it can also be within the normal range but still be too high for the particular eye to tolerate. With time, optic atrophy (expressed as cupping and pallor of the nerve head) is noted, indicating advanced disease. When the pressure is > 21 mm Hg but the patient has no visual field defect, the diagnosis is **ocular hypertension.** The optic nerve usually appears normal. Patients with this condition should be seen at least every 6 mo for visual field testing, but treatment is usually not indicated at this stage.

Prevention

Patients > 40 yr who are in high-risk groups (eg, blacks, persons who have a parent or sibling with glaucoma, and persons receiving long-term corticosteroid therapy) and all patients > 60 yr should have yearly intraocular pressure measurements and ophthalmoscopic examinations. Though not the best method of screening for glaucoma, using pressure measurement alone will detect about half the patients with the disease. Using this measurement and ophthalmoscopy to identify optic nerve head excavation increases the detection rate to about 80%. Performing visual field testing further increases the rate.

Intraocular pressure is measured with the Schiotz or the applanation tonometer. After a topical anesthetic (eg, proparacaine 0.5%) is instilled, the Schiotz tonometer foot plate is gently placed directly on the center of the cornea while the patient is in the supine position, looking at his thumb held straight up at arm's length. The reading in absolute units on the tonometer (reflecting indentation of the cornea by the tonometer's plunger) is recorded and then converted to millimeters of mercury of intraocular pressure using a chart.

Treatment

Whether or not the patient has symptoms, medication is needed to reduce intraocular pressure to prevent irreversible optic nerve damage and thus the loss of peripheral visual fields. **Topical medications** include pilocarpine, a parasympathomimetic drug that can cause brow ache; epinephrine, which may irritate the eye and cause an allergic lid reaction; and levobunolol and timolol, β-adrenergic blockers that may cause cardiopulmonary symptoms in susceptible persons. **Systemic medications** include carbonic anhydrase inhibitors, such as acetazolamide and methazolamide, which may cause slight nausea, tingling, paresthesias, and mental changes. With long-term administration, systemic acidosis or kidney stones (in predisposed patients) may occur. Because these drugs may produce adverse effects and interact with other drugs and because the glaucoma patient needs periodic examinations, they should be prescribed only by an eye care specialist competent to monitor the patient.

Because open-angle glaucoma can be controlled but not cured, treatment is continued indefinitely. A visual field examination should be performed every 6 mo. If medication fails to control progression of the glaucoma, as evidenced by visual field testing, surgery such as laser trabeculoplasty or a filtration procedure is recommended to lower the intraocular pressure to a level at which the disease can be slowed or halted.

SECONDARY GLAUCOMA

Secondary glaucoma, which accounts for about 10% of glaucomas in the USA, *is characterized by a pathologic process that anatomically or functionally blocks the outflow channels*. In diabetes mellitus and central retinal vein occlusion, a fibrovascular membrane may grow over and seal off the outflow channels. In uveitis, or ocular inflammation, inflammatory cells or debris can obstruct the outflow channels. Ocular tumors may also obstruct the outflow channels—either by direct pressure from the tumor in the anterior chamber angle or by tumor cells blocking the channels. Patients with secondary glaucoma usually present with a red, uncomfortable eye, often chronically painful and usually accompanied by decreased vision.

Drug treatment for other disorders may have an adverse impact on incipient or recognized glaucoma. Damage to the optic nerve may result in part from the relationship between the blood pressure within the optic nerve (perfusion pressure) and the intraocular pressure. When the perfusion pressure adequately exceeds intraocular pressure, the optic nerve receives sufficient nutrition. But increased intraocular pressure reduces perfusion pressure. If a hypertensive patient with glaucoma is being treated with antihypertensive medication, the ophthalmologist should be informed so that visual fields can be monitored while the blood pressure is being lowered. The glaucoma medication may need to be increased to further reduce the intraocular pressure.

Drugs with anticholinergic (atropine-like) effects may be dangerous, primarily in patients predisposed to angle-closure glaucoma because the drugs produce chronic pupillary dilation and possibly in patients with open-angle glaucoma because the drugs antagonize the antiglaucoma medication.

Treatment

Treatment is difficult and directed first at removing the underlying cause—eg, treating uveitis with anti-inflammatory drugs, removing a tumor, or changing medications. Antiglaucoma drugs may also be tried to reduce intraocular pressure. If these measures fail, surgery is needed to create a new outflow pathway for the aqueous humor to leave the eye.

DIABETIC RETINOPATHY

Retinopathy associated with diabetes mellitus is the third leading cause of adult blindness, accounting for almost 7% of blindness in the USA. Diabetic retinopathy is associated primarily with the duration of diabetes mellitus; therefore, as the population ages and diabetic patients live longer, its prevalence increases.

Etiology and Pathophysiology

Retinal capillaries have two types of cells—endothelial cells lining the capillary and intramural pericytes or mural cells embedded in the basement membrane of the capillary. For every endothelial cell, there is a mural cell.

In diabetic retinopathy, the first change consistently observed within the retina is a selective loss of mural cells. The initial loss of these cells sets in motion a series of events culminating in the development of diabetic retinopathy. The current hypothesis for explaining this cell loss involves an enzyme, aldose reductase, which is found in mural but not in endothelial cells. As glucose levels increase in diabetes, glucose in mural cells is converted by aldose reductase to its sugar alcohol, sorbitol, which is metabolized slowly and diffuses poorly across cell membranes. Thus, the sorbitol concentration increases within the mural cell, and water moves down its osmotic gradient into the cell, which swells, eventually ruptures, and disappears. It is postulated that this mechanism may be the cause of neuropathy and nephropathy since aldose reductase is localized in the Schwann cells and axoplasm of peripheral nerves and in the kidney.

Because mural cells appear to have contractile properties, their loss results in capillary dilation. The dilated capillaries tend to carry more and more blood because they are wider than adjacent capillaries that still contain a full complement of mural cells. In the dilated capillaries, endothelial cells proliferate and form outpouchings, which become **microaneurysms.** Meanwhile, the adjacent capillaries carry less and less blood, until eventually they carry none at all, becoming ghost vessels without cellular components. Thus, next to clusters of microaneurysms are areas of nonperfused retina.

Eventually, shunt vessels appear between adjacent areas of microaneurysms, and the clinical picture of early diabetic retinopathy with microaneurysms and areas of nonperfused retina is seen. The microaneurysms leak and capillary vessels may hemorrhage, causing exudates and hemorrhages. Once the initial stages of background diabetic retinopathy are established, the condition progresses over a period of years, in some cases developing into proliferative diabetic retinopathy.

Symptoms, Signs, and Diagnosis

An annual ophthalmoscopic examination is indicated in all diabetic patients to detect macular edema and evidence of proliferative diabetic retinopathy. *Since laser photocoagulation can prevent or slow visual loss in the early stages of these conditions, early diagnosis is paramount.*

Usually, little or no evidence of diabetic retinopathy appears until about 3 to 5 yr after the onset of diabetes. Symptoms may be subtle, for example, early and minimal visual loss from macular edema, a shower of spots, or clouded vision from a small vitreous hemorrhage. For those in whom laser treatment would be appropriate, periodic fluorescin angiography should be performed to detect changes when they are most amenable to treatment before advanced retinopathy affects vision.

The first signs of diabetic retinopathy are microaneurysms, seen as red spots with sharp margins in the area around the optic nerve and macula. These lesions disappear after 3 to 6 mo, to be replaced by fresh microaneurysms. Over time, the next stage of **nonproliferative diabetic retinopathy** is seen with the addition of punctate, flame-shaped (linear) or blot-shaped **retinal hemorrhages, soft exudates, hard exudates,** and **intraretinal microvascular abnormalities,** the latter appearing as small areas of dilated capillaries.

An important aspect of nonproliferative diabetic retinopathy is the pooling of fluid in the macula with resulting macular elevation. This **macular edema** is a major cause of reduced vision in nonproliferative diabetic retinopathy and, if allowed to persist, can result in an irreversible loss of vision.

Over time, all these lesions increase, while some areas of the retina continue losing their capillary vessels and become nonperfused. Eventually, about 5% of nonproliferative diabetic retinopathy cases proceed to **proliferative diabetic retinopathy** with the appearance of new vessels on the disk and elsewhere on the retina. These new blood vessels grow into the vitreous and, because they are friable, bleed easily, leading to preretinal hemorrhages. In advanced proliferative diabetic retinopathy, massive vitreous hemorrhage may fill a major portion of the vitreous cavity.

The end stage of diabetic retinopathy is recurrent vitreous hemorrhage, often accompanied by retinal detachment or secondary glaucoma resulting from proliferating new vessels obstructing the outflow channels in the anterior chamber angle (see TABLE 102–1).

Treatment

Laser therapy is beneficial in nonproliferative and proliferative diabetic retinopathy. In 50% of patients with clinically significant macular edema, focal laser treatment of the leaking microaneurysms surrounding the macular area reduces visual loss. In proliferative diabetic retinopathy, the laser scatters several thousand tiny burns throughout the retina (sparing the macular area); this panretinal laser treatment reduces rates of blindness by 60%. Early treatment of macular edema and proliferative diabetic retinopathy prevents blindness for 5 yr in 95% of patients, whereas late treatment prevents blindness in only 50%. Thus, early diagnosis and treatment can virtually eliminate diabetic retinopathy as a major cause of blindness.

Close blood glucose monitoring and regulation should be emphasized to all diabetic patients regardless of age because tight control slows the development of diabetic complications. Clinical trials have not demonstrated that diabetic retinopathy can be prevented or slowed by limiting sorbitol accumulation with aldose reductase inhibitors. However, more potent inhibitors are being developed.

TABLE 102–1. CLASSIFICATION OF DIABETIC RETINOPATHY

Condition	*Description*
Early background diabetic retinopathy	≤ 5 microaneurysms in each eye
Nonproliferative diabetic retinopathy	Multiple microaneurysms, hard exudates, soft exudates, retinal hemorrhages, and intraretinal microvascular abnormalities
Proliferative diabetic retinopathy	New vessels on the disk and elsewhere on the retina, preretinal hemorrhages, and vitreous hemorrhage

AGE-RELATED MACULOPATHY

A series of pathologic changes in the macula accompanied by decreased visual acuity.

Immediately beneath the sensory retina lies a single layer of cells called the **retinal pigment epithelium.** These cells provide nourishment to the portion of the retina in contact with them—the **photoreceptor cells** that contain the visual pigments. For unknown reasons, maintenance of this contact is threatened in the macula of the aging eye. A disruption of this contact between the retinal pigment epithelial cells and photoreceptor cells results initially in distorted vision and eventually in a loss of central visual acuity. Two major processes in the macula can disrupt the retinal pigment epithelium–sensory retina interface.

A small hemorrhage may break through the retinal pigment epithelium from the underlying choroid, which contains a rich vascular bed. Blood accumulates between the retinal pigment epithelium and the sensory retina, and if bleeding resolves quickly, no permanent harm results. However, if new blood vessels grow from the choroid into the clot, they will continue to leak, causing more separation of the retinal pigment epithelium–sensory retina interface. This disrupts the nourishment of the photoreceptor cells and leads to their death, resulting in a loss of central visual acuity. This type of age-related maculopathy is called the **wet type** because of the leaking vessels and the edema or blood that detaches the sensory retina from the retinal pigment epithelium. The **dry type** of age-related maculopathy involves disintegration of the retinal pigment epithelium and a secondary loss of the overlying photoreceptor cells resulting from nutritional loss. The wet type accounts for only 10% of age-related maculopathy cases but results in

90% of cases of legal blindness (visual acuity of 20/200 or less) from macular degeneration in the elderly. The dry type reduces vision but usually only to levels of 20/50 to 20/100.

Symptoms, Signs, and Diagnosis

The patient may notice that central vision is distorted as objects appear larger or smaller, or straight lines appear distorted, bent, or without a central segment. If central vision is distorted in only one eye, the patient is unlikely to notice any change in vision. However, if the patient views a grid of fine lines with each eye alternately, distortion can be quickly detected. Therefore, those considered at high risk for age-related maculopathy are given a grid to view each morning. Following the onset of distortion, visual acuity may decrease, possibly within days.

In the **wet type,** a small detachment of the sensory retina may be noted in the macular area, but the definitive diagnosis of a subretinal neovascular membrane requires fluorescein angiography. In the **dry type, drusen** may disturb the pigmentation pattern in the macular area. Drusen are excrescences of the basement membrane of the retinal pigment epithelium that protrude into the cells, causing them to bulge anteriorly. Through the ophthalmoscope, they appear as small, rounded, yellow-white areas with indistinct borders. Their specific role as a risk factor in age-related maculopathy is still unclear.

Treatment

No treatment is known for the dry type of age-related maculopathy. But laser treatment initially obliterates the neovascular membrane in the wet type and prevents further visual loss in about 50% of patients at 18 mo. By 60 mo, however, only 20% show a substantial benefit. High-risk patients (eg, those who have age-related maculopathy in one eye or a family history of the condition) should view a grid daily to detect early distortion in central vision that could benefit from early laser treatment.

Although patients who have decreased central visual acuity cannot read or drive a car, they can continue to perform many everyday activities. The remainder of the sensory retina is unaffected in these patients, so they can be assured that they will not become completely blind.

For near-vision tasks (eg, reading and watching television), magnifying lenses and high-intensity lighting matched for daylight are often helpful. A telescopic lens may help the patient identify street signs and perform other visual tasks that facilitate travel. Some optometrists and ophthalmologists specialize in fitting such optical aids.

VASCULAR DISEASES

Vascular disorders that affect the eyes include central retinal artery occlusion, central retinal vein occlusion, ischemic optic neuropathy, amaurosis fugax, and occipital lobe vascular accident.

Central Retinal Artery Occlusion

Occlusion of the central retinal artery produces sudden blindness in the affected eye. The typical cause in older patients is an atheroma, usually broken off the carotid artery wall. The atheroma occludes the central retinal artery in the deeper portion of the optic nerve head and thus cannot be seen. Within an hour after loss of vision, the arterial spasm ceases, and some blood flow is restored to the retina, giving the appearance of a relatively normal retina on ophthalmoscopy. However, within several hours, the retina becomes edematous and gray from the death of retinal ganglion cells. Because the retina in the foveal area contains no ganglion cells, the reddish underlying choroid remains visible, accounting for the characteristic central cherry-red spot surrounded by gray retina. In 2 to 3 wk, the cherry-red spot disappears, and as the ganglion cells and their axons die, the optic nerve becomes white, the hallmark of **primary optic atrophy.**

When an atheroma breaks off, passes through the central retinal artery, and lodges in a retinal artery branch, it can usually be seen as a refractile object in the branch and is referred to as a **Hollenhorst plaque.** This finding indicates embolic activity, usually from the carotid system. The portion of the retina supplied by the occluded vessel loses its function and a visual field defect, which may not affect central vision, results.

Intervention is needed within a few minutes of the occlusion to prevent retinal cell death. Acutely reducing intraocular pressure by paracentesis combined with vasodilators may occasionally prevent this complication.

Central Retinal Vein Occlusion

Retinal vein occlusion is probably the most common vascular accident in the eye. About 10% of patients having a central retinal vein occlusion in one eye will also develop one in the other eye. Even after the occlusion occurs, some vision remains.

Ophthalmoscopy reveals distended, tortuous veins with massive hemorrhages and edema throughout the retina. The margins of the optic nerve become blurred and the disk swollen. Complete resorption of the hemorrhages and edema may take months or even years. In the older patient, the prognosis for vision is poor. Also, about 25% of patients develop a fibrovascular membrane that seals the aqueous humor outflow channels in the anterior chamber, resulting in a painful neovascular glaucoma in 3 to 6 mo. If the intraocular pressure remains elevated, blindness results in weeks. Treatment is most often attempted with laser photocoagulation, but its effectiveness is still being assessed.

Branch vein occlusion is also seen when a branch of the central retinal vein becomes obstructed, most often the superior temporal branch. The characteristic exudates and hemorrhages are confined to the involved quadrant of the retina, which has an associated visual field defect. Vision is usually unaffected unless the retinal swelling impinges on the macula. A clinical trial has demonstrated that using laser photocoagulation to treat branch vein occlusion helps preserve vision. Fortunately, the development of neovascular glaucoma is much less common in branch vein occlusion.

ISCHEMIC OPTIC NEUROPATHY

Regardless of the cause, ischemic optic neuropathy almost always occurs in those > 60 yr. Partial or complete loss of vision occurs suddenly, accompanied by swelling of the optic nerve head and often a hemorrhage or two. A visual field defect may produce a loss of half the visual field with a horizontal demarcation. Ischemic optic neuropathy is a medical emergency.

When **temporal arteritis** is the cause, tenderness along the temporal artery may be noted, as well as headache, jaw pain while chewing, and fever. Symptoms are almost always accompanied by an elevated erythrocyte sedimentation rate. Generally, prednisone 60 mg/day should be started as soon as possible, and a temporal artery biopsy should be obtained.

When **atheromatosis** is the cause of ischemic optic neuropathy, pain is uncommon, and decreased vision is soon followed by pallor of the optic disk. The visual loss in the other eye may occur months or years later, and once the ischemic episode has occurred, treatment does not help. In selected older patients with a history of blackouts (amaurosis fugax) suggestive of atheromatosis, long-term anticoagulant therapy may help.

AMAUROSIS FUGAX
(Blackouts)

When unilateral, amaurosis fugax suggests either retinal or optic nerve ischemia. The blackout may present as a dimming of vision with a slow recovery beginning after 5 to 10 min. The restoration of clear vision occurs in the reverse order from the onset pattern. Several episodes of blackout may precede an attack of ischemic optic neuropathy, or episodes may occur for years without serious sequelae. However, patients experiencing such episodes should be under medical care. The blackout can be bilateral if associated with low blood pressure.

Unilateral blackouts are characteristic of carotid artery narrowing, usually at the bifurcation of the common carotid artery. Because atheroma is the major cause of vessel narrowing, patients > 50 yr are most susceptible. Obstruction of the left carotid artery is six times more common than that of the right.

When blackout is accompanied by hemiplegia on the side opposite the affected eye (transient ischemic attack), carotid stenosis on the side of the affected eye should be strongly suspected. Early recognition of serious carotid stenosis is important because many affected patients will develop permanent visual loss or hemiplegia without appropriate medical and surgical intervention.

The aortic arch syndrome may be suspected if increasingly frequent blackouts are related to changes in posture, such as suddenly sitting up or standing.

Occipital Lobe Vascular Accident

A vascular lesion of the occipital lobe, usually the result of a posterior cerebral artery infarction, is usually characterized by sudden homonymous hemianopia. Infarction in one or both occipital lobes may result from local atheromatous disease, vascular insufficiency, or emboli in the vertebral-basilar system. Total blindness occurs suddenly, with some vision returning within minutes in the ipsilateral homonymous visual field. Bilateral posterior occlusions usually occur simultaneously. Thrombosis of the basilar artery also produces a bilateral homonymous hemianopia. In almost all cases of cortical blindness, some vision returns.

MISCELLANEOUS EYE CONDITIONS

Miscellaneous conditions affecting the elderly include acute double vision, diabetic ophthalmoplegia, intracranial tumor, and myasthenia gravis.

Acute Double Vision

The **third cranial nerve** innervates the medial, superior, and inferior rectus muscles, the inferior oblique muscle, and the levator muscle and also carries the parasympathetic nerves constricting the pupil and controlling accommodation. A complete third cranial nerve palsy results in ptosis; a divergence of the eye when looking straight ahead; a dilated fixed pupil; and a lack of upward, inward, and downward eye movement. The main causes of isolated third cranial nerve palsy are intracranial aneurysm, trauma, and diabetic neuropathy. Palsy from diabetes mellitus clears spontaneously in 6 to 12 wk, but palsy from intracranial aneurysm or trauma requires immediate diagnostic and, if indicated, therapeutic intervention.

The **fourth cranial nerve** innervates the superior oblique muscle, and palsy invariably results from a small hemorrhage in the roof of the midbrain, usually from arteriosclerosis. Recovery occurs spontaneously after several weeks.

The **sixth cranial nerve** innervates the lateral rectus muscle and, because it has the longest intracranial course, is often affected by meningitis, skull fracture, and increased intracranial pressure. When the nerve is affected by diabetes mellitus, spontaneous recovery occurs in 6 to 12 wk.

Diabetic Ophthalmoplegia

Severe eye or forehead pain followed by a third cranial nerve palsy that spares the pupil should be considered a manifestation of diabetic neuropathy.

Intracranial Tumor

An intracranial space-occupying mass is often accompanied by increased intracranial pressure and severe headache. Ophthalmoscopy may show papilledema. Prompt referral for a neurosurgical diagnostic evaluation is indicated.

Myasthenia Gravis

Any combination of extraocular muscle palsies, which may vary in severity over days or weeks, along with a normal pupillary response to light and a history of fatigue that waxes and wanes during the day should raise the possibility of myasthenia gravis. An edrophonium chloride (Tensilon) test should help establish the diagnosis.

§3. ORGAN SYSTEMS: EAR, NOSE, AND THROAT DISORDERS

103. EAR DISORDERS

HEARING LOSS

Hearing loss of some sort affects about 1/3 of all adults between 65 and 74 yr of age and about half of those between 75 and 79. In the USA, > 10 million elderly people have a hearing impairment.

Hearing loss may result from dysfunction of any component of the auditory system (see FIG. 103–1). In **conductive hearing loss,** the dysfunction affects the orderly transmission of sound from the external environment to the inner ear and may involve any of the structures lateral to the oval window (eg, the tympanic membrane or stapes). **Sensorineural hearing loss** involves dysfunction of the sensory elements (hair cells) or neural structures (cochlear nerve fibers). In cochlear sensorineural hearing loss, the structures within the cochlea are affected. In retrocochlear hearing loss, any element of the auditory system medial to the cochlea may be affected, although the term refers specifically to disorders of the cochlear nerve, particularly in the internal auditory canal or cerebellopontine angle. A **mixed hearing loss** combines both sensorineural and conductive elements. In **central hearing loss,** the dysfunction is localized to the brain's higher auditory centers.

Besides being categorized according to the anatomy and physiology involved, hearing loss can be categorized by cause. Causes of hearing loss include diseases, noise exposure, ototoxicity, tumors, and injury to the cochlear nerve and brain. Yet, the most common type of hearing loss in elderly persons is **presbycusis,** a term that means "hearing loss of aging" and that describes not a cause but a type of hearing loss whose cause is unknown.

PRESBYCUSIS

A bilaterally symmetric, sensorineural hearing loss that is associated with aging.

The presence, progression, and severity of presbycusis depend upon a variety of factors. Typically, men are more severely impaired than women of the same age. Noise exposure, diet, hypertension, and metabolic and hereditary factors may play a role. Vascular lesions that result

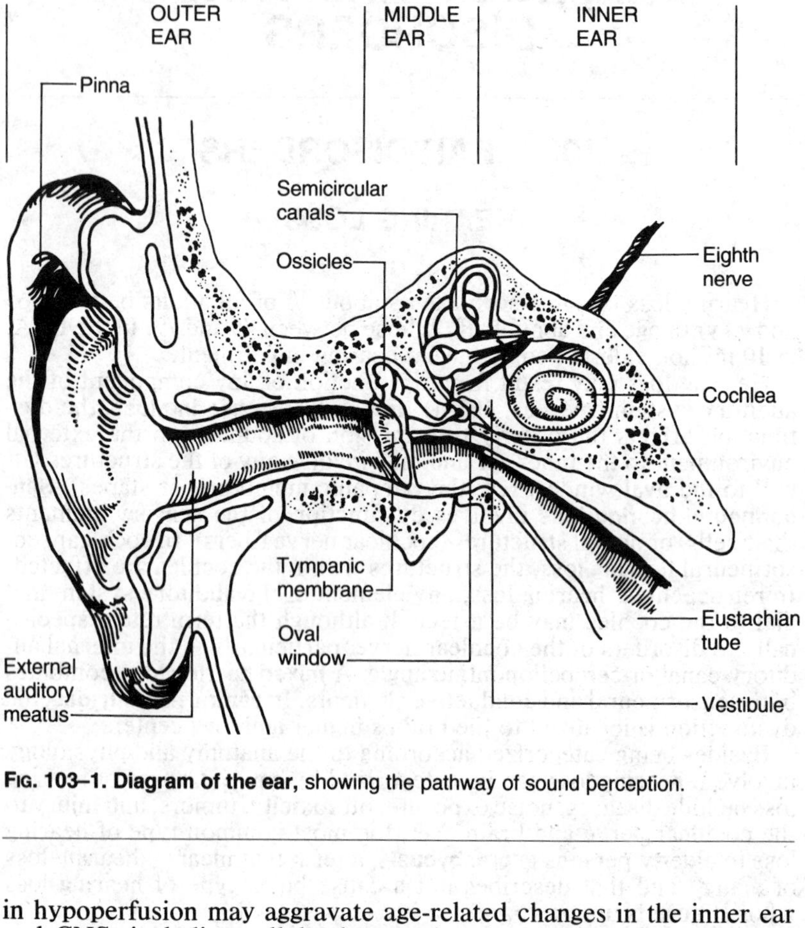

FIG. 103–1. Diagram of the ear, showing the pathway of sound perception.

in hypoperfusion may aggravate age-related changes in the inner ear and CNS, including cellular loss, reduced activity, and depletion of neurotransmitters.

Usually, presbycusis initially affects the very high frequencies, which do not interfere with understanding speech. Difficulty in understanding speech begins when the hearing loss involves the high frequencies that affect consonant discrimination. Patients typically complain of having difficulty understanding persons with higher-pitched voices (eg, women and young children) and conversations in large groups or with background noise (eg, in restaurants or bars). Often, older people complain that others are mumbling rather than admit that they have difficulty hearing. As the hearing loss progresses, communication requires intense effort. The embarrassment of misunderstanding can precipitate withdrawal from social contacts, leading to loneliness, depression, and paranoia.

Types of Presbycusis

Four pathophysiologic types of presbycusis have been described, and typical audiograms are shown in FIG. 103–2.

Sensory presbycusis is marked by atrophy of the organ of Corti. The hearing loss generally begins in middle age and progresses slowly. A loss of cochlear neurons parallels the loss of the organ of Corti. The audiogram generally shows an abrupt, high-frequency hearing loss with good discrimination (see FIG. 103–2*A*).

Neural presbycusis, usually manifested later in life, is ascribed to a loss of cochlear neurons with a relative preservation of the organ of Corti. Neural degeneration is apparently related to genetic factors. Audiometric evaluation shows a predominantly high-frequency hearing loss with very poor discrimination (see FIG. 103–2*B*); a severe loss of speech discrimination (phonemic regression) occurs, but pure tone thresholds are maintained. Rapidly progressing neural presbycusis may be accompanied by other signs of CNS degeneration, including intellectual deterioration, memory loss, and motor incoordination.

Metabolic presbycusis has a familial tendency, onset in middle age, and slow progression. It appears to correlate with patchy atrophy of the stria vascularis, affecting the electrophysiologic function of the organ of Corti. Audiometric evaluation shows a flat threshold pattern, with normal speech discrimination scores until the thresholds exceed 50 dB (see FIG. 103–2*C*).

Cochlear conductive presbycusis usually begins in middle age and is thought to relate to alterations in the motion mechanics of the cochlear duct, such as that caused by stiffening of the basilar membrane, although this has not been proved. Audiometric evaluation shows bilaterally symmetric, linearly descending thresholds; speech discrimination inversely relates to the steepness of the slope of the pure tone curve (see FIG. 103–2*D*).

OTOSCLEROSIS

A disease of the otic capsule and the most common cause of progressive conductive hearing loss in adults with normal tympanic membranes.

Otosclerosis, unique to the human otic capsule, is reported to occur in 10% of whites. About 10% of affected persons actually develop clinically significant conductive hearing loss. A family history of otosclerosis occurs in 50% to 60% of cases.

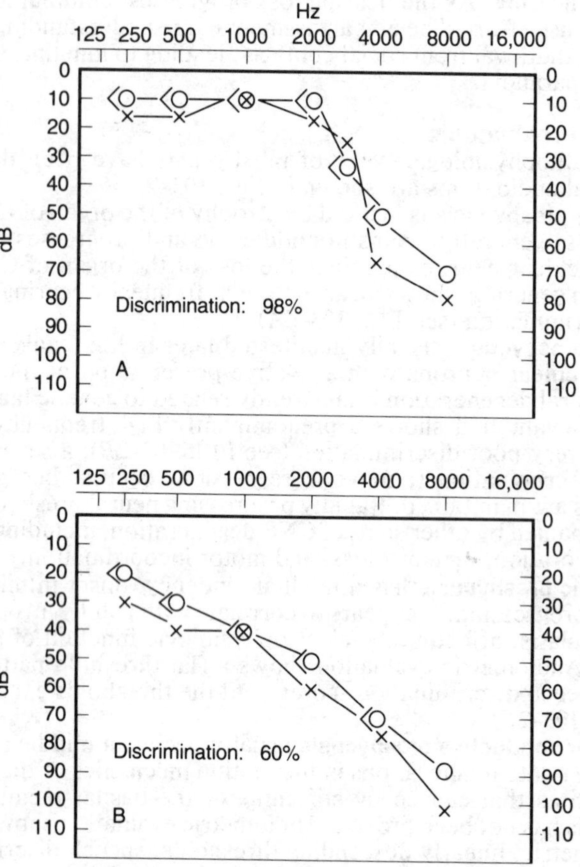

FIG. 103–2. Audiograms in patients with presbycusis. *A*; Abrupt, bilaterally symmetric, high-frequency hearing loss typical of *sensory presbycusis.* Discrimination is excellent. *B*; Downward-sloping sensorineural hearing loss with poor discrimination characteristic of *neural presbycusis*. *C*; Flat sensorineural hearing loss, as seen in *metabolic presbycusis*. Discrimination is unaffected in early stages. *D*; Bilaterally symmetric, downward-sloping, sensorineural hearing loss with excellent discrimination consistent with *cochlear conductive presbycusis*. (Adapted from Wilson WR, Nadol JB, Jr (eds): *Quick Reference to Ear, Nose, and Throat Disorders*. Philadelphia, J.B. Lippincott Company, 1983; used with permission.) *(continued)*

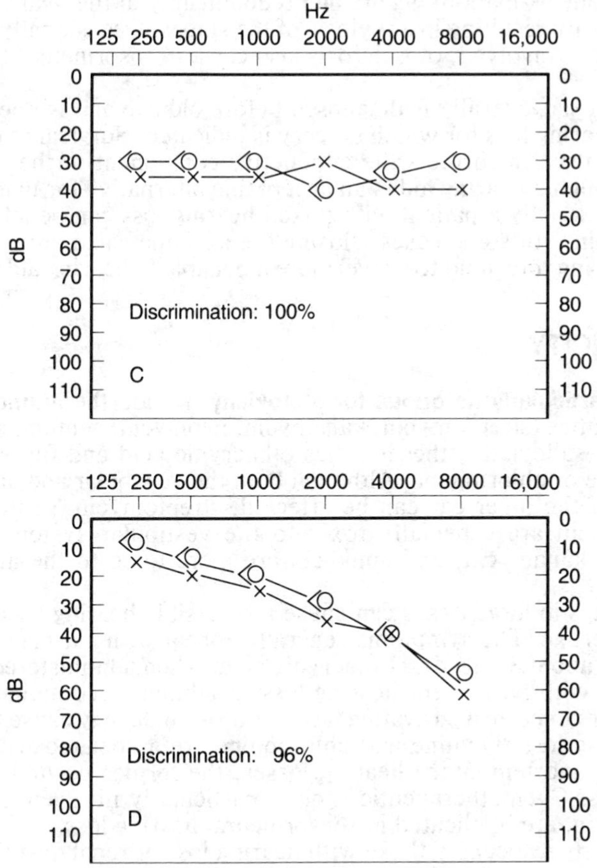

Audiogram code		Unmasked	Masked
Right ear (AD)	Air	○	△
	Bone	<	[
Left ear (AS)	Air	×	□
	Bone	>	]
No response		↓	↓

FIG. 103–2 ***(Continued)*. Audiograms in patients with presbycusis.**

The disease is characterized by irregular areas of bone resorption and new bone formation, occurring predominantly at the oval window and eventually resulting in ankylosis of the stapes. Occasionally, when the cochlea is involved, otosclerosis also causes sensorineural hearing loss.

Otosclerosis generally is diagnosed before old age and is one of the types of hearing loss for which surgery is indicated. Surgical bypass of the stapes usually corrects the conductive component of the hearing loss. Although a hearing aid is an acceptable alternative for many persons, occasionally a patient with mixed hearing loss can benefit from stapedectomy. In some cases, closing the air-bone gap brings the patient's hearing threshold to a level more amenable to hearing aid fitting.

OTOTOXICITY

Drugs particularly notorious for ototoxicity include the aminoglycoside antibiotics (streptomycin, kanamycin, neomycin, gentamicin, and viomycin), salicylates, the diuretics ethacrynic acid and furosemide, and quinine or chloroquine. Although both the vestibular and auditory portions of the inner ear can be affected, streptomycin, gentamicin, and viomycin are especially toxic to the vestibular system, while neomycin, kanamycin, and amikacin are more toxic to the auditory system.

Salicylates in large doses can cause a reversible hearing loss, tinnitus, and vertigo. The symptoms generally appear with plasma concentrations of about 35 mg/dL. Ethacrynic acid, when administered IV, is associated with permanent hearing loss; coadministered aminoglycoside appears to be an aggravating factor. Furosemide may cause temporary hearing loss. Quinine and chloroquine are associated with both permanent and temporary hearing losses, the former occurring with large doses. Chemotherapeutic agents, particularly nitrogen mustard and cisplatin, are implicated in sensorineural hearing loss.

The elderly, especially those with hearing loss or renal dysfunction, should not be treated with ototoxic drugs unless no suitable alternative exists. In such a case, a baseline and follow-up audiogram should be obtained to document any drug-related changes. Vestibular effects may be insidious, particularly when patients are bedridden. A bedside test of the vestibulo-ocular reflex may help in early detection of vestibular dysfunction.

Although the perilymph of the inner ear tends to concentrate and retain certain ototoxic drugs, regular serum monitoring for therapeutic blood levels helps avoid ototoxicity.

TUMORS THAT AFFECT HEARING

Tumors that affect hearing include paraganglioma and vestibular schwannoma.

PARAGANGLIOMA

Tumors of the middle ear and mastoid are rare. Of these, the most common tumors are **paragangliomas,** derived from paraganglion tissue (eg, the carotid body). Otherwise known as **glomus tumors,** these benign lesions generally cause a conductive hearing loss and pulsatile tinnitus. Tumors originating in the middle ear (glomus tympanicum) are clinically evident even when small; those arising in the jugular vein at the mastoid (glomus jugulare) become clinically apparent relatively late and may produce symptoms such as paralysis of cranial nerves IX through XII.

Physical examination may reveal a pulsatile red mass in the middle ear. The integrity of the cranial nerves should be assessed. Audiometric evaluation usually documents a conductive hearing loss; in more widespread tumors, a sensorineural component may also be detected. Because of the multicentricity of these lesions, four-vessel cerebral angiography or magnetic resonance angiography may reveal other, occult growths. Glomus tumors may produce catecholamines, resulting in intermittent hypertension.

Treatment depends on the tumor's size as well as the patient's general medical condition. In the healthy patient, small tumors can be removed relatively easily. In the infirm patient, extensive tumors are probably best managed more conservatively. Relatively low-dose radiation therapy and arteriographic embolization are palliative and may be more appropriate in the elderly.

VESTIBULAR SCHWANNOMA
(Acoustic Neuroma)

A benign tumor that develops from the Schwann cells forming the sheaths of the vestibular nerves. Vestibular schwannomas most commonly arise in or immediately medial to the internal auditory canal; with growth, they present as a cerebellopontine angle mass.

Patients usually complain of a unilateral hearing loss accompanied by tinnitus and, occasionally, disequilibrium. Large tumors may also affect cranial nerves V and lower and may produce hydrocephalus. Since **physical examination** may disclose only a unilateral or asymmetric hearing loss, assessing cranial nerve function is mandatory.

A complete **audiogram** generally shows an asymmetric sensorineural hearing loss with disproportionately poor speech discrimination scores. The acoustic reflex may be absent or may show abnormal decay, and rollover may be found on performance intensity function testing for phonetically balanced words (see under TESTS OF AUDITORY FUNCTION, below). Auditory brain stem response testing shows abnormalities consistent with a retrocochlear lesion. **Radiologic investigation** consists of contrast-enhanced CT scan or MRI directed toward the cerebellopontine angle and the internal auditory canals.

Treatment of acoustic tumors in the elderly is controversial. Complete surgical excision, as performed in younger patients, is recommended by some surgeons, while others believe that a palliative subtotal resection is wiser. Radiation therapy (eg, with a gamma knife or linear accelerator [LINAC]) may be an alternative in selected cases. The tumor's size, its associated symptoms, and the patient's overall medical condition should be considered when deciding on appropriate therapy.

DIAGNOSIS OF HEARING LOSS

Screening for hearing loss is strongly recommended for all elderly persons. Older persons often hide their hearing loss, embarrassed by it and equating it with aging. Those who are not employed and who have few social interactions may remain unaware of mild hearing loss, which places them at risk of injury and further social isolation.

Screening may be conducted at senior centers and can be accomplished in several ways. Questionnaires can augment the traditional review of systems but often must be administered to close social contacts and family members as well as to the patient. Testing is better using standardized instrumentation.

Establishing characteristics of the hearing loss guides the evaluation and helps the physician select the correct treatment. Inquiry should be made into the onset, progression, and severity of the hearing loss. Tinnitus often accompanies presbycusis. Asymmetric, unilateral, or fluctuating hearing losses are not characteristic of presbycusis. Physical examination generally is unrevealing, except when cerumen accumulation is the cause of hearing loss.

Once hearing loss is suspected, referral to an otolaryngologist or audiologist is in order. The minimal diagnostic evaluation entails a medical evaluation and a complete audiogram, including pure tone (an electronically produced sound of a single frequency), speech, and tympanometric testing (see TESTS OF AUDITORY FUNCTION, below). Asymmetry in the audiogram or retrocochlear signs should be pursued with an auditory brain stem response test and a CT or MRI scan to rule out an acoustic neuroma or other cerebellopontine angle tumor.

TESTS OF AUDITORY FUNCTION

A patient's ability to hear should be roughly estimated in a general office setting. In the **Weber test,** a vibrating 512-Hz tuning fork is placed on the midline of the forehead. Patients with normal hearing perceive the vibratory sound as equally loud in each ear. Patients with conductive hearing loss perceive the vibratory sound as louder on the affected side. In the **Rinne test,** the stem of a vibrating tuning fork is placed on the mastoid tip (with firm pressure) and then the tines are held just in front of the external auditory canal. Normally, the vibratory sound is perceived as being louder at the external auditory canal (ie, air conduction is greater than bone conduction). The reverse indicates a significant conductive hearing loss.

A **whisper test,** using a Bárány box to mask the contralateral ear, can crudely estimate auditory thresholds, but most clinicians find it too inaccurate to be useful. An **audioscope** combines both otoscopic visualization and the capacity to check hearing at different frequencies and volumes. Any complaint of hearing loss or any abnormality on office screening tests should be followed up with a complete audiogram.

The **complete audiogram** (see FIG. 103–3) entails a battery of tests for evaluating pure tone and speech reception thresholds and tympanometry. Thresholds for pure tones at octave or half-octave intervals are obtained for frequencies from 250 to 8000 Hz. Testing is done by both air conduction (using earphones) and bone conduction (placing a vibrotactile transducer directly on the mastoid).

The **speech reception threshold** is defined as the intensity at which the patient can correctly identify 50% of a series of spondees (two-syllable words equally accented, eg, cowboy). The speech reception threshold should be within 10 dB of the pure tone average (average threshold in decibels, at 500, 1000, and 2000 Hz). The **speech discrimination score** is determined by presenting a list of monosyllables at levels above the speech reception threshold and having the patient repeat them; the score is the percentage correctly identified.

A specialized test of speech discrimination, the **performance intensity function for phonetically balanced words,** differentiates cochlear from retrocochlear hearing loss. As phonetically balanced words are presented with increased intensity, the speech discrimination score rises and then stabilizes in patients with normal hearing or with a cochlear hearing loss. Patients with retrocochlear hearing loss have an initial rise in the score, followed by a dip (a rollover).

Immittance studies, also called impedance audiometry, consist of tympanometry and acoustic reflex measurements.

Tympanometry (see FIG. 103–4) measures the relative change in acoustic immittance at the plane of the tympanic membrane when air pressure changes are introduced in the external ear canal across a range from high positive to high negative pressure. Normally, the immittance is maximal at atmospheric pressure, where air pressure is about equal on each side of the tympanic membrane. The peak in the tympanogram may shift toward a negative air pressure direction if eustachian tube function is compromised, or the peak may disappear when fluid collects in the middle ear.

The **acoustic reflex threshold** is the lowest sound intensity (between 500 and 4000 Hz) that will produce a reflex contraction of the stapedius muscle. Reflex decay is an abnormal finding involving a decrease in the original reflex amplitude ≥ 50% over a 10-sec test period. Stapes (acoustic) reflex decay suggests a retrocochlear hearing disorder.

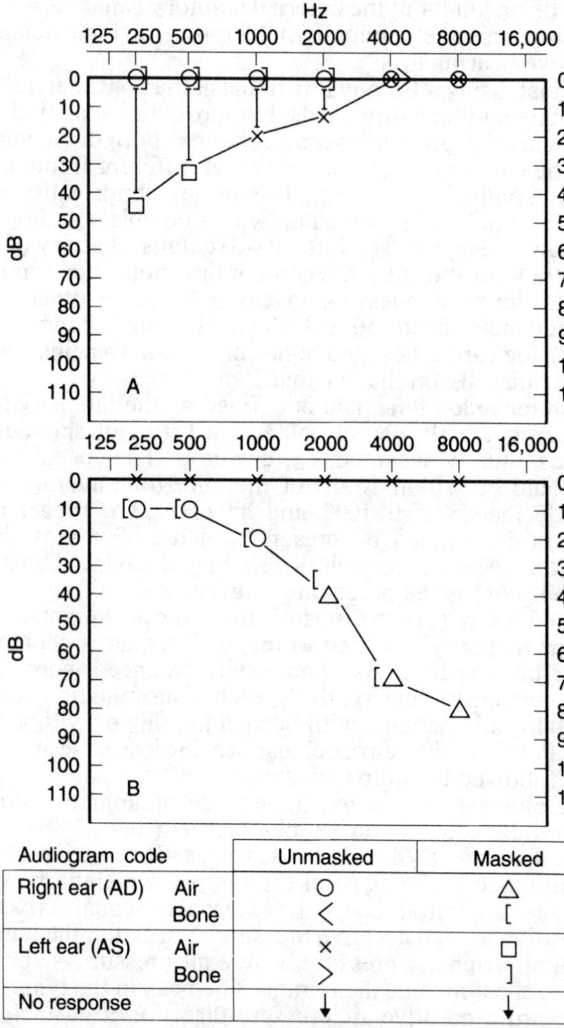

Audiogram code		Unmasked	Masked
Right ear (AD)	Air	○	△
	Bone	<	[
Left ear (AS)	Air	×	□
	Bone	>	]
No response		↓	↓

FIG. 103–3. Audiograms in patients with hearing loss. *A*; A left, low-frequency, conductive hearing loss; the right ear has normal hearing. The air-bone gap between the air curve (□ and ×) and the bone curve ( ]) is indicated by (|–|), demonstrating that the problem is conductive. *B*; The left ear is normal, but the right ear has a downward-sloping, sensorineural hearing loss. The loss of both air and bone hearing indicates that the problem is sensorineural. (Adapted from Wilson WR, Nadol JB, Jr (eds): *Quick Reference to Ear, Nose, and Throat Disorders*. Philadelphia, J.B. Lippincott Company, 1983; used with permission.)

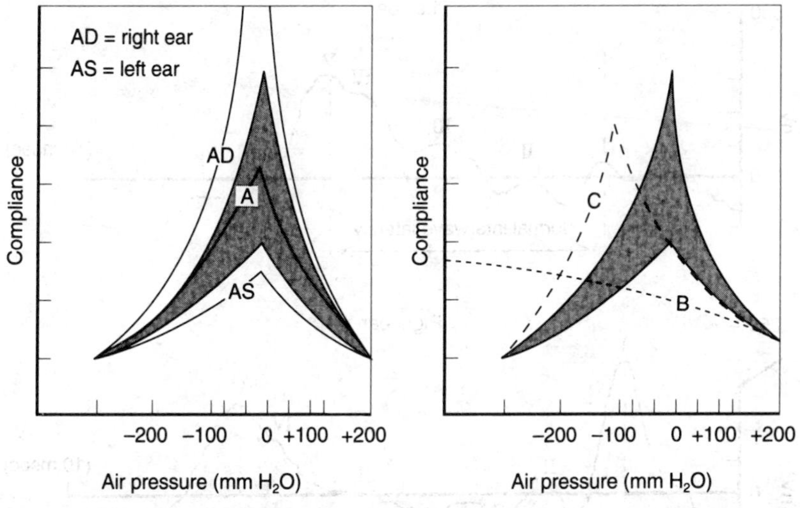

FIG. 103–4. Tympanogram tracings. *Left,* with normal middle ear pressure. AS is a stiffened curve, indicating reduced tympanic compliance. AD is a deep curve, seen with either a flaccid tympanic membrane or ossicular discontinuity. *Right,* curve C is seen with negative middle ear pressure, while curve B is a nonpeaking curve, suggesting middle ear fluid. (Adapted from Wilson WR, Nadol JB, Jr (eds): *Quick Reference to Ear, Nose, and Throat Disorders.* Philadelphia, J.B. Lippincott Company, 1983; used with permission.)

If auditory thresholds are ambiguous, or if the possibility of a retrocochlear disorder exists, appropriate testing includes the **auditory brain stem response.** In this test, recording electrodes are attached to the patient's earlobes and vertex and are connected to a computer that averages responses. Auditory system activity in response to a sound stimulus (a click) is analyzed by the computer and generally results in the delineation of five sequential waves (see FIG. 103–5). Waves I and II are thought to originate from the peripheral and central auditory nerve, wave III from the cochlear nuclei, and wave IV from activity in the superior olivary nucleus. The lateral lemniscus is thought to give rise to wave V. The intensity of the click needed to elicit the characteristic waveforms indicates the auditory threshold, which is determined for each ear individually. Also important is the time at which each wave appears after the sound stimulus (latency). A delay in onset of the entire sequence of waveforms suggests a conductive hearing loss. In the absence of a conductive hearing loss, a delay in onset of wave V strongly suggests a retrocochlear hearing loss.

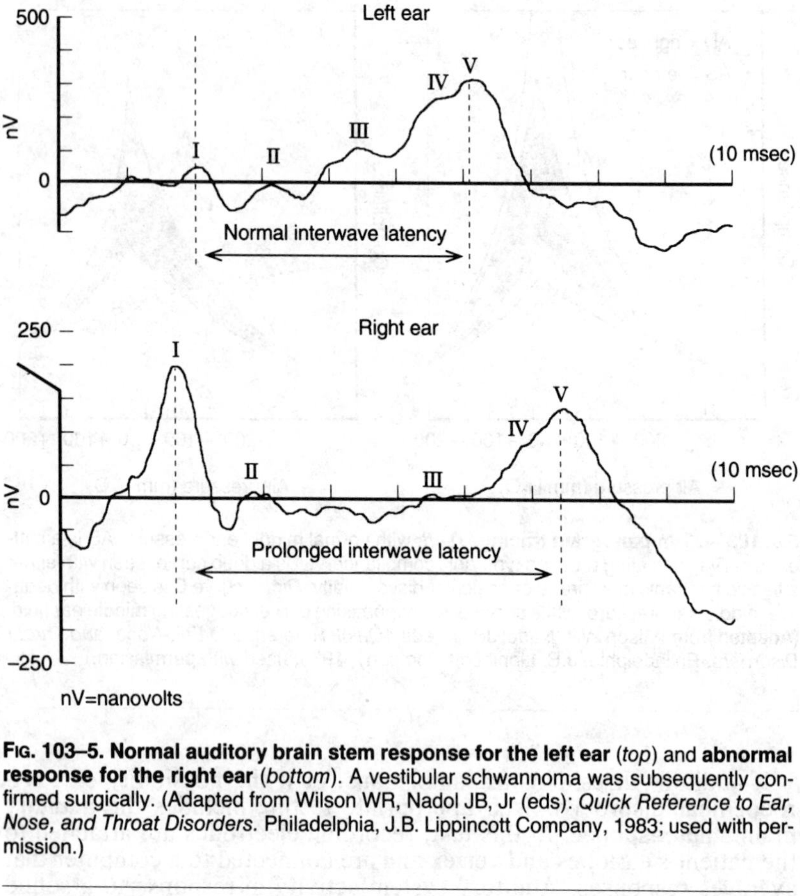

Fig. 103–5. Normal auditory brain stem response for the left ear (*top*) and **abnormal response for the right ear** (*bottom*). A vestibular schwannoma was subsequently confirmed surgically. (Adapted from Wilson WR, Nadol JB, Jr (eds): *Quick Reference to Ear, Nose, and Throat Disorders.* Philadelphia, J.B. Lippincott Company, 1983; used with permission.)

Results of **special tests** to determine central auditory function may be invalidated by a concurrent peripheral hearing loss. In general, these tests evaluate a patient's ability to synthesize distorted or degraded speech signals divided between the two ears, or to detect a specific message in one ear while a competing message is presented in the other ear. In tests using distorted or degraded messages, a cortical (temporal lobe) lesion may cause poor performance in the ear contralateral to the lesion (the **contralateral ear effect**). Inability to fuse binaural information into a meaningful message may indicate a brain stem lesion.

TREATMENT OF HEARING LOSS

Amplification is the best rehabilitative strategy if the hearing loss cannot be treated medically or surgically. A sensorineural hearing loss does not preclude benefit from a hearing aid. Likewise, audiometric configuration (pattern of loss across frequencies), decreased speech discrimination, and the presence of recruitment (an abnormally rapid rise in perceived loudness with increased signal level) do not exclude the possibility of successful hearing aid use.

A person with a sharply sloping pattern on audiometric tracings, severely decreased speech discrimination ability, or greatly reduced dynamic range (difference between the threshold of sensitivity and the threshold of discomfort) may have difficulty adapting to amplification devices. However, no single finding in the history, physical examination, or audiometric evaluation can accurately predict how well a patient with presbycusis will be rehabilitated with amplification. Factors that contribute to successful accommodation to amplification include the patient's desire to communicate (socially and vocationally), expectations and motivation, manual dexterity, and audiometric characteristics. Audiologists experienced in interacting with elderly persons and in dealing with physical and psychologic limitations are most likely to succeed in arranging appropriate amplification.

AMPLIFICATION

Certain guidelines help when communicating with any hearing-impaired person. Communication is most effective when competing environmental sound is absent or minimal. The speaker must first ensure that his face is well illuminated and that the listener is attentive. Optimally, the speaker should be about 3 ft from the listener's better or aided ear, lips and facial expression should be visible, and speech should be slow and clear. Shouting is not necessary and may worsen the patient's ability to discriminate. If the person misunderstands a statement, it should not be repeated word for word; instead, the original statement should be paraphrased.

Assistive Listening Devices

These devices help hearing-impaired persons overcome problems using the telephone, television, or radio and communicating in small or large groups. Portable and nonportable amplifiers boost telephone speaker output, and special devices signal an incoming call with either a louder ring or a flashing light. Other devices can sufficiently amplify television and radio signals for the hearing-impaired person while family members listen at normal volume levels. Telecaptioning may benefit those with good vision whose residual hearing is not sufficient to benefit from amplified sound signals.

For small-group communication (eg, in card games), relatively inexpensive devices that have a portable microphone, amplifier, and headset can be used. For large-group communication (eg, in a concert hall or church), many public facilities have group amplification systems such as infrared transmission, and the person can borrow a special portable receiver.

Hearing Aids

Amplification with hearing aids can help persons with conductive or sensorineural hearing losses. Although hearing aids vary in size and power, they share certain features. A microphone receives the sound, transforms it into electrical energy, and sends this signal to an amplifier that increases its energy. How much the incoming signal is amplified, as manifested in the output of the hearing aid speaker, is known as **gain.** The earmold channels the hearing aid output into the ear canal and affects the acoustic characteristics of the delivered signal.

The hearing aid evaluation matches the patient's auditory thresholds across the frequency band and speech discrimination ability with the type of hearing aid recommended for those characteristics. Some patients with relatively normal pure-tone thresholds demonstrate very poor speech discrimination and are less likely to benefit from a hearing aid. Some patients with hearing loss and recruitment will require a hearing aid with input automatic gain control and output limiters, technologic advances that prevent pain from overamplification.

When the type of hearing aid is selected, the patient should be taught how to adjust the device and how to keep it clean and functional. Important factors in determining whether a patient will be a successful hearing aid user include motivation, the need to communicate, and appropriate expectations for what can be achieved with the hearing aid. The social stigma as well as the expense of the hearing aid may be difficult to overcome.

For a time, the most widely used hearing aid was the **behind-the-ear or postauricular version.** The bulk of the device is hooked above and posterior to the pinna; it is connected to the earmold by flexible tubing. Improvements in technology have made it possible to assemble all the required components into a shell small enough to be inserted in the ear; these **in-the-ear aids** have become popular, in part because they are so unobtrusive. Generally, the smaller the device, the less powerful it is. More important, inserting and adjusting these small devices may be difficult for some elderly persons. **Eyeglass-mounted aids** have diminished in popularity, although they remain useful for some.

The contralateral routing of signals (CROS) aid is for those whose hearing is totally lost in one ear and relatively normal in the other. A microphone directs sound from the poorer-hearing to the better-hearing ear. If the better-hearing ear is also impaired, the signal from the poorer-hearing ear can be amplified; this type of device is called a **BiCROS aid.** Originally, the two devices were connected by cords, but newer models can communicate via FM signals.

A body aid, the most powerful type available (ie, producing the highest gain), may be concealed in a pocket or worn with a body strap and is connected by wires to the earpiece, which is connected to the earmold. The elderly, particularly those with impaired fine motor skills, may find it easier to manage the controls of a body aid. Alternatives include geriatric molds, designed for easier handling, and remote controls similar to a credit card to facilitate adjusting settings.

Hearing aids have various modifications, according to individual need. The T switch enables telephone communication through the hearing aid. Circuitry modifications include automatic gain control, automatic signal processing, and multiple signal processing. Automatic gain control automatically adjusts loud or soft sounds to about the same volume. Automatic signal processing and multiple signal processing attempt to improve the signal (human speech)-to-noise ratio and thus ameliorate hearing ability.

In contrast to air-conduction aids, which require an earmold, the **bone-conduction aid** is placed in direct contact with the head, usually over the mastoid, with a headset. Bone-conduction aids may be appropriate when an in-the-ear aid is contraindicated, as in persistent, uncontrollable otorrhea or canal atresia.

Cochlear Implants

The cochlear implant is approved for profoundly deaf adults who derive no benefit from the most powerful hearing aid. A microphone picks up the incoming sound and sends it to a speech processor; the processor modifies the signal and transmits it to external circuitry, which then relays the information to the receiver in the implanted device. From the internal circuitry, one or more electrodes implanted in the cochlea stimulate the remaining neural elements of hearing.

Implantation generally requires mastoid surgery and brief hospitalization. The device is expensive, and insurance coverage varies. Although it serves a limited population, the cochlear implant can make a tremendous difference in the life of a totally deaf and otherwise isolated person.

Vibrotactile Devices

Vibrotactile devices are alternative modes of rehabilitating profoundly deaf persons; vibrators placed either on the wrist or sternum or around the waist transform speech and environmental sounds into vibrations that can be perceived on the skin. With appropriate training, patients can learn to identify and localize sounds and can use the vibrotactile information to communicate better.

AUDITORY REHABILITATION

The goal of rehabilitation is to achieve the best hearing possible by using a combination of amplification, speech reading, and auditory training.

Speech Reading

The term **speech reading** has replaced **lip reading** because linguistic information is obtained not only by watching the speaker's lips but also by following facial expressions and gestures. Such visual cues may be an adjunct or an alternative to hearing aids. Decreasing visual acuity and poor short-term memory may militate against mastering speech reading.

Auditory Training

Auditory training is often combined with an amplification device to maximize benefit. Auditory training can help patients discriminate between distinctly differing sounds with hearing alone, eventually enabling them to develop schemes for making fine distinctions, particularly between similar speech sounds. In essence, such training makes the patient more aware of subtle auditory clues.

With auditory training, as with any aspect of auditory rehabilitation, having interested family members accompany the geriatric patient is helpful. Family members not only can provide encouragement and support but also may prompt the older patient when short-term memory fails.

CERUMEN ACCUMULATION

Accumulation of cerumen (earwax) may occur in persons of any age but appears to be more common in the elderly. It is a common cause of sudden tinnitus and hearing loss. The accumulation may be rock-hard and, particularly in older men, may contain a generous admixture of exfoliated hairs. The patient may complain of hearing loss and a feeling of fullness in the ear. Obstruction of the external canal is obvious on examination. Because the adnexal elements responsible for cerumen production are located in only the lateral ⅔ of the canal, impaction extending to the medial portion suggests manipulation with instruments such as cotton-tipped applicators.

The cerumen should be removed as gently as possible. In some cases, removal may be accomplished with a cerumen spoon, along with good visualization and an aural speculum. The skin of the external auditory canal can easily be traumatized and is exquisitely sensitive to manipulation. Thus, with hard accumulations, topical therapy with a cerumen-softening agent for several days to a week may be necessary to soften the debris and allow it to be removed atraumatically.

An antibiotic otic solution 4 drops qid for a few days in the affected ear softens the cerumen and quells any smoldering infection. When adequately softened, the cerumen can be easily removed, either with a spoon or by water irrigation. *Irrigation is contraindicated if the tympanic membrane is perforated, since it may provoke an infection.* To avoid perforating the tympanic membrane, the irrigation force should be gentle and directed along the canal wall, *not* directly at the eardrum.

TINNITUS

The perception of a sound in one or both ears without an externally applied stimulus.

The sound may be a ringing, hissing, whistling, or variety of complex sounds. Tinnitus may be subjective (only the patient is able to hear the sound) or objective (the examiner is also able to perceive the sound, eg, a referred carotid bruit). Tinnitus may be described as pulsatile, paralleling the patient's heartbeat, or nonpulsatile. An associated hearing loss, either conductive or sensorineural, is often present.

The mechanism involved in producing tinnitus is not known. One theory likens it to the cross talk of telephone wires: patchy loss of myelin sheaths results in signals crossing over from one auditory fiber to another. Alternatively, tinnitus has been likened to the phantom limb phenomenon in which sensations such as pain are perceived to originate from an amputated limb; loss of hair cells or their innervating fibers in the ear may produce a similar phantom phenomenon. Since the cochlea subserves auditory function, the resulting symptom is the hallucination of sound, or tinnitus.

Etiology

The causes of tinnitus may be local or systemic. Local causes include external auditory canal obstruction (eg, with cerumen or a foreign body); infections of the ear canal, tympanic membrane, middle ear, inner ear, or temporal bone; eustachian tube dysfunction; conductive hearing losses (eg, otosclerosis, Meniere's disease, or cerebellopontine angle tumors); and sensorineural hearing loss, either hereditary, noise induced, or related to trauma of the head or acoustic apparatus. Pulsatile tinnitus may be related to a glomus tumor of the middle ear or mastoid; other causes include vascular obstruction, aneurysmal dilation, and vascular malformation. Palatal myoclonus may be associated with a perception of repetitive clicking sounds, and a patulous eustachian tube results in the perception of breath sounds in the ear. The latter condition often follows loss of fat deposits around the tube, as occurs after significant weight loss.

Systemic causes of tinnitus include syphilis, meningitis, arachnoiditis, drug-induced ototoxicity (eg, from aminoglycoside antibiotics, salicylates, or quinine and its derivatives), hypertension, anemia, and thyroid and cardiovascular diseases, including arteriosclerosis.

Evaluation

After a careful history and thorough physical examination, a complete audiogram and appropriate hematologic testing (eg, CBC, ESR) are required to rule out systemic causes. Unilateral or asymmetric tinnitus demands further evaluation of auditory brain stem response testing or radiologic investigation of the head and brain (eg, with CT or MRI). Pulsatile tinnitus requires evaluating the vascular system; four-vessel cerebral angiography may be indicated.

Treatment

In many instances (eg, tinnitus associated with bilateral sensorineural hearing loss), reassurance that no serious underlying disorder exists may be helpful. Many clinicians recommend avoiding such stimulants as caffeine and chocolate, as well as alcohol, cigarettes, stress, and fatigue. Treating an associated hearing loss or prescribing an amplification device may reduce the perception of tinnitus. Tinnitus maskers have *not* proved practical; however, because many patients complain that the tinnitus is most troublesome when they are trying to fall asleep, playing an FM radio, particularly on interband frequencies, may help mask the tinnitus.

Some patients are driven to distraction by their tinnitus. Psychologic studies suggest that an underlying depression is common. Treatment with biofeedback, antidepressant medication, or both may help. The American Tinnitus Association is a useful support group.

DIZZINESS AND VERTIGO

Dizziness is a *vague term describing a variety of sensations*. **Vertigo** describes *a rotary motion, either of the patient with respect to the environment (subjective vertigo) or of the environment with respect to the patient (objective vertigo); the key element is the perception of motion*. Vertigo may be caused by a lesion anywhere in the labyrinth or its CNS connections. Dizziness, encompassing the sensations of vertigo, disequilibrium, and unsteadiness, is a nearly uniform complaint elicited from up to 90% of patients seen in geriatric outpatient clinics (see also Ch. 6). **Nystagmus,** specifically jerk nystagmus, results from stimulation of the vestibular system. The slow phase of nystagmus is related to the direction of the endolymph flow, while the quick, jerk-like corrective movement is controlled by the CNS. Nystagmus is generally described by the direction of the fast component.

DISEQUILIBRIUM OF AGING

Histologic evaluation of temporal bones from elderly patients gives some indication of the degenerative changes associated with aging. Hair cells are lost, particularly in the cristae of the semicircular canal but also in the maculae of the utricle and saccule. The innervating fibers of the hair cells and neurons in Scarpa's ganglion may also undergo losses. Degenerative changes in the otoconia predominate in the saccule and are observed only occasionally in the utricle.

Lipofuscin appears to accumulate within the labyrinth as in the cochlea. Because the vestibular system and its diffuse interconnections are so complex, correlating the clinical picture with the described histopathologic findings is more difficult than is the case with hearing loss and the cochlea. Nonetheless, four distinct types of disequilibrium have been associated with aging.

1. Cupulolithiasis, leading to **benign paroxysmal positional vertigo**, is characterized by *brief, intense episodes of true spinning vertigo when the head assumes a particular position*. Most commonly, symptoms are precipitated by rolling over in bed to one side or the other (but not both). Occasionally, symptoms are brought on by suddenly moving the head to the left or right, as well as by rapidly extending or (less frequently) flexing the head. Although head injury, ear infection, neurologic disease, ear surgery, or viral infection may precipitate symptoms of cupulolithiasis, usually no specific cause is found. Degeneration of the labyrinth (especially of the otoconia) may result in high specific gravity deposits settling on the cupula of the posterior semicircular canal (see FIG. 103–6). The disorder is generally self-limited but occasionally recurs over months or years.

Positioning testing demonstrates a horizontal-rotary nystagmus toward the lowermost ear that appears within a few seconds of assuming the provocative position (see Clinical Evaluation, below). The nystagmus lasts < 30 sec, and a complementary nystagmus often occurs when resuming the sitting position. Immediately repeating the provocative head position elicits a reduced response, if any; this loss of response is referred to as fatigability. Electronystagmography generally shows a normal bilateral caloric response.

One sensible treatment approach is to avoid the provocative position until the process remits spontaneously. More recently, specific physical therapy positioning maneuvers have been advocated to hasten recovery. Patients debilitated by this disorder may find relief in having the nerve to the posterior semicircular canal sectioned using a middle ear approach, or in undergoing plugging of the posterior semicircular canal using a mastoidectomy approach.

2. Ampullary disequilibrium consists of *vertigo associated with rotational head movements*. Patients note a persistent sensation of motion a few seconds after rapidly turning the head to the right or left; extending or flexing the head may also precipitate the vertigo. A subsequent sensation of unsteadiness may linger for several hours. Histopathologic findings appear to be related to a degenerative change in the ampullae of the semicircular canals.

Physical examination may not document the brief flash of nystagmus precipitated by sudden head rotation. Response to caloric stimulation may be reduced, as documented by electronystagmography. Treatment consists of avoiding abrupt head movements.

3. Macular disequilibrium is characterized by *vertigo brought on when head position changes with respect to gravity*. Typically, patients complain that they can no longer jump out of bed but instead must sit and steady themselves for a few seconds, after which they carry on without

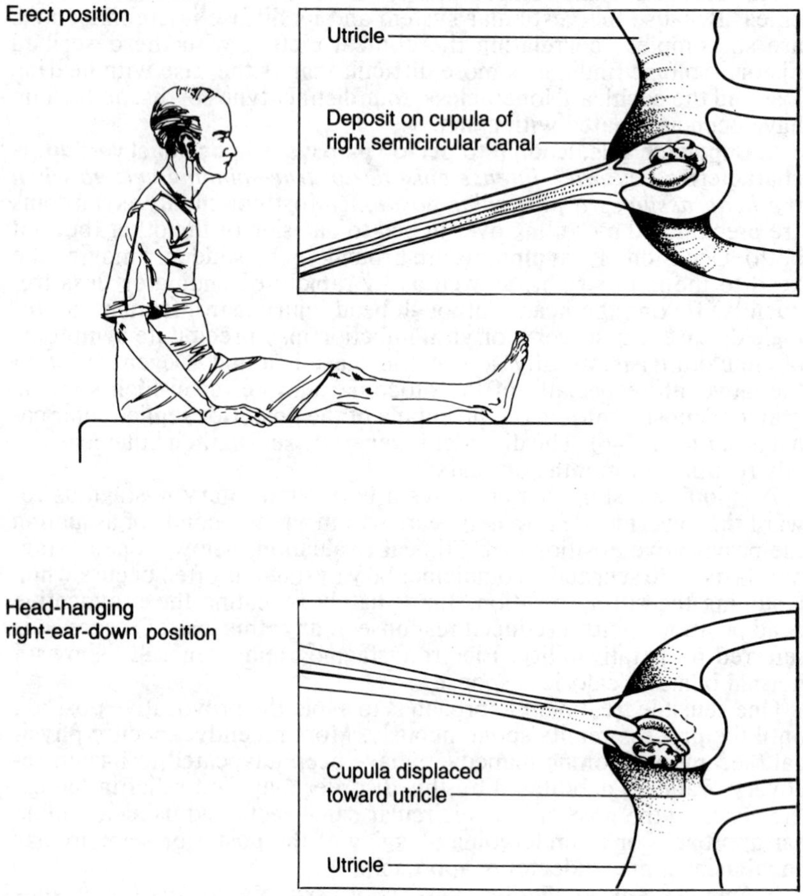

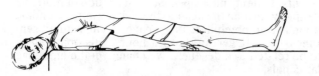

FIG. 103–6. The pathophysiology of cupulolithiasis of aging.

further problems. The histopathologic findings appear to demonstrate degenerative changes in the otolithic membranes or sensory hair cells of the utricle and saccule. Physical examination should seek to exclude possible hypotension. Electronystagmography generally shows normal caloric responses. There is no specific treatment.

4. Vestibular ataxia consists of *a constant sensation of imbalance with ambulation*. The patient has no difficulty with posture while sitting but experiences hesitancy and frequent side stepping when attempting to walk. This disequilibrium may relate to dysfunction of reflex control of the vestibular system over the lower limbs. Vestibular testing is nondiagnostic, and no cure is available.

Clinical Evaluation

The vestibular system can be clinically evaluated in the physician's office, primarily by eliciting or visualizing nystagmus. Bartels (20-diopter) lenses or Frenzel lenses (Bartels lenses with a light source) can eliminate the suppression of nystagmus usually created by visual fixation. Nystagmus that increases with visual fixation suggests central vestibular dysfunction. Spontaneous nystagmus should be sought in both horizontal and vertical planes of gaze. The **fistula test** (or test for **Hennebert's sign**) introduces alternately positive and negative pressure into an ear by means of a Politzer bag while looking for nystagmus.

Positioning testing (see FIG. 103–7) also can be easily performed. Positioning nystagmus is elicited by rapid movement of the patient's head; positional nystagmus is brought on by slow movement to the provocative position. With the patient sitting and his head turned to one side, the physician rapidly lowers him to the supine position with his head hanging over the table edge and notes any nystagmus. This procedure is repeated with the patient's head turned to the opposite side and with his head hanging straight back.

Caloric testing assesses the symmetry of vestibular function. Each ear is stimulated with 250 mL of warm (44° C [111° F]) and then cool (30° C [86° F]) water, each instilled in 40 sec. The less responsive ear (canal paresis, a unilateral reduction in vestibular response) shows a shorter duration or a lower frequency of nystagmus or a slower velocity of the slow component and is presumed to be the diseased ear. Occasionally, ice water stimulation is necessary to elicit a vestibular response.

Laboratory Evaluation

Vestibular testing to determine the severity or location of dysfunction lacks the diagnostic precision of auditory system testing, partly because the functional interconnections of the vestibular system are so complex. **Electronystagmography** is the most common vestibular test. Electrodes are placed around the patient's eyes, and eye movements are recorded on an ECG-like tracing by measuring the corneoretinal potential. Electronystagmography usually consists of tests for horizontal and vertical gaze, pendulum tracking, opticokinetic nystagmus, positional and positioning nystagmus, and caloric stimulation (see above).

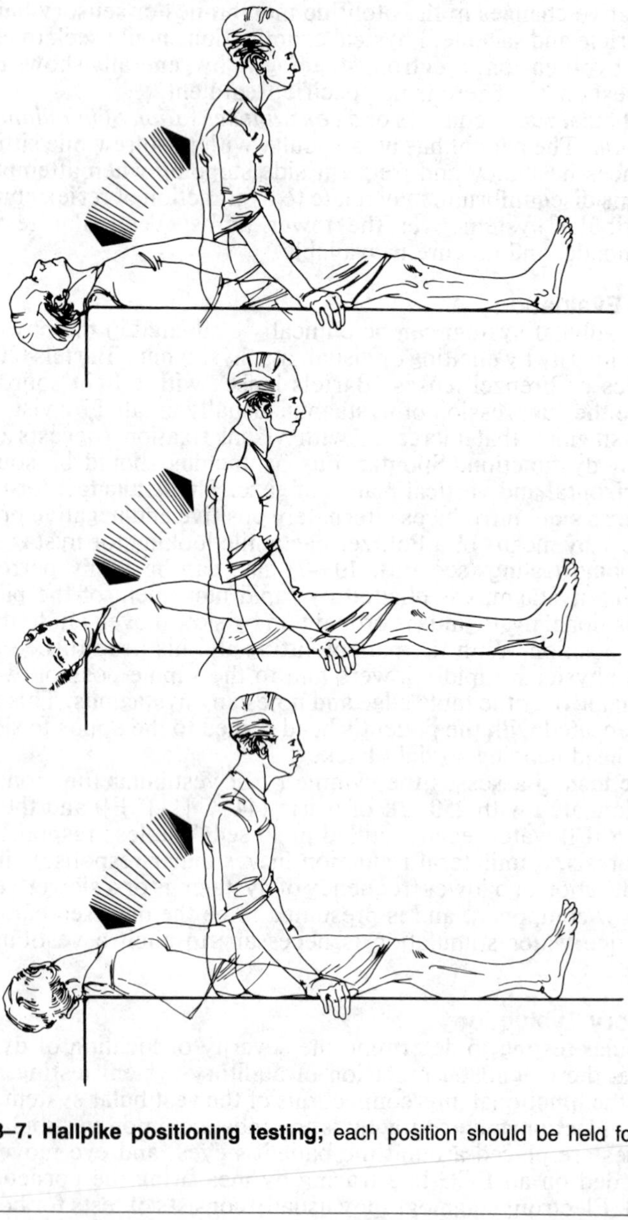

FIG. 103–7. Hallpike positioning testing; each position should be held for at least 10 sec.

Newer tests of vestibular function, including computerized rotational chair testing (sinusoidal harmonic acceleration testing) and posturography, may be indicated in special cases but are not widely available.

Prevention and Treatment

The lack of effective medical therapy for all four types of aging-associated disequilibrium must be emphasized. Vestibular depressants (eg, meclizine or diazepam) do not suppress the burst of vertigo encountered in cupulolithiasis. Worse yet, they may suppress the protective reflexes of elderly patients, rendering them more prone to falls; also their anticholinergic side effects are often severe in the elderly. Because of reduced muscle strength and reflex speed, older persons are particularly prone to falls when dizzy. Providing handrails and adequate lighting, particularly at night, may allow the patient to maximize appropriate proprioceptive and visual orientational clues and thus walk more safely. Vestibular rehabilitation therapy with an appropriately trained physical therapist may be helpful.

ANTERIOR VESTIBULAR ARTERY OCCLUSION

The anterior vestibular artery supplies the lateral and superior semicircular canals as well as the utricle. Acute obstruction results in the sudden onset of severe vertigo without other otologic or CNS manifestations. As in the vertigo of acute viral labyrinthitis, recovery occurs over several weeks. However, positional vertigo develops and may persist for years. Anterior vestibular artery obstruction is thought to cause necrosis of the supplied structures, resulting in deposits of necrotic debris on the cupula of the otherwise unaffected posterior semicircular canal. This disorder is in other ways identical to cupulolithiasis. Aspirin prophylaxis may be helpful.

VERTEBROBASILAR INSUFFICIENCY

The inner ear's blood supply comes either from the internal auditory artery, which arises as a branch of the anteroinferior cerebellar artery, or directly from the basilar artery. Patients with disordered perfusion of the vertebrobasilar system may complain of dizzy spells, usually associated with dysarthria, visual disturbances, or syncope.

The most common cause of vertebrobasilar insufficiency is atherosclerosis of the vertebrobasilar arteries; less often, cervical compression of the vertebral artery results in the insufficiency. The **thyrocervical steal syndrome,** resulting from blockage of the subclavian artery proximal to the vertebral artery, may also be associated with the disorder.

Vestibular tests are nonspecific, and arteriography is often indicated. Therapy depends on the cause and site of the lesion. Hypertension should be controlled, and anticoagulant therapy may be indicated.

MIDDLE EAR DISORDERS

Middle ear disorders include serous otitis media and chronic otitis media.

SEROUS OTITIS MEDIA

An effusion in the middle ear, usually related to eustachian tube obstruction but also observed when acute otitis media is resolving.

The fluid generally is not grossly purulent but may contain low levels of pathogens. Unilateral serous otitis media in the elderly adult has different implications from that in a young child. The former demands evaluation for and exclusion of a nasopharyngeal mass; patients with such lesions commonly have unilateral serous otitis media because the eustachian tube is obstructed at its nasopharyngeal orifice.

The patient perceives a sensation of aural fullness and hearing loss. On physical examination, amber fluid can be visualized medial to the tympanic membrane, causing the malleus handle to appear whiter than usual. Occasionally, air bubbles or an air-fluid level is also seen. The nasopharynx should be examined with a mirror or fiberscope to assess the eustachian tube orifice. Scanning with CT or MRI may be indicated to visualize a more lateral obstruction.

Treatment of any mass lesion depends on the information provided by biopsy. If serous otitis media is accompanied by upper respiratory tract infection or allergy, antibiotic or local vasoconstrictive therapy, or both, may be helpful. Nasal sprays (eg, oxymetazoline HCl 0.05%) can provide local decongestion but should not be used > 5 days in succession. In some cases, myringotomy with aspiration of fluid and, possibly, insertion of a ventilation tube may be necessary.

CHRONIC OTITIS MEDIA

A chronic middle ear infection generally associated with a perforated tympanic membrane and intermittent, purulent otorrhea.

Although not specifically a disorder of the elderly, chronic otitis media may present or recur in this age group. Polypoid hypertrophy of the middle ear mucosa may progress to the extent that it becomes an ear canal mass.

The patient generally complains of ear drainage and hearing loss and may have a history of previous ear surgery. Dizziness is ominous, suggesting erosion of the labyrinthine bone. Facial nerve paralysis, another ominous sign, suggests extensive disease.

One complication of chronic otitis media is **cholesteatoma,** *the accumulation of keratin debris in the middle ear or mastoid.* This debris originates from keratinizing squamous epithelium that has entered these areas from the external auditory canal, generally through a marginal perforation of the tympanic membrane. Symptoms are produced by progressive erosion of middle and inner ear structures. Cholesteatoma may extend through the tegmen into the brain or may involve the lateral venous sinus.

Diagnosis

Physical examination may disclose occlusion of the external auditory canal by purulent debris, which should be gently aspirated and submitted for culture. Otoscopic examination, supplemented by microscopic visualization, can document tympanic membrane perforation and the status of the middle ear mucosa. In other cases, polypoid granulation tissue, representing hypertrophied middle ear mucosa, may preclude adequate examination. The postauricular area may show a scar and depression, indicating previous mastoid surgery.

Plain films of the mastoids can give some idea of the extent of mastoid air cell system development, whether a lytic lesion is present, and whether surgery was previously performed. Alternatively, CT scanning with specific bone-imaging settings visualizes more clearly the status of the middle ear and mastoid structures, as well as the integrity of the tegmen and the otic capsule.

Treatment

Manually removing accumulated debris to the extent safely possible is the initial step. Irrigation with 2 oz 1.5% acetic acid tid helps remove the remaining debris and restore the auditory canal's normal acidic pH. A topical antibiotic solution should be instilled after each irrigation and in the evening.

Preparations containing neomycin, which is ototoxic, should be avoided. A commercially available ophthalmic preparation containing sulfacetamide sodium and prednisolone has not been documented to have any ototoxic properties and does not produce a burning sensation when instilled. Topical therapy can often reduce the size of hypertrophied mucosal lesions.

Polypoid tissue may be gently excised for biopsy. Avulsion of such lesions must be avoided, since their medial attachments may include the stapes or facial nerve. Depending upon the cause of the chronic otitis media and the patient's general condition, surgery may be recommended.

EXTERNAL OTITIS
(Swimmer's Ear)

A painful infection of the external auditory canal.

External otitis is usually precipitated by maceration of the ear canal skin resulting from retained water or by self-initiated attempts to clean the canal. This disorder is particularly significant in elderly diabetic patients, in whom it may progress to a potentially life-threatening *Pseudomonas* osteomyelitis of the temporal bone, commonly referred to as **necrotizing (malignant) external otitis.** Immunodeficiency and diabetic angiopathy may promote an invasive process.

Early examination may disclose only an acute external otitis, but attention should be paid to the posteroinferior aspect of the external auditory canal. Granulation tissue in this region is an ominous sign, demanding further investigation and aggressive therapy. Once the infection penetrates the external auditory canal epithelium, it tends to spread along vascular and fascial planes, resulting in many complications, including facial nerve paralysis, lateral venous sinus thrombosis, paralysis of cranial nerves IX through XII, and extension to the contralateral temporal bone.

If necrotizing external otitis is suspected, **laboratory evaluation** begins with a culture (which almost always reveals *Pseudomonas aeruginosa*) and sensitivity testing. Mastoid x-rays may demonstrate opacification of the mastoid air cell spaces and suggest a more invasive disorder. A technetium 99m diphosphonate bone scan provides early detection of temporal bone osteomyelitis, while scanning with gallium 67 citrate monitors antibiotic response. Temporal bone CT scanning and, more recently, MRI are other diagnostic adjuncts. Biopsy of the granulation tissue helps distinguish necrotizing external otitis from other inflammatory processes.

Treatment of uncomplicated external otitis entails ototopical antibiotics, generally containing a combination of polymyxin, neomycin, and hydrocortisone (eg, Cortisporin Otic), 4 drops in the affected ear qid for 7 to 10 days. For associated tympanic membrane perforation, the suspension form of the topical antibiotic is used. Water entry during bathing is prevented by inserting a cotton ball impregnated with petroleum jelly; otherwise the ear is left open to air.

Occasionally, external otitis is related to a fungal infection, in which case clotrimazole (1% solution) should be substituted for the antibacterial drops. Cresylate is an alternative solution.

Necrotizing external otitis, a potentially lethal disorder, requires hospitalization for administration of antibiotics, usually combination therapy. Some combinations are as follows: aztreonam (1 to 2 gm IV q 6 to 8 h) and clindamycin (600 mg IV q 8 h); ciprofloxacin (500 to 750 mg orally q 12 h) and rifampin (9 mg/kg orally daily); ticarcillin with clavulanate (3.1 gm IV q 4 to 8 h) and an aminoglycoside; ceftazidime (1 to 2 gm IV q 8 to 12 h) and metronidazole (500 mg IV q 6 h). Several weeks of therapy may be required.

Curettage of the granulation tissue with the instillation of wicks containing antibiotics, as well as hyperbaric oxygen therapy, may be useful. Surgery is reserved for cases not responsive to medical therapy. Meticulous management of diabetes is essential.

OTALGIA

Ear pain may result from an ear disorder, or the pain may be referred along neural pathways, including the trigeminal, glossopharyngeal, vagus, and cervical nerves. Inflammation of the pinna, external auditory canal, tympanic membrane, or middle ear leads to a clinically obvious cause of the pain. With eustachian tube obstruction, negative pressure in the middle ear may produce a painful retraction of the tympanic membrane.

A complaint of otalgia without a clearly identified otic source demands complete examination of the head and neck. Pain in the temporomandibular joint may be referred to the ear. More ominously, patients with tumors of head and neck structures (eg, the larynx, pharynx, esophagus, nose, base of the tongue, and base of the skull) may present initially with referred otalgia. Thus, an examination should include visualizing the nasopharynx and hypopharynx and palpating the base of the tongue and tonsillar fossae. Radiographic evaluation of the skull base may be indicated.

Treatment is related to the underlying cause.

EXTERNAL AND INTERNAL LESIONS

Tumors of the external and internal ear include nonmalignant, malignant, and metastatic lesions (see also TUMORS THAT AFFECT HEARING, above).

NONMALIGNANT LESIONS

Gout and **rheumatoid arthritis** may be associated with pinnal lesions. Gouty tophi, most commonly found on the helix, may be painful, occasionally discharging monosodium urate crystals. The nodules of rheumatoid arthritis also may be painful and can develop central necrosis. In both disorders, treatment involves the underlying systemic disease.

Winkler's disease (chondrodermatitis nodularis chronica helicis), particularly prevalent in older men, is characterized by exquisitely painful, firm nodules on the periphery of the pinna. Injection of hydrocortisone acetate (25 mg/mm diameter) may provide some pain relief, or local excision may be necessary.

MALIGNANT LESIONS

The most common malignant tumor of the pinna, **squamous cell carcinoma,** occurs predominantly in older men. The posterosuperior aspect of the pinna is most frequently involved, but in women the tumors tend to occur closer to the external auditory canal. The lesions are generally painless, and diagnosis requires biopsy. Treatment consists of wide local excision by standard techniques or by Mohs' surgery. The prognosis is good for small lesions of the helix, but not for tumors near the opening of the external auditory canal.

Squamous cell carcinoma may occur in the middle ear, generally associated with a chronic ear infection. These tumors may affect hearing, depending on their location. The treatment of choice is surgery, consisting of wide-field resection of the temporal bone, followed by radiation therapy.

The second most common malignant tumor of the pinna, **basal cell carcinoma,** also is most prevalent in older men and appears as a nodule with pearly, heaped-up borders. Biopsy is required for definitive diagnosis. Wide excision is the therapy of choice.

Basal cell carcinoma and, particularly in patients with a history of chronic otitis media, squamous cell carcinoma may involve the external auditory canal. The initial manifestation may be an unrelenting infection that, with disease progression, causes facial nerve paralysis. If the middle ear and facial nerve are not involved, the lateral temporal bone is resected (removing the external auditory canal, tympanic membrane, malleus, and incus), followed by radiation therapy. More extensive lesions have a poor prognosis.

METASTATIC LESIONS

Hematogenous dissemination of cancer may seed the temporal bone with metastatic foci. The most common primary tumors metastasizing to the temporal bone, in descending order of frequency, are those of the breast, kidney, lung, stomach, larynx, prostate, and thyroid.

Symptoms depend on the location of involvement within the temporal bone. Conductive hearing loss and pain are associated with involvement of the external auditory canal, middle ear, mastoid, or eustachian tube. Sensorineural hearing loss, vertigo, and facial paralysis are more characteristic of internal auditory canal involvement.

Appropriate evaluation includes radiographic documentation and confirmation by biopsy. Therapy depends on the lesion detected.

104. NOSE AND THROAT DISORDERS

NOSE AND SINUS DISORDERS

Nasal and paranasal sinus disorders among the elderly include nasal obstruction, rhinorrhea, epistaxis, and nasal fractures.

Nasal Obstruction

The nose gradually changes over a lifetime. The most apparent changes are **gravitational effects,** such as drooping of the tip of the nose. Usually, the angle between the columella of the nose and upper lip is 90° in men and 110° in women. With time, this angle decreases because of laxity of the skin and thinning and softening of the alar cartilage. If this effect is pronounced, nasal obstruction may result.

Elongation of the nose results in narrowing, and many elderly patients experience nasal obstruction because the softened alae close against the septum during inspiration. Such an obstruction can be diagnosed by elevating the tip of the nose with the thumb and noting immediate improvement. The nasal airway can be opened further by placing gentle traction on the cheek. A severe problem can be corrected surgically by lifting the tip, shortening the nasal septum, and correcting the laxity of the skin.

Unilateral obstruction: If a unilateral obstruction is associated with bleeding, neoplasia involving the sinuses or nose is likely. An obstruction may result from nasal swelling or polyps secondary to chronic infection in the maxillary or ethmoidal sinuses, particularly in patients who have had upper jaw dental abscesses or nasogastric or nasotracheal intubation. Among confused patients, unilateral obstruction with discharge may result from a foreign body—commonly a wad of tissue or cotton—pushed into the nose.

The evaluation includes an examination, sinus x-rays, and culture or biopsy, as indicated. Benign sinus disease probably requires limited nasal and sinus surgery. Depending on the biopsy and radiologic findings, malignancy requires radiation, surgery, or both.

Bilateral obstruction: Bilateral obstruction may result from seasonal or perennial nasal allergy. In many patients, the effects of allergic rhinosinusitis seem to be ameliorated with age, but they remain the same in some patients. When an elderly person moves to a new region of the country, allergic symptoms may begin. Bilateral obstruction may also result from bilateral nasal polyps. If the obstruction is associated with unilateral or bilateral hearing loss secondary to serous otitis media, nasopharyngeal tumors such as a carcinoma, lymphoma, or plasmacytoma should be ruled out by sinus x-ray. Occasionally, turbinate congestion is a symptom of hypothyroidism. Nasal congestion may also be caused by certain antihypertensives (especially reserpine) and tricyclic antidepressants. The overuse of nasal decongestant sprays can cause chronic hypertrophic changes of the turbinates, known as rhinitis medicamentosa.

Aging of the Nasal Mucous Membrane

With age, the mucous membrane becomes thinner; elastic fibers and submucosal tissues decrease; and mucus-secreting structures atrophy. The results are decreased mucus production and nasal dryness. Treatment consists of using buffered saline nasal sprays as needed.

Rhinorrhea: The elderly may complain of excessive watery, dripping nasal secretions associated with eating, particularly eating hot or spicy foods. This condition probably results from altered function of the parasympathetic vasomotor secretory fibers in the nose. No satisfactory treatment is available.

Drugs routinely prescribed for nasal congestion or rhinorrhea in younger patients can cause serious side effects in the elderly. Sympathomimetic amines (eg, pseudoephedrine) can cause agitation, confusion, and more commonly, urinary retention. Antihistamines may produce excessive sedation, hypotension, vertigo, syncope, incoordination, constipation, urinary disturbances, and thicker nasal secretions.

Epistaxis (nosebleed): Atrophic changes in the mucous membrane and increased susceptibility of the nasal vasculature to rupture because of thinning vessel walls make epistaxis relatively common in the elderly.

Anterior epistaxis commonly results from ulceration of the mucosa overlying old septal spurs or deviations, particularly in patients taking anticoagulants (eg, daily aspirin for general cardiovascular prophylaxis). Any coagulopathy should be corrected at least temporarily to allow a thrombus to form and the mucous membranes to heal. Acute epistaxis may be treated with oxymetazoline, which has long-acting vasoconstrictive properties and no significant systemic effects. It is applied to the bleeding site with cotton, and the site is then compressed externally until the bleeding stops. Bleeding sites also can be cauterized and protected with a petroleum-based ointment until they heal.

Posterior epistaxis, the more serious type, is most commonly caused by a rupture of a sphenopalatine artery branch in the region of the posterior tip of the inferior turbinate. Usually, nasal packing is needed to control the bleeding, particularly in hypertensive persons. The nose should be anesthetized with a lidocaine-based spray. Next, a vasoconstrictive spray (eg, oxymetazoline) should be used. Then an epistaxis balloon should be inserted into the nose and expanded with water until the bleeding is controlled. (Expanding the balloon with water instead of air prevents softening.) The balloon should be left in place for about 5 days, and a prophylactic antibiotic should be administered to prevent sinusitis. Elderly patients should be hospitalized so that their respiratory status and arterial blood gas levels can be monitored.

Gauze packing causes nasal obstruction and often depresses the palate, resulting in a partial obstruction of the oral airway. In most younger patients, such packing is well tolerated, but in the elderly, hypoxia and carbon dioxide retention can occur.

If epistaxis persists despite balloon therapy, two other approaches may be used, depending on the medical expertise available and the patient's condition. The first is transantral ligation of the sphenopalatine artery in the pterygomaxillary space. The second is angiography and embolization of the internal maxillary artery and sphenopalatine artery. After epistaxis has been treated, a full set of sinus x-rays should be obtained to determine if sinusitis has developed or if an underlying tumor is causing the bleeding.

Nasal Fractures

Relatively common in the elderly, nasal fractures result from falls and age-related thinning of facial bones. Treatment by closed reduction usually suffices; this consists of elevating and positioning the bony fragments with a small, nonobstructive nasal packing for about 1 wk (until the fracture has stabilized). During this period, antibiotic administration is needed to prevent sinus infection.

TASTE AND SMELL DISORDERS

(See also Ch. 2 and GUSTATORY DYSFUNCTION in Ch. 52)

Fine taste, such as distinguishing turkey from chicken, is an olfactory function; crude taste, such as distinguishing sweet from sour, is mediated through the taste buds. Age-related losses of the sense of smell and fine taste start in the sixth decade and progress gradually because of neural degeneration. Years of cigarette smoking may accelerate these age-related losses. The incidence of hyposmia and hypogeusia in the elderly has not been thoroughly studied but may be about 40%. The loss of fine taste does not appear to be related to lingual taste or cognition. In the elderly, loss of fine taste and smell may contribute to a lack of interest in food and in maintaining a proper diet and may lead to the harmful excessive use of salt and sugar to overcome the loss of subtle flavors. More hazardous, certain patients lose the ability to smell ethyl mercaptan, the malodorous additive to natural gas that makes gas leaks apparent. Occasionally, patients complain of **dysgeusia,** *an unpleasant taste in the mouth,* or **dysosmia,** *an unpleasant smell.*

Abrupt changes in olfactory sensation can occur after viral nasal infections that affect the olfactory receptors in the superior region of the nose. These changes are usually permanent, although use of zinc sulfate tablets is a suggested, unproved remedy. Abrupt changes in olfactory sensation may also result from head trauma, particularly if the cribriform plate is fractured, and from brain tumors in the region of the cribriform plate.

LARYNGEAL DISORDERS

Laryngeal disorders among the elderly include atrophic laryngitis and reflux laryngitis.

Atrophic Laryngitis

Besides loss of minor salivary gland tissue and moisture in the larynx, elderly persons experience muscle atrophy with decreased vibratory mass, loss of fibrous tissue support, and squamous metaplasia. These changes may cause a chronic tickle in the throat and a constant urge to clear it. Treatment is symptomatic. Lozenges or sugar-free, citrus hard candies can stimulate salivary flow.

Elderly men often complain of a high, trembling, weakened voice, which may be the first sign of the effects of aging on the larynx. A bowing of the vocal cords related to a decrease in elasticity and muscle mass allows increased air escape with phonation. A weakened voice may also be caused by decreased pulmonary volume and expiratory effort. Patients can be instructed to take a deep breath before they speak; doing so corrects the condition momentarily and confirms the diagnosis. A speech therapist may be able to help the patient.

Reflux Laryngitis

This condition is more common with advancing age because older persons are more likely to have impaired esophageal peristalsis and weakened esophageal sphincter tone. Patients who sleep in the recumbent position may experience a burning sensation in the hypopharynx and larynx caused by nocturnal gastric reflux; this sensation must be differentiated from angina. Sleeping with the head elevated often corrects the condition. An H_2-receptor blocker (eg, ranitidine) or a smooth muscle agonist (eg, metoclopramide) may be beneficial.

CRICOARYTENOIDITIS

Inflammation of the cricoarytenoid joint. This condition occurs in elderly arthritic patients. Usually, only those with the severest forms of arthritis are symptomatic, experiencing chronic pain on swallowing and speaking. Laryngeal examination reveals swelling over the arytenoid cartilage and eventual fixation of the joint so that the vocal cords abduct poorly. This condition can result in respiratory distress and may require arytenoidectomy or tracheostomy.

AGE–RELATED PAIN

Elongation of the styloid process and calcification of the stylohyoid ligament can result in intermittent, sharp pain along the distribution of the glossopharyngeal nerve (ie, in the hypopharynx and base of the tongue), known as **Eagle's syndrome.** Glossopharyngeal neuralgia may be caused by scarring of the tonsillar bed from an old tonsillectomy, but tonsillectomy is usually not a precondition in the elderly. Curative treatment consists of resecting the elongated styloid process.

Carotodynia, *neck pain associated with carotid bulb tenderness,* is intensified by palpation and head movement. This self-limiting disorder may last for months; it responds to anti-inflammatory analgesics.

Cervical arthritis often produces chronic neck and occipital pain along the distribution of C-2 and C-3. However, in the elderly, this pain must be differentiated from atypical angina pectoris (intermittent, intense, exercise-related pain in the neck, throat, or jaw). For the pain of cervical arthritis, analgesics and a cervical collar are helpful.

§4. SPECIAL ISSUES

SPI

§4. SPECIAL ISSUES

105. EPIDEMIOLOGY AND DEMOGRAPHICS

The worldwide population of older persons has grown remarkably during the 20th century. Between 1900 and 1990, the total population of the USA increased threefold, while the number of those ≥ 65 yr old increased tenfold. Current and future population characteristics, as well as patterns of mortality, morbidity, disability, and use of health care services, provide a basis for understanding the enormous impact of aging on society. Worldwide demographic data are given in Ch. 106; this chapter focuses on the older population in the USA.

POPULATION CHARACTERISTICS

Several important aspects of the population growth are illustrated in TABLE 105–1. First, the total number of older persons has risen dramatically and will continue to grow rapidly. In 1990, more than 31 million Americans were ≥ 65 yr old, nearly twice the number as in 1960. By 2020, when a large part of the baby boom generation has passed age 65, there will be more than 50 million older Americans; by 2040, this number will exceed 75 million. Second, the proportion of the total population that is ≥ 65 yr old will increase, so that by 2040 one in five persons in the USA will be ≥ 65 yr old.

Finally, the older population itself is getting older. Of all older persons, about 10% are ≥ 85 yr old, and this proportion is projected to rise to over 17% by 2040. This group, often termed the **oldest old,** is the fastest growing segment of the population. Because per capita costs for medical services and long-term care are highest for persons ≥ 85 yr, the growth of this population subgroup will have a marked impact on the health care system.

Older women outnumber older men, more so now than in the past because the mortality rate for women has declined more rapidly than that for men over the past 40 yr. In 1950, there were 89 men for every 100 women ≥ 65 yr old. In 1990, there were only 67 men for every 100 women ≥ 65 yr old. The ratio is even greater for those ≥ 85 yr old, for whom there are 39 men for every 100 women.

The difference in mortality rates of men and women strongly influence family composition and living arrangements. FIG. 105–1 illustrates the rate of widowhood by age, sex, and race. Of those 75 to 84 yr old, 60% of women are widowed. Among those ≥ 85 yr old, black women have the highest rate of widowhood (86%); white men have the lowest rate (42%). Most older persons live with a spouse in a household with no other persons, but living arrangement varies greatly with age and

TABLE 105–1. ACTUAL AND PROJECTED GROWTH OF THE OLDER POPULATION (NUMBERS IN THOUSANDS)

Year	Total Population (all ages)	≥ 65 yr		≥ 85 yr	
		Number	*Percentage of Total*	*Number*	*Percentage of 65+*
1960	179,323	16,560	9.2	929	5.6
1980	226,546	25,550	11.3	2,240	8.8
1990	248,710	31,079	12.5	3,021	9.7
2000	274,815	34,886	12.7	4,289	12.3
2020	322,602	53,627	16.6	6,480	12.1
2040	364,349	75,588	20.7	13,221	17.5

Sources: US Bureau of the Census. *Current Population Reports,* Special Studies, 823-178, Sixty-Five Plus in America. Washington, DC, US Government Printing Office, 1992; and US Bureau of the Census, *Current Population Reports,* P25-1092, Population Projection of the United States, by Age, Sex, Race, and Hispanic Origin: 1992 to 2050. Washington, DC, US Government Printing Office, 1992.

sex (see FIG. 105–2). Even at the younger old ages, 1/3 of women live alone; after age 75 > 1/2 of women live alone (see Ch. 107). Before age 85, living with relatives other than a spouse or with nonrelatives is uncommon; after age 85, 1/4 of community-dwelling men and 1/3 of community-dwelling women have these living arrangements.

As the proportion of elderly to young persons increases, less financial and social support will be available for older persons. The **elderly support ratio** (the number of persons ≥ 65 yr for every 100 persons age 20 to 64) was 21.3 in 1990. This ratio should remain stable through 2010 and then will begin to increase steadily, a result of both the baby boom generation reaching age 65 and the low birth rates of the 1960s and 1970s. By 2030, the elderly support ratio is projected to reach 40.

As with the total US population, the older population today is more racially diverse and has a greater proportion of Hispanic persons than in the past. The black and white older populations increased by about 20% from 1980 to 1990, compared with a 57% increase for Hispanics and a 150% increase for Orientals. In 1990, 90% of the older population was white; this proportion should decrease to about 80% by 2040.

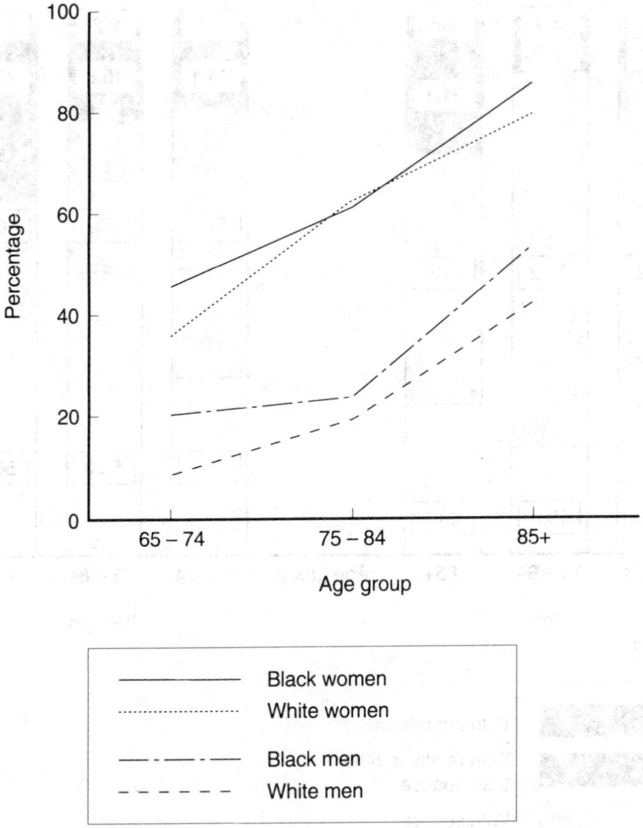

FIG. 105–1. Percentage of persons ≥ 65 yr old who are widowed. (Source: Saluter AF, US Bureau of the Census, Marital status and living arrangements: March 1990, *Current Population Reports,* Series P-20, No. 450. Washington, DC, US Government Printing Office, May 1991.)

The geographic distribution and migration patterns of older persons in the USA have important implications for health and long-term care services. In 1990, > 3 million elderly persons resided in California, > 2 million lived in New York and Florida, and > 1 million lived in Pennsylvania, Texas, Illinois, Ohio, Michigan, and New Jersey. State populations with the highest proportion of persons ≥ 65 yr old (≥ 14%) were Florida, Rhode Island, Pennsylvania, North Dakota, South Dakota, Nebraska, Iowa, Missouri, and Arkansas. Many elderly persons move

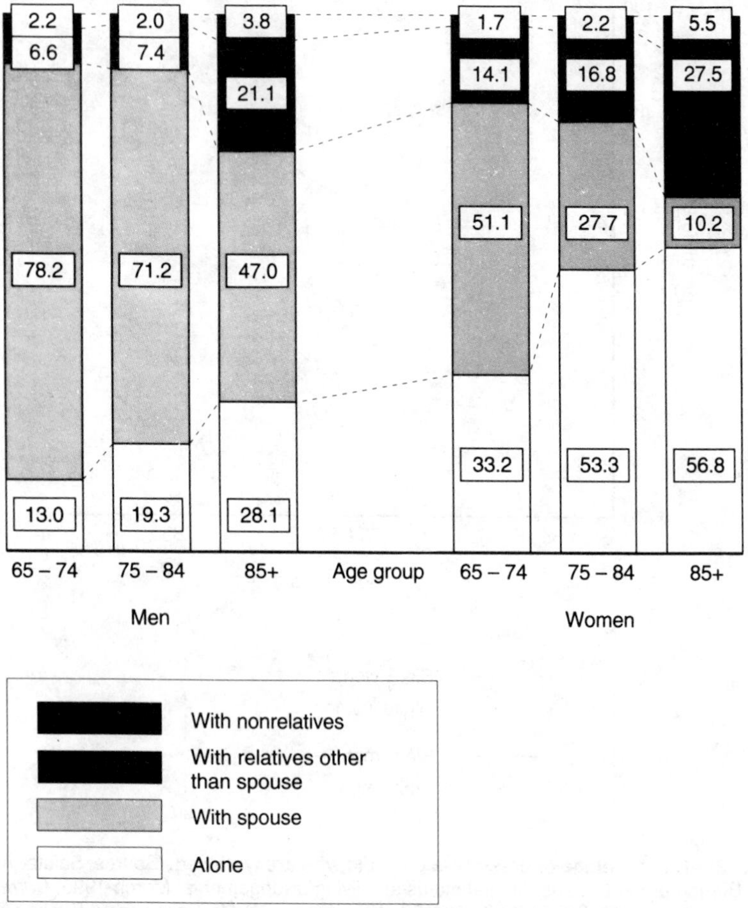

FIG. 105–2. Living arrangements of community-dwelling persons ≥ 65 yr old. (Source: Saluter AF, US Bureau of the Census, Marital status and living arrangements: March 1990, *Current Population Reports,* Series P-20, No. 450. Washington, DC, US Government Printing Office, May 1991.)

to Florida; the high proportion of elderly persons in the other states is primarily the result of younger persons moving out of those states. However, the impact on the need for services is ultimately the same.

The number of older persons in all states increased in the 1980s. Between 1980 and 1990, the greatest proportional increases occurred in

TABLE 105–2. LIFE EXPECTANCY AT SPECIFIED AGES IN 1990

	Male			*Female*		
Age	*All*	*White*	*Black*	*All*	*White*	*Black*
At birth	71.8 yr	72.7 yr	64.5 yr	78.8 yr	79.4 yr	73.6 yr
At 65 yr	15.1 yr	15.2 yr	13.2 yr	18.9 yr	19.1 yr	17.2 yr
At 75 yr	9.4 yr	9.4 yr	8.6 yr	12.0 yr	12.0 yr	11.2 yr
At 85 yr	5.2 yr	5.2 yr	5.0 yr	6.4 yr	6.4 yr	6.3 yr

Source: National Center for Health Statistics. Vital Statistics of the US, 1990, Vol II, Mortality, Part A. Hyattsville, MD, Public Health Service, 1990.

Nevada (94.1%), Alaska (93.7%), Hawaii (64.2%), Arizona (55.8%), New Mexico (40.7%), and Florida (40.4%). The regional relocation of younger elderly to the South and West has occurred since the 1960s and that of older elderly, since the 1970s. Many retirement areas may not have provisions for the kinds of services these people will need as they reach the oldest ages.

MORTALITY AND MORBIDITY

Life expectancy has increased dramatically at all ages, although gains for those ≥ 65 yr old have come mainly since 1940. Between 1900 and 1940, life expectancy at birth rose by nearly 14 yr, whereas life expectancy at age 65 increased by < 1 yr. Life expectancy at age 65 increased nearly 2 yr between 1940 and 1954, remained stable between 1954 and 1968, and rose steadily between 1968 and 1990 from 14.6 yr to 17.2 yr, a remarkable gain of 2.6 yr over this 22-yr period.

TABLE 105–2 shows life expectancy in 1990 according to age, sex, and race. Overall, women live 7 yr longer than men, although this sex differential is 9 yr for blacks. At birth, life expectancy for whites is about 6 to 8 yr longer than for blacks. At age 65, white women can expect to live an additional 19 yr, compared with 15 yr for white men. Life expectancy for blacks at age 65 is about 2 yr less than that for whites, but life expectancy is nearly equal at age 85. Women who reach age 85 can expect to live an additional 6 yr, men an additional 5 yr.

TABLE 105–3. THE TEN LEADING CAUSES OF DEATH AMONG PERSONS AGE ≥ 65 IN 1990

Cause of Death	*Number of Deaths*	*Death Rate (per 100,000 population)*	*Percentage of All Deaths in Those ≥ 65 yr Old*
All causes	1,542,493	4,963.2	100.0
1. Heart disease	594,858	1,914.0	38.6
2. Malignant neoplasms, including neoplasms of lymphatic and hematopoietic tissues	345,387	1,111.3	22.4
3. Cerebrovascular diseases	125,409	403.5	8.1
4. Chronic obstructive pulmonary disease and associated conditions	72,755	234.1	4.7
5. Pneumonia and influenza	70,485	226.8	4.6
6. Diabetes mellitus	35,523	114.3	2.3
7. Accidents and adverse effects	26,213	84.3	1.7
Motor vehicle accidents	7,210	23.2	0.5
All other accidents and adverse effects	19,003	61.1	1.2
8. Nephritis, nephrotic syndrome, and nephrosis	17,306	55.7	1.1
9. Atherosclerosis	17,158	55.2	1.1
10. Septicemia	15,351	49.4	1.0
All other causes, residual	222,048	2,045.9	14.4

Source: National Center for Health Statistics, Advanced report of final mortality statistics, 1990. Monthly Vital Statistics Report Vol. 41, No. 7, Suppl. Hyattsville, MD, Public Health Service, 1993.

The ten leading causes of death in 1990 for persons ≥ 65 yr old are shown in TABLE 105–3. The overall death rate was nearly 5/100/yr. Of the 1.5 million deaths that occurred in this age group, nearly 600,000 (38.6%) were from heart disease, 345,000 (22.4%) were from cancer, and 125,000 (8.1%) were from cerebrovascular diseases. These three diseases account for 69% of all deaths in older persons. Data must be interpreted carefully, especially in the oldest old group, because multiple chronic conditions are common and the physician's designation of the underlying cause of death may be somewhat arbitrary. To increase knowledge of the aging population as life expectancy continues to rise and many more people die at advanced old age, physicians need to be more specific in completing death certificates. For example, a more complete listing of all the diseases contributing to death would allow more thorough analyses of the cause of death. In many cases, an autopsy would help explain the chain of events leading to death.

The importance of heart disease as a cause of death is illustrated in FIG. 105–3. Mortality rates from heart disease rise exponentially after age 55, with heart disease responsible for a greater proportion of deaths at each higher age. Death rates for cerebrovascular diseases and pneumonia and influenza also rise exponentially with age. In contrast, death rates for cancer and chronic obstructive pulmonary disease rise modestly after age 65. In those ≥ 85 yr old, deaths from cerebrovascular diseases nearly equal deaths from cancer; deaths from pneumonia and influenza surpass those from chronic obstructive pulmonary disease and are the fourth leading cause of death.

The increase in life expectancy is largely attributable to substantial declines in the number of deaths from heart disease and stroke since the late 1960s. The mortality rate for stroke has dropped more rapidly than that for heart disease. Declines in mortality rates for heart disease and stroke in the older population have kept pace with those in the total population. Between 1979 and 1990, death rates for ischemic heart disease dropped 33% in those 65 to 74, 29% in those 75 to 84, and 16% in those ≥ 85. Declines in mortality rates for cerebrovascular diseases in these three age groups ranged from 37% to 28%.

In contrast, cancer mortality rates have risen slightly. Between 1979 and 1990, cancer mortality rates increased 3.2% in the total population, 9% in those 65 to 74, 12% in those 75 to 84, and 15% in those ≥ 85. As heart disease and stroke cause fewer deaths, more persons must die at a later age of other diseases, such as cancer.

The incidence of newly diagnosed cancer increases for most cancers through age 85. FIG. 105–4 shows the incidence of the three leading cancers in older men and women. The incidence of prostate cancer exceeds that of all other cancers in men by age 65 and rises to an incidence of > 1/100/yr after age 80. Breast cancer is the leading cancer in women at all older ages. Colon cancer is the second leading cancer in men at age 85 and in women at age 75. Lung cancer incidence peaks in men in the early 80s and in women in the early 70s. This decrease in incidence at the oldest ages may be a cohort effect, since the oldest segments of the population comprise relatively fewer current or past smokers; additionally, smokers may die of cancer and other smoking-related diseases at younger ages.

Although longevity has increased, whether the added years of life are full of health and vigor or disease and disability is unknown. This ques-

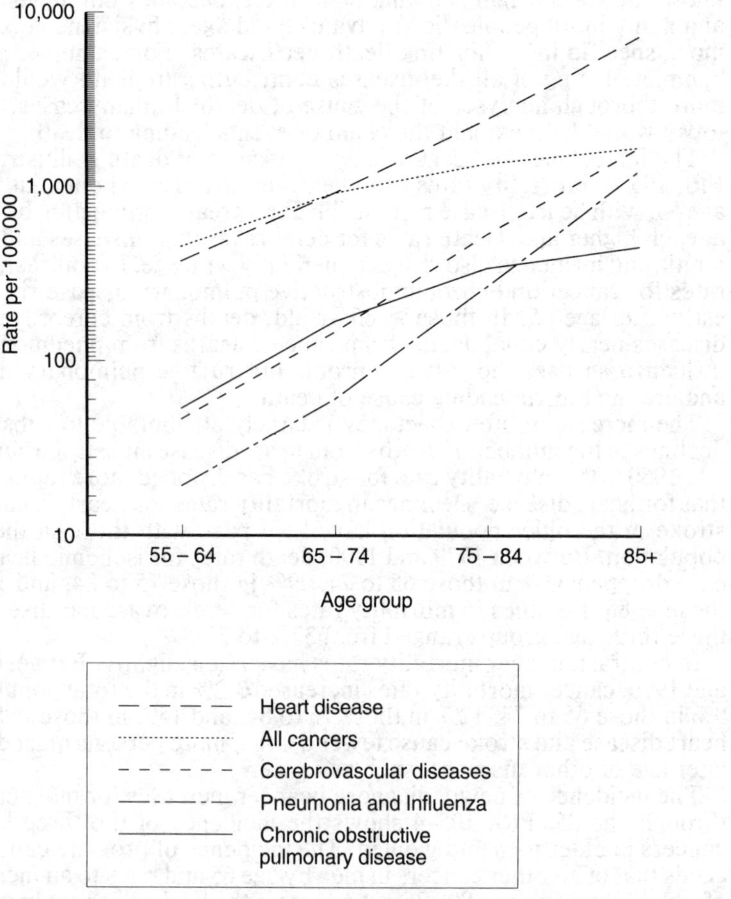

FIG. 105–3. Age-specific mortality rates for five leading causes of death in persons ≥ 55 yr old. (Source: National Center for Health Statistics, Advanced report of final mortality statistics, 1990. Monthly Vital Statistics Report Vol. 41, No. 7, Suppl. Hyattsville, MD, Public Health Service, 1993.)

tion is of particular concern because increases in life expectancy and in the numbers of old and very old persons are expected to continue. The term **compression of morbidity** refers to the theory that with better disease prevention and treatment, the period between the onset of severe disability and death can be compressed into fewer years. This is some-

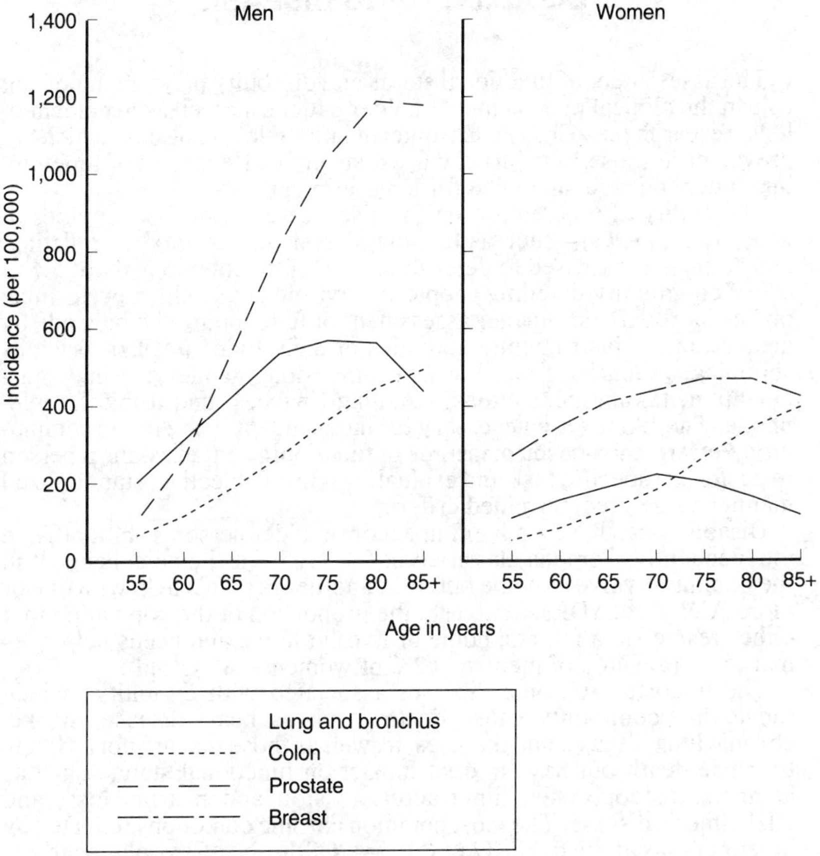

FIG. 105–4. Annual age-specific incidence rates of the three leading cancers in men and women ≥ 55 yr old. (Source: National Cancer Institute SEER Program, 1985–1989.)

times referred to as squaring the morbidity curve. There is contradictory evidence as to whether a compression of morbidity is occurring.

An important tool for evaluating compression of morbidity is what has been termed active, or disability-free, life expectancy. **Active life expectancy** is the average number of years a person is likely to remain in an active or nondisabled state and is calculated using life expectancy table techniques that consider all possible transitions into and out of the disabled state.

DISABILITY AND DISEASE

The assessment of functional status and disability plays an important role in the clinical management of older patients as well as in epidemiologic research (see Ch. 17). Chronic and multiple conditions, which are prevalent in those living to late ages, strongly affect level of functioning, independence, and need for long-term care.

The ability of a person to perform self-care, known as activities of daily living **(ADLs)**—such as bathing, dressing, transferring, toileting, and eating—is assessed to determine level of functioning. About 5% to 8% of community-dwelling people ≥ 65 yr old need help in performing one or more ADLs. Further assessment of functioning can be made by measuring the instrumental activities of daily living **(IADLs)**—such as shopping, preparing food, housekeeping, doing laundry, using transportation, taking medications, handling finances, and using the telephone. The IADLs are necessary for independent living in the community. **Performance-based measures** of functioning entail asking a person to perform a specific task and evaluating it in an objective, standardized manner using predetermined criteria.

Disability can have a major impact on an older person's ability to live independently. Persons classified in FIG. 105–5 as being dependent in the community live at home but need another person's help with one or more ADLs or IADLs. With age, the proportion of the population that either resides in a nursing home or lives at home and needs help rises markedly (eg, 46% of men and 62% of women ≥ 85 yr old).

The important chronic diseases associated with disability include those that commonly cause death, such as heart disease, stroke, chronic lung disease, and diabetes, as well as those that are not as likely to cause death but have a great impact on functional status, such as arthritis, osteoporosis, hip fracture, vision and hearing loss, and Alzheimer's disease. The most common chronic conditions reported by older persons are listed in TABLE 105–4. Of those ≥ 65 yr old, nearly ½ report having arthritis, over ⅓ report having hypertension, and nearly ⅓ report having hearing impairment or heart disease. Some diseases (eg, stroke) are less common but have a profound effect on function.

The prevalence of concurrent multiple chronic diseases **(comorbidity)** increases with age, and at the oldest ages comorbidity occurs in most people. The prevalence of disability increases stepwise with age and the number of chronic conditions. The burden of morbidity and disability is of great concern to society in planning, financing, and delivering health care and social services to the older population. If current prevalence rates of disabling diseases such as arthritis, hip fracture, and Alzheimer's disease remain unchanged, the numbers of older people

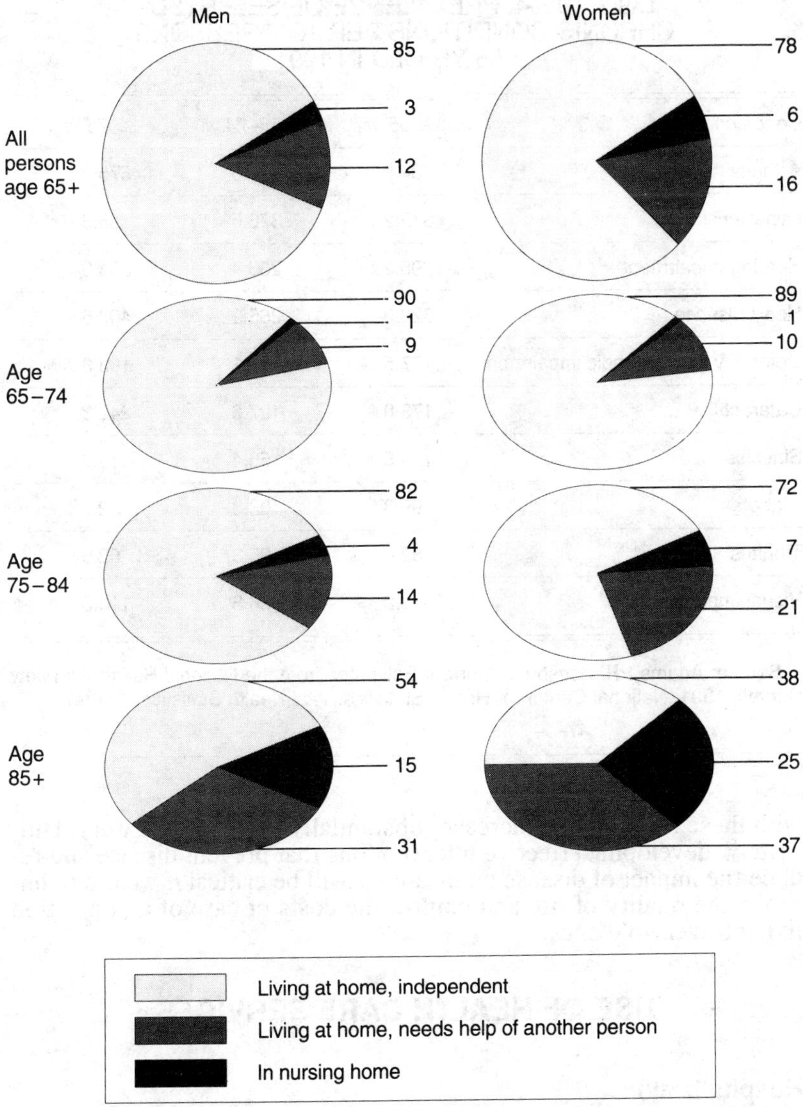

FIG. 105–5. Percentage of the older population that lives at home independently, lives at home but requires the help of another person, or resides in a nursing home. (Source: Schneider EL, Guralnik JM: "The aging of America: Impact on health care costs." *Journal of the American Medical Association* 263:2335–2340; 1990.)

TABLE 105–4. PREVALENCE OF SELECTED CHRONIC CONDITIONS PER 1000 PERSONS ≥ 65 YR OLD IN 1991

Condition	*≥ 65 yr*	*65–74 yr*	*≥ 75 yr*
Arthritis	484.8	425.6	575.2
Hypertension	372.2	376.6	365.5
Hearing impairment	295.2	256.4	354.3
Heart disease	320.5	266.2	403.6
Deformity or orthopedic impairment	177.5	167.1	193.3
Cataracts	173.0	127.6	242.3
Sinusitis	139.5	156.4	113.7
Diabetes	99.3	103.8	92.6
Tinnitus	82.4	95.3	62.6
Visual impairment	79.2	56.8	113.3

Source: Adams PF, Benson V: Current Estimates from the National Health Interview Survey, 1991. National Center for Health Statistics. Vital Health Statistics 10(184).

with these diseases will increase substantially in the next century. Ultimately, developing effective interventions that prevent disease and reduce the impact of disease on disability will be critical if we are to improve the quality of life and control the costs of care of a population living to very old ages.

USE OF HEALTH CARE SERVICES

Hospitalization

Persons ≥ 65 yr old accounted for 1/3 of the 30 million hospitalizations in 1989 and spent over 90 million days in the hospital. TABLE 105–5 shows the six leading causes of hospitalization for men and women ≥ 65 and ≥ 85 yr old. Discharge rates and length of stay are shown for 1981 and 1987. These data include hospitalizations for both those discharged alive and those who died during their hospital stay.

TABLE 105–5. DISCHARGE RATE AND AVERAGE LENGTH OF STAY FOR SIX LEADING DISCHARGE DIAGNOSES IN 1981 AND 1987

	Persons ≥ 65 Yr Old				Persons ≥ 85 Yr Old			
	Discharge Rate (per 1000 population)		*Length of Stay (days)*		*Discharge Rate (per 1000 population)*		*Length of Stay (days)*	
First-Listed Discharge Diagnosis	*1981*	*1987*	*1981*	*1987*	*1981*	*1987*	*1981*	*1987*
Men								
Heart disease	82.2	87.0	9.9	7.3	131.1	119.4	10.7	7.1
Malignant neoplasms	47.9	40.0	12.8	9.3	56.7	43.6	13.4	10.0
Cerebrovascular disease	23.8	22.5	12.2	9.1	45.7	47.0	11.6	8.6
Pneumonia, all forms	13.4	18.4	11.7	9.8	46.4	56.0	11.9	9.6
Hyperplasia of prostate	17.1	17.0	9.3	5.7	18.0	21.5	14.6	8.2
Fractures, all sites	7.6	8.0	16.0	12.0	30.0	24.4	15.9	12.9
Women								
Heart disease	66.8	66.9	10.4	7.6	108.4	104.1	11.5	8.0
Malignant neoplasms	30.8	26.4	12.9	9.5	27.7	22.9	14.1	12.5
Cerebrovascular disease	21.8	22.1	13.4	10.7	43.6	43.2	14.5	10.8
Fractures, all sites	18.6	17.3	16.6	11.7	49.2	46.7	19.4	12.9
Pneumonia, all forms	10.3	12.6	11.3	10.1	27.1	31.6	11.8	10.7
Cholelithiasis	6.3	6.0	12.0	9.2				
Volume depletion, dehydration					10.7	15.9	11.5	12.9

Source: National Center for Health Statistics, National Hospital Discharge Surveys, 1981 and 1987.

For men and women ≥ 65 yr old, heart disease, cancer, and stroke were the leading causes of hospitalization. Heart disease was also the leading cause of hospitalization in those ≥ 85; however, in 1987, the second leading cause of hospitalization was pneumonia in men and fractures in women. Prostate disease and fractures were also important causes of hospitalization in men. Interestingly, volume depletion was the sixth leading cause of hospitalization in 1987 for women ≥ 85 yr old. Length of stay was substantially reduced between 1981 and 1987, a result of changes in methods of reimbursement for Medicare patients.

Cardiac diagnostic and surgical procedures are becoming more common in persons ≥ 65 yr old. For example, between 1981 and 1987, the rate of cardiac catheterization and coronary artery bypass graft surgery increased threefold for both men and women. For men ≥ 65 yr old, the most common hospital procedures were prostatectomy, cardiac catheterization, and coronary artery bypass graft surgery. For women ≥ 65 yr old, the procedures most frequently performed were fracture reduction, cardiac catheterization, and hip replacement. For men ≥ 85 yr old, the leading procedures were prostatectomy, pacemaker insertion, and fracture reduction. For women ≥ 85 yr old, fracture reduction, hip replacement, and pacemaker insertion were most common.

Outpatient Visits

Persons ≥ 65 yr of age made over 150 million visits to physicians' offices in 1989, representing 22% of all visits. Those age 65 to 74 made an average of 4.7 visits per year, and those ≥ age 75 made 5.9 visits per year. General medical examination, postoperative visit, vision dysfunction, blood pressure testing, hypertension, and cough were the most common reasons for visits, according to physicians in the National Ambulatory Medical Care Survey. The most common diagnoses in both the group age 65 to 74 and the group ≥ 75 included hypertension, diabetes, cataract, chronic ischemic heart disease, osteoarthritis and associated disorders, and glaucoma.

Institutionalization

About 5% of the older population resides in nursing homes at any point in time. Only 1% of men and women age 65 to 74 reside in nursing homes, but 15% of men and 25% of women ≥ 85 yr old do so (see FIG. 105–5). However, prevalence rates at a given point do not indicate the chance of being in a nursing home over the course of a lifetime. Among those turning 65, 52% of women and 33% of men will spend some time in a nursing home. Among women who die after age 89, 70% have lived in a nursing home for at least some time. Among all those using nursing homes, 45% will spend < 1 yr and 55% will spend ≥ 1 yr; 21% will spend ≥ 5 yr (see also Chs. 24 and 25).

In 1990, about 1.5 million older persons in the USA lived in nursing homes. Of this population, 75% were women, 16% were age 65 to 74, 39% were age 75 to 84, and 45% were age ≥ 85. Nursing home patients are often cognitively or physically impaired. About 63% of residents are disoriented or have impaired memory, 92% need help with one or more ADLs, 46% have difficulty controlling bowels or bladder, and 47% are confined to a wheelchair or bed.

Risk factors for institutionalization include being widowed; living alone; having reduced family and social support, lower income, mental disorientation or cognitive impairment, and an increased number of medical conditions; being disabled in ADLs or IADLs; and needing an aid for ambulation. Nursing home admission rates for blacks are lower than those for whites, suggesting that factors such as cultural preferences and access to care may be involved.

Use of Services in the Last Year of Life

Over 25% of total Medicare expenditures for a given year go to enrollees who, it turned out, were in the last year of life. In fact, health care expenditures for persons in this group are seven times higher than those for other enrollees. However, Medicare covers only a portion of a person's health care costs. For example, in the last year of life, Medicare pays for only about 1/3 of all care expenses. Expenditures and use of health services in the last year of life are also related to the cause of death. For example, Medicare expenditures in the last year of life are about twice as high for those dying of cancer as for those dying of heart disease or stroke.

106. A CROSS–NATIONAL PERSPECTIVE

The elderly are a challenge to health care providers around the world. Not only is the number of elderly persons rising exponentially, but also health care for this population group is often complicated by many complex clinical problems. Resources, especially in developing countries, are often scarce.

DEMOGRAPHIC ISSUES

Among industrialized countries in 1990, Sweden had the highest proportion of elderly persons, with 17.9% of its population > 65 yr. Other countries with a high proportion of elderly persons were Norway (16.3%), the United Kingdom (15.7%), and Denmark (15.6%). The USA (12.6%) and Canada (11.5%) have a greater proportion of younger persons than Hungary, Germany, Austria, Italy, and Greece. In 1990, the proportion of elderly persons in Japan was 11.5%; Japan will have the greatest proportion of elderly persons by the year 2020 (25.7%). Although the relative number of older persons is higher in developed countries, the number of those in less developed countries is growing rapidly; by the year 2025, > 2/3 of the world's older citizens will reside in poorer regions.

Worldwide, the older population is growing at a rate of 2.4%/yr, much faster than the overall population. Between 1975 and 2025, the percentage of persons > 60 yr old is projected to increase by 224%, compared with only 102% for the general population. For example, in 1950, about 200 million people in the world were > 60 yr of age. In 1975, the number was about 350 million. According to United Nations estimates, the number of older persons is expected to reach 590 million by the year 2000, rising to > 1 billion by the year 2025. Furthermore, in 1985, 23 countries had populations that included > 2 million elders; by 2025, the number of countries with this many older citizens will increase to about 50. They will include Burma, Egypt, Korea, Malaysia, and Zaire, countries not normally considered to be demographically mature.

LIFE EXPECTANCY

The percentage of increased life expectancy at age 65 has surpassed the percentage of that measured from birth, partly because of fewer deaths from heart disease and stroke. For example, in Japan, life expectancy at birth increased 12% between 1960 and 1980 (and in 1985 was the highest in the world at 77.1 yr); during the same period, the life expectancy at age 65 increased 26%, rising to 17.7 yr. Many other countries have seen similar gains in life expectancy, although adult life expectancy in some countries (mainly in Eastern Europe) has actually declined recently. However, much remains to be done to ensure that extra years are spent independently (see CLINICAL ISSUES, below).

THE OLD–OLD POPULATION

Another important demographic index relates to the proportion of elderly persons > 80 yr of age, who are categorized as the **old-old.** The proportion of those > 80 depends in part on the fertility patterns of 60 yr ago. In 1990, 14% of the elderly population worldwide (19% in developed and 11% in developing regions) were > 80 (see TABLE 106–1). Furthermore, the worldwide percentage will rise rapidly over the next 15 yr. Brazil's old-old population will grow fastest, followed by that of China, Japan, and Bulgaria (see TABLE 106–2). However, by the end of this century, the USA will have the largest proportion of old-old population, with 31% of its elderly being > 80 yr old.

The old-old require disproportionately more health and social services. Given the costs of properly caring for all older persons, the challenge to already overburdened societies will be immense. In some African countries, where the AIDS epidemic is ravaging the population of young adults, some authorities believe that within a decade, the very young and the elderly will make up the largest part of the population.

TABLE 106–1. COUNTRIES WITH MORE THAN ONE MILLION OCTOGENARIANS IN 1985

Country	*Population Aged ≥ 80 (000s)*	*Country*	*Population Aged ≥ 80 (000s)*
United States	6,198	Germany (Fed. Rep.)	1,951
China	5,697	France	1,741
Soviet Union	4,610	United Kingdom	1,732
India	2,913	Italy	1,436
Japan	2,000		

From Torrey BB, Kinsella K, Taeuber CM: "An aging world," in *International Population Reports, Series P-95, No. 78*. U.S. Dept. of Commerce, Bureau of the Census, 1987, p 11.

HEALTH CARE EXPENDITURES

Growing health care costs have put pressure on governments around the world. From 1967 to 1987, total health care expenditures as a percentage of gross domestic product nearly doubled—from 3.8% to 7.4%—for the 23 countries represented in the Organization for Economic Cooperation and Development (OECD). In 1987, the mean health care expenditure per person in OECD countries was $934, with $2051 for the USA, $1483 for Canada, $1233 for Sweden, and $1105 for France. Not surprisingly, lower expenditures were reported for poorer countries such as Greece, Turkey, Portugal, and Spain. However, both the United Kingdom and New Zealand had expenditures that were lower than the OECD average.

In contrast to the sharp increases in the USA, health care expenditures as a percentage of gross domestic product have stabilized in Canada and in many European countries. Furthermore, the aging of the population alone does not explain the bulk of the increases in the USA, despite the fact that throughout the developed world, per capita expenses are greater for the elderly than for the younger population. In all developed countries, other factors are at work (eg, increases in the population that is eligible for medical entitlements, as well as a significant increase in real benefits).

TABLE 106–2. COUNTRIES PROJECTED TO HAVE MORE THAN ONE MILLION OCTOGENARIANS IN 2025

Country	*Population Aged ≥ 80 (000s)*	*Country*	*Population Aged ≥ 80 (000s)*
China	25,208	United Kingdom	2,211
India	16,435	France	2,111
United States	14,348	Mexico	1,894
Ex-Soviet Union	9,966	Spain	1,491
Japan	6,531	Poland	1,243
Brazil	3,672	Canada	1,235
Indonesia	3,324	Nigeria	1,135
Germany (Fed. Rep.)	2,855	Turkey	1,043
Italy	2,485	Argentina	1,002

From Torrey BB, Kinsella K, Taeuber CM: "An aging world," in *International Population Reports, Series P-95, No. 78*. U.S. Dept. of Commerce, Bureau of the Census, 1987, p 11.

CLINICAL ISSUES

The elderly tend to suffer disproportionately from many chronic disorders, including cancer, cardiovascular diseases, dementia, incontinence, and musculoskeletal problems. Cross-national comparisons offer insights into the epidemiology and etiology of many conditions as well as into the differences in care patterns. This discussion focuses on two disorders—hip fracture and dementia—and then on quality of life and long-term care issues.

HIP FRACTURE

An estimated 1.66 million hip fractures occurred worldwide in 1990—half of them in Europe and North America. While the numbers

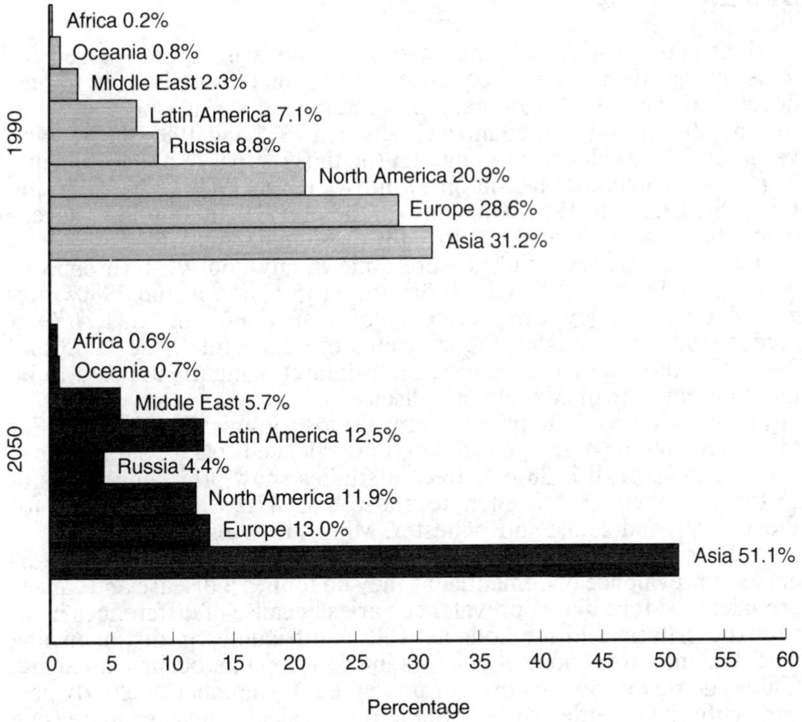

FIG. 106–1. Regional distribution of hip fractures in women ≥ 65 yr of age that occurred in 1990 and are projected to occur in 2050. Russia = the former Soviet Union. (From Cooper G, Campion G, Melton LJ III: "Hip fractures in the elderly: A world-wide projection." *Osteoporosis International* 2:285–289, 1992; used with permission of Springer-Verlag.)

are projected to increase to 3.94 million by 2025 and to 6.26 million by 2050, the geographic distribution of hip fracture is also projected to change significantly. Up to 75% of hip fractures are expected to occur in Asia, Latin America, the Middle East, and Russia (see FIG. 106–1), probably because of age structure, ethnic, dietary, and climate differences. These countries have fewer resources to deal with the problem.

Major interventions such as improvements in nutrition, the widespread use of estrogen replacement therapy, or the development of other treatments are unlikely to be affordable or widely available in less developed regions. Therefore, preventive strategies will have to be applied according to the needs, resources, and cultures of different countries.

DEMENTIA

Alzheimer's disease and the related dementias are already a tremendous burden to developed countries and an increasing burden to less developed regions. A summary of 46 studies done around the world (but mostly in Western countries) between 1945 and 1985 shows wide variation in prevalence of dementia for those ≥ 65 yr of age, ranging from 1.3% (severe dementia only) in Sweden in 1969 to 20.3% in the USA (St. Louis) in 1984. On average, the prevalence of mild to severe dementia worldwide is about 10% for those ≥ 65 yr.

Until recently, few studies were done in any non-Western country other than Japan. Although studies done in China in the 1980s suggested a surprisingly low prevalence of dementia (0.46% to 1.86%), a recent study in Shanghai reports rates of 12.3% for those > 75 and 24.3% for those > 85. In Japan, multi-infarct dementia appears to be more common than Alzheimer's disease.

The prevalence of dementia increases logarithmically with age. For those aged 60 to 64 yr, the estimated prevalence is 0.7%, but for those aged 90 to 95 yr, it is 38.6%. Recent studies show prevalence rates of 28.8% in Gothenberg, Sweden, for those ≥ 85; 47.2% in East Boston for those ≥ 80; and 25.3% in Rochester, Minn., for those ≥ 80.

Biologic and ethnic differences may account for some of the differences in prevalence of dementia, as they do for heart disease and cancer prevalence. More likely, prevalence varies because of differences in diagnostic criteria and methods as well as difficulties in distinguishing true dementia from normal changes in cognition that occur with aging. Unless dementia can be cured or prevented, the number of elderly persons with the disorder will continue to rise, placing an ever-increasing burden on caregivers, societies, and health care systems around the world.

QUALITY OF LIFE

Home and family situations, satisfaction with life, employment and health status, and availability and use of health care services all have an impact on quality of life. A recent study conducted in five countries (Canada, Germany, Great Britain, Japan, and the USA) of 900 elderly people in each country living at home disclosed the following information.

Many older persons live alone. The percentage is highest in Germany at 46%, followed by 40% in Canada, 34% in Britain, and 31% in the USA. In these four countries, 70% of elderly persons reported visiting or being visited by a family member within the previous week. In Japan, most older persons live with their families; only 10% live alone. Interestingly, in Japan, adult children often live in their parents' home rather than vice versa. In all five countries, most of the elderly have close-knit families, and > 80% have children who are still alive.

TABLE 106–3. SETTINGS FOR LONG–TERM CARE SERVICES*

Country	*Service Setting*
Australia	Nursing homes, hostels (residential settings), and home care; emphasis is on home (domiciliary) care
Canada	Chronic care or rehabilitation hospitals, extended care facilities (nursing homes), and home care
China	Hospitals; government, collective, employer-owned, or private institutions; and home care; emphasis is on informal caregiving
England	Long-term geriatric hospitals, nursing homes, residential homes, and home (domiciliary) care
France	Hospitals, including psychiatric, nursing homes, residential facilities, and home care
Germany	General-purpose hospitals, specialty hospitals, nursing homes, old-age homes, and home nursing care
Japan	General-purpose hospitals (used for long stays), geriatric hospitals, geriatric health facilities, and nursing homes
Sweden	Long-term care hospitals, nursing homes, residential settings (service houses), and home care
United States	Rehabilitation hospitals, nursing homes, and home nursing care

*This table shows the array of service settings listed by order of intensity of care rather than by frequency.

From Jazwiecki T, Schwab T: "Conclusion," in *International Models for Long-Term Care, Financing and Delivery*, edited by T Schwab. New York, McGraw-Hill, 1989, p 370; used with permission.

Life satisfaction is high, with 61% of older Americans and 58% of Canadians (compared with 49% of Britons, 40% of Germans, and 28% of Japanese) describing themselves as very satisfied with life. Japan has the highest percentage (28%) of those still employed after age 65, compared with 3% of those in Germany.

Maintaining independence is rated as highly important in all five countries. If they were to become disabled by stroke or another serious illness, most elderly persons would prefer to remain at home: 71% of Americans, 69% of Britons, 59% of Germans, 51% of Canadians, and

48% of Japanese expressed this desire. However, in case of severe disability, < 10% of all respondents want to receive long-term care from a family member.

Satisfaction with health care services was expressed by 55% of elderly Canadians, 45% of Americans, and only 19% of Japanese. However, elderly persons in the USA were the only group to express significant apprehension as to the cost of health care. While < 5% of older persons in Britain, Canada, Germany, and Japan thought that the cost of health care was the most serious threat to their well-being, 27% of Americans expressed this concern.

LONG–TERM CARE

Among industrialized countries, Canada and Sweden have well-developed (although imperfect) systems of long-term care. The USA is unique in that its long-term health care system does not protect the elderly against either chronic disability or impoverishment. The phenomenon of spending down to become eligible for government-paid long-term care is found only in the USA.

TABLE 106–3 lists the long-term care options available in various developed countries. Very few formal arrangements for long-term care exist in less developed countries. TABLE 106–4 depicts variations among the rates of long-term institutionalization in several countries. The percentage of elderly needing institutional care varies from < 2% in Hungary to almost 11% in the Netherlands.

Use of nonmedical facilities (eg, a home for the aged or sheltered housing) also varies significantly. In European countries, commitment to provide nonmedical residential care and coordinated community services contrasts greatly to what is available in much of the USA. Despite cultural and other similarities between the USA and Canada, the two

TABLE 106–4. RATES OF LONG–TERM INSTITUTIONAL USE FOR PERSONS ≥ 65 YR OLD

Country	*Year*	*Total*	*Medical Facilities*	*Nonmedical Facilities*
United States	1985	5.7	4.5	1.2
Canada	1980*	8.7	7.1	1.6
Belgium	1982	6.3	2.6	3.7

(continued)

TABLE 106–4. RATES OF LONG–TERM INSTITUTIONAL USE FOR PERSONS ≥ 65 YR OLD *(Continued)*

Country	*Year*	*Total*	*Medical Facilities*	*Nonmedical Facilities*
Denmark	1984*	7.0	N/A	N/A
France	1982	6.3	5.3	1.0
Federal Republic of Germany	1980	4.1	2.4	1.7
Great Britain†	1981	4.0	N/A	N/A
Hungary	1984	1.9	N/A	N/A
Ireland‡	1982	3.6	N/A	N/A
Netherlands	1982–83	10.9	2.9	8.0
Sweden	1980	9.6	4.6	5.0
Switzerland	1982	8.9	2.8	6.1
Australia	1981	6.4	4.9	1.5
Japan	1981	3.9	3.1	0.8
Israel	1981	4.0	1.4	2.6

* Approximate date.

† 1981 census data indicate that 3% of the elderly were "usually resident" in communal establishments (mainly homes for the elderly but also hospitals, hostels, and hotels); another 1% was present in such places (usually hospitals), though not usually resident.

‡ Excludes elderly in general hospitals.

N/A = not available.

Notes: For reasons of definition, coverage, and temporal reference, rates of institutional use may not be well suited to comparison across nations. Hence, differences between figures in this table should be taken as roughly indicative of different national propensities toward institutional use. Generally, a national use rate reflects the percentage of all elderly persons resident in institutional settings at a particular point in time.

From Suzman R, Kinsella KG, Myers GC: "Demography of older populations in developed countries," in *Oxford Textbook of Geriatric Medicine*, edited by JG Evans and TF Williams. Oxford, Oxford University Press, 1992, p 10; used by permission of Oxford University Press.

countries differ greatly in how they care for the elderly. With respect to payment for long-term care, the average Canadian is far better off than his American counterpart because all Canadians are eligible for such care regardless of income.

Many governments are being pressured to provide more institutional care for the frail elderly. Projections of increases in this population and in the costs of institutionalized care have precipitated an intense debate over the ideal number of beds for such care.

107. LIVING ALONE

About 1/3 of the nearly 30 million noninstitutionalized elderly persons in the USA live alone. The very old are most likely to live alone; almost half of those > 85 yr old do so. Of the elderly living alone, 78% are women. Married men are more likely to die before their wives, and widowed and divorced men are more likely to remarry than are widowed and divorced women.

Elderly persons living alone represent one of the most vulnerable and impoverished segments of American society. Because living alone complicates the aging experience and presents a particular array of challenges and problems, physicians who provide medical care to these elderly persons need to recognize and be sensitive to their nonmedical needs.

PSYCHOSOCIAL ISSUES

Bereavement

The process of living alone usually begins when a spouse dies. Among both men and women, the mortality rate for a spouse left alone rises immediately. In the first week after the death of a spouse, the expected mortality rate doubles, and death usually results from ischemic heart disease. In the first 3 mo after the death of a spouse, the mortality rate increases 48% in men > 65 yr old and 22% in women > 65 yr old. Up to 10 yr after the death of a spouse, men have a higher rate of death than would be expected from infectious diseases, accidents, and suicide. Physicians who provide health care to bereaved elderly persons need to be watchful and supportive. Referral to self-help groups, such as Widow-to-Widow, may be helpful. For frail elderly persons, social support and sources of interaction should be identified and access to vital services secured.

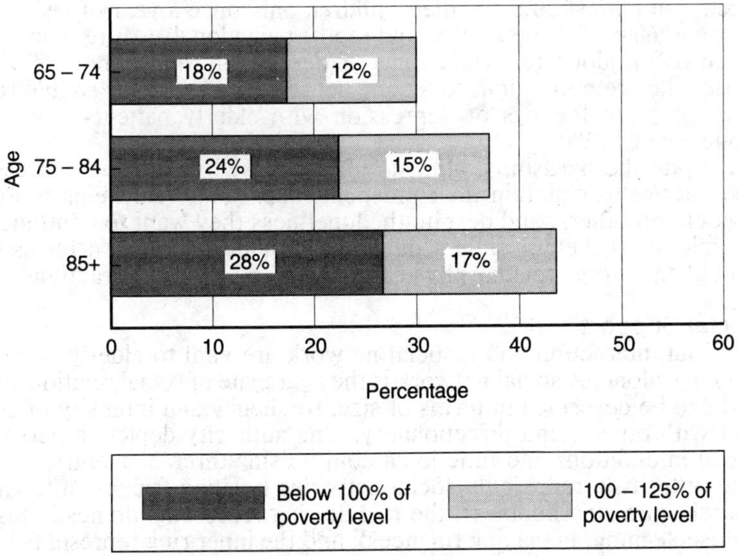

FIG. 107–1. Percentage of elderly persons in 1989 who lived alone and were below or near poverty level. (Source: US Senate Special Committee on Aging, the American Association of Retired Persons, the Federal Council on the Aging, and the US Administration on Aging, *Aging America: Trends and Projections 1991 Edition*, based on Bureau of the Census, 1990.)

Poverty

Many women become impoverished after an illness depletes savings and their husband's death results in the loss of his pension benefits. As age increases, the likelihood of poverty rises (see FIG. 107–1). The poverty rate for those who live alone is 19% for whites, 40% for Hispanics, and 57% for blacks. Those who live in rural areas have a poverty rate of 29%.

In 1989, the median annual income for those who lived alone was $9400, compared with a median income of $22,800 for couples. About 45% of elderly persons living alone survived on < $171/wk. With a limited income and high health care costs, elderly persons often must choose among such basic necessities as food, heat, or medicine.

Loneliness

In addition to not having the social, emotional, and financial support of a spouse, many (> 25%) of elderly persons living alone have no living children. Of those who do have children, most see their children once a week, but almost 20% see their children only once a year or less.

About 60% of those ≥ 75 yr old report being lonely. More than 1/3 of those living alone report feelings of depression, and almost 50% of those who are poor admit to feeling depressed. Physicians should routinely explore feelings of depression with elderly patients who live alone (see Ch. 95).

Despite the hardships, almost 90% of those living alone express a keen desire to maintain their independence. Many fear being too dependent on others, and despite the loneliness they want to continue to live alone. To help a patient maintain his independence, a physician should encourage regular physical activity and social interactions.

Social Support

Social interaction and a social network are vital to elderly persons who live alone. A social network is the aggregate of social relationships and can be described in terms of size, frequency and intensity of contact with others, and directionality. One authority depicts a person's social interactions and functional ability using three concentric rings. The outer ring represents social activities (visiting friends, attending church, pursuing hobbies); the middle ring represents domestic tasks (housecleaning, managing finances); and the inner ring represents personal care activities. By noting changes in the outer ring (eg, no longer attending church or being unwilling to travel to visit friends), the physician may detect an unreported problem and can intervene to prevent further functional decline.

Physicians can help patients assess their social support by asking questions such as "Could someone come to your home and help you during the day if it were necessary?" or "If you came home from the hospital, could someone stay overnight with you?" Of those who live alone and are unable to perform at least one activity of daily living, 74% receive no help at all (see FIG. 107–2). Among people who receive help, 43% rely on paid assistance, 54% rely on unpaid help (usually from family members), and 3% receive both paid and unpaid help. Physicians can encourage those living alone to create a broad support network of friends, neighbors, and family. Mutual dependency pacts—agreements between persons to help each other in times of need—are beneficial.

Older people who live alone are more likely than those living with others to attend senior centers, especially for meals, which can lessen social isolation. In addition, although persons who live alone are less likely than married persons to undertake volunteer activities, those who do report higher rates of satisfaction and enjoyment from these activities. In a program in Florida, volunteer activity is encouraged by having well elderly persons build up "bank accounts" of hours volunteered so that they can draw on the accounts in times of need.

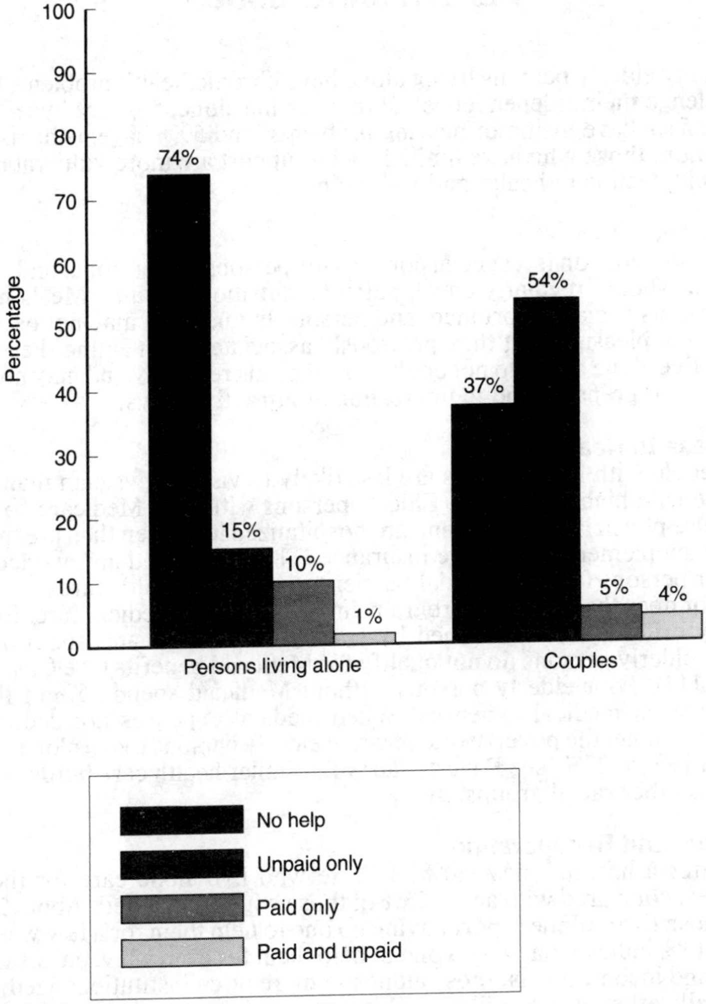

Fig. 107–2. Type of help received by persons > 65 yr of age (couples and those living alone) who have activity limitations. (Source: US Senate Special Committee on Aging, the American Association of Retired Persons, the Federal Council on the Aging, and the US Administration on Aging, *Aging America: Trends and Projections 1991 Edition*, based on Lewin/ICF estimates from the 1984 *Supplement on Aging* and the Brookings/ICF Long-Term Care Financing Model, 1990.)

HEALTH CARE ISSUES

Many elderly persons living alone have chronic health problems that challenge their independence. Of those living alone, 50% are hypertensive, 54% have vision or hearing problems, and 59% have arthritis. In addition, those who have limited social support are more vulnerable to a rapid decline in health and well-being.

Nutrition

Good nutrition is a special concern for persons living alone, and physicians should regularly check patients' nutritional status. Meals have enormous social importance, and persons living alone may not experience the pleasure that they previously associated with eating. Persons who live alone often do not cook and eat meals regularly and may not be willing to prepare food in interesting or attractive ways.

Access to Health Care

People with low incomes are less likely to visit a physician than are those with higher incomes. Elderly persons with only Medicare coverage use physician services and are hospitalized less often than are those with supplementary private insurance. This suggests that low-income older persons face a financial barrier to obtaining health care.

Nor does the Medicaid program ensure access to medical care. Eligibility criteria are determined by state governments, and about 2/3 of poor elderly persons do not qualify for Medicaid benefits (see Chs. 110 and 114). Poor elderly persons without Medicaid spend 25% of their income on medical expenses. When medical expenses are deducted from income, the poverty rate of white elderly persons living alone rises from 19% to 27% (see Poverty, above). Similar health care burdens apply to other racial groups.

Illness and Recuperation

After a hospital stay, 40% of those who live alone care for themselves, compared with about 25% of those who are married. About 25% of those living alone report having no one to help them for a few weeks, and 13% indicate having no one to help them for even a few days. At all age and income levels, those alone are more often institutionalized, especially after a serious illness. Without a social network or community support, they are at the greatest risk for permanent institutionalization and loss of independence if their health declines. Access to social and home care services may be vital to their recuperation.

A physician can order home care services even for those who have not been previously hospitalized (see Ch. 25). Medicare generally covers home care services if skilled nursing services are required intermittently and consistently with the nature and severity of the illness.

Emergency Response Devices

Personal emergency response devices are appropriate for many elderly persons who live alone, especially those who are homebound. The devices are activated by pushing a button on a transmitter that is worn as a pendant or by pressing any one of a number of transmitters placed strategically in the home. Permanently mounted transmitter devices are recommended at the front door and in the bathroom (about 6 in. from the floor). Some devices have special features such as large, soft activation pads for persons with impaired vision or severe arthritis. Portable devices should be light, wireless, and waterproof.

A regional response center monitors any activation of the devices and calls for local medical and emergency services. Devices that hook into existing telephone lines allow two-way communication if activated. Two-way communication allows for better assessment of the situation, and the most appropriate emergency help (eg, police, fire, or ambulance) can be ordered. Furthermore, two-way communication devices enable the monitoring personnel to reassure the elderly person that help is on the way.

Advance Directives

Many elderly patients do not discuss their wishes for resuscitation and heroic live-saving measures with their families or physicians. Because persons living alone usually value their personal autonomy, physicians should initiate discussions about medical treatment and advance directives. A copy of a living will or a durable power of attorney for health care should be in a patient's permanent record and should be readily accessible if emergency care is needed.

108. LEGAL ISSUES

An elderly patient has the same legal rights as any other adult patient who is not congenitally retarded or who has not been declared incompetent by a court. Yet elderly patients are more likely to have their legal rights abrogated because they are more likely to be alone and isolated, poor, demented, and institutionalized. They may be less able to be effective advocates for their personal beliefs and desires. Also, they tend to have less available ancillary support from informal support networks. Because of this vulnerability, health care personnel should identify and support the rights and interests of elderly patients and guard against accidental or planned disempowerment.

An awareness of their personal and ethical interests and vigorous advocacy of their legal rights are critical in our adversary system of justice, which depends largely on individual redress of grievances. This awareness is especially crucial in the medical context, in which patients are often ill-informed or misled about the nature and extent of their individual rights and liberties.

PATIENT RISKS

Because of gradually increasing cognitive deficits, elderly persons are more likely to need help managing financial and personal care plans. They are also more likely to be challenged legally on plans and preferences that may seem strange or bizarre to others or that conflict with the self-interest of prospective heirs or other persons.

Specifically, elderly persons are at risk for **limited guardianship (conservatorship)** or **guardianship (committeeship)** action. Guardianship action is designed to prove incompetence; limited guardianship action attempts to show diminished functional ability in managing property and personal care decisions. The elderly are at risk for these actions because many statutes still stipulate that old age itself is acceptable grounds for instituting such a lawsuit. Physical addiction and mental illness are two other commonly used grounds.

The legal rights of elderly patients are often at risk in medical settings. Physicians and other health care workers have been taught to cure and comfort, but their benevolent mission encourages paternalism. They have been taught to pursue what is in the patient's best interest, which may be at odds with the course of treatment the patient would choose. Thus, the patient's right to choose may be compromised by the physician's benevolent commitment to provide what is seen as appropriate care.

The risk of disempowerment is even greater in acute care settings because the effects of illness or drugs or delirium can remove patients entirely from discussions about preferred care. Therefore, physicians should discuss preferences and future options for care with patients when they are capable of formulating choices and communicating decisions. The patient's expressed preference should be noted in the medical record and recorded in an advance medical directive (see ADVANCE DIRECTIVES, below).

Physicians should be aware that elderly patients are frequently targets of unscrupulous schemes to defraud them of property or money. Many times, lawyers knowledgeable about or dedicated to the legal problems of the elderly can defeat these plots with timely, effective legal intervention. Often, a health care worker is the first person to recognize such a problem and should refer the patient for legal assistance. Offices that provide legal services for the elderly can be located by calling the local agency on aging. Legal services can provide immense support in defending against fraud and pursuing individual rights and benefits.

PATIENT BENEFITS

In most jurisdictions, older patients are eligible for a range of age-based and needs-based services. In every state, the elderly are eligible for Medicare (see FINANCING HEALTH CARE in Ch. 110 and Ch. 114). The type of physician and hospital visits and the range of services (ie, eyeglasses, medications, hearing aids) that Medicare will cover changes regularly with new statutory and regulatory amendments. Physicians should know basic Medicare rules, have materials available that describe the range and extent of benefits, and be able to refer patients to knowledgeable legal and social service resources for further counseling and support. When a patient's Medicare claim is denied, the decision can often be reversed by a prompt individual challenge supported by an appeal in a fair hearing administrative forum. In this administrative procedure, the insurance company handling Medicare claims reviews the case. If unsatisfied with the outcome of that review, the patient has a right to a hearing before a judge.

Poor elderly patients may be entitled to further medical benefits under Medicaid. Only about one third of elderly patients are poor enough to qualify; the exact income and resource levels that qualify a patient for Medicaid vary among states. State departments of social services, local Medicaid offices, and legal services for the elderly or the poor are good sources of information, materials, support, and individual representation.

Also, many states and localities have a bewildering array of special benefits and programs for the elderly, ranging from subsidies for transportation, housing, heating, telephone, and food expenses to discounts at movies. Health care workers are responsible for educating elderly patients about and providing access to benefits and entitlements that may be important to their physical and mental health. Physicians should not attempt to be lawyers, but they should develop an expanded definition of care that includes increased sensitivity to the legal risks of being old and increased knowledge of services available to mitigate those risks.

INFORMED CONSENT AND THE RIGHT TO REFUSE

(See also INFORMED CONSENT in Ch. 109)

Since the early 20th century, the concept that *every adult patient of sound mind shall have the right to decide what shall be done with his own body* has gradually become the rule. This theme, which lawyers call **self-determination** and philosophers call **autonomy,** is the foundation of the legal and ethical doctrine of informed consent.

Historically, the basis of medicine was considered to be touching. Consent in advance of such touching defeated a subsequent action for assault and battery. In the last century, however, negligence replaced assault and battery as the legal rubric governing medicine, and this change has imposed certain positive duties of care on practicing medical professionals. One is the responsibility for providing information and outlining the risks and benefits of alternative treatments so that patients can exercise their right to self-determination and choose in an informed manner.

The constitutional right to privacy, given its first modern articulation in the Supreme Court cases that legalized contraception and used as the basis for a woman's right to an abortion, also supports the right of persons to choose individually appropriate medical care plans. Furthermore, the concepts of personal liberty and the restraints on state interference with independent action and choice also support the legal rights of a person who is capable of making health care decisions to choose among medical care options.

Physicians must, therefore, inform patients of the diagnosis, the prognosis, the available alternative interventions, the risks and benefits of those options, and the risk and probable outcome of no intervention. *The patient then has the right to informed choice;* that is, the patient may consent to or refuse care, even if the likely outcome of the refusal is death. *The physician has an obligation to communicate this right to choose* to help empower the unaware, uninformed, or unsophisticated.

The doctrine of informed consent requires the physician to be more than a passive conduit for technical information. It requires that the physician disclose information in a language and manner appropriate to the individual patient so that the patient can make a personal choice.

A decision to refuse treatment—even if it appears senseless to the physician—does not mean that the patient is incompetent or crazy. Physicians must be aware, however, that *among the most common reasons for a patient's refusal of suggested care is misunderstanding or miscommunication between the physician and patient*. Therefore, physicians should not accept the first sign of reluctance as a refusal of care. Physicians are ethically required to encourage acceptance of the treatment judged to be in the patient's best interest. Most patients' refusals of care will be reversed with attention, extended discussion, and even some cajoling. Advocacy, however, must stop short of coercion, duplicity, or deceit. Some refusals are adamant. They must be respected and can be reversed only by petition to a court. Physicians must not deprive patients of their rights; only a court, after full adversary argument, can order care over a patient's clear and consistent refusal.

A patient's refusal of care is not an attempted suicide. Courts distinguish between a refusal of care and a suicide, which is characterized by behavior begun by and under the control of the person (the inception) and intended to cause death (the intent). Thus, courts readily distinguish between jumping out of a 20th-story window and refusing further painful chemotherapy that may or may not arrest or reverse the progress of a malignancy. Courts regularly protect the right of an adult Jehovah's Witness who has no minor children or disabled dependents to refuse blood transfusions, which are prohibited by religious teaching, even when the attending physician considers them necessary for effective medical care. The individual's right to choose almost always outweighs the physician's responsibility to deliver usual and customary medical care.

Some states do recognize an exception to the informed consent process, called the **therapeutic privilege,** *which allows a physician to withhold information when, in the physician's judgment, the patient would suffer direct and immediate harm as a result of the disclosure.* This doctrine provides a limited exception to the usual rules governing the physician's responsibility to disclose and the patient's right to choose. However, the doctrine is appropriate only infrequently; mere upset or anguish over a grim situation does not qualify. When the doctrine is used, the patient's state of mind should be reevaluated frequently to ensure that disclosure is made as soon as, in the physician's judgment, the risk of serious adverse effects has abated sufficiently.

The theory of informed consent and the rights of patients are regularly violated by well-meaning, benevolent physicians, often acting in concert with concerned family members. Many times, the patient is ill and frightened, and involving loving family members in difficult discussions and decisions seems reasonable, even kind. But family involvement should occur only with the patient's permission and, in general, should not replace the patient's involvement.

Involving the family without the patient's consent violates the patient's right to choose and right to confidential care. Some patients prefer that decisions be made by the family or physician, others refuse to involve the family. Nevertheless, all patients should be given the choice.

Ethical oaths and specific statutes in every state protect the **confidentiality** of the doctor-patient relationship. The relationship is also protected by the **doctrine of privilege,** which provides that the patient has the right to exclude otherwise appropriate, relevant, and admissible testimony in a court of law; this privilege can be invoked only by the patient. Additionally, most states have professional licensing statutes that incorporate professional oaths and make their strictures a clear part of professional practice.

Elderly patients are entitled to confidential care unless they give permission for disclosure or they clearly can no longer express a preference (eg, a patient who is confused or comatose). Even in these cases, personal secrets should be guarded, although decisions about care may need to be discussed with appropriate surrogates. When a patient can no longer make health care decisions, prior expressed preferences should be respected.

COMPETENCE AND DECISIONAL CAPACITY

Competence is both a societal judgment and a legal concept. Historically, persons became competent at age 21, when they were entitled to vote, sign binding contracts, and otherwise participate in the workings of society. The concept of competence thus reflects a societal determination to include or exclude certain persons from full participation. It does not reflect any focused inquiry into the abilities or disabilities of an individual person.

The term **decisional capacity** more accurately reflects the concept of individual capability, which can be assessed by examining mental status, judgment, and short-term memory. Decisional capacity (de facto competence) is a prerequisite for providing legally and morally sufficient informed consent or refusal. The President's Commission for the Study of Ethical Problems in Medicine and Biomedical and Behavioral Research stated: "Decision-making capacity requires, to greater or lesser degree: (1) possession of a set of values and goals; (2) the ability to communicate and to understand information; and (3) the ability to reason and to deliberate about one's choices."

In defining **decision-specific capacity,** many legal scholars, bioethicists, and psychiatrists assert that the greater the risk of the proposed intervention, the greater the need for capacity to understand facts and articulate personal values. Thus, a patient may be capable of choosing between relatively benign alternatives that may have few serious consequences but may not be capable of evaluating and choosing alternatives in a life-threatening circumstance. By a combination of statute, common law, and regulation, all states require that the informed consent of the competent patient precede medical intervention. Yet many elderly patients who are not truly capable of understanding and evaluating alternatives are treated as if they are because they nod in agreement or do not actively oppose a proposed intervention. Such consent is rarely questioned. In many cases, however, this lack of individual scrutiny means that no one is exercising the patient's right to evaluate and choose a medical care plan.

A patient need not have the same level of awareness at all times to provide legally adequate informed consent. For example, a patient who exhibits "sundowning" (increased confusion in the evening) or one who is confused from time to time may still have **windows of lucidity.** During these periods, the patient may be capable of providing informed consent.

Similarly, a patient whose short-term memory is compromised may still be able to judge the appropriateness of a suggested intervention, especially if the patient has shown a long-standing pattern of choice **(a sedimented life preference)** that is supported by the corroborating statements of others. On the other hand, deficits in understanding or reasoning may be so severe that a patient should not bear the responsibility for making informed choices.

In most cases, the care team makes the proper judgment regarding decisional capacity. In acute care institutions and long-term care facilities, the nurses are often most aware of a patient's range of abilities and can provide critical testimony on how momentary capabilities reflect overall functioning.

Formal mental status testing can help determine whether a patient should be considered decisionally capable. However, *a score on a standard examination does not dictate a conclusion about capacity.*

ADVANCE DIRECTIVES

If a patient is no longer able to provide the emotional and intellectual scrutiny the law requires for informed consent, the first alternative should be to refer to any specific documents written or empowerments executed when the patient was capable of choosing and intended to direct future care. These documents, living wills and durable powers of attorney (proxies) for health care decisions, provide the closest approximation of a current evaluation of risks and benefits.

A **living will** is a document that explains what sorts of care the patient would want to accept or reject in the future should the patient be unable to make health care decisions. Despite the fact that living wills are value neutral documents and can be used to refuse or request care, most patients use them to refuse life-sustaining care when the prognosis for recovery or improvement is hopeless and the ability to relate to others is severely diminished or destroyed. Some living wills limit their applicability to terminal illness, a diagnosis that does not apply to a persistent vegetative state and deep coma. Patients desiring to prospectively refuse care in these conditions should not use a living will limited to terminal illness.

In most states, a regular **power of attorney** is a way for a competent person to delegate some of his rights to someone else (eg, the right to sell a car or manage stocks), but this power lapses if the person granting it becomes incompetent. A **durable power of attorney** specifies that the appointee's power begins or continues with the onset of incompetence. A **durable power of attorney for health care decision making** is a document that permits the patient to appoint a person to make health care decisions in case the patient becomes incapacitated. The proxy's decisions should be guided by specific instructions from the patient, by notions of substituted judgment (what the patient would likely want under the circumstances), and by the concept of best interest.

In most states, the legal requirements are so simple that an attorney is not needed to execute such **advance directives,** including living wills and durable powers of attorney for health care decision making.

In 1993, a federal statute, the Patient Self-Determination Act became effective. This statute requires all hospitals, long-term care facilities, and health maintenance organizations receiving federal funds to ask patients on admission whether or not they have an advance directive. If they do, it must be noted in the chart; if they do not, they must be offered the opportunity to consider the options and execute an advance directive.

The schema of most advance directives is as follows: a statement of present capacity to decide; a specification of possible trigger events (eg, hopeless or terminal state, no possibility of returning to sapient existence, inability to relate to others); and a listing of interventions that would not be desired (eg, use of a ventilator, dialysis, intensive care, antibiotics). Advance directives are used almost exclusively to ward off unwanted care and to facilitate what has been labeled death with dignity. However, such a directive can be used to request that all possible care be provided.

The formal requirements for and binding power of living wills and durable powers of attorney vary from state to state. All states now recognize (at least by common law and often by statute) the right of a patient to provide informed consent before a medical intervention. Most states recognize statements made when a patient was capable as evidence of a prior preference that can be applied in the future. Some states have passed laws stipulating the form an advance directive must take and the formal measures required to make it effective. Many of these statutes provide immunity for physicians who withhold or withdraw care in compliance with properly executed and witnessed directives. Other states have developed case law that not only supports written directives but also permits caregivers and others to honor the patient's clear, explicit oral statements.

Without specific statutes indicating when directives may or must be followed, a directive's effectiveness depends greatly on its clarity, specificity, and applicability; the consequences of following the directive; and the legal climate of the locality. A document stating that the patient refuses heroic care provides vague, insufficient guidance for caregivers. Clear, precise statements are more likely to be understood and thus more likely to be followed.

Advance directives are not a perfect substitute for current patient evaluation of a particular situation. Someone can always claim that in this circumstance the patient would or might have felt differently, and such a claim might be true. Nonetheless, these prior statements are legally and morally far superior to the alternative—a decision by others based on their standards rather than on the patient's.

Today, more and more persons are reluctant to permit the extension of organ function beyond sapient and relational existence. Therefore, physicians should raise the issue with patients and provide models of advance directives that are acceptable under state law. Physicians should also document discussions about advance directives and specific decisions on the patient's chart. These admittedly difficult discussions are best done when the patient is not in crisis.

The objection is often made that such discussions depress patients, but there is no evidence to support this objection. As society and the media increasingly focus on these issues, many more people will have already considered them, and a discussion may actually help reduce anxiety. The physician is the best person to explain life-sustaining technologies and interventions to the patient and to help in developing a specific advance directive that reflects the patient's preferences regarding future care.

SURROGATE DECISION MAKING

If the patient is not capable of making a choice and no advance directive provides an alternative basis for consent or refusal, some other person or persons must provide the direction and legally adequate oversight for care. A surrogate decider can be a person chosen by the patient under a proxy designation or a durable power of attorney, a statutorily designated person, or an informally identified person such as a close family member or a friend. The more informal the appointment, the less likely the surrogate will be able to refuse life-sustaining treatment.

In the past, elderly patients were cared for by their physician and family, who were guided by beneficence or personal convictions and respect. Although still the norm, such unreviewed, unsupervised surrogate decision making is increasingly circumscribed by growing legal awareness of the problems involved and the development of rules and regulations to guide and constrain decisions.

In the past decade, courts and legislatures have implemented rules holding that persons who cannot decide about care do not lose their right to consent or refuse. These rights may be exercised by others, based on specific legal standards with procedural safeguards and stipulated possibilities for review.

Most hospitals and physicians accept consent to provide care from a spouse, child, close friend, member of the clergy, or even a distant and uninvolved relative. Yet, in most states, none of these persons is legally empowered to consent on behalf of another. But based on tradition and the supposition that a close relative or friend would care and know most about the patient, accepting the judgment of such a person over that of a total stranger makes practical and ethical sense. Such reasoning does not apply when permission is sought from a distant, uninvolved, or estranged relative. Except in exceedingly rare cases, a decision agreed upon by hospital, physician, and family operates as the basis of care, although it may not be legally adequate if challenged.

For elderly people who have outlived family and friends, a **court-appointed guardian,** who is often uninterested and serves a perfunctory role, may be the only alternative. Some institutions and regions are experimenting with **public guardians** and **patient advocates,** which may prove appropriate and cost-effective.

When **surrogates** attempt to **refuse care** or decide to withhold or withdraw care (an often articulated distinction without any substantial legal or ethical difference), legal concerns increase because the outcome of these actions may be death. Since all courts agree that the state has a fundamental interest in preserving life, these decisions are often legally problematic.

The initial questions in these circumstances are (1) Who decides? and (2) On what basis is the decision made? Answers vary widely among the states. In New Jersey, after a hospital ethics committee (actually a prognosis committee) determines that the prognosis is hopeless and, in the case of elderly residents in long-term care, after the state Office of the Ombudsman determines that the decision does not constitute abuse, a specially appointed guardian may opt for a refusal that will likely permit death. The decisions of surrogates are supposed to be based first on the legal standard of **substituted judgment** (ie, What would this patient want?) and second on the doctrine of best interest. In Massachusetts, such decisions are made by a court after full adversary argument on the issues of patient prognosis, patient preference, and state interest. Other states have formal or informal mechanisms that balance the interests of the state in preserving life, preventing suicide, protecting innocent third parties, and protecting the integrity of the medical profession against the prior wishes of the patient, the desires of family, and the abstract notions of best interest and respect for persons.

In most states, the firmest basis for decision, in the absence of an explicit advance directive, is substituted judgment. If insufficient information is known or can be surmised about the patient and if a decision crisis has been reached, caregivers, family, and sometimes the courts appeal to notions of **best interest.** These discussions often focus on the intrusiveness and burden of the intervention, the likely benefit, the patient's suffering, and the possibility of recovery. As burden and intrusiveness increase and benefit and prognosis dim, the care becomes less likely to be morally or legally mandatory.

Certain types of decisions present special problems—for instance, the decision to discontinue artificial hydration and nutrition. Care providers, legislators, judges, and clergy, as well as legal, medical, religious, and ethical scholars are struggling to analyze the issues and to propose acceptable solutions regarding such life-sustaining interventions. All courts that have considered the issues have held that the mechanical provision of food and fluid is a medical treatment and thus subject to the same strictures that guide other medical decisions. Nonetheless, as a matter of public policy, some state statutes differentiate this intervention from others.

In summary, the protocol for decision making is to use the prior explicit statement made when the patient was decisionally capable, an inference from patterns of preference and from statements and behavior (substituted judgment), or some notion of best interest that precludes unjustified suffering when the treatment is invasive and intrusive, the benefit speculative, and the prognosis hopeless. All courts that have considered the issues have found that under certain circumstances, permitting death is not incompatible with a patient's best interest nor with the state's interest in preserving life.

These decisions are complex for all parties: patient, family, provider, institution, state, legislature, court, and special interest groups. The legal interests of the patient are in self-determination, dignity, and privacy. The family has no legal interest unless specially appointed as proxy or designated by statute, but the family's emotional, moral, and often financial stakes are high. Providers have an interest in maintaining professional integrity, providing legally adequate care, and avoiding civil or criminal challenge (although neither occurs often). Institutions are also concerned about possible liability. The state must safeguard the lives and values of its citizens and the values of its heterogeneous cultures, and it must be aware of its disparate special interests.

DISCHARGE AND PLACEMENT

Discharge planning and placement decisions for elderly patients have received almost no legal focus and only scant scholarly analysis. Many physicians and family members make these decisions without adequate discussion with the patient and often over the patient's objection. Just as patients have the right to consent to or refuse treatment, they also have the right to choose the living arrangements and type of care they want. This right, however, is not as tied to the singular interests of the patient as are the rights of informed consent and refusal of treatment. The legal, practical, and quality-of-life interests of family and neighbors may be compromised by a return to the patient's home in the community or to the home of a family member.

However, the fact that a community placement may entail more risk than a residential placement in a long-term care facility does not mean that the patient must accept the latter. Patients may assume the risks of placement just as they may choose a risky treatment alternative. Many elderly persons choose to return home when caregivers are convinced that residential treatment is medically and socially preferable. Some patients even choose to return home when the possible result is death. *If the patient is decisionally capable, this decision, like a refusal of medically necessary care, can be legally acceptable*. A decisionally capable patient cannot be placed in a residential facility over his objection without a court order. Elderly patients have a right to be obstinate and foolish unless the rights or interests of others are clearly compromised.

Overriding a patient's discharge preference may require petitioning the court for a general or a limited guardianship. Overriding a treatment decision can often be accomplished by an appointment of a special guardian designated for that specific purpose. The ongoing supervision of an elderly person, however, requires a guardian with sustained powers and commitment. Unfortunately, many states provide insufficient education, training, and supervision of such court-appointed guardians, who often opt for the least burdensome alternative for themselves rather than the least restrictive alternative for the patient.

DO–NOT–RESUSCITATE ORDERS

(See also Do-Not-Resuscitate Orders in Ch. 109)

For the last decade, scholars have discussed and institutions have experimented with policies governing special categories of care, especially resuscitation. Many hospitals—and with increasing frequency, long-term care facilities—have policies to guide decisions about resuscitation. These policies vary widely; some reserve the decision for the physician, others empower patients and designated surrogates to make the decision. New York State has legislated the patient's right to decide on resuscitation status.

As with other decisions about care, decisions about resuscitation should be brought to patients' attention when they are lucid. *No matter who decides, some system should exist for recording, communicating, and reviewing the decision.* No legal case has been reported in which a physician or an institution has been found liable for respecting a do-not-resuscitate order that was written after an appropriate discussion with the patient and family and was duly noted on the patient's chart.

LONG–TERM CARE

(See also Chs. 24 and 110)

Long-term care institutions have increasingly come under legal scrutiny, spurred primarily by exposés of neglectful and abusive care of vulnerable, often demented, elderly institutionalized patients. The nature and degree of abuse offended legal, moral, and civic sensibilities. This offense resulted in a framework of federal and state regulations that prescribe staffing patterns, record-keeping procedures, and many aspects of institutional practice. Increasingly, long-term care facilities are being challenged about policies that automatically provide life-sustaining treatment to unknowing patients with no provision for stopping such treatment. Yet, many of these facilities are afraid to adopt policies allowing a resident to die because they may be accused of neglect and abuse. Practitioners should be aware of developments as states struggle to define and regulate these decisions. The legal climate is crucial in discussions with patients and families about possible future care. Many long-term care facilities are adding information about future preference for care and resuscitation status to their postadmission discussions in response to the Patient Self-Determination Act and because of concern for legally supportable decisions.

Federal and state laws and regulations also govern long-term care financing (see also Chs. 110 and 114). Most long-term care is funded by Medicaid, the needs-based cooperative federal and state health reimbursement program. Very little long-term care is funded by Medicare, the age-based federal medical program for the elderly and for some persons with disabilities. Most elderly patients, couples, and families do not understand the complex rules that require spending their income and assets to a level of poverty before Medicaid will assume the cost of long-term care. *In most states, legal advocates can protect a spouse living in the community from impoverishment by appealing to state regulations that permit segregation of funds.* If such an arrangement is not possible, an attorney may file a suit for support in the Family Court or other appropriate state forum. Every state has a long-term care ombudsman whose office is funded by Medicare. These offices can provide information about some of the rights and protections available to residents of long-term care facilities.

RISKS FOR HEALTH CARE PROVIDERS

The US legal system ensures that physicians rarely will be sued for malpractice over an incident relating to the care of an elderly patient. The primary reason is that the measure of recovery—mainly, lost earnings—is very low for elderly persons, whose economically productive work life usually is behind them. Because the prospective calculation of lost earnings is low, the award will be small, and because most malpractice cases are arranged on a contingent fee basis, the lawyer's fee will be small. Therefore, the whole enterprise is usually unattractive to negligence attorneys. The risk of malpractice for other health care providers is even smaller, in part because the legal system assumes that their assets are not as great as those of physicians.

Legal activity is more likely to focus on the propriety of discontinuing treatment and the issues of surrogate decision making. Also, more assault and battery cases are being brought for not discontinuing treatment after it has been refused by a debilitated but decisionally capable patient or by the family. In some nursing home cases, judges or juries have found criminal negligence based generally on patterns of disregard that violate specific regulations for institutional behavior.

FAMILY ISSUES

As a family ages, the physician should recommend that members seek **legal planning,** so that sufficient funds are available for adequate health care or long-term care. Someone, preferably a person who is close and available, must have a durable power of attorney over finances, so that in the event of disability, bills can be paid.

In the event of dementia, the affected person and family should be aware of Medicaid regulations that would deny benefits if a transfer of assets has been made within a specific period of time (usually 2 yr) before the Medicaid application. For many families, denial of Medicaid benefits puts the spouse living in the community at risk of impoverishment. If possible, arrangements should be made for the care of adult dependent or retarded children by appointment of a legal guardian. If any assets are at stake, the person should execute a will and, if the person has strong feelings about the use of life-sustaining care, a living will. For those with substantial assets, trust funds permit the allocation and protection of property.

109. ETHICAL ISSUES

In the course of caring for elderly patients, legal and ethical concerns frequently arise, posing special challenges. Some common challenges involve determining competence, resolving conflicts among decision makers, determining the available treatment options (including withholding or withdrawing treatment), and anticipating future decisions and death. Various factors, including individual and societal determinations of benefits, burdens, resource allocation, and cost containment, influence these ethical issues.

When weighing an ethical issue, the physician should think carefully before relying on age as a rationale for choosing a specific course of action. Generally, the approach to resolving ethical problems is the same for older people as it is for younger people because the two groups are more alike than different. However, differences in physiologic, psychologic, and social reserves may place older people at greater risk of adverse outcomes.

In certain circumstances, age may be an adequate justification for a course of action—for instance, providing Medicare insurance to those over age 65 because they have a substantial need and few resources and because setting age as the criterion for enrollment was administratively easy. In other circumstances, age is merely a substitute for the real rationale for a decision. For example, a line of reasoning may be as follows: People over age 80 are often multiply handicapped; multiply handicapped people are usually poor surgical candidates; therefore, surgery for those over age 80 should be severely restricted. Clearly, the reason for restricting surgery is not age but physical condition. A robust 80-yr-old with strong physiologic, psychologic, and social reserves who could benefit from surgery should not be denied it because of age alone. In contrast, valid reasons may exist for advising a less healthy 80-yr-old not to undergo a potentially beneficial surgical procedure. These reasons should be clearly identified, then explained to the patient, who should understand and agree with them.

ETHICS AND THE LAW

Although physicians may wish they could resolve difficult problems simply by asking if a course of action is legal, the law is not so directive (see also Ch. 108). Only a few actions (such as violent killing and fraud) are always wrong, and only a few (such as informing a patient and referring to another well-qualified physician for consultation) are always legally safe. Nearly everything else is sometimes protected, sometimes penalized, and often ambiguous. Ethical questions are often emotionally charged, and legal precedents may conflict or be ambiguous in their application to a particular case.

With any difficult issue, disagreement arises as to what is unreasonable behavior, and legal developments reflect the disagreement. However, one generalization currently holds true in the USA: *What is considered by professionals and society to be the best medical and ethical practice has usually been upheld when tested in court*. In other words, if a physician proceeds with due care, thorough documentation, and an understanding of the local legal risks, legal considerations will not interfere with good medical and ethical practice. Physicians should learn from reliable sources about the law that affects their practice.

SHARED MEDICAL DECISION MAKING

Rarely is a decision so simple that it depends only on technical and empirical data, especially in older persons or in persons with chronic illness and disability. The patient's perspective and the ethical dimensions of the decision must also be considered, so that the physician can truly treat the patient, not merely the patient's illnesses.

In 1982, the President's Commission for the Study of Ethical Problems in Medicine and Biomedical and Behavioral Research endorsed the model of shared decision making. Such decision making requires relationships among clinicians, patients, and their families that are marked by care, trust, open communication, and collaborative deliberation. The purpose of shared decision making is to determine which treatment alternative will preserve and promote the patient's well-being by providing the best possible future in accordance with the patient's perspectives, preferences, beliefs, and goals.

A patient with a chronic disability or illness may have no chance of being cured or even of experiencing an improvement. Specific diagnostic or therapeutic interventions may even be contraindicated. To make medical decisions, the clinician, patient, and family members must consider the potential length and quality of life and weigh the potential benefits and burdens—both physical and financial. For example, diagnosis and treatment of infection contribute little toward a better future for a nursing home patient who has severe dementia, intractable heart failure, and contractures. In this case, the best approach might be to administer only antipyretics and meticulous skin care, while allowing the patient to die.

Issues of capacity to make decisions, competence, and advance directives are often at the core of ethical decision making and conflicts. Although they are ethical issues, they are usually constrained by state and federal law (see Ch. 108).

CONFLICT AMONG DECISION MAKERS

In some cases, disagreement arises over the choice of treatment. If the physician believes the patient is making a poor choice because of a lack of knowledge or information, the physician must inform the patient more fully. A competent patient can always abandon medical care, but a physician cannot abandon a patient. A competent patient's choice will almost invariably be upheld in court.

Nevertheless, a physician is not required to honor a patient's treatment choice if the physician strongly disagrees with it, even if the patient is competent. If such issues cannot be resolved, the physician can withdraw from the case after examining the risks and benefits of each treatment option, the patient's right to self-determination, and the physician's own commitment to current practice standards and professional integrity. If the physician decides to withdraw, the patient should be notified, perhaps by certified mail. Care should be terminated only upon referral to another physician or after giving the patient ample opportunity to find another physician.

When a patient lacks capacity to make medical decisions or has been declared incompetent by a court, a surrogate decision maker is usually needed. A surrogate is the person who should best know the wishes of the patient and thus is able to speak for the patient. The surrogate may be the next of kin, someone granted durable power of attorney for health care decisions by the patient, or someone appointed by the court. Ch. 108 discusses surrogate decision makers.

INFORMED CONSENT

(See also INFORMED CONSENT AND THE RIGHT TO REFUSE in Ch. 108)

Obtaining informed consent is the formal component of shared decision making by the physician and patient. Unfortunately, the documents developed by institutions to formally record the process of obtaining consent are often substituted for the process itself. Informed consent embodies certain conditions that must be satisfied; these include adequate information, freedom from coercion, and sufficient decision-making capacity. The patient's lifestyle, the likely functional outcome of each choice, and psychosocial factors will affect what the patient needs to know.

The physician should ensure that the patient can comprehend information well enough to make important life choices. Facts about the patient's medical condition and available interventions, including their risks and benefits, should be explained to and understood by the patient. Not all minor or rare risks or benefits need to be articulated, but those that could be expected to affect a particular patient's choice need to be explained. Limiting or forgoing treatment and the consequential risks and benefits ordinarily should be discussed.

Certain attributes of informed consent are especially important with the older patient. The physician must ensure that the patient is not coerced—for instance, by the family or physician imposing goals and values—and that the patient does not acquiesce because of a desire to please others or a perceived loss of self-determination and independence (as may occur with institutionalized or profoundly dependent home-care patients). The process of obtaining informed consent from an older person may require more time because of sensory deficits or slowed cognition.

TREATMENT OPTIONS

Developing a list of treatment options for a patient is a central component of good decision making. Two assumptions help in developing options for a patient. First, although society's financial concerns are an issue, the choices made with a particular patient are ordinarily assumed to have negligible effects upon society as a whole, neither greatly changing costs nor depleting other resources. For example, choosing to dialyze an elderly, disabled patient is usually assumed to have no major effect upon the availability of dialysis to others. Although society's financial concerns usually do not limit the options for a particular patient at a particular time, financial concerns may exclude certain options for everyone. Second, *all* available options, including forgoing specific treatment, should be considered. Thus, a patient with an embolic stroke will have at least the options of (1) having only supportive care for comfort and function, (2) having further diagnostic studies to better assess the risks of recurrence, and (3) receiving anticoagulation therapy. Proceeding directly to full diagnosis and treatment without considering the merits of forgoing specific diagnosis and treatment often is not the best choice.

Decision making may be inappropriately simplified by **either-or choices,** in which one option is held to be unacceptable. An example is the notion that a provider must always give "ordinary" treatments but that "extraordinary" or "heroic" efforts need not be made. One might also be permitted to "allow a patient to die" but not to "kill a patient."

Relying on such either-or choices misleadingly reduces a complex situation to simple moral alternatives. This approach is a poor substitute for one in which choices are made to advance the patient's best interests—as the patient defines them. Advancing the patient's interests may involve stopping a treatment; deciding not to use the usual array of interventions, such as antibiotics or feeding tubes; or giving medications that may lead to an earlier death while relieving symptoms.

Appeal to the common distinction between **ordinary and extraordinary treatments** is made in cases in which some question exists about the obligation to treat. This use of the distinction raises two problems. First, rapidly changing technologies and views about which practices are indicated constantly alter a descriptive definition of ordinary care. Second, and more serious from an ethical point of view, noting that a practice is common is irrelevant to deciding whether it is morally right.

The terms ordinary and extraordinary are used in a variety of ways—to indicate whether treatment is usual, complex, artificial, expensive, or available. Care that is extraordinary in the sense that it is rare might be morally required for a limited time in an unusual case. For example, a patient appropriately may be given ventilator support in dire circumstances precipitated by an unexpected complication of experimental therapy, even though the likelihood of survival is so poor that a ventilator might not be used otherwise.

Ordinary and extraordinary are useful terms to express one's *conclusions* about the ethical evaluation of a situation, but they do not define the appropriateness of treatment. The terms are helpful only when used to indicate whether the burdens imposed by a treatment are disproportionate to its benefits. Thus, when a patient prefers death to prolonged suffering, even treatment with antibiotics may be considered extraordinary.

Many physicians express reservations about **withdrawing treatment** when, all other things being equal, they would not have had doubts about **withholding treatment.** There are often powerful psychological inhibitions against stopping treatment, but there is usually no moral difference between not starting treatment and stopping it once it has started. Attempting a treatment may help determine whether it provides a benefit. Admitting that the treatment is not achieving the desired benefit is more painful (and stopping it often entails more documentation than not starting it would have), but such problems can usually be mitigated by having planned end points of therapeutic trials. Such planning is as necessary for the use of nasogastric feeding tubes as it is for more complicated interventions, such as dialysis or repeated blood transfusions. In each case, the best decision cannot be known until after treatment is initiated. Simply put, a physician need not continue a course of treatment that is not working merely because that treatment was started.

Certain prudent steps should be taken whenever care involves an action that may shorten the patient's life, for example, administering high-dose narcotics for pain or respiratory distress, forgoing antibiotics or feeding tubes, or agreeing to withhold a life-sustaining transfusion or radiation treatment. (1) The physician must be sure that the plan is correctly assessed; for instance, the prognosis should be diligently evaluated. (2) Respected colleagues (including nurses, social workers, and clergy) should be asked to evaluate the situation. If they disagree with the plan, usually it should be reassessed and implementation delayed. (3) The physician must try to determine whether the patient agrees with the plan (or would have agreed were the patient competent). (4) The decision-making process should be carefully documented. (5) The physician might arrange for a formal review by an ethics or patient care committee or for a court review. This last step is emotionally and financially costly and usually unnecessary if the first four steps are followed.

REFUSAL OF SPECIFIC TREATMENT

If a competent patient rejects treatment that the physician believes is in the patient's interest, especially if the treatment would prolong life, the physician should explore the patient's reasons and correct any misunderstandings. However, a physician should not impose treatment if the patient refuses it—even if the treatment could prolong life. Instead, the physician should explore alternatives that might be acceptable to the patient; as discussed earlier, sometimes this involves transferring the patient to the care of a physician or institution that will respect the patient's wishes. In all cases, including those in which a patient refuses a specific treatment, the physician and the institution have an obligation to continue offering supportive care and treatment for pain and suffering.

Physicians and other health care providers should also respect advance directives to refuse treatment given by patients who have become incompetent as well as decisions to refuse treatment made by the patient's appointed representatives (see ADVANCE DIRECTIVES in Ch. 108). If a patient becomes incompetent and no advance directive exists, there is a strong tradition that the next of kin (often an adult child or spouse who is likely to know and share the patient's values) makes decisions for the patient. However, sometimes the next of kin is emotionally distant or hostile, and another person, such as a friend, may be a better surrogate. When someone other than the next of kin is the designated surrogate, the reasons for the choice should be documented.

Often, the surrogate for an elderly person is a group of family members who may disagree with one another. If the controversy threatens to obstruct what seems to be the best course of action, the physician may call upon clergy, nurses, social workers, or the hospital ethics committee to help resolve the conflict. If this approach is unsuccessful, an outside review and court-appointed guardianship may be necessary.

REQUEST FOR SPECIFIC TREATMENT

Just as patients may refuse treatment, they also may request treatment, including treatment to prolong life. Physicians have a strong obligation to respect a competent patient's request, an advance directive, or a surrogate's decision to prolong life. However, certain relevant limitations exist. Physicians are not obliged to provide physiologically futile treatments—that is, treatments that cannot produce the desired physiologic change. Before withholding or withdrawing treatment, physicians should be as sure as possible that it is futile, and they should have a full, open discussion with the patient or the surrogate about the nature and extent of the futility of the treatment. If a requested treatment entails a loss of function, mutilation, or pain disproportionate to benefit, the physician is not obliged to provide it. Also, a physician who has a conscientious objection to a requested treatment is not obliged to provide it. The physician should explain all treatment options and the physician's position regarding them. If the patient wishes, the physician should arrange an orderly transfer to another physician of the patient's choice.

DECISIONS ON DEATH

Just as patients must be informed of their rights to make decisions about treatments and to give advance directives, patients should also have the opportunity to state whether they want to have CPR performed in the event of a cardiopulmonary arrest. In almost all jurisdictions, patients do not have a legal right to euthanasia, but responding to a request for euthanasia poses difficult ethical issues for the physician.

DO-NOT-RESUSCITATE ORDERS

(See also DO-NOT-RESUSCITATE ORDERS in Ch. 108)

Strictly speaking, do-not-resuscitate (DNR) orders mean only that CPR should not be performed for a cardiopulmonary arrest. Other treatment—such as antibiotics, transfusions, dialysis, and ventilator support—may still be given. More specific orders are required to indicate whether the person should be hospitalized or whether a patient should be treated in an intensive care unit.

To assist physicians in managing the care of patients for whom CPR may not be appropriate, the American Medical Association Council on Ethical and Judicial Affairs in 1991 issued the following guidelines.

1. Efforts should be made to resuscitate patients who suffer cardiac or respiratory arrest except when CPR would be futile or not in accordance with the desires or best interests of the patient.

2. Physicians should discuss the possibility of cardiopulmonary arrest with appropriate patients and encourage them to state whether they want CPR. The discussions should include a description of CPR procedures and, when possible, should occur in an outpatient setting when general treatment preferences are discussed or as early as possible during hospitalization, when the patient is likely to be mentally alert. Early discussions before an emergency arises help ensure the patient's participation in the decision-making process. Subsequent peri-

odic discussions can determine if the patient has changed his mind because his circumstances or the treatment alternatives have changed.

3. If a patient is incapable of making a decision about CPR, the surrogate may make it, based on the patient's previously expressed preferences or, if such preferences are unknown, in accordance with the patient's best interests.

4. The physician has an ethical obligation to honor the resuscitation preferences expressed by the patient or the surrogate. Physicians should not allow their personal value judgments about quality of life to affect the implementation of a patient's or surrogate's preferences regarding the use of CPR. However, if in the physician's judgment CPR would be futile, the physician may enter a DNR order into the patient's record. If time permits, the physician must inform the patient or the surrogate of the content of the DNR order and the basis for its implementation. The physician also should be prepared to discuss appropriate alternatives, such as obtaining a second opinion or arranging for a transfer of care to another physician.

5. Resuscitative efforts should be considered futile only if they cannot be expected to restore cardiac or respiratory function or to achieve the patient's expressed goals.

6. The DNR orders, as well as the basis for their implementation, should be entered by the attending physician in the patient's medical record.

7. The DNR orders preclude only resuscitation efforts in the event of cardiopulmonary arrest, not other therapeutic interventions that are appropriate for the patient.

8. Hospital medical staffs should periodically review their experience with DNR orders, revise their DNR policies as appropriate, and inform physicians about their role in the decision-making process for DNR orders.

EUTHANASIA

Requests for euthanasia by competent patients suffering severely and irremediably from an incurable disease are understandable; however, legally they cannot be honored. Physicians are obliged to provide treatment and care that results in a peaceful, dignified, and humane death with minimal physical suffering. Statutory legalization of euthanasia by physicians could have an adverse impact on society. Thoughtful decisions to forgo life-sustaining treatment together with sustained, comprehensive symptom relief and emotional and spiritual support could provide an effective alternative to euthanasia for most dying patients.

However, some physicians and advocacy groups contend that physicians should be allowed to actively assist those who cannot commit suicide because of extreme infirmity and who prefer death to continued suffering. Physicians caring for the elderly have an obligation to be engaged in this policy debate and to seek to ensure safeguards for vulnerable patients and stewardship of the public trust.

110. SOCIAL ISSUES

The social context of geriatric care influences the risk of disease, the experience of illness, and the physician's ability to deliver timely and appropriate care. The social status of the elderly, the changing demographics of health and illness, and evolving social values exert complex pressures on the patchwork of policies, programs, and services that constitute the continuum of care available to the elderly. Thus, the successful practice of geriatric medicine requires an understanding of the broader context in which illness occurs and care is provided.

USE OF HEALTH CARE SERVICES

Older persons are more likely to use health care services than younger persons. While the elderly made up only 12% of the US population in 1990, they accounted for 34% of all hospital stays and 45% of all hospital days. For persons over age 65, the average length of stay was 8.7 days; for persons under age 65, it was 5.3 days. In 1990, older persons averaged nine contacts with physicians, while those under age 65 averaged only five contacts. Per capita spending on health care for those age 65 and older was $5360, compared with $1286 for those under age 65. Persons over age 65 use 34% of all prescription medications, with older Americans taking an average of 4.5 medications at any one time.

Older persons also use institutional services, such as nursing homes, more than younger persons. Evolving social and demographic dynamics have reduced the number of family members available to care for impaired elders. Older persons, particularly women, are likely to be widowed, and when they become very old, their children may be elderly themselves. The increasingly transient and mobile nature of American society and the increased divorce rate have contributed to geographic separation of families and weaker family ties.

The number of single-parent households, most headed by women, continues to grow. This phenomenon as well as new economic and social realities that foster a dependence on two-income households have produced a steady growth of women in the work force—women who in the past would have functioned as caregivers. Today, the demands of a job may diminish a woman's ability to provide the informal support needed by elderly relatives. These factors together with the increased prevalence of disease suggest that the demand for both noninstitutional support systems and institutional services by an expanding population of dependent elderly will continue to grow.

SOCIAL SUPPORTS AND FAMILY CAREGIVING

Although social support includes help from neighbors and friends, family members usually provide most of the physical, emotional, social, and economic support. Family caregivers play a key role in delaying, if not preventing, institutionalization of the chronically ill older person. In fact, about 80% of home health care is provided as informal support by family members (as opposed to purchased services). This care is provided to elderly persons living with adult children or in their own homes.

The amount and type of care depend on economic resources, family structure, quality of relationships, and competing demands on family time and energy. Family caregiving can range from minimal assistance (eg, periodically checking in) to elaborate full-time care. On average, caregivers spend about 4 h a day on caregiving tasks. Women are more likely than men to be both receivers and givers of such care.

Spouses are major providers of care for the frail elderly. While adult children frequently care for mildly or moderately impaired elders, a spouse (usually a wife) is more likely to care for a severely disabled elderly person. Spouse caregivers experience considerable stress and suffer associated health problems. As a group, caregiving couples are disproportionately poor, and the caregiver is usually in poor health.

Recent demographic trends of delayed procreation and increased longevity have created a "sandwich generation" of caregivers who find themselves responsible for care of both their children and their parents. Many of these caregivers who have jobs experience significant conflict between the demands of their job and those of elder care. Although society tends to view families as having special rights and responsibilities in caring for one another, the limits of filial and spousal obligations vary among families and individuals.

Family members' willingness and ability to provide care may be enhanced by services that support family caregivers (technical assistance in learning new skills, counseling services, family mental health services, or personal supports) and services that supplement family caregiving (personal care, home health care, adult day care, meals programs, and social services).

Lack of support or social isolation is associated with an increased risk of mortality. Social supports, however, appear to buffer the elderly from the negative effects of life transitions, such as the departure of children, retirement, and widowhood.

EFFECTS OF LIFE TRANSITIONS

For most elderly persons, late life is a period of transition and adjustment to loss. Transitions include retirement, relocation, and bereavement following the death of a spouse, family members, or friends.

Retirement: Frequently, retirement is the first major transition faced by older persons. About 33% of retirees have difficulty adjusting to certain aspects of retirement, such as reduced income and altered social role and entitlements. Individual circumstances surrounding retirement decisions influence the severity of adjustment problems. Some persons choose to retire and look forward to quitting unpleasant work; others are forced to retire because of health reasons or job loss. These factors help explain the different effects retirement has on retirees' physical and mental health. Appropriate preparation for retirement and counseling for families and retirees who experience difficulties ameliorate many problems.

Relocation: A person or family may experience several transitions in residences in later years, including the sale of the family home and a move to smaller quarters, a move into senior-citizen or retirement housing to minimize the burden of upkeep, and finally a move into a nursing home. Some experts contend that such moves produce relocation trauma; however, recent studies find little or no evidence of increased mortality or other markers of such trauma. Physical and mental status are significant predictors of relocation adjustment. Those who respond poorly to a move are more likely to be men, living alone, socially isolated, poor, and depressed.

However, two factors mediate the stress of moving—the degree of perceived control over the move and the degree of predictability of the new environment. Families should be encouraged to acquaint the older person with the new setting well in advance of moving. For the cognitively impaired elderly, a move away from familiar surroundings may trigger a substantial increase in functional dependence and disruptive behavior. Awareness of the increased vulnerability of a demented elder may help families and staff cope during the adjustment period.

Bereavement: A complex phenomenon, bereavement changes many aspects of the elderly person's life. Loss of companionship is accompanied by a decline in social interaction and a change in social status. The loss of a spouse has different effects on men and women. In the 2-yr period following the death of a spouse, men tend to have higher mortality rates than women. On the other hand, elderly men are much more likely to remarry after the death of a spouse.

Health care workers should be alert to symptoms of stress and depression during the grieving period. A hasty attempt to treat sadness with antidepressant drugs should be avoided because of their potential interference with the process of grieving and adjustment. On the other hand, counseling and supportive services, such as widow-to-widow groups, may ease difficult transitions and facilitate adjustments to new roles and life circumstances. Prolonged and pathologic grief usually requires psychiatric evaluation and treatment.

CONTINUUM OF CARE

(See also Chs. 24, 25, and 26)

The array of health services used by older persons is complex and fragmented. These services have different eligibility requirements and sources of funding, and they are regulated by different agencies.

Acute care hospitals provide services to many older people requiring care for acute illnesses, exacerbations of chronic illnesses, and accidents. Hospitalized elderly persons are at risk for acute confusion (as a result of unfamiliar surroundings, sleep deprivation, and abrupt changes in medication). Efforts to shorten hospital stays have raised concerns that patients are discharged "sicker and quicker." Many elderly fear being sent home too soon with inadequate support.

Psychiatric hospitals were once a major source of care for the elderly, particularly those suffering from dementia. A policy of deinstitutionalization has markedly reduced the populations of such facilities over the past two decades. Unfortunately, for many mentally ill elders, deinstitutionalization has meant reinstitutionalization as patients have been transferred from state mental hospitals to nursing homes, which have been termed the "new back wards." For others, deinstitutionalization has meant release into the community, where care is available through poorly coordinated, underfunded community-based programs or not at all.

Nursing homes are facilities established primarily to provide nursing care. They tend to be classified according to their certification status as providers of care in the Medicare and Medicaid programs. In the USA, about 17,122 nursing homes provide care to 1,249,000 residents over age 65. The rate of nursing home use by the elderly has doubled from 2.5% in 1966 to the current 5%. The typical nursing home resident is an elderly, white widow.

Special housing for the elderly varies widely. **Life-care communities** (or continuing care retirement communities) are the most comprehensive, providing apartments for independent living and a range of services, including skilled nursing care. Most life-care communities have a single campus; some provide services at several sites. With **congregate care,** older persons live in individual apartments or rooms and receive selected services. Congregate care differs from a life-care community in that the residents do not own their units, and there is no commitment to provide care over time as residents' needs change. **Foster, domiciliary, and personal-care homes** generally offer room, board, and some supervision. The availability of these housing options, particularly those providing supervision, is woefully inadequate in most communities.

Hospice care provides services intended to improve the quality of life for terminally ill patients so they can live the remainder of their lives as comfortably and peacefully as possible. Many aspects of hospice care

are being adopted by care providers in the general health system and have been suggested for patients with certain illnesses (eg, Alzheimer's disease), even when death is not imminent.

Respite care refers to services that allow family members time away from caregiving responsibilities. Services range from an in-home visit of a few hours by a volunteer or paid worker to institutional stays of several weeks. Respite care continues to evolve as a valuable resource for those coping with the stresses of providing care to an aged spouse, sibling, or parent.

Community mental health centers provide ambulatory psychiatric care and other services to residents in catchment areas. Generally, the number of elderly persons who actually receive these services is much smaller than the number of persons who need them, but several centers have special outreach programs, nursing home consultation, and other services for geriatric patients.

Adult day care serves persons who need supervision or medical services during the day but who can spend evenings with family members or in other supportive environments. Two types of adult day care exist: the adult day hospital and the multipurpose, social, day-care center. Some adult day hospitals focus specifically on psychiatric patients. Despite significant fragmentation in funding and regulation, adult day-care centers have increased from 800 in 1987 to nearly 3000 in 1992.

Senior centers provide opportunities for social contact and recreational activities. They also serve as convenient sites for health screening, nutrition and education programs, and outreach activities. Most offer meals on weekdays, and some have extensive health and social service programs, including adult day care.

Nutrition programs provide two types of services—congregate meals and home-delivered meals. Congregate meals not only contribute to nutritional health but also provide opportunities for social contact, educational programs, and outreach efforts. Meals for the homebound or meals-on-wheels provides an important service to elders who are unable to shop, prepare meals, or follow special dietary regimens.

Home health care includes a wide range of services, such as skilled nursing care; occupational, physical, and speech therapy; medical social services; physician care; nutritional and dietary services and meals; homemaker services; home health aide services; respiratory and IV therapy; and medical supplies, including drugs and medical appliances.

Monitoring services such as telephone networks and friendly visitors, keep health care systems in touch with chronically impaired or frail persons living at home. These services can be a secondary function of other services.

Access to services: Access occurs through a variety of mechanisms. **Outreach programs** are designed to identify persons with unmet needs. **Information and referral services** are offered by community agencies to answer service-related questions, to make appropriate referrals to service providers, and ideally to follow up on the referrals and determine

Access and Quality Assurance

Outreach
Information and referral
Assessment
Case management
Linkages
Evaluation and quality assurance

Services

Monitoring services
Homemaker
Home health care
Nutrition programs
Legal and protective services
Senior centers
Community medical services
Dental services
Community mental health
Adult day care
Respite care
Hospice care
Life care communities
Congregate care
Domiciliary care
Foster home
Personal-care home
Group home
Intermediate care
Skilled nursing care
Mental hospitals
Acute care hospitals

Home (Monitoring services through Nutrition programs)
Community (Nutrition programs through Respite care)
Institution (Respite care through Acute care hospitals)

FIG. 110–1. Continuum of geriatric care. (Modified from Brody SJ, Masciocchi C: "Data for long-term care planning by health systems agencies." *American Journal of Public Health* 70:1194-1198, 1980; used with permission of the American Public Health Association.)

whether appropriate services have been received. A **comprehensive assessment** is crucial for matching older persons with the appropriate services. **Case management** requires an individualized care plan based on the comprehensive assessment. The case manager coordinates the delivery of services and follows up to determine that the patient received them. Case management has evolved as an integral component of community-based long-term care. Increasingly, case managers find their roles as patient advocates complicated by demands for cost containment and tighter gatekeeping (see also FIG. 110–1).

FINANCING HEALTH CARE

(See also Ch. 114)

An array of federal, state, and private programs finance the services used by the elderly. The cost of geriatric health care is a substantial burden on public programs and on the elderly themselves. Frequently, several sources of funding support the services required by older persons. The major sources are Medicare, Medicaid, the Veterans Administration, private insurance, and certain other federal programs.

Medicare

The principal public health insurance for those ≥ 65 yr, Medicare paid out an estimated $146 billion in 1993. Medicare comprises two complementary but distinct parts: hospital insurance (Part A) and supplementary medical insurance (Part B). About 95% of those ≥ 65 yr are enrolled in Part A; nearly everyone covered by Part A enrolls in Part B, which is a voluntary program.

Part A covers four kinds of care: inpatient hospital care, medically necessary inpatient care in a skilled nursing facility, home health care, and hospice care. Payment for **hospital services** is based on a prospective payment system, using diagnosis related groups (DRGs). Payment for inpatient care in a certified **skilled nursing facility** has restrictive requirements, which change frequently. **Home health care services**—part-time or intermittent skilled nursing care, physical therapy, and speech therapy—are generally covered if the patient is homebound and if a physician develops and certifies a plan of care. **Hospice services** are generally covered if a physician certifies that the patient is terminally ill, the patient chooses to receive hospice care instead of standard Medicare benefits, *and* care is provided by a Medicare-certified hospice program.

Part B covers part of the cost of physician services, outpatient hospital care, outpatient physical and speech therapy services, and some health care services and supplies not covered by Part A. Certain restrictions exist on the types of outpatient care and therapists. Payment may be made to the patient or the physician. In either case, the patient is liable for an annual deductible fee as well as a copayment. If the payment is not made directly to the physician (assignment), the patient may also be billed for some amounts above the "reasonable allowable costs." The 1993 premium for Part B coverage was $36.60 per month. Most state Medicaid programs pay these premiums for persons who qualify for both Medicare and Medicaid benefits.

Several health services widely used by the elderly (routine eye examinations and preventive services) were not covered by Medicare in 1993 and are not projected to be covered in the near future. Drugs and certain dental procedures are covered only if provided during an authorized inpatient hospital stay. Neither intermediate nor long-term nursing care is covered under the Medicare program.

Health maintenance organizations (HMOs) provide an alternative type of care for enrolled Medicare patients. For each Medicare enrollee, the HMO receives 95% of the adjusted average per capita cost for its geographic region. Some authorities believe that HMOs have the potential to improve on the fragmented care provided in the fee-for-service sector by improving management of care and offering a wider array of services.

Medicaid

Funded by a federal-state partnership, Medicaid pays for health services for the aged poor, the blind, the disabled, and low-income families with dependent children. Services covered under the federal guidelines include inpatient and outpatient hospital care, laboratory and x-ray services, physician services, and skilled nursing care and home health services for persons > 21 yr. States may also pay for certain other services and items, including prescription drugs, dental services, eyeglasses, and intermediate-level nursing home care. Eligibility requirements are determined by each state, but cash-assistance recipients (eg, Supplemental Security Income) and certain groups of poor children and pregnant women must be included.

Medicaid is the major public payer for long-term care, contributing about 45% of the $53.1 billion spent for nursing home services in 1990. To qualify for Medicaid reimbursement for such services, the elderly must spend down (ie, pay for care from their own resources until they meet stringent income and asset-related eligibility requirements for the state where they live). Although the Medicaid program was intended to serve the poor, the high cost of long-term care rapidly brings most elderly persons requiring chronic care into this category.

Veterans Administration

Health care is provided to veterans without charge for service-connected disabilities and, on a complicated priority basis, for other conditions. The Veterans Administration operates 172 hospitals, 16 domiciliary facilities, and more than 100 nursing homes; it also contracts for care in community hospitals and nursing homes. The Veterans Administration has launched several innovative geriatric programs, including geriatric assessment units (GAUs), Geriatric Research, Education and Clinical Centers (GRECCs), and hospital-based home health care programs.

Private Insurers

Recently, private insurers have begun to pay more attention to the large market segment made up of those > 65 yr. Many types of private insurance coverage are available to the elderly, most taking the form of Medigap insurance, which pays for some or all of Medicare deductibles and copayments. Very few of these policies cover services such as long-term home health or nursing home care because benefits tend to be tied to Medicare definitions of eligibility and covered services. Recently, however, private insurers have begun offering long-term care insurance. As of 1991, about 1.5 million such policies had been sold. Estimates indicate that the proportion of long-term care expenditures covered by long-term care insurance will slowly increase: in 1990, about 2% of such expenditures were paid by insurance; by 2020, about 6.6% of long-term care expenditures will be paid by insurance. However, it is unknown whether the elderly or their families will pay the relatively high premiums required, or alternatively, whether they will enroll in long-term coverage programs at younger ages, when lower premiums are available. Also, it is not known how much long-term care coverage will be included in new government programs.

Other Federal Programs

Since its enactment in 1965, the **Older Americans Act** (Title III of the Social Security Act) has evolved from a program of small grants and research projects to a network of 57 state, territorial, and Indian tribal units on aging, 664 area agencies on aging, and thousands of community agencies. Its primary purpose is to develop, coordinate, and deliver a comprehensive system of services for older persons at the community level. These services include information and referral, outreach, transportation, senior centers, nutritional programs, advocacy, protective services, senior employment, ombudsman programs, and supportive services. The Older Americans Act also funds research and training. In 1990, the total appropriation for Title III programs was $846,374,000.

Title XX of the Social Security Act authorizes reimbursements to states for social services, including a variety of home health and homemaker services for frail elderly persons. These funds have been shifted to the Social Services Block Grant (SSBG) program, which is designed to prevent or reduce inappropriate institutional care by providing for community-based care and other assistance that allows the elderly to maintain self-sufficiency in the community. The program is defined, administered, and implemented by the states; it focuses on community-based services and does not support institutional care or any service covered by Medicare or Medicaid. Health services are covered only when they are an "integral but subordinate" component of an overall social service program.

Although **Social Security** is not usually considered a health program, as a basic pension system it provides resources that the elderly frequently use to pay for health care. There are two types of payments to the elderly: Old Age and Survivors Insurance (Title II) and Supplementary Security Income (Title VI). Supplementary Security Income provides a guaranteed minimum income to aged, blind, and disabled persons. For the elderly, Supplementary Security Income replaced the state-run old-age assistance programs, in which eligibility and benefits varied widely across the country.

111. ELDER ABUSE AND NEGLECT

Each year, many older Americans are physically injured, psychologically debilitated, financially exploited, or neglected by family members. Much of this abuse and neglect constitutes criminal offenses. Because much of it is perpetrated by spouses, it also must be viewed in the context of domestic violence.

Elderly men and women, whether or not they have impairments or are dependent on family members, are vulnerable to mistreatment. Besides suffering physical injuries, these victims often develop overwhelming feelings of fear, isolation, and anger and need extensive counseling to regain their independence. Given the incidence of mistreatment and the projected growth of the elderly population, the problem is significant enough that those who care for the elderly must learn to recognize mistreatment and intervene. The health professional is well positioned to screen, diagnose, and intervene and may be the only person outside the family who has contact with the elderly victim and established relationships with the victim and family members. However, there may be many barriers to establishing the diagnosis and successfully intervening.

Information about elder abuse and neglect is limited, and more research is needed to better understand the causes and preventive measures as well as the appropriate interventions.

Epidemiology

The epidemiology of elder abuse and neglect has been better understood since the publication of the 1986 survey by the Family Research Laboratory at the University of New Hampshire. In this survey of 2020 randomly selected elderly people living in the Boston metropolitan area, 3.2% reported being abused. Abuse was defined as **physical abuse,** which included hitting, slapping, and pushing; **neglect,** which involved depriving a person of something needed for daily living; and **chronic verbal aggression,** which included verbal threats and insults. Because the survey did not cover all forms of elder mistreatment (eg, financial exploitation), the 3.2% figure underestimates the problem.

Recently, the Women's Initiative of the American Association of Retired Persons categorized elder abuse and neglect as follows: (1) early onset spousal and partner abuse and neglect continuing into later life, (2) late onset spousal and partner abuse and neglect during later life, and (3) abuse and neglect by adult children and other relatives.

The Family Research Laboratory investigators found that most abuse is committed by one spouse against another; 65% of abuse cases were between spouses, and only 23% involved an adult child abusing a parent. Elderly husbands were abused twice as often as elderly wives. It is not known whether the abuse perpetrated by wives is a continuation of early onset spousal abuse done in a spirit of retaliation or self-protection. It is known that elderly wives are more seriously injured by their husbands than elderly husbands are by their wives.

This study also found that the abusers usually were dependent on the person they abused. The study indicates that a significant risk factor for abuse and neglect is a close proximity of living arrangements of victim and abuser. In the study, abuse occurred at all economic levels and in all age groups among the elderly.

Etiology

The four major etiologic theories that help practitioners understand and diagnose elder abuse and neglect focus on psychopathology of the abuser, stress, transgenerational violence, and dependency. Further research is required to substantiate these theories.

Psychopathology of the abuser: Many abusers have been hospitalized repeatedly for serious psychiatric disorders (eg, schizophrenia and other psychoses). Many abuse alcohol or other drugs.

When an adult child has a mental illness requiring inpatient psychiatric care, the parents' home is often the discharge site of last resort. Out of concern that the child will be homeless or have to stay in a shelter, or just out of love, parents often agree to take the child into their home. With the trend toward deinstitutionalization, psychiatrists who discharge a dependent child to the parents' home must be aware of the possible effects on the parents. Patients who are not violent in an institution may be violent in the home. When the potential for domestic violence is not scrutinized and provisions for follow-up are not made, elder abuse may occur.

Stress: Financial problems, death in the family, the responsibilities of caregiving, and other tensions may create frustration and anger that some people express through acts of violence. New studies have investigated the relationships between the care recipient's degree of cognitive impairment and the occurrence of abuse and neglect by the caregiver. A recent study conducted at the University of Medicine and Dentistry of New Jersey associated mistreatment of persons with dementia with the psychologic and physical demands placed on family caregivers. Another study from Cornell University and Louisiana State University found that a caregiver being married to the care recipient is a risk factor as are previous acts of abuse perpetrated by the care recipient on the caregiver.

Transgenerational violence: This theory postulates that violence is a learned response to difficult life experiences and a learned method of expressing anger and frustration. The theory has been hard to substantiate because information about family violence that occurred years ago is difficult to obtain.

Dependency: When family members depend on elders for housing, financial support, emotional support, or other needs, the dependent family members may become resentful and predisposed to abusive and neglectful behavior. This theory also suggests that elders who are functionally or cognitively impaired and dependent on their families for care are at increased risk for abuse and neglect.

Classification

The three general types of abuse and neglect are physical, psychologic, and financial. All can be intentional or unintentional.

Physical abuse and neglect: This type of mistreatment includes striking, shoving, shaking, beating, restraining, or feeding improperly. Sexual assault requires special emphasis, because many health care providers find this form of violence inconceivable when an older person is involved. Sexual assault refers to any form of sexual intimacy without consent or by force or threat of force.

Psychologic abuse and neglect: This type of mistreatment causes emotional stress or injury to an older person. Examples include verbal abuse—threatening remarks, insults, or harsh commands—and remaining silent or ignoring the person. Another form of psychologic abuse is infantilism (a form of ageism), whereby the elderly person is treated as a child, which both patronizes and encourages the person to passively accept a dependent role.

Financial abuse and neglect: This type of mistreatment is defined as the misuse or exploitation of or inattention to an older person's possessions or funds. Abusive behavior includes conning, pressuring the victim to distribute assets, or irresponsibly managing the victim's money.

Diagnosis

The difficulty of detecting abuse and neglect varies, depending on how subtle the signs are and how willing the victim is to talk. Many victims do not disclose abuse. Some tend to hide it out of shame. Others may either feel an obligation to protect the abuser or fear retaliation. Sometimes when elderly victims do seek help, they encounter ageist responses. For example, a health care worker may unquestionably accept a relative's statement that an elderly parent has Alzheimer's disease (supporting the stereotype that everyone > 65 yr has some degree of dementia). Or health care personnel may dismiss the possibility of abuse because they cannot believe that an 80-yr-old husband is capable of beating his 79-yr-old wife.

Health professionals must always be alert to the possibility of elder abuse and neglect—even when the symptoms and signs are not readily apparent. A failure to be alert to these problems may mean missing the diagnosis, even when symptoms and signs are obvious. For example, a relative may bring a patient with a fracture to the emergency department and attribute the injury to a fall caused by poor balance. Although falls and osteoporosis are common in the elderly, each new fracture should be thoroughly assessed, and the possibility of abuse should be considered. Medical personnel should ask specific questions about how the injury occurred and should avoid making assumptions based on an incomplete history or ageist stereotypes.

Isolation of the elderly victim is a common formidable barrier to detection. Factors such as retirement, loss of friends and relatives because of death and relocation, and disabilities that limit mobility tend to leave older people more isolated than younger people. Isolation tends to increase when the person is being abused because the abuser typically limits the victim's access to the outside world (eg, denying visitors, refusing telephone calls). Indeed, the health care worker is often the only person to whom the victim has access, which emphasizes the need to be alert to the possibility of abuse. *For at least part of the interview, the health professional and the elderly patient should be alone, especially if the patient is always accompanied by a relative or caregiver.* This gives the health professional a chance to ask about the patient's life and establish the rapport and confidentiality that are essential for accurate detection.

Several maxims on domestic violence derived from clinical impressions may be helpful in diagnosis. If the severity of the injury does not fit the explanation given by the relative, the health professional must suspect abuse. A relative's resistance to outside intervention (eg, visiting nurse or homemaker services, physical therapy in the home) or reluctance to leave the older person alone with health care personnel may indicate mistreatment. When elderly victims say they are certain no more abuse will occur, health care personnel should question this belief and explore intervention alternatives with them.

Unfortunately, health care workers usually have little or no training in recognizing and intervening in elder abuse and neglect. Therefore, many of them have little therapeutic optimism and so direct little effort toward detection. The lack of exposure, protocols, and well-defined approaches to treating elderly abuse victims contributes to poor detection skills, misdiagnosis, and limited intervention strategies. Nevertheless, there are a number of **signs** that aid in making a correct diagnosis.

Physical mistreatment may be indicated by bruises, burns, welts, lacerations, punctures, fractures, and dislocations; evidence of misuse of medications; malnutrition or dehydration; hair pulling; unexplained venereal disease or unusual genital infections; signs of physical restraint or confinement (eg, rope burns); missing eyeglasses, hearing aids, dentures, or prostheses; or unexpected or unexplained deterioration of health.

Psychologic mistreatment may be indicated by insomnia, sleep deprivation, a need for excessive sleep, unusual weight gain or loss, a change in appetite, tearfulness, unexplained paranoia, low self-esteem, excessive fears, ambivalence, confusion, resignation, or agitation.

Indicators of **financial mistreatment** include a sudden or unexplained inability to pay bills, withdrawal of money from accounts, or disparity between assets and satisfactory living conditions.

Further Assessment

Once the physician determines that abuse or neglect is probably occurring, a number of other specific issues must be assessed before a plan of management is formulated.

Because there is no prototypical abuser of the elderly, the health professional must evaluate the specific cause of abuse in each case. Understanding the cause or causes provides a framework for intervention that can help protect the victim. For example, intervention for a victim with a psychotic family member would be different from that for a recent stroke victim whose caregiver is under extreme stress. The physician should remember that abusers do not abuse continuously; between episodes and when with outsiders, they may exhibit nonabusive behavior.

The medical and psychosocial assessment of the victim should address the following questions (see also FIG. 111–1).

Safety: Is the patient in immediate danger? If so, the physician, in consultation with the patient, should consider hospital admission or law enforcement intervention. Does the patient understand the risks and consequences of the decision to ensure safety? What steps can be taken to increase safety in nonemergency situations?

Access: Do barriers limit or prevent further assessment? If so, the physician may improve access by engaging a trusted family member or friend of the patient, by working with state adult protective services, or, in some cases, by involving law enforcement agencies.

Cognitive status: Is the patient cognitively impaired? Formal, brief instruments such as the Mini–Mental State Examination can provide an objective, reliable assessment. If the patient has cognitive impairment, is it potentially remediable (is it caused by medications, thyroid disease, depression, or other organic causes)? If cognitive impairment is irreversible, is it severe enough to preclude the patient from giving an accurate history? Is it severe enough to impair the patient's decision-making capacity?

Emotional status: Does the patient manifest depression, shame, guilt, anxiety, fear, or anger? If yes, the physician should explore beliefs associated with these emotions. Is the patient reluctant to discuss the possibility of abuse or neglect? If so, the physician should attempt to determine the reason. Does evidence suggest patient denial? Does the patient minimize or rationalize family tension or conflict? If yes, does the denial interfere with the patient's recognition or admission of mistreatment?

Health and functional status: What medical problems exist? Could mistreatment have caused or exacerbated them? If the patient requires help with activities of daily living, who provides it? Does the person have the emotional, financial, and intellectual ability to provide the care? Does the patient have physical limitations that impair self-protection?

Social and financial resources: Does the patient have family or friends able and willing to nurture, listen, and assist with care, if needed? If not, why not? Does the patient have adequate financial resources for basic substantive needs? If yes, but these basic needs are not being met, why?

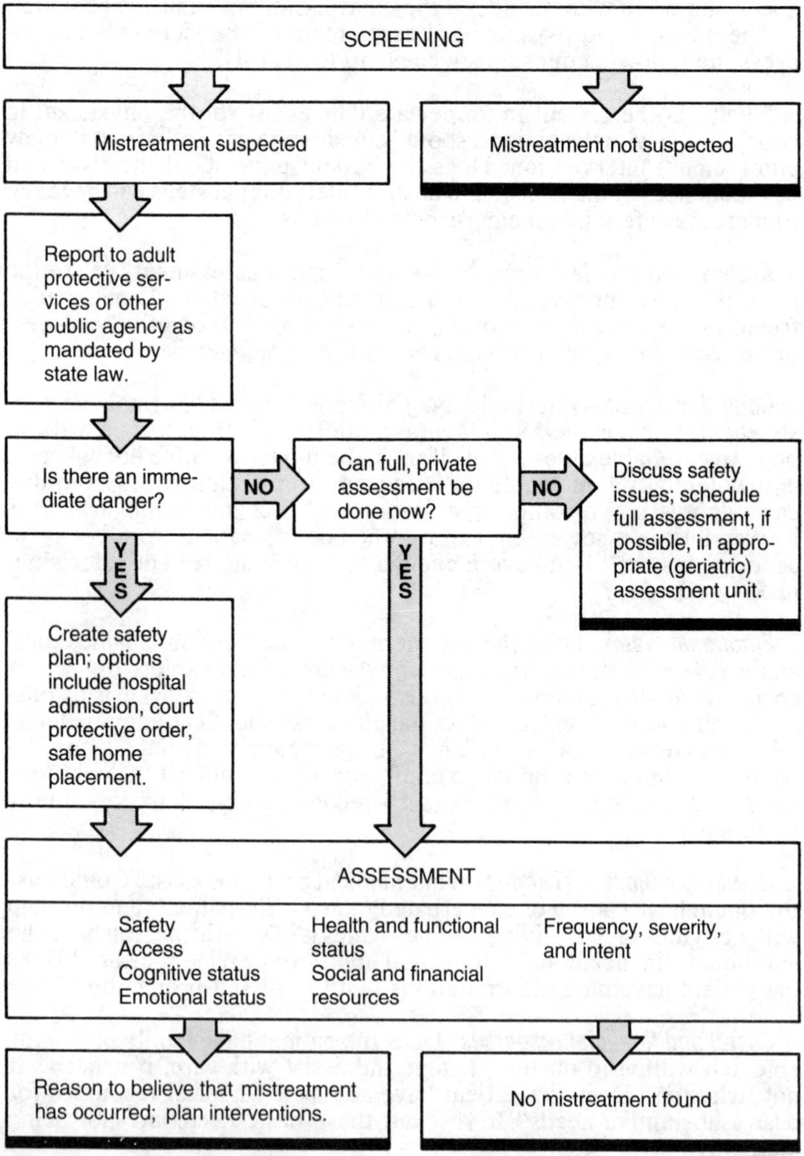

FIG. 111–1. Screening and assessment of elder mistreatment. (Modified from Adelman RD, Breckman R: *Diagnostic and Treatment Guidelines on Elder Abuse and Neglect*. American Medical Association, 1992; used with permission.)

Frequency, severity, and intent: Has mistreatment increased in frequency or severity over time? Although a single violent act can be damaging, elder abuse or neglect is characterized by a pattern of violence increasing in severity and incidence over time. Are there motives or remediable causes for the mistreatment? In some cases, people deliberately mistreat to cause harm; in other cases, the harm is not deliberate. Interventions should vary according to the intent to harm. For example, if a relative administers too much medication because of a misunderstanding of the physician's directions, the only intervention needed may be to give clearer instructions. However, deliberate administration of an excessive dose to control an elder's ability to function independently requires more intensive interventions.

Treatment

After the assessment, an intervention strategy can be developed (see FIG. 111–2). These cases are complicated, and they require a multidisciplinary approach (eg, physicians, nurses, social workers, lawyers, police, and psychiatrists).

First, the health professional must consider whether interventions have been implemented in the past. Information about previous interventions (eg, court orders of protection) and the reasons they failed should be obtained to avoid the same approach.

The health professional must decide whether **emergency intervention,** which usually involves emergency medical attention and law enforcement, is required. Circumstances that dictate such intervention include the urgent need for medical or psychiatric attention and life-threatening mistreatment.

In all cases, interventions may include medical assistance; education (eg, teaching victims about abuse and available options and helping them devise safety plans); psychologic support (eg, individual psychotherapy and support groups); law enforcement and legal intervention (eg, arrest of the abuser and orders of protection and advocacy on behalf of the victim in the criminal justice system); and alternative housing (ranging from sheltered senior housing to nursing home placement). Because counseling the victim usually requires many sessions, the health professional should anticipate incremental progress, not a short-term resolution.

With a competent victim, the health care provider presents options, and the victim decides how to proceed. With a judgmentally impaired victim, the multidisciplinary team should make most decisions. Decisions need to be based on the severity of the violence, the lifestyle choice history of the person, and the legal ramifications. The aim should be to implement the least restrictive plan. Often, there is no single correct decision, and each case must be carefully followed up.

In most states, reporting is mandatory when abuse occurs in the home. In all states, it is mandatory when abuse occurs in an institution. State laws vary as to which agency receives these reports. Thus, health care workers should become familiar with the mandatory reporting laws in their state and the available protective service resources.

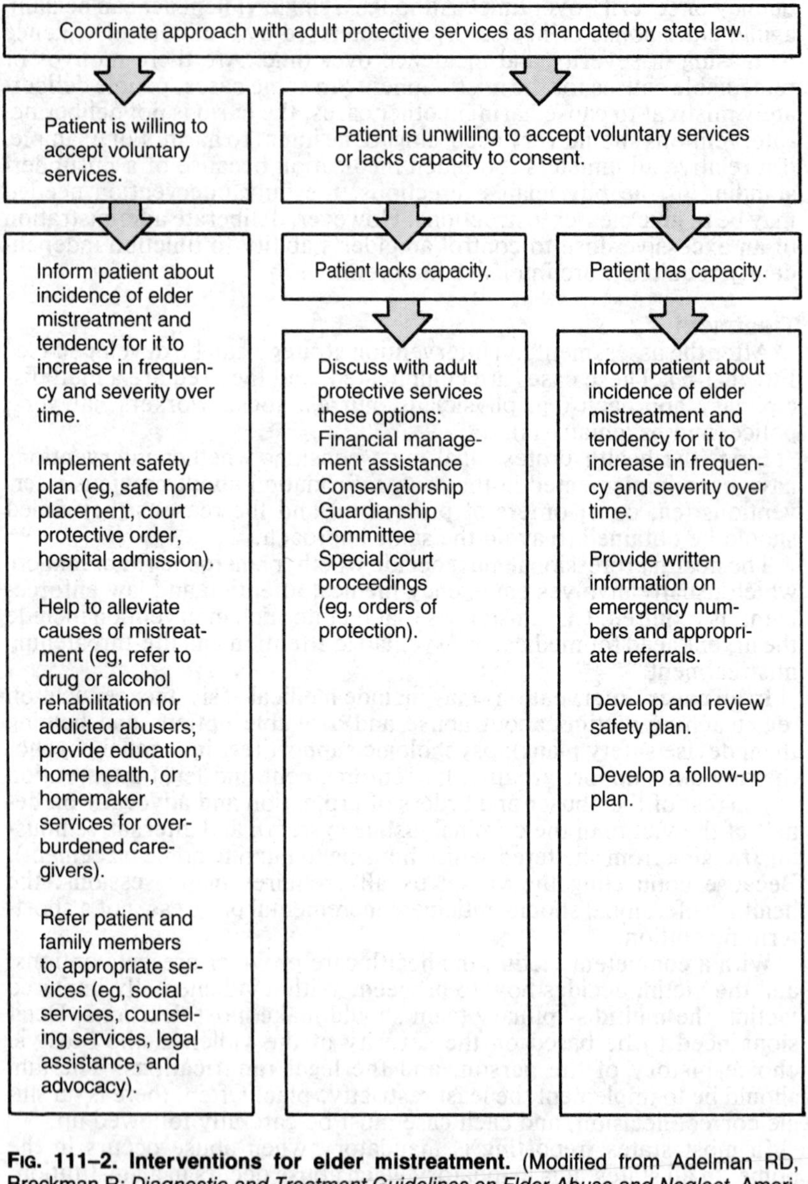

FIG. 111–2. Interventions for elder mistreatment. (Modified from Adelman RD, Breckman R: *Diagnostic and Treatment Guidelines on Elder Abuse and Neglect*. American Medical Association, 1992; used with permission.)

112. THE OLDER DRIVER

Safe driving involves the integration of complex motor, visual, and cognitive activities. A single traffic movement results from many decisions and reactions to myriad visual (and often auditory) stimuli.

In the USA, more than 13% of drivers are over age 65. Despite moderate deterioration of mental, motor, optic, and auditory functions, the elderly usually drive safely, probably because most driving patterns are learned and become second nature. Thus, performance is impaired only after considerable loss of function. Furthermore, the elderly tend to drive fewer miles, shorter distances, less at night, seldom in rush hours, and more slowly and cautiously. Average annual mileage declines steadily with age, decreasing 64% from age 65 to age 85.

Despite these compensations, elderly drivers have higher rates of traffic violations, collisions, and fatalities per mile than younger drivers. Two of the most common violations, failure to yield the right-of-way and failure to obey a traffic sign, probably result from functional deficits and often lead to collisions, mainly at intersections (see FIG. 112–1). Older drivers have higher collision rates per mile than any other age group, except for the youngest drivers (those < 24 yr), as shown in FIG. 112–2. However, these rates do not really begin to increase until age 70; after age 80, they increase rapidly.

Older drivers tend to fare worse in collisions. The collisions are more likely to involve multiple vehicles (which may reflect the patterns of driving, such as more daytime than nighttime driving) and to result in serious injuries and fatalities (which probably reflects underlying frailty, concurrent illnesses, and impaired recovery).

In assessing an elder's ability to drive, the physician must consider both public safety and the patient's independence. Many states have laws concerning the obligation of physicians to report impaired drivers. Yet an inability to drive means a loss of independence because public transportation is usually impractical for essential trips, such as food shopping and medical visits. Elders forced to stop driving rely more on their family for essential trips and reduce their social activities. These elders become depressed more often than those who continue to drive.

The elderly also require careful assessment before undertaking certain other potentially hazardous activities, such as piloting aircraft or boats. These activities are regulated by local, state, and federal authorities. Physicians must be aware of their legal role and their social and medical obligations before advising elderly persons as to their fitness to undertake such activities.

Evaluation of older drivers should include a functional assessment as well as a consideration of the impact of illnesses and medications on driving.

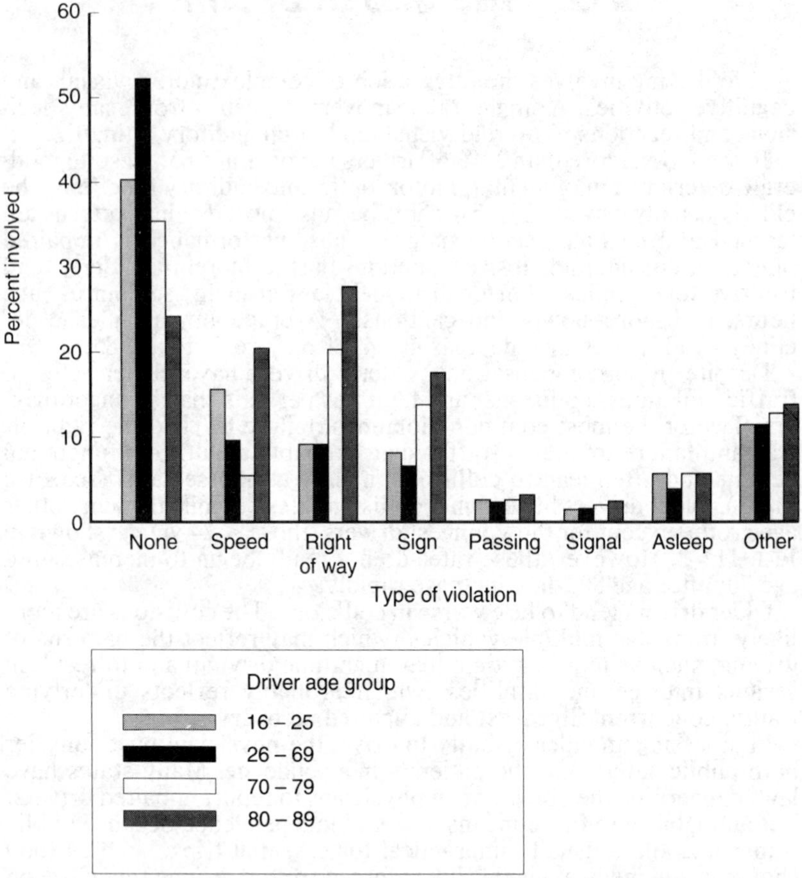

FIG. 112–1. Traffic violations that result in collisions by age group. (From Cerelli E: "Older drivers, the age factor in traffic safety." Department of Transportation HS 807 402. National Highway and Traffic Safety Administration Technical Report, February 1989.)

FUNCTIONAL ASSESSMENT

With age, many functions that affect driving ability may deteriorate, including muscle strength, reaction time, mobility, vision, and cognition (see TABLE 112–1).

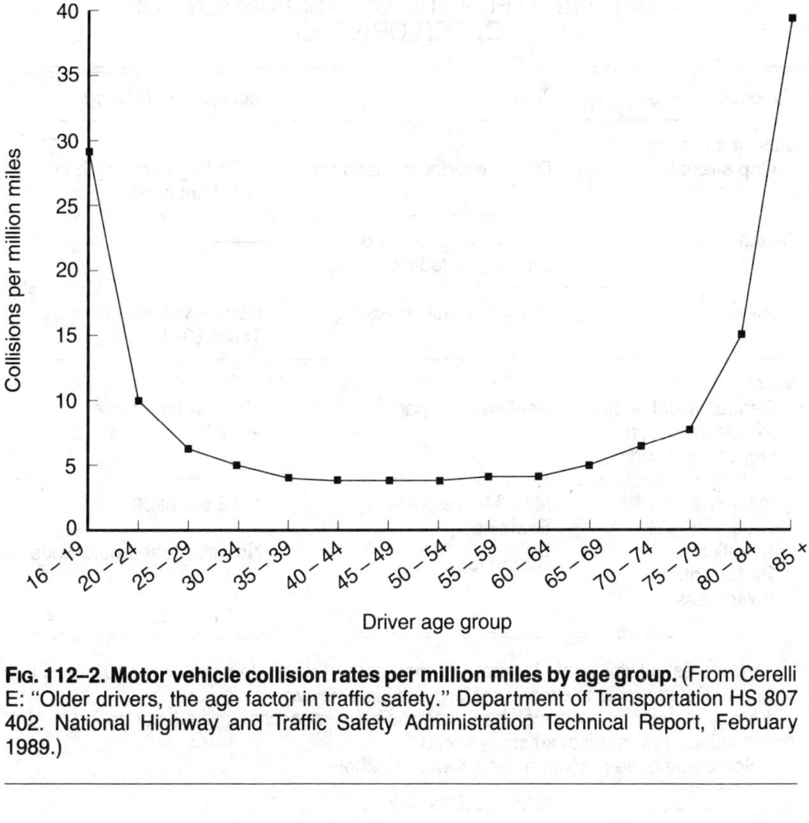

FIG. 112–2. Motor vehicle collision rates per million miles by age group. (From Cerelli E: "Older drivers, the age factor in traffic safety." Department of Transportation HS 807 402. National Highway and Traffic Safety Administration Technical Report, February 1989.)

Muscle Strength and Reaction Time

Decreased muscle strength, particularly decreased grip strength, can pose a problem. Dynamometric values of < 35 lb in the dominant hand should raise concern.

An increased reaction time also is a concern. Reaction time, which increases with the difficulty or number of choices, should be evaluated clinically. No established test exists.

Mobility

Formal evaluation of range of motion by an occupational or physical therapist using a goniometer is usually not required except in unusual circumstances. The neck is often a concern in patients with debilitating rheumatologic conditions because limited mobility may restrict the field of view, especially in critical traffic situations. Restricted mobility of the shoulder, wrist, or elbow can affect the ability to steer, though

TABLE 112–1. FUNCTIONAL ASSESSMENT OF OLDER DRIVERS

Function	*Test*	*Acceptable Findings*
Muscle strength		
Grip strength	Dynamometer for hand grip	≥ 35 lb grip strength in dominant hand*
Reaction time	Clinical judgment; no clinically established test	——
Mobility	Range-of-motion testing	Normal values shown in TABLE 29–1
Vision		
Central visual acuity	Snellen eye chart	20/40 in better eye†
Peripheral vision		≥ 120°†
Light adaptation		
Cognition	Mini–Mental State Examination	≥ 23 out of 30‡
Judgment		
Attention	Stroop test	No established guidelines
Perception		
Awareness		

* Values established only for men; women are estimated to have about 10% less grip strength. Relationship to driving performance is unknown.

† Many states and provinces have specific guidelines; check with local department of motor vehicles or medical advisory board.

‡ Some authorities recommend a lower threshold.

power steering and adaptive devices often can compensate adequately. In many metropolitan areas, body shops can equip vehicles with these devices, but they may be expensive.

Although proprioception is important, measurement is often crude. It should be assessed clinically, particularly in patients with subacute combined degeneration caused by vitamin B_{12} deficiency. Patients with obvious deficits may warrant road testing or other focused evaluations.

Vision

Several age-related changes in vision can affect driving. **Central visual acuity** frequently declines because of physiologic or anatomic changes, such as increasing opacification of the lens, or medical conditions, such as diabetic retinopathy. **Peripheral vision** also declines with age, mostly through the same mechanisms that affect central vision.

The total horizontal peripheral visual field typically declines from 170° in a young adult to 140° by age 50. Because the peripheral retina is less sensitive to low levels of light, twilight can be the most difficult time for driving. Drivers with peripheral vision deficits have twice as many collisions as those with normal vision. Other age-related functional deficits include poor visual adaptation to light changes, increased sensitivity to glare, declining visual accommodation (ie, presbyopia), and diminishing depth perception.

In most states, central visual acuity and peripheral vision are routinely evaluated at the department of motor vehicles. The frequency of evaluations and the minimum acceptable, corrected, central visual acuity depend on state regulations. The most common requirements are visual acuity of 20/40 in the better eye and horizontal peripheral vision of 120°. Medical or surgical therapy, such as cataract surgery, may be helpful.

Cognition

About 3% of community-dwelling elders between ages 65 and 74, 14% between 75 and 84, and > 20% over 85 have moderate degrees of cognitive impairment. Those with such impairment may not fully recognize their limitations, and elderly drivers with mild to moderate dementia have a fivefold greater risk of collisions. To evaluate cognitive impairment, the physician can use the **Mini–Mental State Examination.** Persons who score less than 23 should probably stop driving pending further investigation (see Ch. 89). About 5% to 10% of demented outpatients have reversible components to their dementia.

Although patients with severe dementia should not drive, most older drivers with illness-related dementia do not have severe cognitive impairment. In these patients, **attention deficits** may play a role in motor vehicle collisions. The three major types of attention are selective, divided, and sustained. **Selective attention,** *the ability to shift focus between competing stimuli,* is evaluated using several neuropsychologic tests, such as the dichotic listening test and the Stroop test. Selective attention is important in driving, where stimuli, such as a radio or a cellular phone, interfere with driving tasks. **Divided attention,** *the ability to process two or more stimuli at once and make an appropriate response,* is important when approaching intersections or merging onto freeways. Finally, **sustained attention,** *an endurance in alertness,* may be relevant to a driver with a chronic medical condition (such as heart failure) or to one taking medications that can cause fatigue or drowsiness (such as antidepressants).

ILLNESSES AND MEDICATIONS

Functional assessment is usually considered more relevant than a medical diagnosis in determining a person's fitness to drive. Nonethe-

TABLE 112–2. EFFECTS OF ILLNESSES AND MEDICATIONS ON OLDER DRIVERS

Condition or Medication	*Risks*	*Evaluation*	*Recommendations**
Coronary artery disease	Sudden incapacitating event	Clinical evaluation, ECG, echocardiogram, angiogram, etc	After uncomplicated MI or CABG, no driving for 1 mo; after angioplasty, no driving for 3–4 days
Epilepsy	Sudden incapacitating event	Clinical evaluation, EEG	Seizure-free interval ≥ 6 mo
Transient ischemic attacks	Sudden incapacitating event	Functional assessment	Attack-free interval ≥ 3 mo
Cerebrovascular accident	Sudden incapacitating event	Functional assessment	Attack-free interval ≥ 3 mo
Diabetes mellitus	Sudden hypoglycemic episode affecting awareness	Assessment of glucose control	Episode-free interval ≥ 3 mo
Medications	Side effects: somnolence, slowed reaction time, presyncope, poor judgment	Review of medications	Avoid sedative-hypnotics, long-acting benzodiazepines, more sedating antidepressants

ECG = electrocardiogram; EEG = electroencephalogram; MI = myocardial infarction; CABG = coronary artery bypass graft.

* Many states and provinces have specific guidelines; check with local department of motor vehicles or medical advisory board.

less, some conditions—such as coronary artery disease, neurologic disease, and diabetes mellitus—as well as the use of certain medications warrant special consideration (see TABLE 112–2).

Coronary Artery Disease

Although the incidence of sudden cardiac events while driving accounts for < 1 per 1000 collisions, the quandary for the clinician is estimating the risk in an individual patient. Patients with unstable angina should not drive until symptoms have been treated medically or surgically and the angina is either stabilized or does not occur for at least 1 mo. Some antianginal medications, such as nitroglycerin, can also interfere with driving by causing precipitous drops in blood pressure. Many noncardiac drugs, such as tricyclic antidepressants, also have cardiovascular side effects that can affect driving. Patients should avoid driving for 1 to 2 days after starting such medication.

After an uncomplicated myocardial infarction or a coronary artery bypass graft operation, patients should not drive for about 1 mo. After angioplasty, a delay of 3 to 4 days is warranted. Clinicians should consult local departments of motor vehicles or state medical advisory boards for local regulations and recommendations.

Neurologic Disease

The incidence of **epilepsy** rises with age. About 70% of persons with epilepsy can achieve adequate control with medication, although relapses often occur with a planned withdrawal of anticonvulsant therapy. Drivers with a history of a single episode and no underlying neurologic cause are the least likely to have a recurrence. Each state has adopted regulations for drivers with a seizure history; most require some seizure-free interval such as 6 mo before reinstating driving privileges.

The incidence rates for transient ischemic attacks and strokes are highest among the elderly. An otherwise healthy person who has had a **transient ischemic attack** should have an attack-free interval of ≥ 3 mo before resuming driving. After a **stroke,** the two concerns are residual disability and the likelihood of a recurrence. A functional assessment can help identify residual disability. The probability of recurrence warrants an event-free interval of > 3 mo before resuming driving. One year after a stroke, about 50% of patients have permanently stopped driving.

Other neurologic diseases, such as demyelinating conditions and Parkinson's disease, may also affect driving, but the degree of disability varies widely. Patients should undergo functional assessment before any clinical decision is made.

Diabetes Mellitus

The major risk for patients with insulin-dependent diabetes is sudden hypoglycemia while driving. A diabetic with autonomic neuropathy or one who is using a β-blocker is less able to detect the onset of hypoglycemia.

Otherwise healthy persons with diabetes who have not had a sudden episode affecting awareness for 3 yr should not require driving restrictions. Those who have had such an episode should not drive for at least 3 mo, and diabetic control should be reevaluated before driving is resumed. For insulin-dependent diabetics who have wide fluctuations in glucose levels, including documented hypoglycemia, special scrutiny is warranted. A 3-mo period of good control with no hypoglycemic events is recommended before driving is resumed.

Diabetic patients should also undergo a functional assessment to determine the effects of other diabetic complications, such as retinopathy. Because diabetic complications usually take many years to develop, therapeutic control at higher blood glucose levels is often warranted for an elderly person with diabetes of recent onset. Only extremely high glucose levels are of concern because of potential acute visual impairment.

Medications

Drugs that cause sedation can impair driving. The most common are the benzodiazepines, many of which have extraordinarily long half-lives in the elderly. Other such drugs include diphenhydramine (available over the counter) and other antihistamines, antidepressants, and opioids. Alcohol, either alone or in combination with other sedating drugs, can have a disastrous effect on driving.

LEGAL IMPLICATIONS

The failure to warn a patient of the dangers of driving while taking certain medications or the failure to advise a patient with brittle diabetes or epilepsy or another serious impairment not to drive could result in significant liability. Although the disclosure of a disability to appropriate authorities may violate confidentiality, it is sanctioned when public safety is imperiled. Indeed, the failure to notify such authorities could also result in liability and criminal charges. About 30% of states have laws and policies that mandate the reporting of impaired drivers, and many states have laws to protect physicians' anonymity when reporting such drivers.

The principal legal concern is **foreseeability** (*the ability to predict a risk or threat to public safety and health*), which is particularly relevant for drivers with obvious impairments. If special testing of driving performance is warranted, physicians should report patients to departments of motor vehicles and consult department personnel or the appropriate medical advisory boards for specific guidelines.

§5. REFERENCE GUIDES

REF

§5. REFERENCE GUIDES

113. LABORATORY VALUES

The determination of normal laboratory values in the elderly is complicated by latent or overt disease, multisystem disease, physiologic and anatomic changes associated with aging, and the effect of diet and exercise. These factors exclude many elderly persons from serving as normal controls in determining reference values and confound the determination of age-adjusted normal values.

Reference ranges are determined by using appropriate population samples obtained under precisely defined conditions. Cross-sectional studies provide test results from only one point in a subject's life and therefore cannot demonstrate serial changes. They are not as informative as longitudinal studies, which accumulate data over successive 1-, 2-, or 5-yr periods.

The **normal value** for a laboratory test is *its mean value ± 2 SD in a population of healthy persons*. Thus, in practice, 5% of the abnormal results obtained from healthy persons do not represent anything more than a statistical concept; if each test in a battery of tests is independent, the probability of a healthy person having completely normal results is relatively low.

TABLE 113–1 lists diseases and disorders associated with abnormal results of some common laboratory tests. An abnormal result does not necessarily mean that the disease or disorder is present. The likelihood of disease can be estimated only by knowing the test's sensitivity and specificity and the pretest probability of disease based on clinical findings and prevalence of the disease. A test's **sensitivity** depends on the proportion of patients with a disease in whom the test is positive (ie, percentage *positive in disease*). A test's **specificity** depends on the proportion of disease-free patients in whom the test is negative (ie, percentage *negative in health*). A change in any of these parameters drastically alters a test's usefulness in predicting disease. In addition, clinicians do not always have precise information on the sensitivity and specificity of individual tests in the elderly, and disease prevalence often differs in older populations from that in younger populations. Thus, interpreting test results is often difficult, and inaccurate interpretations tend to overpredict disease.

Drugs may alter the results of laboratory tests by their pharmacologic or toxic actions or by interfering with the testing procedure. For example, isoniazid, levodopa, morphine, vitamin C, nalidixic acid, and penicillin G may lead to false-positive urine glucose reactions. Levodopa may also produce false increases in serum bilirubin and uric acid levels. The possibility of an adverse drug effect or test interference should always be considered when an abnormal test result in an elderly patient is unexplained.

TABLE 113–1. COMMON TESTS AND THEIR ASSOCIATIONS WITH DISEASES AND CONDITIONS

Laboratory Test	*Increase*	*Decrease*
Acid phosphatase	Prostate cancer, prostatic massage, prostatitis, myocardial infarction, excess platelet destruction, bone disease, liver disease	———
Alanine aminotransferase (ALT or SGPT)	Hepatitis, cirrhosis, liver metastases, obstructive jaundice, infectious mononucleosis, hepatic congestion, pancreatitis, renal disease, alcohol ingestion	Pyridoxine (vitamin B_6) deficiency
Albumin	Dehydration, diabetes insipidus	Overhydration, malnutrition, malabsorption, nephrosis, hepatic failure, burns, multiple myeloma, metastatic carcinomas, acute illness
Alkaline phosphatase	Bone growth, bone metastases, Paget's disease, osteomalacia, healing fracture, hyperparathyroidism, hepatic disease, obstructive jaundice, hepatic metastases, pulmonary infarction, heart failure	Pernicious anemia, hypoparathyroidism, hypophosphatasia
α-Fetoprotein	Hepatoma, testicular tumor, hepatitis	———
Amylase	Pancreatitis, GI obstruction, mesenteric thrombosis and infarction, macroamylasemia, parotitis, renal disease, lung carcinoma, acute alcohol ingestion, after abdominal surgery	Massive pancreatic destruction
Aspartate aminotransferase (AST or SGOT)	Myocardial infarction, heart failure, myocarditis, pericarditis, myositis, trauma,	Pyridoxine (vitamin B_6) deficiency, advanced stages of liver disease

(continued)

TABLE 113–1. COMMON TESTS AND THEIR ASSOCIATIONS WITH DISEASES AND CONDITIONS *(Continued)*

Laboratory Test	*Increase*	*Decrease*
Aspartate aminotransferase (AST or SGOT) *(continued)*	hepatic disease, pancreatitis, renal infarction, neoplasia, cerebral damage, seizures, hemolysis, alcohol ingestion	
Bilirubin	Hepatic disease, obstructive jaundice, hemolytic anemia, pulmonary infarction, Gilbert's disease, Dubin-Johnson syndrome	——
Calcium	Hyperparathyroidism, bone metastases, myeloma, sarcoidosis, hyperthyroidism, hypervitaminosis D, malignancy without bone metastases, milk-alkali syndrome	Hypoparathyroidism, renal failure, malabsorption, pancreatitis, hypoalbuminemia, vitamin D deficiency, overhydration
Cholesterol	Hypercholesterolemia, hypothyroidism, obstructive jaundice, nephrosis, diabetes mellitus, pancreatitis	Hyperthyroidism, infection, malnutrition, heart failure, malignancies, severe liver damage (due to chemicals, drugs, hepatitis)
High-density lipoprotein cholesterol	Vigorous exercise, increased clearance of triglyceride (VLDL), moderate alcohol consumption, exogenous intake of insulin or estrogens	Malnutrition, obesity, cigarette smoking, diabetes mellitus, hypothyroidism, liver disease, nephrosis, uremia
Creatine kinase	Myocardial infarction, muscle disease or injury, burns, chest trauma, collagen-vascular disease, meningitis, drug use (eg, lovastatin), status epilepticus, brain infarction, hyperthermia, after surgery	——
Creatinine	Renal failure, urinary obstruction, dehydration, hyperthyroidism, muscle disease	Aging (decreases creatinine clearance but not serum creatinine concentration)

(continued)

TABLE 113–1. COMMON TESTS AND THEIR ASSOCIATIONS WITH DISEASES AND CONDITIONS *(Continued)*

Laboratory Test	*Increase*	*Decrease*
Glucose	Diabetes mellitus, pheochromocytoma, hyperthyroidism, Cushing's syndrome, acromegaly, brain damage, hepatic disease, nephrosis, hemochromatosis, stress (eg, from emotion, burns, shock, anesthesia), acute or chronic pancreatitis, Wernicke's encephalopathy (vitamin B_1 deficiency), chronic hypervitaminosis A, administration of thiazides, corticosteroids, epinephrine, estrogens, ethanol, phenytoin, propranolol, or IV glucose	Excess exogenous insulin, insulinoma, Addison's disease, myxedema, hepatic failure, malabsorption, pancreatitis, glucagon deficiency, extrapancreatic tumors, early diabetes mellitus, postgastrectomy, autonomic nervous system disorders, administration of oral hypoglycemic medications (factitious), malnutrition, alcoholism
Lactate dehydrogenase (LDH)	Myocardial infarction, pulmonary infarction, hemolytic anemia, pernicious anemia, leukemia, lymphoma, other malignancies, hepatic disease, renal infarction, seizures, cerebral damage, trauma, sprue	—
Lipase	Same as amylase (excluding parotitis and macroamylasemia)	—
Magnesium	Renal disease, excess exogenous magnesium	Diarrhea, malabsorption, renal tubular acidosis, acute tubular necrosis, chronic glomerulonephritis, aldosteronism, hyperthyroidism, hypercalcemia, uncontrolled diabetes, dietary deficit, administration of certain drugs (diuretics, antibiotics), alcoholism
Phosphorus	Renal failure, hypoparathyroidism, diabetic	Hyperparathyroidism, osteomalacia,

(continued)

TABLE 113–1. COMMON TESTS AND THEIR ASSOCIATIONS WITH DISEASES AND CONDITIONS *(Continued)*

Laboratory Test	*Increase*	*Decrease*
Phosphorus *(continued)*	acidosis, acromegaly, hyperthyroidism, high phosphate intake (IV or po), vitamin D intoxication, lactic acidosis, leukemia, volume contraction, hyperlipidemia, hyperbilirubinemia, dysproteinemia, heparin sodium contamination, spurious (prolonged refrigeration of sample)	hypokalemia, excess IV glucose, respiratory alkalosis, dietary deficit, ingestion of P-binding antacid, alcoholism, gout, hemodialysis, cirrhosis
Potassium	Hyperkalemic acidosis, diabetic acidosis, hypoadrenalism, hereditary hyperkalemia, hemolysis, myoglobulinuria, renal tubular defect, thrombocytosis, intake of K-retaining diuretic, ACE inhibitors, or large exogenous K load	Cirrhosis, malnutrition, vomiting, metabolic alkalosis, diarrhea, nephrosis, hyperadrenalism, ectopic adrenocorticotropic hormone excess, β-hydroxylase deficiency, administration of diuretics
Prostate-specific antigen (PSA)	Prostate cancer, benign prostatic hyperplasia, prostatic massage, prostatic abscess, prostatitis, cystoscopy	Administration of finasteride
Sodium	Dehydration, diabetes insipidus, excessive salt ingestion, diabetes mellitus with diuresis, diuretic phase of acute tubular necrosis, hypercalcemic nephropathy with diuresis, essential hypernatremia due to hypothalamic lesions	Excess exogenous antidiuretic hormone, nephrosis, hypoadrenalism, myxedema, heart failure, diarrhea, vomiting, diabetic acidosis, adrenocortical insufficiency, hyperlipidemia, hyperglycemia, hyperproteinemia (eg, multiple myeloma), intake of diuretics or mannitol, spurious (serum osmolality is normal or increased—avoid by using direct-reading potentiometry with ion-selective electrode)

(continued)

TABLE 113–1. COMMON TESTS AND THEIR ASSOCIATIONS WITH DISEASES AND CONDITIONS *(Continued)*

Laboratory Test	*Increase*	*Decrease*
Total protein	Multiple myeloma, myxedema, lupus, sarcoidosis, diabetes insipidus, dehydration, collagen-vascular disease	Burns, cirrhosis, malnutrition, nephrosis, malabsorption, overhydration, GI protein loss
Triglyceride	Nephrosis, cholestasis, pancreatitis, cirrhosis, diabetes mellitus, hepatitis, familial hypertriglyceridemia	Malnutrition
Urea nitrogen	Renal disease, dehydration, GI bleeding, leukemia, heart failure, shock, postrenal azotemia, obstruction of urinary tract, acute myocardial infarction	Hepatic failure, overhydration, acromegaly, dietary factors, prolonged IV feedings
Uric acid	Gout, renal failure, diuretic therapy, leukemia, lymphoma, polycythemia, acidosis, psoriasis, hypothyroidism, multiple myeloma, pernicious anemia, tissue necrosis, inflammation, 25% of relatives of patients with gout, cancer chemotherapy (eg, nitrogen mustards, vincristine, mercaptopurine), hemolytic anemia, high-protein weight-reduction diet, lead poisoning, polycystic kidneys, calcinosis universalis and circumscripta, hypoparathyroidism, sarcoidosis, elevated serum triglyceride levels, use of low-dose aspirin	Administration of uricosuric drugs, allopurinol, or large doses of vitamin C; Wilson's disease

ACE = angiotensin converting enzyme; K = potassium; VLDL = very low-density lipoprotein.

Based on material in *Interpretation of Diagnostic Tests,* ed. 4, by J Wallach. Boston, Little, Brown and Company, 1986, pp 41–96; used with permission.

EFFECTS OF PHYSIOLOGIC CHANGES

Population norms, but not individual norms, can be established for any physiologic parameter and its laboratory measurement. Yet, variability is the hallmark of aging, and physiologic change is no exception; as a result, extrapolating from norms to individuals is done with less confidence in the elderly. Many normal elderly persons show little or no physiologic decline in organ function, while many others show significant decline. One of the most useful techniques to establish the presence of disease is to compare current laboratory values with results obtained when disease was not present. Of course, this type of comparison is likely to be possible only for routinely performed tests.

Age-associated declines in cardiac, pulmonary, renal, and metabolic function correlate with changes in normal laboratory values (see TABLE 113–2). For example, systolic blood pressure increases, and maximal cardiac output decreases whether measured invasively or noninvasively. Vital capacity, forced expiratory volume at 1 sec, and maximal breathing capacity decrease progressively with age. Creatinine clear-

TABLE 113–2. EFFECT OF AGING ON LABORATORY VALUES

Increased	*Unchanged*	*Decreased*
Serum copper	Hemoglobin	Creatinine clearance
Serum ferritin	RBC count	Serum calcium
Serum immunoreactive parathormone	WBC count	Serum iron
Serum cholesterol	Serum vitamin A	Serum phosphorus
Serum uric acid	Leukocyte zinc	Serum thiamine
Serum fibrinogen	Serum pantothenate	Serum zinc
Serum norepinephrine	Serum riboflavin	Serum 1,25-dihydroxycholecalciferol
Serum triglycerides	Serum carotene	Serum vitamin B_6
Serum glucose	Erythrocyte sedimentation rate	Serum vitamin B_{12}
Prostate-specific antigen (PSA)	Serum IgM, IgG, IgA	Plasma vitamin C
	Blood urea nitrogen	Serum selenium
	Serum creatinine*	Plasma gammatocopherol (vitamin E)
	Serum alkaline phosphatase	Triiodothyronine (T_3)
		Serum testosterone
		Dihydroepiandrosterone

* Serum creatinine may be normal, even though creatinine clearance is decreased with aging as a result of an age-related decrease in creatinine production.

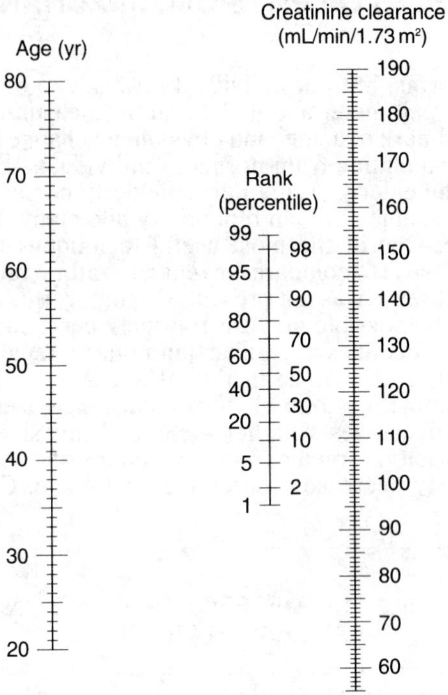

FIG. 113–1. Nomogram for determination of age-adjusted percentile rank in creatinine clearance of normal men. A straight line connecting the subject's age with his observed creatinine clearance intersects the rank scale at his percentile rank. (From *Aging–Its Chemistry,* edited by A Dietz. Washington, DC, American Association for Clinical Chemistry, 1980, p 8; used with permission.)

ance declines (see FIG. 113–1), but serum creatinine level remains stable because elderly persons have less muscle mass. Glucose tolerance, nerve conduction velocity, and maximal muscle strength decline with age.

The functional performance of different organ systems declines at different rates. Nerve conduction velocity diminishes by only about 10% between ages 30 and 70 yr, while renal function decreases on average nearly 40% over the same time period. Nomograms have been developed to illustrate the serial changes in various physiologic functions with age.

EFFECTS OF BIOCHEMICAL CHANGES

Blood and Serum Tests

A study of 150 persons 65 to 80 yr of age and 150 persons > 80 yr of age, selected by history and physical examination to exclude those with apparent disease, showed that most hematologic and biochemical test results for the elderly are the same as for younger adults. Glucose, chloride, and triglyceride levels were elevated in just over 10% of women in one or the other age group. Deviations in results (which, in many cases, were more likely the result of disease than of normal aging) were noted in 5% to 10% of the population for the following: women > 80 yr, a low hematocrit; women 65 to 80 yr, elevated calcium levels; both sexes of both age groups, reduced serum phosphate concentrations and elevated lactic dehydrogenase (LDH) and alkaline phosphatase levels.

Serum electrolyte values are not abnormal because of age alone. **Alkaline phosphatase** values approaching 140 u./L may be found in up to 5% of persons of all ages (normal = 35 to 120 u./L), but elevations may be caused by some drugs (eg, narcotics), eating a fatty meal, and bone abnormalities (including tumors, hyperparathyroidism, Paget's disease, a healing bone fracture, osteomalacia, and renal osteodystrophy). However, the positive predictive value of an elevated alkaline phosphatase level is very low in patients with no prior diagnosis of liver disease, malignancy, or bone disease.

In patients with osteoporosis, levels of serum calcium, phosphate, and alkaline phosphatase and the electrophoretic protein pattern are usually normal. In patients with metastatic cancer and almost always in those with osteomalacia, alkaline phosphatase is increased. Transient increases that do not usually exceed normal limits are noted in osteoporotic women after hip fractures.

A low **serum albumin** level in a healthy person is usually dietary in origin and unrelated to aging. However, serum albumin tends to fall when older persons develop serious disease, especially when accompanied by undernutrition. **Vitamin deficiency**, except for B_{12}, is rare in healthy ambulatory persons; studies have reported vitamin B_{12} deficiency in 12% of hospitalized elderly patients who have no evidence of general malnutrition.

Serum ferritin increases with age, and **serum iron** decreases minimally. Although **fasting blood glucose** increases with age, values remain within the normal range. Glucose tolerance decreases gradually with age. However, lack of exercise, obesity, and the use of some medications may be more important influences on glucose tolerance than age alone. Glucose levels are highest in the nonfasting state after a carbohydrate challenge or during a cortisone-glucose tolerance test. HDL **cholesterol level** tends to rise with age, as does LDL cholesterol, but this is based on values in survivors and, therefore, may not be a general aging trend.

Prostate-specific antigen (PSA) levels rise with age; the levels are typically about 2.5 ng/mL in men 40 to 49 yr of age, increasing to about 6.5 ng/mL by age 70 to 79. PSA levels may increase as a result of conditions other than cancer, such as benign prostatic hyperplasia or a prostatic infection, or briefly as a result of prostatic manipulation.

Age per se has no influence on the **erythrocyte sedimentation rate (ESR).** The sensitivity of an ESR > 20 mm/h in identifying the presence of a clinical disorder is 0.55; however, the specificity is 0.96, and the positive predictive value of an elevated ESR being associated with a clinical disorder is 0.93. Monoclonal gammopathy or elevated fibrinogen level, as well as more common chronic inflammatory diseases, can be a cause of elevated ESR in patients having no other obvious cause. The influence of plasma fibrinogen, total protein, serum globulins, and immunoglobulins on the ESR in older persons is similar to that in younger adults. Therefore, any age-related changes in ESR are best explained by disease rather than by aging itself. Severe anemia or hypoalbuminemia limits the test's usefulness.

A study using agarose gel **electrophoresis and immunofixation** demonstrated a 10% incidence of monoclonal gammopathy in apparently healthy persons ranging in age from 62 to 95 yr. The incidence is 6% in persons < 80 yr and 14% to 19% in those > 90 yr. An unexplained ESR elevation in the elderly warrants investigation for a monoclonal gammopathy, which occurs in about 35% of such persons. These gammopathies may indicate a dysregulation of the immune system occurring with age (ie, impaired T-cell or B-cell function).

Serum levels of the major subsets of **immunoglobulins** (IgG, IgM, and IgA) do not show clinically significant changes with age. A decline in several T-cell functions is the most consistent age-related change in the immune system.

Urine Tests

The incidence of trace proteinuria (defined as **protein excretion** > 80 mg/24 h ± 25 SD) is 40% at age 16, decreases to 2% in the third decade, and rises to 30% in old age. Glomerular and interstitial nephritis are rare in patients with protein excretion < 400 mg/24 h.

The magnitude of proteinuria can be estimated by measuring **protein:creatinine ratios** in single-voided urine samples. These spot measurements correlate with determinations of 24-h urinary proteins and are particularly useful in elderly patients, for whom 24-h specimens may be difficult to obtain. Protein:creatinine ratios > 3.0 indicate massive proteinuria (> 3.5 gm/24 h), while ratios < 0.2 indicate insignificant protein excretion.

Normal values for **white blood cells** and **red blood cells** in the urine do not change with age. **Glucose threshold** decreases so that glucose may be found in the urine of an elderly patient with diabetes, even when the blood glucose is considerably less than 200 mg/dL.

EFFECTS OF HORMONAL CHANGES

Testosterone

An age-dependent decrease in morning and mean 24-h plasma levels of testosterone occurs; free testosterone levels are less affected. A marked decrease occurs only after the seventh decade. Diet does not seem to influence levels significantly at any age. Smokers have higher testosterone levels than nonsmokers in all age groups, but this difference is not significant in the elderly. In response to stress, serum testosterone levels show greater increases in younger than in older men.

Estrogen

Urinary estrogen increases in elderly men, resulting in an increased estrogen:testosterone ratio. The source of this estrogen appears to be androstenedione, which is metabolized to estrogen by peripheral tissues. Estrogen levels in women decrease after the menopause, the consequences of which are discussed in Ch. 83.

Pituitary and Adrenal Hormones

In general, both pituitary and adrenal function decrease slightly. Decreased pituitary function leads to increased levels of gonadotropins secondary to lower levels of gonadal hormones. Growth hormone levels decrease with aging. Decreased adrenal function may lead to lower circulating levels of cortisol, although the diurnal pattern is usually preserved.

Serum renin and aldosterone levels fall with age, causing the so-called hyporeninemic hypoaldosteronism state. Together, these changes make hyperkalemia more likely, especially when potassium supplements or potassium-sparing diuretics are administered. Serum vasopressin levels tend to rise with age.

Endorphin levels increase with age. This may explain the suggestion that elderly persons have a decreased awareness of pain to such events as cardiac ischemia.

Serum concentrations of immunoreactive and bioactive parathyroid hormone increase with age in order to maintain normal serum calcium levels.

Luteinizing hormone (LH) and follicle-stimulating hormone (FSH) concentrations in blood begin to increase in men at about 50 yr of age; the increase is much less pronounced than that in postmenopausal women. In both men and women, the increase in FSH is usually more prominent than the increase in LH. In fact, in elderly men, LH is often not increased despite subnormal plasma bioavailable testosterone, indicating subnormal responsiveness of the pituitary in secreting LH. In confirmation of this, the LH response to luteinizing hormone–releasing hormone (LHRH) decreases with age in men. Serum prolactin also progressively increases in aging men, which may be related to the gradual increase in serum estrogen. In women, the levels of estrogen, prolactin,

LHRH, and FSH eventually fall after menopause, although LHRH may be elevated initially. Dehydroepiandrosterone and its ester, the major secretory products of the adrenal gland, also decrease with age.

Thyroid Hormones

Thyroxine (T_4) is unchanged with age, but triiodothyronine (T_3) tends to decrease by 10% to 15% in patients > 75 yr. Thyroid-stimulating hormone (TSH) may be > 5 μu./mL in 15% to 20% of women > 75 yr and in 4% to 8% of men > 75 yr, indicating mild hypothyroidism, most often without any other clinical manifestations.

VALUE OF SCREENING TESTS

Most patients with diseases that can be detected by biochemical profiles present with clinical symptoms and signs of such significance that laboratory tests usually have little screening value. For example, an increase in lactate dehydrogenase (LDH) levels without symptoms is only weakly predictive of underlying disease.

The sensitivity of a test or the rate of detection is probably more significant. For example, the total serum protein level is not very sensitive for detecting any of the conditions that may alter it; on the other hand, elevated **serum cholesterol** or **blood glucose** levels are virtually always detected in a patient with familial hypercholesterolemia or diabetes, respectively. Because measuring fasting blood glucose is useful and relatively inexpensive, it is a worthwhile screening test for asymptomatic patients with a family history of diabetes or obesity. Also, determining serum cholesterol level is worth the cost, considering the risk for atherosclerosis associated with elevated cholesterol and the evidence that lowering the level may reduce cardiovascular morbidity and mortality (see also Ch. 81). The frequency at which these tests should be repeated has not been determined. Some recommend rechecking cholesterol levels in the elderly every 5 yr if the initial cholesterol level is normal, but others advocate remeasuring cholesterol only if the levels are elevated or borderline. Laboratory variability and an average of 6.1% biologic variation must be accounted for when screening the cholesterol level.

The sensitivity of **creatinine** and **blood urea nitrogen** levels as an indicator of mild to moderate degrees of renal insufficiency is relatively poor. Because serum creatinine levels tend to overestimate renal function in the elderly, a normal value may not reflect the extent of renal disease. Thus, creatinine clearance should be determined to assess renal function. Such a measure is not reasonable for screening unless the following formula is used:

$$\text{Creatinine clearance (mL/min)} = \frac{(140 - \text{age [yr]}) \times \text{body wt (kg)}}{72 \times \text{serum creatinine (mg/dL)}}$$

In women, the calculated value is multiplied by 0.85.

The usefulness of measuring **serum calcium** level as a screening test for hyperparathyroidism is uncertain; both poor sensitivity and poor specificity undermine the test's usefulness. However, the diagnosis of primary hyperparathyroidism has increased since the use of automated biochemical studies has become widespread. The frequent use of diuretics, which increase serum calcium, may unmask hyperparathyroidism.

Measurement of **alkaline phosphatase** is probably useful, since levels are elevated in a number of treatable diseases (see EFFECTS OF BIOCHEMICAL CHANGES, above). Screening for uric acid is not worthwhile if clinical evidence of gout is lacking. Routine screening of **electrolytes** and **hepatic enzymes** is not indicated without a specific clinical indication or a drug history that might affect such tests.

Because elevations of **prostate-specific antigen (PSA)** can occur with benign conditions, its value in screening for prostate cancer is debatable. Men with an abnormal prostate that is detected by rectal examination may have their PSA level checked, although the actual numerical value may be less valuable than the ratio of the PSA level to the gland size, and abnormal results are likely to lead to more expensive and invasive tests. A change in the PSA greater than 5% to 8% in a year may be highly significant and require rectal ultrasound and biopsy.

An abnormal laboratory finding often requires a second test or additional tests, leading to increased costs with a relatively low return. Less than 5% of screening tests yield unanticipated or potentially important findings. In general, unsuspected disease is more prevalent in patients admitted to the hospital than in those undergoing office screening; therefore, the pretest probability for detecting disease is considerably higher in hospitalized patients.

A study of > 9000 tests in 121 elderly patients revealed that 17% of tests were abnormal. Patients received major benefit by having serial CBCs, tests of potassium levels, and BUN measurements. Urinalyses in asymptomatic persons were not cost effective. Recommendations published by the US Preventive Services Task Force in 1990 differ from these findings. The Task Force suggests laboratory screening for cholesterol and fasting blood glucose in patients at risk for diabetes. Of possible benefit are TSH measurement (especially in women > 60 yr old) and urinalysis for detection of bacteriuria (though treating asymptomatic bacteriuria in the elderly has not been shown to be beneficial). The Task Force recommends fecal occult blood testing for high-risk persons. What constitutes appropriate screening in adults is the source of widespread disagreement.

If a disease has a 1% prevalence in the population, the probability of a patient having that disease diagnosed after an abnormal test result (with 70% sensitivity and 65% specificity) is only 16%, and the probability that such a patient does not have the disease is 84%. In general, markedly abnormal test values are more predictive of disease than minimally abnormal values. *In assessing a specific test's value, it is important to consider its discrimination property at each level of abnormal results, to be aware of all of the diseases that might yield an abnormal result, and to consider the probability that several diseases may coexist in a particular person.*

114. HEALTH INSURANCE

(See also FINANCING HEALTH CARE in Ch. 110)

In 1993, health care expenditures in the USA approached $1 trillion; about 33% of this amount was spent on the elderly. The financial implications of providing care for the rapidly increasing elderly population is cause for concern within both political and professional ranks. However, data from geriatrics-oriented research on the delivery and organization of health services, including favorable cost-benefit analyses of preventive care in older persons and biomedical developments of improved diagnosis and treatment, are encouraging.

The core of health insurance for almost all 32 million Americans ≥ 65 yr is Medicare. Additional coverage, ancillary to Medicare, includes supplementary (or Medigap) policies offered by private insurance companies, retirement health benefits offered by employers, veterans' benefits offered by the US Department of Veterans Affairs, and the federally mandated Medicaid welfare programs. Ancillary coverage includes Medicare deductibles, coinsurance, and Part B premiums. Private long-term care insurance is also available.

The USA is undergoing major reform in the financing and organization of health services. Medicare, Medicaid, and other federal programs are being reviewed for potential incorporation into a broad national program that could include long-term care and other improvements in geriatric services. Many components of Medicare are likely to be changed in the process.

MEDICARE

Medicare encompasses hospital benefits (Part A) and medical benefits (Part B) for persons ≥ 65 yr as well as for disabled persons who have been on Social Security disability benefits for at least 2 yr. The program was modeled on employment-based insurance and reflects its acute care focus. Medicare coverage is generally adequate for those who need mainly hospital and medical services for acute conditions, but the 1993 Medicare list of benefits excluded some services that are critically important to the elderly, such as outpatient prescribed drugs, custodial or personal care (except under limited conditions, see below), and most preventive medical services. Preventive coverage recently added includes periodic mammograms, Papanicolaou (Pap) tests, and influenza vaccination (previously, only pneumococcal vaccination was covered). Overall, Medicare covers < 45% of the total health care expenses for the elderly.

Despite its acute care orientation, Medicare provides some coverage of custodial or personal care in certain circumstances. **Custodial care** (care of a medically stable patient who needs assistance with activities of daily living such as eating, dressing, toileting, and bathing) in the home is covered by Medicare only when **skilled care** (the services of a professional nurse or therapist under a physician-authorized plan of home care) is required (see Ch. 25). Medicare covers custodial care in a skilled nursing facility when it is part of posthospital acute and rehabilitation care.

PART A: HOSPITAL INSURANCE

Part A of Medicare is supported by a payroll tax collected during a person's working years. Part A represents paid-up hospital insurance for Medicare-qualified retirees, who pay no premiums during retirement. Generally, only people who are eligible to receive Social Security monthly payments are eligible for Medicare. Persons who never worked or who did not accumulate enough Social Security work quarters are not eligible for Medicare.

In general, a Medicare beneficiary is entitled to **inpatient hospital care** for a maximum number of days (60 days in 1993) during a benefit period. The beneficiary pays a deductible ($690 in 1994), which is established annually by the government. A benefit period begins when the person is admitted to the hospital and ends when the person has been out of the hospital or skilled nursing facility for a given number of consecutive days (60 days in 1993). A readmission in a new benefit period requires that another deductible be paid. If the patient's hospital stay exceeds the maximum number of days in one benefit period, Medicare pays a large part of the recognized costs for days 61 to 90, and the beneficiary pays a daily copayment equal to one fourth of the deductible. This extension is limited to 30 hospital days. In addition, Medicare provides partial coverage for 60 hospital reserve days during a beneficiary's lifetime; after these days are used, they cannot be replaced. The beneficiary pays one half of the deductible for reserve days. Part A provides some coverage for **psychiatric hospital stays.**

Medicare Part A covers virtually all hospital services, including discharge planning and medical social services. It covers the cost of a semiprivate room or, if medically necessary, a private room, but not such amenities as television and telephone.

The amount Medicare pays for hospitalization is predetermined by the **diagnosis related group (DRG)** that covers the beneficiary's principal diagnosis. Some adjustment is made for age and comorbidity. The hospital may make or lose money, depending on how soon the patient is discharged and how many diagnostic and therapeutic services are used. Under this arrangement, the financial pressure for earlier discharge and limited intervention may conflict with medical judgment. When a patient cannot be discharged home safely or to a nursing home because no bed is available, Medicare pays a relatively low per diem for an alternate level of care.

Part A covers posthospital convalescent care and rehabilitative care in a nursing home. However, because Medicare does not pay for custodial or long-term care, coverage ends when the patient is stabilized and skilled professional care is no longer needed.

Hospice care is covered by Part A under certain conditions (see HOSPICE CARE in Ch. 25). The beneficiary pays no deductible or copayment except for part of the costs of outpatient drugs and of **respite care,** a provision to support family members caring for the patient at home (see RESPITE CARE in Ch. 25).

PART B: SUPPLEMENTARY MEDICAL INSURANCE

Part B of Medicare is optional. Social Security beneficiaries are automatically enrolled in Part B, unless they decline the highly subsidized coverage; the federal government pays 75% of Part B costs, and beneficiaries pay 25%. Consequently, 95% of persons aged 65 yr who retire with Social Security benefits elect Part B coverage and agree to have premiums deducted from their monthly checks. Persons who decline coverage but later change their minds must pay a surcharge based on how long they delayed enrollment. Participants may discontinue coverage at any time but must pay a surcharge on the premium if they reenroll.

Part B covers physician services and physician-prescribed services, such as hospital outpatient services, including emergency department care and day surgery; physical, occupational, and speech therapy; diagnostic tests including portable x-ray services in the home; and durable medical equipment for home use. If surgery is recommended for a patient, Part B covers part of the cost of a second and even a third opinion.

In addition, Part B covers medically necessary ambulance services, certain services and supplies (colostomy bags, prostheses) not covered by Part A, drugs and biologicals that cannot be administered by the patient, spinal manipulation by a licensed chiropractor for subluxation demonstrated on x-ray, dental services deemed necessary to medical treatment, optometry services related to providing lenses for cataracts, and the services of physician assistants, nurse practitioners, clinical psychologists, and clinical social workers. Outpatient mental health care, with certain limitations, is covered. A complete description of Part B services and other provisions is available in *The Medicare Handbook,* updated annually.

Under Part B coverage, Medicare determines the allowable charge for each service and pays 80% of the allowable charge, after the annual deductible is paid. If the billed charge equals the allowable charge, the patient pays the remaining 20%. If the billed charge exceeds the allowable Medicare charge, the patient pays 20% of the allowable charge and the amount above the allowable charge, up to a maximum percentage of the allowable charge; in 1993, the maximum was 115%. *Physicians, whether they participate in Medicare Part B or not, whose charges exceed the maximum Medicare fees are subject to fines.*

Physicians may or may not participate in Part B of the Medicare program. A participating physician takes assignment on all Medicare patients. (Assignment means that beneficiaries assign their right to receive payment from Medicare to the physician and that the physician receives payment—80% of allowable charges—directly from the program.) A nonparticipating physician either does not take assignments or takes them selectively. If a physician does not take an assignment, Part B pays the 80% to the patient, who is then responsible for all payments to the physician. Whether participating or not, the physician must send the claim to Medicare and must bill the patient for the Part B deductible ($100 in 1993).

A physician who does not take assignment for elective surgery must give the patient a written estimate in advance if the total charge is more than $500. If the physician does not provide an estimate, the patient can later claim a refund from the physician for any amount paid over the allowable charge.

The Medicare payments to physicians have been criticized for being inadequate compensation for the time involved in giving physical and mental status examinations and obtaining the patient history from family members. A Medicare fee schedule based on a **resource-based relative value scale (RBRVS)** for physician services became effective in January 1992 to address this concern. The effects of the Medicare fee schedule on patient care and on the practice of geriatric medicine remain to be seen.

The services covered by Parts A and B can be provided through a **health maintenance organization (HMO).** Medicare pays the HMO a lump sum per enrollee (capitation) based on the average expenditures for Medicare beneficiaries in the geographic area. If the income from Medicare is greater than the expenses, the HMO must share part of the excess with its Medicare members by providing services not covered by Medicare (eg, preventive medical services) or by eliminating cost sharing.

MEDIGAP INSURANCE

Because of gaps in Medicare's coverage, more than 66% of beneficiaries supplement Medicare with private insurance. Called Medigap, this supplementary insurance pays Medicare deductibles, copayments, and certain charges Medicare does not cover. Most Medigap insurance is purchased individually from private insurers, although it can be provided by employers to retirees.

Congress has restricted Medigap insurance to a basic plan with nine possible expansions. No plan may duplicate Medicare benefits. The basic plan covers hospital copayments, lifetime reserve days, 365 days beyond the total medical hospital benefits provided by Part A, and Part B copayments. The expansion plans, which have higher premiums than the basic plan, may provide additional coverage in a skilled nursing facility and may cover the Part A deductible, the Part B deductible, a percentage of the cost of outpatient prescribed drugs, preventive medical services, and short-term home-based help with activities of daily living during recovery from an illness, injury, or surgery.

LONG–TERM CARE INSURANCE

The greatest single threat to the financial security of older Americans is the cost of long-term care. About 50% of the expenditures for long-term care is paid by patients and their families; private insurance pays about 1%, Medicare pays about 3%, and Medicaid pays the rest. Few persons can afford nursing home care (which averaged about $37,000 per year in 1993) for very long. Many persons admitted to nursing homes have already been impoverished by the costs of personal care, Medicare copayments, prescribed drugs, and other out-of-pocket medical expenses.

MEDICAID

Medicaid encompasses 50 different state programs, mandated by federal law, that cover the health care expenses of poor people, young and old. The federal government pays 50% or more of the costs; states pay from 21% to 50%. About 10% of the elderly receive services under Medicaid, accounting for about 40% of all Medicaid expenditures, chiefly for long-term nursing home care. The growing elderly population and the rapid rise in nursing home expenses have strained state Medicaid budgets.

State Medicaid programs determine eligibility and the payment, duration, and scope of covered services. All programs cover medical, hospital, and custodial nursing home care, and most programs cover prescribed drugs, preventive care, podiatric care, rehabilitation, dental care, dentures, eyeglasses, and physical therapy. In addition, some programs cover personal care at home, adult day care, home-delivered meals, and respite care.

In most states, patients qualify for Medicaid benefits if they are medically needy, ie, if their income minus medical expenses is at poverty level. In some states, eligibility depends on income level without offsetting medical expenses. In addition to this income test, persons must pass an assets test. Equity in a home and certain other assets are excluded. If the remaining assets exceed the limit, the person is not eligible for Medicaid, even if the income test is passed. Thus, patients may need to spend down (use up their resources) to reach the Medicaid qualifying level. Spouses of nursing home patients may keep some income (up to $1,718 per month in some states) and half of the couple's assets (up to about $69,000). The extent to which middle-class persons give away assets to qualify for Medicaid coverage of nursing home care is not known. State Medicaid programs cannot attach assets that are given away, but giving away assets during the 30 mo before entering a nursing home may delay eligibility for Medicaid benefits. Medicaid denies coverage for a period of time determined by the amount of improperly divested funds divided by the average monthly cost of nursing home care in the state. For example, if a person gives away $10,000 in a state where the average monthly cost of care is $3,500, Medicaid coverage is delayed by 3 mo.

PRIVATE INSURANCE

The availability of private insurance for long-term care is relatively recent. The number of policies in existence has grown from < 100,000 in 1980 to > 2 million today. Much private insurance is costly and inadequate in financial protection, range of benefits, and care coordination. Policies usually offer cash benefits of about $50 to $100 per day for nursing home care and a lesser per diem for home care. Premiums are scaled to the desired indemnity level, age of the beneficiary, preexisting conditions, waiting periods, and optional inflation protection (the per diem increases at intervals and, accordingly, the premium). Newer policies with inflation protection and higher indemnity levels are expensive and often unaffordable for most elders.

Under older policies, payment of claims is contingent on a physician's declaration that the services are medically necessary. Under newer, more expensive policies, an evaluation of activities of daily living and cognitive ability is required before payment of claims.

MODELS FOR COMPREHENSIVE COVERAGE

Individually, Medicare, Medicaid, Medigap, and private long-term care insurance have shortcomings in providing comprehensive geriatric care, which includes the medical, nursing, and supportive needs of the elderly patient. Medicare excludes long-term custodial care and many preventive services; Medicaid belatedly intervenes after the patient is impoverished; Medigap, like Medicare, excludes long-term care and outpatient prescribed drugs; and private insurance is unaffordable by most elders, leaves them vulnerable to financial catastrophe, and supports only fragments of long-term care. Collectively, these programs rarely promote integrated acute and long-term care or coordination of health and social services. However, several model projects have demonstrated that with organized delivery of services using combinations of public funding and private insurance, comprehensive geriatric care can be adequately financed.

Social and health maintenance organizations (SHMOs) are demonstration programs conducted by Medicare. They use Medicare, Medicaid, and private patient payments to cover a complete range of care benefits managed by nurses, social workers, and physicians. Patients not eligible for Medicaid benefits use private payments to cover a limited amount of long-term care, principally in the home. Like an HMO, an SHMO is at financial risk for the cost of services and has a stake in frugality.

The Program of All-inclusive Care of the Elderly (PACE) is a federally supported, multisite program of comprehensive care. Its primary objective is to keep patients in the community as long as medically, socially, and financially possible. A professional multidisciplinary team assesses patient needs, develops a care plan, integrates primary care and other services, and arranges for the implementation of services. The project is sponsored by one or more facilities and community groups; the project sponsor receives a preset amount of Medicare, Medicaid, and private funds and guarantees the provision of benefits at a capitated rate. If the costs of benefits exceed the pooled funds, the project covers the loss.

In San Francisco's Chinatown, **On Lok,** the forerunner of PACE, provides prepaid comprehensive care for elderly persons who have a level of impairment that usually requires admission to a nursing home. On Lok provides adult day care and coordinated, comprehensive services, including custodial or personal care, drug treatment, dentistry, and housekeeping services in a community housing project. Fewer than 6% of On Lok participants (who enroll for life) have needed nursing home placement, and hospital admissions and lengths of stay are half those for comparable elders.

The **life-care community** or **continuing care retirement community** is a model for combining housing, health care, and other services under packaged financing and management. These communities may have a clinic, an infirmary, or even a nursing home on the site, and housing is designed to accommodate disabled persons. The most extensive of these communities serve wealthy retirees willing to sign long-term contracts for their housing and care. Some life-care communities have failed when inflation and an aging population caused costs for services to exceed income. Some communities keep costs down by providing housing and minimal services with options to purchase additional services (see also LIFE-CARE COMMUNITIES in Ch. 24).

In 1990, the US Bipartisan Commission on Comprehensive Health Care (the Pepper Commission) developed a model approach to long-term care financing that resembles Social Security. Throughout their working lives, Americans would contribute a portion of earnings to a long-term care fund, with services administered by state government and community organizations. This fund would provide custodial care for as long as a person needed it at home and for 3 mo in a nursing home. The panel also proposed a liberalized Medicaid program for persons who need longer nursing home stays. In consideration of national health reform in the early 1990s, some proposals omitted long-term care on the grounds that the nation could not afford it.

According to one study, long-term care costs will rise substantially if no major changes are made; the $54.7 billion spent on nursing home care and the $20.7 billion spent on home care in 1993 will increase to $126.2 billion and $40 billion, respectively, in 2018. The study also concluded that private insurance was unlikely to have a major effect on individual and Medicaid spending for long-term care and that social insurance was central to the financing and delivery of long-term care (home and community-based care plus 3 mo in a nursing home), with supplementation by private insurance and liberalized Medicaid.

APPENDIX. HIGH-RISK DRUG PRESCRIBING GUIDELINES

Drug	*Prescribing Guideline (Doses are total daily dose)*
Propoxyphene and combination products	Propoxyphene offers few analgesic advantages over acetaminophen, yet has the side effects of a narcotic.
Indomethacin	Indomethacin commonly produces CNS and other side effects.
Phenylbutazone	Phenylbutazone may produce severe hematologic side effects.
Pentazocine	Pentazocine, a narcotic analgesic, produces more CNS side effects, including confusion and hallucinations, than other narcotics. Additionally, it is a mixed agonist-antagonist.
Trimethobenzamide	Trimethobenzamide is one of the least effective antiemetics, yet it can cause extrapyramidal side effects.
Methocarbamol Carisoprodol Oxybutynin Chlorzoxazone Metaxalone Cyclobenzaprine	Most muscle relaxants-antispasmodics are poorly tolerated by the elderly, leading to anticholinergic side effects, sedation, and weakness. Additionally, their effectiveness at doses tolerated by the elderly is questionable.
Flurazepam	This benzodiazepine hypnotic has an extremely long half-life in the elderly (often days), producing prolonged sedation and increasing the incidence of falls and fractures. Medium- or short-acting benzodiazepines are preferable.
Amitriptyline Chlordiazepoxide-amitriptyline Perphenazine-amitriptyline	Because of its strong anticholinergic and sedating properties, amitriptyline is rarely the antidepressant of choice for the elderly.
Doxepin	Because of its strong anticholinergic and sedating properties, doxepin is rarely the antidepressant of choice for the elderly.
Meprobamate	Meprobamate is a highly addictive and sedating anxiolytic that should be avoided in elderly patients. Those using it for prolonged periods may become addicted and may need to be withdrawn slowly.

(continued)

APPENDIX. HIGH-RISK DRUG PRESCRIBING GUIDELINES *(Continued)*

Drug	*Prescribing Guideline (Doses are total daily dose)*
Lorazepam Oxazepam Alprazolam Temazepam Zolpidem Triazolam	Because of increased sensitivity to benzodiazepines in the elderly, smaller doses may be effective as well as safer. Total daily doses should rarely exceed the following suggested maximums (although doses of alprazolam may be higher when used to treat panic disorders): lorazepam—3 mg, oxazepam—60 mg, alprazolam—2 mg, temazepam—15 mg, zolpidem—5 mg, triazolam—0.25 mg.
Chlordiazepoxide Chlordiazepoxide-amitriptyline Clidinium-chlordiazepoxide Diazepam	Chlordiazepoxide and diazepam have a long half-life in the elderly (often several days), producing prolonged sedation and increasing the risk of falls and fractures. Short- and intermediate-acting benzodiazepines are preferred.
Disopyramide	Disopyramide is the most potent negatively inotropic antiarrhythmic and therefore may induce heart failure in the elderly. It is also strongly anticholinergic. Other antiarrhythmics should be used when appropriate.
Digoxin	Because of the decreased renal clearance of digoxin, doses in the elderly should rarely exceed 0.125 mg daily, except when treating atrial arrhythmias.
Dipyridamole	Dipyridamole frequently causes orthostatic hypotension in the elderly. It has been proved beneficial only in patients with artificial heart valves.
Methyldopa Methyldopa-hydrochlorothiazide	Methyldopa may cause bradycardia and may exacerbate depression in the elderly. Alternative treatments for hypertension are preferred.
Reserpine Reserpine-hydrochlorothiazide	Reserpine imposes unnecessary risk in the elderly, inducing depression, impotence, sedation, and orthostatic hypotension.
Chlorpropamide	Chlorpropamide has a prolonged half-life in the elderly and can cause prolonged, severe hypoglycemia. Additionally, it is the only oral hypoglycemic agent that causes SIADH.

(continued)

APPENDIX. HIGH-RISK DRUG PRESCRIBING GUIDELINES *(Continued)*

Drug	*Prescribing Guideline (Doses are total daily dose)*
Dicyclomine Hyoscyamine Propantheline Belladonna alkaloids Clidinium-chlordiazepoxide	Gastrointestinal antispasmodics are highly anticholinergic and generally produce substantial toxicity in the elderly. Additionally, their effectiveness at doses tolerated by the elderly is questionable.
Chlorpheniramine Diphenhydramine Hydroxyzine Cyproheptadine Promethazine Tripelennamine Dexchlorpheniramine Combination products	All nonprescription and many prescription antihistamines have potent anticholinergic properties. Many cough and cold preparations are available without antihistamines and are safer substitutes in the elderly.
Diphenhydramine	Diphenhydramine is potently anticholinergic and usually should not be used as a hypnotic in the elderly. To treat or prevent allergic reactions, it should be used in the smallest possible dose and with great caution.
Ergoloid mesylates Cyclospasmol	Ergoloid mesylates and the cerebral vasodilators have not been shown to be effective, in the doses studied, for the treatment of dementia or any other condition.
Iron supplements above 325 mg	Iron supplements rarely need to be given in doses exceeding 325 mg of ferrous sulfate daily. When doses are higher, total absorption is not substantially increased, but constipation is more likely to occur.
All barbiturates (except phenobarbital used to treat seizure disorders)	Barbiturates cause more side effects in the elderly than most other sedative-hypnotics and are highly addictive. They should not be used as new therapy in the elderly except to control seizures.
Meperidine	Meperidine is not an effective oral analgesic and has many disadvantages compared to other narcotics.
Ticlopidine	Ticlopidine has been shown to be no better than aspirin in preventing clotting and is considerably more toxic.

INDEX

Page numbers followed by *f* indicate FIGURE; by *t*, TABLE

A

IND

B

C

E

F

H

I

J

K

L

M

N

O

P

Q

R

S

T

U

V

X

Y

Z

The Second Edition of THE MERCK MANUAL OF GERIATRICS is set in 10-point English Times with subheads and key words in Helvetica Bold. Tables and Figure legends are set in 8-point Helvetica; the Index is set in 8-point English Times. The manuscript was produced on a DEC Microvax, using MASS-11 software, at the editorial offices of THE MERCK MANUAL OF GERIATRICS in Blue Bell, Pa., and transmitted on diskettes to Alexander Graphics, Ltd., in Indianapolis, Ind., for typesetting. The book was printed on 30-pound Bible paper at National Publishing Co. in Philadelphia, Pa.